Human Cytokines:

Their Role in Disease and Therapy

Human Cytokines:
Their Role in Disease
and Therapy

edited by

Bharat B. Aggarwal, PhD
Professor of Medicine (Biochemistry)
Chief, Cytokine Research Section
University of Texas
M.D. Anderson Cancer Center
Houston, Texas

Raj K. Puri, MD, PhD
Senior Investigator and Acting Chief
Laboratory of Molecular Tumor Biology
Division of Cellular and Gene Therapies
Center for Biologic Evaluation
and Research
Food and Drug Administration
Bethesda, Maryland

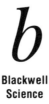

**Blackwell
Science**

Blackwell Science

EDITORIAL OFFICES:
238 Main Street, Cambridge,
  Massachusetts 02142, USA
Osney Mead, Oxford OX2 0EL, England
25 John Street, London WC1N 2BL,
  England
23 Ainslie Place, Edinburgh EH3 6AJ,
  Scotland
54 University Street, Carlton,
  Victoria 3053, Australia
Arnette Blackwell SA, 1 rue de Lille, 75007
  Paris, France
Blackwell-Wissenschaft-Verlag GmbH,
  Kurfürstendamm 57, 10707 Berlin,
  Germany
Blackwell MZV, Feldgasse 13, A–1238
  Vienna, Austria

DISTRIBUTORS:

North America
  Blackwell Science, Inc.
  238 Main Street
  Cambridge, Massachusetts 02142
  (Telephone orders: 800-215-1000 or
            617-876-7000)

Australia
  Blackwell Science, Pty Ltd
  54 University Street
  Carlton, Victoria 3053
  (Telephone orders: 03-347-5552)

Outside North America and Australia
  Blackwell Science, Ltd.
  c/o Marston Book Services, Ltd.
  P.O. Box 87
  Oxford OX2 0DT
  England
  (Telephone orders: 44-865-791155)

Acquisitions: Victoria Reeders
Development: Coleen Traynor
Production: Maria Hight
Manufacturing: Kathleen Grimes

Typeset by Pine Tree Composition, Lewiston, ME

Printed and bound by Braun-Brumfield, Inc., Ann Arbor, MI

© 1995 by Blackwell Science, Inc.

Printed in the United States of America

95 96 97 98 5 4 3 2 1

Library of Congress Cataloging-in-Publication Data

Human cytokines : their role in disease and therapy / edited by Bharat
  B. Aggarwal and Raj Puri.
    p. cm.
  Includes bibliographical references and index.
  ISBN 0–86542–352–0
  1. Cytokines—Pathophysiology, 2. Cytokines—Therapeutic use.
I. Aggarwal, Bharat B., 1950–   . II. Puri, Raj.
  [DNLM; 1. Cytokines, 2. Receptors, Cytokine. 3. Immunity,
Cellular. QW 568 H9178 1994]
QR185.8.C95H88 1995
616.07′1—dc20
DNLM/DLC
for Library of Congress   94–43207
                                                               CIP

Dedicated to our wives Uma and Mara
and our children Rishi, Manoj and Radhika

CONTENTS

CONTRIBUTORS

Eli Y. Adashi, MD
Professor of Obstetrics, Gynecology, and Physiology, Department of Obstetrics and Gynecology, Division of Reproductive Endocrinology, University of Maryland School of Medicine, Baltimore, Maryland

Bharat B. Aggarwal, PhD
Professor of Medicine (Biochemistry), Chief, Cytokine Research Section, University of Texas, M.D. Anderson Cancer Center, Houston, Texas

Anthony C. Allison, DPhil, BM, FRCPath
President and Chief Executive Officer, Dawa Inc., Belmont, California

Edward P. Amento, MD
Clinical Professor of Medicine and Dermatology, Departments of Medicine and Dermatology, Stanford University School of Medicine, Stanford, California; Executive Vice President, Scientific and Medical Affairs, Connective Therapeutics, Inc. Palo Alto, California

Tilo Andus, MD
Department of Internal Medicine, Clinic of the University of Regensberg, Regensberg, Germany

Vivian Barak, PhD
Immunology Laboratory for Tumor Diagnosis, Oncology, Hadassah University Hospital and the Hebrew University, Jerusalem, Israel

Jose Alexandre M. Barbuto, PhD
Section of Hematology and Oncology, Arizona Cancer Center, University of Arizona Health Sciences Center, Tucson, Arizona

Charlotte Behr, PhD
Experimental Parasitology Unit, Institut Pasteur, Paris, France

Izhar Ben-Shlomo, PhD
Division of Reproductive Endocrinology, Departments of Obstetrics and Gynecology and of Physiology, University of Maryland School of Medicine, Baltimore, Maryland

Etty N. Benveniste, PhD
Department of Cell Biology, University of Alabama at Birmingham, Birmingham, Alabama

Maria Carla Bosco, PhD
Macrophage Cell Biology Section, Laboratory of Experimental Immunology, National Cancer Institute, Frederick Cancer Research and Development Center, Frederick, Maryland

Fionula M. Brennan, PhD
The Kennedy Institute of Rheumatology, Hammersmith, London, UK

Hal E. Broxmeyer, PhD
Mary Margaret Walther Professor of Medicine and of Microbiology and Immunology, Indiana University School of Medicine; Scientific Director, Walther Oncology Center, Indianapolis, Indiana

Elmer Brummer, PhD
Research Associate, Division of Infectious Diseases, Department of Medicine, Santa Clara Medical Center, San Jose and Stanford University Medical School, Stanford, California

Parris R. Burd, PhD
Senior Staff Fellow, Laboratory of Cellular Immunology, Division of Cellular and Gene Therapies, Center for Biologic Evaluation and Research, Food and Drug Administration, Bethesda, Maryland

Ronald W. Bussuttil, MD, PhD
Professor of Surgery, Dumont Chair in Transplantation Surgery, Director, Dumont-UCLA Transplant Center, University of California at Los Angeles, California

Larry C. Casey, MD
Associate Professor, Section of Pulmonary and Critical Care Medicine, Department of Internal Medicine, Ruch Medical College, Chicago, Illinois

George W. Cox, PhD
Macrophage Cell Biology Section, Laboratory of Experimental Immunology, National Cancer Institute, Frederick Cancer Research and Development Center, Frederick, Maryland

W. Les Dees, PhD
Department of Veterinary Anatomy, Texas A&M University, College Station, Texas

Michel Denis, PhD
Assistant Professor, Faculty of Medicine, University of Sherbrooke, Quebec, Canada

Kathleen A. Dimock, PhD
Parasite Diseases Branch, Division of Parasitic Diseases, National Center for Infectious Diseases, Centers for Disease Control and Prevention, Atlanta, Georgia

Julie Y. Djeu, PhD
H. Lee Moffitt Cancer Center and Research Institute Immunology Program, University of South Florida College of Medicine, Departments of Medical Microbiology and Biochemistry, Tampa, Florida

Gerard D. Doherty, MD
Department of Surgery, Washington University School of Medicine, St. Louis, Missouri

Michael A. Doukas, MD
Assistant Professor of Medicine, Hematology and Oncology Division, Markey Cancer Center, University of Kentucky, Chandler Medical Center, Lexington, Kentucky

David N. Ernst, PhD
Department of Immunology, The Scripps Research Institute, La Jolla, California

Igor Espinoza-Delgado, PhD
Macrophage Cell Biology Section, Laboratory of Experimental Immunology, National Cancer Institute, Frederick Cancer Research and Development Center, Frederick, Maryland

Elsie M. Eugui, PhD
Syntex Research, Palo Alto, California

Douglas G. Farmer, MD
Senior Resident in General Surgery, University of California, Los Angeles, California

Anthony S. Fauci, MD
Director, National Institute of Allergy and Infectious Diseases, National Institutes of Health, Bethesda, Maryland

Kenneth R. Feingold, MD
Professor of Medicine and Dermatology, Metabolism Section, Department of Veterans Affairs Medical Center, San Francisco, California

Marc Feldmann, PhD
Professor, The Kennedy Institute of Rheumatology, Hammersmith, London, UK

Vincent S. Gallicchio, PhD
Associate Dean for Research, University of Kentucky Medical Center, Professor of Medicine, Microbiology, Immunology, and Clinical Sciences, Lucille P. Markey Cancer Center, University of Kentucky Medical Center Department of Veteran Affairs, Veterans Administration Medical Center, Lexington, Kentucky

Jennifer R. Gamble, PhD
The Hanson Centre for Cancer Research, Adelaide, Australia

Jack Gauldie, MD
Professor and Chairman, Department of Pathology, McMaster University, Hamilton, Ontario, Canada

Martha Gimeno, PhD
CEFYBO-CONICET, Buenos Aires, Argentina

Georges E. Grau, MD, PhD
Department of Pathology, University of Geneva Faculty of Medicine, Geneva, Switzerland

Carl Grunfeld, MD, PhD
Professor of Medicine, Metabolism Section, Department of Veterans Affairs Medical Center, San Francisco, California

Luca Gusella, PhD
Biological Carcinogenesis and Development Program, PRI/DynCorp, Frederick, Maryland

Gabriel P. Haas, MD
Associate Professor and Chief, Section of Urologic Oncology, Department of Urology, Wayne State University School of Medicine, Detroit, Michigan

Evan M. Hersch, MD
Chief, Section of Hematology/Oncology, Professor of Medicine

and of Microbiology and Immunology, Arizona Cancer Center, University of Arizona Health Sciences Center, Tucson, Arizona

Gilda G. Hillman, PhD
Assistant Professor and Director, Tumor Immunology Laboratory, Department of Urology, Wayne State University School of Medicine, Detroit, Michigan

Monte V. Hobbs, PhD
Department of Immunology, The Scripps Research Institute, La Jolla, California

Axel Holstage, MD
Department of Internal Medicine, Clinic of the University of Regensberg, Regensburg, Germany

A. Hurwitz, PhD
Division of Reproductive Endocrinology, Departments of Obstetrics and Gynecology and of Physiology, University of Maryland School of Medicine, Baltimore, Maryland

David K. Imagawa, MD, PhD
Fellow in Liver Transplantation, Clinical Instructor in General Surgery, Department of Surgery, The Dumont UCLA-Transplant Center, Los Angeles, California

Amrita Kamat, PhD
Department of Physiology, Neuropeptide Division, The University of Texas Southwestern Medical Center, Dallas, Texas

Levante Kapas, MD
Department of Physiology and Biophysics, University of Tennessee, Memphis, Tennessee

Sharada Karanth, PhD
Department of Physiology, Neuropeptide Division, The University of Texas Southwestern Medical Center, Dallas, Texas

Tadamitsu Kishimoto, MD
Professor and Chairman, Department of Internal Medicine, Osaka University Medical School, Osaka, Japan

E. Kokia, PhD
Division of Reproductive Endocrinology, Departments of Obstetrics and Gynecology and of Physiology, University of Maryland School of Medicine, Baltimore, Maryland

James M. Kreuger, PhD
Department of Physiology and Biophysics, University of Tennessee, Memphis, Tennessee

Altaf A. Lal, PhD
Malaria Branch, Division of Parasitic Diseases, National Center for Infectious Diseases, Centers for Disease Control and Prevention, Atlanta, Georgia

Patrick J. Lammie, PhD
Parasite Diseases Branch, Division of Parasitic Diseases, National Center for Infectious Diseases, Centers for Disease Control and Prevention, Atlanta, Georgia

Charles H. Lang, PhD
Professor and Director of Surgical Research, Department of Surgery, State University of New York, Stony Brook, New York

John C. Lee, PhD
Smith-Klein Beecham Pharmaceuticals, King of Prussia, Pennsylvania

S. Joseph Leibovich, PhD
Professor, Department of Anatomy, Cell Biology and Injury Sciences, New Jersey Medical School, University of Medicine and Dentistry of New Jersey, Newark, New Jersey

Marek S. Litwin, PhD
The Hanson Centre for Cancer Research, Adelaide, Australia

Jin Hong Liu, MD
H. Lee Moffitt Cancer Center and Research Institute Immunology Program, University of South Florida College of Medicine, Departments of Medical Microbiology and Biochemistry, Tampa, Florida

Michael T. Lotze, MD
Professor of Surgery, Molecular Genetics, and Biochemistry, Chief, Section of Surgical Oncology, Department of Surgery, Pittsburgh Cancer Institute, University of Pittsburgh Medical Center, Pittsburgh, Pennsylvania

Stephen F. Lowry, MD
Department of Surgery, University of Florida School of Medicine, Gainesville, Florida

Krzysztof Lyson, PhD
Department of Physiology, Neuropeptide Division, The University of Texas Southwestern Medical Center, Dallas, Texas

Ravinder N. Maini, BA, MB, BChir, FRCP
The Kennedy Institute of Rheumatology, Hammersmith, London, United Kingdom

Martin M. Matzuk, MD, PhD
Assistant Professor, Department of Pathology, Institute for Molecular Genetics, Baylor College of Medicine, Houston, Texas

Samuel M. McCann, MD
MacGregor Distinguished Professor of Biomedical Science, Department of Physiology, and Director, Neuropeptide Division, The University of Texas Southwestern Medical Center, Dallas, Texas

Grant McFadden, PhD
Professor of Biochemistry, Department of Biochemistry, University of Alberta, Edmonton, Alberta, Canada

Giovanni Melillo, PhD
Macrophage Cell Biology Section, Laboratory of Experimental Immunology, National Cancer Institute, Frederick Cancer Research and Development Center, Frederick, Maryland

Riaz A. Memon, MD, PhD
Research Fellow, Metabolism Section, Department of Veterans Affairs Medical Center, San Francisco, California

Thomas Miethke, MD
Institute of Medical Microbiology and Hygiene, Technical University of Munich, Germany

Lyle L. Moldawer, MD
Department of Surgery, University of Florida College of Medicine, Gainesville, Florida

Walton Montegut, MD
Department of Surgery, University of Florida School of Medicine, Gainesville, Florida

Angus M. Moodycliffe, PhD
Department of Immunology, The University of Texas, M.D. Anderson Cancer Center, Houston, Texas

Gregory R. Mundy, MD
Professor and Head, Department of Medicine, Division of Endocrinology and Metabolism, University of Texas Health Science Center, San Antonio, Texas

T. Musso, PhD
Biological Carcinogenesis and Development Program, PRI/DynCorp, Frederick, Maryland

Arnon Nagler, MD, MSc
Departments of Bone Marrow Transplantation and the Cancer Immunolobiology Research Laboratory, Hadassah University Hospital and the Hebrew University, Jerusalem, Israel

Reiko Namikawa, MD, PhD
DNAX Research Institute for Molecular and Cellular Biology, Palo Alto, California

Faris Nassar, MD
Division of Infectious Diseases, Department of Medicine, Santa Clara Valley Medical Center, San Jose and Stanford University Medical School, Stanford, California: Department Chief of Internal Medicine, Central Emek Hospital, Afula, Israel

Brian J. Nickoloff, MD, PhD
Associate Professor of Pathology and of Dermatology, University of Michigan Medical School, Ann Arbor, Michigan

Jeffrey A. Norton, MD
Professor of Surgery, Chief of Endocrine and Oncologic Surgery, Washington University School of Medicine, St. Louis, Missouri

Donna W. Payne, PhD
Division of Reproductive Endocrinology, Departments of Obstetrics and Gynecology and of Physiology, University of Maryland School of Medicine, Baltimore, Maryland

Gary R. Peplinski, MD
Department of Surgery, Washington University School of Medicine, St. Louis, Missouri

Guido Poli, MD
Divione di Malattie Infecttive, Centro di Ricerca e Cura per le Patologie HIV Correlate, Istituto Scientifico San Raffaele, Milano, Italy

Reuven Porat, PhD
Department of Medicine, Divison of Geographic Medicine and Infectious Diseases, Tufts University, New England Medical Center Hospital, Boston, Massachusetts

Raj K. Puri, MD, PhD
Senior Investigator and Acting Chief, Laboratory of Tumor
Biology, Division of Cellular Gene Therapies, Center for
Biologic Evaluation and Research, Food and Drug
Administration, Bethesda, Maryland

Valerie Rettori, PhD
Department of Physiology, Neuropeptide Division, The
University of Texas Southwestern Medical Center, Dallas,
Texas

Carl D. Richards, MD
Department of Pathology, McMaster University, Hamilton,
Ontario, Canada

Richard .M. Rohan, PhD
Division of Reproductive Endocrinology, Departments of
Obstetrics and Gynecology and of Physiology, University of
Baltimore School of Medicine, Baltimore, Maryland

Johannes A. Romijn, MD, PhD
Endocrinologist, Senior Investigator, Department of Intensive
Care, University of Amsterdam, The Netherlands

G. David Roodman, MD. PhD
Department of Medicine, Division of Hematology, University
of Texas Health Science Center, San Antonio, Texas

Trond Sand, MD
Department of Neurology, University of Trondheim, Norway

Hans-P. Sauerwein, MD, PhD
Professor in Clinical Nutrition, Department of Internal
Medicine and Endocrinology, University of Amsterdam, the
Netherlands

W.J. Scherzer, PhD
Division of Reproductive Endocrinology, Departments of
Obstetrics and Gynecology and of Physiology, University of
Maryland School of Medicine, Baltimore, Maryland

Mohammad K. Sharif, MD, PhD, MRCP
Senior Research Fellow, Miriam Marks Department of
Neurochemistry, Institute of Neurology University of London,
London, UK

Masaaki Shibata, PhD
Department of Physiology and Biophysics, University of
Tennessee, Memphis, Tennessee

Shimon Slavin, MD
Hadassah Medical Organization, Jerusalem, Israel

Cecilia M. Smith, DO
Associate Professor of Medicine, Department of Medicine,
Divisions of Pulmonary and Critical Care Medicine, Allergy
and Immunology, University of California Medical Center, San
Diego, California

Robert M. Smith, MD
Department of Medicine, Divisions of Pulmonary and Critical
Care Medicine, Allergy and Immunology, University of
California Medical Center, San Diego, California

Roger G. Spragg, MD
Professor of Medicine, University of California; Chief, Medical
Service, VA Medical Center, San Diego, California

Sachiko Suematsu, MD, PhD
Division of Immunology, Research Institute, Osaka Medical
Center for Maternal and Child Health, Osaka, Japan

Venkatachalam Udhayakumar, PhD
Malaria Branch, Division of Parasitic Diseases, National Center
for Infectious Diseases, Centers for Disease Control and
Prevention, Atlanta, Georgia

Stephen E. Ullrich, PhD
Department of Immunology, The University of Texas, M.D.
Anderson Cancer Center, Houston, Texas

Elaine N. Unemori, PhD
Group Leader, Cell Biology, Connective Therapeutics, Inc.
Palo Alto, California

Matthew A. Vadas, PhD
The Hanson Center for Cancer Research, Adelaide, Australia

Luigi Varesio, PhD
Head, Macrophage Cell Biology Section, Laboratory of
Experimental Immunology, National Cancer Institute,
Frederick Cancer Research and Development Center,
Frederick, Maryland

Anders Waage, MD
Section of Hematology, Department of Medicine, University of
Trondheim, Norway

Hermann Wagner, PhD, MD
Professor and Director, Institute of Medical Microbiology and
Hygiene, Technical University of Munich, Germany

Claudia Wahl, MD
Institute of Medical Microbiology and Hygiene, Technical
University of Munich, Germany

Stephen I. Wasserman, MD
Chair, Department of Medicine and the Helen M. Ranney
Professor, and Director, Division of Allergy, University of
California, San Diego, California

Eric D. Whitman, MD
Assistant Professor of Surgery, Department of Surgery, Section
of Endocrine and Oncologic Surgery, Washington University
School of Medicine, St. Louis, Missouri

Toshiyuki Yoneda, DDS, PhD
Department of Medicine and Endocrinology, University of
Texas Health Science Center, San Antonio, Texas

PREFACE

Only in 1980 was the structure of the first cytokine, interferon-α, revealed by recombinant DNA methods. Since then as many as 80 distinct cytokines have been identified and their structure determined. In most cases the structure of their receptors has also been elucidated. Not only has the identification and molecular characterization proceeded rapidly, but also their roles in cell biology, physiology, pathology and disease therapy have been delineated. These cytokines provided novel means of both diagnosis and treatment of disease. It appears that virtually every known disease involves some type of imbalance in the cytokine network. The presence of genes for cytokines and their receptors in viruses, where they are most likely used for self-protection as in higher organisms, further shows the significance of these molecules during evolution.

This book is an attempt to provide the reader the latest developments in the field of cytokines with respect to their role in disease and therapy. Every contributor is a pioneer in cytokines research, preeminently qualified to discuss this field. Even though advances in the science of cytokines come so rapidly that staying abreast with the latest is a monumental task, all contributors have enthusiastically provided their best. Without them, this book would not have been possible.

We would like to sincerely thank our chapter contributors, our secretary Ms. Wendy Chaffin and our developmental editor Ms. Coleen Traynor for their patience and aspiration to high standards. We would also like to acknowledge the assistance provided by Dr. Carl Grunfeld, M.D., Ph.D. from the University of California, San Francisco, who helped us in the early stages of the development of this book.

Bharat B. Aggarwal, PhD
Raj K. Puri, MD, PhD

NOTICE

The indications and dosages of all drugs in this book have been recommended in the medical literature and conform to the practices of the general medical community. The medications described do not necessarily have specific approval by the Food and Drug Administration for use in the diseases and dosages for which they are recommended. The package insert for each drug should be consulted for use and dosage as approved by the FDA. Because standards of usage change, it is advisable to keep abreast of revised recommendations, particularly those concerning new drugs.

Human Cytokines:

Their Role in Disease and Therapy

PART **1**

CYTOKINES NETWORK

CHAPTER 1

COMMON AND UNCOMMON FEATURES OF CYTOKINES AND CYTOKINE RECEPTORS: AN OVERVIEW

Bharat B. Aggarwal and Raj K. Puri

In general, cytokines are polypeptide hormones secreted by a cell that affects growth and metabolism either of the same (autocrine) or of another (paracrine) cell. This definition usually excludes the hormones produced by various endocrine organs. Perhaps the first cytokine to be discovered was interferon (IFN); it was discovered in 1957 by Issacs and Lindenmann (1) as a soluble factor produced by cells following exposure to heat-inactivated influenza virus. Within the last decade, there has been a tremendous avalanche of information on cytokines, including identification and characterization of several of these novel proteins.

Even though the term *cytokine* was originally coined to designate the molecules produced by the cells of the immune system and the biological response modifiers of the same system, it quickly became apparent that molecules outside the immune system have similar modes of production and action. Currently, lymphokines and monokines, which are the secreted products of lymphocytes and monocytes, respectively, and the secreted products of neutrophils, mast cells, endothelial cells, fibroblasts, astrocytes, and other cell types are included among the cytokines. Since 1980, when IFN-α became the first cytokine to be isolated, the number has grown to more than 50 distinct molecules (Table 1–1) (2–36). Several reviews have been written on different aspects of cytokines (2,4,37–43). We describe herein some of the general as well as unique features of various cytokines and their receptors.

CYTOKINES ARE PRODUCED EARLY IN DEVELOPMENT

The presence of cytokines early in development suggests their possible role in both embryological growth and differentiation. For instance, tumor necrosis factor (TNF), colony-stimulating factor-1 (CSF-1), interleukin-1 (IL-1), and IL-6 have been shown to be present in oocytes before fertilization (44–49). Levels of these cytokines increase after fertilization and during embryo cleavage from zygote to 8 cells. Leukemia inhibitory factor (LIF) has been demonstrated to have an important role during development of the mouse. It inhibits the differentiation of embryonic stem cells and maintains them in a pluripotent state. LIF has been detected in preimplantation blastocysts and in extraembryonic tissue and placenta. Furthermore, overexpression of LIF complementary DNA (cDNA) in chimeric embryos inhibits gastrulation.

Perhaps the best evidence that cytokines have a role in development has come from the gene "knock out" mouse (50–54). Conventional techniques that rely on microinjecting foreign cytokine genes into fertilized egg introduce genes randomly into the genome. Gene knock out mice, in contrast, are made by cloning a particular gene, disrupting it by introducing a short DNA sequence, and inserting it into a mouse stem cell. The disrupted gene replaces the normal gene by a process called homologous

TABLE 1–1 CYTOKINES WITH MULTIPLE BIOLOGICAL RESPONSES

Cytokine*	Molecular Weight (kd)	mRNA (kb)	Carbohydrate[†]	Reference[‡]
Antiviral				
Interferon-α (IFN-α)	19–29	1.0–2.0	+	(2)
Interferon-β (IFN-β	20	0.7	+	(2)
Interferon-γ (IFN-γ)	20–25	1.2	+	(2)
Interferon-ω (IFN-ω)	24.5	1.0	+	(3)
Inflammation[§]				
Interleukin-1-α (IL-1α)	17.5	2.1	−	(2)
Interleukin-1-β (IL-1β)	17.5	1.6	−	(2)
Interleukin-1 receptor antagonist (IL-1RA)	25	1.8	+	(2)
Interleukin-6 (IL-6)	21–26	1.3	+	(2)
Interleukin-8 (IL-8)	8	1.8	−	(2)
Tumor necrosis factor (TNF)	17	1.7	−	(2)
Lymphotoxin (LT)	20–25	1.3	+	(2)
T cell growth factors				
Interleukin-2 (IL-2)	15–17.2	0.9	+	(2)
Interleukin-4 (IL-4)	15–20	0.9	+	(2)
Interleukin-7 (IL-7)	22–28	1.8,2.4	+	(2)
Interleukin-9 (IL-9)	37–40	0.7	+	(2)
Interleukin-12 (IL-12)	75[‖]	2.4,1.4	+	(2)
Hematopoietic factors				
Interleukin-3 (IL-3)	15–17	1.0	+	(2)
Interleukin-11 (IL-11)	23	2.5	−	(2)
Macrophage colony-stimulating factor (M-CSF)	45–90	4.2[#]	+	(4)
Granulocyte colony-stimulating factor (G-CSF)	19.6	1.6	+	(4)
Granulocyte and macrophage colony-stimulating factor (GM-CSF)	18–32	0.7	+	(4)
Leukemia inhibitory factor (LIF)	32–45	4.2	+	(5)
Stem-cell factor (SCF)	36	6.0	+	(6)
Erythropoietin (EPO)	34–36	1.6	+	(2)
Erythroid differentiation factor (EDF)	14	7.2	+	(7)
CD 27 ligand (CD 27L)	50	1.2	+	(8)
B cell growth factors				
B cell growth factor (BCGF)	12	1.0,1.7	+	(4)
Interleukin-4 (IL-4)	15–20	0.9	+	(2)
Interleukin-5 (IL-5)	18	0.9	+	(2)
Interleukin-6 (IL-6)	21–26	1.3	+	(2)
TNF-related activation protein (TRAP/CD 40 ligand)	29	2.3	+	(9)
Interleukin 14 (IL-14; HMW-BCGF)	53	1.8	+	(10)
Chemotactic factors				
Interleukin-8 (IL-8)	8	1.8	−	(2)
Monocyte chemotactic protein-1 (MCP-1)	15	0.7	+	(2)
Growth factor inducible chemokine (Fic)	11	0.6	+	(11)
Macrophage inflammatory protein-1 (MIP-1α; MIP-1β)	8 8	0.8 0.8	− −	(12) (12)
Regulated on activation, normal T expressed and secreted (RANTES)	8	1.1	−	(13)
Melanoma growth stimulatory activity (MGSA)	13–16	1.1–1.2	−	(14)
Macrophage migration inhibitory factor (MIF)	12	0.7	+	(4)

TABLE 1–1 (*Continued*)

Cytokine*	Molecular Weight (kd)	mRNA (kb)	Carbohydrate[†]	Reference[‡]
Growth inhibitors**				
Tumor necrosis factor (TNF)	17	1.7	–	(2)
Lymphotoxin (LT)	20–25	1.3	+	(2)
Amphiregulin (AR)	9.0–9.8	1.4	+	(15)
Oncostatin M (OM)	20–36	2.0	+	(2)
Mullerian inhibiting substance (MIS)	140[††]	2.1	+	(4)
FAS ligand	38–42	2.0	+	(16)
Growth enhancers				
Platelet-derived growth factor (PDGF)	28[‡‡]	2.8,3.5	+	(17)
Fibroblast growth factor (basic) (bFGF)	16	7.0[§§]	–	(18)
Fibroblast growth factor (acidic) (aFGF)	16	4.2	–	(18)
Epidermal growth factor (EGF)	6.4	4.9	–	(19)
Transforming growth factor-α (TGF-α)	5–20[‖‖]	4.5–4.8	+	(20)
Betacellulin (BTC)	32	3.0	+	(21)
Insulin-like growth factor (IGF-I & II)	6.0	7.6,6.0	–	(22)
Hepatocyte growth factor (HGF)	82[##]	6.0	+	(23)
Autocrine motility factor (AMF)	55	NA	–	(24)
Androgen-induced growth factor (AIGF)	28–32	1.0–1.2	+	(25)
Hergulin (erb B2/HER2 ligand)	45	6.6	+	(26)
Glia activating factor (GAF)	25–30	NA	+	(27)
Glia maturation factor (GMF)	16–17	3.7	–	(28)
Ach receptor–inducing activity (ARIA)	42	7.3,3.0	+	(29)
Pleiotrophin/midkine (PTN/MK)	18	1.5	–	(30)
Osteogenic protein-2 (OP)	32–36	1.8–5.0	–	(31)
Bone morphogenic proteins (BMP)	30	2.8–4.0	–	(32)
Vascular endothelial cell growth factor (VEGF)	46[***]	1.6	+	(4)
Ciliary neurotrophic factor (CNTF)	23	1.2	–	(33)
flt3/flk-2 ligand	24	0.82	+	(34)
Suppressor molecules				
Interleukin-4 (IL-4)	15–20	0.9	+	(2)
Interleukin-10 (IL-10)	17–21	1.0–1.5	+	(2)
Interleukin-13 (IL-13)	9, 17	1.4	+	(35)
Transforming growth factor-β (TGF-β)	11.5–12.5	5.8	–	(1)
Others				
Lymphotoxin-β (LT-β)	25–26	0.9–1.0	+	(36)

*Space limitation permits only commonly used names and abbreviations of cytokines.

[†] + = glycosylated; – = no glycosylation.

[‡] Due to space limitation, only key references are indicated.

[§] TNF, LT, LIF, IL-6, and IL-8 also have inflammatory roles.

[‖] Disulfide-linked heterodimer of 40 and 35 kd subunits.

[#] Due to alternative splicing, mRNA of 1.6, 2.2, and 2.5 kb have been reported.

** TGF-β, IL-1, IL-4, and IL-6 also display growth inhibitory effects on certain cells.

[††] Disulfide-linked homodimer of 72 kd subunit.

[‡‡] Disulfide-linked homo- and heterodimer of A- and B-chain.

[§§] In addition to major mRNA species, minor mRNAs of 1.5, 2.5, 3.7, and 4.5 kb for bFGF, and 0.8, 1.2, 2.7, and 3.2 kb for aFGF are also found.

[‖‖] Molecular weights of secreted forms are indicated.

[##] Heterodimer of α (Mr, 69 kd) and β (Mr, 34 kd). An mRNA of 6.0 kb gives rise to a preprotein, which generates α and β subunits after processing.

[***] Dimer of 23 and 18 kd subunits.

NA = not available.

recombination. These cells are injected into the mouse embryo, yielding mice that are then bred to produce a strain in which all cells carry the knocked out gene. Using these techniques, the function of the missing gene product can be ascertained.

Deletion of genes for specific cytokines has resulted in defective development in the embryo. For instance, deletion of LIF leads to retardation of blastocyst development due to the lack of its implantation (55). A deletion of the IL-10 gene in most animals leads to growth retardation and anemia (56), whereas animals lacking the IL-2 gene develop normally during the first 3 to 4 weeks of age, but some die later, between 4 and 9 weeks after birth (57). However, the immune response of those IL-2–deficient animals who survive is quite normal (58,59).The defects that result from deletion of other cytokine genes, including IL-4, transforming growth factor-β (TGF-β), α-inhibin, IFN-γ, TGF-α, and TNF, are outlined in Table 1–2 (60–81). It clearly documents the importance of various cytokines during early development.

CYTOKINE–LIKE MOLECULES ARE NOT UNIQUE TO VERTEBRATES

The wide-ranging ability of cytokines to initiate and regulate host-defense responses and the critical need of vertebrates for these molecules has led to the suggestion that cytokines are highly conserved through evolution (82). Isolation of epidermal growth factor (EGF), IL-1, and TNF-like molecules from invertebrates supports this hypothesis (83–86). IL-1α-, IL-1β-, IL-2-, IL-6-, and TNF-like molecules have recently been reported in the hemocytes of two molluscs (i.e., *Planobarious corneus* and *Viviparus ater*) (87). These invertebrate cytokines display structural and functional similarities to vertebrate cytokines (83–86). Furthermore, invertebrates have been shown to have receptors for cytokines such as IL-1, IL-2, IL-6, TNF, granulocyte-macrophage colony-stimulating factor (GM-CSF), and EGF (88–93). These cytokine receptors are functional because they lead to biological response (88–95). TNF added to *Trypanosoma musculi* cultured in vitro inhibited their growth (96). Similarly, the growth of *Mycobacterium avium* in culture has been shown to be potentiated by IL-1 and IL-6 (97). In addition to invertebrates, several cytokines, including IL-1, IL-2, and GM-CSF, have been shown to stimulate the growth of *Escherichia coli* (88,90).

Perhaps one of the best-studied examples of invertebrate cytokines is TGF-β and its receptors, for which structural homologues of the vertebrate proteins have been found in invertebrates. TGF-β is a family of proteins that regulate growth and differentiation in a wide variety of organisms in both vertebrates and invertebrates. The

ligands and their receptors have been discovered in vertebrates and in such invertebrates as drosophila and *Caenorhabditis elegans* (98,99). In addition to the *daf-1* gene, which is a member of the TGF-β receptor family, *C. elegans* contains another gene, the cell death gene, CED-3, the predicted amino acid sequence of which is highly homologous to the IL-1β converting enzyme (100,101). The latter is a cysteine protease that can cleave the inactive 31-kd precursor of IL-1β to generate active cytokine. The transcript for CED-3 is most abundant during embryogenesis, the stage during which most programmed cell death occurs (101). These observations suggest that invertebrate organisms are capable of expressing vertebrate cytokines and have receptors to respond to these cytokines.

In addition to bacteria and other invertebrates, in some cases, the viral genome codes for cytokines and cytokine receptor–like molecules (102). For instance, Epstein-Barr virus (EBV), an intracellular human pathogen, has the BCRF1 gene, which is a close functional and structural homolog of the murine and human IL-10 genes. Human IL-10 and BCRF1 are 90% identical in primary amino acid sequence (103). The presence of the IL-10 gene in the EBV genome suggests that this cytokine is important in viral infection. Also, the receptor for a mammalian chemokine, IL-8, which regulates trafficking, activation, and in some cases proliferation of myeloid and lymphoid cells, is remotely related to the gene ECRF3 of the herpesvirus samiri (approximately 30% amino acid identity) (104). This viral gene has been shown to code for the functional IL-8 receptor. The amino acid sequence of the TNF receptor has also been shown to display a high degree of homology to the open-reading frame from the Shope fibroma virus (poxvirus) (105). Cells infected with myxoma virus secrete a 37-kd protein that binds IFN-γ, and it is encoded by the viral gene M-T7 open-reading frame (106). Whether viruses code for cytokine genes in an attempt to protect themselves from the host is not fully understood. It has been suggested, however, that the immunosuppressive effects exerted by many viruses are most likely mediated through inhibitory effects on cytokine production and their action.

SEVERAL NAMES CONTINUE TO BE USED FOR THE SAME CYTOKINE

Several cytokines discovered on the basis of their biological activities were later shown to have identical chemical structures. Thus, one cytokine would have more than one name (4). Lack of a consensus on the nomenclature of cytokines has caused a great deal of confusion in this field. For instance, stem cell growth factor (SCF), c-kit ligand (KL), and mast cell growth factor (MGF) are

TABLE 1–2   EFFECT OF DELETION OF CYTOKINE AND CYTOKINE RECEPTORS ON GROWTH AND DEVELOPMENT

Cytokine/Receptor	Defect	Reference
Cytokines		
IL-2	Animals display normal T- and B-cell development.	(57–59)
	Poor T-cell response to Con A or anti-CD3; 50% of animals die between 4–6 months.	
	Ulcerative colitis develops.	
IL-4	Normal T- and B-cell development.	(60–62)
	Reduced serum IgG1 and IgE levels.	
	No dominance of IgG1 in T-cell dependent.	
	No IgE response to nematode infection.	
	Reduced production of IL-3, IL-5, and IL-10.	
	Resistance to retrovirus-induced immunodeficiency syndrome.	
IL-10	Animals are growth-retarded, anemic, and suffer from chronic enterocolitis.	(56)
TGF-β	Excessive inflammatory response.	(63–65)
	20 days after birth there is rapid wasting syndrome, tissue necrosis, leading to organ failure and early death.	
α-Inhibin	Mixed or incompletely differentiated gonadal stromal tumors develop, either unilaterally or bilaterally.	(66)
IFN-γ	Impaired production of macrophage antimicrobial products.	(67–70)
	Reduced expression of macrophage MHC-II.	
	Animals are killed by *Mycobacterium bovis*.	
	Uncontrolled proliferation of splenocytes.	
SCF*	Encodes membrane stem-cell factor or c-kit ligand.	(71,72)
	Leads to *Steel-Dickie* mutation.	
	Pleiotropic defects similar to those caused by mutations at the W locus.	
	Animals are sterile, anemic, and black-eyed white.	
FAS ligand*	Lymphadenopathy and systemic autoimmunity similar to that in *lpr/lpr* mice develop in mice carrying *gld* mutation.	(73)
M-CSF*	Deficiency of osteoclasts, monocytes.	(74)
	Osteopetrosis (*op*) due to osteoclast defect.	
	Defective in production of M-CSF.	
LIF	Females are fertile, but their blastocysts fail to implant and thus do not develop.	(55)
TGF-α	Abnormalities in hair follicle and eyes.	(75)
CD40L*	X-linked hyper-IgM (*HIgM*) syndrome.	(76)
	Elevated serum IgM levels.	
	Low or no IgG, IgA, and IgE levels.	
Receptors		
(TNF-R) (p55)	Resistance to endotoxin.	(77,78)
	Sensitive to *Listeria monocytogenes* infection.	
IFN-γ R	Defective natural resistance.	(79,80)
	Increased susceptibility to infection by *Listeria monocytogenes*, vaccinia virus, and *Mycobacterium tuberculosis*.	
Fas*	Massive lymphadenopathy develops in mice with *lpr/lpr*, associated with proliferation of aberrant T cells.	(81)
	Systemic autoimmunity.	

*Abnormalities based on natural mutation of the genes.
MHC = major histocompatibility complex; Ig = immunoglobulin.

different names for the same molecule. Similarly, TNF-β and lymphotoxin (LT), and high molecular weight β-cell growth factor (HM-BCGF) and IL-14 (10) are pairs of names for the same cytokine.

MOST CYTOKINES ARE ASSIGNED TO FAMILIES ON THE BASIS OF STRUCTURAL HOMOLOGY

On the basis of homology in primary amino acid sequence, chromosomal localization, and, in some instances, functional homology, several cytokines have been grouped into families. Usually, the name of the family is based on the initial determination of structure of the first member. These families include IL, chemokine, IFN, CSF, TGF-β, TNF, and heregulin. The last group, for example, designates a family of molecules first isolated as specific ligands of human epidermal growth factor receptor-2 (HER2), also called neu or erb B2. A rat homolog was termed *neu differentiation factor* (NDF) because of its ability to induce differentiation of breast cancer cells through its interaction with HER2/neu. Alternatively, spliced forms of the heregulin gene encode two neurotrophic activities—a neural-derived factor termed *acetylcholine receptor–inducing activity (ARIA)* and glial growth factor (GGF). Additional isoforms of the heregulin proteins include p45, gp30, and p75 (107).

TGF-α is another example of a cytokine that binds and activates EGF receptor, and it belongs to a family of peptides that includes EGF, heparin-binding EGF, amphiregulin, cripto, betacellulin, and viral-derived growth factors such as vaccinia virus growth factor. These polypeptides possess six cysteine residues in the same relative position, and the resulting disulfide bonds lead to similar three-dimensional configurations recognized by the EGF receptor.

Similarly, the human TNF family consists of a number of structurally homologous proteins, including LT, LT-β, CD-27L, CD-30L, CD-40L, and fas ligand, showing 36, 22, 18, 16, 25, and 28% homology to human TNF, respectively (16,108). Among 14 members of the IL family, all but IL-4 and IL-13 have distinct structures. These two have 30% homology in their amino acid sequence and compete for the same cell surface receptor (109).

DIVERSE STIMULI REGULATE THE PRODUCTION OF VARIOUS CYTOKINES

It has been shown that most viral, bacterial, and parasitic infections lead to the production of different cytokines. Secretion of cytokines in circulation is also regulated by several physiological and pathological stimuli. Administration of cytokines leads to the production of other cytokines. There are also several examples of feedback autocrine stimulation of cytokines. For instance, production of TNF, IL-1, IL-2, and IL-4 appears to be enhanced by TNF, IL-1, IL-2, and IL-4, respectively (4,110–112). Regulation of a cytokine by other cytokines in most cases is quite complex. For instance, production of TNF from monocytes is down-modulated by IL-10, but TNF up-modulates the production of IL-10 from the same cells (113).

CELLULAR SOURCES OF MOST CYTOKINES ARE DIVERSE

Although there are several cell types reported to produce different cytokines, the cells of the immune system are one major source of most of these polypeptides (Table 1–3). Production of most cytokines by cells is temporary. They are produced transiently and act locally in a combined autocrine and paracrine, rather than endocrine, manner. The transient nature of cytokines has been shown to correlate with the presence of adenine uracil (AU)-rich sequence in the 3' untranslated region of the messenger RNA (mRNA) of different cytokines (114). In addition to cells, cytokines can be observed in various biological fluids, including serum, ascites, and cerebrospinal fluid. Several cytokines and their receptors are excreted in the urine in biological active forms under different physiological conditions (Table 1–4) (115–134). The role of these urinary cytokines and their receptors is not clear, but they appear to reflect physiological or pathological conditions.

MOST CYTOKINES FORM A COMPLEX NETWORK

Cytokines form a network by either inducing or suppressing the expression of other cytokines (135,136). Cells of one type appear to communicate with cells of another type through the production of cytokines. For instance, IL-1 produced by macrophages interacts with lymphocytes to cause production of IL-2, which in turn leads to production of other cytokines, such as IL-3 and GM-CSF. The latter may in turn affect macrophages. The type of cytokine network is specific to the physiological or pathological condition. For example, the molecular network involved in immunoregulation, hematopoiesis, inflammation, atherosclerosis, glomerulonephritis, or reproduction, among others, has begun to be elucidated (48,49,137–139). This cytokine cascade is highly remi-

TABLE 1–3   PRODUCTION OF CYTOKINES BY DIFFERENT CELL TYPES

Cell Type*	Cytokine*
Immune system	
T lymphocytes	
Th1	IL-1, IL-2, IL-9, IFN-γ, LT, G-CSF, M-CSF, GM-CSF
Th2	IL-3, IL-4, IL-5, IL-6, IL-10, IL-13, IL-14, MIP-1α, MIP-1β, RANTES, TNF, LT, LIF, OSM
CTL	TNF, LT, IFN-γ, IL-2
NK	TNF, LT, IFN-γ, IL-3, G-CSF, M-CSF, GM-CSF
B lymphocytes	IL-1, IL-5, IL-6, LT, TNF, GM-CSF, IFN-γ, IFN-α
Macrophages	IL-1α, IL-1β, IL-5, IL-6, IL-8, IL-10, IL-12, IFN-α, TNF, LIF, OSM, PDGF, MIF, MCAF, bFGF, FAF, TGF-α, TGF-β, GRO-α, MIP-1α, MIP-1β, EPO, Thymosine-α1, GM-CSF, G-CSF, M-CSF, β-endorphin, ACTH, NGF, VEGF, HB-EGF
Neutrophils	IL-1α, IL-1β, IL-3, IL-6, IL-8, G-CSF, M-CSF, GM-CSF, IL-1RA, IFN-α, GRO-α
Mast cells	IL-1, IL-3, IL-4, IL-5, IL-6, IL-8, MIP-1α, MIP-1β, TNF, GM-CSF
Eosinophils	IL-3, IL-5, IL-α, IL-6, TNF, MIP-1α, GM-CSF, TGF-α, TGF-β
Platelets	PDGF, TGF-β, EGF, RANTES, IL-1, HGF, GRO-α, PD-ECGF
Endocrine organs	
Placental cells	IL-1, IL-2, IL-6, IFN-α, IFN-β, TNF
Anterior pituitary cells	IL-6, MIF
Granulosa cells	TNF
Oocytes	IL-1, IL-6, M-CSF
Others	
Endothelial cells	GM-CSF, IL-1, IL-6, PDGF
Smooth muscle cells	IL-1α, IL-1β, TNF
Fibroblasts	bFGF, IL-6, IL-1β, G-CSF
Astrocytes	IL-1, TNF

*See Table 1–1 for abbreviations.

niscent of various factors involved in the blood coagulation cascade.

CYTOKINE PROTEINS HAVE DIVERSE PHYSICOCHEMICAL CHARACTERISTICS

Structurally, cytokines are low molecular weight proteins secreted by cells. Their molecular size, glycoprotein or nonglycoprotein nature, and mRNA size are shown in Table 1–1. They range in molecular mass from as low as 5 kd (TGF-α) to as high as 140 kd (Mullerian-inhibiting substance [MIS]). In general, most cytokines consist of a single polypeptide chain, with the exception of TGF-β, IL-12, and MIS, which consist of 2 chains. Both TGF-β and MIS are disulfide-linked homodimers, whereas IL-12

is a heterodimer consisting of 30- and 45-kd chains. Even though most cytokines are glycoproteins, several have been found to lack carbohydrates, including IL-1, IL-8, IL-11, monocyte chemotactic inhibitory protein (MIP-1), RANTES, melanoma growth stimulating activity (MGSA), TNF, FGF, EGF, insulin-like growth factor (IGF), and autocrine motility factor (AMF).

In addition to glycosylation, it has been shown that certain cytokines, such as IL-1 and TNF, are myristylated (140,141). The importance of this acylation is not clear, but the site of myristylation (propiece of the molecule) suggests it has a role in retaining the cytokine in the membrane. Amino-terminal glycine myristyl acylation is a cotranslational modification that affects both protein localization and function. However, TNF and IL-1 both lack amino terminal glycine and acylation occurs at the epsilon amino group of lysine (141). In addition to acylation, some cytokines, such as IFN-γ and IL-6, have been found to exist as phosphoproteins (142–146). Both IFN-γ and

TABLE 1–4 IDENTIFICATION OF CYTOKINES AND THEIR RECEPTORS IN HUMAN URINE

Cytokine/Receptor*	Condition	References
Cytokine		
IL-1	Normal individuals	(114,115)
IL-2	BCG therapy	(115)
	BCG therapy	(116,117)
IL-6	BCG therapy	(115)
	Renal transplant recipient	(118)
TNF	BCG therapy	(115)
IFN-γ	BCG therapy	(119)
M-CSF	Normal individuals	(120–122)
EPO	Aplastic anemia	(123)
AMF	Bladder cancer	(124)
bFGF	Bladder cancer, kidney cancer	(125)
EGF (b-urogastrone)	Normal individuals	(126)
TGF-α	Breast cancer	(127)
Cytokine receptors		
IL-2R	Normal individuals	(128)
IL-6R	Normal individuals	(129)
TNFR	Normal individuals, regular hemodialysis treatment, febrile patients	(130–133)
IFN-γR	Normal individuals	(129)

*See Table 1–1 for abbreviations.

IL-6 are phosphorylated at serine residues 132 and 54, respectively (142–146). Among other cytokines, phosphorylation has been observed in bFGF (147,148). In all these instances, the importance of phosphorylation with regard to either cytokine secretion or its effects on the response of cytokines is not understood. The kinases responsible for their phosphorylation are also not known.

The presence of a signal or a leader sequence in a gene is an indication that its gene product is targeted for secretion from the cell. Most cytokines in general display this type of sequence. However, some cytokines, including endothelial cell growth factor, basic fibroblast growth factor (bFGF), and IL-1β (149–151), lack signal sequence; therefore, the mechanism by which they are secreted is not understood. It has been suggested that specific proteases are responsible for secretion of these cytokines from the cell surface. A calcium-dependent cysteine protease that cleaves protein at an aspartic acid residue and is specific for the cleavage of IL-1 has been identified, and its cDNA has been cloned (152–157). In addition to IL-1 and FGF, there are both secreted and membrane-associated forms of TNF, LT, TGF-α, and SCF. SCF is a transmembrane protein, the secreted form of which lacks the transmembrane domain. In the case of LT, a transmembrane protein with a molecular mass of 33 kd has been identi-

fied; it is referred to as LT-β, to which LT associates noncovalently (36). Very little is known about the mechanism of secretion of either TNF or TGF-α, although the existence of proteases similar to that identified for IL-1 has been postulated.

The crystal structure of several cytokines is now known (Table 1–5) (158–182). The cytokines that display β-sheet structure include hTNF, hLT, IL-1β, IL-1α, bFGF, and IL-8; those with mainly an α-helical structure include IL-2, IL-4, IL-5, IL-10, IFN-β, IFN-γ, GM-CSF, G-CSF, and M-CSF. Interestingly, acidic fibroblast growth factor (aFGF), which has 30% structural homology at the primary amino acid sequence level to IL-1, shows a greater degree of structural similarity at the three-dimensional level (163), as is the case for LT and TNF (161). TNF and LT share a common cell surface receptor, but IL-1 and bFGF bind to distinct receptors. There are very few examples in which the crystal structure of the cytokine-receptor complex is known. Cocrystallization of LT with its receptor revealed that LT interacts as a trimer with its receptor (158).

On the basis of primary, secondary, and tertiary structure, several investigators have begun to synthesize peptides that can mimic the biological effects of intact cytokines (Table 1–6) (183–195). Biologically active peptides analogous to IL-1, IL-6, TNF, and IFN-γ have been

TABLE 1–5   CYTOKINES FOR WHICH THREE-DIMENSIONAL STRUCTURES HAVE BEEN DETERMINED

Cytokine	Characteristics	References
Mainly β-sheet structures		
hTNF	Trimeric molecule.	(159,160)
	Each subunit consists of an anti-parallel B-sandwich.	
	Remarkable similarity to the "jelly-roll" motif found in viral coat proteins.	
hLT	Trimeric molecules.	
	"Jellyroll" B-sheet sandwich.	(161)
hIL-1β	Capped β-barrel consisting of 12 antiparallel β-strands.	(162–164)
	No α-helixes.	
hIL-1α	Similar to IL-1β.	(165)
bFGF	Similar to IL-1β.	(166–167)
hIL-8	Dimeric molecule; each subunit consists of 3 antiparallel β-strands and 1 α-helix.	(168)
Mainly α-helical structures		
hIL-2	Left handed 4-α-helix bundles.	(169)
hIL-4	Left-handed, 4-α-helix bundle plus a short 2-stranded β-sheet.	(170–174)
mIFN-β	Left-handed 4-α-helix bundle plus 1 long α-helix.	(175,176)
hIFN-γ	Dimer of mutually interlocked subunits composed of 5 α-helices.	(177,178)
hGM-CSF	Left-handed, 4-α-helix bundle plus 1 short 2-stranded β-sheet.	(179,180)
hM-CSF	Two GM-CSF–like 4-α-helix bundles connected by a disulfide bond.	(181)
G-CSF	Antiparallel 4-α-helical bundle with up-up-down-down connectivity.	(182)

*See Table 1–1 for abbreviations.
m = murine; h = human; b = basic.

reported. Both agonistic and antagonistic peptides have been sought for various cytokines in an attempt either to achieve a better delivery system (i.e., systemic oral administration) or to suppress the harmful effects of a given cytokine. For instance, in the case of IL-1β, a synthetic peptide corresponding to residues 163–171 of the intact proteins was found to retain the immunomodulatory effects of IL-1, but its pyrogenic effects were abolished (183), suggesting that different activities of the cytokines reside in different domains of the molecule. For antagonistic activity, a hexapeptide has been identified that binds to the receptor for bFGF and blocks its biological effects (193).

A technique commonly used to make a cytokine agonist or antagonist or to alter receptor specificity is site-specific mutagenesis. This process involves a change in one or more amino acid residues from its native structure. Perhaps the best example for this technique is IL-4, in which a single amino acid alteration converts the cytokine from an agonist to an antagonist (196). Replacement of a tyrosine residue at position 124 with aspartic acid

converts this protein into a receptor antagonist and blocks the activity of both IL-4 and IL-13 (196). Similarly, in TNF, which binds to two distinct receptors, site-specific mutagenesis results in mutant TNF protein (referred to as muteins) with specificity for one type of receptor as opposed to the other (197).

MOST CYTOKINE RECEPTORS HAVE COMMON CHARACTERISTICS

Most cytokines interact with cells through specific cell-surface receptors, the density of which may vary from 10 to 10,000 sites/cell. These receptors are usually of high affinity (kd; 10–100 pmol). Some cytokines are distinct in their chemical structure yet share common cell surface receptors (198–200): TNF and LT; IL-4 and IL-13; acidic and basic FGF; EGF and TGF-α; IFN-α and IFN-β; and IL-1α, IL-1β, and IL-1RA. In most instances, cytokine re-

TABLE 1–6   PEPTIDES DERIVED FROM DIFFERENT CYTOKINES THAT DISPLAY AGONISTIC OR ANTAGONISTIC ACTIVITY

Cytokine/Receptor	Peptide Region	Activity	Reference
Cytokine			
IL-1β	163–171	Like IL-1 immunomodulatory in vivo. Unlike IL-1, is not pyrogenic.	(183,184)
IL-1β	Tripeptide	Blocks IL-1β–induced hyperalgesia, body temperature, food intake.	(185)
IL-6	88–121	Blocks IL-6 binding.	(186)
IFN-γ	4–16	Peptide antibody neutralizes antiproliferative activity of IFN-γ.	(187)
IFN-γ	1–39; 95–133	Blocks antiviral activity of IFN-γ and receptor binding.	(188)
TNF-α	31–68	Stimulates fibroblasts chemotaxis.	(189)
	144–157[†]	The peptide has high binding affinity for TNF-α.	(190)
	54–94	Neutrophil stimulation; pyrogenic.	(191)
	10–36; 31–36	Somnogenic and pyrogenic.	(192)
	69–100	Suppressed food intake, fever.	
	44–68	Pyrogenic.	
	31–45	Somnogenic.	
bFGF	13–18	Receptor antagonist.	(193)
	120–125		
Receptors			
TNF-R (p55)	159–178	Binding to TNF and inhibits TNF cytotoxicity.	(194)
IL-1 R	86–93	Binds to IL-1 (α and β), and inhibit IL-1 actions in vitro and in vivo.	(195)

*See Table 1-1 for abbreviations.
[†]This is a complementary peptide to TNF sequence.

ceptors consist of a single polypeptide chain with extracellular, transmembrane, and intracellular domains (Fig. 1–1). Among all the cytokine receptors, IL-8 receptor is the only one that has seven transmembrane domains.

Several instances have been found in which more than one polypeptide chain is needed to constitute a functional receptor. For instance, functional IL-2 receptor consists of three different polypeptide chains: α-, β-, and γ-subunits. Some receptors consist of two different chains; one is specific for binding to the ligand and the other is responsible for signal transduction, as in IL-6, oncostatin M, ciliary neurotrophic factor (CNTF), and LIF. The receptors for cytokines IL-3, GM-CSF, and IL-5 also consist of two distinct subunits. IL-3, GM-CSF, and IL-5 receptors have specific α-subunits, but they share the same β-subunit (Fig. 1–2). Although none of these receptor subunits has intrinsic kinase activity, these cytokines induce protein tyrosine phosphorylation, activation of Ras, Raf-1 and mitogen activated protein (MAP) kinase, and tran-

scriptionally activate nuclear protooncogenes, such as c-myc, c-fos, and c-jun. These signals are mediated through two distinct cytoplasmic regions of the β-subunit (i.e., the membrane proximal region of approximately 60 amino acid residues is essential for c-myc and pim-1 induction, and a distal region of approximately 140 amino acid residues is required for activation of Ras, Raf-1, MAP kinase, and p70 S6 kinase, as well as induction of c-fos and c-jun) (200).

On the basis of their structural characteristics, the receptors for cytokines have been classified into several superfamilies. This classification includes the cytokine receptor superfamily, which is characterized by a common structural design of the extracellular domain, with four conserved cysteine residues in the amino terminal portion and a short motif, WSXWS, proximal to the transmembrane domain. Members of this superfamily can be grouped into three functional categories: single-chain receptors that bind ligand with high affinity and transduce

Cytokine Receptor Families

Common Cell-Signaling Elements of Different Cytokines

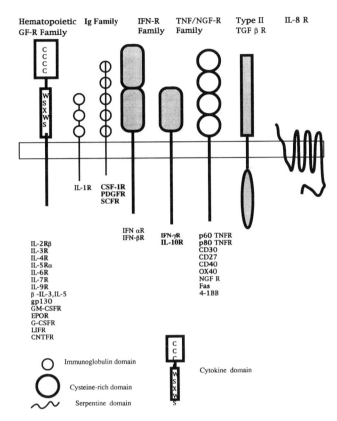

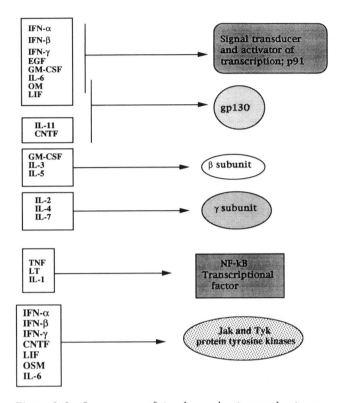

Figure 1–1 Diagrammatic representation of different cytokine receptor families. Different domains of the receptors are also shown. Various cytokines that bind to each type of receptor are also outlined.

Figure 1–2 Convergence of signal transduction mechanisms of several distinct cytokines. Various proteins involved in cellular signaling are shown.

intracellular signals (erythropoietin receptors [EPO-R], G-CSF-R, and IL-4R); a second class of receptors that bind ligand with low affinity and cannot transduce intracellular signals (IL-6-R, GM-CSF-R, and IL-3R); and a third class that constitutes a β-subunit common to several receptors, including IL-3R, IL-5R, and GM-CSF-R, which forms a high affinity receptor when combined with specific α-subunits and then transduces the signal.

Induction of cellular phosphorylation of various proteins is a characteristic feature of most cytokines. Several receptors display kinase activity, mainly the growth factor receptors: M-CSF, SCF, EPO, platelet-derived growth factor (PDGF), FGF, EGF, IGF-1, HGGF, VEGF, and TGF-β. In other instances, the cytokine receptors recruit other proteins that have kinase activity, including (in addition to aforementioned indicated growth factors) IL-2, IL-6, IL-4, and IL-7. The role of phosphatases in the transduction of signals by cytokines is less well understood.

The activity of a cytokine is regulated in part through regulation of their receptors. The cytokine receptors may be modulated by other cytokines and also by several pathological and physiological stimuli. Some cytokines

are capable of modulating their own receptors (e.g., IL-2, IL-4, and TNF) (110–112,201).

MOST CYTOKINES DISPLAY BOTH CELL SURFACE AND SOLUBLE RECEPTORS

In addition to cell surface receptors, soluble receptors corresponding to the ligand binding domains of many polypeptide hormones and cytokine receptors have been described. The function of these soluble receptors is as yet unknown (202,203). The production of soluble low density lipoprotein receptor (sLDL-R) with antiviral activity induced by IFN indicates that such receptors may perform independent functions (204). Previous studies have shown that some viruses code for receptor-like molecules that block their cytokines (e.g., IFN-γ, IL-1, TNF, and IL-8) (104–106,205,206). Such soluble receptors assist virus infection by suppressing host defense mechanisms. From the studies on induction of antiviral sLDL-R by IFNs, it seems that host organisms make use of a similar type of molecule for the opposite role of controlling virus infection.

Down-modulation of the receptors in several instances is due to the shedding of the receptors. Usually, the extracellular domain of the receptor is shed; thus, soluble receptors act as inhibitors of cytokines. The soluble receptors may originate via two separate mechanisms, one involving alternate splicing, in which a receptor gene lacks a transmembrane domain; and a second in which specific enzymes are activated, thus cleaving the receptor from the cell surface. A list of cytokines for which soluble receptors are produced by these mechanisms is shown in Table 1–7 (207–242). The identity of enzymes involved in proteolytic cleavage of the receptors is not known; however, it is a highly regulated process and appears to be controlled by phosphatases and kinases (243–245).The treatment of cells with ligand can also lead to down-modulation of the receptors and their subsequent shedding, thus suggesting activation of specific proteases (246,247). Under normal physiological conditions, these receptors inhibit cytokine response and function in the transport of cytokines (248,249).

Like the soluble and membrane-bound form of cytokine receptors, there are cytokine ligands that also exist in both forms, as in IL-1, TNF, FGF, TFG-α, TGF-β, and SCF. The mechanisms that control conversion of the membrane-bound form to the soluble form have an important role in determination of cytokine activity. In TGF-α, conversion of the membrane to the soluble form has been shown to be a multistep process (250,251).

TABLE 1–7 SOLUBLE RECEPTORS IDENTIFIED FOR VARIOUS CYTOKINES IN BIOLOGICAL FLUIDS

Receptor	Source	Reference
Proteolytic cleavage		
IL-1R	Cellular	(207)
IL-2R	Urine, cellular serum	(208–210)
IL-4R (m)	Serum ascites and urine	(211)
IL-6R	Cellular	(212,213)
IL-6R (gp 130)	Serum	(214)
TNFR	Urine, cellular, serum	(215–221)
IFN-αR	Serum and urine	(223)
IFN-γR	Cellular	(130)
NGFR	Cellular, serum, urine	(240)
MCSFR	Cellular	(225)
Heregulin R	Cellular, serum	(226–229)
EGFR	Cellular	(222)
EPOR	Cellular, serum	(241,242)
PDGFR	Cellular	(230)
Alternative splicing		
IL-4R (m)	Cellular	(231)
IL-5R (m)	Cellular	(232)
IL-7R	Cellular	(233)
LIF-R	Serum	(234)
GM-CSFR	Cellular	(235,236)
G-CSFR	Cellular	(237)
EGFR	Cellular	(238)
c-erbB3	Cellular	(239)
VEGFR	Cellular	(249)

*See Table 1–1 for abbreviations.
m = murine.

DIFFERENT CYTOKINES EXHIBIT OVERLAPPING AND REDUNDANT ACTION

The same activity may be displayed by several structurally distinct cytokines through unrelated cell surface receptors. For instance, it has been shown that IL-1, TNF, IFN, IL-6, and CNTF are intrinsically pyrogenic cytokines that cause fever (252–257). Similarly, growth of certain tumor cells, such as human breast adenocarcinoma MCF-7, can be inhibited by TNF, LT, IL-1, IL-6, TGF-β, amphiregulin, and oncostatin M, all distinct cytokines. In addition to IL-2, proliferation of T lymphocytes is regulated by several other cytokines, including IL-4, IL-7, IL-12, and IL-13. This type of redundancy in the effects of cytokines may explain why animals survive disruption of the IL-2 gene. Wound healing functions have been assigned to several distinct growth factors, including EGF, TGF-α, FGF, PDGF, TNF, and TGF-β (258). Overlapping and redundant actions of cytokines have also been observed during the acute phase response, stimulation of hematopoiesis, septic shock, and cachexia (weight loss) (259).

Why cytokines are so redundant in their biological action is not certain. In most cases, cytokines transmit their signals through distinct pathways, yet the biological response is the same. Examples have been noted, however, in which the molecular basis for overlapping actions may lie in common postreceptor signaling pathways. For instance, IL-6, CNTF, LIF, and oncostatin M, which induce similar responses, mediate their signals through a glycoprotein, gp-130 (recently renamed β-subunit), thus implying that they have a common mechanism of action (see Fig. 1–2). Similarly, the signal transducing apparatus of GM-CSF, IL-3, and IL-5 have a common subunit associated with their specific receptors. Furthermore, it has recently been shown that IL-2, IL-4, and IL-7-mediated T-cell proliferation occurs through a common signaling peptide, the γ-subunit of the IL-2 receptor (260–262).

DIFFERENT CYTOKINES EXHIBIT SYNERGISTIC, ADDITIVE, AND ANTAGONISTIC INTERACTIONS

The cellular response of most cytokines is modulated by other cytokines, either positively or negatively. For instance, the antiproliferative effects of TNF against different tumor cells are potentiated synergistically by IFN-γ and IL-4 (263,264), whereas the proliferative effects of TNF on fibroblasts are antagonized by IFN-γ (265). The latter has also been shown to potentiate the antiviral ef-

fects of IFN-α (266). Exactly how one cytokine modulates the effect of another is not understood. In some instances, it occurs through induction of receptors, but that mechanism is not sufficient to explain the crossmodulation of cellular response observed (267–270).

DIFFERENT CYTOKINES ARE AUTOIMMUNOGENIC AND ACT AS ADJUVANTS

The activities of cytokines in vivo are regulated by several factors. Among those factors that appear to have an important role in this regulation are autoantibodies against cytokines (271). Naturally occurring or therapeutically induced antibodies to cytokines are generally thought to inhibit cytokine functions, and the appearance of such antibodies should result in cytokine deficiency. Autoimmune disease may follow, and the pharmacological action of the cytokine may be inhibited. In contrast, the inhibitory activities of these antibodies may at times be useful; they may also serve as specific carriers of these cytokines in the circulation. For instance, anti-insulin antibodies sometimes prolong the release of active insulin in the tissues, which results in hypoglycemia in nondiabetics and a marked reduction in the requirement for exogenous insulin in diabetic patients (272).

Production of autoantibodies may be associated with a disease, as in patients with systemic lupus erythematosus, who have autoantibodies to IFN-α (273), or patients with the acquired immunodeficiency syndrome (AIDS), who have antibodies against IL-2 (274). The presence of autoantibodies to IL-1α and TNF-α in apparently normal individuals has also been reported (275,276). In vivo, enhancement of cytokine activity appears to occur by a mechanism that retards rapid removal of cytokines from the circulation (277).

Cytokines are known to potentiate cellular and humoral immunity through several different mechanisms, including induction of human leukocyte antigen (HLA) class I molecules; regulation of growth and differentiation of B and T cells; generation of specific cytotoxic T lymphocytes; and activation of macrophages and neutrophils. The growth of genetically modified nonimmunogenic tumors transfected with different cytokines has been shown to be inhibited in vivo. Several cytokines have been exploited to enhance the immunogenic response against tumor cells, including IL-2, IL-4, IL-6, IL-7, IL-10, IL-12, and IFN-γ (278–285). It was suggested that IL-10–transfected cells indirectly suppress tumor growth by inhibiting the infiltration of macrophages that may otherwise promote tumor growth (282).

CYTOKINES ARE THERAPEUTIC DRUGS

Several cytokines have been approved by the Food and Drug Administration (FDA) for human use in the United States, including IFN-α, IFN-β, IFN-γ, G-CSF, GM-CSF, EPO, and IL-2 (Fig. 1–3). IFN-α was the first cytokine to be discovered and also the first approved by the FDA for clinical use in 1986. Its current approved clinical uses include therapy for hairy-cell leukemia, chronic myeloid leukemia, Kaposi's sarcoma, condylomata acuminata, chronic hepatitis C, and chronic hepatitis B. G-CSF was approved for clinical use to decrease the incidence of infection in patients with nonmyeloid malignancies receiving myelosuppressive chemotherapy. GM-CSF was approved for use in patients with non-Hodgkin's lymphoma, Hodgkin's disease, and acute lymphocytic leukemia patients undergoing autologous bone marrow transplantation. It is also used for patients with delayed or failed autologous or homologous bone marrow transplantation. Chronic granulomatous disease and metastatic renal-cell carcinoma are treated with IFN-γ and IL-2, respectively. Erythropoietin is another cytokine that has been approved for anemia associated with chronic renal failure, malignancy, chemotherapy, AIDS, azidothymidine (AZT) treatment, rheumatoid arthritis, anemia of prematurity, autologous blood donation prior to surgery, and for compensation of surgical blood loss. The most recent approval of cytokines has been IFN-β for the treatment of ambulatory patients with relapsing/remitting multiple sclerosis.

Cytokines Approved in United States For Human Use

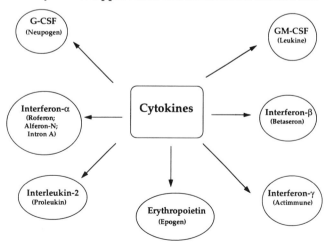

Figure 1–3 Various cytokines and their commercial names recognized for human use in the United States.

CONCLUSION

Cytokines are a new class of molecules discovered within the last decade. These molecules have an important role in both pathogenesis and treatment of disease. Cytokines have already made the transition from concept to clinic and have attracted the attention of a great number of scientists in both academic and industrial settings during the last few years. Because of their importance to homeostasis, therapy, the multiplicity of their interactions, and the complexity of their modulation, it is certain that the cytokine field will continue to expand.

Recently a new interleukin, designated IL-15, with an approximate molecular weight of 14–15 kd, has been discovered. Like IL-2, IL-15 is a growth factor for T cells and it utilizes the beta and gamma chains of the IL-2 receptor for its action (286,287).

ACKNOWLEDGMENTS: This research was conducted in part by The Clayton Foundation for Research, and was supported in part by new program development funds from The University of Texas, M. D. Anderson Cancer Center, Houston, Tex.

REFERENCES

1. Isaacs A, Lindenmann J. Virus interference. I. The interferons. Proc R Soc Lond (Biol) 1957;147:258–267.
2. Aggarwal BB, Pocsik E. Cytokines: from clone to clinic. Arch Biochem Biophys 1992;292:335–359.
3. Roberts RM, Cross JC, Leaman DW. Interferons as hormones of pregnancy. Endocr Rev 1992;13:432–452.
4. Aggarwal BB, Gutterman JU, eds. Human cytokines: a handbook for basic and clinical researchers. Boston: Blackwell Scientific Publications, 1992.
5. Hilton DJ. LIF: lots of interesting functions. Trends Biochem Sci 1992;17:72–76.
6. Witte ON. Steel locus defines new multipotent growth factor. Cell 1990;63:5–6.
7. Schwall RH, Nikolics K, Szonyi E, Gorman C, Mason AJ. Recombinant expression and characterization of human activin A. Mol Endocrinol 1988;2:1237–1242.
8. Goodwin RG, Alderson MR, Smith CA, et al. Molecular and biological characterization of a ligand for CD27 defines a new family of cytokines with homology to tumor necrosis factor. Cell 1993;73:447–456.
9. Hollenbaugh D, Grosmaire LS, Kullas CD, et al. The human T cell antigen gp39, a member of the TNF gene family, is a ligand for the CD40 receptor: expression of a soluble form of gp39 with B cell co-stimulatory activity. EMBO J 1992;11:4313–4321.
10. Ambrus JL, Pippin J, Joseph A, et al. Identification of a cDNA for a human high molecular weight B-cell growth factor. Proc Natl Acad Sci USA 1993;90:6330–6334.
11. Heinrich JN, Ryseck R-P, MacDonald-Bravo H, Bravo R.

The product of a novel growth factor-activated gene, fic, is a biologically active "C-C"-type cytokine. Mol Cell Biol 1993;13:2020–2030.

12. Sherry B, Tekamp-Olson P, Gallegos C, et al. Resolution of the two components of macrophage inflammatory protein 1, and cloning and characterization of one of those components, macrophage inflammatory protein 1β. J Exp Med 1988;168:2251–2259.

13. Schall TJ, Jongstra J, Dyer BJ, et al. A human T cell-specific molecule is a member of a new gene family. J Immunol 1988;141:1018–1025.

14. Richmond A, Balentien E, Thomas HG, et al. Molecular characterization and chromosomal mapping of melanoma growth stimulatory activity, a growth factor structurally related to β-thromboglobulin. EMBO J 1988;7:2025–2033.

15. Plowman GD, Green JM, McDonald VL, et al. The amphiregulin gene encodes a novel epidermal growth factor-related protein with tumor-inhibitory activity. Mol Cell Biol 1990;10:1969–1981.

16. Suda T, Takahashi T, Golstein P, Nagata S. Molecular cloning and expression of the Fas ligand, a novel member of the tumor necrosis factor family. Cell 1993;75:1169–1178.

17. Heldin C-H. Structural and functional studies on platelet derived growth factor. EMBO J 1992;11:4251–4259.

18. Gospodarowicz D. Fibroblast growth factor. Crit Rev Oncog 1989;1:1–26.

19. Carpenter G. EGF: new tricks for an old growth factor. Curr Opin Cell Biol 1993;5:261–264.

20. Derynck R. The physiology of transforming growth factor-α. Adv Cancer Res 1992;58:27–52.

21. Shing Y, Christofori G, Hanahan D, et al. Betacellulin: a mitogen from pancreatic β cell tumors. Science 1993; 259:1604–1607.

22. Daughaday WH, Rotwein P. Insulin-like growth factors I and II. Peptide, messenger ribonucleic acid and gene structures, serum, and tissue concentrations. Endocr Rev 1989;10:68–91.

23. Nakamura T, Nishizawa T, Hagiya M, et al. Molecular cloning and expression of human hepatocyte growth factor. Nature 1980;342:440–443.

24. Watanabe H, Carmi P, Hogan V, et al. Purification of human tumor cell autocrine motility factor and molecular cloning of its receptor. J Biol Chem 1991;266:13442–13448.

25. Tanaka A, Miyamoto K, Minamino N, et al. Cloning and characterization of an androgen-induced growth factor essential for the androgen-dependent growth of mouse mammary carcinoma cells. Proc Natl Acad Sci USA 1992; 89:8928–8932.

26. Marchionni MA, Goodearl ADJ, Chen MS, et al. Glial growth factors are alternatively spliced erbB2 ligands expressed in the nervous system. Nature 1993;362:312–318.

27. Naruo K, Seko C, Kuroshima K, et al. Novel secretory heparin-binding factors from human glioma cells (glia-activating factors) involved in glial cell growth. Purification and biological properties. J Biol Chem 1993;268:2857–2864.

28. Zaheer A, Fionk BD, Lim R. Expression of glia maturation factor β mRNA and protein in rat organs and cells. J Neurochem 1993;60:914–920.

29. Falls DL, Rosen KM, Corfas G, Lane WS, Fischbach GD. ARIA, a protein that stimultes acetylcholine receptor synthesis, is a member of the neu ligand family. Cell 1993; 72:801–815.

30. Li Y-S, Hoffman RM, Le Beau MM, et al. Characterization of the human pleiotrophin gene. Promoter region and chromosomal localization. J Biol Chem 1992;267:26011–26016.

31. Ozkaynak E, Schnegelsberg PNJ, Jin DF, et al. Osteogenic protein-2. A new member of the transforming factor-β superfamily expressed early in embryogenesis. J Biol Chem 1992;267:25220–25227.

32. Wozney JM, Rosen V, Celeste AJ, et al. Novel regulators of bone formation: molecular clones and activities. Science 1988;242:1528–1534.

33. Stockli KA, Lottspeich F, Sendtner M, et al. Molecular cloning, expression and regional distribution of rat ciliary neurotrophic factor. Nature 1989;342:920–923.

34. Lyman SD, James L, Zappone J, Sleath PR, Beckmann MP, Bird T. Characterization of the protein encoded by the flt3 (flk2) receptor-like tyrosine kinase gene. Oncogene 1993; 8:815–822.

35. Minty A, Chalon P, Derocq J-M, et al. Interleukin-13 is a new human lymphokine regulating inflammatory and immune responses. Nature 1993;362:248–250.

36. Browning JL, Ngam-ek A, Lawton P, et al. Lymphotoxin β, a novel member of the TNF family that forms a heteromeric complex with lymphotoxin on the cell surface. Cell 1993;72:847–856.

37. Sporn MB, Roberts AB. Peptide growth factors are multifunctional. Nature 1988;332:217–218.

38. Nathan C, Sporn M. Cytokines in context. J Cell Biol 1991;113:981–986.

39. Balkwill FR, ed. Cytokines: a practical approach. Oxford: Oxford University Press, 1991.

40. Kroemer G, Alboran M, Gonzalo JA, Martinez C. Immunoregulation by cytokines. Crit Rev Immunol 1993; 13:163–191.

41. Elsasser-Beile U, Von Kleist S. Cytokines as therapeutic and diagnostic agents. Tumor Biol 1993;14:69–94.

42. Nicola NA. Hematopoietic growth factors and their receptors. In: Thomas ED, ed. Applications of basic science to hematopoiesis and treatment of disease. New York: Raven, 1993:51–69.

43. Clemens MJ, ed. Cytokines: Oxford: BIOS Scientific Publishers, 1991.

44. Zolte M, Ben-Rafael Z, Meirom R, et al. Cytokine involvement in oocytes and early embryos. Fertil Steril 1991; 56:265–272.

45. Ben-Rafael Z, Orvieto R. Cytokines—involvement in reproduction. Fertil Steril 1992;58:1093–1099.

46. Adamson ED. Growth factors and their receptors in development. Dev Genet 1993;14:159–164.

47. Chen HC, Marcinkiewicz JL, Sancho-Tello M, Hunt JS, Terranova PA. Tumor necrosis factor-α gene expression in mouse oocytes and follicular cells. Biol Reprod 1993; 48:707–714.

48. Mitchell MD, Trautman MS, Dudley DJ. Cytokine networking in placenta. Placenta 1993;14:249–275.

49. Guilbert L, Robertson SA, Wegmann TG. The trophoblast as an integral component of a macrophage-cytokine network. Immunol Cell Biol 1993;71:49–57.

50. Haas W, Kuhn R. Knock out mice as models for immunodeficiency diseases. In: Gergely J, ed. Progress in immunology VIII. Berlin: Springer Hungarica, 1992:561–570.

51. Travis J. Scoring a technical knockout in mice. Science 1992;256:1392–1394.

52. Waldman AS. Targeted homologous recombination in mammalian cells. Crit Rev Oncol 1992;12:49–64.

53. Rajewsky K. A phenotype or not: targeting genes in the immune system. Science 1992;256:483.

54. Castigli E, Pahwa R, Good RA, Geha RS, Chatila TA. Molecular basis of a multiple lymphokine deficiency in a patient with severe combined immunodeficiency. Proc Natl Acad Sci USA 1993;90:4728–4732.

55. Stewart CL, Kaspar P, Brunet LJ, et al. Blastocyst implantation depends on maternal expression of leukaemia inhibitory factor. Nature 1992;359:76–79.

56. Kuhn R, Lohler J, Rennick D, Rajewsky K, Muller W. Interleukin-10-deficient mice develop chronic emterocolitis. Cell 1993;75:263–273.

57. Sadlack B, Merz H, Schorle H, Schimpl A, Feller AC, Horak I. Ulcerative colitis-like disease in mice with a disrupted interleukin-2 gene. Cell 1993;75:253–261.

58. Schorle H, Holtschke T, Hunig T, Schimpl A, Horak I. Development and function of T cells in mice rendered interleukin-2 deficient by gene targeting. Nature 1991; 352:621–624.

59. Horak I. Lymphocyte development and immunoreactivity in IL-2 deficient mice. In: Gergely J, ed. Progress in immunology VIII. Berlin: Springer Hungarica, 1992:305–311.

60. Kanagawa O, Vaupel BA, Gayama S, Koehler G, Kopf M. Resistance of mice deficient in IL-4 to retrovirus-induced immunodeficiency syndrome (MAIDS). Science 1993; 262:240–242.

61. Kopf M, Le Gros G, Bachmann M, Lamers MC, Bluethmann H, Kohler G. Disruption of the murine IL-4 gene blocks TH2 cytokine responses. Nature 1993;362:245–247.

62. Kuhn R, Rajewsky K, Muller W. Generation and analysis of interleukin-4 deficient mice. Science 1991;254:707–710.

63. Shull MM, Ormsbyu L, Kier AB, et al. Targeted disruption of the mouse transforming growth factor-β_1 gene. Nature 1992;359:693–699.

64. Kulkarni AB, Huh C-G, Becker D, et al. Transforming growth factor-β_1 null mutation in mice causes excessive inflammatory response and early death. Proc Natl Acad Sci USA 1993;90:770–774.

65. Kulkarni Ab, Karlsson S. Transforming growth factor-β knockout mice. Am J Pathol 1993;143:3–9.

66. Matzuk MM, Finegold MJ, Su J-GF, Hsueh AJW, Bradley A. α-Inhibin is a tumour-suppressor gene with gonadal specificity in mice. Nature 1992;360:313–319.

67. Barinaga M. Interfering with interferon. Science 1993;259:1693–1694.

68. Cooper AM, Dalton DK, Stewart TA, Griffin JP, Russell DG, Orme IM. Disseminated tuberculosis in interferon γ gene-disrupted mice. J Exp Med 1993;178:2243–2247.

69. Dalton DK, Pitts-Meek S, Keshav S, Figari IS, Bradley A, Stewart TA. Multiple defects of immune cell function in mice with disrupted interferon α-genes. Science 1993; 259:1739–1742.

70. Flynn JL, Chan J, Triebold KJ, Dalton DK, Stewart TA, Bloom BR. An essential role for interferon γ in resistance to Mycobacterium tuberculosis infection. J Exp Med 1993; 178:2249–2254.

71. Brannan CI, Lyman SD, Williams DE, et al. Steel-Dickie mutation encodes a c-kit ligand lacking transmembrane and cytoplasmic domains. Proc Natl Acad Sci USA 1991; 88:4671–4674.

72. Nocka K, Buck J, Levi E, Besmer P. Candidate ligand for the c-kit transmembrane kinase receptor: KL, a fibroblast derived growth factor stimulates mast cells and erythroid progenitors. EMBO J 1990;9:3287–3294.

73. Cohen PL, Eisenberg RA. Lpr and Gld: single gene models of systemic autoimmunity and lymphoproliferative disease. Annu Rev Immunol 1991;9:243–269.

74. Yoshida H, Hayashi S-I, Kunisada T, et al. The murine mutation osteopetrosis is in the coding region of the macrophage colony stimulating factor gene. Nature 1990; 345:442–444.

75. Luetteke NC, Qiu TH, Peiffer RL, Oliver P, Smithies O, Lee DC. TGFα deficiency results in hair follicle and eye abnormalities in targeted and waved-1 mice. Cell 1993;73:263–278.

76. Aruffo A, Farrington M, Hollenbaugh D, et al. The CD40 ligand, gp39, is defective in activated T cells from patients with X-linked hyper-IgM syndrome. Cell 1993;72:291–300.

77. Pfeffer K, Matsuyama T, Kundig TM, et al. Mice deficient for the 55 kd tumor necrosis factor receptor are resistant to endotoxic shock yet succumb to L. monocytogenes infection. Cell 1993;73:457–467.

78. Rothe J, Lessiauer W, Lotscher H, et al. Mice lacking the tumour necrosis factor receptor 1 are resistant to TNF-mediated toxicity but highly susceptible to infection by Listeria monocytogenes. Nature 1993;364:798–802.

79. Huang S, Hendriks W, Althage A, et al. Immune response in mice that lack the interferon-γ receptor. Science 1993;259:1742–1745.

80. Kamuto R, Shapiro D, Le J, Huang S, Aguet M, Vilcek J. Generation of nitric oxide and induction of major histocompatibility complex class II antigen in macrophages from mice lacking the interferon γ receptor. Proc Natl Acad Sci USA 1993;90:6626–6630.

81. Watanabe-Fukunaga R, Brannan CI, Copeland NG, Jenkins NA, Nagata S. Lymphoproliferation disorder in mice explained by defects in fas antigen that mediates apoptosis. Nature 1992;356:314–317.

82. Beck G, Habicht GS. Primitive cytokines: harbingers of vertebrate defense. Immunol Today 1991;12:180–183.

83. Lenard J. Mammalian hormones in microbial cells. Trends Biochem Sci 1992;17:147–150.

84. Raftos DA, Cooper EL, Habicht GS, Beck G. Invertebrate cytokines: tunicate cell proliferation stimulated by an interleukin-1-like molecule. Proc Natl Acad Sci USA 1991;88:9518–9522.

85. Raftos DA, Cooper EL, Stillman DL, Habicht GS, Beck G. Invertebrate cytokines II: release of interleukin-1 like mol-

ecules from tunicate hemocytes stimulated with zymosan. Lymphokine Cytokine Res 1992;11:235–240.

86. Hursh DA, Andrews ME, Raff RA. A sea urchin gene encodes a polypeptide homologous to epidermal growth factor. Science 1987;237:1487–1490.

87. Ottaviani E, Franchini A, Franceschi C. Presence of several cytokine-like molecules in molluscan hemocytes. Biochem Biophys Res Commun 1993;195:984–988.

88. Porat R, Clark BD, Wolff SM, Dinarello CA. Enhancement of growth virulent strains of Escherichia coli by interleukin-1. Science 1991;254:430–432.

89. Treseler CB, Maziarz RT, Levitz SM. Biological activity of interleukin-2 bound to Candida albicans. Infect Immun 1992;60:183–188.

90. Denis M, Campbell D, Gregg EO. Interleukin-2 and granulocyte-macrophage colony-stimulate growth of a virulent strain of Escherichia coli. Infect Immun 1991;59:1853–1856.

91. Shoemaker CB, Ramachandran H, Landa A, Reis MG, Stein LD. Alternative splicing of Schistosoma mansoni gene encoding a homologue of epidermal growth factor receptor. Mol Biochem Parasitol 1992;53:17–32.

92. Malloy PJ, Zhao X, Madani ND, Feldman D. Cloning and expression of the gene from Candida albicans that encodes a high-affinity corticosteroid-binding protein. Proc Natl Acad Sci USA 1993;90:1902–1906.

93. Prosperi M, Ferbus D, Karczinski I, Goubin G. A human cDNA corresponding to a gene overexpressed during cell proliferation encodes a product sharing homology with amoebic and bacterial proteins. J Biol Chem 1993; 15:11050–11056.

94. Hughes TK, Smith EM, Chin R, et al. Interaction of immunoactive monokines (interleukin 1 and tumor necrosis factor) in bivalve moluscs Mytilus edulis. Proc Natl Acad Sci USA 1990;87:4426–4429.

95. Kole HK, Lenard J. Insulin-induced stimulation of protein phosphorylation in Neurospora crassa cells. FASEB J 1991;5:2728–2734.

96. Kongshavn PAL, Ghadirian E. Enhancing and suppressive effects of tumor necrosis factor/cachectin on growth of Trypanosoma musculi. Parasite Immunol 1988;10:581–588.

97. Shiratsuchi J, Johnson JL, Ellner JJ. Bidirectional effects of cytokines on the growth of Mycobacterium avium with human monocytes. J Immunol 1991;146:3165–3170.

98. Childs SR, Wrana JL, Arora K, Attisano L, O'Connor MB, Massague J. Identification of a Drosophila activin receptor. Proc Natl Acad Sci USA 1993;90:9475–9479.

99. Georgi LL, Albert PS, Riddle DL. Daf-1, a C. elegans gene controlling dauer larva development, encodes a novel receptor protein kinase. Cell 1990;61:635–645.

100. Miura M, Zhu H, Rotello R, Hartwieg EA, Yuan J. Induction of apoptosis in fibroblasts by IL-1β-converting enzyme, a mammalian homolog of the C. elegans cell death gene ced-3. Cell 1993;75:653–660.

101. Yuan J, Shaham S, Ledoux S, Ellis HM, Horvitz HR. The C. elegans cell death gene ced-3 encodes a protein similar to mammalian interleukin-1β-converting enzyme. Cell 1993; 75:641–652.

102. Gooding LR. Virus proteins that counteract host immune defenses. Cell 1992;71:5–7.

103. Kurilla MG, Swaminathan S, Welsh RM, Kieff E, Brutkiewicz RR. Effects of virally expressed interleukin-10 on vaccinia virus infection in mice. J Virol 1993;67:7623–7628.

104. Ahuja SK, Murphy PM. Molecular piracy of mammalian interleukin-8 receptor type B by herpes virus saimiri. J Biol Chem 1993;268:20691–20694.

105. Smith CA, Davis T, Anderson D, et al. A receptor for tumor necrosis factor defines an unusual family of cellular and viral proteins. Science 1990;248:1019–1023.

106. Upton C, Mossman K, McFadden G. Encoding of a homolog of the IFN-gamma receptor by myxoma virus. Science 1992;258:1369–1372.

107. Plowman GD, Green JM, Culouscou J-M, Carlton GW, Rothwell VM, Buckley S. Heregulin induces tyrosine phosphorylation of HER4/p180^{erbB4}. Nature 1993;366:473–475.

108. Spriggs MK, Fanslow WC, Armitage RJ, Belmont J. The biology of the human ligand for CD40. J Clin Immunol 1993; 13:373–380.

109. Zurawski SM, Vega F Jr, Huyghe B, Zurawski G. Receptors for interleukin-13 and interleukin-4 are complex and share a novel component that functions in signal transduction. EMBO J 1993;12:2663–2670.

110. Winzen R, Wallach D, Kemper O, Resch K, Holtmann H. Selective up-regulation of the 75-kDa tumor necrosis factor (TNF) receptor and its mRNA by TNF and IL-1. J Immunol 1993;150:4346–4353.

111. Smith KA, Cantrell DA. Interleukin 2 regulates its own receptors. Proc Natl Acad Sci USA 1985;82:864–868.

112. Renz H, Domenico J, Gelfand E. IL-4 dependent up-regulation of IL-4 receptor expression in murine T and B cells. J Immunol 1991;146:3049–3055.

113. Wanidworanun C, Strober W. Predominant role of tumor necrosis factor-α in human monocyte IL-10 synthesis. J Immunol 1993;151:6853–6861.

114. Shaw G, Kamen R. A conserved AU sequence from the 3′ untranslated region of GM-CSF and mRNA mediates selective mRNA degradation. Cell 1986;46:659–667.

115. Kimball E, Pickeral SF, Oppenheim JJ, Rossio JL. Interleukin 1 activity in normal human urine. J Immunol 1984;133:256–260.

116. De Boer EC, De Jong WH, Steerenberg PA, et al. Induction of urinary interleukin-1 (IL-1), IL–2, IL-6, and tumor necrosis factor. Cancer Immunol Immunother 1992;34:306–312.

117. Ratliff TL, Haaff EO, Catalona WJ. Interleukin-2 production during intravesical bacille Calmette-Guerin therapy for bladder cancer. Clin Immunol Immunopathol 1986; 40:375–379.

118. De Jong WH, De Boer EC, Van Der Meijden APM, et al. Presence of interleukin-2 in urine of superficial bladder cancer patients after intravesical treatment with bacillus Calmette-Guerin. Cancer Immunol Immunother 1990; 31:182–186.

119. Van Oers MHJ, Van der Heyden AAPAM, Aarden LA. Interleukin 6 (IL-6) in serum and urine of renal transplant recipients. Clin Exp Immunol 1988;71:115–119.

120. Prescott S, James K, Hargreave TB, Chisholm GD, Smyth

JF. Radio-immunoassay detection of interferon-gamma in urine after intravascular evans BCG therapy. J Urol 1990; 144:1248–1251.

121. Motoyoshi K, Takau F, Mizoguchi H, Miura Y. Purification and some properties of colony-stimulating factor from normal urine. Blood 1978;52:1012–1020.

122. Wang FF, Goldwasser E. Purification of human urinary colony-stimulating factor. J Cell Biochem 1983;21:263–275.

123. Sakai N, Umeda T, Suzuki H, Ishimatsu Y, Shikita M. Macrophage colony-stimulating factor purified from normal human urine. FEBS Lett 1987;222:341–344.

124. Zucali JR, Sulkowski E. Purification of human urinary erythropoietin on controlled-pore glass and silicic acid. Exp Hematol 1985;13:

125. Guirguis R, Schiffmann E, Liu B, Birkbeck D, Engel J, Liotta L. Detection of autocrine motility factor in urine as a marker of bladder cancer. J Natl Cancer Inst 1988; 80:1203–1211.

126. Nguyen M, Watanabe H, Budson AE, Richie JP, Folkman J. Elevated levels of the angiogenic peptide basic fibroblast growth factor in urine of bladder and cancer patients. J Natl Cancer Inst 1993;85:241–242.

127. Mount CD, Lucas TJ, Orth DN. Purification and characterization of epidermal growth factor fragments from large volumes of human urine. Arch Biochem Biophys 1985; 240:33–42.

128. Stromberg K, Hudgins WR, Orth DN. Urinary TGFs in neoplasia: immunoreactive TGF-α in the urine of patients with disseminated breast cancer. Biochem Biophys Res Commun 1987;144:1059–1068.

129. Pizzolo G, Vincenzi C, Vinante F, et al. Highly concentrated urine-purified tac peptide fails to inhibit IL-2 dependent cell proliferation in vitro. Cell Immunol 1992; 141:253–259.

130. Novick D, Engelmann H, Rubinstein M, Wallach D. Soluble cytokine receptors are present in normal human urine. J Exp Med 1989;170:1409–1414.

131. Austgulen R, Liabakk N, Lien E, Espevik T. Increased level of soluble tumor necrosis factor-α receptors in serum from pregnant women and in serum and urine samples from newborns. Pediatr Res 1993;33:82–86.

132. Seckinger P, Isaaz S, Dayer J-M. A human inhibitor of tumor necrosis factor α. J Exp Med 1988;167:1511–1516.

133. Olsson I, Lantz M, Nilsson E, et al. Isolation and characterization of a tumor necrosis factor binding protein from urine. Eur J Haematol 1989;42:270–275.

134. Engelmann H, Aderka D, Rubinstein M, Rotman D, Wallach D. A human tumor necrosis factor-binding protein purified to homogeneity from human urine protects from tumor necrosis factor toxicity. J Biol Chem 1989; 264:11974–11978.

135. Elias JA, Zitnik RJ. Cytokine-cytokine interactions in the context of cytokine networking. Am J Respir Cell Mol Biol 1992; 7:365–367.

136. Balkwill FR, Burke F. The cytokine network. Immunol Today 1989;10:299–303.

137. Ross R. The pathogenesis of atherosclerosis: a perspective for the 1990s. Nature 1993;362:801–809.

138. Elias JA, Freundlich B, Kern JA, Rosenbloom J. Clinical implications of basic research. Chest 1990;97:1439–1445.

139. Johnson R. Cytokine network and the pathogenesis of glomerulonephritis. J Lab Clin Med 1993;121:190–192.

140. Bursten SL, Locksley RM, Ryan JL, Lovett DH. Acylation of monocyte and glomerular mesangial cell proteins. J Clin Invest 1988;82:1479–1488.

141. Stevenson FT, Bursten SL, Locksley RM, Lovett DH. Myristyl acylation of the tumor necrosis factor α precursor on specific lysine residues. J Exp Med 1053;176:1053–1062.

142. Robert-Galliot B, Commoy-Chevalier MJ, Georges P, Chany C. Phosphorylation of recombinant interferon-gamma by kinases released from various cells. J Gen Virol 1985;66:1439–1448.

143. Arakawa T, Parker CG, Lai P-H. Sites of phosphorylation in recombinant human interferon-γ. Biochem Biophys Res Commun 1986;136:679–684.

144. May LT, Santhanam U, Tatter SB, Bhardwaj N, Ghrayeb J, Sehgal PB. Phosphorylation of secreted forms of human β_2-interferon/hepatocyte stimulating factor/interleukin-6. Biochem Biophys Res Commun 1988;152:1144–1150.

145. Fields R, Mariano TM, Stein S, Pestka S. Recombinant rat and murine immune interferons are phosphorylated at a single site, ser[132]. J Interferon Res 1988;8:549–557.

146. May LT, Sehgal PB. Phosphorylation of interleukin-6 at serine[54]: an early event in the secretory pathway in human fibroblasts. Biochem Biophys Res Commun 1992;185:524–530.

147. Feige J-J, Baird A. Basic fibroblast growth factor is a substrate for protein phosphorylation and is phosphorylated by capillary endothelial cells in culture. Proc Natl Acad Sci USA 1989;86:3174–3178.

148. Vilgrain I, Baird A. Phosphorylation of basic fibroblast growth factor by a protein kinase associated with the outer surface of a target cell. Mol Endocrinol 1991;5:1003–1012.

149. Jaye M, Howk R, Burgess W, et al. Human endothelial cell growth factor: cloning nucleotide sequence, and chromosome localization. Science 1986;233:541–545.

150. Abraham JA, Mergia A, Whang JL, et al. Nucleotide sequence of a bovine clone encoding the angiogenic protein, basic fibroblast growth factor. Science 1986;233:545–548.

151. Auron PE, Webb AC, Rosenwasser LJ, et al. Nucleotide sequence of human monocyte interleukin 1 precursor cDNA. Proc Natl Acad Sci USA 1984;81:7907–7911.

152. Kobayashi Y, Yamamoto K, Saido T, Kawasaki H, Oppenheim J, Matsushima K. Identification of calcium-activated neutral protease as a processing enzyme of human interleukin 1α. Proc Natl Acad Sci USA 1990;87:5548–5552.

153. Howard A, Kostura MJ, Thornberry N, et al. IL-1 converting enzyme requires aspartic acid residues for procesing of the IL-1β precursor at two distinct sites and does not cleave 31-kDa IL-1α. J Biol Chem 1991;147:2964–2969.

154. Cerretti DP, Kozloskty CJ, Mosley B, et al. Molecular cloning of the interleukin-1β converting enzyme. Science 1992; 256:97.

155. Thornberry NA, Bull HG, Calaycay JR, et al. A novel heterodimeric cysteine protease is required for interleukin-1 β processing in monocytes. Nature 1992;356:768–774.

156. Kronheim SR, Mumma A, Greenstreet T, et al. Purification

of interleukin-1β converting enzyme, the protease that cleaves the interleukin-1β precursor. Arch Biochem Biophys 1992;296:1.

157. Miller DK, Ayala JM, Eggert LA, et al. Purification and characterization of active human interleukin-1β converting enzyme from THP-1 monocytic cells. J Biol Chem 1993;268:18062–18069.

158. Banner DW, D'Arcy A, Janes W, et al. Crystal structure of the soluble human 55 kd TNF receptor-human TNFβ complex: implications for TNF receptor activation. Cell 1993; 73:431–445.

159. Jones EY, Stuart DI, Walker NP. Structure of tumour necrosis factor. Nature 1989;338:225–228.

160. Eck MJ, Beutler B, Kuo G, Merryweather JP, Sprang SR. Crystallization of trimeric recombinant human tumor necrosis factor (cachectin). J Biol Chem 1988;263:12816–12819.

161. Eck MJ, Sprang SR. The structure of tumor necrosis factor-β at 2.6 A resolution. J Biol Chem 1989;264:17595–17605.

162. Priestle JP, Shar HP, Grutter MG. Crystal structure of cytokine interleukin-1β. Proc Natl Acad Sci USA 1988; 86:9667–9671.

163. Zhang JC, Cousens IS, Barr PJ, Sprang SR. Three dimensional structure of basic fibroblast growth factor, a structure homolog of interleukin 1 β. Proc Natl Acad Sci USA 1991;88:3446–3450.

164. Fintzel BC, Clancy LL, Holland DR, Muchmore SW, Watenpaugh KD. Einspar HM. Crystal structure of recombinant human interleukin-1β at 2.0 A resolution. J Mol Biol 1989;209:779–791.

165. Graves BJ, Hatada MH, Hendrickson WA, Miller JA, Madison VS. Structure of interleukin 1-α at 2.7 A resolution. Biochemistry 1990;29:2679–2684.

166. Eriksson AE, Cousen LS, Weaver LH, Mathews BW. Three-dimensional structure of human basic fibroblast growth factor. Proc Natl Acad Sci USA 1991;88:3441–3445.

167. Ago H, Kitagawa Y, Fujishima A, Matssuura A, Katsube Y. Crystal structure of basic fibroblast factor at 1.6 A resolution. J Biol Chem 1991;110:360–363.

168. Baldwin ET, Weber IT, Charles IS, et al. Crystal structure of interleukin 8: symbiosis of NMR and crystallography. Proc Natl Acad Sci USA 1991;88:502–506.

169. Brandhuber BJ, Boone T, Kenny WC, McKay DB. Three-dimensional structure of interleukin-2. Science 1987; 238:1707–1709.

170. Redfield C, Smith LJ, Boyd J, et al. Secondary structure and topology of human interleukin 4 in solution. Biochemistry 1991;30:11029–11035.

171. Powers R, Garrett DS, March CJ, Frieden EA, Gronenborn AM, Clore GM. Three-dimensional solution structure of human interleukin-4 by multidimensional heteronuclear magnetic resonance spectroscopy. Science 1992;256:1673–1677.

172. Walter MR, Cook WJ, Zhao BG, et al. Crystal structure of recombinant human interleukin-4. J Mol Biol 1992; 267:20371–20376.

173. Wlodawer A, Pavlovsky A, Gustchina A. Crystal structure of human recombinant interleukin-4 at 2.25 A resolution. FEBS Lett 1992;309:59–64.

174. Smith LJ, Redfield C, Boyd J, et al. Human interleukin-4.

The solution structure of a four-helix bundle protein. J Mol Biol 1992;224:899–904.

175. Senda T, Shimazu T, Matsuda S, et al. Three-dimensional crystal structure of murine interferon-β. EMBO J 1992; 11:3193–3201.

176. Senda T, Matsuda S, Kurihara H, et al. Three-dimensional structure of recombinant murine interferon-β. Proc Natl Acad Sci USA 1990;66:77–90.

177. Samudzi CT, Burton IE, Rubin JR. Crystal structure of rabbit interferon-γ at 2.7 A resolution. J Biol Chem 1991; 266:21791–21797.

178. Ealick SE, Cook WJ, Vijay-Kumar S, et al. Three-dimensional structure of human interferon-γ. Science 1991; 252:698–702.

179. Walter MR, Cook WJ, Ealick SE, Nagabhushan TL, Trotta PP, Bugg CE. Three-dimensional structure of recombinant human granulocyte-macrophage colony stimulating factor. J Mol Biol 1992;224:1075–1085.

180. Diederichs K, Boone T, Karplus PA. Novel fold and putative receptor binding site of granulocyte-macrophage colony-stimulating factor. Science 1991;254:1779–1782.

181. Pandit J, Bohm A, Jancarik J, Halenbeck R, Koths K, Kim SH. Three-dimensional structure of dimeric human recombinant macrophage colony-stimulating factor. Science 1992;258:1358–1362.

182. Lovejoy B, Cascio D, Eisenberg. Crystal structure of canine and bovine granulocyte colony-stimulating factor (G-CSF). J Mol Biol 1993;234:640–653.

183. Boraschi D, Nencioni L, Villa L, et al. In vivo stimulation and restoration of the immune response by the noninflammatory fragment 163–171 of human interleukin 1β. J Exp Med 1988;168:675–686.

184. Boraschi D, Volpini G, Villa L, et al. A monoclonal antibody to the IL-1β peptide 163–171 blocks adjuvanticity but not pyrogenicity of IL-1β in vivo. J Immunol 1989; 143:131–134.

185. McLaughlin CL, Rogan CJ, Tou J, Baile CA, Joy WD. Food intake and body temperature responses of rats to recombinant human interleukin-1beta and a tripeptide interleukin-1beta antagonist. Physiol Behav 1992;52:1115–1160.

186. Ekida T, Nishimura C, Masuda S, Itoh S-I, Shimada I, Arata Y. A receptor-binding peptide from human interleukin-6: isolation and a proton nuclear magnetic resonance study. Biochem Biophys Res Commun 1992;189:211–220.

187. Caruso A, Tiberio L, De Rango C, et al. A monoclonal antibody to the NH$_2$-terminal segment of human IFN-γ selectively interferes with the antiproliferative activity of the lymphokine. J Immunol 1993;150:1029–1035.

188. Griggs ND, Jarpe MA, Pace JL, Russell SW, Johnson HM. The N-terminus and C-terminus of IFN-γ are binding domains from cloned soluble IFN-γ receptor. J Immunol 1992;149:517–520.

189. Postlethwaite AE, Seyer JM. Stimulation of fibroblast chemotaxis by human recombinant tumor necrosis factor α (TNF-α) and a synthetic TNF-α 31–68 peptide. J Exp Med 1990;172:1749–1756.

190. Fassina G, Cassani G, Corti A. Binding of human tumor necrosis factor α to multimeric complementary peptides. Arch Biochem Biophys 1992;296:137–143.

191. Rathjen DA, Ferrante A, Aston R. Differential effects of

small tumor necrosis factor-α peptides on tumor cell cytotoxicity, neutrophil activation and endothelial cell procoagulant activity. Immunology 1993;80:293–299.

192. Kapas L, Hong LL, Cady AB, et al. Somnogenic, pyrogenic and anoretic activities of tumor necrosis factor-alpha and TNF-alpha fragments. Am J Physiol 1992;263:R708–R715.

193. Yayon A, Aviezer D, Safran M, et al. Isolation of peptides that inhibit binding of basic fibroblast growth factor to its receptor from a random phage-epitope library. Proc Natl Acad Sci USA 1993;90:10643–10647.

194. Lie B-L, Tunemoto D, Hemmi H, et al. Identification of the binding site of 55kDa tumor necrosis factor receptor by synthetic peptides. Biochem Biophys Res Commun 1992; 188:503–509.

195. Tanihara M, Suzuki Y, Fujiwara C, et al. A synthetic peptide corresponding to 86–93 of the human type I il-1 receptor binds human recombinant IL-1 (α and β) and inhibits IL-1 actions in vitro and in vivo. Biochem Biophys Res Commun 1992;188:912–920.

196. Kruse N, Tony H-P, Sebald W. Conversion of human interleukin-4 into a high affinity antagonist by a single amino acid replacement. EMBO J 1992;11:3237–3244.

197. Loetscher H, Stueber D, Banner D, Mackay F, Lesslauer W. Human tumor necrosis factor α (TNFα) mutants with exclusive specificity for the 55-kDa or 75-kDa TNF receptors. J Biol Chem 1993;268:26350–26357.

198. Miyajma A, Kitamura T, Harada N, Yokota T, Arai K. Cytokine receptors and signal transduction. Ann Rev Immunol 1992;10:295–331.

199. Foxwell BMJ, Barrett K, Feldmann M. Cytokine receptors: structure and signal transduction. Clin Exp Immunol 1992;90:161–169.

200. Dower SK. Cytokine receptor families. Advances in second messenger and phosphoprotein research. Adv Second Messenger Phosphoprotein Res 1993;28:19–25.

201. Obiri NI, Hillman GG, Haas GP, Sud S, Puri RK. Expression of high affinity IL-4 receptors on human renal cell carcinoma cells and inhibition of tumor cell growth in vitro by IL-4. J Clin Invest 1993;91:88–93.

202. Fernandez-Botran R. Soluble cytokine receptors: their role in immunoregulation. FASEB J 1991;5:2567–2574.

203. Heaney ML, Golde DW. Soluble hormone receptors. Blood 1993;82:1945–1948.

204. Fischer DG, Tal N, Novick D, Barak S, Rubinstein M. An antiviral soluble form of the LDL receptor induced by interferon. Science 1993;262:250–253.

205. Alcami A, Smith GL. A soluble receptor for interleukin-1β encoded by vaccinia virus: a novel mechanism of virus modulation of the host response to infection. Cell 1992; 71:153–167.

206. Spriggs MK, Hruby DE, Maliszewski CR, et al. Vaccinia and cowpox viruses encode a novel secreted interleukin-1-binding protein. Cell 1992;71:145–152.

207. Symons JA, Duff GW. A soluble form of the interleukin-1 receptor produced by a human B cell line. FEBS Lett 1990; 272:133–136.

208. Robb RJ, Kutny RM. Structure-function relationships for the IL-2-receptor system. J Immunol 1987;139:855–862.

209. Marcon L, Fritz ME, Kurman CC, Jensen JC, Nelson DL. Soluble Tac peptide is present in the urine of normal indi-

viduals and at elevated levels in patients with adult T cell leukaemia (ATL). Clin Exp Immunol 1988;73:29–33.

210. Damle RN, Advani SH, Gangal SG. Analysis of regulation of T-cell responses by soluble inhibitory factors from the sera of patients with Hodgkin's disease. Int J Cancer 1992; 50:192–196.

211. Fernandez-Botran R, Vitetta ES. A soluble, high-affinity, interleukin-4-binding protein is present in the biological fluids of mice. Proc Natl Acad Sci USA 1990;87:4202–4206.

212. Nakajima T, Yamamoto S, Cheng M, et al. Soluble interleukin-6 receptor is released from receptor-bearing cell lines in vitro. Jpn J Cancer Res 1992;83:373–378.

213. Mullberg J, Schooltink H, Stoyan T, et al. The soluble interleukin-6 receptor is generated by shedding. Eur J Immunol 1993;23:473–480.

214. Narazaki M, Yasukawa K, Saiton T, et al. Soluble forms of the interleukin-6 signal-transducing receptor component gp130 in human serum possessing a potential to inhibit signals through membrane-anchored gp130. Blood 1993; 82:1120–1126.

215. Andus T, Gross V, Holstege A, et al. High concentrations of soluble tumor necrosis factor receptors in ascites. Hepatology 1992;16:749–755.

216. Kalinkovich A, Engelmann H, Harpaz N, et al. Elevated serum levels of soluble tumour necrosis factor receptors (sTNF-R) in patients with HIV infection. Clin Exp Immunol 1992;89:351–355.

217. Gatanaga T, Hwang C, Kohr W, et al. Purification and characterization of an inhibitor (soluble tumor necrosis factor receptor) for tumor necrosis factor and lymphotoxin obtained from the serum ultrafiltrates of human cancer patients. Proc Natl Acad Sci USA 1990;87:8781–8784.

218. Lantz M, Guelberg U, Nillson E, Ollson I. Characterization in vitro of a human tumor necrosis factor-binding protein. A soluble form of a tumor necrosis factor receptor. J Clin Invest 1990;86:1396–1402.

219. Foley N, Lambert C, McNicol M, Johnson N, Rook GAW. An inhibitor of the toxicity of tumour necrosis factor in the serum of patients with sarcoidosis, tuberculosis and Crohn's disease. Clin Exp Immunol 1990;80:395–399.

220. Lantz M, Malik S, Slevin ML, Olsson I. Infusion of tumor necrosis factor TNF causes an increase in circulating TNF-binding protein in humans. Cytokine 1990;2:402–406.

221. Aderka D, Wysenbeek A, Engelmann H, et al. Increased serum levels of soluble receptors for tumor necrosis factor in systemic lupus erythematosus correlate with disease activity. Arthritis Rheum 1993;36:1111–1120.

222. Gunther N, Betzel C, Weber W. The secreted form of the epidermal growth factor receptor. J Biol Chem 1990; 265:22082–22085.

223. Novick D, Cohen B, Rubinstein M. Soluble interferon-α receptor molecules are present in body fluids. FEBS Lett 1993;314:445–448.

224. Mohler KM, Torrance DT, Young DM, Callis G, Roux ER, Jacobs CA. Immunotherapeutic potential of soluble cytokine receptors in inflammatory disease. FASEB J 1992; 6:A1086.

225. Downing JR, Rousesel MF, Sherr CJ. Ligand and protein kinase C downmodulate the colony-stimulating factor 1 re-

ceptor by independent mechanisms. Mol Cell Biol 1989; 9:2890–2896.

226. Alper O, Yamaguchi K, Hitomi J, Honda S, Matsuchima T, Abe K. The presence of c-erb B-2 gene product-related protein in culture medium conditioned by breast cancer cell line SK-BR-3. Cell Growth Differ 1990;1:591–599.

227. Zabrecky JR, Lam T, McKenzie SJ, Carney W. The extracellular domain of p185/neu is released from the surface of human breast carcinoma cells, SK-BR-3. J Biol Chem 1991; 266:1716–1720.

228. Maihle NJ, Flickinger TW, Raines MA, Sanders ML, Kung H-J. Native avian c-erbβ gene expresses a secreted protein product corresponding to the ligand-binding domain of the receptor. Proc Natl Acad Sci USA 1991;88:1825–1829.

229. Leitzel K, Teramoto Y, Sampson E, et al. Elevated soluble c-erbB-2 antigen levels in the serum and effusions of a proportion of breast cancer patients. J Clin Oncol 1992; 10:1436–1443.

230. Tiesman J, Hart CE. Identification of a soluble receptor for platelet-derived growth factor in cell-conditioned medium and human plasma. J Biol Chem 1993;268:9621–9628.

231. Mosley B, Beckmann MP, March CJ, et al. The murine interleukin-4 receptor: a molecular cloning and characterization of secreted and membrane bound forms. Cell 1989; 59:335–348.

232. Takaki S, Tominaga A, Hitoshi Y, et al. Molecular cloning and expression of the murine interleukin-5 receptor. EMBO J 1990;9:4367–4374.

233. Goodwin R, Friend D, Ziegler SF, et al. Cloning of the human and murine interleukin-7 receptors: demonstration of a soluble form and homology to a new receptor superfamily. Cell 1990;60:941–951.

234. Layton MJ, Cross BA, Metcalf D, Ward LD, Simpson RJ, Nicola NA. A major binding protein for leukemia inhibitory factor in normal mouse serum: identification as a soluble form of the cellular receptor. Proc Natl Acad Sci USA 1992;89:8616–8620.

235. Raines MA, Liu L, Quan SG, Joe V, DiPersio JF, Golde DW. Identification and molecular cloning of a soluble human granulocyte-macrophage colony-stimulating factor receptor. Proc Natl Acad Sci USA 1991;88:8203–8207.

236. Sasaki K, Chiba S, Mano H, Yazaki Y, Hirai H. Identification of a soluble GM-CSF binding protein in the supernatant of a human choriocarcinoma cell line. Biochem Biophys Res Commun 1992;183:252–257.

237. Fukunaga R, Seto Y, Mizushima S, Nagata S. Three different mRNAs encoding human granulocyte colony-stimulating factor receptor. Proc Natl Acad Sci USA 1990;87:8702–8706.

238. Petch L, Harris J, Raymond VW, Blasband A, Lee DC, Earp HS. A truncated, secreted form of the epidermal growth factor receptor is encoded by an alternatively spliced transcript in normal rat tissue. Mol Cell Biol 1990;10:2973–2982.

239. Katoh M, Yazaki Y, Sugimura T, Terada M. C-erbB3 gene encodes secreted as well as transmembrane receptor tyrosine kinase. Biochem Biophys Res Commun 1993; 192:1189–1197.

240. DiStefano PS, Johnson EM. Identification of a truncated form of the nerve growth factor receptor. Proc Natl Acad Sci USA 1988;85:270–274.

241. Nagao M, Masuda S, Abe S, Ueda M, Sasaki R. Production and ligand-binding characteristics of the soluble form of murine erythropoietin receptor. Biochem Biophys Res Commun 1992;188:888–897.

242. Baynes RD, Reddy GK, Shih YJ, Skikne BS, Cook JD. Serum form of the erythropoietin receptor identified by a sequence-specific peptide antibody. Blood 1993;82:2088–2095.

243. Aggarwal BB, Eessalu TE. Effects of phorbol esters on down-regulation and redistribution of cell surface receptors for tumor necrosis factor-α. J Biol Chem 1987;262: 16450–16455.

244. Mui AL-F, Kay RJ, Humphries RK, Krystal G. Ligand-induced phosphorylation of the murine interleukin 3 receptor signals its cleavage. Proc Natl Acad Sci USA 1992; 89:10812–10816.

245. Higuchi M, Aggarwal BB. Okadaic acid induces downmodulation and shedding of tumor necrosis factor receptors: comparison with another tumor promoter, phorbol ester. J Biol Chem 1993;268:5624–5631.

246. Chilton PM, Fernandez-Botran R. Production of soluble IL-4 receptors by murine spleen cells is regulated by T cell activation and IL-4. J Immunol 1993;151:5907–5917.

247. Higuchi M, Aggarwal BB. Tumor necrosis factor induces internalization of the p60 receptor and shedding of the p80 receptor. J Immunol 1994;152:3550–3558.

248. Fernandez-Botran R, Vitetta ES. Evidence that natural murine soluble interleukin 4 receptors may act as transport proteins. J Exp Med 1991;174:673–681.

249. Kendall RL, Thomas KA. Inhibition of vascular endothelial cell growth factor activity by an endogenously encoded soluble receptor. Proc Natl Acad Sci USA 1993;90:10705–10709.

250. Ignotz RA, Kelly B, Davis RJ, Massague J. Biologically active precursor for transforming growth factor type α, released by retrovirally transformed cells. Proc Natl Acad Sci USA 1986;83:6307–6311.

251. Teixido J, Wong ST, Lee DC, Massague J. Generation of transforming growth factor-α from the cell surface by an O-glycosylation-independent multistep process. J Biol Chem 1990;265:6410–6415.

252. Shapiro L, Zhang X, Rupp RG, Wolff SM, Dinarello CA. Ciliary neurotrophic factor is an endogenous pyrogen. Proc Natl Acad Sci USA 1993;90:8614–8618.

253. Lesnikov VA, Efremov OM, Simbirtsev AS, Van-Damme J, Billiau A. The pyrogenic activity of native and recombinant human interleukin-1 beta. Vest Ross Akad Med Nauk 1993;2:23–26.

254. Kapas L, Krueger JM. Tumor necrosis factor-beta induces sleep, fever, and anorexia. Am J Physiol 1992;263:R703–R707.

255. Dinarello CA, Cannon JG, Mancilla J, Bishai I, Lees J, Coceani F. Interleukin-6 as an endogenous pyrogen: induction of prostaglandin E_2. Brain Res 1991;562:199–206.

256. Minano FJ, Sancibrian M, Myers RD. Fever induced by macrophage inflammatory protein-1 (MIP-1) in rats: hypothalamic sites of action. Brain Res Bull 1991;27:701–706.

257. Mier JW, Vachino G, van-der Meer JW, et al. Induction of circulating tumor necrosis factor (TNF alpha) as the mechanism for the febrile response to interleukin-2 (IL-2) in cancer patients. J Clin Immunol 1988;8:426–436.

258. Deuel TF, Kawahara RS, Mustoe TA, Pierce AF. Growth factors and wound healing: platelet-derived growth factor as a model cytokine. Annu Rev Med 1991;42:567–584.

259. Lowry SF. Cytokine mediators of immunity and inflammation. Arch Surg 1993;128:1235–1241.

260. Kondo M, Takeshita T, Ishii N, et al. Sharing of the interleukin-2 (IL-2) receptor γ chain between receptors for IL-2 and IL-4. Science 1993;262:1874–1880.

261. Noguchi M, Nakamura Y, Russel SM, et al. Interleukin-2 receptor γ chain: a functional component of the interleukin-7 receptor. Science 1993;262:1877–1880.

262. Russell SM, Keegan AD, Harada N, et al. Interleukin-2 receptor γ chain: a functional component of the interleukin-4 receptor. Science 1993;262:1880–1883.

263. Lee SH, Aggarwal BB, Rinderknecht E, Assisi F, Chiu H. The synergistic antiproliferative effect of γ-interferon and human lymphotoxin. J Immunol 1984;133:1083–1086.

264. Totpal K, Aggarwal BB. Interleukin-4 potentiates the antiproliferative effects of tumor necrosis factor against different tumor cell lines. Cancer Res 1991;51:4266–4270.

265. Sugarman BJ, Aggarwal BB, Hass PE, Figari IS, Palladino MA, Shepard HM. Recombinant human tumor necrosis factor-α: effects on proliferation of normal and transformed cells in vitro. Science 1985;230:943–945.

266. Czarniecki CW, Fennie CW, Powers DB, Estell DA. Synergistic antiviral and antiproliferative activities of Escherichia coli-derived human alpha, beta and gamma interferons. J Virol 1984;49:490–496.

267. Aggarwal BB, Eessalu TE, Hass PE. Characterization of receptors for human tumor necrosis factor and their regulation by γ-interferon. Nature 1985;318:665–667.

268. Aggarwal BB, Eessalu TE. Induction of receptors for tumor necrosis factor-α by interferons is not a major mechanism for their synergistic cytotoxic response. J Biol Chem 1987; 262:10000–10007.

269. Puri PK, Finbloom DS, Leland P, Mostowski H, Siegel JP. Expression of high affinity IL-4 receptors on murine tumor infiltrating lymphocytes and upregulation by IL-2. Immunology 1990;70:492–497.

270. Puri RK, Leland P. Tumor necrosis factor upregulates interleukin-4 receptors on murine sarcoma cell. Biochem Biophys Res Commun 1993;197:1424–1430.

271. Bendtzen K, Svenson M, Jonsson V, Hippe E. Autoantibodies to cytokines—friends or foes. Immunol Today 1990; 11:167–169.

272. Taylor SI, Barbetti F, Accili D, Roth J, Gorden P. Syndromes of autoimmunity and hypoglycemia. Autoantibodies directed against insulin and its receptor. Endocrinol Metab Clin North Am 1989;18:123–143.

273. Panem S, Check IJ, Henricksen D, Vilcek J. Antibodies to alpha-interferon in a patient with systemic lupus erythematosus. J Immunol 1982;129:1–3.

274. Bost KL, Hahn BH, Saag MS, Shaw GM, Weigent DA, Blalock JE. Individuals infected with HIV possess antibodies against IL-2. Immunology 1988;65:611–615.

275. Svenson M, Poulsen LK, Fomsgaard A, Bendtzen K. IgG autoantibodies against interleukin 1 alpha in sera of normal individuals. Scand J Immunol 1989;29:489–492.

276. Fomsgaard M, Svenson M, Bendtzen K. Auto-antibodies to tumour necrosis factor alpha in healthy humans and patients with inflammatory diseases and gram-negative bacterial infections. Scand J Immunol 1989;30:219–223.

277. Rosenblum MG, Unger BW, Gutterman JU, Hersh EM, David GS, Frincke JM. Modification of human leukocyte interferon pharmacology with a monoclonal antibody. Cancer Res 1985;45:2421–2424.

278. Karp SE, Farber A, Salo JC, et al. Cytokine secretion by genetically modified nonimmunogenic murine fibrosarcoma. J Immunol 1993;150:896–908.

279. Golumbek PT, Lazenby AJ, Levitsky HI, et al. Treatment of established renal cancer by tumor cells engineered to secrete interleukin-4. Science 1991;254:713–716.

280. Rosenthal FM, Cronin K, Guarini R, Gansbacher B. Cytokine gene transfer into tumor cells and its application in human cancer. In: Gergely J, ed. Progress in immunology VIII. Berlin: Springer Hungarica, 1992:361–368.

281. Porgador A, Bannerji R, Watanabe Y, Feldman M, Gilboa E, Eisenbach L. Antimetastatic vaccination of tumor bearing mice with two types of IFN-γ gene-inserted tumor cells. J Immunol 1993;150:1458–1470.

282. Richter G, Kruger-Krasagakes S, Hein G, et al. Interleukin 10 transfected into Chinese hamster ovary cells prevent tumor growth and macrophage infiltration. Cancer Res 1993;53:4134–4137.

283. Chang H, Gillet N, Figari I, Lopez AR, Palladino MA, Derynk R. Increased transforming growth factor B expression inhibits cell proliferation in vitro, yet increases tumorigenicity and tumor growth of Meth a sarcoma cells. Cancer Res 1993;53:4391–4398.

284. Tahara H, Zeh HJ III, Storkus WJ, et al. Fibroblasts genetically engineered to secrete interleukin 12 can suppress tumor growth and induce antitumor immunity to a murine melanoma in vivo. Cancer Res 1994;54:182–189.

285. Afonso LCC, Scharton TM, Vieira LQ, Wysocka M, Trinchieri G, Scott P. The adjuvant effect of interleukin-12 in a vaccine against Leishmania major. Science 1994; 263:235.

286. Grabstein KH, Eisenman J, Shanebeck K, et al. Cloning of a T cell growth factor that interacts with the β chain of the interleukin-2 receptor. Science 1994;264:965–968.

287. Giri JG, Ahdieh M, Eisenman J, et al. Utilization of the β and γ chains of the IL-2 receptor by the novel cytokine IL-15. 1994;13:2822–2830.

PART 2

ROLE OF CYTOKINES IN IMMUNO-REGULATION

CHAPTER 2

ROLE OF CYTOKINES IN HEMATOPOIESIS

Hal E. Broxmeyer

BLOOD CELL PRODUCTION

The topic of cytokines and hematopoiesis is a large and rapidly expanding area of investigation, which makes it impossible to cover all areas, and even some of the areas in the depth they deserve. Most of the literature cited is that of the author and his collaborators, but associated studies of others in these areas have been extensively documented in the author's articles cited.

Cytokines, accessory cells, and hematopoietic stem and progenitor cells

The functional blood cells that help to sustain life, including granulocytes (neutrophilic, eosinophilic, basophilic), monocytes/macrophages, erythrocytes, platelets, lymphocytes (T and B cells and their subsets), and natural killer cells, among others, have limited life spans. For sustained health, these end-stage cells must be replenished.

Production of these blood cells (i.e., hematopoiesis) is a dynamic process that must be finely regulated at the cellular and intracellular levels. This regulation, which entails a network of interacting cells and cell-derived biomolecules, has a degree of complexity and redundancy that is slowly becoming unraveled by modern technology. In its simplest description, regulation involves: blood and nonblood cells (termed *accessory cells*), which produce biologically active molecules termed *cytokines* (including monokines and lymphokines); cytokines; and the cells responsive to the actions of the cytokines, which can be other accessory cells or blood-forming elements (i.e., hematopoietic stem and progenitor cells). Accessory cells include differing cell types, such as lymphocytes, monocytes/macrophages, granulocytes, natural killer cells, fibroblasts, endothelial cells, adipocytes, muscle cells, or other stromal cells (1–6).

There are currently more than 40 biochemically purified recombinant and natural cytokines with known activity on hematopoietic cells. These cytokines are listed in Table 2–1, which is not all-inclusive because new cytokines continue to be identified and isolated. These cytokines have stimulating, enhancing (augmenting), or suppressing activities; in fact, most cytokines are characterized by their pleiotrophic, rather than specific, effects. The different biological activities of the same cytokine can relate to target cell responsiveness; in most cases, this responsiveness reflects the capacity of one cytokine to induce or suppress the release of other cytokines from accessory cells (3–5). These latter effects are considered indirect actions.

Direct actions are the effects of cytokines on the blood-producing cells (i.e., stem and progenitor cells). Stem cells are multipotential cells with the capacity to make more of themselves, the elusive process of self-renewal (1,2). A hierarchy appears to exist within the stem-cell compartment: the earliest cells have the greatest capacity

TABLE 2–1   HEMATOPOIETICALLY ACTIVE CYTOKINES

Colony-stimulating factors (CSF)	H-subunit ferritin (i.e., acidic isoferritin)
Granulocyte-macrophage (GM)-CSF	Prostaglandin (PG) E_1 and E_2
Granulocyte (G)-CSF	Tumor necrosis factor (TNF)-α, -β (i.e., lymphotoxin)
Eosinophil (EOS)-CSF (i.e., interleukin-5 [IL-5])	Interferon (IFN)-α, -β, -γ
Macrophage (M)-CSF (i.e., CSF-1)	Transforming growth factor (TGF)-β
Multi-CSF (i.e., IL-3)	Activin
Erythropoietin (EPO)	Inhibin
	Leukemic inhibitory factor
	Oncostatin M
Genetically engineered CSFs	
GM-CSF/IL-3 fusion protein (PIXY321)	
IL-3/GM-CSF fusion protein	Chemokines
	Macrophage inflammatory protein (MIP)-1-α (i.e., stem-cell inhibitor)
Interleukins (IL) (not covered under CSFs or chemokines)	Macrophage inflammatory protein (MIP)-1-β
IL-1, IL-2, IL-4, IL-6, IL-7, IL-9, IL-10, IL-11, IL-12, and IL-13	Macrophage inflammatory protein (MIP)-2-α (i.e., GRO-β)
	GRO-α
	MIP-2-β (i.e., GRO-γ)
Non-CSFs, non-ILs	Platelet factor-4
Steel factor (SLF: c-kit ligand, stem-cell factor, mast cell growth factor)	IL-8
Erythroid potentiating activity (EPA)	Macrophage chemotactic and activating factor
Lactoferrin (LF)	IP-10

for self-renewal, and the more mature cells within this category have a decreased capacity for self-renewal. Marrow-repopulating cells reside in this compartment.

A number of assays appear to detect cells within the stem-cell group. These assays include those for long-term culture-initiating cells (LTC-IC); stem cells (S cells or blast cells); colony-forming unit-spleen (CFU-S); high proliferative potential colony-forming cells (HPP-CFC) (1,2,7,8); and, more recently, even the CFU-granulocyte, erythroid, macrophage, megakaryocytes (CFU-GEMMs), which were previously believed to be confined to a later set of multipotential progenitors, but which has been demonstrated to have stem-cell characteristics, including multipotentiality and self-renewal, the latter as estimated by colony-replating assays (9,10). It is not clear that any of these assays recognize marrow-repopulating cells. This cell type is currently best defined by in vivo competitive repopulation assays (11). Unfortunately, competitive repopulation assays are not applicable for analysis of human cells unless an assay is able in the future to utilize human severe combined immunodeficiency (SCID) mouse models (12).

Stem cells differentiate into the next broad category of cells, the progenitors, which include at least subsets of CFU-GEMM, as well as more lineage-restricted cells (1,2,7), CFU-granulocyte-macrophage (CFU-GM), CFU-granulocyte (CFU-G), the CFU-macrophage (CFU-M),

burst forming unit-erythroid (BFU-E), BFU-megakaryocyte (MK), and the CFU-MK. Progenitors for the lymphoid series have not been as well defined by the type of colony assays used for these myeloid progenitors. Within the progenitor cell compartments, there are also gradations such that the more immature progenitors appear to have the greatest degree of proliferative capacity, and the more mature cells have less of this capacity.

Because stem and progenitor cells are rare populations present in blood-forming tissue at frequencies less than 1/1,000, attempts to demonstrate direct acting effects of cytokines have had to include studies on purified stem-cell and progenitor-cell populations. Physical and immunological approaches have been used to purify stem and progenitor cells (13–15), and these very highly enriched populations of cells have been used to show that a number of actions of cytokines are mediated by direct effects on stem cells and progenitor cells (13,14,16–23). A more rigorous definition of direct actions on stem and progenitor cells has recently revealed effects noted at the single-cell level by sorting a stem or a progenitor cell into a single well in the absence or presence of serum (24–26). The field is not yet at the level of sophistication that allows determination of effects on individual subsets within the hierarchy of stem and progenitor cells expressing more or less self-renewal or proliferative capacity; this determination will no doubt be possible as more selective cluster density (CD) surface antigens are detected, which allow finer dissection of these classes of cells.

Tissue sources of stem and progenitor cells and a use for cytokines

In adults, the major source of stem and progenitor cells is bone marrow, and this source is routinely utilized for allogeneic and autologous engraftment (27). Adult blood contains stem and progenitor cells, and it has also been used as a source of transplantable cells, but almost entirely in the context of an autologous transplantation (28,29).

To get enough cells for transplantation from adult blood, the blood is usually collected after mobilization of stem and progenitor cells using a number of conditioning procedures, including hematopoietic rebound after the cytotoxic effects of chemotherapy drugs; use of growth factors such as granulocyte-macrophage colony-stimulating factor (GM-CSF), granulocyte colony-stimulating factor (G-CSF) interleukin-3 (IL-3); or combinations of these growth factors and drugs (28,29).

Ontologically, however, stem and progenitor cells are found first in the yolk sac, later in fetal liver, then in fetal spleen, and subsequently, in fetal bone marrow (30). Little is known about migration of stem and progenitor cells from fetal organ to organ (31), but these cells are present in high quantity in the fetal circulation. At the birth of a child, the blood contained in the umbilical cord and the placenta is highly enriched with stem and progenitor cells (32,33). On the basis of a laboratory study involving a multi-institutional collaborative effort (32), it was demonstrated that such cells could be used to engraft and save the life of a child with Fanconi's anemia (34). Cord blood has been shown to be efficacious in a number of clinical situations (34–40), and currently, more than 30 transplantations have been performed in children, mainly in an human leukocyte antigen (HLA)-matched sibling setting (40,41).

Encouraging results have also been apparent in partial HLA-matched siblings, and, most recently, the first unrelated cord blood transplantations have been performed. Although there are obviously enough cells in a single collection of cord blood to engraft and repopulate the hematopoietic system of a child, it remains to be determined whether such a collection will suffice for engraftment of adults. The quantity and quality of stem and progenitor cells in cord blood is high (8–10,32,33,42–44), and it has been suggested that single cord blood collections should be able to be utilized for transplantation of adults (33,42–44). However, if collections are small, or if a single collection is desired for transplantations of more than one individual (a possibility also to be considered for adult bone marrow or adult blood), the stem and progenitor cells from these tissue sources would need to be expanded ex vivo.

Herein lies an important application of cytokines, used alone and in combination (because combinations of cytokines are known to synergize in induction of proliferation of stem and progenitor cells) (8,16,25). Moreover, gene transduction efficiency into stem and progenitor cells for gene therapy, a potential option to correct genetic disorders, can be enhanced through the ex vivo use of cytokines (45–47). The actions of some of the important or potentially important clinically useful cytokines listed in Table 2–1 will be focused on below.

CYTOKINES

Colony-stimulating factors: in vivo effects

Cytokines that alone have potent, direct, stimulating effects on proliferation of myeloid progenitor cells include CSFs: IL-3, GM-CSF, G-CSF, IL-5, M-CSF, and erythropoietin (EPO). IL-3 and GM-CSF are considered to be earlier-acting growth factors in the hierarchy of progenitor-cell proliferation, whereas G-CSF, IL-5 (an eosinophilic CSF), M-CSF, and EPO are usually considered to act on later, more lineage-restricted progenitor cells. GM-CSF, G-CSF, M-CSF, IL-3, and EPO have undergone preclinical animal studies and Phase I to III human clinical trials; within the context of their known biological effects in vitro, they have accelerated recovery of hematopoiesis in patients with a variety of disorders (48,49). Effects were dose-dependent, and toxicity was minimal in most patients.

It is not clear yet what the most appropriate clinical context for use will be for most of the CSFs. There is large overlap of in vivo activities for IL-3, GM-CSF, and G-CSF. However, studies on the kinetics of progenitor-cell proliferation in patients administered GM-CSF or G-CSF have noted differing effects.

In a trial aimed at optimizing dose, schedule, and timing of GM-CSF administration that would best abrogate myelosuppression in patients with sarcoma, it was found that GM-CSF enhanced the proliferative rate of marrow CFU-GM, BFU-E, and CFU-GEMM, an effect that was maintained as long as the GM-CSF was infused (50). This effect had been noted previously (51–53), but of most interest was the fact that within one day of discontinuing treatment with GM-CSF, the proliferative status of the progenitors not only decreased to pre-GM-CSF treatment levels, but also decreased to a slow or nonproliferative rate well below that of the pre-GM-CSF values. This state was maintained for at least one week (50).

Increased myeloid mass and quiescent progenitors at

the time of discontinuation of GM-CSF therapy suggest the possibility that chemotherapy may be initiated shortly after GM-CSF to allow dose-rate intensification by shortening the time interval between courses of chemotherapy (50). Progenitor cells from patients receiving G-CSF were in an enhanced rapid cycle (54). However, in sharp contrast to patients receiving GM-CSF, progenitor cells from patients off G-CSF treatment for 2 to 4 days were still rapidly proliferating (54). These latter findings suggest that it may not be prudent to initiate chemotherapy, especially with cell-cycle–active agents, immediately following discontinuation of treatment with G-CSF. Whether these differences in biological effects of G-CSF and GM-CSF on proliferative kinetics of progenitor cells can be utilized for selective therapeutic benefit remains to be determined, but these studies (50,54) highlight subtle differences that may be of use.

Fusion colony-stimulating factors

The CSFs have been shown in preclinical animal models to act in an additive to synergistic (greater than additive) capacity when used in combination (48,55,56). With these types of activities in mind, a number of companies have begun to develop genetically engineered recombinant fusion proteins. One such molecule, a GM-CSF/IL-3 fusion protein called PIXY321, was shown in vitro to be up to 10-fold more active on a weight-to-weight basis than the combination of GM-CSF plus IL-3 (57), an effect also apparent on highly purified human bone marrow progenitor cells (23). The mechanistic reasons for this synergistic proliferation are not clear, but PIXY321 is being studied in a clinical trial (58).

Treatment of patients with sarcoma with PIXY321 produced small but significant increases in leukocytes, platelets, and reticulocytes, and reduced the degree and duration of neutropenia in a chemotherapeutic setting. These patients were also evaluated for the response of their progenitor cells to in vivo administration of PIXY321. Similar to effects with GM-CSF (50), when dosages of up to 750 µg/mm^2/day PIXY321 were given to patients, CFU-GM, BFU-E, and CFU-GEMM in the marrow were placed into an accelerated proliferative state, effects that decreased to below pretreatment values within one day of discontinuing the PIXY321 (59). However, with higher dosages (up to 1,000 µg/mm^2/day) the cycle status of myeloid progenitors increased more quickly; while PIXY321 was still being administered to the patients and the myeloid mass was increased, the progenitors were placed into a noncycling state (59).

PIXY321 rapidly induced mobilization of progenitors into the blood, and the proliferative kinetics of progenitors circulating in the blood were exactly the same as in the marrow (59). It is possible that the phenomenon of PIXY321-decreased proliferative capacity of progenitors while the myeloid mass is high, and even while PIXY321 is being administered, might allow for even shorter time intervals between chemotherapy dosing than that postulated for patients receiving GM-CSF.

It is not at all clear what causes the progenitors from patients administered GM-CSF or PIXY321 to be placed into a slow or nonproliferating state so soon after or during cytokine administration, but several possibilities exist. One is down-modulation of receptors for growth factors; but if this is so, it is not clear why this down-modulation lasts for up to one week after discontinuing cytokine treatment. A possibility the author favors is induced release of suppressor molecules by GM-CSF or PIXY321. The concept of suppressor cytokines in regulation of hematopoiesis will be discussed later.

Enhancing cytokines

A number of cytokines listed in Table 2–1 have little or no capacity to stimulate directly proliferation of hematopoietic stem and progenitor cells, but in combination with a CSF, they enhance (augment) the proliferative effects of the CSFs. Cytokines with this capacity include, but are not limited to, IL-1 (18); IL-4 (60); IL-6 (61); IL-9 (62); IL-11 (63); activin (64); the murine macrophage inflammatory proteins (MIP)-1α, -1β and -2 (21); and steel factor (SLF) (65). Most of these cytokines have been assessed for activity in preclinical animal models. For example, the in vivo effects of activin (66) and IL-11 (67) have been shown to mimic their in vitro activities.

Of these enhancing cytokines, perhaps the most potent costimulating factor available for in vitro assessment thus far is SLF, the ligand for the c-kit protooncogene–encoded receptor (65). SLF has also been termed mast cell growth factor (MGF), stem-cell factor (SCF), and c-kit ligand. SLF is present in both membrane-bound and soluble forms. Although the membrane-bound form may be the most meaningful in vivo, the soluble form has been used most often for analysis. Soluble SLF enhances the numbers and size of CFU-GEMM-, BFU-E-, CFU-GM-, and CFU-G–derived colonies stimulated by EPO, or EPO plus IL-3, GM-CSF, or G-CSF, respectively (20,65). SLF has been associated with enhanced recovery of hematopoiesis in mice (68,69), in dogs after lethal irradiation (70), and with enhancement of stem and progenitor cells in marrow and mobilization of these cells into the blood of baboons (71).

Leukemic clonogenic cells are as responsive to stimulation by the CSFs as normal progenitor cells (1,2). However, assessment of the responsiveness of clonogenic cells from patients with myeloid leukemia and myelodysplasia (MDS) revealed heterogeneity of patients with regard to the in vitro costimulating effects of SLF (72). For example, although bone marrow and blood progenitors from 26 patients with leukemia and MDS all responded to the stimulating effects of GM-CSF, only 9 of 13 patients with acute myeloid leukemia, 2 of 6 patients with chronic myeloid leukemia, and 4 of 7 patients with MDS had responsive cells to the costimulating effects of SLF. Clinical criteria did not readily distinguish between patients with SLF-responsive versus nonresponsive clonogenic cells. It is too early to determine the mechanistic reasons for this heterogeneity in responsiveness, but it may reflect quantity or quality of SLF receptors or defects in intracellular signal transduction.

Mechanisms of intracellular transmission of cytokine signals

Although under the best of circumstances signal transduction studies would be pursued with primary cells from normal donors or patients, in reality this approach is currently not possible due to the rare frequency of the clonogenic cell population in marrow and blood, and to the inability after purification to obtain large enough cell numbers to perform the studies needed. Thus, most mechanistic studies have utilized factor-dependent cell lines, which are cells that will not grow in the absence of growth factor, similar to primary normal and leukemic cells, but that will grow as established cell cultures without differentiating when placed in the presence of the appropriate cytokines.

The human factor–dependent cell line, M07e, proliferates in response to GM-CSF, IL-3, and SLF, and the combination of SLF with either GM-CSF or IL-3 results in synergistic proliferative effects, similar to that of primary progenitor cells (73). This cell line has been used to dissect the signals involved in proliferation and the potential signals involved in synergistic stimulation/costimulation of proliferation. Synergism was not found to be due to SLF-induced upregulation of the numbers or affinity of GM-CSF or IL-3 receptors (73). Although GM-CSF and SLF were found to up-regulate tyrosine or serine/threonine phosphorylation of different or overlapping proteins, such as c-kit, GTPase-activating protein (GAP) and GAP-associated proteins, Raf-1 and MAP kinase, as well as a number of other as yet unidentified proteins, this effect did not appear to explain synergism (74). SLF also synergizes with IL-9 to stimulate M07e cell proliferation (73,75), but this effect also could not be explained merely by protein phosphorylation (75). CD45, a protein tyrosine phosphatase, appeared to be linked to SLF enhancement of primary progenitor cells, but whether this is a direct or an associated event remains to be determined (76).

The expression of immediate-early genes, a more downstream event than phosphorylation, appeared to be more strongly linked to SLF-induced synergism (77).

SLF, GM-CSF, and IL-3 induced/enhanced expression of c-fos, jun-B, egr-1, and c-myc genes. Using optimal dosages for cell proliferation, induction of c-fos and jun-B was greater than additive with SLF plus GM-CSF or IL-3, compared with each factor alone. Using suboptimal amounts of SLF with optimal amounts of GM-CSF or IL-3, induction of these genes was greater than additive. Induction of immediate-early genes was mediated in part at the level of transcription and messenger RNA (mRNA) for c-fos, at the level of mRNA stabilization for jun-B, and at the level of transcription for egr-1 (77).

Evaluation of other signaling pathways noted that during enforced expression of p210bcr-ab1, in which a growth factor–dependent cell line is transformed into a growth factor–independent state, p210bcr-ab1 formed a specific complex (as assessed by immunoprecipitation and immunoblotting with specific antibodies) with Shc p46/p52, a protein containing an src-homology 2 (SH2) domain, and with Grb-2, which contains an SH2 domain that binds phosphotyrosine residues of tyrosine kinase receptors, such as c-kit (78). There appeared to be a higher-order complex containing Shc, Grb-2, and bcr-abl proteins. However, in contrast to p210bcr-abl–transformed cells, in which there was constitutive tight association between Grb-2 and Shc, binding between Grb-2 and Shc was SLF-dependent in an SLF-responsive, nontransformed parent cell line (78). The SLF-dependent association between Grb-2 and Shc in the nontransformed cells involved formation of a complex of Grb-2 with c-kit receptor after SLF treatment.

In addition to intracellular signaling events, receptor down-modulation can also have a role in regulation. In fact, SLF down-modulates the c-kit protein (the SLF receptor) in M07e cells, an event apparently mediated by SLF-induced polyubiquitination of the c-kit receptor protein (79).

There is much yet to be learned regarding the signaling mechanism in normal and leukemic cells, not only for the CSFs and SLF, but also for the other hematopoietically active cytokines listed in Table 2–1.

Suppressing cytokines: chemokines

A number of the cytokines listed in Table 2–1 have been implicated, at least in vitro, as suppressor molecules. These cytokines include lactoferrin; H-subunit (acidic) ferritin; prostaglandins E_1 and E_2; tumor necrosis factor-α and -β (i.e., lymphotoxin); interferon-α, -β, and -γ; transforming growth factor-β; inhibitin; and members of the chemokine family of molecules. Because most of these suppressive cytokines have been discussed in detail elsewhere (1,2,80), this review focuses on the newly identified capacity of MIP-1-α and other members of the chemokine family: MIP-2-α (i.e., GRO-β), IL-8, platelet factor-4 (PF-4), macrophage chemotactic and activating factor (MCAF), and interferon to mediate direct suppression of hematopoietic progenitor cell proliferation in vitro and in vivo.

After it was first noted that murine MIP-1-α, MIP-1-β, and MIP-2 had enhancing activity for more mature subsets of granulocyte-macrophage and macrophage progenitor cells (21,22), it was found that MIP-1-α had suppressor activity for a subset of relatively mature stem cells (day 12 CFU-S) (81), as well as for the more immature subsets of CFU-GEMM, BFU-E, and CFU-GM, those progenitors responsive to stimulation by multiple growth factors, such as EPO plus SLF or GM-CSF plus SLF (22,82). MIP-1-α had myelosuppressive effects in vivo for hematopoietic stem and progenitor cells (83–85), and they appeared to be myeloprotective for the cycle-active drugs, Ara-C and hydroxyurea (84,85).

MIP-1-α, which was known to polymerize, was found to be active in monomeric form and inactive in polymeric form (86). Isolation of monomeric MIP-a-α from the bulk of polymerized MIP-1-α that formed in physiological buffered saline was found to be 1,000-fold more active on a weight-to-weight basis than concentrations previously reported for MIP-1-α (86). This increased specific activity of monomeric MIP-1-α was confirmed in vivo in a murine model (87). However, it is not possible yet to definitively state that the final form of biologically active MIP-1-α interacting with its receptor in vitro in the presence of serum or in vivo is in fact monomeric MIP-1-α .

Efforts to evaluate the mechanistic actions of MIP-1-α are just beginning. MIP-1-α has a suppressive effect on proliferation of M07e cells induced by the combination of GM-CSF or IL-3 with SLF, but this effect is rapidly reversible (88). Currently, the effect of MIP-1-α on M07e cells does not appear to involve changes in protein phosphorylation (Yip-Schneider M, Broxmeyer HE, unpublished observations), but it does appear to influence phosphatidylcholine metabolism in these cells (89). ·

Evaluation of other members of the chemokine family has established that the suppressive effect of MIP-1-α can be reproduced by MIP-2-α, IL-8, PF-4, MCAF, and interferon inducible protein, molecular weight 10 kd (IP-10) (90,91). Moreover, synergistic suppression, as assessed by increased specific activity of these chemokines, is apparent when any two of the six active chemokines are added together at low concentrations at which each chemokine alone is active (90,91). In addition, whereas placing MIP-1-α in an acetylnitrile/TPA (ACN)–containing solution places most or all MIP-1-α in an active, monomeric form (86), placing MIP-2-α, IL-8, PF-4, MCAF, and IP-10 in ACN also increases their specific activity (92). In vivo in mice, MIP-1-α, MIP-2-α, IL-8, PF-4, MCAF, and IP-10 mimic the myelosuppressive effects of MIP-1-α (23).

Although MIP-1-β, GRO-α, and MIP-2-β (i.e., GRO-γ) do not have suppressive effects and do not synergize with MIP-1-α, MIP-2-α, IL-8, PF-4, MCAF, and IP-10 to suppress myeloid progenitor cell proliferation, they do appear to have blocking activity (82,90). Thus, excess of MIP-1-β to MIP-1-α blocks the myelosuppressive effects of MIP-1-α in vitro, and excess of GRO-α and MIP-2-β to PF-4 and IL-8 blocks the myelosuppressive effects of PF-4 and IL-8 in vitro.

It will be of interest to determine if MIP-1-α , MIP-2-α, IL-8, PF-4, MCAF, and IP-10 have myeloprotective effects in vivo, and if so, in what context and against which chemotherapeutic drug or drug combination.

CONCLUSIONS

The complex network of cytokine–cell interactions are slowly unraveling, but it is naive to assume that new interactive cytokines will not be discovered. In this context, it is possible that cord blood plasma, which enhances the replating capacity of CFU-GEMM (10), contains new, as yet unidentified cytokines that may be involved in stem/progenitor cell self-renewal. Cord blood plasma also enhances the ex vivo expansion of cord blood CFU-GEMMS (93). Whether the same factors are involved as in enhancement of CFU-GEMM replating capacity remains to be determined. Also a possibly new low molecular weight suppressor molecule has been identified in mice receiving MIP-1-α, lactoferrin, or H-ferritin that might be a common mediator in vivo of these different suppressor molecules (94).

Many of the cytokines listed in Table 2–1 have the potential for therapeutic usefulness. How to most efficaciously utilize these cytokines remains to be determined. A number of cytokines have shown antimetatastic activity in mouse models (95). How great it would be if these effects could be translated into human clinical use. Unfortunately, treatment of human disease is probably more complicated than that apparent in murine models of tumor metastasis, but we should not lose track of the possibility of using modified approaches, perhaps combination treatments, based on what is learned from studies using mouse models.

ACKNOWLEDGMENTS: Many of the studies reviewed herein were supported by U.S. Public Health Service Grants R37 CA 36464, R01 HL 46549, and R01 HL 49202 from the National Cancer Institute and the National Institutes of Health, and by National Institutes of Health Training Grant DK 07519.

REFERENCES

1. Broxmeyer HE. Update: biomolecule-cell interactions and the regulation of myelopoiesis. In: Murphy MJ Jr, ed. Con-

cise reviews in clinical and experimental hematology. Dayton, OH: Alpha Medical Press, 1992:119–149.

2. Broxmeyer HE, Williams DE. The production of myeloid blood cells and their regulation during health and disease. CRC Crit Rev Oncol Hematol 1988;8:173–226.

3. Falkenburg JHF, Harrington MA, Walsh WK, Daub R, Broxmeyer HE. Gene-expression and release of macrophage-colony stimulating factor in quiescent and proliferating fibroblasts. Effects of serum, fibroblast growth promoting factors and IL-1. J Immunol 1990;144;4657–4662.

4. Harrington MA, Falkenburg JHF, Daub R, Broxmeyer HE. Effect of myogenic and adipogenic differentiation on expression of colony stimulating factor genes. Mol Cell Biol 1990;10:4948–4952.

5. Falkenburg JHF, Harrington MA, de Paus RA, Walsh WK, Daub R, Landegent JE, Broxmeyer HE. Differential transcriptional regulation of gene expression of the colony-stimulating factors by interleukin-1 and fetal bovine serum in murine fibroblasts. Blood 1991;78:658–665.

6. Hangoc G, Daub R, Maze RG, Falkenburg JHF, Broxmeyer HE, Harrington MA. Regulation of myelopoiesis by murine fibroblastic and adipogenic cell lines. Exp Hematol 1993; 21:502–507.

7. Broxmeyer HE. Colony assays of hematopoietic progenitor cells and correlations to clinical situations. CRC Crit Rev Oncol Hematol 1983;1:227–257.

8. Lu L, Xiao M, Shen RN, Grigsby S, Broxmeyer HE. Enrichment, characterization and responsiveness of single primitive CD34+++ human umbilical cord blood hematopoietic progenitors with high proliferative and replating potential. Blood 1993;81:942–949.

9. Carow CE, Hangoc G, Cooper SH, Williams DE, Broxmeyer HE. Mast cell growth factor (c-kit ligand) supports the growth of human multipotential progenitor cells with a high replating capacity. Blood 1993;78:2216–2221.

10. Carow CE, Hangoc G, Broxmeyer HE. Human multipotential progenitor cells (CFU-GEMM) have extensive replating capacity for secondary CFU-GEMM: an effect enhanced by cord blood plasma. Blood 1993;81:942–949.

11. Harrison DE, Jordan CT, Zhong RK, Astle CM. Primitive hematopoietic stem cells: direct assay of most productive populations by competitive repopulation with simple binomial, correlation and covariance calculations. Exp Hematol 1993;21:206–219.

12. Lapidot T, Pflumio F, Doedens M, Murdock B, Williams DE. Cytokine stimulation of multilineage hematopoiesis from immature human cells engrafted in SCID mice. Science 1992;255:1137–1141.

13. Lu L, Walker D, Broxmeyer HE, Hoffman R, Hu W, Walter E. Characterization of adult human marrow hematopoietic progenitors highly enriched by two-color sorting with My10 and major histocompatibility (MHC) class II monoclonal antibodies. J Immunol 1987;139:1823–1829.

14. Williams DE, Straneva JE, Shen R, Broxmeyer HE. Purification of murine bone marrow-derived granulocyte-macrophage colony forming cells. Exp Hematol 1987;15:234–250.

15. Cooper S, Broxmeyer HE. Purification of murine granulocyte-macrophage progenitor cells (CFU-GM) using counterflow centrifugal elutriation. In: Freshney RI, Pragnell I,

16. Williams DE, Stravena JE, Cooper S, et al. Interactions between purified murine colony stimulating factors (natural CSF-1, purified recombinant GM-CSF, and purified recombinant IL-3) on the in vitro proliferation of purified murine granulocyte-macrophage progenitor cells. Exp Hematol 1987;15:1007–1012.

17. Williams DE, Cooper S, Broxmeyer HE. The effects of hematopoietic suppressor molecules on the in vitro proliferation of purified murine granulocyte-macrophage progenitor cells (CFU-GM). Cancer Res 1988;48:1548–1550.

18. Williams DE. Interleukin-1 alpha enhances the in vitro survival of purified murine granulocyte-macrophage progenitor cells in the absence of colony-stimulating factors. Blood 1988;72:1608–1615.

19. Lu L, Lin ZH, Shen RN, Warren DJ, Leemhuis T, Broxmeyer HE. Influence of interleukins 3, 5 and 6 on the growth of eosinophil progenitors in highly enriched human bone marrow in the absence of serum. Exp Hematol 1990;18:1180–1186.

20. Broxmeyer HE, Cooper S, Lu L, et al. Effect of murine mast cell growth factor (c-kit proto-oncogene ligand) on colony formation by human marrow hematopoietic progenitor cells. Blood 1991;77:2142–2149.

21. Broxmeyer HE, Sherry B, Lu L, et al. Myelopoietic enhancing effects of murine macrophage inflammatory proteins 1 and 2 on colony formation in vitro by murine and human bone marrow granulocyte-macrophage progenitor cells. J Exp Med 1989;170:1583–1594.

22. Broxmeyer HE, Sherry B, Lu L, et al. Enhancing and suppressing effects of recombinant murine macrophage inflammatory proteins on colony formation in vitro by bone marrow myeloid progenitor cells. Blood 1990;76:1110–1116.

23. Williams DE, Park LS, Broxmeyer HE, Lu L. Hybrid cytokines as hematopoietic growth factors. Int J Cell Cloning 1991;9:542–547.

24. Bernstein ID, Andrews RG, Zsebo KM. Recombinant human stem cell factor enhances the formation of colonies by CD34+ and CD34+Lin- cells, and the generation of colony-forming cell progeny from CD34-Lin- cells cultures with interleukin-3, granulocyte-colony stimulating factor and granulocyte-macrophage colony stimulating factor. Blood 1991;77:2316–2321.

25. Xiao M, Leemhuis T, Broxmeyer HE, Lu L. Influence of combinations of cytokines on proliferation of isolated single cell-sorted human bone marrow hematopoietic progenitor cells in the absence and presence of serum. Exp Hematol 1992;20:276–279.

26. Lu L, Xiao M, Grigsby S, et al. Comparative effects of suppressive cytokines on isolated single CD34+++ stem/progenitor cells from human bone marrow and umbilical cord blood plated with and without serum. Exp Hematol 1993; 21:1442–1446.

27. Thomas ED. Frontiers in bone marrow transplantation. Blood Cells 1991;17:259–267.

28. Lowry RA, Tabbara IA. Peripheral hematopoietic stem cell transplantation: current concepts. Exp Hematol 1992; 20:937–942.

29. Henon PR. Peripheral blood stem cell transplantation: past, present and future. Stem Cells 1993;11:154–172.

30. Tavassoli M. Embryonic and fetal hematopoiesis: an overview. Blood Cells 1991;17:269–281.

31. Broxmeyer HE. Commentary: self-renewal and migration of stem cells during embryonic and fetal hematopoiesis: important, but poorly understood events. Blood Cells 1991;17;282–286.

32. Broxmeyer HE, Douglas GW, Hangoc G, et al. Human umbilical cord blood as a potential source of transplantable hematopoietic stem/progenitor cells. Proc Natl Acad Sci USA 1989;86:3828–3832.

33. Broxmeyer HE, Hangoc G, Cooper S, et al. Growth characteristics and expansion of human umbilical cord blood and estimation of its potential for transplantation of adults. Proc Natl Acad Sci USA 1992;89:4109–4113.

34. Gluckman E, Broxmeyer HE, Auerbach AD, et al. Hematopoietic reconstitution in a patient with Fanconi's anemia by means of umbilical-cord blood from an HLA-identical sibling. N Engl J Med 1989;321:1174–1178.

35. Wagner JE, Broxmeyer HE, Byrd RL, et al. Transplantation of umbilical cord blood after myeloblative therapy: analysis of engraftment. Blood 1992;79:1874–1881.

36. Kohli-Kumar M, Shahidi NT, Broxmeyer HE, et al. Haematopoietic stem/progenitor cell transplant in Fanconi anemia using HLA-matched sibling umbilical cord blood cells. Br J Haematol 1994;85:419–422.

37. Vowels MR, Tang RLP, Bendoukas V, et al. Correction of x-linked lymphoproliferative disease by cord blood transplantation. N Engl J Med 1994;329:1623–1625.

38. Bogdanic V, Nemet D, Kastelan A, et al. Umbilical cord blood transplantation in a patient with philadelphia chromosome-positive chronic myeloid leukemia. Transplantation 1993;56:477–479.

39. Broxmeyer HE, Kurtzberg J, Gluckman E, et al. Umbilical cord blood hematopoietic stem and repopulating cells in human clinical transplantation. Blood Cells 1991;17:313–329.

40. Wagner JE, Kernan NA, Broxmeyer HE, Gluckman E. Allogeneic umbilical cord blood transplantation: report of results in 26 patients (abstract). Blood 1993;82:86a.

41. Broxmeyer HE, Hangoc G, Cooper S. Clinical and biological aspects of human umbilical cord blood as a source of transplantable hematopoietic stem and progenitor cells. Bone Marrow Transplant 1992;9(suppl 1):7–10.

42. Cardoso AA, Li ML, Bartard P, et al. Release from quiescence of CD34+CD38– human umbilical cord blood cells reveals their potentiality to engraft adults. Proc Natl Acad Sci USA 1993;90:8707–8711.

43. Lansdorp PM, Dragowska W, Mayani H. Ontogeny-related changes in proliferative potential of human hematopoietic cells. J Exp Med 1993;178:787–791.

44. Hows JM, Bradley BA, Marsh JCW, et al. Growth of human umbilical-cord blood in long term haematopoietic cultures. Lancet 1992;340:73–76.

45. Moritz T, Keller DC, Williams DE. Human cord blood cells as targets for gene transfer: potential use in genetic therapies of severe combined immunodeficiency disease. J Exp Med 1993;178:529–536.

46. Lu L, Xiao M, Clapp DW, Li ZH, Broxmeyer HE. High effi-

ciency retroviral mediated gene transduction into single isolated immature and replatable CD34+++ hematopoietic stem/progenitor cells from human umbilical cord blood. J Exp Med 1993;178:2089–2096.

47. Zhou SZ, Broxmeyer HE, Cooper S, Harrington MA, Srivastava A. Adeno-associated virus 2-mediated gene transfer in murine hematopoietic progenitor cells. Exp Hematol 1993;21:928–933.

48. Broxmeyer HE, Vadhan-Raj S. Preclinical and clinical studies with the hematopoietic colony stimulating factors and related interleukins. Immunol Res 1989;8:185–201.

49. Broxmeyer HE, Lu L, Vadhan-Raj S, Shen RN. Haematopoietically active cytokines: roles for therapy of malignant disease with an emphasis on clinical trials with colony stimulating factors. In: Hoffbrand AV, Brenner MK, eds. Recent advances in haematology, vol 6. London: Churchill Livingstone, 1993:195–207.

50. Vadhan-Raj S, Broxmeyer HE, Hittleman WN, et al. Abrogating chemotherapy-induced myelosuppression by recombinant granulocyte-macrophage colony-stimulating factor in patients with sarcoma: protection at the progenitor cell level. J Clin Oncol 1992;10:1266–1277.

51. Broxmeyer HE, Cooper S, Williams DE, Hangoc G, Gutterman JU, Vadhan-Raj S. Growth characteristics of marrow hematopoietic progenitor/precursor cells from patients on a phase I clinical trial with purified recombinant human granulocyte macrophage colony-stimulating factor. Exp Hematol 1988;16:594–602.

52. Broxmeyer HE, Cooper S, Vadhan-Raj S. Cell cycle status of erythroid (BFU-E) progenitor cells from the bone marrows of patients on a clinical trial with purified recombinant human granulocyte-macrophage colony stimulating factor. Exp Hematol 1989;17:455–459.

53. Aglietta M, Piacibello W, Sanavio F, et al. Kinetics of human hemopoietic cells after in vivo administration of granulocyte-macrophage colony stimulating factor. J Clin Invest 1989;83:551–557.

54. Broxmeyer HE, Benninger L, Patel SR, Benjamin RS, Vadhan-Raj S. Kinetic responses of human marrow myeloid progenitor cells to in vivo treatment of patients with G-CSF is different from that with GM-CSF. Exp Hematol 1994;22:100–102.

55. Broxmeyer HE, Williams DE, Hangoc G, et al. Synergistic myelopoietic action in vivo of combinations of purified natural murine colony stimulating factor-1, recombinant murine interleukin-3, and recombinant murine granulocyte-macrophage colony stimulating factor administered to mice. Proc Natl Acad Sci USA 1987;84:3871–3875.

56. Broxmeyer HE, Williams DE, Cooper S, Hangoc G, Ralph P. Recombinant human granulocyte-colony stimulating factor and recombinant human macrophage-colony stimulating factor synergise in vivo to enhance proliferation of granulocyte-macrophage, erythroid and multipotential progenitor cells in mice. J Cell Biochem 1988;38;127–136.

57. Curtis BM, Williams DE, Broxmeyer HE, et al. Enhanced hematopoietic activity of a human GM-CSF/IL-3 fusion protein. Proc Natl Acad Sci USA 1991;88:5809–5813.

58. Vadhan-Raj S, Broxmeyer HE, Bandres J, et al. In vivo biologic effects of PIXY321 (GM-CSF/IL-3 fusion protein) in patients with sarcoma (abstract). Blood 1992;80(suppl 1):87A.

59. Broxmeyer HE, Benninger L, Cooper S, Vadhan-Raj S. Ef-

fects of treatment of patients with sarcoma with PIXY321 (a genetically engineered GM-CSF/IL-3 fusion protein) on proliferation kinetics of marrow and blood myeloid progenitor cells (abstract). Blood 1992;80(suppl 1):87A.

60. Broxmeyer HE, Lu L, Cooper S, et al. Synergistic effects of purified recombinant human and murine B-cell growth factor-1/interleukin-4 on colony formation in vitro by hematopoietic progenitor cells: multiple actions. J Immunol 1988;141:3852–3862.

61. Gentile P, Broxmeyer HE. Interleukin 6 ablates the accessory cell-mediated suppressive effects of lactoferrin on human hematopoietic progenitor cell proliferation in vitro. Ann NY Acad Sci 1991;628:74–83.

62. Williams DE, Morrissey PJ, Mochizuki DY, et al. The T cell growth factor p40 promotes the proliferation of myeloid cell lines and has erythroid potentiating activity by normal human bone marrow cells in vitro. Blood 1990;76:906–911.

63. Paul SR, Bennett F, Calvetti JA, et al. Molecular cloning of a cDNA encoding interleukin-11, a stromal cell-derived lymphopoietic and hematopoietic cytokine. Proc Natl Acad Sci USA 1990;87:7512–7516.

64. Broxmeyer HE, Lu L, Cooper S, Schwall RH, Mason AJ, Nikolics K. Selective and indirect modulation of human multipotential and erythroid hematopoietic progenitor cell proliferation by recombinant human activin and inhibin. Proc Natl Acad Sci USA 1988;85:9052–9056.

65. Broxmeyer HE, Maze R, Miyazawa K, et al. The kit receptor and its ligand, steel factor, as regulators of hemopoiesis. Cancer Res 1991;3:480–487.

66. Broxmeyer HE, Hangoc G, Zucali JR, et al. Effects in vivo of purified recombinant human activin and erythropoietin in mice. Int J Hematol 1991;54:447–454.

67. Hangoc G, Yin T, Cooper S, Schendel P, Yang YC, Broxmeyer HE. In vivo effects of recombinant interleukin-11 on myelopoiesis in mice. Blood 1993;81:965–972.

68. Molineux G, Migdalska A, Szmitkowski M, Zsebo K, Dexter TM. The effects on hematopoiesis of recombinant stem cell factor (ligand for c-kit) administered in vivo to mice either alone or in combination with granulocyte colony-stimulating factor. Blood 1991;78:1954–1962.

69. Ulrich TR, Castillo JD, McNiece IK, et al. Stem cell factor in combination with granulocyte colony stimulating factor (CSF) or granulocyte-macrophage CSF synergistically increases granulopoiesis in vivo. Blood 1991;78:1954–1962.

70. Schuening FG, Appelbaum FR, Deeg JH, et al. Effects of recombinant canine stem cell factor, a c-kit ligand, and recombinant granulocyte colony-stimulating factor on hematopoietic recovery affer otherwise lethal total body irradiation. Blood 1993;81:20–26.

71. Andrews RG, Knitter GH, Bartelman SH, et al. Recombinant human stem cell factor, a c-kit ligand, stimulates hematopoietic in primates. Blood 1991;78:1975–1980.

72. Maze R, Horie M, Hendrie P, et al. Differential responses of myeloid progenitor cells from patients with myeloid leukemia and myelodysplasia to the co-stimulating effects of steel factor in vitro. Exp Hematol 1993;21:545–551.

73. Hendrie PC, Miyazawa K, Yang YC, Langefeld CD, Broxmeyer HE. Mast cell growth factor (c-kit ligand) enhances cytokine stimulation of proliferation of human factor dependent cell line, M07e. Exp Hematol 1991;19:1031–1037.

74. Miyazawa K, Hendrie PC, Mantel C, Wood K, Ashman LK, Broxmeyer HE. Comparative analysis of signalling pathways between mast cell growth factor (c-kit ligand) and granulocyte-macrophage colony-stimulating factor in a human factor-dependent myeloid cell line involves phosphorylation of Raf-1, GTPase-activating protein and mitogen-activated protein kinase. Exp Hematol 1991;19:1110–1123.

75. Miyazawa K, Hendrie PC, Kim YC, Mantel C, Yang YC, Kwon BS, Broxmeyer HE. Recombinant human interleukin-9 induces protein tyrosine phosphorylation and synergises with steel factor to stimulate proliferation of the human factor-dependent cell line, M07e. Blood 1992;80:1685–1692.

76. Broxmeyer HE, Lu L, Hangoc G, et al. CD45 cell surface antigens are linked to stimulation of early human myeloid progenitor cells by interleukin-3 (IL-3), granulocyte/macrophage colony stimulating factor (GM-CSF), a GM-CSF/IL-3 fusion protein, and mast cell growth factor (a c-kit ligand). J Exp Med 1991;174:447–458.

77. Horie M, Broxmeyer HE. Involvement of immediate-early gene expression in the synergistic effects of steel factor in combination with granulocyte-macrophage colony-stimulating factor or interleukin-3 on proliferation of a human factor-dependent cell line. J Biol Chem 1993;268:968–973.

78. Tauchi T, Boswell HS, Leibowitz D, Broxmeyer HE. Coupling between p210 Bcr-abl and Shc and Grb-2 adaptor proteins in hematopoietic cells permits growth factor receptor-independent link to Ras activation pathway. J Exp Med 1994;179:167–175.

79. Miyazawa K, Toyama K, Gotoh A, Hendrie PC, Mantel C, Broxmeyer HE. Ligand-dependent polyubiquintination of c-kit gene product: a possible mechanism of receptor down modulation in M07e cells. Blood 1994;83:137–145.

80. Broxmeyer HE. Suppressor cytokines and regulation of myelopoiesis: biology and possible clinical uses. Am J Pediatr Hematol Oncol 1992;14:22–30.

81. Graham GJ, Wright EG, Hewick R, et al. Identification and characterization of an inhibitor of haematopoietic stem cell proliferation. Nature 1990;344:442–444.

82. Broxmeyer HE, Sherry B, Cooper S, et al. Macrophage inflammatory protein (MIP)-1 beta abrogates the capacity of MIP-1 alpha to suppress myeloid progenitor cell growth. J Immunol 1991;147:2586–2594.

83. Maze R, Sherry B, Kwon BS, Cerami A, Broxmeyer HE. Myelosuppressive effects in vivo of purified recombinant murine macrophage inflammatory protein-1 alpha. J Immunol 1992;149:1004–1009.

84. Lord BI, Dexter TM, Clements JM, Hunter MA, Gearing AJH. Macrophage inflammatory protein protects multipotent hematopoietic cells from the cytotoxic effects of hydroxyurea in vivo. Blood 1992;79:2605–2609.

85. Dunlop DJ, Wright EG, Lorimore S, et al. Demonstration of stem cell inhibition and myeloprotective effects of SCI/rhMIP-1 alpha in vivo. Blood 1992;79:2221–2225.

86. Mantel C, Kim YJ, Cooper S, Kwon BS, Broxmeyer HE. Polymerization of murine macrophage inflammatory protein-1α inactivates its myelosuppressive effects in vitro. The active form is monomer. Proc Natl Acad Sci USA 1993; 90:2232–2236.

87. Cooper S, Mantel C, Broxmeyer HE. Myelosuppressive effects in vivo with very low dosage of monomeric recombi-

nant murine macrophage inflammatory protein-1α. Exp Hematol 1994;22:186–193.

88. Broxmeyer HE, Benninger L, Hague N, et al. Suppressive effects of the chemokine (macrophage inflammatory protein) family of cytokines on proliferation of normal and leukemia myeloid cell proliferation. In: Guigon M, ed. Hematopoietic inhibitors. Paris: Inserm Eurotext Libby, 1994;3:229:141–154.

89. Mantel C, Luo Z, Hendrie PC, Broxmeyer HE. The intracellular signalling effects of GM-CSF, steel factor and macrophage inflammatory protein 1α on phosphatidylcholine metabolism in human cell line M07e (abstract). Blood 1993;82:370a.

90. Broxmeyer HE, Sherry B, Cooper S, et al. Comparative analysis of the suppressive effects of the human macrophage inflammatory protein family of cytokines (chemokines) on proliferation of human myeloid progenitor cells. J Immunol 1993;150:3448–3458.

91. Sarris AH, Broxmeyer HE, Wirthmueller U, et al. Human IP-10: expression and purification of recombinant protein demonstrates inhibition of early human hematopoietic progenitors. J Exp Med 1994;178:1127–1132.

92. Broxmeyer HE, Cooper S, Lu L, Benninger L, Sarris A, Mantel C. Synergistic suppressive interactions and enhanced specific activity of human chemokines on human myeloid progenitor cell proliferation (abstract). Exp Hematol 1993;21:1031.

93. Ruggieri L, Heimfeld S, Broxmeyer HE. Cytokine-dependent ex vivo expansion of early subsets of CD34+ cord blood progenitors is greatly enhanced by cord blood plasma, but expansion of the more mature subsets of progenitors is favored (abstract). Blood 1993;82:16a.

94. Broxmeyer HE, Mantel C, Cooper S, Kreisberg R, Moore RN. Administration of macrophage inflammatory protein 1α, lactoferrin or H-ferritin to mice or rats induces a common non-species specific low molecular weight inhibitor active in vitro and in vivo: biochemical, biological and antigenic characterization (abstract). Blood 1993;82:181a.

95. Shen RN, Lu L, Broxmeyer HE. New therapeutic strategies in the treatment of murine dise'ases induced by virus and solid tumors: biology and implications for the potential treatment of human leukemia, AIDS and solid tumors. CRC Crit Rev Oncol Hematol 1990;10:253–265.

CHAPTER 3

ROLE OF CYTOKINES IN LYMPHOCYTE FUNCTIONS

Gilda G. Hillman and Gabriel P. Haas

Cytokines regulate growth, differentiation, and function of hematopoietic lineages, as well as mediate a large variety of normal and pathological immunological responses. In this chapter, we specifically address the role of cytokines in the immunoregulation of lymphocyte functions. The key to the immune responses elicited by viral, bacterial, protozoan, or neoplastic antigens is the nature of the T-cell activity elicited. Cell-mediated immune responses involve activation of macrophages and induction of CD4+ helper T cells and CD8+ cytotoxic T cells. Helper T cells, B cells, and macrophages respond to antigenic stimulation by production of soluble factors identified as cytokines, which regulate the immune response. These cytokines may stimulate certain effector cells and may inhibit others. The balance of these complex interactions determines the overall response, and any imbalance may result in pathological responses.

EFFECT OF CYTOKINES ON LYMPHOCYTE MATURATION

Different patterns of cytokines are released from the cells of the immune system, including thymocytes, T cells, natural killer (NK) cells, B cells, macrophages, neutrophils, basophils, eosinophils, mast cells, and platelets.

Certain cytokines, including interleukin-1 (IL-1), IL-2, IL-4, and IL-7 may have an important role at an early stage of fetal thymic development (Table 3–1) (1). The thymic anlage is colonized by hematopoietic stem cells from the fetal liver at approximately day 11 of mouse embryonic development (2) and between week 7 and 9 of human development (3). Within the thymus, different thymic stromal cell populations interact with thymocytes at different stages of development and may regulate the coordinated production of cytokines by stromal cells and developing T cells (1).

Experimental in vitro and in vivo studies demonstrated that these cytokines influenced the lineage commitment and proliferative activity of intrathymic T-cell precursors (1,4). IL-1 and IL-7 may mediate the expansion of CD3-TCR-CD4-CD8-thymocyte precursors and differentiation to functionally competent T cells (5,6). Induction of high affinity IL-2 receptor by IL-2 in human thymocyte precursors results in cellular proliferation and may regulate the proliferative phase of T-cell development (7). IL-2 can induce T-cell differentiation (8). Cytokine receptor studies in developing thymocytes revealed that receptors for IL-1, IL-2, and IL-4 are regulated developmentally and that their expression is coordinated with production of IL-1 by stromal cells and IL-2 and IL-4 by thymocytes (1). The T-cell receptor (TCR) rearrangement phase, which is associated with later differentiation of the T-cell lineage, is also influenced by cytokines (1).

Mature T cells respond to antigenic stimulation with production of cytokines. In both humans and mice, helper T cells can be subdivided further into Th1 and Th2

TABLE 3–1 EFFECTS OF CYTOKINES ON IMMUNE CELL PRECURSOR MATURATION

Cytokines	Target	Activity
IL-1	Thymic T-cell precursors B-cell precursors	Maturation Maturation
IL-2	Thymocyte T-cell precursors	Proliferation and differentiation
IL-3	Multipotential hematopoietic stem cells and committed progenitor cells	Proliferation and differentiation
IL-4	Thymocytes	Role in development
IL-5	Eosinophil and basophil lineages	Proliferation and differentiation
IL-6	Mitogen-stimulated thymocytes Hematopoietic stem cells	Proliferation Synergy with IL-3 for maturation
IL-7	Thymocyte T-cell precursors Pro-B- and pre-B-cell precursors	Expansion and differentiation into competent T cells Proliferation
IL-9	Early erythroid progenitors	Differentiation
IL-10	Murine thymocytes	Proliferation and differentiation
IL-11	Hematopoietic progenitors	Synergy with IL-3 and IL-4
TNF-α	Thymocytes	Proliferation in the presence of IL-1, IL-2, and IL-7
TGF-β	Immature hematopoietic cells and thymocytes	Suppression of growth

IL = interleukin; TNF = tumor necrosis factor; TGF = transforming growth factor.

distinct subsets based on the spectrum of cytokines that they secrete (9). Th1 cells produce interferon-γ (IFN-γ) and IL-2, as well as granulocyte-macrophage colony-stimulating factor (GM-CSF), tumor necrosis factor-α (TNF-α) and TNF-β. Th2 cells secrete GM-CSF, IL-3, IL-4, IL-5, IL-6, IL-10, and IL-13. A third subset, Th0, can secrete a combination of cytokines characteristic to both Th1 and Th2 subsets. CD8+T cells have a Th1-like cytokine pattern.

Th cell functions are mediated by the cytokines they secrete. Consequently, Th1 and Th2 cells have distinct functions because each subset induces and regulates effector functions targeted at specific types of antigens and pathogens. Th1 cells mediate macrophage activation via IFN-γ, TNF, and GM-CSF, as well as delayed-type hypersensitivity reactions (10,11). Th2 cells are important in the regulation of humoral immunity, antibody responses, and allergic diseases (12). Cytokines produced by Th1

and Th2 subsets reciprocally regulate the functions of each other. IFN-γ inhibits the proliferation of Th2 cells, but not Th1 cells (13), and IL-10 inhibits the synthesis of cytokines by Th1 cells (14). Like T helper cells, macrophages are also an important source of regulatory cytokines. Following stimulation by antigen, macrophages can exert a profound influence on the immune reaction by the production of cytokines.

B lymphocytes differentiate in fetal liver or adult bone marrow. The earliest steps of B-cell lineage development occur during a pro-B-cell stage defined by B220-negative precursors in which immunoglobulin (Ig) genes are in a germ-line configuration, and at a pre-B-cell stage, during which precursors are B220-positive and begin rearrangement and expression of cytoplasmic μ-heavy chain. These two B-cell precursors proliferate in response to IL-7 produced by bone marrow stromal cells (Table 3–1). The pre-B cells are precursors of immature B cells (B220-positive and surface IgM-positive [sIgM]), which give rise to mature B cells (B220-positive, sIgM-positive, sIgD-positive).

Cytokines function through a cytokine network and exert their function through their receptors on target cells (15). Among others, lymphocytes are the primary target cells of cytokines, which regulate their immune functions (Tables 3–2 and 3–3).

B lymphocytes represent 5 to 15% of the lymphocytes circulating in peripheral blood. They are responsible for the humoral response to foreign antigens by producing immunoglobulins (Ig) in response to specific immunogenic determinants. Several cytokines have an important role in B-cell maturation. Following contact with a foreign antigen, mature B cells are activated and become antibody-secreting plasma cells in a process involving the participation of several cytokines, including IL-4, IL-5, IFN-γ, and transforming growth factor-β (TGF-β). These cytokines exert control over immunoglobulin regulation, including isotype switching (16).

T lymphocytes (approximately 80% of the circulating lymphocytes) are characterized by the expression of the T cell antigen receptor (TCR). The majority of T cells express TCR-αβ, and only 5% of T cells express TCR-γδ. TCR is associated with the CD3 molecular complex. T cells consist of phenotypically and functionally distinct subpopulations: T helper (Th) cells (positive for CD4 marker), T suppressor (Ts) cells, and T cytotoxic (Tc) cells (positive for CD8 marker). Th cells regulate or modulate interactions among multiple cell types (T cells, B cells, macrophages) through the secretion of lymphokines, as detailed. Cytotoxic T cells (CTL or Tc) are able to lyse specific target cells, including tumors. T cells recognize antigen in association with major histocompatibility complex (MHC) molecules present on the surface of the antigen-presenting cell, and their response is therefore restricted by MHC antigens.

A third population of lymphocytes, the natural killer (NK) cells, account for 5 to 15% of the circulating lymphocytes and are defined by morphology as large granular lymphocytes. They do not express TCR or immunoglobulin markers, but they are characterized by the presence of CD16 (Fc receptor for IgG) and CD56 (homologous to neural cell adhesion molecule) antigens; they also express the adhesion molecule, CD2, which is also present on T cells. NK cells are able to mediate cytotoxicity against certain tumor cell lines and virus-infected cells without requiring prior sensitization or activation. The cytotoxicity of NK cells is not MHC-restricted, and it is not specific for a particular target.

In this review, we discuss the role of each cytokine in the regulation of immune functions mediated by the different lymphocytic populations. Tables 3–2 and 3–3 summarize the activating and suppressing effects of cytokines on lymphocyte functions. The synergistic or antagonistic effects of cytokine combinations are presented in Table 3–4.

INTERLEUKIN-1

Interleukin-1 (IL-1), also called hematopoietin-1, is a 14- to 17-kd polypeptide primarily produced by macrophages, although epidermal, epithelial, lymphoid, and vascular tissues may also synthesize IL-1 (17,18). Two forms of IL-1 (IL-1α and IL-1β) have been described, but they recognize the same cell surface receptors and share various biological activities (19). IL-1 acts on a broad spectrum of target cells involved in immune or inflammatory responses. IL-1 is a chemoattractant for lymphocytes, and it regulates various aspects of T- and B-lymphocyte development, including maturation of thymic T- and B-cell precursors and induction of lymphokine and lymphokine receptor synthesis and expression (18). IL-1 stimulates the production of other cytokines, such as IL-2, IFNs, IL-3, IL-6, and CSF hematopoietic growth factors.

IL-1, TNF, and IL-6 share the ability to stimulate T and B lymphocytes, augment cell proliferation, and initiate or suppress gene expression for several proteins (19). Unlike TNF, IL-1 can stimulate lymphocytes both by direct activation and by the induction of other cytokines. IL-1 increases the proliferation and activation of resting T cells by inducing IL-2 and IL-2 receptor (IL-2R) expression (17,19). Activation of T cells by IL-1 is increased by IL-6, and both are synergistic in IL-2 production (19). IL-1 synergizes with various B cell growth factors, probably including IL-4, IL-6, and IL-2, for proliferation, activation, and antibody production of B lymphocytes (19). IL-1 augments NK cell binding to tumor targets and synergizes with IL-2 and IFN for NK activity (17,19). IL-1 is also synergistic with several other lymphokines, such as TNF, IL-3, IL-8, and CSFs. Thus, IL-1 is an important element of the cytokine network that induces augmentation or suppression of biological responses during host responses to infection or inflammation.

INTERLEUKIN-2

IL-2, probably the most extensively studied lymphokine in preclinical and clinical settings, has profound influence on development, expansion, and activation of T cells, NK cells, and B cells (20–23). IL-2 is a 15.5-kd glycoprotein that is produced by activated T lymphocytes, and it is critical for normal immune responsiveness. Following binding to cell surface IL-2 receptors (IL-2R), IL-2 stimulates all lymphoid cells to proliferate and differentiate (21,23). IL-2R affinity determines IL-2 effect. Three IL-2R sub-

TABLE 3–2 ACTIVATING EFFECTS OF CYTOKINES ON LYMPHOCYTES

Cytokines	Target	Activity
IL-1	Lymphocytes	Chemoattractant; induction of IL-2 and IL-2R; stimulation of production of IL-2, IFN-α, IL-3, IL-6, and CSFs
	Resting T cells	Proliferation and activation
	NK cells	Synergy with IL-2 and IFN for NK activity; increase in NK cell binding to tumor targets
	B cells	Synergy with IL-4, IL-6, and IL-2 for proliferation, activation, and antibody production
IL-2	Stimulated T cells	Induction of proliferation, cytokine production, cytolytic molecules production; differentiation of naive to memory T cells
	Stimulated B cells	Proliferation, antibody production
	NK cells	Activation of NK cells: increase proliferation, cytotoxic activity, and production of IFN-γ, GM-CSF, and TNF-α, -β
	LAK cells	Generation of LAK cells, with increased non-MHC-restricted cytotoxicity
	TIL	Activation and proliferation of TIL; synergy with IL-4, TNF-α, or anti-CD3 for TIL expansion
IL-4	B cells	Increase proliferation response to anti-IgM or LPS; increase expansion of class II MHC antigens, CD23, IL-4R; production of IgE in mice
	T cells	Autocrine factor for murine Th2 cell lines
	CD8+ CTL	Increase proliferation, differentiation of CTL precursor IL-2+IL-4 cause expansion of CD8$^+$ T cells
IL-5	Activated B cells	Mouse: increase synthesis of IgM, IgG1, and IgA; synergy with IL-4 for IgE secretion
		Human: IgA secretion
IL-6	Activated B cells	Differentiation, increase antibody production
	Resting T cells	Activation, induction of IL-2R, production of IL-2
	CTL	Proliferation and differentiation
	NK	Increase NK activity, but not LAK
IL-7	T cells	Costimulation with anti-CD3 or lectin for proliferation; increase CTL activity of stimulated CD8$^+$ T cells
	LAK cells	Generation of LAK cells from NK cells, synergy with IL-2 and IL-12
IL-8	T cells	Chemoattractant
IL-9	Murine Th clones	Proliferation in presence of IL-4
	B cells	Synergy with IL-4 for antibody production
IL-10	B cells	Proliferation and antibody production
IL-12	T and NK cells	Increase proliferation of activated cells and production of IFN-γ; synergy with IL-2 for CTL and NK/LAK activity; Th1 differentiation
IL-13	B cells	Up-regulation of class II MHC antigens, sIgM, CD23, CD17, and CD72; switch factor for IgE synthesis; enhance proliferation of activated B cells
	LGL (NK) cells	IFN-γ synthesis
IL-14	Activated B cells	Proliferation

TABLE 3–2   (*Continued*)

Cytokines	Target	Activity
IFN-α	NK cells	Increase NK cell cytotoxicity; synergy with IL-2 for NK activity
	B cells	Ig isotype selection
IFN-γ	CTL and NK cells	Required for induction of proliferative and cytotoxic responses; promotes cell-mediated immunity
	B cells	Regulation of Ig isotype switching
TNF-α	Activated T cells	Increase in IL-2R and proliferation to IL-2; increase in IL-2 and IFN-γ production
	NK and LAK cells	Increase response to IL-2, IL-2R, and cytolytic activity
	Stimulated B cells	Growth and maturation
TGF-β	B cells	Isotype switching to IgA in cooperation with IL-2 and IL-5

IL = interleukin; IFN = interferon; CSF = colony-stimulating factor; NK = natural killer; TNF = tumor necrosis factor; LAK = lymphokine-activated killer; MHC = major histocompatibility complex; TIL = tumor-infiltrating lymphocyte; Ig = immunoglobulin; LPS = lipopolysaccharide; CTL = cytotoxic T cell; LGL = large granular lymphocyte; TGF = transforming growth factor.

units, IL-2Rα (55 kd, Tac), IL-2Rβ (70/75 kd), and IL-2Rγ (64 kd) have been identified (22). IL-2Rα, a low affinity receptor with a short cytoplasmic domain, has no signaling capacity, whereas IL-2Rβ, an intermediate affinity receptor with a large cytoplasmic domain, is responsible for signal transduction. High affinity receptors are formed when all subunits are noncovalently associated in a receptor complex. IL-2Rγ has a pivotal role in facilitating IL-2 binding by IL-2Rβ and in receptor signaling (22). Most resting T cells, B cells, and NK cells do not express IL-2Rα and lack high affinity receptors, but these receptors are rapidly expressed after activation. NK cells constitutively express IL-2Rβ and IL-2Rγ, and a small NK subset expresses both CD56 and IL-2Rα (21).

Addition of IL-2 to NK cells enhances NK cell cytotoxic activity and leads to the generation of lymphokine-activated killer (LAK) cells (24,25). IL-2 activation of NK cells also augments their ability to release cytokines, including IFN-γ, GM-CSF, TNF-α, and TNF-β (21,26). These cytokines, in conjunction with microbial agents, stimulate monocytes and macrophages, which in turn release large amounts of IL-1, IL-6, IL-8, and TNF-α, resulting in the formation of a cytokine network in response to infection (21).

IL-2 incubation of human peripheral blood lymphocytes (PBL) or murine splenocytes for 4 to 7 days induces the generation of LAK cells. LAK cells mediate enhanced cytotoxic activity against NK-resistant tumor cell lines and freshly isolated tumor cells (24,25,27) with lower levels of killing against normal cells (28). The majority of human LAK cell activity is mediated by IL-2–activated NK cells characterized by the expression of CD56 and CD16 markers (20,29,30). A small subset of T cells, which are CD3+/CD56+, are also capable of mediating non-MHC–restricted cytotoxic activity. The major role of IL-2 in activation of cytotoxic cells has led to clinical trials for cancer therapy using IL-2 infusions alone or combined with autologous LAK cells (20). Following IL-2 therapy, in vivo generation of LAK activity with IL-2–activated NK-cell phenotype was demonstrated (20,30).

T and B cells both require antigenic stimulation for IL-2R expression (31). Once activated, the cells respond to IL-2 by proliferating and secreting effector molecules as cytokines, cytolytic molecules, or antibodies (21). Therefore, IL-2 is critical in the generation of the primary immune response. IL-2 derived from antigen-activated T cells stimulates the switch from secretory IgM and J-chain expression necessary for the formation of secreted IgM molecules that constitute most of the primary immune response (32). IL-2 also promotes the differentiation of naive to memory T cells and the ability to express cytokine genes other than IL-2 in response to secondary stimulation (21). Thus, IL-2 also has a major role in secondary responses as T cells are primed to secrete cytokines. IL-2 is also important in delayed-type hypersensitivity reactions (21). A selective defect in IL-2 production leads to severe combined immunodeficiency (SCID) due to a functional defect in T cells and low levels of Igs (33). IL-2 toxicity reported in high-dose IL-2 therapy and manifested by capillary leak syndrome may be attributed to

TABLE 3–3 SUPPRESSING EFFECTS OF CYTOKINES ON LYMPHOCYTES

Cytokines*	Target	Activity
IL-4	NK cells	Inhibition of NK activation and proliferation
	LAK	Inhibition of IL-2–induced LAK activity; inhibition of IL-8 production; suppresses Th1 cell development, favors Th2 cells
IL-10	Mouse Th1 clones	Inhibition of cytokine production
	Stimulated human PBMC	Inhibition of IFN-γ, TNF-α, GM-CSF, and LT synthesis
	Monocyte/macrophage	Inhibition of APC function affects T-cell proliferation and cytokine synthesis
	IL-2 stimulated NK cells	Inhibition of IFN-γ and TNF-α production, but not LAK generation
	Accessory cells	Inhibition of IL-12 synthesis
IL-13	Helper T cells	Suppress development of Th1 cells, favor Th2 cells by down-regulation of IL-12 production by monocytes
IL-14	B cells	Inhibition of antibody secretion
IFN-α	NK cells	Inhibition of IL-2–mediated LAK activity
IFN-γ	Th2 cells	Inhibition of Th2 cell proliferation
TGF-β	T cells	Inhibition of proliferation
	NK cells	Suppression of activity
	LAK cells and CTL	Inhibition of generation of LAK and CTL, but not their activity
	B cells	Suppression of IgG and IgM from B cells; inhibition of proliferation

*See Table 3–2 for abbreviations.
PBMC = peripheral blood mononuclear cell; LT = lymphotoxin.

TNF-α release from IL-2–activated NK cells and monocytes (21). Therefore, the levels of IL-2 are critical for maintaining a balance in immune responses.

IL-2 has also been used extensively for activation and selective expansion of tumor-infiltrating lymphocytes (TIL) isolated from enzymatically digested tumor specimens (20). TIL mediate cytotoxic activity against autologous and allogeneic tumor targets in vitro. TIL isolated from melanomas often demonstrate MHC-restricted cytotoxicity against the autologous melanoma tumor mediated by specific T cells (34). These TIL were effective when combined with IL-2 therapy for the treatment of melanoma. We and others have shown that IL-2 can be combined with IL-4 or TNF-α to enhance the expansion of selective lymphocyte subsets from TIL obtained from human tumor specimens (35–37). IL-4 has been shown to inhibit IL-2–induced, non-MHC–restricted LAK cell activity (38). IL-2 combined with IL-4 can promote the growth of melanoma T-cell TIL specific for the autologous tumor (36). TNF-α was found to up-regulate expression of MHC antigens and IL-2R and to synergize with IL-2 for the expansion of T cells (35,37). This finding reflects on the coordinated effect of various cytokines on lymphocytic expansion.

INTERLEUKIN-3 AND INTERLEUKIN-5

Initially described as hematopoietic growth factors, IL-3 and IL-5, together with GM-CSF, also regulate inflammation, allergic reactions, and cell adherence (39). IL-3 is a T-cell–derived 28-kd glycoprotein. IL-3 acts as a hematopoietic growth factor that promotes proliferation and differentiation of multipotential hematopoietic stem cells and committed progenitor cells of granulocytes, macrophages, megakaryocytes, mast cells, and erythroid cell lineages (18). IL-3 produced during immune reactions may recruit additional hematopoietic cells to sustain or

TABLE 3–4   COORDINATED ACTIVITIES OF CYTOKINES

Cytokine Combination*	Synergy (Augmentation)	Antagonism (Inhibition)
IL-1		
IL-1+IL-2/IFN	NK activity	
IL-1+IL-6	IL-2 production	
IL-1+IL-4/IL-6/IL-2	B-cell activity	
IL-1+IL-7		Pre-B-cell proliferation by IL-7
IL-2		
IL-2+IL-4	Expansion of TIL or CD8+ T cells	
IL-2+TNF-α	Expansion of T cells	
IL-4		
IL-4+IL-2		IL-2–induced IFN-γ production
IL-4+IFN-γ		IgG$_{2a}$ production by B cells
IL-4+IL-10		Antibody production
IL-6		
IL-6+IL-7	Thymocyte proliferation	
IL-7		
IL-7+IL-2/IL-6/TNF-α	Thymocyte proliferation	
IL-7+IL-2	Increase CTL activity	
IL-7+IL-2/IL-12	Increase LAK generation	
IL-7+IL-4/TGF-β		LAK induced by IL-7
IL-9		
IL-9+IL-4	B cell antibody production	
IL-10		
IL-10+IL-4	B-cell proliferation	
IL-12		
IL-12+IL-2	Increase CTL and NK/LAK activities	
IL-13		
IL-13+IL-2	IFN-γ synthesis by LGL	
IFN-γ		
IFN-γ+IL-2	LAK-cell generation	
IFN-γ+IL-4		Antibody production and class II MHC antigens induced by IL-4
TNF-α		
TNF-α+IL-2	NK and LAK activities	
TGF-β		Antagonizes effects of IL-1, IL-2, IL-3, TNF, and IFN
		IL-8 production
TGF-β+IL-7		Pre-B cell and thymocyte growth induced by IL-7

*See Table 3–2 for abbreviations.

amplify these responses. In experimental tumor systems, IL-3 has been shown to indirectly enhance the activity of cytotoxic T cells (CTL) by stimulating the release of T cell growth factors (40).

IL-5 is a 45-kd glycoprotein secreted by T cells and mast cells. IL-5 is a more restricted hematopoietic growth factor than IL-3; it controls mainly the eosinophil and the basophil lineages (39). It stimulates proliferation and differentiation in vitro of activated murine B cells, CD5+ B cells, and eosinophils. IL-5 enhances the synthesis of IgM, IgG1, and IgA in cultures of lipopolysaccharide (LPS)-stimulated cells (16,18). IL-5 also synergizes with IL-4 to promote IgE secretion (16). Conflicting reports have been published regarding the role of IL-5 on human B cells. IL-5 has been implicated in IgA secretion by human B cells in the presence of T cells (16).

INTERLEUKIN-4

IL-4 is a species-specific glycoprotein of 15 to 19 kd first described in 1982 as a B cell growth factor (BCGF) (41–43). IL-4 is primarily produced by activated helper T cells and mast cells (44,45), and it has demonstrated multiple stimulatory and regulatory effects. IL-4 can promote growth and differentiation of B cells, T cells, and mast cells, as well as mediate regulatory effects on macrophages (43). IL-4 also affects a wide variety of other cell types, including NK cells, LAK cells, mast cells, eosinophils, basophils, fibroblasts, endothelial cells, and various human solid and lymphoproliferative tumors (43). IL-4 exerts its effect by interacting with cell surface high affinity IL-4R, which are present on hematopoietic as well as non-hematopoietic cells. IL-4R are present in relatively low numbers (<300) on both murine and human T and B cells, but they can be up-regulated by IL-2 and IL-4 (46–48).

IL-4 is essential for various aspects of the humoral immune response. IL-4 may act at a very early step of B-cell development. Preculture of resting B cells with IL-4 enhance their proliferative response to anti-IgM antibody or to the B-cell mitogen LPS. IL-4 induces or increases expression of class II MHC antigens, low affinity receptor for IgE (CD23), and IL-4R on the surface of B cells (42). IL-4 action of costimulant of B-cell proliferation has been less striking in humans than in mice. IL-4 is responsible for the production of IgE in mice in response to stimuli inducing Ig class switching (42). IL-4 transgenic mice have elevated levels of serum IgE and IgG$_1$, thus confirming the role of IL-4 on production of these antibodies by B cells. IL-4 and IFN-γ mutually regulate Ig class expression that they induce. IFN-γ inhibits B-cell production of IgE and IgG$_1$ in response to LPS and IL-4, whereas IL-4 inhibits IgG$_{2a}$ production by B cells treated with LPS and IFN-γ (42).

IL-4 also has potent effects on T lymphocytes. IL-4 acts as an autocrine factor for murine Th2 cell lines and their growth in response to mitogens, IL-1, or antigen can be inhibited by anti-IL-4 antibodies. The growth of normal T-cell populations in the presence of IL-4 and mitogens, or IL-4 combined with IL-2 favors the preferential expansion of CD8+ T cells (49). IL-4 enhances the proliferation of precursors of CTL and their differentiation into active CTL (50,51). These findings corroborate the effect of IL-4 on human lymphocytes, showing that IL-4 regulates IL-2 activation and proliferation of NK cells and inhibits the IL-2–induced non-MHC–restricted LAK cell activity (38,52). Therefore, IL-4 is utilized to expand specific CTL from TIL cultures in the presence of IL-2 while inhibiting the growth of nonspecific killer cells (36).

IL-4 is capable of inducing a potent antitumor response in murine tumor models (53–55). These studies demonstrated that tumor cells transduced with IL-4 gene were not tumorigenic when inoculated subcutaneously into animals, and tumor inhibition correlated with IL-4 production. Whether the IL-4 effect is due to T-cell induction of systemic immunity or to induction of a local inflammatory response in the tumor primarily involving eosinophil and macrophage remains a matter of controversy (53–55).

INTERLEUKIN-6

IL-6 is a 21- to 28-kd glycoprotein, and it is a pleiotropic lymphokine also known as B cell differentiation factor (BCDF), B cell stimulatory factor 2 (BSF-2), interferon-β_2 (IFN-β_2), hybridoma/plasmacytoma growth factor (HPGF), hepatocyte-stimulating factor (HSF), and monocyte-granulocyte inducer type 2 (MGI-2) (56–58). Originally described as a T-cell–derived lymphokine that induces the final maturation of activated B cells into antibody-producing cells, IL-6 is also produced by T cells, monocytes, and a number of tissues and interacts with a wide variety of cell types. IL-6 has a central role in defense mechanisms, including the immune response, acute phase reactions, and hematopoiesis (56). IL-6 synergistically enhances the IL-3–induced multipotential colony cell formation in hematopoietic stem cells and the maturation of megakaryocytes (57).

IL-6 functions as a B cell differentiation factor and augments the production of IgM, IgG, and IgA in pokeweed mitogen–stimulated human PBL (56,58,59). Anti-IL-6 antibodies inhibited this activity (59). IL-6R are not expressed by resting B cells, but by activated B cells, indicating that IL-6 acts on the final stage of maturation of B cells. However, resting T cells do express IL-6R and are responsive to IL-6 activation (56). IL-6 induces expression of IL-2R and production of IL-2 and promotes the growth of mitogen-stimulated thymocytes and T cells (60). IL-6 induces the proliferation and differentiation of cytotoxic T cells (CTL), probably through the induction of serine esterases required for the expression of cytotoxic function (61). IL-6 can also enhance NK activity of purified large granular lymphocyte (LGL) cells, but, unlike IL-2, it does not induce LAK activity from LGL cells (62).

Elevated levels of IL-6 have also been observed in a number of pathological conditions, including bacterial and viral infections, human immunodeficiency virus (HIV) infection, autoimmune diseases, trauma, and certain neoplasias (57). Viral infections may induce IL-6 production, and latent viral infections may be involved in the deregulated expression of the IL-6 gene through the activation of nuclear factor regulating IL-6 gene expression (NF-IL6).

INTERLEUKIN-7

IL-7, a 25-kd protein (previously called lymphopoietin-1), is produced by bone marrow stromal cells and is capable of supporting the growth of pre-B cells in the absence of other cytokines or stromal cells. Distribution studies demonstrate the presence of IL-7R on pre-B cells, thymocytes, some T-cell lines, and bone marrow–derived macrophages, but not mature B-lineage cells (63). The cloning of IL-7R complementary DNA (cDNA) resulted in its classification within the "hematopoietin receptor superfamily" that includes the receptors for IL-2, IL-3, IL-4, IL-6, erythropoietin, G-CSF, and GM-CSF. These receptors are characterized by the presence of pairs of cysteine residues, a Trp-Ser-X-Trp-Ser motif as part of the extracellular domain, and the absence of intrinsic tyrosine kinase activity (63,64).

IL-7 causes proliferation of early B-cell progenitors as the pro-B and pre-B cell precursors of immature B cells, but it has no effect on immature or mature B cells and plasma cells (63). These later cells do not express the IL-7 receptor. IL-1α and TGF-β inhibit IL-7–induced proliferation of pre-B cells. There is evidence that IL-7 may have a role in the regulation of a common B- and T-lymphocyte precursor. Takai and colleagues (65) identified and cloned untransformed IL-7–dependent immature bone marrow lymphoid cells that rearrange and express both Ig heavy chain and TCR-γ genes.

IL-7 is a growth factor for immature and mature thymocytes, and it is likely to interact with other cytokines in the thymus to regulate proliferation and differentiation of thymocytes. IL-7 messenger RNA (mRNA) levels are high early in murine fetal thymic development; they then decline (66). IL-7 synergizes with low concentrations of IL-2 to promote the growth of TCR-positive thymocytes (67). IL-7 alone or in combination with IL-2, IL-6, or

TNF-α supports thymocyte proliferation (63). This activity of IL-7 is inhibited by TGF-β. IL-7 has a role in the differentiation of thymocytes as CD3–CD4–/CD8–TCR– cells develop into CD3+TCR-γ/δ+ cells and premature CD4+CD8+ cells develop into CD4+CD8– cells under the influence of IL-7 (68,69).

Mature lymph node T cells are costimulated by IL-7 in the presence of concanavalin A (CON A), and they demonstrate increased IL-2 production and IL-2R expression (70). Human peripheral T cells proliferate in response to IL-7 combined with anti-CD3 or lectin in short-term cultures, but in long-term cultures, IL-7 alone is sufficient to promote growth (63).

IL-7 augments the cytotoxic activity of human CD8+ CTL stimulated with CON A and IL-2 or antigen, and CTL activity may be blocked by neutralizing antiserum to IL-7 (71). Similar effects in the mouse may be partially diminished by antibodies to IL-2 and IL-6, but not to IL-4 (63). IL-7–generated murine CTL are highly effective in reducing tumor burden when adoptively transferred into mice (72–74). A recent article shows that IL-7 promotes the long-term in vitro growth of antitumor-specific cytotoxic CD8+ T lymphocytes from tumor draining lymph nodes in the absence of stimulator tumor cells (75). These CTL retain their antitumor ability in vivo (75).

IL-7 has been shown to generate LAK cells in both murine (75) and human systems (76), albeit with delayed and lower activity compared with LAK cells generated with IL-2. IL-7–induced LAK activity from human PBL is IL–2–independent and is regulated by IL-4 and TGF-β (63). This activity is mediated by CD3–CD56+ NK cells and can be improved by the addition of low concentrations of IL-2 (76). IL-7 and IL-12 have an additive effect on proliferation of CD56+ NK cells (63).

Subcutaneous administration of IL-7 into normal mice causes an increased cellularity of the spleen, bone marrow, and lymph nodes; an increase of precursor, immature, and mature B and T cells in the spleen; but no change in the thymic composition (63). All these studies support the role of IL-7 in B- and T-cell development. On the basis of its effects on CTL and LAK activity, IL-7 may also be an important addition to current strategies of adoptive immunotherapy.

INTERLEUKIN-8

IL-8 belongs to a family of chemoattractant, heparin-binding polypeptide cytokines of 8 to 10 kd (77). IL-8 is produced massively and rapidly by various kinds of cells in response to inflammatory stimuli. Monocytes, macrophages, T cells, and a variety of nonlymphoid cell types can produce IL-8 in response to IL-1 or TNF-α, as well as mitogens, lectins, and viruses (77). IL-8 expression and secretion can also be induced from NK cells by the synergistic effect of IL-2 and anti-CD16 monoclonal antibody (MAB) (78). IL-4, TGF-β, and glucocorticoids inhibit IL-8 production at the transcriptional level.

IL-8 displays an important chemotactic activity for T cells, basophils, and neutrophils in vitro. IL-8 is also responsible for the release of lysosomal enzymes by neutrophils and has a role in adhesion and migration of neutrophils through vascular endothelium (77). IL-8 binds to target cells via specific receptors. Normal human T lymphocytes have approximately 300 binding sites per cell and respond to 10 times lower concentrations of IL-8 than neutrophils (77). IL-8 down-regulates its own receptor expression by internalization of the ligand-receptor complex into the cell, as observed for various other cytokines. The receptors are rapidly re-expressed in the absence of de novo protein synthesis, and this recycling is essential for signal transmission by IL-8 (77).

The major role of IL-8 in inflammation is confirmed by the findings that it is produced in neoplastic and infectious diseases of the human central nervous system and that it may determine the leukocyte infiltrates found in these diseases (79).

INTERLEUKIN-9

Originally described as a p40 mouse T cell growth factor, IL-9 activities extend to erythroid progenitors, B cells, mast cells, and fetal thymocytes (80). The cloned human homolog of the IL-9/p40 gene shares a similar genomic organization with murine IL-9. Murine helper T-cell lines and fresh T cells are capable of secreting IL-9 on activation by lectins or allogenic spleen cells (80). Human IL-9 is expressed by peripheral blood T lymphocytes after activation by lectins or anti-CD3 antibodies. IL-2 is the major signal required for IL-9 expression because the induction of IL-9 can be completely blocked by anti-IL-2 antibodies (80). IL-9R have been described on murine T-cell clones (81), and IL-9 has a role in promoting early erythroid progenitor differentiation (80,82). Certain murine helper T-cell clones proliferate in response to IL-9, whereas murine CTL clones are not affected (80). In helper T-cell clones, the presence of IL-4 is required for the development of responsiveness to IL-9; subsequently, these clones will proliferate in response to IL-9 alone. IL-9–transfected T-cell clones can induce T-cell tumor formation in syngeneic mice (80).

Human IL-9 can also synergize with IL-4 to induce IgE and IgG production or IgG and IgM production by B cells. IL-9 supports activation and proliferation of mast cell, and it may be involved in allergic responses (80).

INTERLEUKIN-10

IL-10, a 18-kd polypeptide, was originally described as a cytokine synthesis inhibitory factor (CSIF) produced by Th2 helper clones because it inhibits IFN-γ production from Th1 clones (83,84). Like IL-6, IL-10 is also expressed by a variety of cells, including Th0 and Th1 subsets, monocytes, macrophages, and B cells (83). IL-10 has a major role in the regulation of immune responses because it blocks activation of cytokine synthesis, and it is an inhibitor of macrophage, T cell, and NK cell effector functions (83). Murine IL-10 (mIL-10) inhibits production of cytokines by mouse Th1 clones in response to antigen (84). Human IL-10 (hIL-10) also inhibits synthesis of the cytokines IFN-γ, TNF-α, GM-CSF, and lymphotoxin (LT) by human PBMC stimulated by phytohemagglutinin antigen (PHA) or anti-CD3 antibodies (83). IL-10 inhibits antigen presenting cell (APC)-dependent stimulation of cytokine synthesis by Th0 and Th2 clones. Inhibition of monocyte/macrophage APC function by IL-10 affects both cytokine synthesis and proliferation of human T cells and T-cell clones (85,86). This effect may be due partly to down-regulation of monocyte/macrophage class II MHC antigens (85). IL-10 may act by inhibiting the function of B7/BB1, a membrane-bound costimulator required for activation of Th1 and NK cells (83).

IL-10 inhibits monocyte/macrophage–dependent IFN-γ and TNF-α synthesis by human NK cells stimulated by IL-2 (87). However, IL-10 does not inhibit proliferation and generation of LAK cells by IL-2 in this system (87). This property may be of importance for the use of IL-10 in conjunction with IL-2 in LAK therapy as an inhibitor of the cytokine-mediated side effects of the therapy. Recently, IL-10 has been shown to suppress the synthesis of the NK stimulatory factor, NKSF/IL-12, a powerful inducer of IFN-γ, in accessory cells (88).

In addition to its suppressing activity, IL-10 seems to be involved in T-cell differentiation, and it can induce proliferation of thymocytes in the presence of IL-2 and IL-4 in the mouse system (89), but not in humans. IL-10 has demonstrated an immunostimulatory effect on murine B cells as up-regulation of MHC class II antigens and increase in proliferation and production of Ig (83). Human IL-10 has a comparable costimulatory activity to IL-4 on B cells, and together they induce a considerable increase in B-cell proliferation (83). IL-10 is a differentiation factor for human B cells activated by anti-CD40 antibodies causing production of large amounts of IgM, IgG, and IgA (90), but this activity is antagonized by IL-4.

The Epstein-Barr virus genome encodes a homolog of IL-10, designated viral IL-10 genome, which shares many of the cytokine's biological activities and may have a role in host-virus interaction (83).

INTERLEUKIN-11

IL-11 is produced by stromal fibroblasts and trophoblasts. IL-11 synergizes with IL-3 and IL-4 for the growth of hematopoietic progenitors, and it has no effect on lymphocytes.

INTERLEUKIN-12

IL-12, first described as NK cell stimulatory factor (NKSF) or cytotoxic lymphocyte maturation factor, is a disulfide-linked heterodimer cytokine consisting of 40- and 35-kd subunits, and it is produced by macrophages and B lymphocytes (91–93). IL-12 stimulates the production of IFN-γ from T cells and NK cells (92,94), and it exerts a variety of biological effects on human T cells and NK cells in vitro. IL-12 is a growth factor for activated human T cells and NK cells. IL-12 can augment the proliferation of PHA-activated lymphoblasts, including activated T cells of the CD4+ and CD8+ subsets (95), independently of IL-2. IL-12 can also promote the expansion of IL-2–activated CD56+ NK cells, whereas IL-12 has no effect on resting lymphocytes similar to IL-4 (95). IL-12 synergizes with IL-2 in augmenting allogeneic CTL response (93,96) and NK/LAK cytolytic activity (92,96–98).

Recently, using naive CD4+ T cells from TCR-αβ transgenic mice, Hsieh and associates (99) demonstrated that IL-12 produced by macrophages induces differentiation of Th1 cells from uncommitted T cells in response to the pathogen *Listeria,* which is associated with increased IFN-γ production. In contrast to IL-12, IL-4 drives the differentiation of T cells toward the Th2 type (91). Similarly, in the human system, addition of IL-12 to a mixed T-cell population from patients with allergies will shift the phenotype from the normally dominant Th2 population to Th1 cells (100). Thus, IL-12 may have a potential role in the treatment of allergic reactions, HIV infections associated with Th1 cell loss, and malignancies that could be better controlled by cell-mediated immunity.

Recently, injection of mice with recombinant IL-12 augmented NK activity, enhanced allogeneic CTL responses, and induced secretion of IFN-γ, thus confirming the in vitro activities of IL-12 (101). On the basis of these findings, IL-12 has been recently evaluated in murine tumor models and was shown to have a potent in vivo antitumor effect mediated by IL-12 (102). CD8+ T cells have a critical role in this activity as well (102). IL-12 gene therapy of murine tumors in which IL-12 was delivered locally at the tumor site by IL-12–transfected fibroblasts could induce an immune response against poorly immunogenic tumors (103).

INTERLEUKIN-13

IL-13 is a recently described protein secreted by activated T cells that regulates human monocyte and B-cell functions (104). It is specifically produced by activated T cells, including CD8+, Th0, Th1, and Th2 T-cell clones in humans (104), and by Th2 cells in mice (105). It can induce proliferation of the human premyeloid cell line, TF-1 (105).

IL-13 shares some regulatory biological functions with IL-4. IL-13 and IL-4 genes are closely linked on chromosome 5q 23–31 (106), and there is a sequence homology between their proteins (104). Although it does not bind IL-13, the functional receptor of IL-4 shares a common subunit with the IL-13 receptor that is important for signal transduction (104).

Similar to IL-4, IL-13 has various effects on human monocytes. In the presence of IL-13, human monocytes undergo a marked change in morphology and in cell surface phenotype, including increased expression of certain integrin molecules, MHC class II antigens, and low affinity receptor for IgE (105). In addition, monocytes have increased survival time when cultured in the presence of IL-13 (105). However, like IL-4, IL-13 inhibits the production of proinflammatory cytokines from monocytes stimulated by LPS (106). IL-13 may act like IL-4 to suppress the development of Th1 cells through down-regulation of IL-12 production by monocytes, thus favoring Th2 cell development. In addition to being a monocyte deactivator, IL-13 can up-regulate the capacity of monocytes to present antigen (104).

IL-13 induces expression of CD23 on purified human B cells and up-regulation of MHC class II, sIgM, CD17, and CD72 molecules (107). IL-4 has similar effects on B-cell phenotype, but it is generally more potent than IL-13. Both IL-13 and IL-4 enhance the proliferative responses of human B cells, which have been preactivated by anti-IgM antibodies or through ligation of surface CD40 (105). Human IL-4 induces human B cells to switch to production of IgG4 and IgE, but this process requires costimulatory signals delivered by activated CD4+ T helper cells (104). Interactions between CD40L (transiently expressed on activated CD4+ T helper cells) and CD40 (constitutively expressed on B cells) have an essential role in productive T cell–B cell interactions, which result in switching of Ig isotype. Thus, IL-13 acts as a switch factor directing synthesis of IgE-like IL-4, but it acts independently of IL-4, because neutralizing anti-IL-4 antibodies do not affect this activity (107). Moreover, IL-13 switch factor activity is not augmented by IL-4, indicating that both cytokines use common signaling pathways for the induction of these Ig isotypes (107). IL-13 may have an important role in the regulation of enhanced IgE synthesis in allergic patients.

IL-13, in contrast to IL-4, fails to activate human T cells or PHA-activated T-cell blasts (104). IL-13 induces IFN-γ synthesis by LGL and synergizes with IL-2 for this activity, whereas IL-4 inhibits IL-2–induced IFN-γ production (106).

Although the biological activities of IL-13 are more restricted than those of IL-4, because it does not act on human and mouse T cells or mouse B cells, IL-13 may be critical in regulating inflammatory and immune responses.

INTERLEUKIN-14

IL-14, previously defined as high molecular weight B cell growth factor (HMW-BCGF), is produced by malignant B cells and normal and malignant T cells (108). IL-14 is a human B cell growth factor based on its ability to induce proliferation of activated B cells. IL-14 does not stimulate resting B cells, and it does not induce antibody synthesis or secretion by B cells. IL-14 inhibits antibody secretion and acts predominantly on normal and malignant B cells (108).

INTERFERONS

Interferons are glycoproteins that are produced and released from virally infected cells; they were originally characterized for their antiviral properties (109). IFNs bind to IFN receptors on other cells and induce synthesis of antiviral proteins, thus protecting the cells against further viral infection. Three major classes of IFNs have been described and characterized. IFN-α is produced by leukocytes; IFN-β is produced by fibroblasts, epithelial cells, macrophages, and lymphoblastoid cells; and IFN-γ is produced by activated lymphocytes. Twenty-six IFN-α genes with common structures have been identified, and they encode for at least 22 distinct proteins consisting of 20 kd single polypeptide chains (110). These different IFN-αs mediate distinct biological activities in different cells. In contrast, there is only a single form of IFN-β encoded by a distinct gene located next to the IFN-α locus in both humans and mice (111). IFN-β shares only limited antigenic relatedness to IFN-α. IFN-γ is unrelated to the type I IFNs, and it is encoded by a single gene (111). The mature human IFN-γ protein, which displays biological activity, consists of two polypeptides associated in a homodimer of 34 kd. IFN-α and IFN-β, originally known as type I IFN, bind to a common IFN-α/-β (type I) recep-

tor, whereas IFN-γ, known as type II IFN, binds to a different (type II) receptor (112).

IFNs have demonstrated antiproliferative effects, resulting in decreased multiplication of tumor cells. IFN can also induce an increase in the expression of MHC and tumor-associated antigens of the target cells and thus render them more susceptible to destruction by immune cells. In addition to this direct antitumor effect, IFN can act as biological response modifiers (BRMs) to increase NK cell cytotoxic activity, antibody-dependent cellular cytotoxicity (ADCC), or lysis by specifically sensitized lymphocytes (20,109).

IFN-α has been shown to augment NK cell cytotoxicity against a variety of neoplastic cells, including those from several hematological malignancies (109,113,114). IFN-α acts synergistically with IL-2 to augment NK activity, but it inhibits the induction of IL-2–mediated LAK activity (115,116). IFN-α may have a role in directing Ig isotype selection in B cells, because injection of mice with murine IFN-α suppresses IgE secretion while enhancing IgG2a secretion (117).

IFN-γ is considerably more active as an immunomodulator than other classes of interferons, but its antiviral activity is lower. IFN-γ is produced by all CD8+ T-cell populations and by the Th1 and Th0 subsets of CD4+ T cells following antigenic or T cell mitogen stimulation (111,118). IFN-γ is also produced by NK cells after exposure to mitogens and IL-2 (119), to TNF-α (produced by macrophages), and to microbial products (120). IFN-γ production from T cells or NK cells is stimulated by IL-12, which can act synergistically with alloantigens, mitogens, or IL-2 (93). In contrast, IL-10 inhibits IFN-γ production by T cells and NK cells (84).

INF-γ is a pleiotropic cytokine instrumental in the regulation of immune and inflammatory processes. IFN-γ has a major role in differentiation and function of monocytes/macrophages (111,121). It promotes the antigen-presenting activity in macrophages by induction of MHC antigen expression and by increasing the levels of intracellular enzymes and adherent molecules (ICAM-1), which are required during the interaction between macrophages and T cells (111). IFN-γ has a critical role in up-regulation of MHC class I and II antigens on a variety of other cells, including endothelial and epithelial cells, but it inhibits class II expression in B cells (111). IFN-α and IFN-β can also up-regulate class I antigens, but not class II antigens. IFN-γ enhances MHC class I expression on cells that constitutively express these antigens, and it is capable of inducing class II antigens on cells negative for them. These effects are exerted by IFN-γ regulation of MHC gene transcription, and they are of importance for promoting antigen presentation during the inductive phase of immune responses (111). IFN-γ can activate the cytotoxic activity of macrophages against parasites and neoplastic cells by promoting the elaboration of cytocidal compounds, such as reactive oxygen and nitrogen intermediates and TNF-α (122). IFN-γ participates in inflammatory responses through its ability to enhance TNF production and its activity.

IFN-γ is required in the early phases of induction of proliferative and cytotoxic responses of human CTL and NK cells elicited in PBL by alloantigens, IL-2, and anti-CD3 antibody (123). IFN-γ and IL-2 collaborate to generate LAK cells in the human system (124). In the mouse, IFN-γ appears to provide a signal for CTL and LAK maturation (125,126).

On B cells, IFN-γ regulates immunoglobulin isotype switching directly (127) and controls the development of specific T helper subsets indirectly. IFN-γ inhibits the proliferation of Th2, but not Th1 subsets; it is therefore a key element in determining the type of immune effector function that develops during an immune response (118). By inhibiting the expansion of Th2 cells, it eliminates the source of IL-10 and thus promotes cell-mediated immunity. IFN-γ antagonizes the ability of IL-4 to induce MHC class II expression on murine B cells (128).

On the basis of their direct antitumor effects and their biological response modifier (BRM) properties, recombinant IFNs have been utilized in several clinical trials involving many types of cancer (20).

TUMOR NECROSIS FACTOR

TNF (also called cachectin), originally defined by its antitumor activity, is a mediator of inflammation and cellular immune responses (129). Two distinct TNF molecules, TNF-α and TNF-β, have been described, and although TNF-α shows only 30% homology with TNF-β (also called lymphotoxin[LT]), both share the same receptors and have similar activity. Macrophages stimulated by LPS are a major source of TNF (129). IFN-γ potentiates LPS-induced TNF release. TNF induces its own synthesis and release by monocytes. IL-2, GM-CSF, and CSF-1 can also induce TNF release from monocytes (130–132). A membrane form of TNF not released from activated macrophages but present on their surface has been described.

T cells activated by anti-CD3 and IL-2 or mitogens can also produce TNF (133,134). B lymphocytes produce TNF when stimulated to proliferate (135). NK and LAK can release TNF following culture in IL-2 or after contact with NK targets and virally infected cells (129). Among other sources of TNF are masts cells, polymorphonuclear leukocytes, keratinocytes, and tumor cells (129).

TNF receptors (TNF-R) are found on most types of cells; therefore, TNF has profound effects on a wide variety of cells and organ systems (129). A major function mediated by TNF is activation and differentiation of monocytes and macrophages. TNF synergizes with IFN-γ for activation of macrophages cytotoxic to parasites and tumor cells (129,136).

In the presence of other cytokines, such as IL-1, IL-2, or IL-7, TNF increases thymocyte proliferation (137). Resting T cells do not bear TNF-R and are not responsive to TNF, whereas activated T cells express TNF-R. TNF causes an increase in high affinity IL-2R expression on stimulated T cells and consequently augments their proliferative response to IL-2, as well as IL-2 and IFN-γ production (138,139). TNF is produced in mixed lymphocyte culture (MLC), and addition of TNF to MLC can augment the generation of CTL (140). TNF augments the response of NK and LAK cells to IL-2 by increasing IL-2R expression and cytolytic activity. This effect probably involves some autocrine step because these cells produce TNF (141). TNF also seems to enhance the growth and maturation of stimulated B cells (142,143). TNF may induce the secretion of other cytokines, including GM-CSF, G-CSF, IL-1, and IL-6 by endothelial cells (129,144). TNF influences leukocyte traffic by enhancing the expression of adhesion molecules on endothelial cells (129).

High levels of TNF characterize numerous pathological conditions, including inflammatory conditions, cachexia, vascular permeability, and shock. TNF causes hemorrhagic necrosis in tumors in vivo. It has direct and indirect effects on both the tumor cells and the immune effectors of the antitumor response.

TRANSFORMING GROWTH FACTOR-β

TGF-β1, a 25-kd peptide homodimer first purified from human platelets (145), was defined based on its ability to induce normal rat kidney fibroblasts to grow and to form colonies in soft agar in the presence of epidermal growth factor (146). Four additional forms of TGF-β (β2, β3, β4, β5) have been identified following the cloning of TGF-β1, and they show 60 to 80% homology with TGF-β 1 in their amino acid sequences (146). These five forms of TGF-β share similar biological activities. Almost all cells, regardless of their origin, express TGF-β receptors and bind TGF-β with high affinity (146). TGF-β is therefore a multifunctional growth factor and it has a major role in the regulation of normal and pathological physiology.

TGF-β 1 and TGF-β2 are immunoregulatory agents that enhance monocyte function and suppress lymphocyte proliferation and function. TGF inhibits proliferation of T and B lymphocytes at femtomolar concentrations (147,148). TGF-β functions as an autoregulatory lymphokine that limits T cell clonal expansion. Activation of T cells with PHA increases TGF-βR expression and a delayed secretion of TGF-β1 peptide, suggesting a role for

TGF-β in ending T-cell activation (148). TGF-β also suppresses the activity of NK cells (149). TGF-β inhibits the in vitro generation of LAK cells and allospecific CTL, but not their activity (150). TGF-β antagonizes the effects of several cytokines, including IL-1, IL-2, IL-3, IFN, and TNF-α (146). TGF-β inhibits the production of TNF-α in mixed lymphocyte cultures (151) and inhibits the production of IFN-γ and TNF during LAK generation by IL-2 (152). TGF-β suppresses the effect of IFN-γ on induction of class II MHC antigens in both lymphoid and non-lymphoid cells (153). TGF-β can also suppress immune cell function in vivo (146).

TGF-β suppresses the secretion of IgG and IgM from B cells, even in the presence of IL-2 (147). However, TGF-β has a critical role in isotype switching, and it cooperates with IL-2 and IL-5 to up-regulate the secretion of IgA by splenic lymphocytes (154). TGF-β also suppresses the growth of thymocytes and less mature hematopoietic cell populations in bone marrow culture systems (146).

In contrast to its effects on lymphocytes, TGF-β activates several functions of monocyte/macrophages, but it deactivates the release of H_2O_2. Therefore, TGF-β suppresses the destructive aspects of the inflammatory response while facilitating the anabolic effects of macrophage-derived growth factors on tissue repair (146).

ACKNOWLEDGMENTS: This work was supported in part by the American Cancer Society, Veterans Administration Research Funds, and the Pardee Foundation. We thank Emily Montecillo and Esa Ali for their valuable help.

REFERENCES

1. Carding SR, Hayday AC, Bottomly K. Cytokines in T-cell development. Immunol Today 1991;12:239–245.

2. Owen JJT, Jenkinson EJ. Early events in T lymphocyte genesis in the fetal thymus. Am J Anat 1984;170:301–310.

3. Haynes BF, Martin ME, Kay HH, Kurtzberg J. Early events in human T cell ontogeny. Phenotypic characterization and immunohistologic localization of T cell precursors in early human fetal tissues. J Exp Med 1988;168:1061–1080.

4. Foon KA. The cytokine network. Oncology 1993;7:11–15.

5. DeLuca D, Mizel SB. I-A-positive nonlymphoid cells and T cell development in murine fetal thymus organ cultures: Interleukin 1 circumvents the block in T cell differentiation induced by monoclonal anti-I-A antibodies. J Immunol 1986;137:1435–1441.

6. Watson JD, Morrissey PJ, Namen AE, Conlon PJ, Widmer MB. Effect of IL-7 on the growth of fetal thymocytes in culture. J Immunol 1989;143:1215–1222.

7. Toribio ML, Gutierrez-Ramoz JC, Pezzi L, Marcos MAR, Martinez AC. Interleukin-2 dependent autocrine proliferation in T cell development. Nature 1989;342:82–85.

8. Carding SR, Jenkinson EJ, Kingston R, Hayday AC, Bottomly K, Owen JJT. Developmental control of lymphokine gene expression in fetal thymocytes during T cell ontogeny. Proc Natl Acad Sci USA 1989;86:3342–3345.

9. Powrie F, Coffman RL. Cytokine regulation of T-cell function: potential for therapeutic intervention. Immunol Today 1993;14:270–274.

10. Murray HW, Spitalny GL, Nathan CF. Activation of mouse peritoneal macrophages in vitro and in vivo by interferon-γ. J Immunol 1985;134:1619–1622.

11. Cher DJ, Mosmann TR. Two types of murine helper T cell clone. II. Delayed-type hypersensitivity is mediated by Th1 clones. J Immunol 1987;138:3688–3694.

12. Mosmann TR, Coffman RL. Th1 and Th2 cells: different patterns of lymphokine secretion lead to different functional properties. Ann Rev Immunol 1989;7:145–173.

13. Gajewski TF, Fitch FW. Anti-proliferative effect of IFN-γ in immune regulation. I. IFN-γ inhibits the proliferation of Th2 but not Th1 murine helper T lymphocyte clones. J Immunol 1988;140:4245–4252.

14. Fiorentino DF, Zlotnik A, Mosmann TR, Howard M, O'Garra A. IL-10 inhibits cytokine production by activated macrophages. J Immunol 1991;147:3815–3822.

15. Masuda ES, Naito Y, Arai KI, Arai N. Expression of lymphokine genes in T cells. Immunologist 1993;1:198–203.

16. Callard RE, Turner MW. Cytokines and Ig switching: evolutionary divergence between mice and humans. Immunol Today 1990;11:200–205.

17. Dinarello CA. Biology of interleukin 1. FASEB J 1988;2:108–115.

18. Mizel SB. The interleukins. FASEB J 1989;3:2379–2388.

19. Dinarello CA. Interleukin-1 and interleukin-1 antagonism. Blood 1991;77:1627–1652.

20. Hillman GG, Haas GP, Wahl W, Callewaert DM. Adoptive immunotherapy of cancer: biological response modifiers and cytotoxic cell therapy. Biotherapy 1992;5:119–129.

21. Kaplan G, Cohn ZA, Smith KA. Rational immunotherapy with interleukin-2. Biotechnol 1992;10:157–162.

22. Waldmann TA. The IL-2/IL-2 receptor system: a target for rational immune intervention. Immunol Today 1993;14:264–269.

23. Smith KA. The interleukin 2 receptor. Ann Rev Cell Biol 1989;5:397–425.

24. Trinchieri G, Matsumoto-Kobayshi M, Clark SC, Seehra J, London L, Perussia B. Response of resting peripheral blood natural killer cells to interleukin 2. J Exp Med 1984;160:1147–1169.

25. Rosenstein M, Yron I, Kaufman Y, Rosenberg SA. Lymphokine-activated killer cells: lysis of fresh syngeneic natural killer-resistant murine tumor cells by lymphocytes cultured in interleukin 2. Cancer Res 1984;44:1946–1953.

26. Ritz J, Schmidt RE, Michon J, Hercend T, Schlossman SF. Characterization of functional surface structures on human natural killer cells. Adv Immunol 1988;42:181–211.

27. Grimm EA, Mazumder A, Zhang HA, Rosenberg SA. The lymphokine activated killer cell phenomenon: lysis of NK resistant fresh solid tumor cells by IL-2 activated autologous human peripheral blood lymphocytes. J Exp Med 1982;155:1823–1841.

28. Sondel PM, Hank JA, Kohler PC, Chen PB, Minkoff DZ,

Molenda JA. Destruction of autologous human lymphocytes by interleukin-2 activated cytotoxic cells. J Immunol 1986;137:502–511.

29. Phillips JH, Lanier LL. Dissection of the lymphokine-activated killer phenomenon. Relative contribution of peripheral blood natural killer cells and T lymphocytes to cytolysis. J Exp Med 1986;164:814–825.

30. Weil-Hillman G, Fisch P, Prieve AF, Sosman JA, Hank JA, Sondel PM. Lymphokine-activated killer activity induced by in vivo interleukin 2 therapy: predominant role for lymphocytes with increased expression of CD2 and Leu19 antigens but negative expression of CD16 antigens. Cancer Res 1989;49:3680–3688.

31. Smith KA. Interleukin 2: inception, impact, and implications. Science 1988;240:1169–1176.

32. Blackmen MA, Tigges MA, Minie ME, Koshland ME. A model system for peptide hormone action in differentiation: interleukin 2 induces a B lymphoma to transcribe the J chain gene. Cell 1986;47:609–617.

33. Weinberg K, Parkman R. Severe combined immunodeficiency due to a specific defect in the production of interleukin-2. N Engl J Med 1991;322:1718–1723.

34. Aebersold P, Hyatt C, Johnson S, et al. Lysis of autologous melanoma cells by tumor-infiltrating lymphocytes: association with clinical response. J Natl Cancer Inst 1991; 83:932–937.

35. Hillman GG, Sud S, Dybal EJ, Pontes JE, Haas GP. Combinations of lymphocyte activating agents for expansion of tumor infiltrating lymphocytes from renal cell carcinoma. In: Goldstein AL, Garaci E, eds. Combination therapies: biological response modifiers in the treatment of cancer and infectious diseases. New York: Plenum Press, 1992;39–48.

36. Kawakami Y, Rosenberg SA, Lotze MT. Interleukin 4 promotes the growth of tumor-infiltrating lymphocytes cytotoxic for human autologous melanoma. J Exp Med 1988;168:2183–2191.

37. Yi Li W, Lusheng S, Kanbour A, et al. Lymphocytes infiltrating human ovarian tumors: synergy between tumor necrosis factor alpha and interleukin 2 in the generation of CD8+ effectors from tumor-infiltrating lymphocytes. Cancer Res 1989;49:5979–5985.

38. Nagler A, Lanier LL, Phillips JH. The effects of IL-4 on human natural killer cells: a potent regulator of IL-2 activation and proliferation. J Immunol 1988;141:2349–2351.

39. Lopez AF, Elliott MG, Woodcock J, Vadas MA. GM-CSF, IL-3 and IL-5: cross-competition on human haemopoietic cells. Immunol Today 1992;13:495–498.

40. Pulaski BA, McAdam AJ, Hutter EK, Bigger S, Lord EM, Frelinger JG. IL-3 enhances development of tumor reactive cytotoxic cells by a CD4 dependent mechanism. Cancer Res 1993;53:2112–2117.

41. Howard M, Farrar J, Hilfiker M, et al. Identification of a T cell derived B cell growth factor distinct from interleukin-2. J Exp Med 1982;155:914–923.

42. Paul WE. Interleukin-4: a prototypic immunoregulatory lymphokine. Blood 1990;77:1859–1870.

43. Puri RK, Siegel JP. Interleukin-4 and cancer therapy. Cancer Invest 1993;11:473–486.

44. Milanese C, Richardson NER, Reinherz EL. Identification of T helper cell-derived lymphokine that activates resting T lymphocytes. Science 1986;231:1118–1122.

45. Plaut M, Pierce JH, Watson CJ, et al. Mast cell lines produce lymphokines in response to cross lineage of FC$_\varepsilon$R1 or to calcium ionophores. Nature 1989;6219:64–67.

46. Ohara J, Paul WE. Upregulation of interleukin 4/B cell stimulatory factor-1 receptor expression. Proc Natl Acad Sci USA 1988;85:8221–8225.

47. Puri RK, Finbloom DS, Leland P, et al: Expression of high affinity IL4 receptors on murine tumor infiltrating lymphocytes and their upregulation by IL2. Immunology 1990;70:492–497.

48. Armitage RJ, Beckmann MP, Idzerda RL, et al. Regulation of interleukin 4 receptors on human T cells. Int Immunol 1990;2:1039–1045.

49. Hu-Li J, Shevac EM, Mizuguchi J, Ohara J, Mosmann T, Paul WE. B cell stimulatory factor-1 (interleukin 4) is a potent costimulant for normal resting T lymphocytes. J Exp Med 1987;165:157–172.

50. Widmer MB, Grabstein KH. Regulation of cytolytic T-lymphocyte generation by B-cell stimulatory factor. Nature 1987;326:795–798.

51. Trenn G, Takayama H, Hu-Li J, Paul WE, Sitkovsky MV. B cell stimulatory factor 1 (IL-4) enhances the development of cytotoxic T cells from Lyt-2+ resting murine T lymphocytes. J Immunol 1988;140:1101–1108.

52. Kawakami Y, Custer MC, Rosenberg SA, Lotze MT. IL-4 regulates IL-2 induction of lymphokine-activated killer activity from human lymphocytes. J Immunol 1989; 142:3452–3461.

53. Tepper RI, Pattengale PK, Leder P. Murine interleukin-4 displays potent anti-tumor activity in vivo. Cell 1989; 57:503–512.

54. Tepper RI, Coffman RL, Leder P. An eosinophil-dependent mechanism for the antitumor effect of IL-4. Science 1992; 257:548–551.

55. Golumbek PT, Lazemby AJ, Levitsky HI, et al. Treatment of established renal cancer by tumor cells engineered to secrete interleukin-4. Science 1991;254:713–716.

56. Kishimoto T. The biology of interleukin-6. Blood 1989;74:1–10.

57. Hirano T, Akira S, Taga T, Kishimoto T. Biological and clinical aspects of interleukin-6. Immunol Today 1990; 11:443–449.

58. Kishimoto T, Hibi M, Murakami M, Narazaki M, Saito M, Taga T. The molecular biology of interleukin-6 and its receptor. In: Ciba Foundation symposium 167, polyfunctional cytokines: IL-6 and LF. New York: John Wiley & Sons, 1992:5–23.

59. Muraguchi A, Hirano T, Tang B, et al. The essential role of B-cell stimulatory factor 2 (BSF-2/IL-6) for the terminal differentiation of B cells. J Exp Med 1988;167:332–344.

60. Lotz M, Jirik F, Kabouridis R, et al: BSF-2/IL-6 is costimulant for human thymocytes and lymphocytes. J Exp Med 1988;167:1253–1258.

61. Takai Y, Wong GG, Clark SC, Burakoff SJ, Herrmann SH. B cell stimulatory factor-2 is involved in the differentiation of cytotoxic T lymphocytes. J Immunol 1988;140:508–512.

62. Smyth MJ, Ortaldo JR. Comparison of the effect of IL-2 and IL-6 on the lytic activity of purified human peripheral blood large granular lymphocytes. J Immunol 1991; 146:1380–1384.

63. Appasamy PM. Interleukin-7: biology and potential clinical applications. Cancer Invest 1993;11:487–499.

64. Goodwin RG, Friend D, Ziegler SF, et al. Cloning of the human and murine interleukin-7 receptors: demonstration of a soluble form and homology to a new receptor superfamily. Cell 1990;60:941–951.

65. Takai Y, Sakata T, Iwagami S, et al. Identification of IL-7-dependent bone marrow-derived Thy-1 B220-lymphoid cell clones that rearrange and express both Ig and T cell receptor genes. J Immunol 1992;148:1329–1337.

66. Montgomery RA, Dallman MJ. Analysis of cytokine gene expression during fetal thymic ontogeny using the polymerase chain reaction. J Immunol 1991;147:554–560.

67. Okazaki H, Ito M, Sudo T, et al. IL-7 promotes thymocyte proliferation and maintains immunocompetent thymocytes bearing α/β or γ/δ T-cell receptors in vitro: synergism with IL-2. J Immunol 1989;143:2917–2922.

68. Groh V, Fabbi M, Strominger JL. Maturation of differentiation of human thymocyte precursors in vitro? Proc Natl Acad Sci USA 1990;87:5973–5977.

69. Uckun FM, Tuel-Ahlgren L, Obuz V, et al. Interleukin 7 receptor engagement stimulates tyrosine phosphorylation, inositol phospholipid turnover, proliferation, and selective differentiation to the CD4 lineage by human fetal thymocytes. Proc Natl Acad Sci USA 1991;88:6323–6327.

70. Morrissey PJ, Goodwin RG, Nordan RP, et al. Recombinant interleukin-7, pre-B cell growth factor, has costimulatory activity on purified mature T cells. J Exp Med 1989;169:707–716.

71. Hickman CJ, Crim JA, Mostowski HS, et al. Regulation of human cytotoxic T lymphocyte development by IL-7. J Immunol 1990;145:2415–2420.

72. Jicha DL, Schwarz S, Mule JJ, Rosenberg SA. Interleukin-7 mediates the generation and expression of murine allosensitized and antitumor CTL. Cell Immunol 1992;141:71–83.

73. Jicha DL, Mule JJ, Rosenberg SA. Interleukin-7 generates anti-tumor cytotoxic T lymphocytes against murine sarcomas with efficacy in cellular adoptive immunotherapy. J Exp Med 1991;174:1511–1515.

74. Lynch DH, Miller RE. Interleukin 7 promotes long-term in vitro growth of antitumor cytotoxic T lymphocytes with immunotherapeutic efficacy in vivo. J Exp Med 1994;179:31–42.

75. Lynch DH, Miller RE. Induction of murine lymphokine-activated killer cells by recombinant IL-7. J Immunol 1990;145:1983–1990.

76. Naume B, Espevic T. Effects of IL-7 and IL-2 on highly enriched CD56+ natural killer cells. A comparative study. J Immunol 1991;147:2208–2214.

77. Mukaida N, Harada A, Yasumoto K, Matsushima K. Properties of pro-inflammatory cell type-specific leukocyte chemotactic cytokines, interleukin 8 (IL-8) and monocyte chemotactic and activating factor (MCAF). Microbiol Immunol 1992;36:773–789.

78. Smyth MJ, Zachariae COC, Norihisa Y, Ortaldo JR, Hishinuma A, Matsushima K. IL-8 gene expression and reproduction in human peripheral blood lymphocyte subsets. J Immunol 1991;146:3815–3823.

79. Van Meir E, Ceska M, Effenberger F, et al. Interleukin-8 is produced in neoplastic and infectious diseases of the human central nervous system. Cancer Res 1992;52:4297–4305.

80. Renauld JC, Houssiau F, Druez C. Interleukin-9. Int Rev Exp Pathol 1993;34A:99–109.

81. Druez C, Coulie P, Uyttenhove C, Van Snick J. Functional and biochemical characterization of mouse P40/IL-9 receptors. J Immunol 1990;145:2494–2499.

82. Holbrook ST, Ohls RK, Schribler KR, Yang YC, Christensen RD. Effect of interleukin-9 on clonogenic maturation and cell-cycle status of fetal and adult hematopoietic progenitors. Blood 1991;77:2129–2134.

83. Moore KW, O'Garra A, de Waal-Malefyt R, Vieria P, Mosmann T. Interleukin-10. Ann Rev Immunol 1993;11:167–190.

84. Fiorentino DF, Bond MW, Mosmann TR. Two types of mouse helper T cell. IV. Th2 clones secrete a factor that inhibits cytokine production by Th1 clones. J Exp Med 1989;170:2081–2095.

85. de Waal-Malefyt R, Haanen J, Spits H, et al. IL-10 and viral IL-10 strongly reduce antigen-specific human T cell proliferation by diminishing the antigen-presenting capacity of monocytes via down-regulation of class II MHC expression. J Exp Med 1991;174:915–924.

86. Taga K, Tosato G. IL-10 inhibits T cell proliferation and IL-2 production. J Immunol 1992;148:1143–1148.

87. Hsu D-H, Moore KW, Spits H. Differential effects of interleukin-4 and -10 on interleukin-2 induced interferon-γ synthesis and lymphokine-activated killer activity. Int Immunol 1992;4:563–569.

88. D'Andrea A, Miguel A-A, Valiante NM, Ma X, Kubin M, Trinchieri G. Interleukin 10 (IL-10) inhibits human lymphocyte interferon γ-production by suppressing natural killer cell stimulatory factor/IL-2 synthesis in accessory cells. J Exp Med 1993;178:1041–1048.

89. MacNeil I, Suda T, Moore KW, Mosmann TR, Zlotnik A. IL-10: a novel cytokine growth cofactor for mature and immature T cells. J Immunol 1990;145:4167–4173.

90. Rousset F, Garcia E, Defrance T, et al. IL-10 is a potent growth and differentiation factor for activated human B lymphocytes. Proc Natl Acad Sci USA 1992;89:1890–1893.

91. Scott P. IL-12: initiation cytokine for cell-mediated immunity. Science 1993;260:496–497.

92. Kobayashi M, Fitz L, Ryan M, et al. Identification and purification of natural killer cell stimulatory factor (NKSF), a cytokine with multiple biological effects on human lymphocytes. J Exp Med 1989;170:827–845.

93. Stern AS, Podlaski FJ, Hulmes JD, et al. Purification to homogeneity and partial characterization of cytotoxic lymphocyte maturation factor from human B-lymphoblastoid cells. Proc Natl Acad Sci USA 1990;87:6808–6812.

94. Chan SH, Perussia B, Gupta JW, et al. Induction of interferon γ production by natural killer cell stimulatory factor: characterization of the responding cells and synergy with other inducers. J Exp Med 1991;173:869–879.

95. Gately MK, Desai BB, Wolitzky AG, et al. Regulation of human lymphocyte proliferation by a heterodimeric cytokine, IL-12 (cytolytic lymphocyte maturation factor). J Immunol 1991;147:874–882.

96. Gately MK, Wolitzky AG, Quinn PM, Chizzonite R. Regu-

lation of human cytolytic lymphocyte responses by inter-leukin-12. Cell Immunol 1992;143:127–142.

97. Robertson MJ, Soiffer RJ, Wolf SF, et al. Responses of human natural killer (NK) cells to NK cell stimulatory factor (NKSF): cytolytic activity and proliferation of NK cells are differentially regulated by NKSF. J Exp Med 1992; 175:779–788.

98. Naume B, Gately M, Espevik T. A comparative study of IL-12 (cytotoxic lymphocyte maturation factor)-, IL-2-, and IL-7-induced effects on immunomagnetically purified CD56+ NK cells. J Immunol 1992;148:2429–2436.

99. Hsieh C-S, Macatonia SE, Tripp CS, et al. Development of Th1 CD4+ T cells through IL-12 produced by Listeria-induced macrophages. Science 1993;260:547–549.

100. Manetti R, Parronchi P, Giudizi MG, et al. Natural killer cell stimulatory factor (interleukin 12 [IL-12]) induces T helper type 1 (Th1)-specific immune responses and inhibits the development of IL-4-producing Th cells. J Exp Med 1993;177:1199–1204.

101. Gately MK, Warrier RR, Honasoge S, et al. Administration of recombinant IL-12 to normal mice enhances cytolytic lymphocyte activity and induces production of IFN-γ in vivo. J Immunol 1994 (in press).

102. Brunda MJ, Luistro L, Warrier R, et al. Antitumor and anti-metastatic activity of interleukin-12 against murine tumors. J Exp Med 1993;178:1223–1230.

103. Tahara H, Zeh III HJ, Storkus WJ, et al. Fibroblasts genetically engineered to secrete interleukin 12 can suppress tumor growth and induce antitumor immunity to a murine melanoma in vivo. Cancer Res 1994;54:182–189.

104. Zurawski G, de Vries JE. Interleukin-13, an interleukin-4–like cytokine that acts on monocytes and B cells, but not on T cells. Immunol Today 1994;15:19–26.

105. McKenzie ANJ, Culpepper JA, de Waal-Malefyt R, et al. Interleukin-13, a T-cell derived cytokine that regulates human monocyte and B-cell function. Proc Natl Acad Sci USA 1993;90:3735–3739.

106. Minty A, Chalon P, Derocq JM, et al. Interleukin-13 is a new human lymphokine regulating inflammatory and immune responses. Nature 1993;362:248–250.

107. Punnonen J, Aversa G, Cocks BG, et al. Interleukin 13 induces interleukin 4-independent IgG4 and IgE synthesis and CD23 expression by human B cells. Proc Natl Acad Sci USA 1993;90:3730–3734.

108. Amburs JL, Pippin J, Joseph A, et al. Identification of a cDNA for a human high-molecular-weight B-cell growth factor. Proc Natl Acad Sci USA 1993;90:6330–6334.

109. Pestka S. Langer JA, Zoon KC, Samuel CE. Interferons and their actions. Ann Rev Biochem 1987;56:727–777.

110. Zoon KC, Miller D, Bekisz J, et al. Purification and characterization of multiple components of human lymphoblastoid interferon-α. J Biol Chem 1992; 267:15210–15216.

111. Farrar MA, Schreiber RD. The molecular cell biology of interferon-γ and its receptor. Ann Rev Immunol 1993; 11:571–611.

112. Langer JA, Pestka S. Interferon receptors. Immunol Today 1988;9:393–400.

113. Oshimi K, Oshimi Y, Motoji T, et al. Lysis of leukemia and lymphoma cells by autologous and allogenic interferon-activated blood mononuclear cells. Blood 1983;61:790–798.

114. Lee SH, Kelly S, Chiu H, Stebbihg N. Stimulation of natural killer cell activity and inhibition of proliferation of various leukemic cells by purified human leukocyte interferon subtypes. Cancer Res 1982;42:1312–1316.

115. Brunda MJ, Tarnowski D, Davatelis V. Interaction of recombinant interferons with recombinant interleukin 2: differential effects on natural killer cell activity and interleukin-2-activated killer cells. Int J Cancer 1986;37:787–793.

116. Sone S, Utsugi T, Nii A, Ogura T. Differential effects of recombinant interferons α, β and γ on induction of human lymphokine (IL-2)-activated killer activity. J Natl Cancer Inst 1988;80:425–431.

117. Finkelman FD, Svetic A, Gresser I, et al. Regulation by interferon α of immunoglobulin isotype selection and lymphokine production in mice. J Exp Med 1991; 174:1179–1188.

118. Gajewski TF, Schell SR, Nau G, Fitch FW. Regulation of T cell activation: differences among T cell subsets. Immunol Rev 1989;111:79–110.

119. Handa K, Suzuki R, Matsui H, Shimizu Y, Kumagai K. Natural killer (NK) cells as a responder to interleukin 2 (IL-2). II. IL-2-induced interferon gamma production. J Immunol 1983;130:988–992.

120. Wherry JC, Schreiber RD, Unanue ER. Regulation of gamma interferon production by natural killer cells in scid mice: roles of tumor necrosis factor and bacterial stimuli. Infect Immunol 1991;59:1709–1715.

121. Schreiber RD, Celada A. Molecular characterization of interferon gamma as a macrophage activating factor. Lymphokines 1985;11:87–118.

122. Ding AH, Nathan CF, Stuehr DJ. Release of reactive nitrogen intermediates and reactive oxygen intermediates from mouse peritoneal macrophages: comparison of activating cytokines and evidence for independent production. J Immunol 1988;141:2407–2412.

123. Novelli F, Giovarelli M, Reber-Liske R, Virgallita G, Garotta G, Forni G. Blockade of physiologically secreted IFN-γ inhibits human T lymphocyte and natural killer cell activation. J Immunol 1991;147:1445–1452.

124. Itoh K, Siba K, Shimizu Y, Suzuki R, Kumagai K. Generation of activated killer cell (AK) cells by recombinant interleukin-2 (rIL-2) in collaboration with interferon-γ. J Immunol 1985;134:3124–3129.

125. Landolfo S, Cofano F, Giovarelli M, et al. Inhibition of interferon-gamma may suppress allograft reactivity by T lymphocytes in vitro and in vivo. Science 1985;229:176–179.

126. Giovarelli M, Santoni A, Jemma C, et al. Obligatory role of IFN-γ in induction of lymphokine-activated and T lymphocyte killer activity, but not in boosting of natural cytotoxicity. J Immunol 1988;140:2831–2836.

127. Snapper CM, Paul WE. Interferon-gamma and B cell stimulatory factor-1 reciprocally regulate Ig isotype production. Science 1987;236:944–947.

128. Finkelman FD, Holmes J, Katona IM, et al. Lymphokine control of in vivo immunoglobulin isotype selection. Ann Rev Immunol 1990;8:303–333.

129. Vassalli P. The pathophysiology of tumor necrosis factors. Ann Rev Immunol 1992;10:411–452.

130. Economou JS, McBride WH, Essner R, et al. Tumour necrosis factor production by IL-2-activated macrophages in vitro and in vivo. Immunology 1989;67:514–519.

131. Cannistra SA, Rambaldi A, Spriggs DR, Herrmann F, Kufe D, Griffin JD. Human granulocyte-macrophage colony-stimulating factor induces expression of the tumor necrosis factor gene by the U937 cell line and by normal human monocytes. J Clin Invest 1987;79:1720–1728.

132. Warren MK, Ralph P. Macrophage growth factor CSF-1 stimulates human monocyte production of interferon, tumor necrosis factor, and colony stimulating activity. J Immunol 1986;137:2281–2285.

133. Snug S, Bjorndahl J, Wang C, Kao H, Fu S. Produciton of tumor necrosis factor/cachectin by human T cell lines and peripheral blood T lymphocytes stimulated by phorbol myristate acetate and anti-CD3 antibody. J Exp Med 1988;167:937–953.

134. Steffen M, Ottmann O, Moore M. Simultaneous production of tumor necrosis factor-α and lymphotoxin by normal T cells after induction with IL-2 and anti-T3. J Immunol 1988;140:2621–2624.

135. Sung S, Jung L, Walters J, Chen W, Wang C, Fu S. Production of tumor necrosis factor/cachectin by human B cell lines and tonsillar B cells. J Exp Med 1988;168:1539–1551.

136. Liew F, Li Y, Millott S. Tumor necrosis factor-α synergizes with IFN-γ in mediating killing of Leishmania major through the induction of nitric oxide. J Immunol 1990;145:4306–4310.

137. Ranges G, Zlotnik A, Espevic T, Dinarello C, Cerami A, Palladino M. Tumor necrosis factor α/cachectin is a growth factor for thymocytes. Synergistic interactions with other cytokines. J Exp Med 1988;167:1472–1478.

138. Scheurich P, Thoma B, Ucer U, Pfizenmaier K. Immunoregulatory activity of recombinant human tumor necrosis factor (TNF)-α: induction of TNF-α mediated enhancement of T cell responses. J Immunol 1987;138:1786–1790.

139. Yokota S, Geppert T, Lipsky P. Enhancement of antigen- and mitogen-induced human T lymphocyte proliferation by tumor necrosis factor-α. J Immunol 1988;140:531–536.

140. Shalaby M, Espevic T, Rice G, et al. The involvement of human tumor necrosis factors-α and -β in the mixed lymphocyte reaction. J Immunol 1988;141:499–503.

141. Ostensen M, Thiele D, Lipsky P. Tumor necrosis factor-α enhances cytolytic activity of human natural killer cells. J Immunol 1987;138:4185–4191.

142. Kehrl JH, Miller A, Fauci AS. Effect of tumor necrosis factor alpha on mitogen-activated human B cells. J Exp Med 1987;166:786–791.

143. Jelinek D, Lipsky P. Enhancement of human B cell proliferation and differentiation by tumor necrosis factor-α and interleukin 1. J Immunol 1987;139:2970–2976.

144. Jirik FR, Podor TJ, Hirano T, et al. Bacterial lipopolysaccharide and inflammatory mediators augment IL-6 secretion by human endothelial cells. J Immunol 1989;142:144–147.

145. Assoian RK, Komoriya A, Meyers CA, Miller DM, Sporn MB. Transforming growth factor-beta in human platelets. J Biol Chem 1983;258:7155–7160.

146. Roberts AB, Sporn MB. The transforming growth factor-βs. In: Sporn MB, Roberts AB, eds. Peptide growth factors and their receptors I. New York: Springer-Verlag, 1990:419–472.

147. Kehrl JH, Roberts AB, Wakefield LM, Jakowlew SB, Sporn MB, Fauci AS. Transforming growth factor beta is an important immunomodulatory protein for human B-lymphocytes. J Immunol 1986;137:3855–3860.

148. Kehrl JH, Wakefield LM, Roberts AB, et al. Production of transforming growth factor beta by human T lymphocytes and its potential role in the regulation of T cell growth. J Exp Med 1986;163:1037–1050.

149. Rook AH, Kehrl JH, Wakefield LM, et al. Effects of transforming growth factor β on the functions of natural killer cells: depressed cytolytic activity and blunting of interferon responsiveness. J Immunol 1986;136:3916–3920.

150. Mule JJ, Schwarz SL, Roberts AB, Sporn MB, Rosenberg SA. Transforming growth factor-beta inhibits the in vitro generation of lymphokine-activated killer cells and cytotoxic T cells. Cancer Immunol Immunother 1988;26:95–100.

151. Ranges GE, Figari IS, Espevik T, Palladino MA. Inhibition of cytotoxic T cell development by transforming growth factor β and reversal by recombinant tumor necrosis factor alpha. J Exp Med 1987;166:991–998.

152. Espevik T, Figari IS, Ranges GE, Palladino MA. Transforming growth factor-β1 (TGF-β1) and recombinant human tumor necrosis factor-alpha reciprocally regulate the generation of lymphokine-activated killer cell activity. J Immunol 1988;140:2312–2316.

153. Czarniecki CW, Chiu HH, Wong GHW, McCabe SM, Palladino MA. Transforming growth factor-β1 modulates the expression in class II histocompatability antigens on human cells. J Immunol 1988;140:4127–4223.

154. Coffman RL, Lebman DA, Shrader B. Transforming growth factor-β specifically enhances IgA production by lipolysaccharide-stimulated murine B lymphocytes. J Exp Med 1989;170:1039–1044.

CHAPTER 4

ROLE OF CYTOKINES
IN THE ACTIVATION OF MONOCYTES

Luigi Varesio, Igor Espinoza-Delgado, Luca Gusella, George W. Cox,
Giovanni Melillo, Tiziano Musso, and Maria Carla Bosco

Mononuclear phagocytes derive from primordial immune defense mechanisms designed to engage pathogens in a frontal and direct combat. Mononuclear phagocytes evolved as an essential component of a complex multicell immune system; hence, they acquired the ability to communicate with it, to decipher and respond to endogenous signals, among which cytokines are important components. Mononuclear phagocytes are an important source of cytokines that can act in an autocrine manner by modulating the stage of activation of the cell or in a paracrine fashion by delivering information and providing support and control to the cells of the immune system and surrounding tissues.

The lymphoid component of the immune system communicates with the mononuclear phagocyte via cytokines that are powerful regulators of macrophage and monocyte functions. In this context, "activation" is defined as the process by which macrophages and monocytes modify their phenotype and acquire new functional activities in response to environmental stimulation. Activation of mononuclear phagocytes is controlled by inhibitory (deactivating) signals of autocrine or paracrine nature that limit the duration and the magnitude of the response. The feedback inhibitory circuits are very important to prevent potential damage caused by the activated mononuclear phagocytes that are not endowed with fine specificity for the target and that can attack the host tissues.

One important feature of macrophage biology relevant to understand the physiology of these cells in the cytokine network is that proliferation is not required for, and it is not part of, the activation program of the cell. As opposed to B or T lymphocytes, macrophage activation is not dependent on clonal expansion or mitotic activity. Conversely, the proliferative capacity conferred to macrophages by retrovirus-transduced oncogenes does not affect their molecular or functional response, which remains comparable to that of fresh peritoneal macrophages (1–7). This property renders macrophage cell lines a relevant model to study macrophage biology at a single-cell level.

Under physiological conditions, expression of the activated phenotype is a transient event that is followed by a return of macrophages to a resting state (8). The magnitude of the macrophage-mediated response is determined mainly by the number of responding cells or by the accumulation of the macrophages into the inflammatory region, and it is modulated by cellular feedback mechanisms and by the extent and nature of the environmental stimulation (9–12).

Proliferation is important to maintain an adequate supply of circulating monocytes that are ready to extravasate to the tissues in response to chemoattractants released during the inflammatory response. Monocytes can undergo some proliferation in the circulation and in the tissues (13). However, the majority of circulating monocytes originates in the bone marrow from the proliferation of stem cells and their differentiation along the monocytic lineage. The proliferative ability of precursor cells decreases progressively during differentiation (14). Thus, the majority of mitotic activity is restricted to the bone marrow, and the levels of peripheral cells are dictated by cell death and replenishment from the bone marrow. The critical event in determining the extent of the macrophage-mediated defense mechanism is the recruitment of mononuclear cells at the site of injury and the activation of every individual cell.

The recognition that proliferation is not part of the genetic program of a macrophage poses interesting questions about the function and biology of growth factor receptor on these cells. Macrophages express receptors for a variety of growth factors specific for monocytic cells, such as the colony-stimulating factor-1 receptor (CSF-1R) (5,15,16), or typical of other lineages, such as the interleukin-2 receptor (IL-2R) (17,18). However, macrophages respond to stimulation by growth factors with functional changes. The CSF-1 receptor induces proliferation of bone marrow–derived macrophage precursors (19). In monocytes and macrophages, CSF-1 induces secretory activity (20,21), resistance to viral infection, and sustains cell viability and cytotoxic responses (16,22–24). The CSF-1R is modulated by cytokines and other signals (15,16,25). Stimulation of the IL-2R causes activation of mononuclear phagocytes, which is discussed extensively. These considerations indicate that one cannot extrapolate easily information from lymphocytes to mononuclear phagocytes, even when dealing with a cytokine acting on both cell types.

There is an overwhelming amount of literature on cytokines and mononuclear phagocytes that cannot be covered herein. We present selected topics in this growing field of cytokine/mononuclear phagocytes–research. We focus our discussion on the activation of tumoricidal human monocytes by interferon-γ (IFN-γ), a ubiquitous and potent stimulus, and by IL-2, whose monocyte-activating properties have been recently characterized. In an attempt to focus on human cytokines, we do not refer systematically to the literature on murine macrophages.

ACTIVATION OF MONONUCLEAR PHAGOCYTES TO A TUMORICIDAL STAGE

Mononuclear phagocytes can be activated by cytokines to express cytocidal activity against tumor cells. This function may be of relevance in host defense against tumors, and it is often considered the ultimate expression of the activated phenotype. Activation to express cytotoxic activity will be taken as a reference in discussing the effects of cytokines on mononuclear phagocytes to organize the presentation.

Human monocytes and murine macrophages respond to IFN-γ or IL-2 with expression of tumoricidal activity. However, murine macrophages respond to IFN-γ alone only under specific conditions (26,27), and optimal cytotoxic activity is achieved by combining IFN-γ with a costimulus, such as endotoxin (lipopolysaccharide [LPS]) or picolinic acid (28,29). IL-2 does not activate murine macrophages to express tumoricidal activity or other functions by itself, but it can function as a costimulus in cells treated with IFN-γ (17). In contrast, human monocytes can be fully activated by treatment with IFN-γ or IL-2 alone, providing an important model to study the mechanism of action of these cytokines (29).

The reasons for the differences between murine macrophages and human monocytes in their requirement for activation signals are unclear. It could be that murine and human cells differ in their response to cytokines. However, it seems more likely that the differences between human monocytes and murine macrophages are due to the different stage of differentiation of the two-cell populations: circulating or tissue-resident, respectively. IL-2 and IFN-γ utilize different pathways to activate monocytes, because IL-2 but not IFN-γ up-regulates IL-6 messenger RNA (mRNA) and protein (30), IL-2Rβ mRNA (31), c-fms mRNA and protein (32), and IL-8 mRNA and protein (33). In contrast, IFN-γ but not IL-2 induces IL-2Rα mRNA (31). Furthermore, protein kinase inhibitors block IL-2–induced, but not IFN-γ–induced, monocyte cytotoxicity (Espinoza-Delgado I., unpublished observations).

IFN-γ is probably the most potent and studied activator of mononuclear phagocytes that can stimulate effector functions and immunoregulatory activities of these cells. This literature has been reviewed often (25,28,29,34–45), and this information will not be summarized herein.

IL-2 was originally discovered and studied for its mitogenic effects on T lymphocytes (46). Subsequent studies demonstrated that other cell types can respond to IL-2, including B lymphocytes (47), natural killer cells, lymphokine-activated killer cells (48–50), glioma cells (51), and polymorphonuclear cells (52–54). The ability of IL-2 to activate monocytes and macrophages demonstrates that pleiotropic effects of this cytokine extend beyond proliferative control. IL-2 can activate human monocytes to express tumoricidal (18,31,55) and bactericidal activity (56), hydrogen peroxide, superoxide anion (57–60), prostaglandin E_2 (PGE$_2$), and tromboxane production (61). Treatment of human monocytes with IL-2 in vitro results in their increased expression of several genes. IL-2 induces the mRNA expression of IL-1β (62,63), tumor necrosis factor-α (TNF-α)(64), CSF-1R (16), IL-6 (65), IL-8 (33), CSF-1 (66), and granulocyte-macrophage CSF (GM-CSF) (67).

Several features differentiate the murine macrophage or macrophage cell lines from human monocytes regarding IL-2 responsiveness (29,68). It has been shown that murine macrophage cell lines or bone marrow–derived macrophages express constitutive levels of IL-2Rα on their surface and that IL-2Rα protein is increased by treatment of the cells with IFN-γ (17,57). This finding is in sharp contrast to what has been observed in human monocytes which are negative for IL-2Rα. Although murine macrophages express IL-2Rα constitutively, IL-2 alone does not induce murine macrophage activation (17,57,69). Indeed, experiments designed to examine the ability of IL-2 to induce tumoricidal activity demonstrated that IL-2 is a costimulator of murine macrophages (17). Murine peritoneal macrophages or murine macrophage cell lines (3,5) treated with IL-2 in combination with IFN-γ, but not IL-2 alone, expressed cytolytic activity. Moreover, IL-2 and IFN-γ participate in the induction of macrophage resistance to intracellular parasites via their cooperative activities on TNF-α production (57).

IL-2 AND IFN-γ RECEPTORS ON MONONUCLEAR PHAGOCYTES

Modulation of cytokine receptors is an important mechanism to control the actions of the cytokine network. For example, the stimulatory effects of IFNs on TNF-αR expression (70) may contribute to the synergism between IFN-γ and TNF-α (71). Although IFN-γ and IL-2 are both potent activators of monocytes, their respective receptors are controlled by different mechanisms and signals.

One single type of IFN-γR is ubiquitously expressed on cells other than erythrocytes (39). IFN-γR does not possess any identifiable kinase, phosphatase, SH2, or SH3 domain characteristics, and the mechanisms of signal transduction in human monocytes are largely unknown. Receptor-mediated ligand internalization is important, although not sufficient, to induce biological responses (39). IFN-γR recycling has been described in some cell types; however, its occurrence on mononuclear phagocytes is still controversial because reports exist of both degradation (72) and recycling in primary or cultured human monocytes (73). Evidence exists that the IFN-γR on human monocytes consists of multiple distinct subunits (74) and that in vitro culture of human monocytes with GM-CSF results in enhancement of IFN-γR (75). However, the biological significance of such changes remains to be determined because it was found that the increased receptor expression in GM-CSF–cultured monocytes is associated to a diminished, rather than augmented, response to IFN-γ (75).

IL-2R was initially demonstrated on T and B lymphocytes, and the molecular structure of the IL-2R on lymphoid cells has been extensively studied (76). The lymphocyte IL-2R is composed of at least three protein subunits—IL-2Rα, IL-2Rβ, and IL-2Rγ—with molecular masses of 55, 70 to 75, and 65 kd, respectively. Different combinations of the three chains form three classes of IL-2 binding sites. IL-2Rα alone binds with low affinity, the

heterodimer of IL-2Rβ and IL-2Rγ binds with intermediate affinity, and the combination of the three subunits forms a high affinity receptor. Studies of the IL-2R on lymphoid cells and receptor reconstitution experiments in fibroblasts indicated that a simple α/β structure could not account for IL-2 binding, internalization, and signal transduction by the IL-2R (77–81); the existence of other lymphoid cell-specific components was postulated (82–86). The third subunit, termed IL-2Rγ chain, was identified in human lymphocytes and natural killer cells (85,87), and the complementary DNA (cDNA) for this molecule was cloned (88). Transfection experiments with the IL-2Rγ chain cDNA showed that the IL-2Rγ subunit is essential for the achievement of full ligand binding and receptor-mediated internalization (49,87–89), probably through its direct interaction with IL-2, and that it may have a critical role in intracellular signal transduction (89,90).

Fresh human monocytes purified by elutriation express constitutively IL-2Rβ and IL-2Rγ membrane proteins and mRNAs (18,31,91,92). The IL-2Rα is not constitutively expressed (18,58,93), but it is inducible by IFN-γ (31,94) or LPS (58). However, little information exists on the binding properties of IL-2 on monocytes. Determination of the number of binding sites and affinities is technically complex because of high background binding of iodinated IL-2 to fresh human monocytes (Espinoza-Delgado I, unpublished observations). Some studies indicate the existence of a very small number of binding sites expressed on monocytes (58,95). However, the question of the affinity of IL-2 binding to monocytes is not fully addressed.

MODULATION OF IL-2R BY CYTOKINES

An interesting and important characteristic of the IL-2R on human monocytes is the independent regulation of the expression of the three subunits by different cytokines and intracellular mechanisms. Differential regulation of the two subunits of the TNF-α receptor has also been reported (96). The differential expression of the various subunits can be very important for controlling the reactivity of monocytes to IL-2 during an inflammatory process because it will determine the affinity of the receptor and therefore the susceptibility of monocytes to the levels of IL-2 in the environment. Furthermore, the IL-2Rγ chain may be involved in the formation of the receptor for other cytokines (97,98), and modulation of its expression may affect the activation of monocytes at multiple levels.

IL-2 does not induce the expression of the IL-2Rα (31). However, treatment of monocytes with IL-2 causes up-regulation of the constitutive levels of IL-2Rβ mRNA

(31). The constitutive transcriptional activity of the IL-2Rβ gene is not modified by IL-2, whereas the half-life of the message is significantly increased, indicating stabilization of the message following IL-2 stimulation (31). Similar results were reported when expression of the IL-2Rγ chain was studied. IL-2 induced up-regulation of the constitutive levels of the IL-2Rγ chain through posttranscriptional stabilization of the message (92). However, expression of the total cellular IL-2Rγ chain, measured by Western blot, was increased by IL-2, whereas expression of the membrane IL-2Rβ chain, assessed by flow cytometry, was not affected (91,92).

It is possible that the total content of IL-2Rβ protein increased proportionally to the mRNA levels, similarly to the γ-chain. However, the fraction of IL-2Rβ exposed to the membrane may not have increased because of slower processing, increased internalization, and shedding of the binding structure that includes the β-chain. If the latter was the case, one would also expect that the membrane IL-2Rγ was constant in IL-2–treated cells because both subunits would be involved in the binding site. However, the levels of IL-2Rγ chain on the membrane of IL-2–treated monocytes have not been determined yet. In summary, IL-2 induces replenishment/augmentation of the structures constitutively present on the membrane of resting monocytes (γ- and β-subunits), perhaps augmenting the number of binding sites, but without changing the affinity of the binding because the α-chain is not induced by IL-2. Recent studies of binding of fluorescent-labeled IL-2 support the notion that the number of binding sites is indeed increased in IL-2–treated monocytes (91). The association of IL-2Rβ and IL-2Rγ subunits is absolutely required for the formation of a functionally competent receptor in lymphoid cells (49,79,85,87,88,90), and it is tempting to speculate that in monocytes the γ-chain is also involved in the formation of functional IL-2 binding sites. Monocytes may express a constitutively low, limiting level of the γ-protein that is augmented by IL-2 or IFN-γ. The number of functional IL-2R should increase, thereby allowing greater IL-2 binding and increased cell response.

IFN-γ is very effective in modulating the expression of the α- and γ-subunits of the IL-2R on human monocytes, but it does not affect the constitutive expression of the IL-2Rβ chain. The IL-2Rα subunit is not constitutively expressed (18,58,93) or modulated by IL-2 (31), but it is inducible by IFN-γ (94) or LPS (58). Induction of IL-2Rα by IFN-γ is associated with an increase in the transcriptional activity of the gene and in the levels of mRNA (31). Low amounts of IFN-γ are sufficient to induce IL-2Rα, indicating that this event is likely to occur in vivo during an inflammatory response. Moreover, such low amounts of IFN-γ released by contaminating lymphocytes could induce IL-2Rα on monocytes following prolonged in vitro culture (99). The constitutive IL-2Rγ mRNA levels are greatly augmented by incubation of monocytes with

IFN-γ (91,92). Induction of IL-2Rγ required relatively low amounts of IFN-γ, similar to those needed for the induction of the α-chain. In opposition to the induction of the α-chain, one mechanism by which IFN-γ induces IL-2Rγ chain accumulation is posttranscriptional, through stabilization of the message (91).

The promoters of the IL-2Rγ and IL-2Rβ genes are similar to those of other genes constitutively expressed in the cell in that they lack classic TATA motifs (100). In addition, IL-2Rγ and IL-2Rβ promoters do not contain the NF-kB and CArG motifs (101) that are present in the IL-2Rα promoter (102–104) and that are involved in its transcriptional inducibility by IFN-γ (105). The constitutive expression of IL-2Rβ and IL-2Rγ genes in resting monocytes may provide a constant supply of membrane subunits capable of forming a functional receptor for IL-2. The increase in β- and γ-chain mRNA in response to IL-2 could be important to balance the loss of receptors that should follow the interaction with the ligand and subsequent internalization or shedding of the complex (106).

Up-regulation of IL-2Rγ expression following activation of monocytes with IFN-γ is coupled to the induction of IL-2Rα (18,31,99), and it may be a critical mechanism for the formation of the high affinity configuration. Indirect evidence that induction of the IL-2Rα chain increases the affinity of the binding of IL-2 to human monocytes is provided by the demonstration that pretreatment of monocytes with low doses of IFN-γ, which did not elicit tumoricidal response but induced IL-2Rα expression (18,31,99) and augmented IL-2Rγ mRNA levels (91), increased the sensitivity of monocytes to activation by suboptimal doses of IL-2 (31). Modulation of IL-2R on monocytes is summarized in Fig. 4–1.

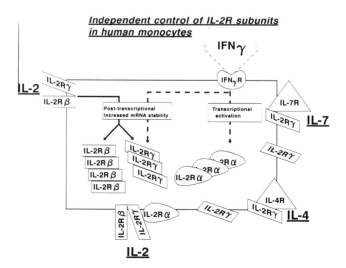

Figure 4–1   Control of IL-2 receptor subunits in human monocytes. Modulation of IL-2R subunits on human monocytes stimulated by IL-2 or IFN-γ, and potential association of the IL-2Rγ subunit with IL-4 or IL-7 receptors.

An exciting recent development in the IL-2R field is the demonstration that the IL-2Rγ chain is a functional component of other cytokine receptors. The suggestion that the IL-2Rγ chain may control the response to several lymphokines stems from the observation that humans with a mutated IL-2Rγ chain have X-linked severe combined immunodeficiency characterized by virtual absence of T cells (107). The depletion of T cells is not fully accounted for by loss of response to IL-2 because knock out mice, in which the IL-2 gene was inactivated by targeted gene disruption, exhibited relatively normal T-cell development (108), suggesting that the IL-2Rγ chain is used by other cytokine receptors. So far, it has been shown that the binding sites of IL-4 and IL-7 receptors in lymphoid cells can involve the IL-2Rγ chain (109,110). IL-2, IL-4, and IL-7 affect B- and T-cell development and proliferation, thereby explaining why the mutation of the IL-2Rγ chain, by disrupting the response to multiple cytokines, caused a dramatic T-cell deficiency.

These findings have profound implications for the biology of mononuclear phagocytes, because both IL-4 and IL-7 are active on monocytes. It can be speculated that the different association of the IL-2Rγ chain with distinct receptors may influence the specificity or the extent of the response of monocytes to IL-2, IL-4, or IL-7. The choice of responding to one of these lymphokines may be critical for the kind of functional activity of the monocyte. In fact, IL-7 and IL-2 have similar, although not equal, activating properties on monocytes, whereas IL-4 can be inhibitory for monocyte activity and antagonize IL-2–induced responses. Because of the IL-2Rγ connection, we discuss the main effect of IL-7 and IL-4 on mononuclear phagocytes, although it should be emphasized that the potential role of IL-2Rγ as a master switch for the response of monocytes to these lymphokines is attractive but still totally speculative.

THE IL-2Rγ CONNECTION: IL-7 AND IL-4

IL-7, mostly known for its stimulatory activity on lymphopoiesis, is also biologically active on mononuclear phagocytes (111). IL-7 induces in human monocytes the expression of macrophage inflammatory protein-1β (MIP-1β) mRNA (112), IL-8 (113), IL-6, IL-1α, IL-1β, and TNF-α (114). The stimulatory activity of IL-7 seems similar to that of IL-2, suggesting the existence of a positive agonistic relationship between these cytokines. Interestingly, activation of monocytes by IL-7 is susceptible to inhibition by IL-4, demonstrating an antagonistic relationship between IL-4 and IL-7 (112). In turn, IL-7 can inhibit in macrophages the expression of transforming growth factor-β (TGF-β) (115). TGF-β is a potent inhibi-

tor of leukocyte functions (116), and some of the proliferative and immunostimulating activities mediated by IL-7 may involve a decrease in macrophage-derived TGF-β. The property of TGF-β to inhibit IL-2–induced activation of monocytes is discussed later.

IL-4 is a cytokine that exerts a dual role on mononuclear phagocytes (117). IL-4 can stimulate monocytic functions. For example, IL-4 can induce antigen presentation; expression of MHC class II antigens (118,119) and CD23 (120); and production of granulocyte colony-stimulating factor (G-CSF), macrophage colony-stimulating factor (M-CSF) (121), and the C2 complement protein (122). However, IL-4 has inhibitory properties on several cell types, including lymphokine-activated killer cells (123), T cells (124), and B cells (125–128). IL-4 can also down-regulate the activation of mononuclear phagocytes (129–131) and antagonize the responses induced by IFN-γ, IL-2, and IL-7. IL-4 inhibits the induction of MIP-1β by IL-7 (112), as well as several activities triggered by IL-2 or IFN-γ, including production of IL-1 (133), TNF-α and IL-6 (128,134–137); hydrogen peroxide (129), superoxide (130), and Fc receptor expression (134); and anti-Leishmania activity (129). Moreover, IL-4 inhibits the costimulatory activity of IL-2 on IFN-γ–treated murine macrophages in the induction of tumoricidal activity (131).

IL-4 demonstrated some degree of selectivity in this system because it did not affect activation of macrophages by IFN-γ plus LPS (131). A possible mechanism by which IL-4 inhibits activation by IFN-γ plus IL-2 is by impairing IL-2Rα induction by IFN-γ and preventing the binding of IL-2 (131). Inhibition of IL-2Rα expression by IL-4 has been documented in macrophages and other cell types (124,131,138,139). The initial report that IL-4 activates cytotoxic macrophages (140) has not been confirmed in several macrophage activation systems (131,141,142), and it contrasts with the inhibitory activity of IL-4 on macrophage activation.

In human monocytes and monocytic cell lines, it was demonstrated that IL-4 attenuates the transcriptional activation of both IFN-α– and IFN-γ–induced cellular genes (143). Furthermore, IL-4 is a potent inhibitor of IFN-γ–induced indoleamine 2,3-dioxygenase (IDO) activity in human monocytes (144). IDO is a flavin-dependent enzyme that catalyzes the conversion of tryptophan to kynurenine. These results provide the first evidence that a cytokine can provide a negative signal for IDO expression and that IL-4 can influence the catabolism of tryptophan. The connection between tryptophan metabolism, cytokines, and macrophage activation is discussed in detail.

Because IL-4, IL-7, and IL-2 share the IL-2Rγ chain, we speculate that the relative concentration of the cytokines in the extracellular environment may determine the type of response. IL-4, IL-2, and IL-7 will compete with each other for the cytokine binding in their attempt to sequester the IL-2Rγ chain and to transduce a signal. Each of these cytokines delivers a different signal, the specificity of which may be conferred by IL-2Rβ, IL-4R, or IL-7R. Furthermore, the dual role of IL-4 on macrophage activation may be due to two different effects of this cytokine. First, competition between IL-4 and IL-2 causes inhibition of IL-2–induced functions; second, activation of the IL-4 receptor delivers a true activation signal. Competition could explain the reason why, in some experimental systems, IL-4 seems to inhibit selectively IL-2–induced, but not IFN-γ- or LPS-induced, macrophage activation (131).

INHIBITORY CIRCUITS: IFN-γ AND TGF-β INTERPLAY

Inhibitory factors or negative regulatory mechanisms should exist to prevent the potentially deleterious consequence of prolonged or excessive activation of monocytes. The inhibitory activity that IFN-γ exerts on monocytes is intriguing because IFN-γ is at the same time a powerful monocyte activator. This fact can be rationalized by considering that it may be advantageous for the host that macrophages express the several functions associated with the activated phenotype in a timely and controlled way. For example, the chemokine IL-8 (145) is produced by monocytes in response to IL-2, IL-1 (33), TNF-α, and IL-7 (113,146). IFN-γ not only does not induce IL-8, but also it inhibits the stimulation of IL-8 by IL-2 at the level of gene transcription (33). IL-4 (147) or IL-10 (148) can also inhibit IL-8 production, not only in monocytes but also in TNF-α–stimulated fibroblasts (149). In contrast, IFN-γ is synergistic with TNF-α for the induction of IL-8 in human keratinocytes (150).

These results suggest that the positive or negative nature of the effects on IL-8 expression depend on the cell lineage. Furthermore, differential expression control may exist even within the same cell lineage, because IFN-γ induces IL-8 in the human promonocytic cell line U937 by augmenting the levels of mRNA through stabilization of the message (151). Activated lymphocytes contribute to leukocyte recruitment by releasing IL-2, which stimulates IL-8 secretion by monocytes. A delayed production of IFN-γ by inflammatory lymphocytes might act as negative feedback that decreases the extent of recruitment at later stages of inflammation. Perhaps, further recruitment of inflammatory mediators by IL-8 in an environment saturated with cytokines would be detrimental for the host.

Transforming growth factor-β1 (TGF-β1) (116) is a 25-kd polypeptide growth hormone produced by transformed cells as well as normal cells, including platelets, activated T cells, B cells, macrophages, and monocytes (152–154). Originally defined by its ability to induce an-

chorage-independent growth in nonmalignant cells (155), TGF-β1 can inhibit the growth of a variety of cell types (156) and decrease the expression of IL-1R on lymphoid and myeloid cells (157). TGF-β1 is also a powerful chemotactic factor for monocytes (158), and it has an important role in wound healing and inflammation (159). TGF-β1 suppresses several immune responses, including T cell, B cell, and large granular lymphocyte functions (153,160,161). In addition, TGF-β1 may act as a monocyte-macrophage deactivating factor by decreasing hydrogen peroxide production (162), as well as IL-6 (30) and TNF-α production (163).

The dual role of IFN-γ on monocyte activation and the inhibitory effects of TGF-β on such activity raised questions about the effects of these cytokines on receptors. Studies on the production of IL-6 by monocytes revealed the existence of different and complex inhibitory circuits dimming the response of monocytes to IL-2, in which IFN-γ and TGF-β are both inhibitory, but at different levels. IL-2 can induce IL-6 without, and before, induction of an IL-1β primary response (30). However, IL-1β will be induced by IL-2 at later time points (63) and will in turn induce IL-6, thereby generating a loop to increase IL-6 production by IL-2–stimulated monocytes via the secretion of IL-1β. At least two inhibitory molecules, IFN-γ and TGF-β, can down-regulate IL-6 production (30,164). However, the inhibitory signals delivered by these cytokines are different depending on the IL-6 inducer. IFN-γ inhibits IL-6 induction by IL-1β, but not by IL-2, whereas TGF-β down-regulates IL-6 production induced by both stimuli (30). Thus, the inhibitory activity of IFN-γ seems to be targeted to decrease, but not to block, IL-6 production because it does not affect the direct response of monocytes to IL-2, but it will inhibit the positive amplifying loop mediated by IL-1β. In contrast, TGF-β acts in a more nonspecific way by inhibiting IL-6 production, whether induced by IL-1β or IL-2.

Studies on the expression of tumoricidal activity indicated the existence of an important relationship between IFN-γ and TFG-β that is manifested at the level of receptor expression. It was found that TGF-β₁ selectively inhibited IL-2- but not IFN-γ–induced tumoricidal activity in human monocytes (105). Dose-response experiments demonstrated that as little as 0.1 ng/mL of TGF-β₁ was sufficient to decrease IL-2–induced tumoricidal activity. A possible target of the inhibitory effects of TGF-β₁ on IL-2–dependent activation could have been IL-2R expression. TGF-β₁ not only did not inhibit but it increased IL-2Rβ mRNA expression by IL-2. However, TGF-β₁ decreased IL-2γ R mRNA induced by IL-2 but not by IFN-γ (92,105). These results suggest that one mechanism by which TGF-β₁ suppressed IL-2–induced tumoricidal activity may be by inhibiting the expression of the IL-2Rγ chain.

Resistance of the activation of human monocytes to the inhibitory activity of TGF-β was ascribed to the fact that

IFN-γ down-modulated the receptor for TGF-$β_1$. IFN-γ significantly decreased the expression of type I TGF-$β_1$R (65 kd) (105,165), thereby preventing the interaction between monocytes and TGF-$β_1$. Thus, a possible mechanism by which IFN-γ-, but not IL-2–treated monocytes, were resistant to the effects of TGF-$β_1$ was related to the ability of IFN-γ, not of IL-2, to down-modulate the expression of TGF-$β_1$R. TGF-β should also inhibit the response of monocytes to IL-7 and IL-4 because the IL-2Rγ chain is shared with these receptors. In fact, it was shown that IL-7 can inhibit TGF-β expression in human monocytes (115), thereby ascertaining a possible autocrine inhibitory loop.

IFN-γ seems to have developed several strategies to counteract cytokines that may inhibit monocyte activation. It has been reported that IFN-γ can inhibit the production of IL-10 (166) by monocytes. IL-10 is a cytokine secreted also by macrophages endowed with suppressor activity on cytokine secretion and accessory functions (148,167–170). Inhibition of IL-10 production by IFN-γ will contribute to the manifestation of the activated phenotype.

CYTOKINE AND AMINO ACID METABOLISM: ARGININE AND TRYPTOPHAN CONNECTION

The catabolism of two enzymes, tryptophan and arginine, generates metabolites of major biological relevance for the pathophysiology of the organism. Recent data demonstrate that the catabolism of these two enzymes is under cytokine control, which occurs in mononuclear phagocytes, and that it is associated with their activation. We review some aspects of this vast and complex literature because of the potential relevance of tryptophan and arginine metabolites in the ability of mononuclear phagocytes to express effector functions and to communicate with other tissues.

The catabolism of arginine leads to the formation of nitric oxide (NO), which has been identified as a very important bioregulatory molecule. Murine macrophages synthesize reactive nitrogen intermediates (RNI), such as nitric oxide, nitrite, and nitrate from the terminal guanidino nitrogen atom of L-arginine after exposure to IFN-γ alone or IFN-γ plus either microbial products (i.e., LPS or muramyl dipeptide) or cytokines (i.e., TNF-α or TNF-β)(171,172).

Production of NO, from the L-arginine metabolic pathway, is controlled by an inducible enzyme, nitric oxide synthase (NOS), the activity of which can be inhibited by the L-arginine analog N^G-monomethyl-L-arginine (NMMA) (173). At least three different forms of NOS have been isolated, characterized, and cloned from brain

tissue, endothelial cells, and macrophages, and, comparing across species, they have approximately 50 to 60% homology at the amino acid level (174–180). NOS is constitutively expressed in endothelial cells and in the brain, and its activity is dependent on exogenous Ca^{2+} and calmodulin. In contrast, the macrophage NOS is independent of exogenous Ca^{2+} and calmodulin, and it is inducible by IFN-γ alone or IFN-γ in combination with several agents, including LPS, TNF, and IL-2 (171,172,181–185). A body of literature has been accumulating during the past several years on the involvement of ·NO in the generation of tumoricidal activity by murine macrophages (28,32,171–190). Indeed, NO binds to and inhibits iron-sulfur–containing enzymes, including those present in the mitochondrial electron transport chain and the citric acid cycle, and thereby impairs oxidative metabolism in target cells (191,192). Although much information has been accumulated regarding the role of NOS in the production of ·NO by activated murine macrophages, the molecular mechanisms underlying this process are still poorly understood.

Evidence exists that the catabolism of tryptophan is connected to the biological effects of IFN (65,187). The first and rate-limiting enzymatic step in the degradation of tryptophan is conversion of tryptophan to formylkynurenine (65). Two different enzymes are involved in this function. Tryptophan 2,3-dioxygenase (TDO) is found only in the liver, is very specific for tryptophan, and is induced by several amino acids (including tryptophan) and by glucocorticoids (193). The second enzyme, IDO, is found in all the tissues examined thus far. IDO is less specific for tryptophan because it can use other indoleamine derivatives (e.g., tryptamine, serotonin) as a substrate, and it is inducible preferentially by IFN and IFN inducers, such as LPS and viruses (193). Induction of IDO is associated with the antitumor and antimicrobial effects of IFN (65,187), antiproliferative activity (65,194), and tumor cell rejection (195).

Tryptophan catabolism (Fig. 4–2) can be demon-

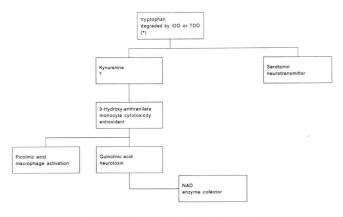

Figure 4–2 Generation of bioactive molecules from tryptophan catabolism.

strated in vivo in LPS- or IFN-β–treated mice (196,197) and humans (198–200). IDO activity has been demonstrated in human monocytes activated by IFN-γ (187, 201–206). Moreover, the monocytic leukemia cell line, THP-1, can also be induced to express IDO activity in response to IFN-γ (207). Tryptophan metabolites may be relevant for macrophage activation. For example, hydroxyanthranilic acid is produced by activated human monocytes, and it may be involved in macrophage defense mechanisms (208). 3-Hydroxykynurenine and 3-hydroxyanthranilic acid scavenge peroxide radicals, and they may represent a local antioxidant defense in inflammatory diseases (209).

Evidence of a connection between the catabolism of tryptophan and arginine was provided by the observation that picolinic acid, a terminal metabolite of L-tryptophan, is a potent costimulatory agent for the activation of murine macrophages (29,34,86,210). Picolinic acid was identified in body fluids (210,211), and it is biologically active when administered to animals and humans (212–218). Synergistic interaction between picolinic acid and IFN-γ were demonstrated in vitro for activation of peritoneal macrophages (219), as well as in mouse macrophage cell lines derived from mice responsive or nonresponsive to LPS (4,131). Furthermore, the macrophage-activating properties (212,220) and the antitumor activity (213, 220) of picolinic acid were demonstrated in vivo in experimental murine systems. The demonstration that a catabolite of tryptophan is a costimulus for the induction of L-arginine–dependent RNI production in murine macrophages (132) provided the first evidence of a possible connection between tryptophan and arginine metabolism. Activation of NOS gene expression by IFN-γ plus picolinic acid is due to increased rate of transcription (221), similar to what was shown previously for the mouse macrophage cell lines RAW 264.7 (178,182) and ANA-1 (221) following stimulation with IFN-γ plus LPS.

Picolinic acid is a naturally occurring molecule and could be the physiological mediator of the interaction between arginine and tryptophan metabolism. Elevated levels of tryptophan metabolites, such as kynurenine and quinolinic acid, have been detected in vivo in cerebrospinal fluid in pathological conditions (13,222), as well as in cancer patients treated with IL-2 (223). Although there is only one report of RNI production in vitro by human monocyte–derived macrophages (224), elevation of nitrate levels in urine and plasma of IL-2–treated patients has also been demonstrated (225). Therefore, in pathological conditions or following therapy with cytokines, an increased production of IFN-γ might be responsible for the concomitant activation of tryptophan and arginine metabolic pathways. Under the same conditions, activation of IDO activity by IFN-γ might lead to accumulation of picolinic acid, which in localized compartments could feed back on macrophages amplifying production of RNI.

IL-4 down-regulated, although did not completely abolish, IFN-γ plus picolinic acid–induced NOS mRNA expression (221). In addition to IL-4 (226), other cytokines, such as TGF-β (227), have been described to exert a negative influence on NO_2^- production by murine macrophages. The induction of IDO by IFN-γ in human monocytes was also susceptible to inhibition by IL-4 (144). It is intriguing that one of the enzymes catabolizing tryptophan and one of those catabolizing arginine are susceptible to the same kind of cytokine control. Both are induced by IFN-γ and inhibited by IL-4. Thus, one of the common events associated with the response of the organism to IFN-γ is the induction of tryptophan- and arginine-degrading enzymes and the release of many catabolites mediating a variety of biological effects on different tissues in addition to macrophages. The demonstration that picolinic acid can exert synergistic activity in combination with IFN-γ, although it does not induce RNI production by itself, suggests the existence of a network of amino acid catabolites that are important for activation and expression of effector functions by macrophages, and it provides a good indication that the spectrum of action of the biological effects of cytokines may be extended to amino acid metabolism.

CONCLUSIONS

Cytokines provide a wealth of positive and negative signals that modulate the function of macrophages. Most of the available information is derived from experimental systems in which monocytes are isolated from their natural setting and tested in vitro. Such an approach is relevant to establish the potential interaction between signals and monocytes, to dissect the mechanisms of action of cytokines, as well as to obtain insights into the regulation of the biological response of monocytes. However, great caution should be used in an attempt to predict the behavior of the monocyte in a more complex setting comprised of multiple cytokines and target cells.

The function of cytokines is to serve as signals in intercellular communication. "Biological communication is the act on the part of one organism or cell that alters the probability pattern of behavior in another organism or cell . . . " is Wilson's definition of communication in sociobiology (228). Thus, communication among the cells of the immune system is not the cytokine or the macrophage response in itself, but it is the relationship between the two within the context of the whole body. Genetic engineering will help progress in this direction. For example, expression of the cytokine receptor subunits in extraneous cells helped to decipher their role in the response to the ligand. Still, the challenge will be to predict, in a given inflammatory situation, whether the net result of the cytokine signaling will favor lymphocytes or monocytes, proliferative response or activation process. Analysis of knock out mice will also help generate experimental systems to analyze the intricacy of cytokines in cell communication.

The demonstration that cytokines carry signals that affect amino acid metabolism adds a new dimension to the potential targets of cytokine control and expands the connection between the cells of the immune system and other types. Nitric oxide serves a variety of functions in different tissues, including vascular endothelium, immune cells, neurons, smooth muscle, and cardiac muscle, among others (229). Tryptophan catabolites can affect similar targets and have a broad spectrum of biological effects. Accumulation of the metabolites from the tryptophan/kynurenine pathway may have a role in the etiology of inflammatory neuronal diseases (13). Furthermore, tryptophan can be metabolized to serotonin in the brain and influence mood. Thus, control of such pathways by the cytokine network could have profound implications not only on the immune response, but also theoretically on the behavior of individuals. Because of the relevance of the catabolism of these two amino acids, there is redundancy in the degradation pathways. Each of the amino acids can be catabolized by two sets of enzymes distinct in regulation and tissue distribution. Nevertheless, dramatic changes in tryptophan catabolism in vivo following systemic immunostimulation were reported.

Strictly from the mononuclear phagocyte point of view, efforts should be made to study and understand the relationship between human monocytes and murine macrophages in their response to cytokines. Combinations of species and differentiation stage differences are blamed for discordant results often reported in the literature. Conversely, extrapolations from one experimental system to the other are not always justified. We are among the scientists who believe the process of extravasation of the monocyte into the tissue has changed irreversibly the phenotype of monocytes that now respond to cytokines with different outcomes. However, more comparative information on mononuclear phagocytes from the same species is needed to be confident in adapting the vast information of murine macrophages to the human situation.

REFERENCES

1. Gandino L, Varesio L. Immortalization of macrophages from mouse bone marrow and fetal liver. Exp Cell Res 1990;188:192.

2. Blasi E, Radzioch D, Merletti L, et al. Generation of macrophage cell line from fresh bone marrow cells with a myc/raf recombinant retrovirus. Cancer Biochem Biophys 1989; 10:303.

3. Cox GW, Mathieson BJ, Gandino L, et al. Heterogeneity of hematopoietic cells immortalized by v-myc/v-raf recombinant retrovirus infection of bone marrow or fetal liver. J Natl Cancer Inst 1989;81:1492.

4. Blasi E, Radzioch D, Varesio L. Inhibition of retroviral

mRNA expression in the murine macrophage cell line GG2EE by biologic response modifiers. J Immunol 1988; 141:2153.

5. Blasi E, Radzioch D, Durum SK, et al. A murine macrophage cell line, immortalized by v-raf and v-myc oncogenes, exhibits normal macrophage functions. Eur J Immunol 1987;17:1491.

6. Blasi E, Mathieson BJ, Varesio L, et al. Selective immortalization of murine macrophages from fresh bone marrow by a raf/myc recombinant murine retrovirus. Nature 1985; 318:667.

7. Blasi E, Farinelli S, Varesio L, et al. Augmentation of GG2EE macrophage cell line-mediated anti-Candida activity by gamma interferon, tumor necrosis factor, and interleukin-1. Infect Immun 1990;58:1073.

8. Taffet SM, Pace JL, Russell SW. Lymphokine maintains macrophage activation for tumor cell killing by interfering with the negative regulatory effect of prostaglandin E_2. J Immunol 1981;127:121.

9. Rosen H, Gordon S. Adoptive transfer of fluorescence-labeled cells shows that resident peritoneal macrophages are able to migrate into specialized lymphoid organs and inflammatory sites in the mouse. Eur J Immunol 1990; 20:1251.

10. Rosen H, Gordon S. The role of the type 3 complement receptor in the induced recruitment of myelomonocytic cells to inflammatory sites in the mouse. Am J Respir Cell Mol Biol 1990;3:3.

11. Crocker PR, Morris L, Gordon S. Novel cell surface adhesion receptors involved in interactions between stromal macrophages and haematopoietic cells. J Cell Sci (Suppl) 1988;9:185.

12. Perry VH, Gordon S. Macrophages and microglia in the nervous system. Trends Neurosci 1988;11:273.

13. Saito K, Crowley JS, Markey SP, et al. A mechanism for increased quinolinic acid formation following acute systemic immune stimulation. J Biol Chem 1993;268:15496.

14. Metcalf D. The molecular biology and functions of the granulocyte-macrophage colony-stimulating factor. Blood 1986;67:257.

15. Gusella GL, Ayroldi E, Espinoza-Delgado I, et al. LPS but not IFN gamma down regulates c-fms protooncogene expression in murine macrophages. J Immunol 1990;145: 1137.

16. Espinoza-Delgado I, Longo DL, Gusella GL, et al. Interleukin 2 enhances c-fms expression in human monocytes. J Immunol 1990;145:1719.

17. Cox GW, Mathieson BJ, Giardina SL, et al. Characterization of IL-2 receptor expression and function on murine macrophages. J Immunol 1990;145:1719.

18. Espinoza-Delgado I, Ortaldo JR, Winkler-Pickett R, et al. Expression and role of p75 interleukin 2 receptor on human monocytes. J Exp Med 1990;171:1821.

19. Roth P, Stanley ER. The biology of CSF-1 and its receptor. Curr Top Microbiol Immunol 1992;181:141.

20. Moore RN, Larsen HS, Horohov DW, et al. Endogenous regulation of macrophage proliferative expansion by colony stimulating factor induced interferon. Science 1984; 223:178.

21. Warren MK, Ralph P. Macrophage growth factor CSF-1 stimulates human monocytes production of interferon,

tumor necrosis factor, and colony stimulating activity. J Immunol 1986;137:2281.

22. Ralph P, Nakoinz I. Stimulation of macrophage tumoricidal activity by the growth and differentiation factor CSF-1. Cell Immunol 1987;105:270.

23. Lee MT, Warren K. CSF-1 induced resistance to viral infection in murine macrophages. J Immunol 1987;138:3019.

24. Sherr CJ. Colony-stimulating factor-1 receptor. Blood 1990; 75:1.

25. Downing R, Roussel MF, Sherr CJ. Ligand and protein kinase C downmodulate the colony stimulating factor 1 receptor by independent mechanisms. Mol Cell Biol 1989;9:2890.

26. Pace JL, Varesio L, Russell SW, et al. The strain of mouse and assay conditions influence whether MuIFN-gamma primes or activates macrophages for tumor cell killing. J Leuk Biol 1985;37:475.

27. Varesio L, Blasi E, Thurman GB, et al. Potent activation of mouse macrophages by recombinant interferon-gamma. Cancer Res 1984;44:4465.

28. Varesio L, Radzioch D, Bottazzi B, et al. Ribosomal RNA metabolism in macrophages. Curr Top Microbiol Immunol 1992;181:209.

29. Varesio L, Cox GW, Pulkki K, et al. Activation of macrophages and monocytes by interferon-gamma and interleukin-2. In: Klostergaard J, Lopez-Berestein G, eds. Mononuclear phagocytes in cell biology. Boca Raton, Fla: CRC Press, 1993;119–146.

30. Musso T, Espinoza-Delgado I, Pulkki K, et al. IL-2 induces IL-6 production in human monocytes. J Immunol 1992; 148:795.

31. Espinoza-Delgado I, Longo DL, Gusella GL, et al. Regulation of IL-2 receptor subunit genes in human monocytes. Differential effects of IL-2 and IFN-gamma. J Immunol 1992;149:2961.

32. Moncada S, Palmer RM, Higgs EA. Nitric oxide: physiology, pathophysiology, and pharmacology. Pharmacol Rev 1991;43:109.

33. Gusella GL, Musso T, Bosco MC, et al. IL-2 up-regulates but IFN-gamma suppresses IL-8 expression in human monocytes. J Immunol 1993;151:2725.

34. Varesio L, Cox GW, Pulkki K, et al. Arginine and tryptophan catabolism: the picolinic acid connection. In: Ishiguro I, Kido R, Nagatsu T, Nagamura Y, Otha Y, eds. Advances in tryptophan research. Toyoake, Japan: Fujita Health University Press, 1992;309–313.

35. Adams DO, Johnson SP, Uhing RJ. Early gene expression in the activation of mononuclear phagocytes. In: Grinstein S, Rothstein OD, eds. Mechanisms of leukocyte activation. 1990:587–601.

36. Adams DO, Koerner TJ. Gene regulation in macrophage development and activation. In: Cruse JM, Lewis RE Jr, eds. The year in immunology 1988. Cellular, molecular and clinical aspects. Basel: Karger, 1989;159–180.

37. Hamilton TA, Adams DO. Molecular mechanisms of signal transduction in macrophages. Immunol Today 1987;8:151.

38. Varesio L. Molecular bases for macrophage activation. Ann Inst Pasteur Immunol 1986;137:235.

39. Farrar WL, Schreiber RD. The molecular and cell biology of interferon-gamma and its receptors. Annu Rev Immunol 1993;11:571.

40. Adams DO, Hamilton TA. The cell biology of macrophage activation. Annu Rev Biochem 1984;2:283.

41. Hamilton JA. Colony stimulating factors, cytokines and monocyte-macrophages—some controversies. Immunol Today 1993;14:18.

42. Varesio L. Induction and expression of tumoricidal activity by macrophages. In: Dean RT, Jessup W, eds. Mononuclear phagocytes: physiology and pathology. Amsterdam: Elsevier Science Publishers, 1985:381–407.

43. Drysdale BE, Agarwal S, Shin HS. Macrophage-mediated tumoricidal activity: mechanisms of activation and cytotoxicity. Prog Allergy 1988;40:111.

44. Mantovani A. Cytotoxic killing of tumor cells by monocytes. In: Zembala M, Asherson GL, eds. Human monocytes. New York: Academic Press, 1989:304.

45. Hoover DL, Meltzer MS. Lymphokines as monocyte activators. In: Zembala M, Asherson GL, eds. Human monocytes. New York: Academic Press, 1989:152.

46. Morgan DA, Ruscetti FW, Gallo RC. Selective in vitro growth of T lymphocytes from normal human bone marrow. Science 1976; 193:1007–1008.

47. Waldmann TA, Goldman CK, Robb RJ, et al. Expression of interleukin-2 receptors on activated human B cells. J Exp Med 1984;160:1450.

48. Phillips JH, Takeshita T, Sugamura K, et al. Activation of natural killer cells via the p75 interleukin 2 receptor. J Exp Med 1989;170:291.

49. Trinchieri G, Kobayashi MM, Clark SC, et al. Response of resting human peripheral blood natural killer cells to interleukin 2. J Exp Med 1984;160:1147.

50. Radzioch D, Hudson T, Boule M, et al. Genetic resistance/susceptibility to mycobacteria: phenotypic expression in bone marrow derived macrophage lines. J Leuk Biol 1991;50:263.

51. Okamoto Y, Minamota S, Shimizu K, et al. Interleukin-2 receptor beta chain expressed in an oligodendroglioma line binds interleukin 2 and delivers growth signal. Proc Natl Acad Sci USA 1990;87:6584.

52. Rand TH, Silberstein DS, Kornfeld H, et al. Human eosinophils express functional interleukin-2 receptors. J Clin Invest 1991;88:825.

53. Wei S, Blanchard DK, Liu JH, et al. Activation of tumor necrosis factor alpha production from human neutrophils by IL-2 via IL-2R beta. J Immunol 1993;150:1979.

54. Djeu JY, Liu JH, Wei S, et al. Function associated with IL-2 receptor beta on human neutrophils. J Immunol 1993; 150:960.

55. Malkovsky M, Loveland B, North M, et al. Recombinant interleukin-2 directly augments the cytotoxicity of human monocytes. Nature 1987;325:262.

56. Wahl SM, McCartney-Francis N, Hunt DA, et al. Monocyte interleukin-2 receptor gene expression and interleukin-2 augmentation of microbicidal activity. J Immunol 1987; 139:1342.

57. Belosevic M, Finbloom DS, Meltzer MS, et al. IL-2 cofactor for induction of activated macrophage resistance to infection. J Immunol 1990;145:831.

58. Holter W, Goldman CK, Casabo L, et al. Expression of functional IL 2 receptors by lipopolysaccharide and interferon-γ stimulated human monocytes. J Immunol 1987; 138:2917.

59. Wahl SM, McCartney-Francis N, Hunt DA, et al. Monocyte interleukin 2 receptor gene expression and interleukin 2 augmentation of microbicidal activity. J Immunol 1987; 139:1342.

60. Belosevic M, Davis CE, Meltzer MS, et al. Regulation of activated macrophage antimicrobial activities. Identification of lymphokines that cooperate with IFN-τ for induction of resistance to infection. J Immunol 1988;141:890.

61. Remick DG, Larrick JW, Nguyen DT, et al. Stimulation of prostaglandin E_2 and thromboxane B_2 production by human monocytes in response to interleukin-2. Biochem Biophys Res Commun 1987;147:86.

62. Herrmann F, Cannistra SA, Lindemann A, et al. Functional consequences of monocyte IL-2 receptor expression. Induction of IL–1β secretion by IFN and IL-2. J Immunol 1989;142:139.

63. Kovacs EJ, Brock B, Varesio L, et al. IL-2 induction of IL-1 beta mRNA expression in monocytes. Regulation by agents that block second messenger pathways. J Immunol 1989; 143:3532.

64. Strieter RM, Remick DG, Lynch JPI, et al. Interleukin-2-induced tumor necrosis factor-alpha (TNFα) gene expression in human alveolar macrophages and blood monocytes. Am Rev Respir Dis 1989;139:335.

65. Taylor MW, Feng GS. Relationship between interferon-gamma, indoleamine 2,3-dioxygenase, and trytophan catabolism. Faseb J 1991;5:2516.

66. Brach MA, Arnold C, Kiehntopf M, et al. Transcriptional activation of the macrophage colony-stimulating factor gene by IL-2 is associated with secretion of bioactive macrophage colony-stimulating factor protein by monocytes and involves activation of the transcription factor NF-kB. J Immunol 1993;150:5535.

67. Epling-Burnette PK, Wei S, Blanchard DK, et al. Coinduction of granulocyte-macrophage colony-stimulating factor release and lymphokine-activated killer cell susceptibility in monocytes by interleukin-2 via interleukin-2 receptor beta. Blood 1993;81:3130.

68. Nelson BJ, Belosevic M, Green SJ, et al. Interleukin-2 and the regulation of activated macrophage cytotoxic activities. In: Friedman H, ed. Microbial infection. New York: Plenum Press, 1992;77–88.

69. Narumi S, Finke JH, Hamilton TA. Interferon τ and interleukin 2 synergize to induce selective monokine expression in murine peritoneal macrophages. J Biol Chem 1990; 265:7036.

70. Aggarwal BB. Structure of tumor necrosis factor and its receptor. Biotherapy 1991;3:113.

71. Aggarwal BB, Eessalu TE, Hass PE. Characterization of receptors for human tumor necrosis factor and their regulation by gamma-interferon. Nature 1985;318:665.

72. Fisher DG, Novick D, Orchaansky P, et al. Two molecular forms of the human interferon-gamma receptor. Ligand binding, internalization and down regulation. J Biol Chem 1988;263:2632.

73. Celada A, Schreiber RD. Internalization and degradation of receptor bound interferon gamma by murine macrophages. Demonstration of receptor recycling. J Immunol 1987;139:147.

74. Finbloom DS, Wahl LM, Winestock KD. The receptor for interferon-gamma on human peripheral blood monocytes

75. consists of multiple distinct subunits. J Biol Chem 1991; 266:22545.

75. Finbloom DS, Larner AC, Nakagawa Y, et al. Culture of human monocytes with granulocyte-macrophage colony-stimulating factor results in enhancement of IFN-gamma receptors but suppression of IFN-gamma-induced expression of the gene IP-10. J Immunol 1993;150:2383.

76. Waldman TA. The multi-subunit interleukin-2 receptor. Annu Rev Biochem 1989;58:875.

77. Hatakeyama M, Mori H, Doi T, et al. A restricted cytoplasmic region of IL-2-beta chain is essential for growth and signal transduction but not for ligand binding and internalization. Cell 1989;59:837.

78. Hatakeyama M, Tsudo M, Minamoto S, et al. Interleukin-2 receptor-beta chain gene: generation of three receptor forms by cloned human alpha and beta cDNAs. Science 1989;244:551.

79. Voss SD, Robb RJ, Weil-Hilman G, et al. Increased expression of the interleukin 2 (IL-2) receptor beta chain (p70) on CD56+ natural killer cells after in vivo IL-2 therapy: p70 expression does not alone predict the level of intermediate affinity IL-2 binding. J Exp Med 1990;172:1101.

80. Tsudo M, Karasuyama H, Kitamura F, et al. The IL-2R-beta chain (p70): ligand binding ability of the cDNA-encoding membrane and secreted forms. J Immunol 1990;145:599.

81. Minamoto S, Mori H, Hatakeyama M, et al. Characterization of the heterodimeric complex of human IL-2 receptor alpha/beta chain reconstituted in a mouse fibroblast cell line, L929. J Immunol 1990;145:2177.

82. Herrmann T, Diamanstein T. The high affinity interleukin 2 receptor: evidence for three distinct polypeptide chains comprising the high affinity IL-2 receptor. Mol Immunol 1988;25:1201.

83. Saragovi H, Malek TR. Evidence for additional subunits associated to the mouse interleukin 2 receptor p55/p75 complex. Proc Natl Acad USA 1990;87:11.

84. Saito Y, Tada H, Sabe H, et al. Biochemical evidence for a third chain of the interleukin-2 receptor. J Biol Chem 1991;266:22186.

85. Takeshita T, Ohtani K, Asao H, et al. An associated molecule, p64, with IL-2 receptor beta chain. Its possible involvement in the formation of the functional intermediate-affinity IL-2 receptor complex. J Immunol 1992;148:2154.

86. Sharon M, Gnarra JR, Leonard WJ. A 100-kilodalton protein is associated with the murine interleukin 2 receptor: biochemical evidence that p100 is distinct from the α and β chains. Proc Natl Acad Sci USA 1990;87:4869.

87. Voss SD, Sondel PM, Robb RJ. Characterization of the interleukin 2 receptors (IL-2R) expressed on human natural killer cells activated in vivo by IL-2: association of the p64 IL-2R gamma chain with the IL-2R beta chain in functional intermediate-affinity IL-2R. J Exp Med 1992; 176:531.

88. Takeshita T, Asao H, Ohtani K, et al. Cloning of the gamma-chain of the human IL-2 receptor. Science 1992; 257:379.

89. Arima N, Kamio M, Imada K, et al. Pseudo-high affinity interleukin 2 (IL-2) receptor lacks the third component that is essential for functional IL-2 binding and signaling. J Exp Med 1992;176:1265.

90. Asao H, Takeshita T, Ishii N, et al. Reconstitution of functional interleukin 2 receptor complexes on fibroblastoid

cells: involvement of the cytoplasmic domain of the gamma chain in two distinct signaling pathways. Proc Natl Acad Sci USA 1993;90:4127.

91. Bosco MC, Espinoza-Delgado I, Schwabe M, et al. Regulation by IL-2 and IFN-gamma of IL-2Rgamma gene expression in human monocytes. Blood 1994:83:2993–3002.

92. Bosco MC, Espinoza-Delgado I, Schwabe M, et al. The gamma subunit of the IL-2R is expressed in human monocytes and modulated by IL-2, IFNgamma, and TGFbeta. Blood 1994;83:3462–3467.

93. Hancock WW, Muller WA, Cotran RS. Interleukin 2 receptors are expressed by alveolar macrophages during pulmonary sarcoidosis and are inducible by lymphokine treatment of normal human lung macrophages, blood monocytes, and monocyte cell lines. J Immunol 1987; 138:185.

94. Wahl SM, McCartney-Francis N, Hunt DA, et al. Monocyte interleukin 2 receptor gene expression and interleukin 2 augmentation of microbicidal activity. J Immunol 1987; 139:1342.

95. Stanakova J, Dupuis G, Gagnon N, et al. Priming of human monocytes with leukotriene B4 enhances their sensitivity in IL-2-driven tumor necrosis factor alpha production. J Immunol 1993;150:4041.

96. Aggarwal BB, Graff K, Samal B, et al. Regulation of two forms of the TNF receptors by phorbol ester and dibutyryl cyclic adenosine 3′,5′-monophosphate in human histiocytic lymphoma cell line U-937. Lymphokine Cytokine Res 1993;12:149.

97. Noguchi M, Nakamura Y, Russell S, et al. Interleukin-2 receptor gamma chain: a functional component of the interleukin-7 receptor. Science 1993;262:1877–1880.

98. Russell S, Keegan AD, Harada N, et al. Interleukin-2 receptor gamma chain: a functional component of the interleukin-4 receptor. Science 1993;262:1880–1883.

99. Holter W, Grunow R, Stockinger H, et al. Recombinant interferon-gamma induces interleukin 2 receptors on human peripheral blood monocytes. J Immunol 1986;136:2171.

100. Noguchi M, Adelstein S, Cao X, et al. Characterization of the human interleukin-2 receptor gamma chain gene. J Biol Chem 1993;268:13601.

101. Gnarra JR, Otani H, Ge Wang M, et al. Human interleukin 2 receptor beta-chain gene: chromosomal localization and identification of 5′ regulatory sequences. Proc Natl Acad Sci USA 1990;87:3440.

102. Pomerantz JL, Mauxion F, Yoshida M, et al. A second sequence element located 3′ to the NF-kB binding site regulates IL-2 receptor-alfa gene induction. J Immunol 1989; 143:4275.

103. Toledano MB, Roman DG, Halden NF, et al. The same target sequences are differentially important for activation of the interleukin 2 receptor alpha chain gene in two distinct T-cell lines. Proc Natl Acad Sci USA 1990;87:1830.

104. Kuang AA, Novak KD, Kang SM, et al. Interaction between NF-kB- and serum response factor-binding elements activates an interleukin-2 receptor-alpha-chain enhancer specifically in T lymphocytes. Mol Cell Biol 1993;13:1536.

105. Espinoza-Delgado I, Bosco MC, Musso T, et al. Inhibitory cytokine circuits involving transforming growth factor-beta, interferon-gamma, and interleukin-2 in human monocyte activation. Blood 1994;83:3332–3338.

106. Johnson KW, Smith KA. cAMP regulation of IL-2 receptor

107. Noguchi M, Yi H, Rosenblatt HM, et al. Interleukin-2 receptor gamma chain mutation results in X-linked severe combined immunodeficiency in humans. Cell 1993; 73:147.

108. Schorle H, Holtschke T, Huning A, et al. Development and function of T cells in mice rendered interleukin-2 deficient by gene targeting. Nature 1991;352:621.

109. Russell SM, Keegan AD, Harada N, et al. Interleukin-2 receptor-gamma chain: a functional component of the interleukin-4 receptor. Science 1993;262:1880.

110. Noguchi M, Nakamura Y, Russell SM, et al. Interleukin-2 receptor-gamma chain: a functional component of the interleukin-7 receptor. Science 1993;262:1877.

111. Appasamy PM. Interleukin-7: biology and potential clinical applications. Cancer Invest 1993;11:487.

112. Ziegler SF, Tough TW, Franklin RJ, et al. Induction of macrophage inflammatory protein-1beta gene expression in human monocytes in lipopolysaccharide and IL-7. J Immunol 1991;147:2234.

113. Standiford TJ, Strieter RM, Allen R, et al. IL-7 up-regulates the expression of IL-8 from resting and stimulated human peripheral blood monocytes. J Immunol 1992;149:2035.

114. Alderson MR, Tough TW, Ziegler SF, et al. Interleukin 7 induces cytokine secretion and tumoricidal activity by human peripheral blood monocytes. J Exp Med 1991; 173:923.

115. Dubinett SM, Huang M, Dhnani S, et al. Down-regulation of macrophage transforming growth factor-beta messenger RNA expression by IL-7. J Immunol 1993;151:6670.

116. Ruscetti FW, Varesio L, Ochoa A, et al. Pleiotropic effects of transforming growth factor-beta on cells of the immune system. Ann NY Acad Sci 1993;685:488.

117. Puri RK, Siegel JP. Interleukin-4 and cancer therapy. Cancer Invest 1993;11:473.

118. Stuart PM, Zlotnick A, Woodward JG. Induction of class I and class II MHC antigen expression on murine bone marrow derived macrophages by IL-4 (B-cell stimulatory factor). J Immunol 1988;140:1542.

119. te Velde AA, Klolmp JPG, Yard BA, et al. Modulation of phenotype and functional properties of human monocytes by IL-4. J Immunol 1988;140:1548.

120. Vercelli D, Jabara HH, Lee BW, et al. Human recombinant interleukin-4 induced FcR3/CD23 on normal human monocytes. J Exp Med 1988;167:1406.

121. Weiser M, Bonifer R, Oster W, et al. Interleukin-4 induces secretion of CSF for granulocytes and CSF for macrophages by peritoneal blood monocytes. Blood 1989; 73:1105.

122. Littman BH, Davstan FF, Carlson PL, et al. Regulation of monocyte/macrophage C2 production and HLA-DR expression by IL-4 (BSF-1) and IFN gamma. J Immunol 1989; 142:520.

123. Spits H, Yssel H, Paliard X, et al. IL-4 inhibits IL-2-mediated induction of human lymphokine-activated killer cells, but not the generation of antigen-specific cytotoxic T lymphocytes in mixed leukocyte cultures. J Immunol 1988; 141:29.

124. Martinez OM, Gibbons RS, Garovoy MR, et al. IL-4 inhibits

IL-2 receptor expression and IL-2 dependent proliferation of human T cells. J Immunol 1990;144:2211.

125. Jelinek DF, Lipsky PE. Inhibitory influence of IL-4 on human B cell responsiveness. J Immunol 1988;141:164.

126. Karray S, DeFrance T, Merle-Bëral H, et al. Interleukin 4 counteracts the interleukin 2-induced proliferation of monoclonal B cells. J Exp Med 1988;168:85.

127. DeFrance T, Vandervliet B, Aubry JP, et al. Interleukin 4 inhibits the proliferation but not the differentiation of activated human B cells in response to interleukin 2. J Exp Med 1988;168:1321.

128. McBride WH, Economou JS, Nayersina R, et al. Influences of interleukins 2 and 4 on tumor necrosis factor production by murine mononuclear phagocytes. Cancer Res 1990; 50:2949.

129. Lehn M, Weiser WY, Engelhorn S, et al. IL-4 inhibits H_2O_2 production and antileishmanial capacity of human cultured monocytes mediated by IFN-gamma. J Immunol 1989; 143:3020.

130. Abramson SL, Gallin JI. IL-4 inhibits superoxide production by human mononuclear phagocytes. J Immunol 1990; 144:625.

131. Cox GW, Chattopadhyay U, Oppenheim JJ, et al. IL-4 inhibits the costimulatory activity of IL-2 or picolinic acid but not of lipopolysaccharide on IFN-gamma-treated macrophages. J Immunol 1991;147:3809.

132. Melillo G, Cox GW, Radzioch D, et al. Picolinic acid, a catabolite of L-tryptophan, is a costimulus for the induction of reactive nitrogen intermediate production in murine macrophages. J Immunol 1993;150:4031.

133. Donnelly RP, Fenton MJ, Finbloom DS, et al. Differential regulation of IL-1 production in human monocytes by IFN-gamma and IL-4. J Immunol 1990;145:569.

134. te Velde AA, Huijbens RJ, de Vries JE, et al. IL-4 decreases Fc gamma R membrane expression and Fc gamma R-mediated cytotoxic activity of human monocytes. J Immunol 1990;144:3046.

135. te Velde AA, Huijbens RJ, Heije K, et al. Interleukin-4 (IL-4) inhibits secretion of IL-1 beta, tumor necrosis factor alpha, and IL-6 by human monocytes. Blood 1990;76: 1392.

136. Parodi MT, Varesio L, Tonini GP. Morphological change and cellular differentiation induced by cisplatin in human neuroblastoma cell lines. Cancer Chemother Pharmacol 1989;25:114.

137. Cheung DL, Hart PH, Vitti GF, et al. Contrasting effects of interferon-gamma and interleukin-4 on the interleukin-6 activity of stimulated human monocytes. Immunology 1990; 71:70.

138. Nakanishi K, Matsui K, Hirose S, et al. Lymphokine-regulated differential expression of mRNA for p75kDa-IL-2R and p55kDa-IL-2R in a cloned B lymphoma line (BLC1-CL-3 cells). J Immunol 1990;145:1423.

139. Karray S, Dautry-Varsat A, Tsudo M, et al. IL-4 inhibits the expression of high affinity IL-2 receptors on monoclonal human B cells. J Immunol 1990;145:1152.

140. Crawford RM, Finbloom DS, Ohara J, et al. B cell stimulatory factor-1 (interleukin 4) activates macrophages for increased tumoricidal activity and expression of Ia antigens. J Immunol 1987;139:135.

141. Ralph P, Nakoinz I, Rennick D. Role of interleukin 2, interleukin 4, and alpha, beta, and gamma interferon in stimu-

lating macrophage antibody-dependent tumoricidal activity. J Exp Med 1988;167:712.

142. Stout RD, Bottomly K. Antigen-specific activation of effector macrophages by IFN-gamma producing (TH1) T cell clones. Failure of IL-4-producing (TH2) T cell clones to activate effector function in macrophages. J Immunol 1989;142:760.

143. Larner AC, Petricoin EF, Nakagawa Y, et al. IL-4 attenuates the transcriptional activation of both IFN-alpha and IFN-gamma-induced cellular gene expression in monocytes and monocytic cell lines. J Immunol 1993;150:1944.

144. Musso T, Gusella GL, Brooks A, et al. Interleukin-4 inhibits indoleamine 2,3-dioxygenase expression in human monocytes. Blood 1994;83:1408–1411.

145. Matsushima K, Baldwin ET, Mukaida N. Interleukin-8 and MCAF: novel leukocyte recruitment and activating cytokines. In: Kishimoto T, ed. Interleukins: molecular biology and immunology. Basel: S. Karger, 1992:263–265.

146. Matsushima K, Morishita K, Yoshimura T, et al. Molecular cloning of human monocyte derived neutrophil chemotactic factor (MNDCF) and the induction of MNDCF mRNA by interleukin 1 and tumor necrosis factor. J Exp Med 1988; 167:1883.

147. Standiford TJ, Strieter RM, Chensue SW, et al. IL-4 inhibits the expression of IL-8 from stimulated human monocytes. J Immunol 1990;145:1435.

148. de Waal Malefyt R, Abrams J, Bennett B, et al. Interleukin 10 (IL-10) inhibits cytokine synthesis by human monocytes: an autoregulatory role of IL-10 produced by monocytes. J Exp Med 1991;174:1209.

149. Oliveira IG, Sciavolino PJ, Lee TH, et al. Downregulation of interleukin 8 gene expression in human fibroblasts: unique mechanism of transcriptional inhibition by interferon. Proc Nat Acad Sci USA 1992;89:9049.

150. Barker JNWN, Sarma V, Mitra RS, et al. Marked synergism between tumor necrosis factor-α and interferon-τ in regulation of keratinocyte-derived adhesion molecules and chemotactic factors. J Clin Invest 1990;85:605.

151. Bosco MC, Gusella GL, Espinoza-Delgado I, et al. Interferon-gamma upregulates interleukin-8 gene expression in human monocytic cells by a posttranscriptional mechanism. Blood 1994;83:537.

152. Assoian RK, Komoriya A, Meyers CA, et al. Transforming growth factor β in human platelets. Identification of a major storage site, purification, and characterization. J Biol Chem 1983;258:7155.

153. Kehrl JH, Wakefield LM, Roberts AB, et al. Production of transforming growth factor-β by human T lymphocytes and its potential role in the regulation of T cell growth. J Exp Med 1986;163:1037.

154. Deryck R, Jarret JA, Chen EY, et al. Human transforming growth factor-β complementery DNA sequence and expression in normal and transformed cells. Nature 1985; 316:701.

155. Roberts AB, Anzano MA, Wakefield LM, et al. Type beta transforming growth factor: a bifunctional regulator of cellular growth. Proc Natl Acad Sci USA 1985;82:119.

156. Roberts AB, Frolik CA, Anzano MA, et al. Transforming growth factors from neoplastic and nonneoplastic tissues. Fed Proc 1983;42:2621.

157. Dubois CM, Ruscetti FW, Palaszynski EW, et al. Transforming growth factor beta is a potent inhibitor of interleu-

kin 1 (IL-1) receptor expression: proposed mechanism of inhibition of IL-1 action. J Exp Med 1990;172:737.

158. Wahl SM, Hunt DA, Wakefield LM, et al. Transforming growth factor type B induces monocyte chemotaxis and growth factor production. Proc Natl Acad Sci USA 1987; 84:5788.

159. Wahl SM, McCartney-Francis N, Mergenhagen SE. Inflammatory and immunomodulatory roles of TGF-beta. Immunol Today 1989;10:258.

160. Kehrl JH, Roberts AB, Wakefield LM, et al. Transforming growth factor β is an important immunomodulatory protein for human B lymphocytes. J Immunol 1986;136:3916.

161. Rook AH, Kehrl JH, Wakefield LM, et al. Effects of transforming growth factor β on the function of natural killer cells: depressed cytolytic activity and blunting of interferon responsiveness. J Immunol 1986;136:3916.

162. Tsunawaki S, Sporn M, Ding A, et al. Deactivation of macrophages by transforming growth factor-β. Nature 1988; 334:260.

163. Espevik T, Figari IS, Shalaby MR, et al. Inhibition of cytokine production by cyclosporin A and transforming growth factor B. J Exp Med 1987;166:571.

164. Musso T, Espinoza-Delgado I, Pulkki K, et al. Transforming growth factor beta downregulates interleukin-1 (IL-1)-induced IL-6 production by human monocytes. Blood 1990;76:2466.

165. Brandes ME, Wakefield LM, Wahls SM. Modulation of monocyte type I transforming growth factor-β receptors by inflammatory stimuli. J Biol Chem 1991;266:19697.

166. Chomarat P, Rissoan MC, Banchereau J, et al. Interferon gamma inhibits interleukin 10 production by monocytes. J Exp Med 1993;177:523.

167. Moore KW, O'Garra A, de Waal Malefyt R, et al. Interleukin-10. Annu Rev Immunol 1993;11:165.

168. Spits H, De Waal Malefyt R. Functional characterization of human IL-10. Int Arch Allergy Immunol 1992;99:8.

169. de Waal Malefyt R, Yssel H, Roncarolo MG, et al. Interleukin-10. Curr Opin Immunol 1992;4:314.

170. Howard M, O'Garra A, Ishida H, et al. Biological properties of interleukin 10. J Clin Immunol 1992;12:239.

171. Drapier JC, Wietzerbin J, Hibbs JB Jr. Interferon-gamma and tumor necrosis factor induce the L-arginine-dependent cytotoxic effector mechanism in murine macrophages. Eur J Immunol 1988;18:1587.

172. Ding AH, Nathan CF, Stuehr DJ. Release of reactive nitrogen intermediates and reactive oxygen intermediates from mouse peritoneal macrophages. J Immunol 1988;141:2407.

173. Hibbs JB Jr, Vavrin Z, Taintor RR. L-arginine is required for expression of the activated macrophage effector mechanism causing selective metabolic inhibition in target cells. J Immunol 1987;138:550.

174. Bredt DS, Hwang PM, Glatt CE, et al. Cloned and expressed nitric oxide synthase structurally resembles cytochrome p-450 reductase. Nature 1991;351:714.

175. Lamas S, Marsden PA, Li GK, et al. Endothelial nitric oxide synthase: molecular cloning and characterization of a distinct constitutive enzyme isoform. Proc Natl Acad Sci USA 1992; 89:6348.

176. Janssens SP, Shimouchi A, Quertermoust T, et al. Cloning and expression of a cDNA encoding human endothelium-derived relaxing factor/nitric oxide synthase. J Biol Chem 1992;267:14519.

177. Sessa WC, Harrison JK, Barber CM, et al. Molecular cloning and expression of a cDNA encoding endothelial cell nitric synthase. J Biol Chem 1993;267:15274.

178. Xie Q, Cho HJ, Calaycay J, et al. Cloning and characterization of inducible nitric oxide synthase from mouse macrophages. Science 1992;256:225.

179. Lyons CR, Orloff GJ, Cunningham JM. Molecular cloning and functional expression of an inducible nitric oxide synthase from a murine macrophage cell line. J Biol Chem 1992;267:6370.

180. Lowenstein CJ, Glatt CS, Bredt DS, et al. Cloned and expressed macrophage nitric oxide synthase contrasts with the brain enzyme. Proc Natl Acad Sci USA 1992;89:6711.

181. Stuehr DJ, Marletta MA. Mammalian nitrate biosynthesis: mouse macrophages produce nitrite and nitrate in response to E. coli lipopolysaccharide. Proc Natl Acad Sci USA 1985;82:7738.

182. Ding AH, Nathan CF, Stuehr DJ. Release of reactive nitrogen intermediates and reactive oxygen intermediates from mouse peritoneal macrophages: comparison of activating cytokines and evidence for independent production. J Immunol 1988;141:2407.

183. Stuehr DJ, Marletta MA. Induction of nitrite/nitrate synthesis in murine macrophages by BCG infection, lymphokines, or interferon-gamma. J Immunol 1987;139:518.

184. Drapier JC, Hibbs JB Jr. Differentiation of murine macrophages to express non-specific cytotoxicity for tumor cells results in L-arginine dependent inhibition of mitochondrial iron-sulfur enzymes in the macrophage effector cells. J Immunol 1988;140:2829.

185. Cox GW, Melillo G, Chattopadhyay U, et al. Tumor necrosis factor-alpha-dependent production of reactive nitrogen intermediates mediates IFN-gamma plus IL-2-induced murine macrophage tumoricidal activity. J Immunol 1992; 149:3290.

186. Marletta MA. Nitric oxide: biosynthesis and biological significance. Trends Biochem Sci 1989;14:488.

187. Carlin JM, Ozaki Y, Byrne GI, et al. Interferons and indoleamine 2,3-dioxygenase: role in antimicrobial and antitumor effects. Experientia 1989;45:535.

188. Nathan C. Nitric oxide as a secretory product of mammalian cells. Faseb J 1992;6:3051.

189. Hibbs JB Jr, Taintor RR, Vavrin Z. Macrophage cytotoxicity: role for L-arginine deaminase activity and imino nitrogen oxidation to nitrite. Science 1987;235:473.

190. Nathan CF, Hibbs JB Jr. Role of nitric oxide synthesis in macrophage antimicrobial activity. Curr Opin Immunol 1991;3:65.

191. Hevel JM, White KA, Marletta MA. Purification of the inducible murine macrophage nitric oxide synthase. Identification as a flavoprotein. J Biol Chem 1991;266:22789.

192. Stuehr DJ, Cho HJ, Kwon NS, et al. Purification and characterization of the cytokine-induced macrophage nitric oxide synthase: an FAD- and FMN-containing flavoprotein. Proc Natl Acad Sci USA 1991;88:7773.

193. Hayaishi O, Ryotaro Y, Takikawa O, et al. Indoleamine-dioxygenase. A possible biological function. In: Progress in tryptophan and serotonin research. Berlin: Walter De Gruyter, 1984;33.

194. Feng GS, Taylor MW. Interferon gamma-resistant mutants are defective in the induction of indoleamine 2,3-dioxygenase. Proc Natl Acad Sci USA 1989;86:7144.

195. Yoshida R, Park SW, Yasui H, et al. Tryptophan degradation in transplanted tumor cells undergoing rejection. J Immunol 1988;141:2819.

196. Yoshida R, Hayaishi O. Induction of pulmonary indoleamine 2,3-dioxygenase by intraperitoneal injection of bacterial lipopolysaccharide. Proc Natl Acad Sci USA 1978; 75:3998.

197. Byrne GI, Lehmann LK, Kirschbaum JG, et al. Induction of tryptophan degradation in vitro and in vivo: a gamma-interferon-stimulated activity. J Interferon Res 1986;6:389.

198. Yasui H, Takai K, Yoshida R, et al. Interferon enhances tryptophan metabolism by inducing pulmonary indoleamine 2,3-dioxygenase: its possible occurrence in cancer patients. Proc Natl Acad Sci USA 1986;83:6622.

199. Carlin JM, Borden EC, Byrne GI. Enhancement of indoleamine 2,3-dioxygenase activity in cancer patients receiving interferon-beta. Ser J Interferon Res 1989;9:167.

200. Byrne GI, Lehmann LK, Kirschbaum JG, et al. Induction of tryptophan degradation in vitro and in vivo: a gamma-interferon-stimulated activity. J Interferon Res 1986;6:389.

201. Werner-Felmayer G, Werner ER, Fuchs D, et al. Characteristics of interferon induced tryptophan metabolism in human cells in vitro. Biochim Biophys Acta 1989; 1012:140.

202. Carlin JM, Borden EC, Sondel PM, et al. Intereferon-induced indoleamine 2,3-dioxygenase activity in human mononuclear phagocytes. J Leuk Biol 1989;45:29.

203. Werner ER, Hirsch-Kauffmann M, Fuchs D, et al. Interferon-gamma-induced degradation of tryptophan by human cells in vitro. Biol Chem Hoppe Seyler 1987; 368:1407.

204. Ozaki Y, Edelstein MP, Duch DS. The actions of interferon and antiinflammatory agents of induction of indoleamine 2,3-dioxygenase in human peripheral blood monocytes. Biochem Biophys Res Commun 1987;144:1147.

205. Carlin JM, Borden EC, Byrne GI. Interferon-induced indoleamine 2,3-dioxygenase activity inhibits Chlamydia psittaci replication in human macrophages. J Interferon Res 1989;9:329.

206. Murray HW, Szuro-Sudol A, Wellner D, et al. Role of tryptophan degradation in respiratory burst-independent antimicrobial activity of gamma interferon-stimulated human macrophages. Infect Immun 1989;57:845.

207. Werner-Felmayer G, Werner ER, Fuchs D, et al. Induction of indoleamine 2,3-dioxygenase in human cells in vitro. Adv Exp Med Biol 1991;294:505.

208. Werner ER, Bitterlich G, Fuchs D, et al. Human macrophages degrade tryptophan upon induction by interferon-gamma. Life Sci 1987;41:273.

209. Christen S, Peterhans E, Stocker R. Antioxidant activities of some tryptophan metabolites: possible implication for inflammatory diseases. Proc Natl Acad Sci USA 1990; 87:2506.

210. Rebello T, Lonnerdal B, Hurley LS. Picolinic acid in milk, pancreatic juice and intestine: inadequate for role in zinc absorption. Am J Clin Nutr 1982;35:1.

211. Evans GW, Johnson PE. Characterization and quantitation of a zinc binding ligand in human milk. Pediatr Res 1980; 14:867.

212. Ruffmann R, Welker RD, Saito T, et al. In vivo activation of macrophages but not natural killer cells by picolinic acid (PLA). J Immunopharmacol 1984;6:291.

213. Leuthauser SWC, Oberley LW, Oberley TD. Antitumor activity of picolinic acid in CBA/J mice. J Natl Cancer Inst 1982;68:123.

214. Krieger I, Statter M. Tryptophan deficiency and picolinic acid: effect on zinc metabolism and clinical manifestations of pellagra. Am J Clin Nutr 1987;46:511.

215. Seal CJ, Heaton FW. Effect of dietary picolinic acid on the metabolism of exogenous and endogenous zinc in the rat. J Nutr 1985;115:986.

216. Evans GW, Johnson EC. Zinc absorption in rats fed a low-protein diet and supplemented with tryptophan or picolinic acid. J Nutr 1980;110:1076.

217. Menard MP, Cousins RJ. Effect of citrate, glutathione and picolinate on zinc transport by brush border membrane vesicles from rat intestine. J Nutr 1983;113:1653.

218. Hurley LS, Lonnerdal B. Zinc binding in human milk: citrate versus picolinate. Nutr Rev 1982;40:65.

219. Varesio L, Clayton M, Blasi E, et al. Picolinic acid, a catabolite of tryptophan, as the second signal in the activation of IFN-gamma primed macrophages. J Immunol 1990;145: 4265.

220. Ruffmann R, Schlick R, Chirigos MA, et al. Antiproliferative activity of picolinic acid due to macrophage activation. Drugs Exp Clin Res 1987;13:607.

221. Melillo G, Cox GW, Biragyn A, et al. Regulation of nitric oxide synthase mRNA expression by interferon-gamma and picolinic acid. J Biol Chem 1994;269:8128–8133.

222. Heyes MP, Saito K, Jacobowitz D, et al. Poliovirus induces indoleamine-2,3-dioxygenase and quinolinic acid synthesis in macaque brain. Faseb J 1992;6:2977.

223. Brown RR, Lee CM, Kohler PC, et al. Altered tryptophan and neopterin metabolism in cancer patients treated with recombinant interleukin 2. Cancer Res 1989;49:4941.

224. Denis M. Tumor necrosis factor and granulocyte macrophage colony-stimulating factor stimulate human macrophages to restrict growth of virulent Mycobacterium avium and to kill avirulent M. avium: killing effector mechanism depends on the generation of reactive nitrogen intermediates. J Leuk Biol 1991;49:380.

225. Hibbs JB Jr, Westenfelder C, Taintor R, et al. Evidence for cytokine-inducible nitric oxide synthesis from L-arginine in patients receiving interleukin-2-therapy. J Clin Invest 1992;89:867.

226. Liew FY, Li Y, Severn A, et al. A possible novel pathway of regulation by murine T helper type-2 (Th2) cells of a Th1 cell activity via the modulation of the induction of nitric oxide synthase on macrophages. Eur J Immunol 1991; 21:2489.

227. Ding A, Nathan CF, Graycar J, et al. Macrophage deactivating factor and transforming growth factors-beta 1, -beta 2, and -beta 3 inhibit induction of macrophage nitrogen oxide synthesis by IFN-gamma. J Immunol 1990;145:940.

228. Wilson EO. Sociobiology. Cambridge, MA: The Belknap Press of Harvard University Press, 1976:176.

229. Madison DV. Pass the nitric oxide. Proc Natl Acad Sci USA 1993;90:4329.

CHAPTER 5

ROLE OF CYTOKINES IN NEUTROPHIL FUNCTIONS

Jin Hong Liu and Julie Y. Djeu

The mammalian immune system is essential for surviving infections with a great range of potential pathogens. The protective effect produced is dependent on many types of cells that require flexible and independent production and regulation. In particular, the polymorphonuclear neutrophils (PMN) have long been regarded as major effector cells against pathogenic microbes. The participation of neutrophils at the sites of inflammation is associated with activation, resulting in phagocytosis and the release of reactive oxygen metabolites and proteolytic enzymes. As the acute inflammatory process evolves, neutrophil accumulation exceeds emigration of monocytes. Activated PMN are thought to be especially important for controlling infectious diseases and are also important in the pathogenesis of tissue damage in certain noninfectious diseases (1–3). The importance of PMN in host defense is dramatically illustrated by the consequences of neutropenia and severe neutrophil dysfunction. Either condition can result in severe, recurrent, and often life-threatening bacterial and fungal infections (4,5). Activated PMN are also believed to be involved in neoplastic processes (1,6,7). Infiltrating PMN at inflammatory and tumor sites can be primed by a variety of cytokines to have enhanced functional activity.

Cytokines represent essential soluble transmitters of cell-to-cell communication, and they coordinate immune and inflammatory responses. Cytokines have a crucial role in transmitting signals for proliferation, differentiation, and function of various target cells, including PMN,

through interaction with specific cell surface receptors. Most cytokines can be released by a range of cell types, such as mononuclear leukocytes, lymphocytes, endothelial cells, and some local tissue cells, following interaction with microbial components of bacterial, viral, or parasite origin, or stimulation with antigen or mitogens. By interaction with these cytokines, PMN may be educated in their search for as well as destruction of microorganisms and neoplasm in body tissues. Alterations in neutrophil function in response to cytokines, which may be released during a humoral or a cellular immune reaction, suggest that PMN may participate as effector cells in both B and T lymphocyte–directed immunity.

However, accumulated evidence now suggests that PMN are not only activated by cytokines but can also produce many cytokines that may have important autocrine and paracrine effects. These cytokines can bring about changes in the rate of bone marrow production and release of PMN, enhance the ability of PMN to localize at sites of inflammation, increase neutrophil phagocytic activity, stimulate further cytokine production of PMN and local induction of vascular endothelial cell adhesion molecules, and promote further PMN accumulation, thereby resulting in enhanced cytocidal activity and bacteriocidal activity of PMN. The cytokines produced by PMN may also have stimulatory function on lymphocytes. Thus, PMN may serve as important immunoregulating cells involved in modulating both cellular and humoral immunity, particularly via synthesis and secretion of cytokines

(3). These roles of PMN would be in addition to their established role as an important component of the first line of defense against infectious agents. The potential impact of PMN as immunoregulatory cells is further supported by the fact that they are produced in large numbers, are continuously regenerated from the bone marrow, and constitute the vast majority of infiltrating cells at acute inflammatory sites.

FUNCTIONAL ACTIVATION OF NEUROPHIL BY CYTOKINES

Activation and recruitment of PMN have been shown to be regulated by a variety of cytokines, including colony-stimulating factor (CSF), interleukin-1 (IL-1), IL-2, IL-6, IL-8, tumor necrosis factor (TNF), and interferon-γ (IFN-γ). By interacting with specific cell receptors on the PMN surface, these cytokines are capable of altering a wide range of neutrophil functions essential in the evolution of the inflammation response, as well as in the tissue damage that accompanies this response. This damage includes adherence and chemotaxis, which promotes cellular infiltration in tissue; increased oxygen-dependent respiratory activity, leading to the production of reactive oxygen intermediates; and release of lysosomal enzymes and proteins.

Production of reactive oxygen species is an important component of PMN activation, and it is responsible for many of the microbicidal, tumoricidal, and inflammatory activities of these cells. Intracellular killing is dependent on the initiation of an oxidative burst and the subsequent generation of reactive oxygen species. This is particularly true for anaerobic pathogens, which lack superoxide dismutase, but it is also important for efficient elimination of other pathogens. In contrast, lysosomal enzymes and other proteins released from PMN are important for elimination of extracellular pathogens that cannot be phagocytosed.

To study the functional activities of cytokines on PMN, it is important to identify the cytokine receptors on the neutrophil surface. Low numbers of cell receptors on PMN have been reported for many cytokines (e.g., IL-1α and -β, IL-2, IL-3, IL-8, TNF, granulocyte-macrophage CSF [GM-CSF], and IFN-γ). With the advent of recombinant DNA technique, may of the cytokine genes have been isolated, thus allowing evaluation of the direct effect of individual factors on neutrophils.

Colony-stimulating factors

Hematopoietic growth factors are low molecular weight glycoprotein cytokines that regulate maintenance, repli-cation, and differentiation of blood progenitor cells. Human-derived GM-CSF, granulocyte CSF (G-CSF), and multi-CSF (IL-3) are three major growth factors that have been sequenced and cloned. The numbers of GM-CSF and G-CSF receptors on the surface of PMN are low, and they decrease to a few hundred during cell maturation. Despite the low numbers of receptors, GM-CSF and G-CSF binding to PMN has been shown to be specific (8–10).

In the low picomolar range, all of the CSFs stimulate hematopoietic progenitor cells to form colonies in soft agar culture. GM-CSF is identified by its capacity to induce myeloid precursors to proliferate and differentiate into neutrophils, eosinophils, or monocytes (11–13). G-CSF is postulated to support growth, proliferation, and differentiation of only relatively late progenitor granulocytes already committed to their respective lineage (14,15). IL-3 is a multipotent CSF that controls differentiation of all cells of the immune system (16). As hematopoietic growth factors, these CSFs are all known to influence granulocytopoiesis. Initial clinical trials indicated that the CSFs were valuable agents in stimulating hematopoiesis, either following chemotherapy or marrow transplants or in stimulating resistance to life-threatening infections (17).

PMN have the shortest half-life among leukocytes. It is generally accepted that in vivo PMN meet their fate in site because there is little evidence that they can return from tissues to blood. In vitro, PMN die rapidly, with changes characteristic of cells undergoing programmed cell death or apoptosis (18,19). Recently, it has been postulated that both GM-CSF and G-CSF can support the survival of mature neutrophils by inhibition of programmed cell death (14,20,21). Because mature circulating PMN are short-living cells, incapable of proliferation and of self-renewal, regulation of PMN survival in inflammatory sites may represent, in addition to recruitment from blood, a major mechanism through which functional PMN are accumulated in inflammatory sites.

In addition to their effects on hematopoiesis, recombinant GM-CSF, G-CSF, and IL-3 have been shown to activate mature neutrophil functions both in vitro and in vivo. Although recombinant human GM-CSF (rhGM-CSF) has not been shown to directly induce nonadherent neutrophil superoxide production, degranulation, or phagocytosis, it can prime neutrophils to increase these functions in response to a second stimulus, including N-Formyl-met-leu-phe (FMLP), the complement component C_{5a}, leukotriene B_4, phorbol myristate acetate (PMA), and opsonized zymosan (22–29). Enhancement of respiratory burst activity induced by rhGM-CSF is due to both recruitment of previously unresponsive PMN and intensification of the response of the responding cells (27). Thus, GM-CSF may be an endogenous regulator of PMN inflammatory responses induced by the major physiological chemoattractants. However, GM-CSF directly stimulates the oxidative activity of PMN adhered to proteins derived from serum or plasma, or to the basement membrane protein, laminin (30). The rhGM-CSF can also directly enhance antibody-dependent cell-mediated cytotoxicity (ADCC) against ^{51}Cr-labeled p815 mouse mastocytoma cells (22,24,31) and fungicidal activity against *Candida albicans* (32). It has been shown that PMN can respond to GM-CSF readily within 2 hours of activation, and they may utilize any of the three antifungal pathways (i.e., oxidative radical production, enzyme degranulation, and lactoferrin release) to control *Candida,* which serves as a second stimulus (32,33). GM-CSF has also been shown to have a chemotactic property on PMN (34). Thus, the cytokine has bifunctional roles for PMN; it not only activates them but also mobilizes them to the site of inflammation.

G-CSF has also been shown to modulate certain functions of neutrophils. As with GM-CSF, rhG-CSF has not been shown to directly affect the chemotactic response, superoxide production, or degranulation responses of neutrophils. It apparently primes the neutrophil, because the oxidative metabolic burst of PMN, as measured by superoxide production in response to both FMLP and opsonized blastoconidia, is enhanced after preincubation with G-CSF (29,35), but the rhG-CSF exerts a much smaller effect on PMN superoxide release than rhGM-CSF (29).

Like GM-CSF, G-CSF is capable of directly stimulating a respiratory burst of adherent human PMN (30). In particular, G-CSF enhances the antibacterial but not the antifungal activities of normal and defective human PMN in vitro. Bacterial phagocytosis and bactericidal activity against *Staphylococcus aureus* are significantly enhanced after preincubation of PMN with G-CSF. However, G-CSF enhances neither phagocytosis nor fungicidal activity of normal PMN against *C. albicans* blastoconidia (36).

PMN can be induced to synthesize and release lysosomal enzymes, prostaglandins (PG), thromboxanes (TX), and lipoxygenase products that may be involved in PMN aggregation responses during inflammatory reactions. GM-CSF alone does not cause any significant increases in aggregation of the PMN. However, prior exposure of PMN to GM-CSF markedly increased the aggregation induced by FMLP, as opposed to that detected with PMN stimulated with FMLP alone. This finding suggests that GM-CSF facilitates the action of FMLP on the adhesion-dependent cellular functions of the inflammatory response, and that it may serve as an important cofactor in neutrophil aggregation (37). PMN can be stimulated to synthesize PGE_2 from endogenous and exogenous arachidonic acid on exposure to GM-CSF and G-CSF. However, treatment of PMN with rhM-CSF and IL-3 does not result in detectable PGE_2 synthesis (38).

The potential mechanisms to account for the priming effect of PMN by both GM-CSF and G-CSF are still not completely understood. Both GM-CSF and G-CSF have no detectable immediate effects on the resting levels of calcium, the internal pH, or the resting transmembrane electrical potential of mature PMN (39,40). A few recent studies have shown that the selective recognition of PMN-activating agents, such as FMLP and GM-CSF, is achieved by ligand-specific cell membrane receptors on neutrophils, which are coupled to intracellular signal transduction pathways (including activation of tyrosine phosphorylation and phospholipases) that initiate cell activation (3,41–43). Preincubation of the neutrophil with GM-CSF results in an increase in the magnitude of the calcium transients and in the cytoplasmic acidification that follows stimulation of the cells with chemotactic factors (i.e., FMLP, leukotriene B_4, or PMA). The neutrophil priming mechanism by GM-CSF may be through internal signaling to increase the concentration of free calcium and by the changes in the internal pH in combination with cofactors.

These results show the effects of GM-CSF on the cellular physiology of PMN and provide insights into the mechanism of action of this factor, as well as into the excitation-response coupling sequence activated by chemotactic factors (39). It has also been reported that although either GM-CSF or G-CSF does not induce translocation of protein kinase C or stimulate significant degranulation, they each directly cause prompt release of arachidonic acid from plasma membrane phospholipids, an event that may represent the receptor-mediated activation of membrane phospholipases and that may contribute to priming of the cells for enhancement of their functional responsiveness (40).

IL-3 has been proven to be a priming factor for mature human eosinophils (i.e., ingestion, ADCC, superoxide anion production). However, it has little effect on mature human PMN activity (29,31).

Interleukin-1

Production of IL-1 is part of the host's response to challenges, such as microbial ingestion, injury, immunological reactions, neoplastic changes, and inflammatory processes. During these processes, IL-1 is released from a variety of cells in two distinct forms, Il-1α and IL-1β (44). There are approximately 900 IL-1 receptors per cell on human PMN with a dissociation constant of 3.0×10^{10} M. Binding of ^{125}I-IL-1α to human PMN is inhibited by both human IL-1α and IL-1β, indicating that both IL-1α and IL-1β bind to the same receptor on these cells (45). By expressing IL-1 receptors on their surface, neutrophils may be educated by IL-1 in their search for microorganisms in body tissues, as well as by destruction of these organisms.

Studies by Seow and colleagues (46) showed that treatment of human neutrophils with rhIL-1α decreases their adherence to dacron fiber and depresses enhancement of adherence induced by both FMLP and phorbol myristate acetate. Although initial studies using leukocyte-derived purified IL-1 showed it to be chemotactic (47), further studies with rhIL-1α indicated that it was not chemotactic, using the migration-under-agarose method (48) and modified Boyden chambers employing a polycarbonate membrane (49). Further experiments definitely confirmed that IL-1α is not a chemoattractant for human peripheral blood neutrophils (50).

Pretreatment of neutrophils with rhIL-1α results in an increase in phagocytic activity for opsonized paraffin oil droplets and enhanced production of superoxide anion and H_2O_2, as well as release of lactoferrin in the presence of opsonized zymosan (48). The rhIL-1α pretreatment of human neutrophils also results in augmented azurophilic granule release in response to cytochalasin B-FMLP stimulation (48). Enhancement of FMLP-induced PMN H_2O_2 production requires at least 30 minutes of preincubation with rhIL-1α (48,50). These results suggest that IL-1α can prime PMN in response to a second stimulus, but that it has no direct effect on the function of mature PMN. It has been suggested that IL-1 might stimulate PMN via the second messenger because extracellular Ca^{2+}, but not Mg^{2+}, is required for maximal lactoferrin release induced by rhIL-1α (51). It is not surprising that resting Ca^{2+} concentrations are unaffected by IL-1β because IL-1β does not affect neutrophil function in vitro (52).

Interleukin-2

The PMN responses to many cytokines are well documented, but the distribution of IL-2 receptors on neutrophils has only been studied very recently. Djeu and associates (53) were able to show that freshly isolated human PMN constitutively express detectable surface levels of IL-2Rβ, but not IL-2Rα, with intermediate IL-2 binding affinity. More importantly, PMN are able to respond functionally to IL-2 by enhanced growth inhibitory activity against an opportunistic fungal pathogen C, albicans. Seow and coworkers (54) also reported that IL-2 depresses basal neutrophil adherence and FMLP- and PMA-induced adherence response. Studies examining the chemotactic activity of IL-2 in migration under agarose failed to demonstrate activity using both a leukocyte-purified human IL-2 and recombinant IL-2. However, IL-2–treated neutrophils show inhibited migration randomly and toward FMLP. IL-2 is also found to modulate the granule release response of neutrophils. IL-2–treated neutrophils are induced to release constituents of specific but not azurophilic granules. However, IL-2 enhances release from both granules in response to opsonized zymosan

(55). These data support the evidence that IL-2 is also a neutrophil modulator and that PMN may have a central role in the generation of IL-2–induced immunomodulation.

Interleukin-8

Acute inflammation either local or systemic is often associated with infiltration and sequestration of PMN at the inflammatory loci. This process is mediated by secretion of chemoattractants, accumulation of PMN by adhesion to endothelial cells, and increased microvascular permeability. Emigration of PMN from the vascular compartment to the site of tissue inflammation is a complex and dynamic process. The significance of neutrophil chemotaxis in response to an acute inflammatory event is accentuated by the number of redundant factors that have been shown to mediate this response, including formyl methionyl peptides, split products of the fifth component of complement, and leukotriene B_4.

In addition to these traditional neutrophil chemotactic/activating factors, a new neutrophil chemotactic/activating factor, IL-8, distinct from IL-1 and TNF, was first purified from the supernatant of human monocytes stimulated with lipopolysaccharide (LPS) (56). It has been isolated, purified, cloned, and expressed recently (57–59).

The specific receptors for IL-8 have been detected on human PMN and some other cell types. Binding of IL-8 to human PMN is not inhibited by IL-1α, TNF-α, insulin, and epidermal growth factor. In addition, chemoattractants, such as C5a, FMLP, leukotriene B_4, and platelet-activating factor, fail to inhibit binding, suggesting that IL-8 utilizes a unique receptor. Steady-state binding experiments indicate kd values of 4 nmol/L and receptor numbers of 75,000 for human PMN (60). PMN express receptors for IL-8 that are coupled to guanine nucleotide binding proteins.

A cDNA clone from HL-60 promyelocytic tumor cells has now been isolated that encodes a human IL-8 receptor (61). IL-8 bound to human PMN is rapidly internalized and subsequently released from cells (60). Binding of IL-8 to its receptor induces an increase in cytosolic calcium concentrations by enhancement of membrane calcium permeability and mobilization of intracellular calcium stores (62).

The movement of leukocytes from blood into tissues is a characteristic feature of inflammation. IL-8 has potent chemotactic activity on PMN, but not on monocytes, and its potency approaches that of FMLP (56,63,64). IL-8 can either up-regulate or down-regulate neutrophil adhesion to the endothelium, depending on the in vitro experimental conditions (65). IL-8 enhances the adhesiveness of human neutrophils to plastic, extracellular matrix proteins, and both unstimulated and tumor necrosis factor (TNF)-stimulated endothelial monolayers in vitro. This adhesion is inhibited by antibodies to the neutrophil adhesion molecule CD11b/CD18. CD11b/CD18 is a member of the β_2-integrin family, which are adhesion molecules involved in neutrophil-endothelial interaction and PMN recruitment (66).

In vivo, the first adhesion step results in PMN rolling along the surface of endothelial cells. To strengthen their adhesion and to permit emigration, PMN have to establish additional adhesive contact with endothelial cells through interaction of the CD11/CD18 integrin heterodimer with the intercellular adhesion molecule 1 on endothelial cells. IL-8 is responsible for this second step of B_2-integrin–mediated neutrophil-endothelial cell adhesion. By binding to endothelial cells, IL-8 induces both translocation of CD11a/CD18 from the intracellular storage pool onto the neutrophil surface and its activation (65,67). Thus, IL-8 may contribute to PMN adhesion to endothelial cells and further recruitment by converting the β-integrins into a high avidity state. Endothelial surface-bound IL-8 can also directly induce neutrophil transendothelial migration and increased permeability of monolayers. This process results in a high rate of PMN transmigration, which may correlate with increased permeability of vessels at inflammatory sites in vivo. The property of IL-8 to stimulate movement of neutrophils across endothelial monolayers in vitro supports the concept of a central role for this molecule on the accumulation of neutrophils at inflammatory lesions in vivo (66,68).

Although IL-8 has been characterized primarily as a chemoattractant, there is a controversial report that indicated IL-8 has an inhibitory effect on PMN-endothelial adhesive interactions in vitro. Stimulation of circulating PMN by soluble IL-8 inhibits their binding to the endothelium. In addition to inhibiting attachment of freshly isolated peripheral blood neutrophils to cytokine-activated human endothelial cell monolayers, soluble IL-8 also promotes rapid detachment of tightly adherent PMN from activated endothelial cells and abolishes PMN transendothelial migration (65,69). Thus, IL-8 may exert a wide range of modulatory effects on neutrophil-endothelial interactions. It can either induce or inhibit PMN emigration in vitro, depending on whether IL-8 is bound to the endothelial surface.

Evidence is accumulating to indicate that IL-8 may also functionally activate PMN, in addition to chemoattract PMN to the inflammatory sites, as characterized by shape change, degranulation, and respiratory burst (63,66,70). IL-8 acts via a selective receptor, and it appears to share, at least in part, the signal transduction system that operates for agonists such as FMLP and $C5_a$ (59). PMN exposed to IL-8 express increased amounts of CD11b/CD18, as well as CD11c/CD18 and complement

receptor-1 (CR-1), on their cell surface due to translocation of these molecules from their intracellular pool to the cell surface. Increased CD11b/CD18 and CD11c/CD18 levels appear to correspond with the release of specific granules by IL-8. These CR-1 receptors are involved in the binding and phagocytosis of C3 breakdown products (C3b)–coated particles (70–73). Finally, host antifungal defenses are dependent on PMN competence. IL-8, similar to FMLP, has been shown to exert an effect on this PMN function by enhancing PMN-mediated anti-*Candida* activity via release of azurophilic enzymes via a glutamyl transpeptidase (GTP) binding protein rather than oxygen-dependent pathways (74).

In addition, IL-8 has been found to be a potent priming agent for human PMN, and it enhances superoxide release stimulated by FMLP, similar to other cytokines, such as TNF, GM-CSF, and G-CSF. The potency of the maximal priming effect on FMLP-induced O_2^- release is TNF > GM-CSF > IL-8 > G-CSF (75). These findings suggest that IL-8 has an important role in controlling the movements of PMN through the extravascular space to the inflammatory site. Once localized, the PMN ingest and phagocytize particles, such as bacteria and immune complexes bearing immunoglobulin G (IgG) via Fc receptor, or complement C3b via CR-1.

Tumor necrosis factor

Thus far, two different forms of TNFs have been described: TNF-α (cachectin), a soluble nonglycosylated protein (17 kd); and TNF-β (lymphotoxin), a secreted glycoprotein (25 kd). The TNFs are products of different genes and are produced by different cell types, but they have approximately 30% amino acid homology and similar functions (76). The action of TNFs on PMN requires binding to surface receptors. Receptors of TNFs on the surface of PMN have been demonstrated. PMN contain a single class of specific, high-affinity receptors that are internalized and degraded after TNF binding (77,78). Approximately 6,000 TNF receptors per cell are indicated by Scatchard analysis of competitive binding studies, and the dissociation constant is approximately 10^{-9} to 10^{-10} mol/L. Both TNF-α and TNF-β compete for the same cellular receptor, which is consistent with the finding of the strong amino acid homology between TNF-α and TNF-β (77,79,80).

TNFs, especially TNF-α, remain the most highly studied cytokines with respect to regulation of neutrophil function. Pretreatment with TNF-α for 15 minutes and TNF-β for 20 minutes increases phagocytic activity of PMN (80,81). In other reports, both TNFs strongly activate PMNs within 2 hours of incubation; significant effects are evident at 1 to 10 U/mL, as shown by weak induction of lysosomal enzyme release and stimulation of superoxide production (48,77,82). Both TNF-α and TNF-β are able to increase antibody-mediated neutrophil cytoxicity. Augmentation of neutrophil ADCC occurs rapidly in the presence of TNF-α and TNF-β compared with IFN-γ. The effects of TNFs on ADCC are short-lived and are probably independent of protein synthesis (82,83). The antitumor activity of TNF has been well established, although the exact mechanisms mediating in vitro and in vivo cytolytic activities of TNF-α and TNF-β are not well characterized. The ability of these cytokines to activate neutrophils and to increase their adherence and postadhesion activities on vascular endothelial cells has been implicated as one possible mechanism that mediates part of the hemorrhagic necrosis of solid tumors and the associated inflammation (77,81,84).

Regarding antimicrobial activity, it has been observed that TNF-α and TNF-β can prime human neutrophils for increased amoebicidal, fungicidal, and bactericidal activities (85–87). Human PMN treated with TNF-α show significant increased growth inhibition or killing of the fungal pathogens, *C. albicans* and *Torulopsis glabrata*. Its continued presence is not required following a short pulse of PMN with TNF (88,89). TNF-β also increases the fungicidal and bactericidal activity of neutrophils; however, TNF-α always causes greater augmentation of the fungicidal activity than TNF-β (90). TNF-α or TNF-β significantly increases the damage of parasites such as *Plasmodium falciparum* and *Entamoeba histolytica* by neutrophils (91,92). TNF-α, TNF-β, and IFN-γ at very high concentrations are not toxic to *P. falciparum* in culture. It is postulated that the basis for cytokine-modulated anti-Plasmodial activity of PMN is increased expression of Fc and complement receptors, which leads to more efficient interaction between the parasite and the PMN (91).

In addition to their direct activating effect on PMN, TNFs are also instrumental in attracting PMN by a variety of mechanisms. Although IL-1 and IL-2 depress neutrophil adherence to dacron fiber, TNF-α enhances neutrophil adherence. The T-lymphocyte product, TNF-β, shows similar enhancement of neutrophil adherence as TNF-α. Only a few minutes' treatment of leukocytes with these cytokines is adequate to achieve optimal depression (with IL-1 and IL-2) or optimal enhancement (with TNF) of adherence (46,54).

TNF-β enhances FMLP- and PMA-induced neutrophil adherence (54). In addition, rhTNF-α also influences adherence-related events of PMN during the attachment stage of phagocytosis (80,81). TNF-α regulates affinity and response of PMN to FMLP (93). Both TNF-α and TNF-β are reported to possess chemotactic property for human neutrophils and monocytes in vitro, which indicates that TNFs may have bifunctional roles for PMN (i.e., not only activating PMN but also attracting them into inflammatory sites). The level of chemotaxis induced by TNF-α is comparable to that elicited by standard chemotactic agents, FMLP and $C5_a$ (94,95).

By promoting a wide variety of functions of the neutrophil essential in the evolution of the inflammatory response and in the tissue damage that accompanies this response, TNF-α and TNF-β may be the main cytokines involved in regulating neutrophil-mediated tissue damage (96). Both TNF-α and TNF-β have been shown to cause cartilage injury by enhancing neutrophil-mediated proteoglycan degradation in cartilage (97,98). TNF-α induces expression of neutrophil surface receptors, such as CR-1 and CR-3 (99,100), which may be related to its ability to increase proteoglycan degradation by neutrophils. These increased receptors promote increased adherence to targets (54,100) and thereby promote the effective delivery of neutrophil mediators on the tissue surface. Neutrophils treated with TNF-α display increased adherence to monolayers of endothelial cells or tumor cells in culture, which may be subsequently damaged (100–103). In addition, TNF-α can activate PMN to produce PGE_2 via the same mechanism as CSF, discussed earlier (38).

Interferon-γ

Interferon was originally described as a protein mediator released from virus-infected cells that prevented viral replication in a target cell. It is a heterogeneous family of proteins (i.e., IFN-α, -β, -γ; IFN-γ has the unique ability to exert more generalized immunoregulatory functions. Considerable recent interest has focused on determining whether these immunomodulatory properties may lead to a role for IFN-γ in clinical practice. IFN-γ exerts its action by binding to high-affinity, membrane-associated receptors (104), and the ligand-receptor complex is internalized and ultimately degraded, an event referred to as down-regulation of receptors (105).

Many of the effects of IFN-γ on PMN have only recently been elucidated. Human PMN have been shown to express the IFN-γ receptors on their surface (106). Binding of IFN-γ to specific receptors on the surface of mature PMN primes various aspects of neutrophil function. The rhIFN-γ increases adhesion of neutrophils to endothelial cells (84), decreases neutrophil random migration (107), and chemoattracts PMN (94). IFN-γ promotes PMN accumulation at the inflammatory site by attracting them and inhibiting their egress. Thus, this process may contain the infection by keeping the PMN at the site of cytokine production.

Phagocytosis can be facilitated by the presence of a specific antibody attached to the foreign antigen. IFN-γ increases expression of high-affinity IgG receptors (FcR_{high}, FcRI, CD64) on the PMN surface (83,108,109), which mediate binding and ingestion of IgG-coated particles (82,107,108). FcR-mediated phagocytosis of IgG red blood cells by PMN is enhanced by IFN-γ (108). Normally, PMN do not express FcR_{high} receptor, but, as a process of differentiation, they acquire low-affinity (FcR_{low})

receptor that bind aggregated IgG. The enhanced expression of FcR_{high} on mature PMN in response to rhIFN-γ is dependent on neutrophilic de novo RNA and protein synthesis, as determined by use of inhibitors of these cellular processes (104). In addition to immunoglobulin-dependent binding, phagocytosis may be facilitated by nonspecific attachment via complement opsonin, C3b. Incubation of human PMN with IFN-γ for 24 hours significantly increases expression of C3b receptor, CR-3 (108). Preincubation of normal PMN with IFN-γ has been reported to increase neutrophil-mediated ADCC (82,83,110,111). This enhancement of neutrophilic ADCC by rhIFN-γ against target cells appears also to be dependent on the increased expression of FcR_{high}. Neutrophil FcR engagement of the Fc portion of antibody-coated cells results in a nonphagocytic cytolysis of selected target cells (83,112).

IFN-γ by itself has minimal but direct effects on neutrophilic degranulation (106,107), oxidative metabolism, and production of superoxide anion (83,95,113–116), which may have a role in diapedeses. More importantly, IFN-γ enhances oxidative burst in response to LPS, FMLP, blastoconidia, and pseudohyphae of C. albicans (35,116,117). This priming effect can be abolished by inhibitors of protein synthesis (118). Modulation of PMN oxidative metabolism by IFN-γ appears to be dependent on transcriptional increase of cytochrome B heavy chain (pg91-phox), a key component of the oxidase. The light chain gene transcripts are less affected (119,120). Not only are the metabolic responses of PMN increased by preincubation with IFN-γ, IFN-γ also prolongs PMN survival by preventing programmed cell death and protects PMN from deterioration on storage (20,121). This functional activation of PMN by IFN-γ may be important for microbicidal activity in IFN-γ–stimulated PMN, including killing enhancement of bacteria, such as *Staphylococcus aureus* and *Mycobacterium fortuitum* (122,123); fungi, such as *C. albicans*, *C. tropicalis*, and *Blastomyces dermatitidis* (88,124); and parasites, such as *E. histolytica* trophozoite (92).

IFN-γ–activated PMN in local tissues are known to cause tissue damage. PMN participate in articular cartilage destruction and predominate in the synovial fluid of inflamed joints during the early stages and acute exacerbation of the disease. Cartilage proteoglycan degradation by PMN is augmented by IFN-γ, but it has no effect on the inhibition of proteoglycan synthesis by PMN (125).

Although IFN-α has little effect on PMN, it should be noted that IFN-α is shown to inhibit neutrophil colony formation in vitro (126), and it may have a similar action in clinical use (127). Thus, IFN-α may have a role in the feedback inhibitory regulation of neutropoiesis, because blood PMN are normally maintained at very precise levels. Elevated levels accompanying bacterial or fungal infection rapidly return to normal when the infection is eliminated.

Cytokine synergism

Because polypeptide cytokines most likely occur as a mixture in body fluids, it is more relevant to study their combined function on cells. Studies of antibody-dependent neutrophil cytotoxicity and neutrophil phagocytosis show that either IFN-γ or TNF-β increase these neutrophil functions. However, enhancement by treatment with a combination of IFN-γ and TNF-β exceeds enhancement caused by either agent alone, suggesting that IFN-γ and TNF-β have a synergistic effect on PMN function (82). Addition of both TNF and IFN-γ also has a synergistic effect on neutrophil growth inhibition of C. albicans in that TNF and IFN-γ, at a concentration that does not activate PMN, cause potent stimulation of PMN function (88). Similarly, studies with the protozoa, E. histolytica, show that although IFN-γ–activated neutrophils are stimulated to kill these amoebae, TNF-α is ineffective. However, killing of E. histolytica by human neutrophils is augmented by the combined treatment of the leukocytes with IFN-γ and TNF-α (92). Addition of two cytokines, GM-CSF and TNF-α, which act on distinct receptors on neutrophils, does not result in a synergistic effect (90). IL-8 becomes a more potent priming agent in combination with the suboptimal concentration of TNF, GM-CSF, or G-CSF, and to enhance O_2^- release stimulated by FMLP (75).

REGULATION OF CYTOKINE GENE EXPRESSION IN NEUTROPHILS

Traditionally, PMN have been considered as terminally differentiated cells incapable of protein synthesis. Definitive studies of RNA and protein production by PMN have been hampered by the low level of detectable product, and by the difficulties in obtaining highly purified PMN free of contaminating peripheral blood mononuclear cells and immature granulocytes. Despite the historical view of neutrophils as the primary scavenger cells, a growing body of evidence now suggests that PMN contribute significantly to the inductive phase of the immune response by modulating both cellular and humoral immunity via cytokine production.

Although IL-1, IL-6, IL-8, TNF-α, and CSF are secreted mainly by activated macrophages, circulating PMN have also been shown to synthesize and release these immunoregulatory cytokines (i.e., IL-1, IL-6, IL-8, TNF-α, GM-CSF, G-CSF, M-CSF) in response to appropriate cytokine or noncytokine stimuli, including bacterial products, such as FMLP, LPS, and the fungal pathogen, C. albicans. The mechanisms involved in regulation of cytokine production in PMN are quite complicated. It is important to bear in mind that gene expression can be controlled at many levels. Accumulation of mRNA often may not be due to transcription activation of the gene. For example, evidence for the effect of cycloheximide in modulation of a specific mRNA degradation pathway has been provided. Thus, ongoing transcription does not always correlate with accumulation of mRNA transcripts.

The ability to produce cytokines after various stimulation supports a role for PMN as part of the cytokine network of regulation/autoregulation among tissue cells. Although the cytokines produced by PMN are approximately 10-fold less than those produced by peripheral blood lymphocytes, the physiological roles of the secretion of these cytokines are supported by the quantitative predominance of PMN both in the peripheral blood and at sites of acute inflammation. Thus, accumulation of limited protein synthesis from individual PMN may result in a biologically significant tissue concentration of cytokines.

Another important factor to consider is that although PMN have a short half-life of 24 hours, this half-life is extended under the influence of many cytokines, such as GM-CSF, IFN-γ, and IL-1β (20,21,121). These cytokines produced by PMN may have important autocrine /paracrine effects, which can be divided into five categories. First, they may bring about changes in the rate of bone marrow cell production and release of new PMN. The best examples are G-CSF and GM-CSF (17). Second, they may help PMN ingest and destroy microbes or express direct tumoricidal activity, as well as antibody-mediated cell cytotoxicity. Examples of this response are numerous and are indicated by GM-CSF, IL-1, IL-8, TNF-α, and IFN-γ (7,23,48,58,74,82,88,102,128). Third, PMN, by the release of chemokines, may be involved in the recruitment of other PMN to the local site. The best known cytokine for this process is IL-8 (58,70,74). Fourth, PMN, by the release of cytokines such as TNF-α, IL-1α, and IL-1β, may be involved in the inflammatory process. These cytokines may induce adherence of PMN via adhesion molecules to vascular endothelial cells, which leads to both hemorrhagic necrosis and inflammation (130,131). Finally, and most importantly, PMN, via a cytokine release, may contribute significantly to the afferent or inductive limb of the immune response by modulation of both T and B cells to affect cellular and humoral immune responses (3).

IL-1 production

IL-1α and IL-1β mRNA can be transcribed in PMN within 1 to 6 hours of stimulation by LPS, TNF, or GM-CSF. Recombinant IL-1α and IL-1β can also stimulate neutrophil-derived IL-1α and IL-1β gene expression in an autocrine fashion (131–136). Furthermore, these stimuli cause the release of protein with IL-1 activity in the culture supernatants, which is found to be exclusively IL-1β (133,134). Virtually all PMN show diffuse staining with both IL-1α

and IL-1β–specific antisera, indicating that all, or nearly all, PMN can produce cell-associated IL-1. The absence of secreted IL-1α is at least partially due to an inhibition of translation (133). With IL-1 or TNF as stimulus, IL-1β mRNA accumulation in PMN peaks at 1 hour and returns to near unstimulated levels by 2 hours.

When treated with the combination of IL-1 plus TNF, IL-1β mRNA levels are sustained for up to 3 hours in PMN. In addition, IL-1β protein accumulation correlates with IL-1β mRNA (i.e., cell-associated antigen is first detected at 1 hour and peaks at 2 hours). Furthermore, relative levels of IL-1β antigen induction follow the pattern of relative levels of IL-1β mRNA induction in that TNF plus IL-1 > TNF > IL-1. Therefore, there is a cooperative effect of IL-1 and TNF on the kinetics of induction of IL-1β mRNA (134,135).

Marucha and colleagues (134) studied whether protein synthesis is required for induction of IL-1β gene expression by treating PMN simultaneously with cytokines and cycloheximide. Cycloheximide enhances accumulation of IL-1–induced IL-1β mRNA, but it abrogates accumulation of IL-1β mRNA by TNF- or TNF plus IL-1–treated PMN, indicating that TNF and IL-1 may regulate PMN functions through different regulatory pathways. Abrogation of TNF-induced IL-1β mRNA accumulation is not caused by inhibition of induction of IL-1β transcription, because TNF induction of transcription of IL-1β is not affected by simultaneous treatment with cycloheximide. Thus, IL-1 and TNF regulate IL-1β gene expression via both transcriptional and posttranscriptional mechanisms in vitro.

During the inflammatory process, IL-1 produced by PMN may serve numerous functions, including stimulation of synthesis and release of acute-phase reactants; augmentation of monocyte, T-, and B-cell activation; accumulation of inflammatory cells; and induction of other regulatory cytokines, such as IL-6, IL-8, and GM-CSF (137). IL-1 also has a costimulatory role, along with GM-CSF and IL-6, on growth and differentiation of hemopoietic progenitors (138,139). In addition, IL-1 production from PMN may have important autocrine and paracrine effects, including stimulation of further IL-1 production and local induction of vascular endothelial cell adhesion molecules, thereby promoting further PMN accumulation. Thus, PMN may regulate their own activation and replication by establishing a positive feedback loop via release of IL-1.

IL-6 production

The potential for PMN to regulate the cellular and humoral immune response is further demonstrated by the finding that PMN are able to produce IL-6, because PMN, through the production of IL-6, may be able to participate in the modulation of several T- and B-lymphocyte responses. Unstimulated PMN have been shown to produce some IL-6–specific mRNA using Northern blotting analysis, reverse-transcriptase polymerase chain reaction, and in situ hybridization (136,140). This expression is rapidly down-regulated after removal of the cells from the circulating blood. This abolished IL-6 expression can be reactivated by addition of GM-CSF to the culture medium (140). The degree of IL-6 gene transcription in PMN is also greatly augmented by LPS after 1 hour of activation; the peak of IL-6 protein production is reached later (136).

Immediate stimulation of highly purified PMN with GM-CSF, and to a lesser extent with TNF-α, also leads to rapid accumulation of IL-6 mRNA. IL-6 protein was detected by a biological assay that can be specifically inhibited by anti-IL-6 polyclonal antibodies (141). PMN accumulating at sites of acute inflammation may release IL-6 to induce acute-phase proteins and to stimulate the terminal maturation of T and B cells, thereby augmenting cytotoxic function in T cells and antibody production of B cells (142,143).

IL-8 production

Although IL-8, a neutrophil chemoattractant, was initially believed to be primarily a product of monocytes, it is now known that PMN are another important source of IL-8. PMN freshly isolated from whole blood are not found to constitutively express IL-8 mRNA. In contrast, when these leukocytes are cultured on plastic, they are activated, leading to significant expression of de novo steady-state levels of IL-8 mRNA. Either LPS or cytokines, such as TNF-α and IL-1, can further activate PMN to express IL-8 mRNA and antigen in both a time- and a dose-dependent manner. PMN stimulated with traditional chemotactic/activating factors, such as C5a, FMLP, and LTB$_4$, do not produce significant antigenic IL-8, as compared with unstimulated controls. In contrast, when PMN are exposed to either of these neutrophil agonists in the presence of LPS, the production of antigenic IL-8 is significantly elevated, as compared with either of the stimuli alone, suggesting a synergistic response (144,145). In contrast, one opposing study (146) indicated that, in addition to cytokines and LPS, chemotactic/activating factors, such as FMLP, C5a, and platelet-activating factor, are able to induce a transient gene expression and release of IL-8 by PMN through a pertussis toxin-sensitive pathway.

Phagocytic challenge also induces IL-8 synthesis from PMN. After phagocytosis of yeast opsonized with IgG, PMN progressively express high levels of IL-8 mRNA and release considerable amounts of IL-8 peptide, which remain elevated after 18 hours (147). In contrast, IFN-γ down-regulates the constitutive IL-8 mRNA levels expressed by resting PMN (148). This down-modulation occurs rapidly, is not dependent on new protein synthesis, and is not caused by an increased rate of degradation of IL-8 mRNA. Preincubation of PMN with IFN-γ significantly inhibits their ability to express IL-8 gene and to subsequently release the protein after stimulation with TNF, LPS, FMLP, and phagocytizable particles (yeast IgG), suggesting that IL-8 synthesis in human PMN is precisely controlled (148). In addition, in human PMN, degradation of IL-8 mRNA is also finely regulated. When PMN are treated with cycloheximide, an inhibitor of protein synthesis, there is evidence for superinduction of steady-state levels of mRNA for IL-8 in a dose- and time-dependent manner (145,148).

PMN only express mRNA for IL-8, but not for monocyte chemotactic activation factor. By the release of IL-8, PMN have the capacity to amplify recruitment of additional nearby neutrophils to the sites of inflammation. IL-8 may also cause further autocrine and paracrine activation of additional PMN. Apart from its predominant role in neutrophil chemotaxis, IL-8 has also been shown to stimulate chemotaxis of a small proportion of resting T cells. IL-8 has a 10- to 100-fold increase in potency as a lymphocyte chemotoxin. This finding suggests that PMN may also have the potential to regulate recruitment of T cells to the site of an immune response (149). Production of IL-8 by PMN at in vivo sites of acute inflammation may have prolonged biological activity for the recruitment/activation of neutrophils, and it provides a further means to orchestrate the conventional immune response at sites of inflammation. Thus, PMN can no longer be viewed as only phagocytes or a warehouse for proteolytic enzymes, but as pivotal effector cells that are able to respond to mediators in their environment and to generate cytokines.

TNF production

Circulating PMN have been shown to be an excellent source of one of the most important immunoregulatory cytokines, TNF-α, albeit at a lower level than that produced by natural killer cells or monocytes. Medium-cultured PMN only have low, but detectable, TNF-α mRNA levels. Many stimulatory agents, such as IL-2 (150), IL-8 (150), GM-CSF (150,151), C. albicans (152), and LPS (152,153), are known to induce rapid TNF mRNA accumulation in human PMN, followed by TNF release. Incubation of PMN with C. albicans for 3 hours is sufficient for detection of TNF release by a biological lytic assay. The kinetics of TNF induction from PMN by C. albicans is the same as that from monocytes, with a steady increase from 8 to 18 hours. The release of TNF is by de novo synthesis because actinomycin D, which inhibits RNA synthesis, and blockers of protein synthesis (i.e., emetine and cycloheximide) can interfere with TNF production from PMN stimulated with *C. albicans*. The cytokine is typed to be TNF-α by specific neutralizing antibodies (152).

Recently, purified human peripheral blood PMN have been identified to express surface receptors for IL-2, but only IL-2Rβ and not IL-2Rα are present (53). PMN can therefore respond to stimulation by IL-2 with the induction of TNF-α. This IL-2–induced transcription in PMN peaks at 3 hours, is maintained for at least 18 hours, and is associated with release of TNF-α protein in the culture supernatant (150). Although the levels of TNF-α induced by IL-2 in PMN are much less than those detected in stimulated monocytes and large granular lymphocytes (154,155), they are in the range known to activate PMN function against microbes, pointing to the possible physiological importance of this cytokine in the neutrophil microenvironment. Enhancement of TNF-α gene expression induced by these stimuli is also affected by cycloheximide. Combination of GM-CSF with cycloheximide decreases the level of TNF-α mRNA by almost 90%, compared with that in cells treated with only GM-CSF. In contrast, cycloheximide slightly increases TNF-α mRNA in IL-8–treated PMN, but cycloheximide combination with *C. albicans* results in a significant superinduction of mRNA for TNF-α. These investigations indicate that modulation of TNF production by various stimuli is through different pathways.

TNF has been reported to have chemotactic property for PMN (94). Therefore, the finding of TNF production by PMN indicates that PMN may respond to stimuli by rapid TNF release at a level that may not be toxic, which cannot only activate PMN in an autocrine loop, but can also recruit neighboring PMN to the sites of inflammation. In addition, production of TNF-α by PMN may fulfil immunomodulatory functions similar to, and in concert with, IL-1, including induction of acute-phase proteins and stimulation of T cells.

Colony-stimulating factors

After stimulation with the calcium inophore, ionomycin, PMN can produce IL-3 and GM-CSF, although the amounts are less than those produced by monocytes and eosinophils. Thus, PMN may have a role in allergic inflammation, because IL-3 and GM-CSF are known to induce eosinophilopoiesis and to activate mature peripheral blood eosinophils in vitro (156). Stimulation of PMN with GM-CSF has also been shown to induce synthesis and release of G-CSF and M-CSF (132). Functional assays demonstrate that G-CSF and M-CSF produced from PMN are immunologically and biologically active. However, expression of these cytokines is dependent on stimulation by exogenous signals, preferentially provided by the T cell–derived lymphokine, GM-CSF. Stimulation of hema-

topoiesis and amplification of defense mechanisms after T-cell activation therefore might involve not only monocytes but also PMN. PMN arriving early at an inflammatory site may release M-CSF, thereby activating the more slowly invading monocytes, thus enhancing their survival and cytotoxic potential (8,157) and stimulating monocyte production of TNF-α (158). G-CSF production by PMN may further augment the proposed autoregulatory loop, thus increasing the pool of PMN progenitor cells, in addition to stimulating mature neutrophil functions, including phagocytosis and superoxide generation (138).

Interferon-α

Although IFN-α is generally known to be produced from viral-stimulated lymphoblastoid cells (159), a possibility still remains that IFN-α may also be produced by neutrophils, as suggested by the report that IFN-α can be produced by chronic myelogenous leukemia cells (160). This possibility has now been proven by Shirafuji and associates (161). Northern blot analysis shows that mRNA for human IFN-α becomes detectable in PMN stimulated with highly purified recombinant human G-CSF, but not with either LPS or FMLP. In addition, use of radioimmunoassay for human IFN-α shows that its level in culture medium of the rhG-CSF–treated PMN increases markedly in a time-dependent way. Blood neutrophils are normally maintained at very precise levels; elevated levels accompanying bacterial or fungal infection rapidly return to normal when the infection is eliminated. This phenomenon may be logically explained by the presence of inhibitors, such as IFN-α, that are triggered by increased neutropoiesis. Because IFN-α is shown to inhibit neutrophil colony formation (122,123), these findings suggest that the G-CSF/IFN-α system may participate in the feedback regulatory loop of neutropoiesis.

Interleukin-1 receptor antagonist

After appropriate stimulation, mononuclear phagocytes express a specific inhibitor of IL-1, now renamed IL-1 receptor antagonist (IL-1Ra), which serves as a negative regulator of inflammation. Following molecular cloning of the IL-1Ra (162), purified human peripheral blood PMN have been shown to express low but detectable levels of IL-1Ra mRNA, which can be considerably augmented after treatment with LPS, IL-4, GM-CSF, G-CSF, and TNF (163,164). The levels of induced IL-1Ra mRNA are comparable with those observed in LPS-stimulated human monocytes. In contrast, IL-1β, IL-8, IFN-γ, and FMLP fail to promote IL-1Ra expression in PMN. In addition, PMN also produce IL-1Ra protein. Secretion of IL-1Ra is induced in PMN treated with LPS, IL-4, and GM-CSF, but not by IL-1β, IFN-γ, and FMLP, thus yielding results that parallel those seen in Northern blot experiments (164). IL-1Ra has also been shown to be up-regulated in vivo during acute inflammation (165). As IL-1Ra blocks IL-1 activity both in vitro and in vivo, PMN, although exerting a series of proinflammatory activities, may also modulate the inflammatory potential of IL-1 in tissue and may possess the capacity to inhibit an established IL-1–mediated inflammatory response.

SUMMARY

This chapter outlines current evidence of the role of cytokines in neutrophil function. Cytokines selectively affect some of the following functions of the neutrophil: adherence, cell migration, phagocytosis, antibody-mediated neutrophil phagocytosis, respiratory burst, nonspecific and specific lysosomal enzyme release, cell surface receptor expression, and production of proteins, including other cytokines. These changes in PMN seem to be closely correlated with increased fungicidal, bactericidal, tumoricidal, and protozoacidal activity of cytokine-activated or primed neutrophils.

There is little doubt that a high degree of communication observed during an immune response occurs via sophisticated cell-to-cell, cell-to-cytokine, and cytokine-to-cytokine mediator circuits. A coordinated expression of specific signals is needed to orchestrate inflammation as the lesion is initiated, maintained, and finally resolved. The interaction of PMN and cytokines is much more complex than has been conventionally accepted. PMN can not only be activated by cytokines, but can also produce cytokines. These cytokines in turn affect function of local and neighboring PMN and many other immune and non-immune cells, including T cells, B cells, monocytes, and endothelial cells. Taken together, neutrophils are not only an end effector cell population, waiting for outside signals to mobilize and activate them, but are also active participants in the afferent phase of the immune response. This growing evidence suggests that PMN contribute significantly to both the afferent and the efferent limbs of the immune response.

REFERENCES

1. Steinbeck MJ, Roth JA. Neutrophil activation by recombinant cytokines. Rev Infect Dis 1989;2:549–567.

2. Kessel KPM, Verhoef J. A view to a kill: cytotoxic mechanisms of human polymorphonuclear leukocytes compared with monocytes and natural killer cells. Pathobiology 1990;58:249–264.

3. Lloyd AR, Oppenheim JJ. Poly's lament: the neglected role of the polymorphonuclear neutrophil in the afferent limb of the immune response. Immunol Today 1992;13:169–172.

4. Malech HL, Gallin JI. Neutrophils in human diseases. N Engl J Med 1987;317:687–694.

5. Rotrosen D, Gallin JI. Disorders of phagocyte function. Ann Rev Immunol 1987;5:127–150.

6. Cavallo F, Giovarelli M, Gulino A, et al. Role of neutrophils and CD4$^+$ T lymphocytes in the primary and memory response to nonimmunogenic murine mammary adenocarcinoma made immunogenic by IL-2 gene. J Immunol 1992;149:3627–3635.

7. Fady C, Reisser D, Martin F. Non-activated rat neutrophils kill syngeneic colon tumor cells by the release of a low molecular weight factor. Immunobiology 1990;181:1–12.

8. Clark SC, Kamen R. The human hematopoietic colony-stimulating factors. Science 1987;236:1229–1237.

9. Dipersio J, Billing P, Kaufman SE, Eghtesady P, Williams RE, Gasson JC. Characterization of the human granulocyte-macrophage colony-stimulating factor receptor. J Biol Chem 1988;263:1834–1841.

10. Gasson JC, Kaufman SE, Weibart RH, Tomonaga M, Golde DW. High-affinity binding of granulocyte-macrophage colony-stimulating factor to normal and leukemic human myeloid cells. Proc Natl Acad Sci USA 1986;83:669–673.

11. Clark SC. Biological activities of human granulocyte-macrophage colony-stimulating factor. J Cell Cloning 1988; 6:365–377.

12. Metcalf D. The granulocyte-macrophage colony-stimulating factors. Science 1985;229:16–22.

13. Metcalf D. The molecular biology and functions of the granulocyte-macrophage colony-stimulating factors. Blood 1986;67:257–267.

14. Metcalf D, Nicola NA. Proliferative effects of purified granulocyte colony-stimulating factor (G-CSF) on normal mouse hemopoietic cells. J Cell Physiol 1983;116:198–206.

15. Nomura H, Imazeki I, Oheda M, et al. Purification and characterization of human granulocyte colony-stimulating factor (G-CSF). EMBO J 1986;5:871–876.

16. Schrader JW. The panspecific hemoprotein of activated T lymphocytes (interleukin-3). Ann Rev Immunol 1986; 4:205–230.

17. Metcalf D. Colony stimulating factors and hemopoiesis. Ann Acad Med 1988;17:166–170.

18. Savill JS, Henson PM, Haslett C. Phagocytosis of aging human neutrophils by macrophages is mediated by a novel charge-sensitive recognition mechanism. J Clin Invest 1989;84:1518–1527.

19. Savill J, Dransfield I, Hogg N, Haslett C. Vitronectin receptor-mediated phagocytosis of cells undergoing apoptosis. Nature 1990;343:170–173.

20. Colotta F, Re F, Polentarutti N, Sozzani S, Mantovani A. Modulation of granulocyte survival and programmed cell death by cytokines and bacterial products. Blood 1992; 80:2012–2020.

21. Brach MA, deVos S, Gruss H-J, Herrmann F. Prolongation of survival of human polymorphonuclear neutrophils by granulocyte-macrophage colony-stimulating factor is caused by inhibition of programmed cell death. Blood 1992;80:2920–2924.

22. Lopez AF, Williamson DJ, Gamble JR, et al. Recombinant human granulocyte-macrophage colony-stimulating factor stimulates in vitro mature human neutrophil and eosino-

phil function, surface receptor expression, and survival. J Clin Invest 1986;78:1220–1228.

23. Weisbart RH, Golde DW, Clark SC, Wong GG, Gasson JC. Human granulocyte-macrophage colony-stimulating factor is a neutrophil activator. Nature 1985;314:361–363.

24. Metcalf D, Begley CJ, Johnson GR, et al. Biological properties in vitro of a recombinant human granulocyte-macrophage colony-stimulating factor. Blood 1986;67:37–45.

25. Kowanko IC, Ferrante A, Harvey DP, Carmen KL. Granulocyte-macrophage colony-stimulating factor augments neutrophil killing of Torulopsis glabrata and stimulates neutrophil respiratory burst and degranulation. Clin Exp Immunol 1991;83:225–230.

26. Weisbart RH, Kwan L, Golde DW, Gasson JC. Human GM-CSF primes neutrophils for enhanced oxidative metabolism in response to the major physiological chemoattractants. Blood 1987;69:18–21.

27. Jaswon MS, Khwaja A, Roberts PJ, Jones HM, Linch DC. The effects of rhGM-CSF on the neutrophil respiratory burst when studied in whole blood. Br J Hematol 1990; 75:181–187.

28. Watson F, Robinson JJ, Edwards SW. Neutrophil function in whole blood and after purification: changes in receptor expression, oxidase activity and responsiveness to cytokines. Biosci Rep 1992;12:123–133.

29. Sullian GW, Carper HT, Mandell GL. The effect of three human recombinant hematopoietic growth factors (granulocyte-macrophage colony-stimulating factor, granulocyte colony-stimulating factor, and interleukin-3) on phagocyte oxidative activity. Blood 1993;81:1863–1870.

30. Nathan CF. Respiratory burst in adherent human neutrophils: triggering by colony-stimulating factors GM-CSF and G-CSF. Blood 1989;73:301–306.

31. Lopez AF, To LB, Yang Y-C, et al. Stimulation of proliferation, differentiation, and function of human cells by primate interleukin 3. Proc Natl Acad Sci USA 1987;84:2761–2765.

32. Blanchard DK, Michelini-Norris MB, Djeu JY. Production of granulocyte-macrophage colony-stimulating factors by large granular lymphocytes stimulated with Candida albicans: role in activation of human neutrophil function. Blood 1991;77:2259–2265.

33. Djeu JY. Cytokines and anti-fungal immunity. Adv Exp Med Biol 1992;319:217–223.

34. Wang JM, Colella S, Allavena P, Mantovani A. Chemotactic activity of human recombinant granulocyte-macrophage colony stimulating factor. Immunology 1987;60:439–444.

35. Roilides E, Uhlig K, Venzon D, Pizzo PA, Walsh TJ. Neutrophil oxidative burst in response to Blastoconidia and pseudohyphea of Candida albicans: augmentation by granulocyte colony-stimulating factor and interferon-γ. J Infect Dis 1992;166:668–673.

36. Rolides E, Walsh TJ, Pizzo PA, Rubin M. Granulocyte colony-stimulating factor enhances the phagocytic and bactericidal activity of normal and defective human neutrophils. J Infect Dis 1991;163:579–583.

37. Conti P, Reale M, Barbacane RC, et al. Granulocyte-macrophage colony stimulating factor potentiates human polymorphonuclear leukocyte aggregation responses to formyl-methionyl-leucyl-phenylalanine. Immunol Lett 1992; 32:71–79.

38. Herrmann F, Lindemann A, Grauss J, Mertelsmann R. Cytokine-stimulation of prostaglandin synthesis from endogenous and exogenous arachidonic acids in polymorphonuclear leukocytes involving the activation and new synthesis of cyclooxygenase. Eur J Immunol 1990;20: 2513–2516.

39. Naccache PH, Faucher N, Borgeat P, Gasson JC, Dipersio JF. Granulocyte-macrophage colony stimulating factor modulates the excitation-response coupling sequence in human neutrophils. J Immunol 1988;140:3541–3546.

40. Sullivan R, Griffin JD, Simons ER, et al. Effects of recombinant human granulocyte and macrophage colony-stimulating factors on signal transduction pathways in human granulocytes. J Immunol 1987;139:3422–3430.

41. Gomez-Cambronero J, Huang CK, Gomez-Cambronero TM, Waterman WH, Becker EL, Sha'afi RI. Granulocyte-macrophage colony-stimulating factor-induced protein tyrosine phosphorylation of microtubule-associated protein kinase in human neutrophils. Proc Natl Acad Sci USA 1992;89:7551–7555.

42. Berkow RL. Granulocyte-macrophage colony-stimulating factor induces a staurosporine inhibitable tyrosine phosphorylation of unique neutrophil proteins. Blood 1992; 79:2446–2454.

43. Uings IJ, Thompson NT, Randall RW, et al. Tyrosine phosphorylation is involved in receptor coupling to phospholipase D but not phospholipase C in the human neutrophil. Biochem J 1992;281:597–600.

44. Dower SK, Kronheim SR, Hopp TP, et al. The cell surface receptor for interleukin-1 alpha and interleukin-1 beta are identical. Nature 1986;324:266–268.

45. Parker KP, Benjamin WR, Kaffka KL, Kilian PL. Presence of IL-1 receptors on human and murine neutrophils. Relevance to IL-1 mediated effects in inflammation. J Immunol 1989;142:537–542.

46. Seow WK, Thong YH, Ferrante A. Macrophage-neutrophil interactions: contrasting effects of the monokine interleukin-1 and tumor necrosis factor (cachectin) on human neutrophil adherence. Immunology 1988;82:357–361.

47. Sauder DN, Mounessa NL, Katz SI, Dinarello CA, Gallin JI. Chemotactic cytokines: the role of leukocytic pyrogen and epidermal cell thymocyte-activating factor in neutrophil chemotaxis. J Immunol 1984;132:828–832.

48. Ferrante A, Nandoskar M, Walz A, Goh DHB, Kowanko IC. Effects of tumor necrosis factor α and interleukin-1 α and β on human neutrophil migration, respiratory burst and degranulation. Int Arch Allergy Appl Immunol 1988; 86:82–91.

49. Figari IS, Mori NA, Palladino MA Jr. Regulation of neutrophil migration and superoxide production by recombinant tumor necrosis factor-α and β: comparison to recombinant interferon γ and interleukin-1α. Blood 1987;79:979–984.

50. Kharazmi A, Nielsen H, Bendtzen K. Recombinant interleukin-1α and beta prime human monocyte superoxide production but have no effect on chemotaxis and oxidative response of neutrophils. Immunobiology 1988;177:32–39.

51. Ozaki Y, Ohashi T, Kume S. Potentiation of neutrophil function by recombinant DNA-produced interleukin-1α. J Leukocyte Biol 1987;42:621–627.

52. Georgilis K, Schaefer C, Dinarello CA, Klempner MS. Human recombinant interleukin-1 β has no effect on intra-

cellular calcium or on functional responses of human neutrophils. J Immunol 1987;138:3403–3407.

53. Djeu JY, Liu JH, Wei S, et al. Function association with IL-2 receptor-β on human neutrophils. J Immunol 1993;150: 960–970.

54. Seow WK, Thong YH, McCormack JG, Ferrante A. Lymphocyte-neutrophil interactions: opposite effects of interleukin-2 and tumor necrosis factor-β on human neutrophil adherence. Int Arch Allergy Appl Immunol 1988;85:63–68.

55. Kowanko IC, Ferrante A. Interleukin-2 inhibits migration and stimulates the respiratory burst and degranulation of human neutrophils in vitro. Immunol Lett 1987;15:285–289.

56. Yoshimura T, Matsushima K, Oppenheim JJ, Leonard EJ. Neutrophil chemotactic factor produced by lipopolysaccharide (LPS)-stimulated human blood mononuclear leukocytes: partial characterization and separation from interleukin-1 (IL-1). J Immunol 1987;139:788–793.

57. Matsushima K, Oppenheim JJ. Interleukin-8 and MCAF: novel inflammatory cytokines inducible by IL-1 and TNF. Cytokine 1989;1:2–13.

58. Baggiolini M, Walz A, Kunkel SL. Neutrophil-activating peptide-1/interleukin-8, a novel cytokine that activates neutrophils. J Clin Invest 1989;84:1045–1049.

59. Westwick J, Li SW, Camp RD. Novel neutrophil-stimulating peptides. Immunol Today 1989;10:146–147.

60. Grob PM, David E, Warren TC, Deleon RP, Farina PR, Homon CA. Characteristic of a receptor for human monocyte-derived neutrophil chemotactic factor/interleukin-8. J Biol Chem 1990;265:8311–8316.

61. Murphy PM, Tiffany HL. Cloning of complementary DNA encoding a functional human interleukin-8 receptor. Science 1991;253:1280–1283.

62. Liu JH, Blanchard DK, Wei S, Djeu JY. Recombinant interleukin-8 induces changes in cytosolic Ca²⁺ in human neutrophils. J Infect Dis 1992;166:1089–1092.

63. Peveri P, Walz A, Dewald B, Baggiolini M. A novel neutrophil-activating factor produced by human mononuclear phagocytes. J Exp Med 1988;167:1547–1559.

64. Yoshimura T, Matsushima K, Robinson EA, Appella E, Oppenheim JJ, Leonard EJ. Purification of a human monocyte-derived neutrophil chemotactic factor that has peptide sequence similarity to other host defense cytokine. Proc Natl Acad Sci USA 1987;84:9233–9237.

65. Rot A. Endothelial cell binding of NAP-1/IL-8: role in neutrophil emigration. Immunol Today 1992;13:291–294.

66. Carveth HJ, Bohnsack JF, McIntyre TM, Baggiolini M, Prescott SM, Zimmerman GA. Neutrophil activating factor (NAF) induces polymorphonuclear leukocyte adherence to endothelial cells and to subendothelial matrix proteins. Biochem Biophys Res Commun 1989;162:387–393.

67. Stoolman LM. Adhesion molecules involved in leukocytes recruitment and lymphocyte circulation. Chest 1993; 103:79s–86s.

68. Smith WB, Gamble JR, Clark-Lewis I, Vadas MA. Interleukin-8 induces neutrophil transendothelial migration. Immunology 1991;72:65–72.

69. Luscinskas FW, Kiely JM, Ding H, et al. In vitro inhibitory effect of IL-8 and other chemoattractants on neutrophil-endothelial interactions. J Immunol 1992;149:2163–2171.

70. Detmers PA, Lo SK, Olsen-Egbert E, Walz A, Baggiolini M, Cohn ZA. Neutrophil-activating-protein 1/interleukin 8 stimulates the binding activity of the leukocyte adhesion receptor CD11b/CD18 on human neutrophils. J Exp Med 1990;171:1155–1162.

71. Paccaud JP, Schifferli JA, Baggiolini M. NAP-1/IL-8 induces up-regulation of CR-1 receptors in human neutrophil leukocytes. Biochem Biophys Res Commun 1990;166:187–192.

72. Fearon DT. Identification of the membrane glycoprotein that is the C3b receptor of the human erythrocyte, polymorphonuclear leukocyte, B lymphocyte, and monocyte. J Exp Med 1980;152:20–30.

73. Fearon DT, Collins LA. Increased expression of C3b receptors on polymorphonuclear leukocytes induced by chemotactic factors and by purification procedures. J Immunol 1983;130:370–375.

74. Djeu JY, Matsushima K, Oppenheim JJ, Shiotsuki K, Blanchard DK. Functional activation of human neutrophils by recombinant monocyte-derived neutrophil chemotactic factor/IL-8. J Immunol 1990;144:2205.

75. Yuo A, Kitagawa S, Kasahara T, Matsushima K, Saito M, Takaku F. Stimulation and priming of human neutrophils by interleukin-8: cooperation with tumor necrosis factor and colony-stimulating factors. Blood 1991;78:2708–2714.

76. Pennica D, Nedwin GE, Hayflick, JS, et al. Human tumor necrosis factor: precursor structure, expression and homology to lymphotoxin. Nature 1984;312:724–729.

77. Shalaby MR, Palladin MA, Hirabayashi SE, et al. Receptor binding and activation of polymorphonuclear neutrophils by tumor necrosis factor-alpha. J Leukocyte Biol 1987; 41:196–204.

78. Tsujimoto M, Yip YK, Vilcek J. Tumor necrosis factor: specific binding and internalization in sensitive and resistant cells. Proc Natl Acad Sci USA 1985;82:7626–7630.

79. Beutler B, Mahoney J, Le Trang N, Pekala P, Cerami A. Purification of cachectin, a lipoprotein lipase-suppressing hormone secreted by endotoxin-induced RAW 264.7 cells. J Exp Med 1985;161:984–995.

80. Picheangkul S, Schick D, Jia F, Berent S, Bollon A. Binding of tumor necrosis factor alpha (TNFα) to high-affinity receptors on polymorphonuclear cells. Exp Hematol 1987;15:1055–1059.

81. Klebanoff SJ, Vadas MA, Harland JM, et al. Stimulation of neutrophils by tumor necrosis factors. J Immunol 1986; 136:4220–4225.

82. Shalaby MR, Aggarwal BB, Rinderknecht E, Svedersky LP, Finkle BS, Palladino MA Jr. Activation of human polymorphonuclear neutrophil functions by interferon-gamma and tumor necrosis factors. J Immunol 1985;135:2069–2073.

83. Perussia B, Kobayashi M, Rossi ME, Anegon I, Trinchieri G. Immune interferon enhanced properties of lymphotoxin, tumor necrosis factor, and granulocyte macrophage colony-stimulating factor. J Immunol 1987;138:765–774.

84. Naworth PP, Stern DM. Modulation of endothelial cell hemostatic properties by tumor necrosis factor. J Exp Med 1986;163:740–745.

85. Ferrante A, Abell TJ. Conditioned medium from stimulated mononuclear leukocyte augments human neutrophil mediated-killing of a virulent Acantheamoeba. Infect Immun 1986;51:607–617.

86. Ferrante A, Harvey D, Bates EJ. Staphylococcus aureus stimulated PMN conditioned medium increases the neutrophil bactericidal activity, and augments the oxygen radical production and degranulation in response to the bacteria. Clin Exp Immunol 1989;78:366–371.

87. Ferrante A. Augmentation of neutrophil responses to Neagleria fowleri by tumor necrosis factor alpha. Infect Immun 1989;57:3110–3115.

88. Djeu JY, Blanchard DK, Halkias H, Friedman H. Growth inhibition of Candida albicans by human polymorphonuclear neutrophils: activation by interferon-γ and tumor necrosis factor. J Immunol 1986;137:2980–2984.

89. Ferrante A. Tumor necrosis factor alpha potentiates neutrophil antimicrobial activity: increased fungicidal activity against Torulopsis glabrata/Candida albicans and associated increases in oxygen radical production and lysosomal enzyme release. Infect Immun 1989;57:2115–2122.

90. Ferrante A. Activation of neutrophils by interleukins-1 and -2 and tumor necrosis factors. Immunol Series 1992; 57:417–436.

91. Ferrante A, Kumaratilake L, Rzepczyk CM, Dayer JM. Killing of Plasmodium falciparum by cytokine activated effector cells (neutrophils and macrophages). Immunol Lett 1990;25:179–187.

92. Denis M, Chadee K. Human neutrophils activated by interferon-γ and tumor necrosis factor-α kill Entamoeba histolytica trophozoite in vitro. J Leukocyte Biol 1989; 46:270–274.

93. Beutler B, Cerami A. The biology of cachectin/TNF—a primary mediator of the host response. Ann Rev Immunol 1989;7:625–655.

94. Wang JM, Bersani L, Mantovani A. Tumor necrosis factor is chemotactic for monocytes and polymorphonuclear leukocytes. J Immunol 1987;138:1469–1474.

95. Figari IS, Mori NA, Palladino MA Jr. Regulation of neutrophil migration and superoxide production by recombinant tumor necrosis factors-α and β: comparison to recombinant interferon-γ and interleukin-1α. Blood 1987;70:979–984.

96. Ferrante A, Kowanko IC, Bates EJ. Mechanisms of host tissue damage by cytokine-activated neutrophils. Immunol Series 1992;57:499–521.

97. Kowanko IC, Bates EJ, Ferrante A. Tumor necrosis factor-β modulates human neutrophil-mediated cartilage damage. Scand J Immunol 1988;28:591–598.

98. Kowanko IC, Bates EJ, Ferrante A. Neutrophil-mediated cartilage injury in vitro is enhanced by tumor necrosis factor α. Rheumatol Int 1990;10:85–90.

99. Berger M, Wetzler EM, Wallis RS. Tumor necrosis factor is the major monocyte product that increases complement receptor expression on mature human neutrophils. Blood 1988;71:151–158.

100. Gamble JR, Harlan JM, Klebanoff SJ, Vadas NA. Stimulation of the adherence of neutrophils to umbilical vein endothelium by human recombinant tumor necrosis factor. Proc Natl Acad Sci USA 1985;82:8667–8671.

101. Lo SK, Detmers PA, Levin SM, Wright SD. Transient adhesion of neutrophils to endothelium. J Exp Med 1989; 169:1779–1793.

102. Shau H. Characteristics and mechanism of neutrophil-mediated cytostasis induced by tumor necrosis factor. J Immunol 1988;141:234–240.

103. Varani J, Bendelow MJ, Sealey DE, et al. Tumor necrosis factor enhances susceptibility of vascular endothelium to neutrophil mediated killing. Lab Invest 1988;59:292–295.

104. Williams JG, Jurkovich GJ, Maier RV. Interferon-γ: a key immunoregulatory lymphokine. J Surg Res 1993;54:79–93.

105. Zoon KC, Arnheiter H, Fitzgerald D. Procedures for measuring receptor-mediated binding and internalization. Methods Enzymol 1986;119:332–339.

106. Finbloom DS. The interferon-gamma receptor on human monocytes, monocyte-like cells and polymorphonuclear leukocytes. Biochem Soc Trans 1990;18:222–224.

107. Bielefeldt Ohmann H, Babiuk LA. Alteration of some leukocyte functions following in vivo and in vitro exposure to recombinant bovine alpha- and gamma-interferon. J Interferon Rev 1986;6:123–136.

108. Petroni KC, Shen L, Guyre PM. Modulation of human polymorphonuclear leukocyte IgG Fc receptors and Fc-mediated functions by IFN-γ and glucocorticoids. J Immunol 1988;140:3467–3472.

109. Perussia B, Dayton ET, Lazarus R, Fanning V, Trinchieri G. Immune interferon induces the receptor for monomeric IgG1 on human monocytic and myeloid cells. J Exp Med 1983;158:1092–1113.

110. Hokland P, Berg K. Interferon enhances the antibody-dependent cellular cytotoxicity (ADCC) of human polymorphonuclear leukocytes. J Immunol 1981;127:1585–1588.

111. Basham TY, Smith WK, Merigan TC. Interferon enhances antibody-dependent cellular cytotoxicity when suboptimal concentrations of antibody are used. Cell Immunol 1984; 88:393–400.

112. Shen L, Guyre PM, Fanger MW. Polymorphonuclear leukocyte function triggered through the high affinity Fc receptor for monomeric IgG. J Immunol 1987;139:534–538.

113. Kowanko IC, Ferrante A. Stimulation of neutrophil respiratory burst and lysosomal enzyme release by human interferon-gamma. Immunology 1987;62:149–151.

114. Cassatella MA, Cappelli R, Della Bianca V, Grzeskowiak M, Dusi S, Berton G. Interferon-gamma activates human neutrophil oxygen metabolism and exocytosis. Immunology 1988;63:499–506.

115. Humphreys JM, Hughes V, Edwards SW. Stimulation of protein synthesis in human neutrophils by γ-interferon. Biochem Pharmacol 1989;38:1241–1246.

116. Suzuki K, Furui H, Kaneko M, Takagi K, Satake T. Priming effect of recombinant human interleukin-2 and recombinant human interferon-gamma on human neutrophil superoxide production. Arzneimittelforschung 1990; 40:1176–1179.

117. Perussia B, Kobayashi M, Rossi ME, Anegon I, Trinchieri G. Immune interferon enhances functional properties of human granulocytes: role of Fc receptors and effect of lymphotoxin, tumor necrosis factor, and granulocyte-macrophage colony-stimulating factor. J Immunol 1987; 138:765–774.

118. Berton G, Zeni L, Cassatella MA, Rossi F. Gamma interferon is able to enhance the oxidative metabolism of human neutrophils. Biochem Res Commun 1986; 138: 1276–1282.

119. Newburger PE, Ezekowitz RAB, Whitney C, Wright J, Orkin SH. Induction of phagocyte cytochrome b heavy chain gene expression by interferon γ. Proc Natl Acad Sci USA 1988;85:5215–5219.

120. Newburger PE, Ezekowitz RAB. Cellular and molecular effects of recombinant interferon gamma in chronic granulomatous disease. Hematol Oncol Clin North Am 1988; 2:267–276.

121. Klebanoff SJ, Olszowski S, Van Voorhis WC, Ledbetter JA, Waltersdorph AM, Schlechte KG. Effects of γ-interferon on human neutrophils: protection from deterioration on storage. Blood 1992;80:225–234.

122. Edwards SW, Say JE, Hughes V. Gamma interferon enhances the killing of Staphylococcus aureus by human neutrophils. J Gen Microbiol 1988;134:37–42.

123. Geertsma MF, Nibbering PH, Pos O, van Furth R. Interferon-γ activated human granulocytes kill ingested Mycobacterium fortuitum more efficiently than normal granulocytes. Eur J Immunol 1990;20:869–873.

124. Morrison CJ, Stevens DA. Enhanced killing of Blastomyces dermatitidis by gamma interferon-activated murine peripheral blood polymorphonuclear neutrophils. Int J Immunopharmacol 1989;11:855–862.

125. Kowanko IC, Ferrante A. Interferon-gamma increases human neutrophil-mediated cartilage proteoglycan degradation. Clin Exp Rheumatol 1992;10:123–129.

126. Greenberg PL, Mosny SA. Cytotoxic effects of interferon in vitro on granulocytic progenitor cells. Cancer Res 1977; 37:1794–1799.

127. Gutterman JU, Blumenschein GR, Alexanian R, et al. Leukocyte interferon-induced tumor regression in human metastatic breast cancer, multiple myeloma, and malignant lymphoma. Ann Intern Med 1980;93:399–406.

128. Fady C, Reisser D, Martin F. Non-activated rat neutrophils kill syngeneic colon tumor cells by the release of a low molecular weight factor. Immunobiology 1990;181:1–12.

129. Barker E, Reisfeld RA. A mechanism for neutrophil-mediated lysis of human neutroblastoma cells. Cancer Res 1993; 53:362–367.

130. Naworth PP, Stern DM. Modulation of endothelial cell hemostatic properties by tumor necrosis factor. J Exp Med 1986;163:740–745.

131. Cominelli F, Nast CC, Clark BD, et al. IL1 gene expression, synthesis and effect of specific IL1 receptor blockade in rabbit immune complex colitis. J Clin Invest 1990;86:972–980.

132. Tiku J, Tiku ML, Skosey JL. Interleukin-1 production by human polymorphonuclear neutrophils. J Immunol 1986; 136:3677–3685.

133. Lindemann A, Riedel D, Oster W, et al. Granulocyte/macrophage colony-stimulatory factor induces interleukin-1 production by human polymorphonuclear neutrophils. J Immunol 1988;140:837–839.

134. Lord PCW, Wilmoth LMG, Mizel SB, McCall CE. Expression of interleukin-1 α and β genes by human blood polymorphonuclear leukocytes. J Clin Invest 1991;87: 1312–1321.

135. Marucha PT, Zeff RA, Kreutzer DL. Cytokine regulation of IL-1β gene expression in the human polymorphonuclear leukocytes. J Immunol 1990;145:2932–2937.

136. Marucha PT, Zeff RA, Kreutzer DL. Cytokine-induced IL-1β gene expression in the human polymorphonuclear leukocyte. J Immunol 1991;147:2603–2608.

137. Palma, C, Cassone A, Serbousek D, Perason CA, Djeu JY. Lactoferrin release and interleukin-1, -6, and tumor necrosis factor production by human polymorphonuclear cells stimulated by various lipopolysaccharide: relationship to growth inhibition of Candida albicans. Infect Immun 1992; 60:4604–4611.

138. Dinarello CA. Interleukin-1 and interleukin-1 antagonism. Blood 1991;77:1627–1652.

139. Nicola NA. Hemopoietic cell growth factors and their receptors. Annu Rev Biochem 1989;58:45–77.

140. Ikebuchi K, Wong GG, Clark SG, Ihle JN, Hirai Y, Ogawa M. Interleukin-6 enhancement of interleukin 3-dependent proliferation of multipotential hemopoietic progenitors. Proc Natl Acad Sci USA 1987;84:9035–9039.

141. Melani C, Mattia GF, Silvani A, et al. Interleukin-6 expression in human neutrophil and eosinophil peripheral blood granulocytes. Blood 1993;81:2744–2749.

142. Cicco NA, Lindemann A, Content J, et al. Inducible production of interleukin-6 by human polymorphonuclear neutrophils: role of granulocyte; macrophage colony-stimulatory factor and tumor necrosis factor-alpha. Blood 1990;75:2049–2052.

143. Van Snick J. Interleukin-6: an overview. Ann Rev Immunol 1990;8:253–278.

144. Kishimoto T. The biology of interleukin-6. Blood 1989; 74:1–10.

145. Strieter RM, Kasahara K, Allen RM, Showell HJ, Standiford TJ, Kunkel SL. Human neutrophils exhibit disparate chemotactic factor gene expression. Biochem Biophys Res Commun 1990;173:725–730.

146. Strieter RM, Kasahara K, Allen RM, et al. Cytokine-induced neutrophil-derived interleukin-8. Am J Pathol 1992; 141:397–407.

147. Cassatella MA, Bazzoni F, Ceska M, Ferro I, Baggiolini M, Berton G. IL-8 production by human polymorphonuclear leukocytes. The chemoattractant formyl-methionyl-leucyl-phenylalanine induces the gene expression and release of IL-8 through a pertussis toxin-sensitive pathway. J Immunol 1992;148:3216–3220.

148. Bazzoni F, Cassatella MA, Rossi F, Ceska M, Dewald B, Baggiolini M. Phagocytosing neutrophils produce and release high amounts of the neutrophil-activating peptide-1/interleukin 8. J Exp Med 1991;173:771–774.

149. Cassatella MA, Guasparri I, Ceska M, Bazzoni F, Rossi F. Interferon-gamma inhibits interleukin-8 production by human polymorphonuclear leukocytes. Immunology 1993;78:177–184.

150. Larsen CG, Anderson AO, Appella E, Oppenheim JJ, Matsushima K. Neutrophil activating protein (NAP-1) is also chemotactic for T-lymphocytes. Science 1989; 243:1464–1466.

151. Wei S, Blanchard DK, Liu JH, Leonard WJ, Djeu JY. Activation of tumor necrosis factor-α production from human neutrophils by IL-2 via IL-2Rβ. J Immunol 1993; 150:1979–1987.

152. Lindemann A, Riedel D, Oster W, Ziegler-Heitbrock HW, Mertelsmann R, Herrmann F. Granulocyte-macrophage colony-stimulating factor induces cytokine secretion by

human polymorphonuclear leukocytes. J Clin Invest 1989; 83:1308–1312.

153. Djeu JY, Serbousek D, Blanchard DK. Release of tumor necrosis factor by human polymorphonuclear leukocytes. Blood 1990;76:1405–1409.

154. Dubravec DB, Spriggs DR, Mannick JA, Rodrick ML. Circulating human peripheral blood granulocytes synthesize and secrete tumor necrosis factor α. Proc Natl Acad Sci USA 1990;87:6758–6761.

155. Djeu JY, Blanchard DK, Richards AL, Friedman H. Tumor necrosis factor induction by Candida albicans from human natural killer cells and monocytes. J Immunol 1988; 141:4047–4052.

156. Michelini-Norris MB, Blanchard DK, Friedman H, Djeu JY. TNF induction by Mycobacterium avium intracellular: involvement of HLA-DR⁺ large granular lymphocytes and monocytes. J Leukocyte Biol 1991;50:529–538.

157. Kita H, Ohnishi T, Okubo Y, Weiler D, Abrams JS, Gleich GJ. Granulocyte/macrophage colony-stimulating factor and interleukin 3 release from human peripheral blood eosinophils and neutrophils. J Exp Med 1991;174:745–748.

158. Tushinski RJ, Oliver IT, Guilbert LJ, Tynan PW, Warner JR, Stanley ER. Survival of mononuclear phagocytes depends on a lineage-specific growth factor that the differentiated cells selectively destroy. Cell 1982;28:71–81.

159. Warren MK, Palph P. Macrophage growth factor CSF-1 stimulates human monocyte production of interferon, tumor necrosis factor, and colony stimulating activity. J Immunol 1986;137:2281–2285.

160. Cantell K, Hirvonen S, Kauppinen H-L, Myllyla G. Production of interferon in human leukocytes from normal donors with the use of Sendai virus. Meth Enzymol 1981;78:29–38.

161. Rubinstein M, Levy WP, Moschera JA, et al. Human leukocyte interferon: isolation and characterization of several molecular forms. Arch Biochem Biophys 1981;210:307–318.

162. Shirafuji N, Matsuda S, Ogura H, et al. Granulocyte colony-stimulating factor stimulates human mature neutrophilic granulocytes to produce interferon α. Blood 1990;75:17–19.

163. Eisenberg SP, Evans RJ, Arend WP, et al. Primary structure and functional expression from complementary DNA of a human interleukin-1 receptor antagonist. Nature 1990; 343:341–343.

164. Ulich TR, Guo K, Yin S, et al. Endotoxin-induced cytokine gene expression in vivo. IV. Expression of interleukin-1 alpha/beta and interleukin-1 receptor antagonist mRNA during endotoxemia and during endotoxin-initiated local acute inflammation. Am J Pathol 1992;141:61–68.

165. Re F, Mengozzi M, Muzio M, Dinarello CA, Mantovani A, Collotta F. Expression of interleukin-1 receptor antagonist (IL-1Ra) by human circulating polymorphonuclear cells. Eur J Immunol 1993;23:570–573.

166. Ulich TR, Yin SM, Guo KZ, del Castillo J, Eisenberg SP, Thompson RC. The intratracheal administration of endotoxin and cytokines. III. The interleukin-1 receptor antagonist inhibits endotoxin- and IL-1–induced acute inflammation. Am J Pathol 1991;138:521–524.

CHAPTER 6

ROLE OF CYTOKINES
IN MAST CELL FUNCTIONS

Parris R. Burd

Mast cell–associated mediators have been divided historically into preformed mediators, such as histamine and proteases, which are stored in cytoplasmic granules and released upon cellular activation, and the newly synthesized mediators, such as the sulfidopeptide leukotrienes and prostaglandins, which are not preformed and stored but rather are produced and secreted following cellular activation (1,2). During the past few years, however, the immunoregulatory functions of mast cells have undergone a radical reassessment. It is now well established that mast cells possess the biological capability to initiate or modulate a wide variety of immunological processes through production of an array of multifunctional cytokines that act on diverse targets throughout the body. The combined biological potentials for these cytokines argue that mast cells have important roles in many adaptive or pathological responses. Examples of such responses include regulation of mast-cell proliferation and phenotype; contributing or responding to microenvironmental influences; modulation of leukocyte effector function; regulation of immunoglobulin E (IgE) production; and numerous aspects of inflammation, clotting, angiogenesis, wound repair, tissue and bone remodeling, and pathological fibrosis.

This review focuses on identification of cytokines produced by mast cells and basophils of rodent and human origin in response to signals delivered through IgE and other receptors and presents recent advances in our understanding of the possible ways mast cells may participate in immunoregulation.

ORIGIN, DISTRIBUTION, AND FUNCTION OF MAST CELLS AND BASOPHILS

Mast cells and basophils arise from hematopoietic precursors, and they express on their surfaces a high affinity receptor for binding the Fc portion of the IgE antibody, termed $Fc_{\epsilon}RI$ (3). Expression of $Fc_{\epsilon}RI$ was initially thought to be restricted to mast cells and basophils, but recent studies indicate that other cell types may express it, including Langerhans cells, eosinophils, monocytes, and macrophages (4–6).

When IgE antibodies bound to $Fc_{\epsilon}RI$ on mast cells and basophils encounter specific multivalent antigen, a signaling cascade is initiated, which results in characteristic morphological and biochemical changes, termed *anaphylactic degranulation*. Although the panel of biologically active mediators released by each type of cell is similar, but not identical, they differ in their responses to some activating agents and in many aspects of their morphology, natural history, and cell surface structures (Table 6–1) (3).

Mast cells are found throughout the body, but espe-

TABLE 6–1 NATURAL HISTORY, MAJOR MEDIATORS, AND SURFACE-MEMBRANE
STRUCTURES OF MAST CELLS AND BASOPHILS*

Characteristic	Mast Cells	Basophils
Natural history		
Origin of precursor cells	Bone marrow	Bone marrow
Site of maturation	Connective tissue	Bone marrow
Mature cells in circulation	No	Yes (usually <1% blood, leukocytes)
Recruitment of mature cells into tissue from circulation	No	Yes (during inflammatory or immunological responses)
Residence of mature cells in connective tissues	Yes	No
Proliferative response of mature cells	Yes, but only under certain circumstances	No
Life span	Weeks to months (rodent studies)	Days (like other granulocytes)
Mediators		
Mediators preformed and stored in granules	Histamine, heparin, chondroitin sulfate, neutral proteases, acid hydrolases, cathepsin G, carboxypeptidase, vasoactive intestinal peptide, TNF-α	Histamine, chrondroitin sulfate, neutral protease with bradykinin-generating activity, β-glucuronidase, elastase, cathepsin G-like enzyme, major basic protein, Charcot-Leyden crystal protein, vasoactive intestinal peptide
Major lipid mediator following activation	Prostaglandin D_2, leukotriene C_4, platelet-activating factor	Leukotriene C_4
Cytokines released following activation	Many (see text and Table 6–2)	IL-4, IL-8
Surface structures		
Ig receptors	$Fc_\varepsilon RI$, $Fc_\gamma RIIb1$, $Fc_\gamma RIIb2$, $Fc_\gamma RIII$	$Fc_\varepsilon RI$, $Fc_\gamma RII$ (CD32)
Cytokine receptors	Receptors for IL-3, IL-4, IL-9, IL-10, c-kit (CD117), β-chemokines	Receptors for IL-2, IL-3, IL-4, IL-5, IL-8, α- and β-chemokines
Integrin** and other receptors	Functional integrin receptors for LN, FN, VN (CD29, CD49d, e, CD61, CD51), LFA-2, LFA-3, ICAM-1 (CD54), CD44, CD40 ligand, endothelin receptor A, CD21	Functional receptors for LM, CO, FN (CD29, CD49b, d, e, CD11a, b, c, CD18), CD40 ligand

*Adapted from (84)
Galli SJ. New concepts about the mast cell. N Engl J Med 1993; 328:257.
**LN = laminin; FN = fibronectin; CO = collagen; VN = vitronectin.

cially at sites of environmental contact: connective tissues and especially beneath the skin; respiratory, gastrointestinal, and urogenital tracts; adjacent to blood and lymphatic vessels; and near or within peripheral nerves. This distribution places mast cells near parasites, pathogens, and environmental antigens that come in contact with the skin or mucosa. In turn, mast-cell products are then available to a wide range of cells within these organ systems.

Mast cells exhibit heterogeneity not only when com-

pared at different anatomical sites, but also within individual anatomical sites and over time. This phenotypic plasticity includes differences in mediators and individual granule constituents and responsiveness to particular pharmacological agents. Many factors may modulate this heterogeneity and include effects of cytokines and components of the particular microenvironment. Thus, the mast cell is able to respond to and modify its functions in response to microenvironmental influences.

MAST CELLS AS A SOURCE
OF MULTIFUNCTIONAL CYTOKINES

The first direct evidence that mast cells could produce a cytokine was obtained from studies of the ability of the v-abl oncogene to immortalize cell lines capable of growth in the absence of exogenously added growth factor (7). Following transformation of hematopoietic multilineage colonies with Abelson murine leukemia virus (A-MuLV), several of the resultant transformed mast-cell lines were found to contain messenger RNA (mRNA) for granulocyte-macrophage colony-stimulating factor (GM-CSF) and to release bioactive GM-CSF, as demonstrated by growth of FDC-P1 cells in the presence of excess neutralizing anti-interleukin-3 (IL-3) antibody. IL-3 mRNA or bioactivity was not observed in these cell lines.

Subsequent studies showed that nine of 15 fetal liver-derived mouse mast-cell lines arising spontaneously or following infection with A-MuLV constitutively expressed mRNA for IL-4 and that some of them constitutively released bioactive IL-4 (8). In contrast, only several of the lines expressed mRNA for GM-CSF or IL-3. IL-4 mRNA but not bioactivity was also detected at low levels in five IL-3–dependent mast-cell lines. Further characterization of the A-MuLV–transformed mast-cell lines showed that some of these lines constitutively produced IL-3 and GM-CSF mRNA and bioactivities, as well as a bioactivity similar to that of IL-6 and another substance with growth factor activity for pre-B cells (9). Thus, many individual virally transformed mast-cell lines constitutively produced IL-4, but these lines varied in their ability to produce IL-3 or GM-CSF.

The first cytokine bioactivity to be associated clearly with normal mast cells was tumor necrosis factor-α (TNF-α)/cachectin and was based on the initial observation that purified murine peritoneal mast cells were cytotoxic for certain specific target cells (10). Subsequent investigators defined the specificity of mast cell–mediated killing using IL-3–dependent bone marrow–derived cultured mast cells (BMMC) and mouse peritoneal mast cells as a natural cytotoxic activity, rather than a natural killer activity based on the ability of these cells to lyse WEHI-164 but not YAC-1 target cells (11,12). Augmentation of killing was shown to occur following crosslinkage of surface IgE receptors (13).

IL-3–dependent mouse natural cytotoxic cells generated in vitro were subsequently shown to be similar to IL-3–dependent mast cells isolated by similar culture conditions (14–16). Following the realization that mast cell- and TNF-α–mediated cytotoxicities were similar, anti-TNF-α antibodies were found to block partially mast-cell cytotoxicity, and new protein synthesis was not required for expression of this cytotoxicity. Thus, mast cell natural cytotoxicity appeared to be mediated through a TNF-α–like molecule that was preformed and stored in the cytoplasmic compartment.

Confirmation of this finding was obtained by several groups (17–20). Young and colleagues (17) demonstrated that mouse peritoneal mast cells, as well as IL-3–dependent and IL-3–independent mouse mast-cell lines contained cytoplasmic granule-associated TNF-α–like activity, which could be released following stimulation with phorbol 12-myristate 13-acetate (PMA) and concanavalin A or lipopolysaccharide (LPS). Immunoblot analysis and affinity purification with anti-TNF-α antibodies demonstrated a single band of 50 kd, consistent with the size of trimeric TNF-α. Definitive proof of the identity of TNF-α as the mediator of mast cell natural cytotoxicity was achieved when resident mouse peritoneal mast cells were shown to contain constitutively large amounts of TNF-α bioactivity, which was released immediately in response to IgE-dependent activation and was followed by secretion of newly synthesized TNF-α (21). Thus, mast cells possess the ability to release TNF-α immediately following activation as a preformed product, followed by sustained and prolonged secretion of newly synthesized protein. In fact, mouse peritoneal mast cells contain approximately twice as much preformed TNF-α bioactivity as LPS-stimulated mouse peritoneal macrophages. In addition, mast cells produce nitric oxide through constitutive nitric oxide synthase, which augments TNF-α–mediated cytotoxicity by approximately one third (22).

Elucidation of the potential roles mast cell TNF-α production might have in vivo comes from studies of mast cell–deficient mice. Gordon and Galli (23) showed that TNF-α mRNA levels were significantly higher at sites of passive cutaneous anaphylaxis in normal animals compared with mast cell–deficient mice (WBB6F$_1$–W/W^v). Wershil and associates (24) demonstrated that this response could be repaired by adoptive transfer of normal mast cells into the mast cell–deficient animals and that mast cells were essential for both early and late phases of tissue swelling and neutrophil infiltration associated with IgE-dependent reactions in the skin. They further demonstrated that local administration of anti-TNF-α antibodies inhibited 50% of this infiltration, indicating that TNF-α is a primary but not the only component leading to leukocyte infiltration during passive cutaneous anaphylaxis.

Zhang and coworkers (25) showed that neutrophil recruitment during immune complex peritonitis is mediated by mast cells through production of TNF-α. Induction of an IgG-mediated, reverse passive Arthus reaction in the peritoneum of normal mice, but not mast cell–deficient mice, resulted in rapid (within 5 minutes) release of TNF-α, followed by infiltration of neutrophils and subsequent high level TNF-α production. Repair of the mast-cell deficiency by adoptive transfer of normal mast cells reconstituted the effect in the mast cell–deficient mice.

Moreover, use of a specific leukotriene synthesis inhibitor suggested that mast-cell leukotrienes are also required, in addition to TNF-α, for subsequent neutrophil-mediated TNF-α production.

CYTOKINE PRODUCTION IN RESPONSE TO IGE-MEDIATED SIGNALS

The demonstration that the IL-3, IL-4, and GM-CSF genes were transcriptionally active and that bioactivity was secreted from a variety of mast-cell lines led various investigators to embark on an examination of the transcriptional responsiveness of cytokine genes in mast cells to signals transduced through the high affinity IgE receptor (Fc$_\epsilon$RI) or pharmacological agents. In most cases, steady-state levels of mRNA were examined rather than determining the contributions of de novo transcription rates versus message stabilization to mRNA accumulation (26). For most of these studies, the primary goal was to determine the spectrum of cytokines that could be expressed in mast cells to begin a determination of the mast cell's role in immunoregulatory processes. The accumulated results of these studies (Table 6–2) indicate that the mast cell represents a biologically important source of multifunctional cytokines that may augment or even supplant other immunological sources of these im-

TABLE 6–2 CYTOKINES DETECTED IN HUMAN AND RODENT MAST CELLS

Cytokine	mRNA Detected	Bioactivity
IL-1α	Yes	Yes
IL-1β	Yes	Yes
IL-2	Yes	No
IL-3	Yes	Yes
IL-4	Yes	Yes
IL-5	Yes	Yes
IL-6	Yes	Yes
IL-7	Yes	ND
IL-8 (α-chemokine)	Yes	Yes
IL-9	?	?
IL-10	Yes	ND
IL-11	Yes	ND
IL-12	No	ND
IL-13	Yes	Yes
GM-CSF	Yes	Yes
LIF	Yes	Yes
TNF-α	Yes	Yes
IFN-γ	Yes	ND
α-chemokines		
MIG	Yes	ND
IP-10	Yes	ND
β-chemokines		
MCP-1/JE	Yes	ND
MIP-1α	Yes	ND
MIP-1β	Yes	ND
TCA-3/I309	Yes	ND
RANTES	Yes	ND
MARC/FIC	Yes	ND
Endothelin-1	Yes	Yes
TGF-β	Yes	ND

ND = not done.
See text for abbreviations.

munoregulatory molecules under certain circumstances. Currently, however, little information exists regarding regulation and production of these factors in vivo.

Following the realization that TNF-α–like activity could be released from mast cells after challenge with IgE, several groups rapidly established that the cytokine gene repertoire transcribed in mast cells was indeed quite broad. Wodnar-Filipowicz and associates (27) demonstrated that IL-3 and GM-CSF were rapidly and transiently induced and secreted in response to IgE receptor crosslinkage in BMMC cultured for 3 weeks in the presence of IL-3. Plaut and colleagues (28) demonstrated that IgE-mediated or calcium ionophore stimulation of long-term IL-3–dependent mouse mast-cell lines resulted in increased levels of mRNA for IL-3, IL-4, IL-5, and IL-6, and they detected released bioactivity for IL-3, IL-4, and IL-6. Low level mRNA expression was also detected for IL-2 and IFN-γ, but not bioactivity. TNF-α mRNA was not detected in the cell lines examined. Stimulation also resulted in the ability of several subclones to proliferate in the absence of exogenous growth factor, and the response was sensitive to the immunosuppressive drug cyclosporin A or the blocking effects of antibodies for IL-3 and IL-4.

Burd and co-workers (29) demonstrated that stimulation of murine mast cells through IgE, calcium ionophore, or phorbol ester resulted in transcription of a broad range of cytokine genes. In one study, which examined cytokine transcription and secretion in several different IL-3–dependent and IL-3–independent long-term cell lines, mRNAs were identified for IL-1, IL-3, IL-5, IL-6, GM-CSF, IFN-γ, and the β-chemokines marcrophage inflammatory protein (MIP)-1α, MIP-1β, JE, and TCA3, as well as bioactivity for IL-1, IL-4, and IL-6 (29). Subsequent studies demonstrated receptor-mediated accumulation of transcripts for these cytokines (30), as well as IL-7, IL-10, and IL-11 (Burd PR, unpublished observation) in primary 6-week cultures of IL-3–dependent, bone marrow-derived cultured mast cells activated through IgE. In addition, TGF-β mRNA levels (originally described in dog mastocytoma cell lines [31]) were found to be constitutively expressed and relatively unchanged in response to stimulation.

Further studies have expanded the list of mast cell–derived cytokines. In addition to producing IL-3, IL-4, IL-5, and GM-CSF, mast cells also transcribe and secrete high levels of IL-13 in response to IgE or chemical signals (Burd PR, Mills FC, unpublished observations). This finding is in contrast to the other members of this chromosomally colocalized group of structurally related genes, whereby expression is observed in response to IgE stimulation, but is of a more restricted nature, both temporally and quantitatively. IL-13 and IL-4 share many biological properties; however, they are fundamentally distinguished by their target populations. Whereas IL-4 acts on

a variety of cells, including T cells, IL-13 has no known activity on T cells (32).

Mast cells store significant quantities of preformed endothelin-1 within the cytoplasmic compartment and transcribe and secrete endothelin-1 in response to pharmacological or IgE-mediated signals (33). Unlike TNF-α, however, release of preformed endothelin-1 is not directly related to mast-cell degranulation and occurs only after a pronounced delay (after 5 hours). In addition, mast cells were found to possess endothelin type A receptors, although the functional significance of their presence is not known, because endothelin-1 binding did not result in histamine release, autoregulation of the receptor, or augment proliferation. Marshall and associates (34) identified constitutive levels of leukemia inhibitory factor (LIF) mRNA and bioactivity in rat mast-cell lines and in peritoneal mast cells and showed increased levels in response to calcium ionophore treatment (production of LIF in response to IgE-mediated signals was not examined).

Mast cells stimulated via IgE are an unusually rich source of chemokines (previously called intercrines), a two-branched family of structurally related cytokines that possess potent chemoattractant and activating properties for leukocytes or their precursors (35,36). Members of the "CXC" or α-branch of the family are primarily neutrophil or basophil chemoattractants, whereas members of the "CC" or β-branch are chemoattractive for neutrophils, macrophages, eosinophils, and subsets of T cells. Members of this cytokine family were initially identified through screening procedures designed to isolate early inducible genes in a variety of cell types (e.g., T cells, fibroblasts, macrophages), usually in response to cytokine or other receptor-mediated activation, and thus may be thought of as components of a cytokine cascade operative in many biological processes.

Moeller and co-workers (37) identified the α-chemokine IL-8 mRNA and immunoreactive protein in the immature human mast-cell line HMC-1, as well as immunoreactive IL-8 protein in IgE-stimulated human skin mast cells, and they demonstrated that the secreted protein possessed neutrophil chemotactic properties. Mast cells may also express other α-chemokines, including MIG (38) and IP-10 (35), two IFN-γ–inducible genes originally described in macrophages (Burd PR, unpublished observations). In addition to the four β-chemokines previously described by Burd and colleagues (29) in mast cells, two recently described members of the β-chemokine family are also transcribed in murine mast cells in response to IgE-mediated signals: RANTES (Burd PR, unpublished observation) and MARC. MARC is transcribed in response to IgE or PMA plus ionophore stimulation and was identified by differential screening of activated mast cells (39). Also identified as an immediate-early gene in serum-stimulated quiescent fibroblasts termed FIC (40), MARC has been shown to be chemotactic for monocytes

TABLE 6–3 MAST-CELL PRODUCTS INVOLVED IN CELL RECRUITMENT/INFLAMMATION

Product	Function/Responding Cells
Preformed, released after IgE stimulation	
Histamine	Induction of P selectin
TNF-α	Induction of E selectin
Heparin	Bind and augment biological activity of cytokines, chemokines in particular
Newly synthesized chemoattractants	
TNF-α	Neutrophils
α-chemokines	
IL-8	Neutrophils, basophils
MIG	
β-chemokines	
JE/MCP-1	Monocytes, neutrophils, basophils, eosinophils, subpopulations of T lymphocytes
MIL-1α	
MIP-1β	
TCA3	
RANTES	
MARC/FIC	
Products of arachidonate and phosphatidylcholine metabolism	Monocytes, eosinophils, neutrophils
Nitric oxide (NO), constitutive form, G protein–regulated	Endothelial cells, macrophages, neurons, many other cell types

and is most related to monocyte chemotactic protein (MCP)-1/JE and to two other related chemokines, MCP-2 and MCP-3 (41), the murine homologs of which have not yet been identified.

The combined spectrum of cytokines produced by mast cells is quite broad (see Table 6–2), although the response of an individual cell line may be a subset of the total aggregate response. This finding suggests a clonal basis for the different patterns of cytokine gene induction seen in response to IgE or chemically mediated signaling. To this end, several groups examined the individual cellular response from mixed populations of mast cells. In situ hybridization showed that individual BMMC activated through IgE were heterogenous in their production of IL-6; approximately 50% of the cells contained detectable levels of IL-6 mRNA, and individual cells differed markedly in the relative amounts of IL-6 mRNA (42). Polymerase chain reaction analysis of individual cells showed that BMMC in contact with fibroblasts as a source of stem-cell factor (SCF) variably expressed IL-3 mRNA; some expressed undetectable levels (43). Inasmuch as the mast cells distributed throughout the body represent a heterogenous population of cells, information derived from culture of BMMC may more closely reflect the spectrum of potential responses observed in the intact animal. However, production of a given cytokine at a particular ana-

tomical site may be influenced or even determined by microenvironmental factors, which may change over time or respond to other influences (3).

MAST-CELL RESPONSES TO NON-FCεRI SIGNALS

Recent studies have begun to examine the responsiveness of mast cells to signals delivered by non-FcεRI receptors. Other receptors present on mast cells include cytokine receptors; the low affinity IgG receptors FcγRII (CD32) and FcγRIII (CD16) (44,45) (which are capable of binding both IgG and IgE [46]); the receptor encoded by the c-kit protooncogene (CD117); members of the seven transmembrane G-protein–coupled family of receptors for histamine, chemokines, neuropeptides, endothelins, and other proteins; and adhesion receptors, including integrins. Mast cell effector function is under the control of a wide range of receptors. These receptor systems allow mast cells to either initiate or participate distally in leukocyte-cytokine cascades.

It is now well established that integrins represent a means by which cells are able to interact with other cells, as well as with the extracellular environment, and to receive signals in response to changes in the extracellular compartment (47). Thompson and coworkers (48) established that functional activation of integrin receptors for laminin, fibronectin, and matrigel results from IgE-mediated or PMA signals and that such activation results in mast-cell migration on these various materials. However, these effects may be viewed as secondary effector functions associated with the postactivation program of mast cells and may reflect some of the mast cell's roles in wound and tissue repair. The secondary or effector nature of this response is underscored in that in the absence of IgE-mediated signals, mast cells do not significantly attach to surfaces coated with laminin, collagen, or fibronectin. The dispersed distribution of mast cells suggests, however, that mast cells are able to localize specifically to various anatomical sites and thus should be able to monitor the extracellular environment independently of IgE-mediated signals and respond accordingly. Moreover, integrin expression by mast cells is subject to environmental influences, including modulation by cytokines (49,50).

Evidence for such a mechanism was provided through use of a proliferation augmentation assay to detect integrin-mediated signals in the absence of IgE signals (51). This approach was based on the supposition that integrin-mediated signals, which result in changes in intracellular calcium (52) but do not necessarily possess direct mitogenic capabilities, nevertheless may be detected by augmentation of mitogenic responses in a variety of cell types. Applied to mast cells, this approach indicates that engagement of the vitronectin receptor by plate-bound but not soluble vitronectin in the absence of IgE-mediated signals augments the maximal IL-3 proliferative response of 3-week cultures of BMMC. This finding demonstrates that mast cell environmental surveillance occurs in part through the vitronectin receptor. Furthermore, functional binding of vitronectin receptors transduces a signal that functions independently of IgE receptor–mediated signals, and which is available to interact with the proliferation-differentiation pathway. By analogy with other cell types, vitronectin receptor-mediated signals, and perhaps other integrin-mediated signals, may function in a variety of cell processes, including cell differentiation and function, migration, and augmentation of the transcriptional response. What effects such signals may have on mast cell cytokine production are currently unknown, but they are certainly intriguing.

Functional studies suggest that mast cells express members of a family of structurally related receptors possessing seven transmembrane spanning domains, which are coupled to signal transduction pathways through G-proteins. Examples of this receptor family (approaching 1,000 members) include but are not limited to receptors for odorants; neuropeptides, including substance P and neuropeptide Y; endothelins and other vasoactive peptides; chemokines; formylpeptides; C5a; thrombin; and histamine. Recent studies have begun to examine the function of these receptors in mast cells and basophils. Ehrenreich and associates (33) showed that BMMC possess pertussis toxin–sensitive type A endothelin receptors, which show a marked preference for endothelin-1; however, the functional significance of these receptors on mast cells was not determined, because treatment of the cells with endothelin-1 did not result in autoregulation of the receptor, cause histamine release, augment proliferation, or induce a limited panel of cytokine genes. However, both neuropeptide Y (53) and substance P (54) binding to their respective pertussis toxin–sensitive receptors have been shown to cause histamine release from mast cells. Furthermore, Ansel and coworkers (55) showed that substance P selectively activated secretion and gene expression of TNF-α but not IL-1, IL-3, IL-4, IL-5, or GM-CSF. However, it was not determined whether the secreted TNF-α represented preformed, newly synthesized, or both, although the latter is most likely, because TNF-α, unlike endothelin-1, does not appear to be compartmentalized separately from other preformed mediators.

Mast cells and basophils not only produce chemokines, but also possess chemokine receptors, and many individual chemokines are able to cause histamine release from mast cells (56,57) or basophils (58–61) alone or following priming by IL-3, IL-5, or GM-CSF. Insight into the mechanism of chemokine action on basophils in vitro has come from receptor binding, competition, and desensitization studies (60), as well as from cloning the receptor for MIP-1α (62,63). These studies indicate that basophils possess at least three (pertussis toxin–sensitive) β-chemokine receptors binding different subsets of β-chemokines and resulting in mediator release, chemotaxis, or both, and that multiple chemokines interact with each of the receptors, although receptor affinity does not predict signaling efficacy of each chemokine/receptor pair.

Similar effects have been reported for mast cells in vivo (57), whereby injections of human MCP-1 or MIP-1α into mouse footpads resulted in mast-cell degranulation, footpad swelling, and cellular infiltration consistent with their known chemotactic activities. However, although MCP-1 is a much more potent activator of basophils than MIP-1α, MIP-1α appears to be a much more potent activator of mast-cell degranulation in vivo than MCP-1.

Thus, one of the functions of chemokines may be to regulate mast-cell activation independently of IgE signals. The ability of various chemokines to cause chemotaxis or degranulation of basophils and mast cells suggests that mast cells not only may participate in the initial stages of a cytokine cascade through IgE-mediated activation, but also may serve as effectors to amplify the cytokine response downstream in such a cascade. The ability of various cytokines to affect chemokine response (e.g., priming of basophils by IL-3, IL-5, or GM-CSF) adds a further level of specificity to this response. However, extrapolation of these findings to function in vivo must be placed within the context that chemokines do not arise singly during immunological processes, but rather are produced as groups of related chemokines, with each able to interact with multiple chemokine receptors. What differences these panels of chemokines or microenvironmental factors (e.g., cytokines or proteoglycans) may have on chemokine receptor signaling and function in vivo is poorly understood.

Studies of mast cell–deficient mice have shown that the signals delivered through the c-kit protooncogene (CD117), a receptor tyrosine kinase, are of primary importance in the development and function of the mast cell in vivo. Mice with mutations at both copies of the W/c-kit locus or with mutations at the Sl/SCF locus (the ligand for c-kit) are profoundly deficient in mast cells. Signals delivered via c-kit share some common elements with the IL-3–induced signal transduction pathway (64), but this commonality does not extend to the transcriptional regulation level because each signal pathway results in distinct patterns of gene expression for members of the AP-1 family of transcription factors (65), secretory granule proteases (66), and IL-3 (43).

In addition to their involvement in growth and differentiation of mast cells from hematopoietic precursors, signals delivered via c-kit also appear to effect mediator release (67). Short-term exposure of lung and skin mast cells and basophils to submitogenic doses of SCF enhances the release of histamine and newly formed mediators in response to IgE-mediated signals, but not to G-protein–coupled receptor signals (68–70), whereas long-term exposure to SCF does not potentiate mediator release in response to IgE (69,71). Similarly, short-term in vivo administration of SCF results in dermal mast-cell activation and a mast cell–dependent inflammatory response (68). These studies indicate that although c-kit signals may indeed potentiate mediator release during short-term assays, their in vivo function may be somewhat different. Nevertheless, they indicate that the c-kit signaling pathway affects mast cell effector function and points the way toward a role for SCF isoforms in the microenvironment.

Signals delivered by growth factor receptors also modulate the expression of granule-associated proteases and cytokines. IL-3 but not IL-4 potentiates the inducible cytokine response of mast cells to IgE receptor crosslinkage (72). Introduction of other cytokine receptors into mast cells by transfection followed by specific ligand stimulation does not result in cytokine production; however, the signals generated are able to enhance cytokine production following IgE stimulation (72). Similarly, IL-3—but not IL-5, GM-CSF, or nerve growth factor, all of

which are able to function as priming agents for enhanced release of preformed mediators—acts in a costimulatory manner to induce IL-4 production by human basophils in response to IgE stimulation (73).

Cytokines that are able to augment IL-3–mediated growth of mast cells include IL-4, IL-9, IL-10, and SCF. Signals transduced via receptors for each of these cytokines also affect other cellular processes, because each of these cytokines also modulates expression of mast cell granule–associated protease genes. In the absence of other cytokines, IL-3 does not induce expression of proteases associated with the mature phenotype. SCF, IL-9, and IL-10 induce, but IL-4 suppresses induction of mature phenotype protease genes (66,74,75). Moreover, these effects are reversible (74): Induced expression of a particular protease gene may be lost following removal of the inducing cytokine, demonstrating that the mast-cell phenotype is not fixed and that cytokine levels in the microenvironment may reversibly affect mast-cell phenotype and perhaps function (76).

Mast cells possess the low affinity IgG receptors Fc$_\gamma$RII and Fc$_\gamma$RIII (44,45) and release their granules and arachidonic acid metabolites in response to receptor crosslinkage (46,77). Functional activity of these receptors in vivo has been implied through study of immune complex peritonitis in normal and mast cell–deficient mice (25), suggesting that, as with Fc$_\epsilon$RI, IgG receptor–mediated signals result in cytokine production. Mast cells also express CD21 (78), an endogenous galactose-binding lectin that binds CD23, the low affinity IgE receptor found on B cells. Although CD21 may be considered an adhesion molecule, with its binding to CD23 constituting an important regulatory mechanism in IgE production by B cells (79), its role in mast cell–mediated function is unknown.

Thus, mast cell effector function is under the control or influence of a wide range of receptors. Ligands for some of these receptors may constitute important components of the microenvironment, and their regulation may be critical to induction, maintenance, or progression of certain pathological states.

REGULATION OF MAST CELL CYTOKINE PRODUCTION

Fc$_\epsilon$RI-mediated cytokine gene induction falls into one of two major response patterns (30). The first group is characterized by relatively high levels of mRNA induction, appearing within a short time (by 30 minutes) after activation, and includes TNF-α, IL-6, the α-chemokine MIG, and the β-chemokines TCA3, MIP-1α, MIP-1β, JE (MCP-1), RANTES, and MARC. Members of this group also share predominantly proinflammatory and chemotactic properties. Induction of these genes does not appear to be inhibited by pretreatment of cells with cycloheximide, but cyclosporin A pretreatment completely blocks induction of TCA3, MIP-1α, and MIP-1β and markedly inhibits induction of TNF-α.

The second group of cytokines induced in BMMC by IgE-mediated signals represents immunomodulatory and hematopoietic cytokines and includes IL-1, IL-3, IL-4, IL-5, and GM-CSF. In contrast to the high level and rapid induction of the proinflammatory cytokine group, this latter group is characterized by delayed and lower level expression. In addition to their roles as growth factor–type cytokines, members of this group possess priming capability for histamine release from basophils in response to other agents (e.g., chemokines).

Activation of mast cells via the FcεRI initiates an activation program composed of (at least) three parts. The immediate result of receptor engagement is the release of preformed granules containing stores of preformed products (e.g., proteases, histamine, heparin, vasoactive intestinal peptide, and TNF-α), followed by release of newly synthesized metabolites of phosphatidylcholine and arachidonic acid metabolism. This release is followed within 30 minutes by high-level transcription (and secretion) of a variety of proinflammatory cytokines, including TNF-α, IL-6, and the chemokines. Bioactivity of many of these newly synthesized factors may be enhanced through release into the immediate environment of mast-cell heparin and proteoglycans, which are capable of binding and enhancing the biological activity of secreted chemotactic factors, particularly the chemokines. These two early phases may be considered a recruitment phase for inflammatory cells, which is then followed by an effector phase characterized by production of immunomodulatory and hematopoietic-like cytokines, including IL-1, IL-3, IL-4, IL-5, and GM-CSF, as well as changes in affinities of adhesion molecules for substrate and in cell motility, induction of cell surface receptors, and secretion of endothelin-1, an important regulator of smooth muscle tone in the vasculature.

Signals transduced through the IgE receptor result in mobilization of intracellular Ca²⁺ and activation of protein kinase C (80), events shared by other receptor signaling pathways, such as antigen receptors on T and B cells. Unlike that found in T and B cells, in which both events are required for induction of most early genes, stimulation of mast cells by agents that specifically activate one or the other of these pathways produces distinct patterns of mast cell cytokine expression. Activation of protein kinase C through the action of PMA results in high level (but delayed relative to IgE induction) accumulation of TNF-α, IL-6, and β-chemokine genes, but not IL-2, IL-3, IL-4, IL-5, GM-CSF, or IFN-γ; is not associated with granule exocytosis; and is inhibited by pretreatment with cycloheximide, but not by cyclosporin A. In contrast, activation of the Ca²⁺ pathway through calcium ionophore closely resembles the pattern seen with antigen stimulation; both mRNA increases and histamine release are inhibited by cyclosporin A, but not by cycloheximide. Optimal induction of IL-2, IL-3, IL-5, and GM-CSF requires both PMA and ionophore for maximal induction. In one mast-cell line, however, IL-3 mRNA is constitutively transcribed and regulated by Ca²⁺, primarily at the level of mRNA stability (26).

Although expression of most of these genes in T cells requires both protein kinase C and calcium pathways, different regulatory mechanisms exist for the transcription of these cytokines in mast cells. The ability to express high levels of cytokine mRNA in response to either protein kinase C or calcium pathways poses interesting questions for the interactions of these pathways with microenvironmental influences. For example, protein kinase C–affecting agents could lead to the release of proinflammatory cytokines, whereas IgE-dependent signals would lead to immunomodulatory and hematopoietic cytokines, in addition to proinflammatory factors. Augmentation or diminution of these signals via other receptor-mediated means could further alter the pattern or relative amounts of cytokines produced by mast cells at a given site.

It should also be mentioned that although FcεRI-mediated signals induce a pattern of early gene expression similar to IL-3- or SCF-mediated signals in primary cultures of mast cells and which appears similar to early gene expression in activated T cells or fibroblasts, these signals do not result in mast-cell proliferation (65). Moreover, regulation of this effect appears to be fundamentally different from the regulatory processes at work (at least) in fibroblasts, in which control of this process is regulated in part through junD (81). Thus, activation of mast cells via the IgE receptor would appear to result in inhibition of autocrine growth through IL-3 or SCF.

MAST CELLS AS CRITICAL COMPONENTS OF LEUKOCYTE CYTOKINE CASCADES AND THE IMMUNOLOGICAL SYNAPSE

The ability of mast cells to initiate recruitment of leukocytes to sites of mast-cell activation has led to the proposal of a mast cell leukocyte cascade (82–84). This hypothesis is based on the observation that many of the cell types recruited by mast cells (Table 6-3) are capable of producing multifunctional cytokines, thereby amplifying or diversifying the cytokine response at a given locale and over time. For example, neutrophils recruited during IgE-mediated cutaneous reactions or during immune complex peritonitis in the mouse contribute to TNF-α production at these sites. Eosinophils recruited during IgE-mediated reactions in humans are capable of producing TNF-α, MIP-1α (85), IL-1, IL-5, TGF-β, and TGF-α (84). Basophils recruited to sites of late-phase reactions are potent sources of IL-4, IL-8, and other factors.

At its simplest, this hypothesis emphasizes the potential contributions of cytokines to responses associated with mast-cell activation leading to leukocyte infiltration (86). However, as shown by the responsiveness of mast cells to β-chemokines, mast cells need not function solely as initiators of this process, but may also act at later amplification steps. It is also important to emphasize that mast cells and recruited leukocytes may have complex effects during persistent inflammatory conditions (84). These effects will reflect activities of both cytokines and other products, which may change over time and in response to local conditions.

Do mast cells modulate the functions of other cells through direct contact? Although this question has not been extensively examined, circumstantial evidence suggests that mast cells may indeed participate in a form of the immunological synapse. Much like its neurological counterpart, the immunological synapse can be thought of as the opposing surfaces of two functionally distinct cells, through which the interactions of specific cell surface ligand-receptor complexes are tethered to each other. These closely associated cell surfaces are the sites of receptors for additional factors (e.g., cytokines) that are secreted (perhaps preferentially) into the synaptic space, resulting in localized high level delivery and signaling to their cognate receptors (87). The immunological paradigm for this hypothesis is T- and B-cell interactions, whereby T cell surface structures, including the T-cell antigen receptor complex and costimulatory structures such as CD28 and CD40 ligand, stably bridge B cells via major histocompatibility complex (MHC) class II plus antigen-derived peptide and cell surface structures, including B-7 and CD40 (88). Secreted across this junction are T-cell cytokines, which act on different stages of B-cell growth and differentiation (87). Formation of such a structure allows very specific targeting of multifunctional cytokines and their resultant responses.

Much like T cells, mast cells produce not only a broad range of multifunctional cytokines, but also express a number of cell surface structures capable of stably joining them to other cells, including intercellular adhesion molecule-1 (ICAM-1), leukocyte function-associated molecule (LFA-2), LFA-3, c-kit, and other adhesion molecules (89). They also express other cell surface proteins, which act as ligands or bind receptors, such as CD40 ligand (90), antigen presenting MHC class II (91), and CD21 (92). Moreover, the presence of some of these structures or their affinity for ligand are subject to change in response to activation signals, providing a means by which

the mast cell may selectively interact with cell populations, depending on its activation state or vice versa. For example, there is intriguing evidence that, following activation, mast cells and basophils may be able to direct B cell immunoglobulin class switching to IgG4 and IgE through the direct interactions of B-cell CD23 and CD40 and mast cell CD21, CD40 ligand IL-4, and IL-13 (90) (Burd PR, Mills FC, unpublished observations). Such a process may operate independently of T cells and could result in antigen nonspecific amplification of the IgE response.

Similar speculations may be advanced for mast-cell interactions with a wide range of cells, including monocytes/macrophages, fibroblasts, and cells of the nervous system. Although much remains to be done before firm conclusions can be drawn, it is tempting to speculate that disregulation of such mast cell–mediated interactions may be an important component of certain pathological states.

CONCLUSIONS

Much progress has been made in elucidating the potential of mast cells to participate in normal and pathologic processes through elaboration of multifunctional cytokines and interactions with other cells through cell surface and other structures. Mast cells can no longer be regarded as mere initiators of acute allergic reactions through their release of histamine and products of arachidonic acid metabolism. They are responsible for initiating leukocyte infiltration and, through production of cytokines and other factors, modulating the effects of infiltrating effector cells. Mast cells also may be recruited to participate in leukocyte cytokine cascades at later steps, amplifying or diversifying immunological responses according to dynamic conditions. However, much remains to be discovered about the roles mast cells play in a wide range of host processes associated with normal and pathological states.

REFERENCES

1. Ishizaka T. Mechanisms of IgE-mediated hypersensitivity. In: Middleton E Jr, Reed CE, Ellis EF, Adkinson NF Jr, Yuninger JW, eds. Allergy: principles and practice. St. Louis: Mosby, 1988:71–93.
2. Galli SJ, Lichtenstein LM. Biology of mast cells and basophils. In: Middleton E Jr, Reed CE, Ellis EF, Adkinson NF Jr, Yuninger JW, eds. St. Louis: Mosby, 1988:106–134.
3. Galli SJ. New insights into "the riddle of the mast cells": microenvironmental regulation of mast cell development and phenotypic heterogeneity. Lab Invest 1990;62:5.
4. Rieger A, Wang B, Kilgus O, et al. FcεRI mediates IgE binding to human epidermal Langerhans cells. J Invest Dermatol 1992;99:30S.

5. Maurer D, Fiebiger E, Reininger B, et al. Expression of functional high affinity immunoglobulin E receptors (Fc$_\varepsilon$RI) on monocytes of atopic individuals. J Exp Med 1994;179:745.

6. Abdelilah SG, Lamkhioued B, Ochiai K, et al. High affinity IgE receptor on eosinophils is involved in defence against parasites. Nature 1994;367:183.

7. Chung SW, Wong PMC, Shen-Ong G, Ruscetti S, Ishizaka T, Eaves CJ. Production of granulocyte-macrophage colony-stimulating factor by Abelson virus-induced tumorigenic mast cell lines. Blood 1986;69:1071.

8. Brown MA, Pierce JH, Watson CJ, Falco J, Ihle JN, Paul WE. B-cell stimulatory factor-1/interleukin-4 mRNA is expressed by normal and transformed mast cells. Cell 1987; 50:809.

9. Humphries RK, Abraham S, Krystal G, Lansdorp P, Lemoine F, Eaves CJ. Activation of multiple hemopoietic growth factor genes in Abelson virus-transformed myeloid cells. Exp Hematol 1988;16:774.

10. Farram E, Nelson DS. Mouse mast cells as anti-tumor effector cells. Cell Immunol 1980;55:294.

11. Ghiara P, Boraschi D, Villa L, Scapigliati G, Taddei C, Tagliabue A. In vitro generated mast cells express natural cytotoxicity against tumour cells. Immunology 1985; 55:317.

12. Ernst PB, Petit A, Lee TGE, Befus AD, Bienenstock J. Mast cell mediated cytotoxicity resembles natural cytotoxic (NC) activity (abstract). Fed Proc Fed Am Soc Exp Biol 1985;44:584.

13. Okuno T, Yakagaki Y, Pluznik DH, Djeu JY. Natural cytotoxic (NC) cell activity in basophilic cells: release of NC-specific cytotoxic factor by IgE receptor triggering. J Immunol 1986;136:4652.

14. Stutman O, Paige CJ, Figarella EF. Natural cytotoxic cells against solid tumors in mice. I. Strain and age distribution and target cell susceptibility. J Immunol 1978;121:1819.

15. Paige CJ, Figarella EF, Cuttito MJ, Cahan A, Stuttman O. Natural cytotoxic cells against solid tumors in mice. II. Some characteristics of the effector cells. J Immunol 1978; 121:1827.

16. Jadus MR, Schmunk G, Djeu JY, Parkman R. Morphology and lytic mechanisms of interleukin 3-dependent natural cytotoxic cells: tumor necrosis factor as a possible mediator. J Immunol 1986;137:2774.

17. Young JD-E, Liu C-C, Butler G, Cohn ZA, Galli SJ. Identification, purification, and characterization of a mast cell-associated cytolytic factor related to tumor necrosis factor. Proc Natl Acad Sci USA 1987;84:9175.

18. Kasper C, Tharp M. Mast cells are cytotoxic against TNF-sensitive and TNF-resistant targets (abstract). Fed Proc Fed Am Soc Exp Biol 1987;46:1225.

19. Richards AL, Okuno T, Takagaki Y, Djeu JY. Natural cytotoxic cell-specific cytolytic factor produced by IL-3-dependent basophilic/mast cells. Relationship to TNF. J Immunol 1988;141:3061.

20. Bissonnette EY, Befus AD. Inhibition of mast cell-mediated cytotoxicity by IFN-α/β and -γ. J Immunol 1990;145:3385.

21. Gordon JR, Galli SJ. Mast cells as a source of preformed and immunologically inducible TNFα/cachectin. Nature 1990;346:274.

22. Bissonnette EY, Hogaboam CM, Wallace JL, Befus AD. Potentiation of tumor necrosis factor-α-mediated cytotoxicity of mast cells by their production of nitric oxide. J Immunol 1991;147:3060.

23. Gordon JR, Galli SJ. Release of both preformed and newly synthesized tumor necrosis factor α (TNFα)/cachectin by mouse mast cells stimulated via the Fc$_\varepsilon$RI. A mechanism for the sustained action of mast cell-derived TNFα during IgE-dependent biological responses. J Exp Med 1991; 174:103.

24. Wershil BK, Wang Z-S, Gordon JR, Galli SJ. Recruitment of neutrophils during IgE-dependent cutaneous late phase reactions in the mouse is mast cell-dependent. J Clin Invest 1991;87:446.

25. Zhang Y, Ramos BF, Jakschik BA. Neutrophil recruitment by tumor necrosis factor from mast cells in immune complex peritonitis. Science 1992;258:1957.

26. Wodnar-Filipowicz A, Moroni C. Regulation of interleukin 3 mRNA expression in mast cells occurs at the post-transcriptional level and is mediated by calcium ions. Proc Natl Acad Sci USA 1990;87:777.

27. Wodnar-Filipowicz A, Heusser CH, Moroni C. Production of the haemopoietic growth factors GM-CSF and interleukin-3 by mast cells in response to IgE receptor-mediated activation. Nature 1989;339:150.

28. Plaut M, Pierce JH, Watson CJ, Hanley-Hyde J, Nordan RP, Paul WE. Mast cell lines produce lymphokines in response to cross-linkage of Fc$_\varepsilon$RI or to calcium ionophores. Nature 1989;339:64.

29. Burd PR, Rogers HW, Gordon JR, et al. Interleukin-3-dependent and-independent mast cells stimulated with IgE and antigen express multiple cytokines. J Exp Med 1989; 170:245.

30. Costa JJ, Burd PR, Siebenlist U, Metcalfe DD. Primary mouse bone marrow mast cell (BMMC) cultures transcribe multiple cytokines in response to Fc$_\varepsilon$RI crosslinking (abstract). FASEB J 1990;4:A1943.

31. Pennington DW, Lopez AR, Gold WW. Transforming growth factor-β production by canine mastocytoma cells (abstract). FASEB J 1989;3:A1213.

32. Zurawski G, de Vries JE. Interleukin-13, an interleukin-4-like cytokine that acts on monocytes and B cells, but not on T cells. Immunol Today 1994;15:19.

33. Ehrenreich H, Burd PR, Rottem M. Endothelins belong to the assortment of mast cell-derived and mast cell-bound cytokines. The New Biologist 1992;4:147.

34. Marshall JS, Gauldie J, Nielsen L, Bienenstock J. Leukemia inhibitory factor production by rat mast cells. Eur J Immunol 1993;23:2116.

35. Oppenheim JJ, Zachariae CC, Mukaida N, Matsushima K. Properties of the novel proinflammatory supergene "intercrine" cytokine family. Ann Rev Immunol 1991;9:617.

36. Schall TJ. Biology of the RANTES/SIS cytokine family. Cytokine 1991;3:165.

37. Moeller A, Lippert U, Lessman D, Human mast cells produce IL-8. J Immunol 1993;151:3261.

38. Farber JM. A macrophage mRNA selectively induced by g-interferon encodes a member of the platelet factor 4 family of cytokines. Proc Natl Acad Sci USA 1990;87:5238.

39. Kulmburg PA, Huber NE, Scheer BJ, Wrann M, Baumruker

T. Immunoglobulin E plus antigen challenge induces a novel intercrine/chemokine in mouse mast cells. J Exp Med 1992;176:1773.

40. Heinrich JA, Ryseck R-P, MacDonald-Bravo H, Bravo R. The product of a novel growth factor-activated gene, fic, is a biologically active "C-C"-type cytokine. Mol Cell Biol 1993;13:2020.

41. VanDamme J, Proost P, Lenaerts J-P, Opdenakker G. Structural and functional identification of two human, tumor-derived monocyte chemotactic proteins (MCP-2 and MCP-3) belonging to the chemokine family. J Exp Med 1992; 176:59.

42. Gurish MF, Ghildyal N, Arm J, et al. Cytokine mRNA are preferentially increased relative to secretory granule protein mRNA in mouse bone marrow-derived mast cells that have undergone IgE-mediated activation and degranulation. J Immunol 1991;146:1527.

43. Razin E, Leslie KB, Schrader JW. Connective tissue mast cells in contact with fibroblasts express IL-3 mRNA. Analysis of single cells by polymerase chain reaction. J Immunol 1991;146:981.

44. Katz HR, Arm JP, Benson AC, Austen KF. Maturation-related changes in the expression of Fc$_\gamma$RII and Fc$_\gamma$RIII on mouse mast cells derived in vitro and in vivo. J Immunol 1990;145:3412.

45. Benhamou M, Bonnerot C, Fridman WH, Daeeron M. Molecular heterogeneity of murine mast cell Fc$_\gamma$R receptors. J Immunol 1990;145:3412.

46. Takizawa F, Adamczewski M, Kinet J-P. Identification of the low affinity receptor for immunoglobulin E on mouse mast cells and macrophages as Fc$_\gamma$RII and Fc$_\gamma$RIII. J Exp Med 1992;176:469.

47. Hynes RO. Integrins: versatility, modulation, and signalling in cell adhesion. Cell 1992;69:11.

48. Thompson HL, Thomas L, Metcalfe DD. Murine mast cells attach to and migrate on laminin-, fibronectin-, and matrigel-coated surfaces in response to Fc$_\epsilon$RI-mediated signals. Clin Exp Immunol 1993;23:270.

49. Gurish MF, Bell AF, Smith TJ, Ducharme LA, Wang R-K, Weis JH. Expression of murine β7, α4, and β1 integrin genes by rodent mast cells. J Immunol 1992;149:1964.

50. Ducharme LA, Weis JH. Modulation of integrin expression during mast cell differentiation. Eur J Immunol 1992; 22:2603.

51. Bianchine PJ, Burd PR, Metcalfe DD. IL-3-dependent mast cells attach to plate-bound vitronectin: demonstration of augmented proliferation in response to signals transduced via cell surface vitronectin receptors. J Immunol 1992; 149:3665.

52. Leavesley DI, Schwartz MA, Rosenfeld M, Cheresh DA. Integrin β1- and β3-mediated endothelial cell migration is triggered through distinct signalling mechanisms. J Cell Biol 1993;121:163.

53. Arzubiaga C, Morrow J, Roberts LJ, Biaggioni I. Neuropeptide Y, a putative cotransmitter in noradrenergic neurones, induces mast cell degranulation but not prostaglandin D$_2$ release. J Allergy Clin Immunol 1991;87:88.

54. Ebertz JM, Hirschman CA, Kettelman NS, Uno H, Hanifin JM. Substance P induced histamine release in human cutaneous mast cells. J Invest Dermatol 1987;88:682.

55. Ansel JC, Brown JR, Payan DG, Brown MA. Substance P selectively activates TNFα gene expression in murine mast cells. J Immunol 1993;150:4478.

56. Alam RA, Forsythe PA, Stafford S, Lett-Brown MA, Grant AJ. Macrophage inflammatory protein-1α activates basophils and mast cells. J Exp Med 1992;176:781.

57. Alam R, Kumar D, Anderson-Walters D, Forsythe PA. Macrophage inflammatory protein-1α and monocyte chemoattractant peptide-1 elicit immediate and late cutaneous reactions and activate murine mast cells in vivo. J Immunol 1994;152:1298.

58. Kuna P, Reddigari SR, Schall TJ, Rucinski D, Viksman MY, Kaplan AP. RANTES, a monocyte and T lymphocyte chemotactic cytokine releases histamine from human basophils. J Exp Med 1992;149:636.

59. Kuna P, Reddigari SR, Rucinski D, Oppenheim JJ, Kaplan AP. Monocyte chemotactic and activating factor is a potent histamine-releasing factor for human basophils. J Exp Med 1992;175:489.

60. Dahinden CA, Geiser T, Brunner T, et al. Monocyte chemotactic protein 3 is a most effective basophil- and eosinophil-activating chemokine. J Exp Med 1994;179:751.

61. Kuna P, Reddigari SR, Schall TJ, Rucinski D, Sadick M, Kaplan AP. Characterization of the human basophil response to cytokines, growth factors, and histamine releasing factors of the intercrine/chemokine family. J Immunol 1993;150:1932.

62. Neote D, DiGregorio D, Mak JY, Horuk R, Schall TJ. Molecular cloning, functional expression, and signalling characteristics of a C-C chemokine receptor. Cell 1993;72:415.

63. Gao J-L, Kuhns DB, Tiffany HL, et al. Structure and functional expression of the human macrophage inflammatory protein 1α/RANTES receptor. J Exp Med 1993; 177:1421.

64. Welham MJ, Schrader JW. Steel factor-induced tyrosine phosphorylation in murine mast cells. J Immunol 1992; 149:2772.

65. Tsai M, Tam S-Y, Galli SJ. Distinct patterns of early response gene expression and proliferation in mouse mast cells stimulated by stem cell factor, interleukin-3, or IgE and antigen. Eur J Immunol 1993;23:867.

66. Gurish MF, Ghildyal N, McNeil HP, Austen KF, Gillis S, Stevens RL. Differential expression of secretory granule proteases in mouse mast cells exposed to interleukin 3 and c-kit ligand. J Exp Med 1992;175:1003.

67. Galli SJ, Tsai M, Wershil BK. The c-kit receptor, stem cell factor, and mast cells: what each is teaching us about the others. Am J Pathol 1993;142:965.

68. Wershil BK, Tsai M, Geissler EN, Zsebo KM, Galli SJ. The rat c-kit ligand, stem cell factor, induces c-kit receptor-dependent mouse mast cell activation in vivo. Evidence that signalling through the c-kit receptor can induce expression of cellular function. J Exp Med 1992;175:245.

69. Bischoff SC, Dahinden CA. c-kit ligand: a unique potentiator of mediator release by human lung mast cells. J Exp Med 1992;175:237.

70. Columbo M, Horowitz EM, Botana LM, et al. The human recombinant c-kit receptor ligand, rhSCF, induces mediator release from human cutaneous mast cells and enhances IgE-dependent mediator release from both skin mast cells and peripheral blood basophils. J Immunol 1992;149:599.

71. Coleman JW, Holliday MR, Kimber I, Zsebo KM, Galli SJ.

Regulation of mouse peritoneal mast cell secretory function by stem cell factor, IL-3 or IL-4. J Immunol 1993; 150:556.

72. Keegan AD, Pierce JH, Artrip J, Plaut M, Paul WE. Ligand stimulation of transfected and endogenous growth factor receptors enhances cytokine production by mast cells. EMBO J 1991;10:3675.

73. Brunner T, Heusser CH, Dahinden CA. Human peripheral blood basophils primed by interleukin 3 (IL-3) produce IL-4 in response to immunoglobulin E receptor stimulation. J Exp Med 1993;177:605.

74. Ghildyal N, Nicodemus CF, Austen KF, Stevens RL. Reversible expression of mouse mast cell protease 2 mRNA and protein in cultured mast cells exposed to IL-10. J Immunol 1993;151:3206.

75. Eklund KK, Ghildyal N, Austen KF, Stevens RL. Induction by IL-9 and suppression by IL-3 and IL-4 of the levels of chromosome 14-derived transcripts that encode late-expressed mouse mast cell proteases. J Immunol 1993; 151:4266.

76. Pejler G, Karlstroem A. Thrombin is inactivated by mast cell secretory granule chymase. J Biol Chem 1993; 268:11817.

77. Katz HR, Raizman MB, Gartner CS, Scott HC, Benson AC, Austen KF. Secretory granule mediator release and generation of oxidative metabolites of arachidonic acid via Fc-IgG receptor bridging in mouse mast cells. J Immunol 1992; 148:868.

78. Cherayil BJ, Weiner SJ, Pillai S. The Mac-2 antigen is a galactose-specific lectin that binds IgE. J Exp Med 1989; 170:1959.

79. Bonnefoy J-Y, Pochon S, Aubry J-P, et al. A new pair of surface molecules involved in human IgE regulation. Immunol Today 1993;14:1.

80. Beaven MA, Metzger H. Signal transduction by Fc receptors: the $Fc_\varepsilon RI$ case. Immunol Today 1993;14:222.

81. Pfarr CM, Mechta F, Spyrou G, Lallemand D, Carillo S, Yaniv M. Mouse junD negatively regulates fibroblast growth and antagonizes transformation by ras. Cell 1994; 76:747.

82. Gordon JR, Burd PR, Galli SJ. Mast cells as a source of multifunctional cytokines. Immunol Today 1990;11;458.

83. Galli SJ, Gordon JR, Wershil BK. Cytokine production by mast cells and basophils. Curr Opin Immunol 1991;3:865.

84. Galli SJ. New concepts about the mast cell. N Engl J Med 1993;328:257.

85. Costa JJ, Matossian K, Resnick MB, et al. Human eosinophils can express the cytokines tumor necrosis factor-alpha and macrophage inflammatory protein-1 alpha. J Clin Invest 1993;91:2673.

86. Springer T. Traffic signals for lymphocyte recirculation and leukocyte emigration: the multistep paradigm. Cell 1994;76:301.

87. Paul WE, Seder RA. Lymphocyte responses and cytokines. Cell 1994;76:241.

88. Clark EA, Ledbetter JA. How B and T cells talk to each other. Nature 1994;367:425.

89. Hamawy MM, Mergenhagen SE, Siraganian RP. Adhesion molecules as regulators of mast-cell and basophil function. Immunol Today 1994;15:62.

90. Gauchat J-F, Henchoz S, Mazzei G, et al. Induction of human IgE synthesis in B cells by mast cells and basophils. Nature 1993;365:340.

91. Frandji P, Oskeritzian C, Cacaraci F, et al. Antigen-dependent stimulation by bone marrow-derived mast cells of MHC class II-restricted T cell hybridoma. J Immunol 1993; 151:6318.

92. Frigeri LG, Liu F-T. Surface expression of functional IgE binding protein, an endogenous lectin, on mast cells and macrophages. J Immunol 1992;148:861.

CHAPTER 7

ROLE OF CYTOKINES
IN ENDOTHELIAL CELL FUNCTIONS

Marek S. Litwin, Jennifer R. Gamble, and Mathew A. Vadas

Vascular endothelium, consisting of the cells and the extracellular matrices (ECM) that line the blood vessels, displays two characteristic properties: (a) endothelial renewal and angiogenesis, and (b) interactions with blood molecules and leukocytes. The turnover of endothelial cells (ECs) in most adult tissues is exceedingly slow, varying from just under 100 days in lung, liver, and mesentery to 1,000 days in brain, but replication periods may shorten 20 to 2,000 times during wound healing, inflammation, and malignancy, and are even faster in uteroplacental tissue and embryogenesis (1,2). Established endothelium regulates the blood coagulation system (3), the lumenal diameter of its vessel (4), attachment of leukocytes to its surface and their migration into interstitium (5), and antigen presentation to lymphocytes (6).

Each of the endothelial functions described is coordinated by cytokines. These soluble, small molecular weight proteins are directed at ECs and their neighbors from adjoining mast cells, T cells, and macrophages, from other ECs, and from distant sites upstream in the circulation. Many cytokines possess binding sites on the ECM or endothelial surface, which prevent them from being washed away in the axial blood stream, potentially creating an important periendothelial cytokine reservoir (7,8). We discuss the cytokines involved in EC proliferation and interactions with the blood, with an emphasis on their contribution to pathophysiological mechanisms.

RENEWAL AND ANGIOGENESIS

Endothelial renewal entails EC multiplication and migration (9,10). However, in addition to local EC division, there may be a role in vivo for a circulating pool of EC precursors, the existence of which has been implied by the finding of ECs in the bloodstream (11).

Angiogenesis, in contrast, summarizes a myriad of activities leading to the formation of an entire new blood vessel. It may be divided into component stages, using models such as cultured ECs on a three-dimensional (3D) gel or the growth of vessels on cornea or chorioallantoic membrane. New capillaries begin the process by sprouting from venules as ECs move in response to a migratory stimulus through basement membrane that has been locally degraded. The motile ECs elongate and align to create a solid sprout, which lengthens, canalizes, and joins other sprouts to form a loop. Pericytes adjoin the ECs, and the mature, stable capillary is formed (12). The place of cytokines in each stage may be studied.

Fibroblast growth factor

BACKGROUND: Fibroblast growth factor (FGF) comprises a family of at least seven heparin binding growth factors sharing 35 to 55% amino acid identity.

FGF-1 and FGF-2 (acidic and basic FGF) are the best characterized isoforms and are the subject of this review, in which they are generally viewed synonomously. Each is a 154 amino acid polypeptide and together they are produced by most cell types, including ECs (13).

FGF is thought by some to be the principal cytokine involved in the in vivo induction of angiogenesis (9,14). It is expressed ubiquitously in normal adult tissues, but a paradox is raised in that endothelial proliferation in these tissues is generally quiescent, except in the female reproductive organs and at sites of pathology. This inactivity is not accounted for by FGF's lack of a classic signal sequence for secretion, because it is found extracellularly, possibly due to a truncated receptor, which serves as a secretory carrier (15). A more likely explanation is that the cellular responses to FGF are mediated by a receptor complex comprising heparin sulfate moieties, rather than by a single protein, which is subject to considerable polymorphism (16).

EFFECTS ON ECS IN VITRO:
FGF stimulates proliferation and migration of cultured ECs (9,14,17), but, in addition to promitotic actions, it has several other effects that are likely to be important. One of the phenotypic hallmarks of migrating ECs is expression of plasminogen activator (PA), a central mediator of extracellular proteolysis. FGF up-regulates the synthesis of PA and collagenase (17–19). Wounding of an EC monolayer triggers a marked, rapid, and sustained increase in expression of a specific high-affinity receptor for the urokinase-type PA (u-PA) on the surface of migrating cells, the postulated role of which is to mediate efficient and spatially restricted extracellular proteolytic activity by migrating ECs (20,21). Increases in u-PA and u-PA receptor are both dependent on endogenous FGF.

EC invasiveness and formation of patent capillaries in fibrin and collagen gels is stimulated by FGF (22). It increases expression of the $\alpha v\beta 3$ integrin, which correlates with an increased ability of microvascular ECs to bind to vitronectin, but not to fibronectin-coated surfaces (23). There is up-regulated biosynthesis of the collagen/laminin receptor, the $\alpha 2\beta 1$ integrin and the $\alpha 5$-chain, which conjugates with $\beta 1$ to form a fibronectin receptor. These effects of FGF may provide ECs with an enhanced capacity to attach to, or migrate through, both their underlying basement membrane and the interstitial matrix (24).

FGF INTRACELLULAR SIGNALING:
The signaling pathway of FGF appears to involve both a membrane receptor and a direct nuclear site of action. There are two FGF receptors, one of high affinity, which possesses an intracellular tyrosine kinase domain (25), and the other of low affinity, a heparan sulfate proteoglycan (HSPG) (26,27). It appears that binding to cell surface HSPG is a prerequisite for high-affinity binding and mitogenic activity (16). Studies employing peptide mutants of FGF and anti-FGF antibodies to regulate the FGF-receptor interaction suggest that the mitogenic and PA-inducing activities of FGF depend on different domains of the FGF high-affinity receptor and different intracellular transduction pathways (28). Mitogenic activity involves triggering of protein kinase C (PKC), whereas plasminogen activation is independent of PKC, but requires a calcium flux (29).

FGF translocates to and accumulates in the nucleolus of ECs, independent of its high affinity receptor binding (30). It appears to stimulate the transcription of ribosomal genes during the transition from G_0 to G_1 phases of the cell cycle, a step closely linked to ribosome assembly and cell proliferation (31). Confluent ECs, in contrast to growing cells, contain no nuclear FGF (32). A mutant FGF lacking a nuclear translocation sequence fails to induce DNA synthesis and EC proliferation at concentrations sufficient to give rise to receptor-mediated tyrosine phosphorylation and c-fos expression (33).

A long-lasting interaction between FGF and cultured ECs with prolonged activation of PKC has been thought by others to be required to induce cell proliferation (34). Because high-affinity receptors lead to rapid internalization of FGF, and the low affinity sites mediate a slow internalization of FGF (35), the HSPG binding sites may be essential for FGF's growth factor activity.

FGF-HEPARAN SULFATE PROTEOGLYCAN INTERACTIONS:
Heparan sulfate proteoglycans (HSPGs) are ubiquitous constituents of mammalian cell surfaces and most extracellular matrices. EC surface heparan sulfates facilitate the interaction of FGF with its receptor by concentrating FGF at the cell surface, possibly through phosphorylation of FGF at its receptor-binding domain because this process is associated with increased receptor affinity (16,36,37). FGF binding to HSPGs offers protection against proteolytic degradation and creates a reservoir of growth factor in tissues (8,38). Degradative enzymes may not be needed to release FGF from the heparan sulfates in instances where receptors and heparan sulfate–bound FGF are in close proximity because dissociation from heparan sulfates occurs rapidly enough to allow FGF to bind to unoccupied receptors by laws of mass action (36).

In a model of neuroepithelial embryogenesis that may hold clues for the endothelial scenario, Nurcombe and colleagues (39) showed that by sequentially binding different forms of FGF, differentially glycosylated HSPG species regulate development. This regulatory mechanism does not rely on changes in cell surface receptor expression or cessation of growth factor production and allows for rapid changes in cell signaling during development (39).

FGF INHIBITORS: The activities of FGF are limited by transforming growth factor-β (TGF-β), interferon-γ (IFN-γ), and platelet factor-4 (PF-4). TGF-β can be activated from its latent, secreted form by plasmin, which is activated by FGF. TGF-β then limits the PA-inducing activity of FGF through increased synthesis of PA inhibitor-1 (PAI-1) and decreased transcription of the u-PA gene (18). IFN-γ inhibits EC growth possibly by decreasing FGF receptor expression (40). PF-4 blocks the binding of FGF to its receptor and therefore inhibits the migration and tube formation of bovine capillary ECs in culture (41).

A bacterially derived sulfated polysaccharide inhibits the growth and chemotaxis of ECs stimulated by FGF possibly by preventing the binding of FGF at both its low and high affinity binding sites (42). Chloroquine, a drug used to treat malaria and inflammatory diseases, inhibits FGF-stimulated EC growth in a dose-dependent fashion (43).

EFFECTS IN VIVO: Antisense oligonucleotides complementary to FGF messenger RNA (mRNA) illustrate the significant role of FGF as an endothelial growth promoter in an in vitro environment (44). In vivo experiments confirm that FGF has a critical part in the formation of new blood vessels.

Nanogram amounts of FGF induce angiogenesis in the chick embryo chorioallantoic membrane and in the cornea (45). Nabel and colleagues (46) used a eukaryotic expression vector encoding a secreted form of FGF-1 and introduced it by direct gene transfer into porcine arteries. In this somatic transgenic model, FGF-1 expression induced intimal thickening and angiogenesis within 21 days, in comparison with control arteries transfected with an *Escherichia coli* β-galactosidase gene. The neointimal ECs appeared to originate from adjacent arterial luminal ECs because both were negative for von Willebrand factor (46).

Using rabbit ear excision wounds and introducing various cytokines, Pierce and associates (47) showed that FGF induces an angiogenic response with a marked increase in ECs and neovessels. This effect appears to delay wound maturation. In contrast, platelet-derived growth factor (PDGF) augments early glycosaminoglycan and fibronectin deposition and induces greater amounts of collagen, whereas TFG-β1 rapidly enhances collagen synthesis and maturation. Each agent appears to have complementary actions (47).

Villaschi and Nicosia (48) found that addition of purified FGF increases both the number and the length of microvessels sprouting from the explants in a rat aortic injury model and prevents microvessel regression. Neutralizing anti-FGF antibodies cause a 40% reduction of angiogenesis (48).

Vascular endothelial growth factor/vascular permeability factor

BACKGROUND AND EC EFFECTS: Vascular endothelial growth factor (VEGF) and vascular permeability factor (VPF) are two terms for an identical 46-kd protein related to PDGF and produced by several tumor cells, luteal cells, renal glomerular visceral epithelial cells, and vascular smooth muscle cells (VSMCs) (49–51). It is a selective and potent EC mitogen both in vitro and in vivo (50,52); it has no proliferative activity on VSMCs, fibroblasts, and epithelial cells (49). VEGF is angiogenic in vitro, and it causes microvascular ECs grown on 3D collagen gels to invade the underlying matrix and to form capillary-like tubules (52).

VEGF promotes vascular leakage, causes von Willebrand factor release, and synergizes with tumor necrosis factor-α (TNF-α) to promote procoagulant activity on ECs (49). In addition, it induces expression of the only metalloproteinase that can initiate the degradation of interstitial collagen types I to III under normal physiological conditions (53).

VEGF SIGNALING: Several tyrosine kinase receptors have been described for VEGF, including flt and flk-1 (2,54). These receptors are detected only on ECs. Flk-1 in particular is found on ECs during embryogenesis; it is especially abundant in blood islands of the yolk sac, where EC progenitors originate, and on vascular sprouts and branching vessels of developing brain. In contrast, flk-1 transcripts are drastically reduced in adult brain, in which vascular proliferation has ended (2). These findings contrast with the lack of detectable FGF receptors on ECs during embryogenesis (55).

VEGF binds heparin via a nonreceptor binding domain, which strongly potentiates its binding to flt, whereas α2-macroglobulin, a major serum protein, inactivates the receptor binding ability of VEGF (50). Akin to FGF, VEGF induces an angiogenic response via a direct effect on endothelial cells, and, when acting in concert, these two cytokines have a potent synergistic effect on the induction of angiogenesis in vitro (52).

VEGF IN ANGIOGENESIS, MALIGNANCY, AND WOUND HEALING: VEGF mRNA is expressed in cells surrounding an expanding vasculature in embryonic implantation sites, ovarian follicles, corpus luteum, and at sites of repair of endometrial vessels. It predominates in tissues that acquire a new capillary network, but its binding activity is found on both quiescent and proliferating ECs. VEGF expression may be hormonally regulated because it increases with the acquisition of cellular steroidogenic activity and varies with the ovarian cycle in the endometrium. During the early proliferative phase, it is found in the estrogen-responsive, secretory columnar epithelium. Under the influence of progesterone in the secretory phase, when new blood vessel development is maximal, VEGF expression shifts to cells of the underlying stroma comprising the functional endometrium (56).

A particular role for VEGF in tumor angiogenesis is apparent. Expression of VEGF on Chinese hamster ovary (CHO) cells confers on them the ability to form tumors in nude mice (57). Monoclonal antibodies to VEGF inhibit the growth of rhabdomyosarcoma, glioblastoma multiforme, and leiomyosarcoma cell lines in nude mice, but they have no effect on the growth rate of these tumor cells in vitro, implying a direct effect on reducing the vascular density in antibody-treated tumors (57).

In situ analysis of glioblastoma multiforme brain tumor specimens shows that VEGF production is specifically induced in a subset of glioblastoma cells distinguished by their proximity to necrotic foci. Capillaries appear to cluster alongside these VEGF-producing tumor cells. VEGF mRNA levels are dramatically responsive to their O_2 milieu, suggesting a mechanism for these findings. Within a few hours of exposing glioma and muscle cell cultures to hypoxia, VEGF mRNA levels increase and return to background when a normal O_2 supply is restored (58). Comparison of astrocytomas with the more malignant glioblastoma, which is characterized by necrosis and vascular proliferation, reveals that more VEGF is expressed in the latter. Flt is not expressed in normal brain ECs, but it is found in these tumor ECs (59).

The other activity of VEGF on ECs—increased permeability—is a characteristic feature of normal wound healing. Persistent microvascular permeability to plasma proteins, even after cessation of injury, results in extravasation of fibrinogen, and the resultant fibrin serves as a provisional matrix that promotes angiogenesis and scar formation. VEGF mRNA levels in keratinocytes at wound edges are greatly increased, and they correlate with the permeability of wound tissue vessels (60).

Hepatocyte growth factor/scatter factor

Hepatocyte growth factor (HGF) and scatter factor (SF) are identical, basic, heparin-binding glycoproteins that share 38% amino acid identity with plasminogen (61,62). They are produced by fibroblasts and VSMCs. HGF induces renal epithelial cells to form branching networks of tubules in a collagen matrix (63), whereas SF disperses cohesive epithelial colonies and stimulates cell motility (64,65). The receptor for HGF/SF is c-met, a transmembrane tyrosine kinase (66), which is expressed and stimulated by HGF on ECs (67).

HGF stimulates EC growth and motility in vitro and promotes wound repair in EC monolayers. ECs assume a

dendritic phenotype. HGF does not induce procoagulant activity or platelet-activating factor (67), but EC secretion of plasminogen activators and urokinase, which are required during the early stages of angiogenesis when ECs degrade ECM, are induced by SF (68). In a corneal model, HGF produced angiogenesis (67). Immunoreactive SF is present in a perivascular distribution surrounding sites of blood vessel formation in the skin of psoriatic plaques, but not in normal skin, in which angiogenesis is not a feature (68).

Transforming growth factor-β

TGF-β is unlike other cytokines with proangiogenic effects. Some investigators have found that TGF-β induces tube formation by ECs in 3D collagen gels without affecting cell proliferation (69,70), but in other in vitro systems, it is a potent inhibitor of EC proliferation, migration, tube formation, and protease synthesis (71–75). Dramatic increases in collagen and fibronectin synthesis and inhibition of matrix-degrading enzyme production (76,77), brought about by TGF-β, may modulate its effects on endothelial phenotype and explain differences between various in vitro models (69). In vivo TGF-β is angiogenic, although it has been suspected that this action is not directly on ECs but rather on other cells (e.g., fibroblasts and macrophages, whose many products may potentiate the angiogenic response) (78,79).

TGF-β may signal resolution of the angiogenic process begun by factors that are principally initiating stimuli, such as FGF and VEGF. Wound studies in vivo show that FGF produces marked increases in new vessels and persistence of the provisional ECM, whereas TGF-β accelerates maturation of the provisional ECM through rapidly enhanced collagen synthesis, leading to coverage of wound defects with fibrous tissue (47,80). In chorioallantoic membranes, FGF induces primarily small blood vessels, whereas the vessels formed in response to TGF-β are large and bear intercellular junctional complexes (70,79). TGF-β1 also promotes the differentiation of ECs into VSMCs in vitro (81) and stimulates intimal VSMCs to synthesize increased amounts of lipoprotein-binding proteoglycans (82).

TGF-β is secreted constitutively by ECs as a high molecular weight inactive complex, with a latency-associated peptide and a latent TGF-β binding protein. Activation of latent TGF-β occurs in cocultures of ECs with VSMCs or pericytes and is thought to be at least in part mediated by plasmin cleavage of the aminoterminal propeptide. This process is facilitated by FGF, which increases plasminogen activator activity (18,72). Thus, the presence and effectiveness of TGF-β are determined by proximal cell types and the ability to activate the latent form.

Hematopoietic colony-stimulating factors

The colony-stimulating factors (CSFs) are characterized by their profound effects on the proliferation of blood cell precursors. ECs and hematopoietic cells share surface markers such as PECAM-1 (83,84), CD34 (85,86), CD36 (87), and CD45 (88), and they closely interact in the bone marrow, suggesting the common ancestry of their lineages and the possible effectiveness of the CSFs upon the former.

Granulocyte and granulocyte-macrophage CSFs (G-CSF, GM-CSF) have been shown to induce human ECs to migrate and proliferate, without altering their hemostatic or inflammatory phenotypes. In comparison to FGF, induction of migration was of a similar order of magnitude, although the extent of proliferation was less (89,90). In the corneal model, G-CSF induced neovascularization. An inability to repeat these results, however (91), and in particular the lack of demonstrable receptors for GM-CSF on human umbilical vein ECs (HUVECs) by binding analysis, surface expression, and receptor mRNA analysis (92,93), leave the significance of the original observations unclear.

In the last year, it has emerged that resting HUVECs express mRNA for the α- and β-chains of the interleukin-3 (IL-3) receptor (90,91,94). This receptor is functional in mediating IL-3 stimulation of HUVEC DNA synthesis and proliferation (92). Furthermore, use of recombinant human IL-3 and GM-CSF after high-dose cancer chemotherapy is associated with expansion of the vascular network of the bone marrow and an increase in the proportion of CD34-expressing ECs (95). Erythropoietin is also reported to possess mitogenic and chemotactic activity on ECs (96).

Other cytokines affecting EC renewal and angiogenesis

ONCOSTATIN M: Oncostatin M is a glycoprotein of 196 amino acids produced by activated T cells that inhibits the growth of several human tumor cell lines. It also inhibits the growth of normal bovine aortic ECs, while stimulating the growth of a number of fibroblast cell lines (97).

INTERLEUKIN-4: IL-4 is a potent EC mitogen (98), and it also stimulates the expression of u-PA (99), suggesting that it has a role in angiogenesis. Both these effects of IL-4 occur preferentially in microvascular, rather than in macrovascular, endothelium.

INTERLEUKIN-8: IL-8 has been reported to stimulate the chemotaxis of HUVECs with effects comparable to FGF. TNF-α or IL-8 antibodies reduce the chemotactic response for HUVECs to conditioned media from lipo-polysaccharide-stimulated peripheral blood monocytes or synovial tissue macrophages. Antisense RNA oligonucleotide to IL-8 blocks the production of angiogenic activity by monocytes. IL-8 binds to heparin, as do the well characterized angiogenic factors, such as FGF and VEGF (100).

EPIDERMAL GROWTH FACTOR: Epidermal growth factor (EGF) is a mitogenic polypeptide that accelerates angiogenesis (101). EGF and EGF receptor immunoreactivity is present at the cytoplasmic interdigitations between ECs and pericytes in the angiogenic immature capillaries of human granulation tissue, but it is absent in mature capillaries (102).

PLATELET-DERIVED GROWTH FACTOR: PDGF is a mitogen and a chemotaxin for VSMCs and fibroblasts (103), and it has roles in wound healing and angiogenesis (47,104,105). It stimulates fibroblasts to synthesize collagen and collagenase, which leads to modification of the ECM; it is also a potent vasoconstrictor (101). PDGF is stored in platelet α-granules, ECs, VSMCs, and macrophages, in particular those in newly formed atherosclerotic plaques (101,106). Two receptors, α and β, are ligand-activated tyrosine kinases (107). IL-1, TNF-α, lipopolysaccharide, and blood flow induce accumulation of PDGF mRNA in ECs, whereas IFN-γ and nitric oxide have the opposite effect (108,109).

INSULIN-LIKE GROWTH FACTOR: Insulin-like growth factor-1 is secreted by ECs from their basal abluminal surface. It supports VSMC and fibroblast growth in vitro (110,111).

INTERLEUKIN-1: IL-1 inhibits the proliferation of ECs in vitro, particularly when combined with FGF (112). It promotes growth of VSMCs and fibroblasts, possibly via increased PDGF release (106).

ENDOTHELIN-1: Endothelin-1 (ET-1) is a 21 amino acid peptide released from the endothelium. It elicits a variety of biological effects that include VSMC contraction and proliferation (113). ET-1 production by ECs is augmented by thrombin, G-CSF, TGF-β, and IL-1 (114–116). Fluid shear stress induces rapid and significant down-regulation of ET-1 mRNA and peptide release (117).

Summary of the pathophysiological effects of endothelial mitogens

Knowledge of the actions, structures, and encoding genes of the endothelial mitogenic factors has been applied to pathophysiology, and examples of the in vivo relevance of each cytokine have been given. A range of studies, including those of cytokine or cytokine-induced mediator expression in pathological specimens and those of direct addition of a cytokine (e.g., by gene transfection) or its withdrawal (e.g., by antisense oligonucleotide), permit increasing levels of confidence with regard to conclusions of causality.

The descriptive method, which is more suited to human samples, is exemplified by work on VEGF expression in the uterus (56) and the role of angiogenic factors in rheumatoid arthritis. Synovial pannus tissue in rheumatoid arthritic joints is invasive and destructive of adjacent cartilage and bone. Its formation is accompanied by ingrowth of new vascular networks, and the level of angiogenic activity correlates with infiltration of inflammatory cells, synovial hyperplasia, and clinical score (118,119). FGF expression has been shown in ECs of the rheumatoid pannus and in streptococcal-induced arthritis in rats (120,121). EGF and PDGF localization is also associated with areas of new vessel growth (122). Agents effective in the therapy of rheumatoid arthritis inhibit EC proliferation (123,124).

A study of injured rat aorta implicates FGF more conclusively in endothelial cell responses, but its application in human disease has not been established. Immunohistochemical staining of rat aorta shows FGF in the cytoplasm of endothelial and smooth muscle cells. Endogenous FGF is demonstrable by Western blot analysis in aorta-conditioned medium after ring dissection. Neutralizing anti-FGF antibodies inhibit the increased numbers and length of sprouting microvessels provoked by injury, suggesting that the FGF present is functional. Purified FGF increases both the number and the length of microvessels sprouting from the explants, particularly late after the injury, when release of endogenous FGF is minimal. FGF release by vascular cells thus appears to have a role in the autoregulation of angiogenesis after vascular injury (48).

Surgical interventions, such as bypass grafting, atherectomy, or endarterectomy, involve similar vascular injury, but they are also often complicated by intimal hyperplasia of VSMCs. The increased rate of migration and turnover of VSMCs in response to injury is dependent on the presence of dividing ECs. VSMC proliferation is maximal when the ECs are proliferating. When the ECs stabilize and cover the lumenal surface, VSMC proliferation slows. The relationship of this phenomenon to EC-derived FGF or PDGF is not clear (125), although the failure of confluent ECs to localize FGF to their nuclei is interesting (32). TGF-β also decreases VSMC proliferation (72). This effect may explain why VSMC proliferation slows when ECs cover an injury.

A recent innovation of in vitro assays—coculturing ECs with their supporting stromal cells to parallel the in vivo situation—provides another demonstration of interactions between ECs with their neighboring pericytes or VSMCs. Pericytes grown in coculture with ECs inhibit EC proliferation (126), on the basis of the ability of cocultures but not homocellular cultures to produce activated TGF-β (72). Angiogenesis in the fetal retina ceases as mural pericytes appear, and pathological neovascularization in diabetic retinopathy is associated with loss of pericytes (127).

EC cocultures with keratinocytes shed light on the common dermatological disease psoriasis, which is characterized by hyperproliferation of keratinocytes and abnormally extensive dermal capillary networks. Keratinocytes produce TGF-α, which in an autocrine manner leads to their hyperproliferation. TGF-α also stimulates human omental microvascular ECs in type I collagen gels to form tubular-like structures. When keratinocytes are cocultured with omental ECs, tubular-like EC structures appear in collagen gels, which are inhibitable by anti-TGF-α antibodies (128). It thus appears that TGF-α acts in an autocrine fashion on keratinocytes and in a paracrine manner on ECs, therefore appearing to facilitate the neovascularization required to allow for the increased surface keratinocyte population.

Angiogenesis appears to be closely related to malignancy (129). Angiogenic agents have been isolated from tumors, and neovascularization is present in most malignancies at the time of their detection, thus appearing to be directly related to malignant grade and prognosis. The malignant progression of melanoma from normal skin to dysplastic melanocytic nevus, to cutaneous malignant melanoma, and finally to metastatic malignant melanoma is associated with increasing vascularity (130). Horak and associates (131) showed that the number of microvessels in primary breast cancers is directly correlated with pathological indicators of an increasingly poor prognosis. The association of VEGF with rhabdomyosarcoma, glioblastoma multiforme, and leiomyosarcoma is an example of the role of cytokine-induced angiogenesis in malignancy (57). Tumor-cell hypoxia is believed to stimulate production of VEGF. In acquired immunodeficiency syndrome–related Kaposi's sarcoma, the malignant cells also express cytokines with autocrine and paracrine growth effects, which foster growth of this vascular tumor (132–134). Coculture of ECs with human glioblastoma cells demonstrates how angiogenic cytokines may be working. In contact with glioma cells, ECs form tubes, an in vitro surrogate for capillaries. Only glioma-cell lines that possess high levels of FGF mRNA induce such tube formation, and this process can be blocked by coadministration of anti-FGF antibody (135).

Because EC renewal and angiogenesis are key events in important pathological processes such as wound healing, inflammation, and malignancy, but are not a feature of normal tissues except in the female reproductive system, attempts to define angiogenic inhibitors have been in progress. Physiological inhibitors of angiogenesis are present in blood and urine, and they include cortisol metabolites that lack glucocorticoid and mineralocorticoid activities (136). These metabolites may act by increasing the synthesis of PAI-1 (137). Heparin potentiates their action, and it is believed to function by virtue of its high affinity for angiogenic factors, such as FGF and VEGF (138).

IFN-α has been used successfully in pulmonary hemangiomatosis with an associated decrease in the density of abnormal vessels (139). Derivatives of *Aspergillus fumigatus* products are effective inhibitors of angiogenesis in vitro, as well as in tumors and collagen-induced arthritis in rats, with minimal toxicity (140,141). A number of other compounds inhibit angiogenesis in vitro, including antiestrogens (142), cyclosporine (143), ribonuclease inhibitors (144), protein kinase inhibitors (145), and calcium channel blockers (146). In vitro experimentation has shown that changes in the constitution of ECM or monoclonal antibodies directed to β1 and β3 integrins, which mediate EC-matrix interactions, can alter the type and number of capillary tubes formed (147,148). This finding offers prospects for the development of targeted inhibitors of angiogenesis.

ENDOTHELIAL CELL INTERACTIONS WITH BLOOD MOLECULES AND LEUKOCYTES

In this section, the roles of cytokines acting on or produced by endothelia, which affect its relationship with the elements of blood, are considered. It appears that specific, separate mechanisms exist that deal with the arrest of mobile leukocytes, their secure attachment to the endothelial surface, and finally their passage between surface ECs into the interstitium. These inflammatory processes and others leading to thrombosis or immune recognition are controlled by specific cytokines with both facilitatory and inhibitory actions.

Tumor necrosis factor-α and interleukin-1

TNF-α and IL-1 are proinflammatory cytokines with effects on multiple biological systems. Both act on ECs, most often with a similar outcome; thus, they are considered together, but mention will be made of each individually when their effects differ.

IL-1 is a 17-kd peptide with two biologically active forms, IL-1α and IL-1β (149). TNF-α is a trimer of three 17-kd subunits. Its main source is the monocyte-macrophage when it is stimulated by lipopolysaccharide (LPS), IL-1, IFN-α, IFN-γ, OR GM-CSF (150). The mast cell may be another important source of TNF-α in vivo (151). Peripheral blood lymphocytes, natural killer (NK) cells, and

polymorphs produce a relatively small amount of TNF-α (150). VSMCs adjacent to the endothelium express TNF-α mRNA and protein on exposure to inflammatory signals, and this process is superinduced by protein synthesis inhibitors (152). Sources of IL-1 are extensive and include blood monocytes, neutrophils, T and B lymphocytes, tissue macrophages, VSMCs, and ECs. The most common stimulus for IL-1 transcription is endotoxin (149).

In general, TNF-α promotes selective cytotoxicity and catabolism. There are changes in ECM through induction of collagenases, which lead to bone resorption, and of plasminogen activator, which leads to angiogenesis (153). On blood cells, TNF-α and IL-1 have a proinflammatory effect. Neutrophils and monocytes gain an increased capacity for phagocytosis, antibody-dependent cellular cytotoxicity, degranulation, and production of reactive oxygen species. T cells express more IL-2 receptor and major histocompatibility complex (MHC) class II antigens. They achieve a greater proliferative potential in synergy with IL-2, and they produce more IFN-γ. B cells also augment their proliferation, differentiation, and production of antibodies (149,150). The general proinflammatory effects of these cytokines, however, also depend on their endothelial functions, as well as on these leukocyte changes.

COAGULATION: TNF-α and IL-1 regulate the coagulation system through actions on the endothelium. Procoagulant activity of ECs is induced (3,154). The production of thrombomodulin, a surface glycoprotein on ECs that controls intravascular coagulation cascades through interactions with proteins C and S, is suppressed (154,155). Arachidonate metabolism is activated; in particular, prostacyclin synthesis in cultured vascular ECs is induced (156). TNF-α induces expression of an EC plasminogen activator inhibitor (157–159). Effects on plasminogen activator are recognized, but both increases and decreases have been reported (153,157). In patients treated with recombinant human TNF-α in a Phase I cancer trial, induction of endothelial-derived tissue-type plasminogen activator, recognized by the presence of fibrin degradation products in plasma, occurred within one hour of the initiation of TNF-α (160).

The surface of TNF-α-activated ECs elicits a hemostatic response when exposed to flowing nonanticoagulated blood. Tissue factor is expressed, and deposition of fibrin, platelet aggregates, and leukocytes follows; in an experimental model, 63% of the EC surface became covered. Resting ECs, in contrast, show no or little fibrin, platelet, and leukocyte deposition. The addition of antibodies against tissue factor to TNF-α-activated ECs abrogates fibrin and platelet deposition, but it allows leukocyte adherence to occur to the same extent. Thus, the endothelial effects of TNF-α on hemostasis and leukocyte capture involve related but dissociated mechanisms (161).

ADHESION: TNF-α and IL-1 increase the adhesiveness of endothelium for bloodstream leukocytes by an EC-specific mechanism (162). They also modulate the interactions between adjoining ECs. This process involves induction, up-regulated expression, or activation of molecules on the endothelial surface, which interact with ligands on leukocytes and ECs. The main groups of such regulated adhesins are the selectins, the L-selectin ligands, the immunoglobulin superfamily, and the integrins.

SELECTINS: E-selectin (ES; ELAM-1) and P-selectin (PS; GMP-140; CD62) are endothelial, lectin-bearing glycoproteins that mediate the initial contacts between leukocyte and endothelium as leukocytes move away from the axial bloodstream and roll over the endothelial surface, prior to their firm attachment (163–165). Their leukocyte ligands are sialylated, fucosylated oligosaccharides (166).

ES is found in low to undetectable quantities on resting ECs in vitro and in vivo. Both IL-1 and TNF-α induce ES mRNA and protein synthesis. Surface expression in vitro reaches a maximal level at 4 hours, after which it declines to background by 24 hours, despite the continued presence of the agonists (167–170). Mast-cell degranulation leads to the display of ES on adjacent ECs in vivo. Antiserum to TNF-α abrogates this potentially important pathway of induction (151). Surface ES is lost by internalization and external release, processes not known to be controlled by cytokines (171). The rate of internalization of ES is comparatively higher than that of intercellular adhesion molecule (ICAM)-1; therefore, its pro-adhesive effects may be relatively acute (1.7% of membrane-bound ES/min vs < 0.1% of membrane-bound ICAM-1/minute) (172,173).

PS is expressed in varying levels on resting ECs, which maintain a large stock of PS in cytoplasmic granules (Weibel-Palade bodies). This store is rapidly transferred to the EC membrane in response to histamine and thrombin, but expression is brief, and its functional aspect is lost within 30 minutes (174,175). PS is inducible by TNF in mouse and bovine ECs at both mRNA and cell surface protein levels. The PS protein increase is 2- to 4-fold, and it is maximal at 3 to 4 hours (176).

L-SELECTIN LIGANDS: CD34 is a highly glycosylated, negatively charged, sialomucin-like transmembrane molecule better known for its presence on hematopoietic progenitor cells, which has recently been recognized as an endothelial ligand for L-selectin (LS; LAM-1; LECAM-1), the leukocyte adhesion molecule (177,178). It has a broad EC distribution, including high endothelial venules, but it is absent from most large vessels and placental sinuses (178). The function of CD34 is likely to be controlled by differential vessel-specific glycosylation, as well as translocation to and oligomerization at the EC surface. Vessel-specific glycosylation may explain why leukocytes only adhere to postcapillary venules, even though CD34 appears to be expressed on capillaries and venules (162). TNF-α, IL-1β, and IFN-γ have been reported to decrease the expression of CD34 on cultured ECs (179).

Glycam-1 (or Sgp50) is a 50-kd, mucin-like glycoprotein that also serves as an LS ligand. It is restricted, however, to lymph node high endothelial venules, and it is not known to be influenced by cytokines (180). Both CD34 and Glycam-1 were characterized by precipitation with a chimeric molecule containing the extracellular domain of mouse LS and human immunoglobulin.

A third endothelial ligand for LS must be proposed on the basis of older evidence describing an antigen on HUVECs that is optimally induced by TNF-α and IL-1β, but also to a lesser extent by IFN-γ and IL-4 (181). This ligand is a neuraminidase-sensitive molecule, which implies that it bears sialic acid, as do CD34 and Glycam-1. It is expressed between 2 and 4 hours after HUVEC stimulation, and it persists for at least 24 hours (181). Its induction by cytokines is thus unlike CD34, and its distribution is wider than that known for Glycam-1.

Soluble LS is shed from the surface of leukocytes after their stimulation by cytokines such as TNF-α. Soluble LS inhibits LS-specific attachment of lymphocytes to TNF-α–activated ECs (182). Fluid-phase PS also inhibits adhesion of TNF-α–activated neutrophils to resting ECs, through inhibition of a CD18-dependent process. The control of soluble PS production is not currently understood (183).

IMMUNOGLOBULIN SUPERFAMILY ENDOTHELIAL ADHESINS: Intercellular adhesion molecule-1 and -2 (ICAM-1, 2), vascular cell adhesion molecule-1 (VCAM-1), and platelet endothelial cell adhesion molecule-1 (PECAM-1; CD31) are members of the immunoglobulin superfamily. ICAM-1, and ICAM-2 and VCAM-1 interact with leukocyte β2 and β1 integrins respectively, to serve a shear-resistant adhesion between ECs and leukocytes, which follows and stabilizes the rolling attachment initiated by the selectins (148). ICAM-1, the ligand for CD11a-CD11b/CD18, is constitutively expressed on ECs. TNF-α or IL-1 increase its expression, with a plateau at 24 to 72 hours (169). ICAM-2 is also constitutively expressed on ECs, but it is not subject to regulation (184).

VCAM-1 expression is absent on resting ECs. TNF-α or IL-1 induce it within 2 hours (peak, 12–24 hours), and levels substantially higher than baseline persist for at least 72 hours (185,186). There are two isoforms of VCAM-1 with 6 and 7 Ig-like domains and subtlely different binding characteristics (187). The former is expressed earlier than the latter, which then becomes the main EC isoform. VSMCs are normally devoid of adhesion proteins in vivo, and they express only small amounts of VCAM-1 in culture. TNF-α and IL-1 induce human saphenous vein SMCs to express VCAM-1 (Gamble JR, et al., unpublished observations).

PECAM-1 is constitutively expressed in a homogeneous pattern on EC membranes in vivo, but it concentrates predominately at points of cell-to-cell contact on cultured ECs (188,189). It appears to have a role in EC-to-EC contacts and in leukocyte transmigration through the intercellular junctions of ECs (190). Using tissue specimens from breast, skin, stomach, colon, uterine cervix, endometrium, myometrium, and bronchus incubated with TNF-α for up to 6 hours, as well as a dermal ragweed antigen injection model, Ioffreda and colleagues (191) showed that TNF-α leads to a redistribution of PECAM-1 from its original uniform pattern on EC surfaces to one localized to areas of contact between adjacent ECs (191). Thus, TNF-α–stimulated molecules, ES and PECAM-1, may sequentially enhance leukocyte-EC binding in postcapillary venules, direct adherent cells to sites most conducive to transvascular diapedesis, and lead to transmigration.

INTEGRINS: ECs express a number of integrins believed to function as interendothelial adhesins or as ECM receptors. TNF-α and IFN-γ decrease EC β3 integrins, and they induce α1β1. The α1β1 integrin is normally absent from HUVECs, but is present on capillary ECs. The laminin receptor α6β1 is strongly decreased by TNF-α or IL-1β, whereas α2β1, α3β1, and α5β1 are not altered. Laminin adhesion by ECs is consequently decreased (192).

MAJOR HISTOCOMPATIBILITY COMPLEX GENES: Class I MHC is expressed on ECs, but at a level relatively lower than that on macrophages or lymphocytes. This expression is increased 2- to 4-fold over 24 hours by TNF-α (but not by IL-1) through an increase in transcription. There is a synergistic elevation in class I antigen with IFN-γ or IFN-β, without any alteration in TNF receptor number due to a multiplicative increase in transcriptional rate (193,194). Synthesis and expression of transporter in antigen processing-1 (TAP-1), an MHC-encoded gene product that is required for efficient association of intracellular peptide antigen with nascent human leukocyte antigen (HLA) class I H-chain and β2-microglobulin, are increased in human ECs by TNF-α, IFN-β, or IFN-γ (195). TNF-α does not induce class II expression de novo in human ECs (193), and neither TNF-α nor IL-1 alters MHC on VSMCs (196). TNF-α thus allows ECs to present class I–restricted antigens to T cells, which may propagate the inflammatory response.

ENDOTHELIAL PERMEABILITY TO MACRO-MOLECULES: The permeability of endothelial surfaces to macromolecules such as albumin is an important feature of edematous processes. TNF-α, IL-1, and IFN-γ increase EC monolayer permeability to albumin in vitro,

and this effect is augmented by combining these cytokines (197,198). The ECs undergo parallel changes in morphology, from cobblestone to elongated cells, with formation of prominent intercellular gaps and actin stress fibers. There is an accompanying loss of fibronectin and remodeling of the ECM (199). ECs from different sites show varying susceptibility to this change: HUVECs require prolonged exposures of 72 hours, whereas bovine ECs demonstrate a change within 1 to 3 hours after exposure (198,200).

Endothelial glycosaminoglycans (GAGs) are important in regulating vascular permeability as well as cell interactions with soluble factors and resistance to thrombosis. IL-1 and TNF-α alter GAG metabolism in cultured HUVECs, causing a marked increase in culture supernatant GAGs and a decrease in cell-associated GAGs that is detectable after 12 to 48 hours of coincubation. There is a concomitant increase in GAG synthesis. Histochemically, these changes are associated with marked reduction and redistribution of endothelial surface anionic sites. Such changes may contribute to the disturbances of vascular endothelial homeostasis associated with inflammatory states (201).

LEUKOCYTE TRANSMIGRATION: HUVECs incubated with TNF-α or IL-1 for 4 hours do not display morphological changes or increased albumin permeability, but they do show an increase in leukocyte transmigration (202). Migration occurs across EC junctions, and it is dependent on the ECs being biosynthetically active. Neutrophils are polarized but not degranulated, and there are no signs of ECM lysis. Because the number of traversing neutrophils is no greater when cytokine stimulation is joined by a chemotactic gradient in some systems, it is suggested that both operate through this mechanism (203–205).

Conditioned media of TNF-α- or IL-1–stimulated ECs induce transmigration of neutrophils when added to the basal EC compartment. IFN-γ, IL-2, PDGF, and platelet-activating factor (PAF) are unable to mimic this effect. Antisera to IL-6, G-CSF, and GM-CSF, all products of stimulated ECs, do not diminish the chemotactic activity of the conditioned medium. IL-8, a member of the chemokine family, is present in this conditioned medium (206), and it acts as a chemoattractant for granulocytes. Other products of activated ECs, such as macrophage inflammatory protein-1 (MIP-1) and monocyte chemotactic protein-1 (MCP-1), are selective for lymphocyte and monocyte chemotaxis. Adhesion to ECs and transmigration through EC monolayers by leukocytes are thus both facilitated by TNF-α or IL-1 in separate, sequential processes (204).

EFFECTS ON CYTOKINE PRODUCTION: TNF-α and IL-1 foster EC production of a number of cytokines that often have proinflammatory actions (e.g., IL-1 itself)

(106,207), the chemokines (207), and G-CSF and GM-CSF (208,209). They mediate the release of PDGF from cultured ECs, and they augment IL-6 secretion (106, 210–212). IL-1 increases EC production of ET-1 (116).

Synthesis and release of the signaling phospholipid PAF is stimulated by TNF-α or IL-1α treatment of ECs (213). Such ECs support adhesion of neutrophils that are unactivated and do not adhere to plastic, suggesting that PAF may be a proadhesion signal from ECs to neutrophils. Although PAF antagonists inhibit adhesion, the time course for adhesion and PAF production are not strictly concordant. Acetyl coenzyme A raises PAF levels, but it has no effect on adhesion, and although both IL-1α and IL-1β stimulate adhesion, only the former results in PAF production (214).

TNF-α also decreases expression of endothelial antigens. Westphal and associates (215) reported a monoclonal antibody recognizing a 180-kd molecule expressed on the EC luminal surface, which is down-regulated by TNF-α and is possibly endoglin, a TGF-β–binding cell surface protein.

EFFECTS ON LIPOPROTEIN METABOLISM:
TNF-α or IL-1 increase low density lipoprotein (LDL) receptor expression on microvascular ECs in culture. There is a parallel increase in internalization and degradation of LDL (216). Because ECs oxidize LDLs, and because LDLs are atherogenic, cytokines produced by adherent monocytes found in early atherosclerosis may facilitate this pathological process.

INTRACELLULAR SIGNALING

TNF-α Receptors: TNF-α acts on cells via two receptors, p55 and p75, which are partially homologous in their extracellular domains, but lack any intracytoplasmic similarity. The role of these two moieties is still controversial, and it varies with the analytical method (217). ECs possess both receptors (218). Using TNF-α mutants with preferential binding to either p55 or p75, Barbara and colleagues (219) showed that the p55 receptor is necessary for induction of ES, neutrophil transmigration across EC monolayers, and EC IL-8 secretion. The p75 receptor only facilitates an increase in the potency of TNF (219,220). N-terminal amino acids of TNF-α are also critical for both receptor binding and biological activity on ECs (221).

Postreceptor Pathways: TNF-α increases EC monolayer permeability via a G-protein intermediary (200), but activators of the stimulatory or inhibitory guanine nucleotide–dependent binding proteins do not affect TNF-α–induced surface expression of ES or VCAM-1 (222).

There is partial evidence of protein kinase C and A (PKC, PKA) involvement in the induction of ES expres-

sion and IL-6 production. PMA and forskolin, both agonists of these respective protein kinases, can mediate these effects, and appropriate kinase inhibitors impede them. These kinase inhibitors, however, do not block the effects of TNF-α, and other cyclic adenosine monophosphate agonists are not effective (193,222).

Absence of PKC translocation from cytosol to the plasma or nuclear membrane particulate fractions of HUVECs after TNF-α exposure, has argued against a significant PKC-mediated pathway for the actions of TNF-α. The β-1 PKC isozyme, however, becomes activated without translocation, and it is sufficient for expression of ES and VCAM-1. This evidence from Harlan's group (223) suggests that PKC may mediate some effects of TNF-α. PKC is also strongly implicated in TNF-α induction of tissue plasminogen activator, because this substance is interdicted by the PKC inhibitors, H7 and staurosporine, and it is stimulated by 4β phorbol, 12 myristate, 13 acetate (PMAs) (153).

IL-1β–mediated endothelial cell phospholipase A2 activity and prostacyclin synthesis occur via a novel transducing pathway that does not involve early activation of phospholipase C, phospholipase D, or adenylate cyclase (224).

Activation of Transcription Factors: TNF-α and IL-1 signaling on ECs involves activation of the transcription factors AP-1, NF-kappa B (NF-kB), interferon regulatory factor 1, cAMP response element (CRE), and TRE (PMA response element) (193,225). This level of the signaling pathway offers some explanation for the selective endothelial induction of ES. Two proximal ES promoter elements, in addition to NF-kB, are essential for cytokine induction of ES transcription. One of these elements, however, is not endothelial-specific, because it can function as a T-cell enhancer, as well as cooperate with NF-kB to yield cytokine induction of ES gene transcription in ECs (226). DNA methylation of the ES promoter represses NF-kB transactivation in nonendothelial cells, and, in comparison, the ES promoter in ECs is undermethylated, suggesting that methylation could have a role in cell-type–specific expression of this gene (227).

The cytokine-responsive regions of the VCAM-1 promoter are functional NF-kB and GATA elements (228). A comparison of the transcriptional control of VCAM-1 in muscle and ECs is enlightening. Muscle cells display high basal VCAM-1 expression that is not cytokine-inducible; a position-specific enhancer overrides other promoter elements. ECs have octamer binding sites that act as silencers, thus dampening VCAM-1 expression in unstimulated cells. TNF-α overcomes this inhibition through two adjacent NF-kB sites (229).

NF-kB induction by IL-1α, TNF-α, and LPS is inhibited by I-kappa Bα (IKBα or MAD-3), which sequesters NF-kB to the cytoplasm. Cell stimuli, such as TNF-α or

PMA, cause rapid degradation of IKBα, thus relieving this inhibition and allowing NF-kB to translocate to the nucleus and transactivate its target genes. Following this process, there is a dramatic increase in IKBα mRNA and protein synthesis. Expression of IKBα is also inversely regulated by NF-kB in a negative-feedback mechanism: NF-kB down-regulates its own activity after transient activation of target genes has been achieved (230,231).

DISEASE ASSOCIATIONS

ENDOTHELIAL DAMAGE: Several diseases are associated with elevated serum or tissue levels of TNF-α or IL-1, such as idiopathic pulmonary fibrosis (232), systemic vasculitis (233,234), rheumatoid arthritis (235), psoriasis (236), cerebral malaria (237), and sepsis (238). All these disorders have some form of vascular pathology.

There is ex vivo evidence that supports the role of TNF-α and IL-1 in EC injury in Kawasaki's disease (KS). KS histopathology shows panvasculitis with endothelial necrosis and Ig deposition. Sudden death stemming from coronary arteritis is well recognized in this condition. Circulating antibodies in patients with KS display complement-dependent cytotoxic activity against IL-1 or TNF-α–inducible EC antigens, but not against resting ECs (239).

In vitro models of endothelial injury also suggest that these cytokines may bring about EC damage. After IL-1 activation, for instance, EC monolayers coincubated with unstimulated neutrophils show extensive EC detachment and loss of monolayer integrity. This process is mimicked by neutrophil elastase exposure, and it is prevented by serine protease inhibitors or avoidance of direct EC-neutrophil contact (240).

ADHESION MOLECULE EXPRESSION IN TISSUES: Examination of the tissue expression of adhesion molecules confirms their association with inflammatory diseases, and it indirectly implies that TNF-α and IL-1 exhibit widespread endothelial activity.

Normal peripheral lymph node and mucosa-associated lymphoid endothelium show no VCAM-1, but they do exhibit ICAM-1. VCAM-1 is present in follicular centers and interfollicular zones. ECs in most other normal tissues express little or no VCAM-1, but focal reactivity is seen in arterial vasa vasorum, hepatic Kupffer's cells, and some renal tubular epithelial cells (241). ES is absent from normal capillaries, but it is found on large vessel and umbilical vein endothelium (242).

In acute appendicitis or diverticulitis, strong VCAM-1 and ES staining is seen in ECs of dilated serosal venules. Lymphadenitis (sarcoid or toxoplasmal) shows focal venular VCAM-1, but there is little or no ES. VCAM-1 staining is stronger and more widespread in cat-scratch lymphadenitis, and ES is also present. In most dermatoses, VCAM-1 and ES show venular endothelial expression. Vascular pericytes in inflamed skin may also stain for VCAM-1; ECs in the same vessel sometimes stain negative. This finding is consistent with our in vitro observations of the induction of VCAM-1 staining on VSMCs by TNF-α or IL-1.

VCAM-1 is abundant in the synovitis of rheumatoid arthritis. It is present in venules associated with chronic inflammatory cell infiltrates and also on hyperplastic synovial lining cells. ES is also present; it varies in intensity according to disease activity, and it is localized to ECs. The level of expression of both adhesins is far less in the synovium of osteoarthritis, a condition with fewer inflammatory features (241,243). Psoriatic arthritis, usually indistinguishable from rheumatoid disease with regard to the degree of clinical inflammatory joint findings, also shows less EC ES (244).

VCAM-1 is expressed on venular ECs in cardiac and renal allografts, and its presence correlates with T cell infiltrates (245,246). During rejection of human liver transplants, there is increased expression of ICAM-1 on target structures, such as bile ducts and venous endothelium, as well as on lymphocytes infiltrating the graft (247).

Human coronary arteries and abdominal aortas affected by diffuse intimal thickening and atheromatous plaques show a marked increase in expression of ICAM-1, ES, and, to a lesser extent, HLA-DR/DP on ECs adjacent to subendothelial infiltrates of T lymphocytes and macrophages. This effect contrasts with lower or absent expression of these markers at sites without prominent inflammatory cell infiltrates, and it suggests that cytokines produced by these subintimal infiltrates may activate the endothelium in a manner similar to that observed in the microvasculature at sites of immune inflammation (248).

IN VIVO ACTIONS: Subcutaneous injections of TNF-α in baboon skin attempt to stimulate the natural release of this cytokine in vivo. These experiments show that ES, ICAM-1, and VCAM-1 expression are induced at postcapillary sites, which concurs with results seen in cultured ECs. Expression of ES at such sites is evident 2 hours after injection, and it correlates highly with neutrophilic exudates. ICAM-1 and VCAM-1 are seen 24 to 48 hours after TNF-α exposure, and they correlate with mononuclear infiltration. Such results support the hypothesis that selective adhesion molecule expression contributes to selective leukocyte extravasation (249,250).

The tissue injury that accompanies hypoxemia and reoxygenation has features of the host response in inflammation, suggesting that cytokines such as IL-1 may act as mediators in this setting. Human ECs subjected to hypoxia elaborate IL-1 activity. There is an increase in the level of IL-1α mRNA, followed by induction of ES and enhanced expression of ICAM-1 during reoxygenation.

Adherence of leukocytes is increased 3- to 5-fold, and it is partly blocked by antibodies to ES and ICAM-1. Suppression of endothelial-derived IL-1, using antibodies to IL-1α, specific, antisense oligonucleotides, or the IL-1 receptor antagonist, decreases leukocyte adherence to reoxygenated ECs, thus emphasizing the integral role of IL-1 in the adherence phenomenon.

Mice subjected to hypoxia display increased plasma levels of IL-1α, induction of IL-1α mRNA in lung, and enhanced expression of ICAM-1 in pulmonary tissue compared with normoxemic control mice. Thus, hypoxia is a stimulus that induces EC synthesis and release of IL-1α, and it may result in an autocrine enhancement of adhesion molecule expression (251,252).

Plasmodium falciparum–infected erythrocytes isolated from a patient with severe complicated malaria bound to TNF-α–treated human vascular ECs via ES, ICAM-1, and VCAM-1. Attachment of infected erythrocytes to blood vessel walls is understood to be the primary step in the vascular occlusion underlying this disease, in which serum TNF-α levels are characteristically high. ES and VCAM-1 are expressed on brain microvascular endothelium of postmortem brain tissue from patients dying of cerebral malaria (253).

A role for IL-1 and ECs in the neuronal mechanisms related to β-amyloid protein deposition in senile plaques in patients with Alzheimer's disease is suspected. The protein precursor of β-amyloid is expressed on ECs in senile plaques. Its mRNA in human endothelial, neuronal, and brain-derived murine ECs increases when these cells are exposed to IL-1β (254).

Pancreatic carcinoma cells are among a group of neoplastic cells that express the ES ligand, sialyl Lewis (a). Their attachment to activated ECs is thus regulated by cytokines such as IL-1β and TNF-α, which induce endothelial ES (255).

Finally, EC activation by cytokines can also be beneficial. Congenital toxoplasmosis involves infection of umbilical cord vessels as a major route of transmission. IL-1β and TNF-α, in cooperation, inhibit EC replication of *T. gondii*, an obligate intracellular parasite. IFN-γ has a similar retardive effect (256).

Chemokines

Chemokines are a group of 8- to 11-kd proteins produced by ECs as well as leukocytes, fibroblasts, and keratinocytes (206,257). Their primary function is chemoattraction, but stimulation of leukocyte microbicidal activity and the respiratory burst become evident at higher concentrations. They are divided into two families on the basis of their leukocyte predilection and structure. The α-subfamily, exemplified by IL-8 (neutrophil-activating protein-1), has an amino acid intervening between the first two cysteines of its amino terminus (i.e., C-X-C), whereas the β-subfamily, exemplified by MCP-1, does not (i.e., C-C) (258,259).

Each chemokine shows some selectivity for a leukocyte species both in vitro and in vivo. IL-8 acts on neutrophils, although there is also some evidence for T cell and eosinophil activity (259–261). MCP-1 is a chemoattractant for human monocytes (262). MIP-1 attracts activated T cells, whereas RANTES (regulated on activation, normal T expressed and secreted) acts on unstimulated T cells, monocytes, and eosinophils (263–265). Furthermore, MIP-1α acts preferentially on CD8+ lymphocytes, whereas MIP-1β attracts CD4+ cells (263). This chemotactic discrimination, plus that offered by the adhesion molecules, provides the means to selectively control extravasation of each leukocyte subset.

IL-8 AND NEUTROPHIL TRANSMIGRATION:

Endothelia treated with IL-1 or TNF-α bring about neutrophil transmigration. This effect appears to be at least partly due to stimulation of the endothelium's endogenous production of IL-8, which acts as a chemoattractant if added to the basal EC compartment in an in vitro model of the vessel wall (205,206). Antisera to IL-8 markedly inhibit neutrophil transmigration across activated EC monolayers, and washing the basilar compartment of the vessel wall, which depletes IL-8 from the subendothelial matrix, also prevents neutrophil invasion unless IL-8 is readded (205). IL-8 is less effective in a chemokinetic role (i.e., when placed on both sides of the endothelium) (202).

Given that neutrophils must contact the endothelium for transmigration to occur, it is suggested that IL-8 creates not only a chemotactic gradient, but also a haptotactic gradient of IL-8 molecules over the EC surface, along which neutrophils may move (7,204). Consistent with this proposal, IL-8 binding sites exist on ECs of postcapillary and collective venules and small veins, but they are not found on arteries or capillaries (266). Immunohistochemical analysis of IL-1β–stimulated ECs in vivo reveals IL-8 in association with both the EC monolayer and the underlying interstitium (205). IL-8 may reach these sites by diffusion from perivascular tissues or through local production by endothelium. A soluble chemotactic mechanism alone would be an unlikely method for neutrophil transmigration, because soluble IL-8 inhibits neutrophil-endothelial interactions, it leads neutrophils to shed L-selectin (a molecule involved in their primary rolling attachment to ECs), and it would be continually eroded by virtue of flow dilution (7,267).

Desensitization of neutrophils to IL-8 confirms the existence of another factor involved in the control of transendothelial migration. The procedure decreases neutrophil transmigration through cytokine-stimulated ECs totally. Desensitization to another chemotactic agent, N-formyl-methionyl-leucyl-phenylalanine (FMLP), creates neutrophils that still respond to an IL-8 gradient, suggesting that the desensitization process does not prevent neutrophil migration. They are, however, inhibited from transmigrating across cytokine-stimulated ECs by 74%, through a putative second, IL-8–independent pathway (268). TNF-α and IL-8 have additive effects on transmigration, which further suggests the existence of an IL-8–independent mechanism (202).

Chemotactic desensitization also demonstrates the dichotomy between adhesion and transmigration. Neutrophils desensitized to IL-8 adhere avidly to ECs due to activation of their CDIIb/CD18, but they do not migrate (269). Furthermore, lymphocytes will adhere to TNF-α–treated EC monolayers, but they do not migrate through them (204).

IL-8 AND NEUTROPHIL ADHESION: Neutrophils that have established adhesive contact on the endothelium display activation of their β_2-integrins, and they lack L-selectin (7). Soluble IL-8 also causes nonadherent neutrophils to shed L-selectin, and as a result of further, as yet uncertain means, it decreases neutrophil-endothelial interactions (267). Intravenous IL-8 administration to nonhuman primates results in granulocytosis and neutrophil margination in lung, liver, and spleen, but no tissue infiltration (270). Thus, depending on whether more IL-8 is bound or free, neutrophils are either stimulated to or are inhibited from adhering.

Because neutrophil contact with cytokine-activated endothelium may lead to EC damage, IL-8 steers the interactions of these two cells through three possible courses: (a) diapedesis and transmigration, (b) expulsion of granule contents and EC damage, or (c) detachment via soluble IL-8 to reenter the circulating pool (240). The levels of soluble, intravascular IL-8 at a site of inflammation are controlled by the availability of free binding sites, blood flow washing away soluble factors, circulating antibodies to IL-8 (271), and red blood cells, which bind IL-8, rendering it incapable of stimulating neutrophils (272).

MONOKINES: MCP-1, MIP-1, and RANTES are the mononuclear cell chemoattractant equivalents of IL-8. Their synthesis is induced in ECs by IL-1, TNF-α, LPS, and thrombin (273,274). IFN-γ also induces MCP-1 mRNA, but to a lesser extent (274). MCP-1 protein steadily accumulates from ECs exposed to IL-1β over 48 hours. It has chemoattractant properties for monocytes, and it can activate monocyte β_2-integrins (274,275).

Akin to IL-8, MIP-1β is also present on lymph node endothelium in an immobilized form, and thus it is resistant to loss in the flow of the bloodstream. In vitro immobilization of MIP-1β on proteoglycans assists the binding of T cells to VCAM-1 (276). MIP-1β may therefore control not only the chemotaxis of T cells, but also their ad-

hesion to endothelial VCAM-1. This process is similar to IL-8 activation of neutrophil β_2-integrin, although the mechanism of this effect of MIP-1β is unresolved.

DISEASE ASSOCIATIONS: The chemokines are associated with both acute and chronic disease processes. IL-8 appears in the circulation in patients with septic shock, endotoxemia, and after IL-1 administration (277). Bronchioloalveolar lavage IL-8 levels are higher in patients with acute respiratory illnesses in whom the adult respiratory distress syndrome subsequently develops (278), than in those in whom it does not develop. Acute asbestos-induced pleurisy is characterized by an influx of neutrophils. Introduction of crocidolite asbestos or TNF-α into the pleural space leads to the appearance of chemotactic activity for neutrophils, which is inhibited by anti-IL-8 and is accompanied by rapid induction of IL-8 mRNA in mesothelial cells (279).

Extracts of synovium from joints afflicted by rheumatoid arthritis possess diverse chemotactic activities to monocytes, T cells, and neutrophils. mRNA for IL-8, MCP, RANTES, and GRO is expressed in synovial fluid cells and synovial macrophages and fibroblasts. The chemotactic activity can be adsorbed by anti-IL-8 and anti-MCP-1 antibodies. MCP-1 levels are significantly higher in synovial fluid from patients with rheumatoid arthritis than those with osteoarthritis, which is consistent with the relative components of inflammation in the two disorders. The concentration of IL-8 and RANTES mRNA in blood is also less than in synovial fluid cells, which is consistent with the central site of inflammatory activity (280–285).

Circulating antibodies to IL-8 have been demonstrated in patients with rheumatoid arthritis; they correlated strongly with C-reactive protein, number of arthritic joints, and disease activity (271). IL-8 immunostaining is also noted on ECs in the minor salivary glands of patients with Sjögren's syndrome (286).

Minimally modified low density lipoprotein (LDL) induces MCP-1 in human endothelial and smooth muscle cells, and a role in atherosclerosis is further suggested by expression of MCP-1 mRNA and protein in atherosclerotic lesions of rabbits, but not from the intima or the media of normal animals. MCP-1 can be extracted and hybridized from lesional foam cells, but not from alveolar macrophages, sublesional VSMCs, or normal arteries (287,288).

Interferon-γ

IFN-γ is a T-cell product that steers ECs toward a phenotype consistent with chronic inflammation; they express class I and II MHC antigens, and they resemble a high endothelial venule (289). Its intracellular signaling involves phospholipase D–dependent triphasic activation of PKC (290).

EFFECTS ON ADHESION MOLECULES: The effects of IFN-γ on the EC adhesion molecule profile differ from those of IL-1 and TNF-α. IFN-γ stabilizes the surface expression of ES, but it does not induce or prolong its period of synthesis (291). It does not increase PS expression, but ICAM-1 is up-regulated (169,292). IFN-γ has a minor part in the induction of the L-selectin ligand compared with TNF-α and IL-1β (181), but it decreases EC expression of CD34, another L-selectin ligand (179).

IFN-γ has not been found to induce VCAM-1 on cultured ECs (185), but it does lead to a marked up-regulation of endothelial and dermal dendritic cell VCAM-1 after intradermal injection. In comparison to normal skin, in which VCAM-1 is present on perivascular dendritic cells and some follicular keratinocytes only, VCAM-1 is variably up-regulated on dermal endothelial and dendritic cells in allergic contact dermatitis, atopic dermatitis, lichen planus, and psoriasis, all conditions with increased local IFN-γ (293).

EFFECTS ON MHC EXPRESSION: Class I MHC appears on ECs exposed to IFN-γ (169); the ECs then become antigen-presenting cells for lymphocytes (294). IFN-γ increases TAP-1 expression, thus permitting assembly and normal surface expression of the class I MHC molecules. Both class I MHC and TAP-1 are synergistically increased by combinations of TNF-α with IFN-γ (196).

Class II HLA-DR antigens are uniquely induced on ECs by IFN-γ; they selectively increase the adhesion of CD4+ lymphocytes to ECs over other leukocyte populations (289,295,296). Serially passaged EC cultures will stimulate highly purified peripheral blood CD4+ T cells to proliferate if the EC cultures are pretreated with IFN-γ to induce de novo expression of MHC class II molecules (297). T-cell production of IFN-γ correlated with the intensity of EC expression of MHC antigen in a rat model of insulitis (298).

OTHER ENDOTHELIAL EFFECTS: Human recombinant IFN-γ increases HUVEC monolayer permeability to [^{125}I]-labeled bovine serum albumin in a time- and dose-dependent manner. IFN-γ and TNF-α or IL-1 produce an increase in permeability greater than that seen with each cytokine alone (299). Migration of lymphocytes through endothelial cell monolayers is also augmented by an endothelial-specific effect of IFN-γ. This augmentation affects even prebound lymphocytes; it therefore affects migration and not just adhesion (300). The mechanism is not resolved, although IFN-γ increases MCP-1 production.

IFN-γ decreases EC αvβ3-integrin (the vitronectin re-

ceptor), and it induces α1β1 (192,301). It decreases EC mRNA and protein levels of PDGF and GM-CSF, it increases IL-1 mRNA, and it weakly induces IL-6 production (106,154,302).

Hematopoietic CSFs

IL-3 acts directly on hematopoietic and endothelial cells, and it favors their proliferation, as discussed. Proinflammatory effects of excess levels of CSFs have been evident in clinical practice and in animal models (303,304), but they have been ascribed to actions on mature leukocytes, such as those favoring their adhesion to endothelium (305,306) and activation (307–310). ECs have been seen as a source of G-CSF, GM-CSF, and M-CSF when activated by other cytokines (e.g., IL-1, TNF-α, oncostatin-M) (311–313). Modified LDLs produce a similar effect, and because M-CSF binds preferentially to type V collagen (a collagen reported in atherosclerosis), this effect has led to suggestions that CSFs thus produced and acting on leukocytes may have a role in atherosclerosis (314,315).

We and others have observed that resting HUVECs express mRNA for the α- and β-chains of the IL-3 receptor, and that this is a functional mediator of endothelial interactions with leukocytes (90–92). Previous reports had generally concluded that CSFs do not influence these endothelial properties (e.g., procoagulant activity; production of PAF; expression of ES, PA, or PAI-1) (88,89). Positive reports (e.g., G-CSF augmenting ET-1 production (316), and GM-CSF and M-CSF weakly increasing endothelial ICAM-1 expression) (292,317) are controversial in light of the absence of demonstrable receptors for these cytokines on ECs.

IL-3, however, induces ES surface expression on resting HUVECs, as well as those treated with TNF-α. It supports neutrophil and CD4+ lymphocyte adhesion (90,92). IL-8 production and neutrophil transmigration across TNF-α–activated HUVEC monolayers are also increased by IL-3 (90). Thus, at least one CSF clearly alters endothelial interactions with leukocytes in vitro.

Transforming growth factor-β

TGF-β is a 25-kd dimer that appears to be a vital anti-inflammatory factor. Three isoforms are known in humans, but consideration is given in this discussion only to TGF-β1. At the cellular level, TGF-β has pleiotropic effects on morphogenesis, proliferation, and differentiation (318,319). Lin and Lodish (320) categorize its effects as (a) interruption of cell cycle in mid-to-late G1-phase, thus preventing induction of DNA synthesis and progression into S-phase; (b) induction of ECM and decreased synthesis of matrix-degrading proteinases; and (c) modulation of the secretion of other growth factors and their receptors (320).

Endothelium secretes latent TGF-β which undergoes activation in heterotypic co-cultures with other cell types such as pericytes or VSMCs (18,72). Its production in addition appears to be under positive autocrine control and is increased by TNF-α and IL-1 in a synergistic manner (321,322).

ENDOTHELIAL EFFECTS OF TGF-β1: TGF-β is recognized as a fundamental protein given the multifocal inflammatory disease seen in mice with targeted deletion of the TGF-β1 gene. At birth, these animals show no gross developmental abnormalities, but approximately 20 days later, they succumb to a wasting syndrome accompanied by a mixed inflammatory infiltrate, leading to organ failure in heart, stomach, liver, lung, pancreas, salivary gland, and striated muscle. There are increased numbers of neutrophils and monocytes in peripheral blood, and analysis of cytokine mRNAs from spleen, liver, and lung show increased IFN-γ, MIP-1α, TNF-α, and IL-1β levels (323,324).

Although the mechanisms behind this pathology are not entirely certain and may not be directly applicable to humans, experimental data demonstrate that TGF-β negatively modulates the interactions between human ECs and leukocytes therefore contribute to the inflammatory homeostasis of the organism. The basal and TNF-α/IL-1–induced adhesiveness of ECs for neutrophils (325), T lymphocytes (326), monocytes (Litwin MS, et al., unpublished observations), and tumor cells (327) are decreased by TGF-β. This decrease is accompanied by a reduction in the EC surface expression of ES; there is no change in VCAM-1 or ICAM-1 (328). Neutrophil transmigration across basal and cytokine-stimulated EC monolayers is also inhibited by TGF-β, with an accompanying reduction in EC IL-8 secretion (Smith WC, et al., unpublished observations).

Expression of VCAM-1 on VSMCs in their basal state or after TNF-α stimulation is also inhibited by TGF-β. Because active TGF-β is produced as a result of coculture of VSMCs and ECs, this close cellular association may be responsible for the lack of VCAM-1 expression on in situ normal VSMCs. Interruption of this contact in atheroma and loss of active TGF-β may be important pathogenic events (Gamble JR, et al., unpublished observations).

TGF-β RECEPTORS AND SIGNALING: There are three cell surface TGF-β binding proteins, each reported to be expressed on ECs (74,329). Type I and III receptors are thought to capture TGF-β and present it to type II receptors, which are functional transmembrane serine/threonine kinases (320,330). In addition, there are a number of other binding proteins that exist as soluble forms or in the ECM. α$_2$-Macroglobulin and β-glycan are believed to

deliver TGF-β to its signal transduction receptors, whereas decorin neutralizes TGF-β (8). The effects of TGF-β on ECs, however, may relate more to expression of downstream components of the signaling pathway than to the type of receptor expressed, because these receptors are found even on TGF-β–unresponsive ECs. On other cell types, divergent responses are produced despite expression of the same receptors (331,332).

DISEASE ASSOCIATIONS: In several experimental animal diseases modeling human illnesses marked by a significant inflammatory component, administration of TGF-β leads to amelioration of both disease and tissue infiltration. In experimental allergic encephalomyelitis TGF-β appears to protect against disease relapses. Anti-TGF-β antibody increases the incidence and severity of relapses, whereas anti-TNF-α antibody decreases them. TGF-β treatment does not influence the appearance of sensitized cells in peripheral blood and lymph nodes, but it does prevent accumulation of T cells in brain and spinal cord (333). Similar benefits from TGF-β are claimed in myocardial ischemia/reperfusion injury (334,335), as well as acute and chronic streptococcal-induced arthritis. Histopathological examination of the latter shows reduced inflammatory cell infiltration, pannus formation, and joint erosion (336).

Lipoprotein(a) (Lp[a]) is an LDL-like particle that contains apolipoprotein(a), a molecule with homology to plasminogen. Epidemiological studies have shown significant correlation between blood levels of Lp(a) and coronary/cerebral vascular disease. Lp(a) inhibits generation of TGF-β in cocultures of ECs with VSMCs by competing with plasminogen for EC surface binding, thus decreasing the EC plasmin-generating activity. This process may lead to down-regulation of TGF-β activation, and, because TGF-β is an inhibitor of EC proliferation, adhesiveness for leukocytes, VSMC migration, and VCAM-1 expression, Lp(a) may use this mechanism in the generation of atheromatous lesions (337).

ECs from skin affected by psoriasis show specific unresponsiveness to the inhibitory effects of TGF-β on baseline, IL-1-, and TNF-α–induced increases in lymphocyte adhesion, compared with cultured normal dermal microvascular ECs (338). If this finding reflects only swamping of the relatively weak negative signal of TGF-β by other more powerful proinflammatory influences, it is still a demonstration of the finely balanced forces in inflammation.

Interleukin-4

IL-4 is a product of T cells, mast cells, and bone marrow stroma cells. It has a dominant role in the development of undifferentiated T helper (Th) cells into Th1 and Th2 cells, favoring the Th2 phenotype (339). It also inhibits several monocyte functions in vitro, including the respiratory burst; adhesion to endothelium and IL-1, TNF-α, IL-6, and IL-8 (340–343).

IL-4 assists endothelial induction of VCAM-1 by IL-1, TNF-α, or IFN-γ. Expression of basal and cytokine-induced ES and, to some extent, ICAM-1, is decreased, however, and together with TGF-β there is additive inhibition of ES (328,344,345). Through these changes, IL-4 increases EC adhesiveness for T cells, eosinophils, and basophils, but not for neutrophils, because the former express very-late antigen (VLA-4); a ligand for VCAM-1, but neutrophils do not (346,347). Furthermore, eosinophils (but not neutrophils) from individuals with atopic dermatitis migrate through IL-4–pretreated EC monolayers (348).

Both IL-4 and TNF-α increase intracellular cyclic AMP in ECs, but only IL-4 uses this pathway to mediate lymphocyte adhesion. Elevation of cAMP in ECs does not induce VCAM-1, the only identified adhesion molecule induced by IL-4, indicating that an increase in cAMP in EC promotes an as yet unidentified adhesion pathway (349).

IL-4 increases resting endothelial MCP-1 production. It does not further increase IL-1 or TNF-induced MCP-1 mRNA, but there is an increase in secreted MCP-1 with these factors in combination; therefore, monocytes that adhere to the vascular wall by IL-4–induced VCAM-1 may be uniquely positioned to respond to EC-produced MCP-1 (350–352). IL-4 decreases IL-8 production by endothelium (Smith WB, et al., unpublished observations), which further suggests its activity favors mononuclear rather than neutrophil transmigration.

IL-4 may alone be insufficient to mediate leukocyte extravasation in vivo. Studies of monocyte morphology after adhesion to IL-4–treated, VCAM-1–bearing endothelium show that although there are more adherent monocytes, they do not stretch over the surface of ECs, which is thought to be a precursor of their transmigration. In contrast, stimulation of ECs with IL-1α for 24 hours increases surface expression of both ICAM-1 and VCAM-1, enhances binding of monocytes to ECs, and increases the percentage of EC-bound monocytes with a stretched morphology (353).

IL-4 induces IL-6 production by ECs in synergy with IFN-γ, IL-1, and TNF-α (354,355).

Interleukin-6

IL-6 is a T-cell cytokine that acts as a B-cell differentiator, a plasmacytoma growth factor, and a stimulator of hepatic acute-phase reactants. It increases endothelial ICAM-1 expression (292). IL-6 is produced by ECs stimulated with a variety of proinflammatory cytokines, such as IL-1, IL-4, TNF, and IFN-γ (221,352,356). Exposure of ECs to mouse hepatitis virus leads to their production of IL-6 (357).

Endothelial monocyte-activating polypeptide II

Endothelial monocyte-activating polypeptide II (EMAP-II) is a 22-kd polypeptide purified to homogeneity from the conditioned medium of murine fibrosarcoma cells based on its ability to induce tissue factor activity in ECs. In addition to procoagulant activity, it induces monocyte migration, and it is chemotactic for granulocytes. Injection into foot pads of mice leads to tissue swelling, with neutrophil infiltration (358).

SUMMARY

The major functions of the endothelium (i.e., renewal, angiogenesis, and interactions with blood components) are subject to the influence of many cytokines (Table 7–1) that often have overlapping, generally redundant effects, but nevertheless a wide spectrum of different actions.

Redundancy and pleiotropism among cytokines

Redundancy among these cytokines is well exemplified by the control of surface adhesion molecules by TNF-α, IL-1, IFN-γ, IL-3, and IL-4, or of EC proliferation by FGF, VEGF, SF, IL-3, and TGF-β. For instance, TNF-α, IL-1, and IL-4 each encourage interaction of ECs with mononuclear cells by increasing endothelial expression of VCAM-1. TNF-α and IL-1 have the additional capacity to induce the display of ES by ECs and, consequently, their attachment of neutrophils. In direct contrast, IL-4 decreases ES expression by the endothelium, and it restricts its interactions to mononuclear cells and eosinophils.

Stimulation of angiogenesis by FGF and TGF-β is another example. Both enhance angiogenesis, but, as described, they appear to have opposite effects on EC division and deposition of ECM. They appear to act in a complementary manner as respective initiators and completors of this process. Therefore, what appears to be redundancy is in fact also specificity and complementary activity created through the varying actions of diverse agents.

Pleiotropism among the cytokines acting on endothelium is also evident. TNF-α and TGF-β provide a clear example. Amid their many actions on endothelium is, however, a consistent pattern. TNF-α is the proinflammatory agent that encourages coagulation, adhesion, and chemokine production, whereas TGF-β prevents these changes or acts to restore the status quo. A clear aid in defining the understanding of pleiotropic agents, such as TGF-β, has been the study of animals with cytokine gene deletions. The multiinflammatory disease of TGF-β–deficient mice now awaits further work to determine to what

TABLE 7–1 CYTOKINE ACTIONS ON ENDOTHELIUM

EC Actions	TNF-α, IL-1	IFN-γ	TGF-β	IL-4	FGF	VEGF	CSF
Mitosis	↓	↔	↓	↑	↑	↑	↑
Migration	↔	↔	↓	↔	↑	↑	↑
Plasminogen activation	↑	ND	↓	ND	↑	ND	ND
Integrin expression	↑	↑	↔	↔	↑	ND	ND
Angiogenesis	↓	↔	↑	ND	↑	↑	↑
Coagulation	↑	↔	↔	ND	↔	ND	ND
Adhesion molecules	↑	↑	↓	↑↓	↔	↔	↑
Permeability to molecules	↑	↑	ND	↔	↔	↑	↔
Permeability to leukocytes	↑	↑	↓	↔	↔	↔	↑
Cytokine production	↑	↑↓	↓	↑	↔	ND	↔
MHC expression	↑	↑	↔	↔	↔	ND	↔

TNF = tumor necrosis factor; IFN = interferon; TGF-β = transforming growth factor-β; IL = interleukin; FGF = fibroblast growth factor; VEGF = vascular endothelial growth factor; CSF = colony-stimulating factor; MHC = major histocompatibility complex; ND = not done.

extent the endothelial effects of TGF-β contribute to its overall phenotype. Transgenic methods have not yet been applied to endothelial biology due to the lack of endothelial-specific promoters. Study of the control of ES transcription, which is uniquely expressed on endothelium, offers hope in this direction.

Local availability of cytokines acting on endothelium

The local availability and source of cytokines are key factors in their relative importance to endothelium. Activated monocytes or lymphocytes, which produce many of the cytokines discussed, are generally features of established, chronic inflammation; thus, their cytokine production would not be expected to begin the first endothelial changes. Mast cells, by virtue of their ubiquity, secretory granule storage (i.e., holding TNF-α), and responsiveness to neural stimuli, are suspected of being the key initiating cell. In delayed-type hypersensitivity reactions in human skin, degranulation of mast cells situated about superficial vessels is the first ultrastructural change seen; it precedes inflammatory cell accumulation by 16 hours (151).

Cytokine availability is influenced by the ECM, which may provide binding sites that function as reservoirs or aids to receptor interaction (8). The presence of binding sites is clearly important for the chemokines; as bound surface molecules, they favor leukocyte haptotaxis, but as free molecules, they inhibit leukocyte adhesion to ECs. ECM–EC interactions can also trigger the same intracellular signals evoked by cytokines, and the ECM is another area in which endothelial cell biologists will find fertile ground.

Signaling

Although cytokines are important signals for ECs, other means of communication are increasingly being understood. Molecules assigned one particular function have been discovered to have a second signaling function. For example, CD31 (PECAM-1) was viewed only as an intercellular junction molecule with a role in leukocyte transmigration, but its ligation selectively assists interaction between the α4β1-integrin found on leukocytes and VCAM-1 (359). Mechanical displacements from the bloodstream lead to changes in cell biochemistry. Flow or shear stress is transduced by ECs into the induction of c-fos, PDGF, and activated factor X expression. Circumferential tensile stress due to blood pressure leads to thickening of the vascular wall (360–362).

The signaling pathways of cytokines, as well as the signals that follow ligation of surface molecules or perceptible displacement of cell membranes, are likely to assume increasing importance. The cyclosporine revolution in clinical medicine has clearly shown that the pathways for intracellular communication are central to an understanding of cytokine actions, and that they are likely to be promising sites for clinically oriented interventions. TNF receptor-binding mutants with decreased endothelial proinflammatory actions that retain antitumor properties offer the promise of isolating the actions of other pleiotropic cytokines and potentially applying these findings selectively to clinical practice (219).

REFERENCES

1. Denekamp J. Vasculature as a target for tumour therapy. Prog Appl Microcirc 1984;4:28–38.

2. Millauer B, Wizigmann-Voos S, Schnurch H, et al. High affinity VEGF binding and developmental expression suggest FLK-1 as a major regulator of vasculogenesis and angiogenesis. Cell 1993;72:835–846.

3. Bevilacqua MP, Pober JS, Majeau GR, Fiers W, Cotran RS, Gimbrone MA Jr. Recombinant tumor necrosis factor induces procoagulant activity in cultured human vascular endothelium: characterisation and comparison with the actions of interleukin 1. Proc Natl Acad Sci USA 1986; 83:4533–4537.

4. Palmer RMJ, Ferrige AG, Moncada S. Nitric oxide release accounts for the biological activity of endothelium-derived relaxing factor. Nature 1987;327:524–526.

5. Moser R, Schleiffenbaum B, Groscurth P, Fehr J. Interleukin 1 and tumor necrosis factor stimulate human vascular endothelial cells to promote transendothelial neutrophil passage. J Clin Invest 1989;83:444–455.

6. Pober JS, Collins T, Gimbrone MA, et al. Lymphocytes recognise human vascular endothelial and dermal fibroblast Ia antigens induced by recombinant immune interferon. Nature 1983;305:726–729.

7. Rot A. Endothelial cell binding of NAP-1/IL-8: role in neutrophil emigration. Immunol Today 1992;13:291–294.

8. Ruoslahti E. Yamaguchi Y. Proteoglycans as modulators of growth factor activities. Cell 1991;64:867–869.

9. Schweigerer L, Neufeld G, Friedman J, Abraham JA, Fiddes JC, Gospodarowicz D. Capillary endothelial cells express basic fibroblast growth factor, a mitogen that promotes their own growth. Nature 1987;325:257–295.

10. Itoh H, Mukoyama M, Pratt RE, Dzau VJ. Specific blockade of basic fibroblast growth factor gene expression in endothelial cells by antisense oligonucleotide. Biochem Biophys Res Commun 1992;188:1205–1213.

11. George F, Sampol J. Circulating endothelial cells: a marker of vascular lesion. Nouv Rev Fr Hematol 1993;35:259–261.

12. Folkman J, Haudenschild C. Angiogenesis in vitro. Nature 1980;288:551–556.

13. Folkman J, Klagsbrun M. Angiogenic factors. Science 1987;235:442–447.

14. Shing Y, Folkman J, Haudenschild C, Lund D, Crum R, Klagsbrun M. Angiogenesis is stimulated by a tumor-derived endothelial cell growth factor. J Cell Biochem 1985; 29:275–287.

15. Eisemann A, Ahn JA, Graziani G, Tronick SR, Ron D. Alternative splicing generates at least five different isoforms of the human basic-FGF receptor. Oncogene 1991;6:1195–1202.

16. Klagsbrun M, Baird A. A dual receptor system is required for basic fibroblast growth factor activity. Cell 1991:67–229–231.

17. Sato Y, Rifkin DB. Autocrine activities of basic fibroblast growth factor: regulation of endothelial cell movement, plasminogen activator synthesis and DNA synthesis. J Cell Biol 1988;107:1199–1205.

18. Flaumenhaft R, Abe M, Mignatti P, Rifkin DB. Basic fibroblast growth factor-induced activation of latent transforming growth factor β in endothelial cells: regulation of plasminogen activator activity. J Cell Biol 1992;118:901–909.

19. Mostacelli D, Presta M, Rifkin DB. Purification of a factor from human placenta that stimulates capillary endothelial cell protease production, DNA synthesis and migration. Proc Natl Acad Sci USA 1986;83:2091–2095.

20. Mignatti P, Mazzieri R, Rifkin DB. Expression of the urokinase receptor in vascular endothelial cells is stimulated by basic fibroblast growth factor. J Cell Biol 1991;113:1193–1201.

21. Pepper MS, Sappino AP, Stocklin R, Montesano R, Orci L, Vassalli JD. Upregulation of urokinase receptor expression on migrating endothelial cells. J Cell Biol 1993;122:673–684.

22. Montesano R, Vassalli JD, Baird A, Guillemin R, Orci L. Basic fibroblast growth factor induces angiogenesis in vitro. Proc Natl Acad Sci USA 1986;83:7297–7301.

23. Swerlick RA, Brown EJ, Xu Y, Lee KH, Manos S, Lawley TJ. Expression and modulation of the vitronectin receptor on human dermal microvascular endothelial cells. J Invest Dermatol 1992;99:715–722.

24. Enenstein J, Waleh NS, Kramer RH. Basic FGF and TGF-beta differentially modulate integrin expression of human microvascular endothelial cells. Exp Cell Res 1992; 203:499–503.

25. Lee PL, Johnson DE, Cousens LS, Fried VA, Williams LT. Purification and complementary DNA cloning of a receptor for basic fibroblast growth factor. Science 1989;245:57–60.

26. Moscatelli D. High and low affinity binding sites for basic fibroblast growth factor on cultured cells: absence of a role for low affinity binding in the stimulation of plasminogen activator production by bovine capillary endothelial cells. J Cell Physiol 1987;131:123–130.

27. Roghani M, Moscatelli D. Basic fibroblast growth factor is internalized through both receptor-mediated and heparan sulfate-mediated mechanisms. J Biol Chem 1992; 267:22156–22162.

28. Isacchi A, Statuto M, Chiesa R, et al. A six-amino deletion in basic fibroblast growth factor dissociates its mitogenic activity from its plasminogen activator-inducing capacity. Proc Natl Acad Sci USA 1991;88:2628–2632.

29. Presta M, Maier JAM, Ragnotti G. The mitogenic signalling pathway but not the plasminogen activator-inducing pathway of basic fibroblast growth factor is mediated through protein kinase C in fetal bovine aortic endothelial cells. J Cell Biol 1989;109:1877–1884.

30. Dell'Era P, Presta M, Ragnotti G. Nuclear localisation of endogenous fibroblast growth factor in cultured endothelial cells. Exp Cell Res 1991;192:505–510.

31. Bouche G, Gas N, Baldin V, et al. Basic fibroblast growth factor enters the nucleolus and stimulates the transcription of ribosomal genes in ABAE cells undergoing G_0–G_1 transition. Proc Natl Acad Sci USA 1987;84:6770–6774.

32. Baldin V, Roman AM, Bosc-Bierne I, Amalric F, Bouche G. Translocation of bFGF to the nucleus is G_1 phase cell cycle specific in bovine aortic endothelial cells. EMBO J 1990; 9:1511–1517.

33. Imamura T, Engelka K, Zhan X, et al. Recovery of mitogenic activity of a growth factor mutant with a nuclear translocation sequence. Science 1990;249:1567–1570.

34. Presta M, Tiberio L, Rusnati M, Dell'Era P, Ragnotti G. Basic fibroblast growth factor requires a long lasting activation of protein kinase C to induce cell proliferation in transformed fetal bovine aortic endothelial cells. Cell Reg 1991;2:719–726.

35. Rusnati M, Urbinati C, Presta M. Internalization of basic fibroblast growth factor (bFGF) in cultured endothelial cells: role of the low affinity heparin-like bFGF receptors. J Cell Physiol 1993;154:152–161.

36. Mostacelli D. Basic fibroblast growth factor (bFGF) dissociates rapidly from heparan sulfates but slowly from receptors. Implications for mechanisms of bFGF release from pericellular matrix. J Biol Chem 1992;267:25803–25809.

37. Feige JJ, Bradley JD, Fryburg K, et al. Differential effects of heparin, fibronectin and laminin on the phosphorylation of basic fibroblast growth factor by protein kinase C and the catalytic subunit of protein kinase A. J Cell Biol 1989; 109:3105–3114.

38. Schubert D. Collaborative interactions between growth factors and the extracellular matrix. Trends Cell Biol 1992; 2:63–66.

39. Nurcombe V, Ford MD, Wildschut JA, Bartlett PF. Developmental regulation of neural response to FGF-1 and FGF-2 by heparan sulfate proteoglycan. Science 1993;260:103–106.

40. Friesel R, Komoriya A, Maciag T. Inhibition of endothelial proliferation by gamma-interferon. J Cell Biol 1987; 104:689–696.

41. Sato Y, Waki M, Ohno M, Kuwano M, Sakata T. Carboxyl-terminal heparin-binding fragments of platelet factor 4 retain the blocking effect on the receptor binding of basic fibroblast growth factor. Jpn J Cancer Res 1993;84:485–488.

42. Nakayama Y, Iwahana M, Sakamoto N, Tanaka NG, Osada Y. Inhibitory effects of a bacteria-derived sulfated polysaccharide against basic fibroblast growth factor-induced endothelial cell growth and chemotaxis. J Cell Physiol 1993; 154:1–6.

43. Healy AM, Herman IM. Preparation of fluorescent basic fibroblast growth factor: localization in living retinal microvascular endothelial cells. Exp Eye Res 1992;55:663–669.

44. Itoh H, Mukoyama M, Pratt RE, Dzau VJ. Specific blockade of basic fibroblast growth factor gene expression in endothelial cells by antisense oligonucleotide. Biochem Biophys Res Commun 1992;188:1205–1213.

45. Lobb RR, Alderman EM, Fett JW. Induction of angiogenesis by bovine brain derived class 1 heparin-binding growth factor. Biochemistry 1985;24:4969–4973.

46. Nabel EG, Yang ZY, Plautz G, et al. Recombinant fibroblast growth factor-1 promotes intimal hyperplasia and angiogenesis in arteries in vivo. Nature 1993;362:844–846.

47. Pierce GF, Tarpley JE, Yanagihara D, Mustoe TA, Fox GM, Thomason A. Platelet-derived growth factor (BB homodimer), transforming growth factor-β1 and basic fibroblast growth factor in dermal wound healing. Neovessel and matrix formation and cessation of repair. Am J Pathol 1992; 140:1375–1388.

48. Villaschi S, Nicosia RF. Angiogenic role of endogenous basic fibroblast growth factor released by rat aorta after injury. Am J Pathol 1993;143:181–190.

49. Dvorak HF, Nagy JA, Dvorak AM. Structure of solid tumours and their vasculature: implications for therapy with monoclonal antibodies. Cancer Cells 1991;3:77–85.

50. Soker S, Svahn CM, Neufeld G. Vascular endothelial growth factor is inactivated by binding to α2-macroglobulin and the binding is inhibited by heparin. J Biol Chem 1993;268:7685–7691.

51. Brown LF, Berse B, Tognazzi K, et al. Vascular permeability factor mRNA and protein expression in human kidney. Kidney Int 1992;42:1457–1461.

52. Pepper MS, Ferrara N, Orci L, Montesano R. Potent synergism between vascular endothelial growth factor and basic fibroblast growth factor in the induction of angiogenesis in vitro. Biochem Biophys Res Commun 1992;189:824–831.

53. Unemori EN, Ferrara N, Bauer EA, Amento EP. Vascular endothelial growth factor induces interstitial collagenase expression in human endothelial cells. J Cell Physiol 1992; 153:557–562.

54. De Vries C, Escobedo JA, Ueno H, Houck K, Ferrara N, Williams LT. The fms-like tyrosine kinase, a receptor for vascular endothelial growth factor. Science 1992;255:989–991.

55. Peters KG, Werner S, Chen G, Williams LT. Two FGF receptor genes are differentially expressed in epithelial and mesenchymal tissues during limb formation and organogenesis in the mouse. Development 1992;114:233–243.

56. Shweiki D, Itin A, Neufeld G, Gitay-Goren H, Keshet E. Patterns of expression of vascular endothelial growth factor (VEGF) and VEGF receptors in mice suggest a role in hormonally regulated angiogenesis. J Clin Invest 1993;91: 2235–2243.

57. Kim KJ, Li B, Winer J, et al. Inhibition of vascular endothelial growth factor-induced angiogenesis suppresses tumour growth in vivo. Nature 1993;362:841–844.

58. Shweiki D, Itin A, Soffer D, Keshet E. Vascular endothelial growth factor induced by hypoxia may mediate hypoxia-initiated angiogenesis. Nature 1992;359:843–845.

59. Plate KH, Breier G, Weich HA, Risau W. Vascular endothelial growth factor is a potential tumour angiogenesis factor in human gliomas in vivo. Nature 1992;359:845–848.

60. Brown LF, Yeo KT, Berse B, et al. Expression of vascular permeability factor (vascular endothelial growth factor) by epidermal keratinocytes during wound healing. J Exp Med 1992;176:1375–1379.

61. Weidner KM, Arakaki N, Vandekerckhove J, et al. Evidence for the identity of human scatter factor and human hepatocyte growth factor. Proc Natl Acad Sci USA 1991; 88:7001–7005.

62. Nakamura T, Nishizawa T, Hagiya M, et al. Molecular cloning and expression of human hepatocyte growth factor. Nature 1989;342:440–443.

63. Monteasano R, Matsumoto K, Nakamura T, Orci L. Identification of a fibroblast-derived epithelial morphogen as hepatocyte growth factor. Cell 1991;67:901–908.

64. Rosen EM, Goldberg ID, Kacinski DM, Buckholz T, Vinter DW. Smooth muscle releases an epithelial cell scatter factor which binds to heparin. In Vitro Cell Dev Biol 1989; 25:163–173.

65. Stoker M, Gheradi E, Perryman M, Gray J. Scatter factor is a fibroblast-derived modulator of epithelial cell mobility. Nature 1987;327:238–242.

66. Weidner KM, Sachs M, Birchmeier W. The met receptor tyrosine kinase transduces motility, proliferation and morphogenic signals of scatter factor/hepatocyte growth factor in epithelial cells. J Cell Biol 1993;121:145–154.

67. Bussolino F, Di Renzo MF, Ziche M, et al. Hepatocyte growth factor is a potent angiogenic factor which stimulates endothelial cell motility and growth. J Cell Biol 1992; 119:629–641.

68. Grant DS, Kleiman HK, Goldberg ID, et al. Scatter factor induces blood vessel formation in vivo. Proc Natl Acad Sci USA 1993;90:1937–1941.

69. Madri JA, Pratt BM, Tucker AM. Phenotypic modulation of endothelial cells by transforming growth factor-beta depends upon composition and organisation of the extracellular matrix. J Cell Biol 1988;106:1375–1384.

70. Merwin JR, Anderson JM, Kocher O, van Itallie CM, Madri JA. Transforming growth factor β1 modulates extracellular matrix organisation and cell-cell junctional complex formation during angiogenesis. J Cell Physiol 1990;142:117–128.

71. Frater-Schroder M, Muller G, Birchmeier W, Bohlen P. Transforming growth factor-beta inhibits endothelial cell proliferation. Biochem Biophys Res Commun 1986;137:295–302.

72. Antonelli-Orlidge A, Saunders K, Smith S. D'Amore PA. An activated form of transforming growth factor-β is produced by co-cultures of endothelial cells and pericytes. Proc Natl Acad Sci USA 1989;86:4544–4548.

73. Heimark RL, Twardzik DR, Schwart SM. Inhibition of endothelial regeneration by type-β transforming growth factor from platelets. Science 1986;223:1078–1080.

74. Muller G, Behrens J, Nussbaumer U, Bohlen P, Birchmeier W. Inhibitory action of transforming growth factor β on endothelial cells. Proc Natl Acad Sci USA 1987;84:5600–5604.

75. Saksela O, Moscatelli D, Rifkin DB. The opposing effects of basic fibroblast growth factor and transforming growth factor beta on the regulation of plasminogen activator activity in capillary endothelial cells. J Cell Biol 1987;105:767–775.

76. Ignotz RA, Massague J. Transforming growth factor-β stimulates the expression of fibronectin and collagen and their incorporation into the extracellular matrix. J Biol Chem 1986;261:4337–4345.

77. Edwards DR, Murphy G, Reynolds JJ, et al. Transforming growth factor beta modulates the expression of collagenase and metalloproteinase inhibitor. EMBO J 1987;6:1899–1904.

78. Roberts AB, Sporn MB, Assoian RK, et al. Transforming growth factor type β: rapid induction of fibrosis and angiogenesis in vivo and stimulation of collagen formation in vitro. Proc Natl Acad Sci USA 1986;83:4167–4171.

79. Yang EY, Moses HL. Transforming growth factor β1-induced changes in cell migration, proliferation and angiogenesis in the chick chorioallantoic membrane. J Cell Biol 1990:111:731–741.

80. Gonzlez T, Gutirrez R, Diaz-Flores L. Transforming growth factor β1 and basic fibroblast growth factor in articular cartilage defects. Rev Esp Reumatol 1993;20:S1.

81. Arciniegas E, Sutton AB, Allen TD, Schor AM. Transforming growth factor beta 1 promotes the differentiation of en-

82. Merrilees MJ, Sodek J. Synthesis of TGF-beta 1 by vascular endothelial cells is correlated with cell spreading. J Vasc Res 1992;29:376–384.

83. Muller WA, Ratti CM, McDonnell SL, Cohn ZA. A human endothelial cell-restricted, externally disposed plasmalemmal protein enriched in intercellular junctions. J Exp Med 1989;170:399–414.

84. Ohto H, Maed H, Shibata Y, et al. A novel leukocyte differentiation antigen: two monoclonal antibodies TM2 and TM3 define a 120-kd molecule present on neutrophils, monocytes, platelets and activated lymphoblasts. Blood 1985;66:873–881.

85. Fina L, Molgaard HV, Robertson D, et al. Expression of the CD34 gene in vascular endothelial cells. Blood 1990;75:2417–2426.

86. Baumhueter S, Singer MS, Henzel W, et al. Binding of L-selectin to the vascular sialomucin CD34. Science 1993;262:436–438.

87. Kudo E, Hirose T, Sano T, Hizawa K. Epitopic heterogeneity of the CD36 antigen expressed by normal and neoplastic endothelial cells. An immunohistochemical study with a novel monoclonal antibody 8C9. Acta Pathol Jpn 1992;42:807–817.

88. Forsyth KD, Chua KY, Talbot V, Thomas WR. Expression of the leukocyte common antigen CD45 by endothelium. J Immunol 1993;150:3471–3477.

89. Bussolino F, Wang JM, Defilippi F, et al. Granulocyte- and granulocyte-macrophage colony stimulating factor induce human endothelial cells to migrate and proliferate. Nature 1988;337:471–473.

90. Bussolino F, Ziche M, Wang JM, et al. In vitro and in vivo activation of endothelial cells by colony stimulating factors. J Clin Invest 1991;87:986–995.

91. Yong K, Cohen A, Khwaja A, Jones HM, Linch DC. Lack of effect of granulocyte-macrophage and granulocyte colony-stimulating factors on cultured human endothelial cells. Blood 1991;77:1675–1680.

92. Korpelainen EI, Gamble JR, Smith WB, et al. The receptor for interleukin 3 is selectively induced in human endothelial cells by tumor necrosis factor-α and potentiates interleukin 8 secretion and neutrophil transmigration. Proc Natl Acad Sci USA 1993;90:11137–11141.

93. Colotta F, Bussolino F, Polentarutti N, et al. Differential expression of the common β and specific α chains of the receptors for GM-CSF, IL-3, and IL-5 in endothelial cells. Exp Cell Res 1993;206:311–317.

94. Brizzi MF, Garbarino G, Rossi PR, et al. Interleukin 3 stimulates proliferation and triggers endothelial-leukocyte adhesion molecule 1 gene activation of human endothelial cells. J Clin Invest 1993;91:2887–2892.

95. Orazi A, Cattoretti G, Sciro R, et al. Recombinant human interleukin 3 and recombinant human granulocyte-macrophage colony stimulating factor administered in vivo after high dose cyclophosphamide cancer chemotherapy: effect on hematopoiesis and microenvironment in human bone marrow. Blood 1992;79:2610–2619.

96. Anagnostou A, Lee ES, Kessiman N, Levinson R, Steiner M. Erythropoietin has a mitogenic and positive chemotactic

activity on endothelial cells. Proc Natl Acad Sci USA 1990; 87:5978–5982.

97. Bruce AG, Hoggatt IH, Rose TM. Oncostatin M is a differentiation factor for myeloid leukemia cells. J Immunol 1992;149:1271–1275.

98. Toi M, Harris AL, Bicknell R. Interleukin-4 is a potent mitogen for capillary endothelium. Biochem Biophys Res Commun 1991;174:1287–1293.

99. Wojta J, Gallicchio M, Zoellner H, Filonzi EL, Hamilton JA, McGrath K. Interleukin-4 stimulates expression of urokinase-type-plasminogen activator in cultured human foreskin microvascular endothelial cells. Blood 1993; 81:3285–3292.

100. Koch AE, Polverini PJ, Kunkel SL, et al. Interleukin-8 as a macrophage-derived mediator of angiogenesis. Science 1992;258:1798–1801.

101. Buckley A, Davidson JM, Kamerath CD, Wolt TB, Woodward SC. Sustained release of epidermal growth factor accelerates wound repair. Proc Natl Acad Sci USA 1985; 82:7340–7344.

102. Wakui S. Epidermal growth factor receptor at endothelial cell and pericyte interdigitation in human granulation tissue. Microvasc Res 1992;44:255–262.

103. Ross R, Raines EW, Bowen-Pope DF. The biology of platelet-derived growth factor. Cell 1986;46:155–169.

104. Risau W, Drexler H, Mironov V, et al. Platelet-derived growth factor is angiogenic in vivo. Growth Factors 1992; 7:261–266.

105. Nabel EG, Yang Z, Liptay S, et al. Recombinant PDGF B gene expression in porcine arteries induces intimal hyperplasia in vivo. J Clin Invest 1993;91:1822–1829.

106. Ross R, Masuda J, Raines EW, et al. Localisation of PDGF-B protein in macrophages in all phases of atherogenesis. Science 1990;248:1009–1012.

107. Hart CE, Forstrom JW, Kelly JD, et al. Two classes of PDGF receptor recognise different isoforms of PDGF. Science 1988;240:1529–1531.

108. Suzuki H, Shibano K, Okane M, et al. Interferon-γ modulates mRNA levels of c-sis (PDGF-B chain), PDGF-A chain and IL-1β genes in human vascular endothelial cells. Am J Pathol 1989;134:35–43.

109. Kourembanas S, McQuillan LP, Leung GK, Faller DV. Nitric oxide regulates the expression of vasoconstrictors and growth factors by vascular endothelium under both normoxia and hypoxia. J Clin Invest 1993;92:99–104.

110. Gajdusek CM, Luo Z, Mayberg MR. Sequestration and secretion of insulin-like growth factor-I by bovine aortic endothelial cells. J Cell Physiol 1993;154:192–198.

111. Taylor WR, Nerem RM, Alexander RW. Polarized secretion of IGF-I and IGF-I binding protein activity by cultured aortic endothelial cells. J Cell Physiol 1993;154:139–142.

112. Cozzolino F, Torcia M, Aldinucci D, et al. Interleukin-1 is an autocrine regulator of human endothelial cell growth. Proc Natl Acad Sci USA 1990;87:6487–6491.

113. Janakidevi K, Fisher MA, Del-Vecchio PJ, Tiruppathi C, Figge J, Malik AB. Endothelin-1 stimulates DNA synthesis and proliferation of pulmonary artery smooth muscle cells. Am J Physiol 1992;263:C1295–1301.

114. Namiki A, Hata Y, Fukazawa M, et al. Granulocyte-colony stimulating factor stimulates immunoreactive endothelin-1 release from cultured bovine endothelial cells. Eur J Pharmacol 1992;227:339–341.

115. Emori T, Hirata Y, Imai T, et al. Cellular mechanism of thrombin on endothelin-1 biosynthesis and release in bovine endothelial cell. Biochem Pharmacol 1992;44:2409–2411.

116. Maemura K, Kurihara H, Morita T, Oh-hashi Y, Yazaki Y. Production of endothelin-1 in vascular endothelial cells is regulated by factors associated with vascular injury. Gerontology 1992;38(suppl 1):29–35.

117. Malek AM, Greene AL, Izumo S. Regulation of endothelin 1 gene by fluid shear stress is transcriptionally mediated and independent of protein kinase C and cAMP. Proc Natl Acad Sci USA 1993;90:5999–6003.

118. Fassbender HG, Simmling-Annefield A. The potential aggressiveness of synovial tissue in rheumatoid arthritis. J Pathol 1983;139:399–406.

119. Rooney M, Condell D, Quinlan W, et al. Analysis of the histologic variation in rheumatoid arthritis. Arthritis Rheum 1988;31:956–963.

120. Sano H, Forough R, Maier JAM, et al. Detection of high levels of heparin binding growth factor 1 (acidic fibroblast growth factor) in inflammatory arthritic joints. J Cell Biol 1990;110:1417–1426.

121. Ou Z, Planck R, Hart CE, Rosenbaum JT. Distribution pattern of basic fibroblast growth factor in synovial tissue from patients with rheumatoid arthritis. Arthritis Rheum 1990;33(suppl):75.

122. Shiozawa S. Shiozawa K, Tanaka Y, et al. Human epidermal growth factor for the stratification of synovial lining layer and neovascularisation in rheumatoid arthritis. Ann Rheum Dis 1989;48:820–828.

123. Hirata S, Matsubara T, Saura R, Tateishi H, Hirohata K. Inhibition of in vitro vascular endothelial cell proliferation and in vivo neovascularisation by low dose methotrexate. Arthritis Rheum 1989;32:1065–1073.

124. Matsubara T, Ziff M. Inhibition of endothelial cell proliferation by gold compounds. J Clin Invest 1987;79:1440–1446.

125. Williams SK. Regulation of intimal hyperplasia: do endothelial cells participate? Lab Invest 1991:64:721–723.

126. Orlidge A, D'Amore PA. Inhibition of capillary endothelial cell growth by pericytes and smooth muscle cells. J Cell Biol 1987;105:1455–1462.

127. Kuwubara T, Cogan DG. Retinal vascular patterns. Arch Ophthalmol 1963;69:114–124.

128. Ono M, Okamura K, Nakayama Y, et al. Induction of human microvascular endothelial tubular morphogenesis by human keratinocytes: involvement of transforming growth factor-alpha. Biochem Biophys Res Commun 1992; 189:601–609.

129. Folkman J, Shing Y. Angiogenesis. J Biol Chem 1992;267: 10931–10934.

130. Barnhill RL, Fandrey K, Levy MA, Mihm MC, Hyman B. Angiogenesis and tumor progression of melanoma. Quantification of vascularity in melanocytic nevi and cutaneous malignant melanoma. Lab Invest 1992;67:331–337.

131. Horak ER, Leek R, Klenk N, et al. Angiogenesis, assessed

by platelet/endothelial cell adhesion molecule antibodies, as indicator of node metastases and survival in breast cancer. Lancet 1992;340:1120–1124.

132. Ensoli B, Nakamura S, Salahuddin S, et al. AIDS-Kaposi's sarcoma-derived cells express cytokines with autocrine and paracrine growth effects. Science 1989;243:223–226.

133. Miles SA, Rezai AR, Salazar-Gonzalez JF, et al. AIDS Kaposi sarcoma-derived cells produce and respond to interleukin-6. Proc Natl Acad Sci USA 1990;87:4068–4072.

134. Corbeil J, Evans LA, Vasak E, Cooper DA, Penny R. Culture and properties of cells derived from Kaposi sarcoma. J Immunol 1991;146:2972–2976.

135. Abe T, Okamura K, Ono M, et al. Induction of vascular endothelial tubular morphogenesis by human glioma cells. A model system for tumor angiogenesis. J Clin Invest 1993;92:54–61.

136. Folkman J. Successful treatment of an angiogenic disease. N Engl J Med 1989;320:1211–1212.

137. Blei F, Wilson EL, Mignatti P, Rifkin DB. Mechanism of action of angiostatic steroids: suppression of plasminogen activator activity via stimulation of plasminogen activator inhibitor synthesis. J Cell Physiol 1993;155:566–578.

138. Folkman J, Shing Y. Control of angiogenesis by heparin and other sulfated polysaccharides. Adv Exp Med Biol 1992;313:355–364.

139. White CW, Sondheimer HM, Crouch EC, Wilson H, Fan LL. Treatment of pulmonary hemangiomatosis with recombinant interferon alpha-2a. N Engl J Med 1989;320:1197–1200.

140. Ingber D, Fujita T, Kishimoto S, et al. Synthetic analogues of fumagillin that inhibit angiogenesis and suppress tumour growth. Nature 1990;348:555–557.

141. Peacock DJ, Banquerigo ML, Brahn E. Angiogenesis inhibition suppresses collagen arthritis. J Exp Med 1992;175:1135–1138.

142. Gagliardi A, Collins DC. Inhibition of angiogenesis by anti-estrogens. Cancer Res 1993;53:533–535.

143. Norrby K. Cyclosporine is angiostatic. Experientia 1992;48:1135–1138.

144. Polakowski IJ, Lewis MK, Muthukkaruppan VR, Erdman B, Kubai L, Auerbach R. A ribonuclease inhibitor expresses anti-angiogenic properties and leads to reduced tumor growth in mice. Am J Pathol 1993;143:507–517.

145. Fotsis T, Pepper M, Adlercreutz H, et al. Genistein, a dietary-derived inhibitor of in vivo angiogenesis. Proc Natl Acad Sci USA 1993;90:2690–2694.

146. Kaneko T, Nagata I, Miyamoto S, et al. Effects of nicardipine on tube formation of bovine vascular endothelial cells in vitro. Stroke 1992;23:1637–1642.

147. Ingber DE, Folkman J. Mechanochemical switching between growth and differentiation during fibroblast growth factor-stimulated angiogenesis in vitro: role of extracellular matrix. J Cell Biol 1989;109:317–330.

148. Gamble JR, Matthias L, Meyer G, et al. Regulation of in vitro capillary tube formation by anti-integrin antibodies. J Cell Biol 1993;121:931–943.

149. Dinarello CA. Interleukin-1 and interleukin-1 antagonism. Blood 1991;77:1627–1652.

150. Jaattela M. Biologic activities and mechanisms of action of tumor necrosis factor-α/cachectin. Lab Invest 1991;64:724–742.

151. Klein LM, Lavker RM, Matis WL, Murphy GF. Degranulation of human mast cells induces an endothelial antigen central to leukocyte adhesion. Proc Natl Acad Sci USA 1989;86:8972–8976.

152. Warner SJC, Libby P. Human vascular smooth muscle cells: target for and source of tumour necrosis factor. J Immunol 1989;142:100–109.

153. Niedbala MJ, Stein-Picarella M. Role of protein kinase C in TNF induction of endothelial cell urokinase-type plasminogen activator. Blood 1993;81:2608–2617.

154. Hashimoto Y, Hirohata S, Kashiwado T, Itoh K, Ishii H. Cytokine regulation of hemostatic property and IL-6 production of human endothelial cells. Inflammation 1992;16:613–621.

155. Miyake S, Ohdama S, Tazawa R, Aoki N. Retinoic acid prevents cytokine-induced suppression of thrombomodulin expression on surface of human umbilical vein vascular endothelial cells in vitro. Thromb Res 1992;68:483–487.

156. Kawakami M, Ishibashi S, Ogawa H, Murase T, Takahu F, Shibata S. Cachectin/TNF as well as interleukin-1 induces prostacyclin synthesis in cultured vascular endothelial cells. Biochem Biophys Res Commun 1986;141:482–487.

157. Schleef RR, Bevilacqua MP, Sawdey M, Gimbrone MA Jr. Cytokine activation of vascular endothelium. Effects on tissue-type plasminogen activator and type 1 plasminogen activator inhibitor. J Biol Chem 1988;263:5797–5809.

158. Dosne AM, Dubor F, Lutcher F, Parant M, Chedid L. Tumor necrosis factor (TNF) stimulates plasminogen activator inhibitor (PAI) production by endothelial cells and decreases blood fibrinolytic activity in the rat. Thromb Res 1988;51:115–122.

159. Van Hinsbergh VWM, Kooistra T, Vanderberg EA, Princer HMG, Fiers W, Emeis JJ. Tumor necrosis factor increases the production of plasminogen activator inhibitor in human endothelial cells in vitro and in rats in vivo. Blood 1988;72:1467–1473.

160. Logan TF, Virji MA, Gooding WE, Bontempo FA, Ernstoff MS, Kirkwood JM. Plasminogen activator and its inhibitor in cancer patients treated with tumor necrosis factor. J Natl Cancer Inst 1992;84:1802–1810.

161. Kirchhofer D, Sakariassen KS, Clozel M, et al. Relationship between tissue factor expression and deposition of fibrin, platelets and leukocytes on cultured endothelial cells under venous blood flow conditions. Blood 1993;81:2050–2058.

162. Gamble JR, Harlan JM, Klebanoff SJ, Vadas MA. Stimulation of the adherence of neutrophils to umbilical vein endothelium by recombinant tumor necrosis factor. Proc Natl Acad Sci USA 1985;82:8667–8671.

163. Lawrence MB, Springer TA. Leukocytes roll on a selectin at physiological flow rates: distinct from and prerequisite for adhesion through integrins. Cell 1991;65:859–873.

164. von Adrian UH, Chambers JD, McEvoy LM, Bargatze RF, Arfors KE, Butcher EC. Two-step model of leukocyte-endothelial cell interaction in inflammation: distinct roles for LECAM-1 and the leukocyte β2 integrins in vivo. Proc Natl Acad Sci USA 1991;88:7538–7542.

165. Mayadas TN, Johnson RC, Rayburn H, Hynes RO, Wagner DD. Leukocyte rolling and extravasation are severely com-

promised in P selectin-deficient mice. Cell 1993;74:541–554.

166. Picker LJ, Warnock RA, Burns AR, Doerschuk CM, Berg EL, Butcher EC. The neutrophil selectin LECAM-1 presents carbohydrate ligands to the vascular selectins ELAM-1 and GMP-140. Cell 1991;66:921–933.

167. Pober JS, Bevilacqua MP, Mendrick DL, Lapierre LA, Fiers W, Gimbrone MA. Two distinct monokines, interleukin-1 and tumor necrosis factor, each independently induce biosynthesis and transient expression of the same antigen on the surface of cultured human endothelial cells. J Immunol 1986;136:1680–1687.

168. Bevilacqua MP, Stengelin S, Gimbrone MA, Seed B. ELAM-1. An inducible receptor for neutrophils related to complement regulatory proteins and lectins. Science 1989;243:1160–1165.

169. Pober JS, Gimbrone MA, Lapierre LA, et al. Overlapping patterns of activation of human endothelial cells by interleukin 1, tumor necrosis factor and immune interferon. J Immunol 1986;137:1893–1896.

170. Messadi DV, Pober JS, Fiers W, Gimbrone MA, Murphy GF. Induction of an activation antigen on post-capillary venular endothelium in human skin organ culture. J Immunol 1987;139:1557–1562.

171. Leeuwenberg JFM, Smeets EF, Neefjes JJ, et al. E-selectin and intercellular adhesion molecule-1 are released by activated human endothelial cells in vitro. Immunology 1992;77:543–549.

172. Smeets EF, de Vries T, Leeuwenberg JFM, van den Eijnden, Buurman WA, Neefjes JJ. Phosphorylation of surface E-selectin and the effect of soluble ligand (Sialyl Lewis^x) on the half-life of E-selectin. Eur J Immunol 1993;23:147–151.

173. von Asmuth EJU, Smeets EF, Ginsel LA, Onderwater JJM, Leeuwenberg JFM, Buurman WA. Evidence for endocytosis of E-selectin in human endothelial cells. Eur J Immunol 1992;22:2519–2526.

174. Geng J-G, Bevilacqua MP, Moore KL, et al. Rapid neutrophil adhesion to activated endothelium mediated by GMP-140. Nature 1990;343:757–760.

175. Sugama Y, Tiruppathi C, Janakidevi K, Andersen TT, Fenton JW II, Malik AB. Thrombin-induced expression of endothelial P-selectin and intercellular adhesion molecule-1: a mechanism for stabilising neutrophil adhesion. J Cell Biol 1992;119:935–944.

176. Weller A, Isenmann S, Vestweber D. Cloning of the mouse endothelial selectins. Expression of both E- and P-selectin is inducible by tumor necrosis factor α. J Biol Chem 1992;267:15176–15183.

177. Fina L, Molgaard HV, Robertson D, et al. Expression of the CD34 gene in vascular endothelial cells. Blood 1990;75:2417–2426.

178. Baumhueter S, Singer MS, Henzel W, et al. Binding of L-selectin to the vascular sialomucin CD34. Science 1993;262:436–438.

179. Delia D, Lampugnani MG, Resnati M, et al. CD34 expression is regulated reciprocally with adhesion molecules in vascular endothelial cells in vitro. Blood 1993;81:1001–1008.

180. Lasky LA, Singer MS, Dowbenko D, et al. An endothelial ligand for L-selectin is a novel mucin-like molecule. Cell 1992;69:927–938.

181. Spertini O, Luscinskas FW, Kansas GS, et al. Leukocyte adhesion molecule-1 (LAM-1, L-selectin) interacts with an inducible endothelial cell ligand to support leukocyte adhesion. J Immunol 1991;147:2565–2573.

182. Schleiffenbaum B, Spertini O, Tedder TF. Soluble L-selectin is present in human plasma at high levels and retains functional activity. J Cell Biol 1992;119:229–238.

183. Gamble JR, Skinner MP, Berndt MC, Vadas MA. Prevention of activated neutrophil adhesion to endothelium by soluble adhesion protein GMP-140. Science 1990;249:414–417.

184. Nortamo P, Li R, Renkonen R, et al. The expression of human intercellular adhesion molecule-2 is refractory to inflammatory cytokines. Eur J Immunol 1991;21:2629–2632.

185. Osborn L, Hession C, Tizard R, et al. Direct expression cloning of vascular cell adhesion molecule 1, a cytokine-induced endothelial protein that binds to lymphocytes. Cell 1989;59:1203–1211.

186. Wellicome SM, Thornhill MH, Pitzalis C, et al. A monoclonal antibody that detects a novel antigen on endothelial cells that is induced by TNF, IL-1 or lipopolysaccharide. J Immunol 1990;144:2558–2565.

187. Vonderheide RH, Springer TA. Lymphocyte adhesion through very late antigen 4: evidence for a novel binding site in the alternatively spliced domain of vascular cell adhesion molecule 1 and an additional α4 integrin counter-receptor on stimulated endothelium. J Exp Med 1992;175:1433–1442.

188. Lampugnani MG, Renati M, Raiteri M, et al. A novel endothelial-specific membrane protein is a marker of cell-cell contacts. J Cell Biol 1992;118:1511–1522.

189. Muller WA, Ratti CM, McDonnell SL, Cohn ZA. A human endothelial cell-restricted, externally disposed plasmalemmal protein enriched in intercellular junctions. J Exp Med 1989;170:399–414.

190. Muller WA, Weigl SA, Deng X, Phillips DM. PECAM-1 is required for transendothelial migration of leukocytes. J Exp Med 1993;178:449–460.

191. Ioffreda MD, Albelda SM, Elder DE, et al. TNF-α induces E-selectin expression and PECAM-1 (CD31) redistribution in extracutaneous tissues. Endothelium 1993;1:47–54.

192. Defilippi P, Silengo L, Tarone G. α6β1 integrin (laminin receptor) is down-regulated by tumor necrosis factor-α and interleukin-1β in human endothelial cells. J Biol Chem 1992;267:18303–18307.

193. Johnson DR, Pober JS. Tumor necrosis factor regulation of major histocompatibility complex gene expression. Immunol Res 1991;10:141–155.

194. Johnson DR, Pober JS. TNF and immune interferon synergistically increase transcription of HLA class I heavy- and light-chain genes in vascular endothelium. Proc Natl Acad Sci USA 1990;87:5183–5187.

195. Epperson DE, Arnold D, Spies T, Cresswell P, Pober JS, Johnson DR. Cytokines increase transporter in antigen processing-1 expression more rapidly than HLA class I expression in endothelial cells. J Immunol 1992:149:3297–3301.

196. Warner SJ, Friedman GB, Libby P. Regulation of major histocompatibility gene expression in human vascular smooth muscle cells. Arteriosclerosis 1989;9:279–288.

197. Burke-Gaffney A, Keenan AK. Modulation of human endothelial cell permeability by combinations of the cytokines interleukin-1 alpha/beta, tumor necrosis factor-alpha and interferon-gamma. Immunopharmacology 1993;25:1–9.

198. Stolpen AH, Guinan EC, Fiers W, Pober JS. Recombinant tumor necrosis factor and immune interferon act singly and in combination to reorganise human vascular endothelial cell monolayers. Am J Physiol 1986;123:16–24.

199. Partridge CA, Horvath CJ, Del-Vecchio PJ, Phillips PG, Malik AB. Influence of extracellular matrix in tumor necrosis factor-induced increase in endothelial permeability. Am J Physiol 1992;263:L627–633.

200. Brett J, Gerlach H, Nawroth P, Steinberg S, Godman G, Stern D. Tumor necrosis factor/cachectin increases permeability of endothelial cell monolayers by a mechanism involving regulatory G proteins. J Exp Med 1989;169:1977–1991.

201. Klein NJ, Shennan GI, Heyderman RS, Levin M. Alteration in glycosaminoglycan metabolism and surface charge on human umbilical vein endothelial cells induced by cytokines, endotoxin and neutrophils. J Cell Sci 1992;102:821–832.

202. Smith WB, Gamble JR, Clark-Lewis I, Vadas MA. Interleukin-8 induces neutrophil transendothelial migration. Immunology 1991;72:65–72.

203. Furie MB, McHugh DD. Migration of neutrophils across endothelial monolayers is stimulated by treatment of the monolayers with interleukin-1 or tumor necrosis factor-α. J Immunol 1989;143:3309–3317.

204. Moser R, Scheiffenbaum B, Groscurth P, Fehr J. Interleukin 1 and tumor necrosis factor stimulate human vascular endothelial cells to promote transendothelial neutrophil passage. J Clin Invest 1989;83:444–455.

205. Huber AR, Kunkel SL, Todd RF, Weiss SJ. Regulation of transendothelial neutrophil migration by endogenous interleukin-8. Science 1991;254:99–102.

206. Strieter RM, Kunkel SL, Showell HJ, Marks RM. Monokine-induced gene expression of a human endothelial cell-derived neutrophil chemotactic factor. Biochem Biophys Res Commun 1988;156:1340–1345.

207. Warner SJC, Auger KR, Libby P. Interleukin 1 induces interleukin 1. II. Recombinant human interleukin 1 induces interleukin 1 production by adult human vascular endothelial cells. J Immunol 1987;139:1911–1917.

208. Broundy VC, Kaushansky K, Segal GM, Harlan JM, Adamson JW. Tumor necrosis factor α stimulates human endothelial cells to produce granulocyte/macrophage colony-stimulating factor. Proc Natl Acad Sci USA 1986;83:7467–7471.

209. Broundy VC, Kaushansky K, Harlan JM, Adamson JW. Interleukin 1 stimulates human endothelial cells to produce granulocyte-macrophage colony-stimulating factor. J Immunol 1988;139:464–468.

210. Hajjar KA, Hajjar DP, Silverstein RL, Nachman RL. Tumor necrosis factor-mediated release of platelet-derived growth factor from cultured endothelial cells. J Exp Med 1987;166:235–245.

211. Jirik FR, Podor TJ, Hirano T, et al. Bacterial lipopolysaccharide and inflammatory mediators augment IL-6 secretion by human endothelial cells. J Immunol 1989;142:144–147.

212. Sironi M, Breviario F, Proserpio P, et al. IL-1 stimulates IL-6 production in endothelial cells. J Immunol 1989;142:549–553.

213. Bussolino F, Camussi G, Baglioni C. Synthesis and release of platelet-activating factor by human vascular endothelial cells treated with tumor necrosis factor or interleukin-1α. J Biol Chem 1988;263:11856–11861.

214. Breviario F, Bertocchi F, Dejana E, Bussolino F. Interleukin-1 induced adhesion of polymorphonuclear leukocytes to cultured human endothelial cells. J Immunol 1988;141:3391–3397.

215. Westphal JR, Willems HW, Schalkwijk CJ, Ruiter DJ, deWaal RM. A new 180-kd dermal endothelial cell activation antigen: in vitro and in situ characteristics. J Invest Dermatol 1993;100:27–34.

216. Hamanaka R, Kimitoshi K, Seguchi T, et al. Induction of low density lipoprotein receptor and a transcription factor SP-1 by tumor necrosis factor in human microvascular endothelial cells. J Biol Chem 1992;267:13160–13165.

217. Tartaglia LA, Goeddel DV. Two TNF receptors. Immunol Today 1992;13:151–153.

218. Shalaby MR, Sundan A, Loetscher H, Brockhaus M, Lesslauer W, Espevik T. Binding and regulation of cellular functions by monoclonal antibodies against human TNF receptors. J Exp Med 1990;172:1517–1520.

219. Barbara AJ, Smith WB, Gamble JR, et al. Dissociation of TNF-α cytotoxic and proinflammatory activities by p55 receptor- and p75 receptor-selective TNF-α mutants. Embo J 1994;13:843–850.

220. Van Ostade X, Vandenabeele P, Everaerdt B, et al. Human TNF mutants with selective activity on the p55 receptor. Nature 1993;361:266–269.

221. Tchorzewski H, Zeman K, Paleolog E, et al. The effects of tumor necrosis factor (TNF) derivatives on TNF receptors. Cytokine 1993;5:125–132.

222. Deisher TA, Garcia I, Harlan JM. Cytokine-induced adhesion molecule expression on human umbilical vein endothelial cells is not regulated by cyclic adenosine monophosphate accumulation. Life Sci 1993;53:365–370.

223. Deisher TA, Sato TT, Pohlman TH, Harlan JM. A protein kinase C agonist, selective for the beta I isozyme, induces E-selectin and VCAM-1 expression on HUVECs but does not translocate PKC. Biochem Biophys Res Commun 1993;193:1283–1290.

224. Garcia JG, Stasek JE, Bahler C, Natarajan V. Interleukin 1-stimulated prostacyclin synthesis in endothelium: lack of phospholipase C, phospholipase D, or protein kinase C involvement in early signal transduction. J Lab Clin Med 1992;120:929–940.

225. Schutze S, Potthoff K, Machleidt T, et al. TNF activates NF-kB by phosphatidylcholine-specific phospholipase c-induced "acidic" sphingomyelin breakdown. Cell 1992;71:765–776.

226. Hooft van Huijsduijnen R, Whelan J, Pescini R, Becker-Andre M, Schenk AM, DeLarmarter JF. A T cell enhancer cooperates with NF-kB to yield cytokine induction of E-selectin gene transcription in endothelial cells. J Biol Chem 1992;267:22385–22391.

227. Smith GM, Whelan J, Pescini R, Ghersa P, DeLamarter JF, Hooft van Huijsduijnen R. DNA-methylation of the

E-selectin promoter represses NF-kappa B transactivation. Biochem Biophys Res Commun 1993;194:215–221.

228. Neish AS, Williams AJ, Palmer HJ, Whitley MZ, Collins T. Functional analysis of the human vascular cell adhesion molecule 1 promoter. J Exp Med 1992;176:1583–1593.

229. Iademarco MF, McQuillan JJ, Dean DC. VCAM-1: contrasting transcriptional control mechanisms in muscle and endothelium. Proc Natl Acad Sci USA 1993;90:3943–3947.

230. de-Martin R, Vanhove B, Cheng Q, Hofer E, Csizmadia V. Cytokine-inducible expression in endothelial cells of an I kappa B alpha-like gene is regulated by NF kappa B. EMBO J 1993;12:2773–2779.

231. Brown K, Park S, Kanno T, Franzoso G, Siebenlist U. Mutual regulation of the transcriptional activator NF-kB and its inhibitor, IkB-α. Proc Natl Acad Sci USA 1993;90:2532–2536.

232. Nash JRG, McLaughlin PJ, Butcher D, Corrin B. Expression of tumour necrosis factor-α in cryptogenic fibrosing alveolitis. Histopathology 1993;22:343–347.

233. Deguchi Y, Shibata N, Kishimoto S. Enhanced transcription of TNF in systemic vasculitis. Lancet 1989;2:745–746.

234. Grau GE, Roux-Lombard P, Gysler C, et al. Serum cytokine changes in systemic vasculitis. Immunology 1989;68:196–198.

235. Arend WP, Dayer JM. Cytokines and cytokine inhibitors or antagonists in rheumatoid arthritis. Arthritis Rheum 1990;33:305–315.

236. Nickoloff BJ, Karabin GD, Barker JNWN, et al. Cellular localisation of interleukin-8 and its inducer tumor necrosis factor-alpha in psoriasis. Am J Pathol 1991;138:129–140.

237. de Kossodo S, Grau GE. Role of cytokines and adhesion molecules in malaria immunopathology. Stem Cells 1993;11:41–48.

238. Casey LC, Balk RA, Bone RC. Plasma cytokine and endotoxin levels correlate with survival in patients with the sepsis syndrome. Ann Intern Med 1993;119:771–778.

239. Leung DYM, Geha RS, Newburger JW, et al. Two monokines, interleukin 1 and tumor necrosis factor, render cultured vascular endothelial cells susceptible to lysis by antibodies circulating Kawasakisyndrome. J Exp Med 1986;164:1958–1972.

240. Westlin WF, Gimbrone MA. Neutrophil-mediated damage to human vascular endothelium. Role of cytokine activation. Am J Pathol 1993;142:117–128.

241. Rice GE, Munro JM, Corless C, Bevilacqua MP. Vascular and nonvascular expression of INCAM-110. A target for mononuclear leukocyte adhesion in normal and inflamed human tissues. Am J Pathol 1991;138:385–393.

242. Page C, Rose M, Yacoub M, Pigott R. Antigenic heterogeneity of vascular endothelium. Am J Pathol 1992;141:673–683.

243. Koch AE, Burrows JC, Haines GK, Carlos TM, Harlan JM, Leibovich SJ. Immunolocalisations of endothelial and leukocyte adhesion molecules in human rheumatoid and osteoarthritic synovial tissues. Lab Invest 1991;64:313–320.

244. Veale D, Yanni G, Rogers S, Barnes L, Bresnihan B, Fitzgerald O. Reduced synovial membrane macrophage numbers, ELAM-1 expression, and lining layer hyperplasia in psori-

atic arthritis as compared with rheumatoid arthritis. Arthritis Rheum 1993;36:893–900.

245. Briscoe DM, Schoen FJ, Rice GE, Bevilacqua MP, Ganz P, Pober JS. Induced expression of endothelial leukocyte adhesion molecules in cardiac allografts. Transplantation 1991;51:537–539.

246. Briscoe DM, Pober JS, Harmon WE, Cotran RS. Expression of vascular cell adhesion molecule-1 in human renal allografts. J Am Soc Nephrol 1992;3:1180–1185.

247. Adams DH, Mainolfi E, Elias E, Neuberger JM, Rothlein R. Detection of circulating intercellular adhesion molecule-1 after liver transplantation; evidence of local release within the liver during graft rejection. Transplantation 1993;55:83–87.

248. van der Wal AC, Das PK, Tigges AJ, Becker AE. Adhesion molecules on the endothelium and mononuclear cells in human atherosclerotic lesions. Am J Pathol 1992;141:1427–1433.

249. Briscoe DM, Cotran RS, Pober JS. Effects of tumor necrosis factor, lipopolysaccharide and IL-4 on the expression of vascular cell adhesion molecule-1 in vivo. Correlation with CD3+ T cell infiltration. J Immunol 1992;149:2954–2960.

250. Munro JM, Pober JS, Cotran RS. Tumor necrosis factor and interferon-γ induce distinct patterns of endothelial activation and associated leukocyte accumulation in skin of Papio Anubis. Am J Pathol 1989;135:121–133.

251. Shreeniwas R, Koga S, Karakurum M, et al. Hypoxia-mediated induction of endothelial cell interleukin-1 alpha. An autocrine mechanism promoting expression of leukocyte adhesion molecules on the vessel surface. J Clin Invest 1992;90:2333–2339.

252. Ala Y, Palluy O, Favero J, Bonne C, Modat G, Dornand J. Hypoxia/reoxygenation stimulates endothelial cells to promote interleukin-1 and interleukin-6 production. Effects of free radical scavengers. Agents Actions 1992;37:134–139.

253. Ockenhouse CF, Tegoshi T, Maeno Y, et al. Human vascular endothelial cell adhesion receptors for plasmodium falciparum-infected erythrocytes: roles for endothelial leukocyte adhesion molecule 1 and vascular cell adhesion molecule 1. J Exp Med 1992;176:1183–1189.

254. Forloni G, Demicheli F, Giorgi S, Bendotti C, Angeretti N. Expression of amyloid precursor protein mRNAs in endothelial, neuronal and glial cells: modulation by interleukin-1. Brain Res Mol Brain Res 1992;16:128–134.

255. Iwai K, Ishikura H, Kaji M, et al. Importance of E-selectin (ELAM-1) and sialyl Lewis(a) in the adhesion of pancreatic carcinoma cells to activated endothelium. Int J Cancer 1993;54:972–977.

256. Dimier IH, Bout DT. Il-1β and TNF-α activation of HUVECs co-operatively inhibits Toxoplasma gondii replication. Immunology 1993;79:336–338.

257. Larsen CG, Anderson AO, Oppenheim JJ, Matsushima K. Production of interleukin-8 by human dermal fibroblasts and keratinocytes in response to interleukin-1 or tumor necrosis factor. Immunology 1989;68:31–36.

258. Bischoff SC, Krieger M, Brunner T, et al. RANTES and related chemokines activate human basophil granulocytes through different G protein-coupled receptors. Eur J Immunol 1993;23:761–767.

259. Baggloini M. Walz A, Kunkel SL. Neutrophil-activating

peptide-1/interleukin 8, a novel cytokine that activates neutrophils. J Clin Invest 1989;84:1045–1049.

260. Collins PD, Web VB, Faccioli LH, Watson ML, Moqbel R, Williams TJ. Eosinophil accumulation induced by human interleukin-8 in the guinea pig in vivo. Immunology 1993; 79:312–318.

261. Larsen CG, Anderson AO, Appella E, Oppenheim JJ, Matsushima K. The neutrophil-activating protein (NAP-1) is also chemotactic for T lymphocytes. Science 1989;243: 1464–1466.

262. Leonard EL, Yoshimura T. Human monocyte chemoattractant protein-1 (MCP-1). Immunol Today 1990;11: 97–101.

263. Taub DD, Conlon K, Lloyd AR, Oppenheim JJ, Kelvin DJ. Preferential migration of activated CD4+ and CD8+ T cells in response to MIP-1α and MIP-1β. Science 1993;260:355–358.

264. Schall T, Bacon K, Toy K, Goedell D. Selective attraction of monocytes and T lymphocytes of the memory phenotype by cytokine RANTES. Nature 1990;347:669–671.

265. Rot A, Krieger M, Brunner T, Bischoff SC, Schall TJ, Dahinden CA. RANTES and macrophage inflammatory protein 1α induce the migration and activation of normal human eosinophil granulocytes. J Exp Med 1992;176: 1489–1495.

266. Rot A. Binding of neutrophil attractant/activation protein-1 (interleukin 8) to resident dermal cells. Cytokine 1992;4: 347–352.

267. Luscinskas FW, Kiely JM, Ding H, et al. In vitro inhibitory effect of IL-8 and other chemoattractants on neutrophil-endothelial adhesive interactions. J Immunol 1992:149: 2163–2171.

268. Smith WB, Gamble JR, Clark-Lewis I, Vadas MA. Chemotactic desensitisation of neutrophils demonstrates interleukin-8 (IL-8)-dependent and IL-8-independent mechanisms of transmigration through cytokine-activated endothelium. Immunology 1993;78:491–497.

269. Detmers PA, Lo SK, Olsen-Egbert E, et al. Neutrophil activating protein 1/IL 8 stimulates the binding activity of the leukocyte adhesion receptor CD11b/CD18 on human neutrophils. J Exp Med 1990;171:1155–1162.

270. Van Zee KJ, Fischer E, Hawes AS, et al. Effects of intravenous IL-8 administration in nonhuman primates. J Immunol 1992;148:1746–1752.

271. Peichl P, Ceska M, Broell H, Effenberger F, Lindley IJD. Human neutrophil activating peptide/interleukin 8 acts as an autoantigen in rheumatoid arthritis. Ann Rheum Dis 1992;51:19–22.

272. Darbonne WC, Rice GC, Mohler MA, et al. Red blood cells are a sink for interleukin 8, a leukocyte chemotaxin. J Clin Invest 1991;88:1362–1369.

273. Strieter RM, Wiggins R, Phan SH, et al. Monocyte chemotactic protein gene expression by cytokine-treated human fibroblasts and endothelial cells. Biochem Biophys Res Commun 1989;162:694–700.

274. Rollins BJ, Yoshimura T, Leonard EJ, Pober JS. Cytokine-activated human endothelial cells synthesize and secrete a monocyte chemoattractant, MCP-1/JE. Am J Pathol 1990; 136:1229–1233.

275. Jiang Y, Beller DI, Frendl G, Graves DT. Monocyte

chemoattractant protein-1 regulates adhesion molecule expression and cytokine production in human monocytes. J Immunol 1992;148:2423–2428.

276. Tanaka Y, Adams DH, Hubscher S, Hirano H, Siebenlist U, Shaw S. T-cell adhesion induced by proteoglycan-immobilized cytokine MIP-1 beta. Nature 1993;361:79–82.

277. Van Zee KJ, DeForge LE, Fischer E, et al. IL-8 in septic shock, endotoxemia and after IL-1 administration. J Immunol 1991;146:3478–3482.

278. Donnelly SC, Strieter RM, Kunkel SL, et al. Interleukin-8 and development of adult respiratory distress syndrome in at-risk patient groups. Lancet 1993;341:643–647.

279. Boylan AM, Ruegg C, Jin Kim K, et al. Evidence of a role for mesothelial cell-derived interleukin 8 in the pathogenesis of asbestos-induced pleurisy in rabbits. J Clin Invest 1992; 89:1257–1267.

280. Koch AE, Kunkel SL, Harlow LA, et al. Enhanced production of monocyte chemoattractant protein-1 in rheumatoid arthritis. J Clin Invest 1992;90:772–779.

281. Seitz M, Dewald B, Gerber N, Bagglioni M. Enhanced production of neutrophil-activating peptide-1/interleukin-8 in rheumatoid arthritis. J Clin Invest 1991;87:463–469.

282. Koch AE, Kunkel SL, Burrows JC, et al. Synovial tissue macrophage as a source of the chemotactic cytokine IL-8. J Immunol 1991;147:2187–2195.

283. Hachicha M, Rathanaswami P, Schall TJ, McColl SR. Production of monocyte chemotactic protein-1 in human type b synoviocytes. Synergistic effect of tumor necrosis factor-α and interferon-γ. Arthritis Rheum 1993;36:26–34.

284. Akahoshi T, Kondo H. PCR analysis of intercrine superfamily gene expression in rheumatoid arthritis. Rev Esp Reumatol 1993;20(suppl 1):210.

285. Nishiura H, Matsubara S, Tanaka J, et al. Role of chemotactic cytokines in the leukocyte recruitment into the synovium of rheumatoid arthritis. Rev Esp Reumatol 1993; 20(suppl 1):M06.

286. Cauli A, Yanni G, Challacombe S, Panayi G. Patterns of cytokine expression and mononuclear cell infiltration in the minor salivary glands of patients with Sjögren's syndrome. Br J Rheumatol 1993;32(suppl 1):331.

287. Cushing SD, Berliner JA, Valente AJ, et al. Minimally modified low density lipoprotein induces monocyte chemotactic protein (MCP-1) in human endothelial and smooth muscle cells. Proc Natl Acad Sci USA 1990;87:5134–5138.

288. Yla-Herttuala S, Lipton BA, Rosenfeld ME, et al. Expression of monocyte chemoattractant protein 1 in macrophage-rich areas of human and rabbit atherosclerotic lesions. Proc Natl Acad Sci USA 1991;88:5252–5256.

289. Duijvestijn A, Hamann A. Mechanisms and regulation of lymphocyte migration. Immunol Today 1989;10:23–28.

290. Mattila P, Renkonen R. IFN-gamma induces a phospholipase D dependent triphasic activation of protein kinase C in endothelial cells. Biochem Biophys Res Commun 1992;189:1732–1738.

291. Doukas J, Pober JS. IFN-γ enhances endothelial activation induced by tumor necrosis factor but not IL-1. J Immunol 1990;145:1727–1733.

292. Buchsbaum ME, Kupper TJ, Murphy GF. Differential induction of intercellular adhesion molecule-1 in human

skin by recombinant cytokines. J Cutan Pathol 1993; 20:21–27.

293. Groves RW, Ross EL, Barker JN, MacDonald DM. Vascular cell adhesion molecule-1: expression in normal and diseased skin and regulation in vivo by interferon gamma. J Am Acad Dermatol 1993;29:67–72.

294. Pober JS, Collins T, Gimbrone MA, et al. Lymphocytes recognise human vascular endothelial and dermal fibroblast Ia antigens induced by recombinant immune interferon. Nature 1983;305:726–729.

295. Masuyama J, Minato N, Kano S. Mechanisms of lymphocyte adhesion to human vascular endothelial cells in culture. T lymphocyte adhesion to endothelial cells through endothelial HLA-DR antigens induced by γ-interferon. J Clin Invest 1986;77:1596–1605.

296. Hughes CCW, Male DK, Lantos PL. Adhesion of lymphocytes to cerebral microvascular cells: effects of interferon-γ, tumour necrosis factor and interleukin-1. Immunology 1988;64:677–681.

297. Savage CO, Hughes C, McIntyre BW, Picard JK, Pober JS. Human CD4+ T cells proliferate to HLA-DR+ allogeneic vascular endothelium. Identification of accessory interactions. Transplantation 1993;56:128–134.

298. Doukas J, Mordes JP. T lymphocytes capable of activating endothelial cells in vitro are present in rats with autoimmune diabetes. J Immunol 1993;150:1036–1046.

299. Burke-Gaffney A, Keenan AK. Modulation of human endothelial cell permeability by combinations of the cytokines interleukin-1 alpha/beta, tumor necrosis factor-alpha and interferon-gamma. Immunopharmacology 1993;25:1–9.

300. Oppenheimer-Marks N, Ziff M. Migration of lymphocytes through endothelial cell monolayers; augmentation by interferon-γ. Cell Immunol 1988;114:307–323.

301. Defilippi P, Truffa G, Stefanuto G, Altruda F, Silengo L, Tarone G. Tumor necrosis factor α and interferon γ modulate the expression of the vitronectin receptor (integrin β3) in human endothelial cells. J Biol Chem 1991;266:7638–7645.

302. Akahane K, Pluznik DH. Interferon-gamma destabilizes interleukin-1-induced granulocyte-macrophage colony-stimulating factor mRNA in murine vascular endothelial cells. Exp Hematol 1993;21:878–884.

303. Brandt SJ, Peters WP, Atwater SK, et al. Effect of recombinant granulocyte-macrophage colony stimulating factor on hematopoietic reconstitution after high-dose chemotherapy and autologous bone marrow transplantation. N Engl J Med 1988;318:869–873.

304. Metcalf D. The consequences of excess levels of haemopoietic growth factors. Br J Haematol 1990;75:1–3.

305. Elliott MJ, Vadas MA, Cleland LG, Gamble JR, Lopez AF. IL-3 and granulocyte-macrophage colony stimulating factor stimulate two distinct phases of adhesion in human monocytes. J Immunol 1990;145:167–176.

306. Yong KW, Rowles PM, Patterson KG, Linch DC. Granulocyte-macrophage colony-stimulating factor induces neutrophil adhesion to pulmonary vascular endothelium in vivo: role of β2 integrins. Blood 1992;80:1565–1575.

307. English D, Graves V. Simultaneous mobilisation of Mac-1 (CDIIb/CD18) and formyl peptide chemoattractant receptors in human neutrophils. Blood 1992;80:776–787.

308. Yong KL, Linch DC. Differential effects of granulocyte- and granulocyte-macrophage colony-stimulating factors (G- and GM-CSF) on neutrophil adhesion in vitro and in vivo. Eur J Haematol 1992;49:251–259.

309. Vadas MA, Nicola NA, Metcalf D. Activation of antibody-dependent cell-mediated cytotoxicity of human neutrophils and eosinophils by separate colony-stimulating factors. J Immunol 1983;130:795–799.

310. DeNicholo MO, Stewart AG, Vadas MA, Lopez AF. Granulocyte-macrophage colony-stimulating factor is a stimulant of platelet-activating factor and superoxide anion generation by human neutrophils. J Biol Chem 1991;266:4896–4902.

311. Broudy VC, Kaushansky K, Harland JM, Adamson JW. Interleukin-1 stimulates human endothelial cells to produce granulocyte-macrophage colony-stimulating factor and granulocyte colony-stimulating factor. J Immunol 1987;139:464–468.

312. Broudy VC, Kaushansky K, Segal GM, Harlan JM, Adamson JW. Tumor necrosis factor type alpha stimulates human endothelial cells to produce granulocyte-macrophage colony-stimulating factor. Proc Natl Acad Sci USA 1986;83:7467–7471.

313. Brown TJ, Liu J, Brashem-Stein C, Shoyab M. Regulation of granulocyte colony-stimulating factor and granulocyte-macrophage colony-stimulating factor expression by oncostatin M. Blood 1993;82:33–37.

314. Rajavashisth TB, Andalibi A, Territo MC, et al. Induction of endothelial cell expression of granulocyte and macrophage colony-stimulating factors by modified low-density lipoproteins. Nature 1990;344:254–257.

315. Suzu S, Ohtsuki T, Makishima M, et al. Biological activity of a proteoglycan form of macrophage colony-stimulating factor and its binding to type V collagen. J Biol Chem 1992; 267:16812–16815.

316. Namiki A, Hirata Y, Fukazawa M, et al. Granulocyte-colony stimulating factor stimulates immunoreactive endothelin-1 release from cultured bovine endothelial cells. Eur J Pharmacol 1992;227:339–341.

317. Chin YH, Cai JP, Johnson K. Lymphocyte adhesion to cultured Peyer's patch HEV cells is mediated by organ-specific homing receptors and can be regulated by cytokines. J Immunol 1990;145:3669–3677.

318. Massague J. The TGF-β family of growth and differentiation factors. Cell 1987;49:437–438.

319. Sporn MB, Roberts AB. Transforming growth factor-β: recent progress and new challenges. J Cell Biol 1992;119:1017–1021.

320. Lin HY, Lodish HF. Receptors for the TGF-β superfamily: multiple polypeptides and serine/threonine kinases. Trends Cell Biol 1993;3:14–19.

321. Das SK, White AC, Fanburg BL. Modulation of transforming growth factor-β1 antiproliferative effects on endothelial cells by cysteine, cystine and n-acetylcysteine. J Clin Invest 1992;90:1649–1656.

322. Phan SH, Gharakee-Kermani M, McGarry B, Kunkel SL, Wolber FW. Regulation of rat pulmonary endothelial cell transforming growth factor-β production by IL-1β and tumor necrosis factor-α. J Immunol 1992;149:103–106.

323. Shull MM, Ormsby I, Kier AB, et al. Targeted disruption of

the mouse transforming growth factor-β1 gene results in multi-focal inflammatory disease. Nature 1992;359:693–699.

324. Kulkarni AB, Huh CG, Becker D, et al. Transforming growth factor-β1 null mutation in mice causes excessive inflammatory response and early death. Proc Natl Acad Sci USA 1993;90:770–774.

325. Gamble JR, Vadas MA. Endothelial adhesiveness for blood neutrophils is inhibited by transforming growth factor-β. Science 1988;242:97–99.

326. Gamble JR, Vadas MA. Endothelial cell adhesiveness for human T lymphocytes is inhibited by transforming growth factor-β. J Immunol 1991;146:1149–1154.

327. Bereta J, Bereta M, Coffman F, Cohen S, Cohen MC. Inhibition of basal and tumor necrosis factor-enhanced binding of murine tumor cells to murine endothelium by transforming growth factor-β. J Immunol 1992;148:2932–2940.

328. Gamble JR, Khew-Goodall Y, Vadas MA. TGF-β inhibits E-selectin expression on human endothelial cells. J Immunol 1993;150:4494–4503.

329. Fafeur V, Terman BJ, Blum J, Bohlen P. Basic FGF treatment of endothelial cells down-regulates the 85-kDa TGF-β receptor subtype and decreases the growth inhibitory response to TGF-β1. Growth Factors 1990;3:237–245.

330. Lin HY, Wang XF, Ng-Eaton E, Weinberg RA, Lodish HF. Expression cloning of the TGF-β type II receptor, a functional transmembrane serine/threonine kinase. Cell 1992; 68:775–785.

331. Fafeur V, O'Hara B, Bohlen P. A glycosylation-deficient endothelial cell mutant with modified responses to transforming growth factor-β and other growth inhibitory cytokines: evidence for multiple growth inhibitory signal transduction pathways. Mol Cell Biol 1993;4:135–144.

332. Kataoka R, Sherlock J, Lanier SM. Signaling events initiated by transforming growth factor-β1 that require $G_{i\alpha1}$. J Biol Chem 1993;268:19851–19857.

333. Santambrogio L, Hochwald GM, Saxena B. Studies on the mechanisms by which transforming growth factor-beta (TGF-beta) protects against allergic encephalomyelitis. Antagonism between TGF-beta and tumor necrosis factor. J Immunol 1993;151:1116–1127.

334. Lefer AM, Tsao P, Aoki N, Pallidino MA Jr. Mediation of cardioprotection by TGF-β. Science 1990;249:61–63.

335. Lefer AM, Ma XL, Weyrich AS, Scalia R. Mechanism of the cardioprotective effect of transforming growth factor-β1 in feline myocardial ischemia and reperfusion. Proc Natl Acad Sci USA 1993;90:1018–1022.

336. Brandes ME, Allen JB, Ogawa Y, Wahl SM. Transforming growth factor β1 suppresses acute and chronic arthritis in experimental animals. J Clin Invest 1991;87:1108–1113.

337. Kojima S, Harpel PC, Rifkin DB. Lipoprotein (a) inhibits the generation of transforming growth factor B: an endogenous inhibitor of smooth muscle migration. J Cell Biol 1991;113:1439–1445.

338. Cai JP, Falanga V, Taylor JR, Chin YH. Transforming growth factor-beta differently regulates the adhesiveness of normal and psoriatic dermal microvascular endothelial cells for peripheral blood mononuclear cells. J Invest Dermatol 1992;98:405–409.

339. Abehsira-Amar O, Gibert M, Joliy M, Theze J, Jankovic DJ.

IL-4 plays a dominant role in the differential development of Th0 and Th1 and Th2 cells. J Immunol 1992;148:3820–3829.

340. Abramson SL, Gallin JL. IL-4 inhibits superoxide production by human mononuclear phagocytes. J Immunol 1990; 144:625–630.

341. Hart PH, Vitti GF, Burgess DR, Whitty GA, Piccoli DS, Hamilton JA. Potential antiinflammatory effects of interleukin 4: suppression of human monocyte tumor necrosis factor alpha, interleukin 1 and prostaglandin E_2. Proc Natl Acad Sci USA 1989;86:3803–3807.

342. te Velde AA, Huijbens RJF, Heije K, de Vries JE, Figdor CG. Interleukin-4 inhibits secretion of IL-1β, tumor necrosis factor α and IL-6 by human monocytes. Blood 1990; 76:1392–1397.

343. Standiford TJ, Strieter RM, Chensue SW, Westwick J, Kasahara K, Kunkel SL. IL-4 inhibits the expression of IL-8 from stimulated human monocytes. J Immunol 1990; 145:1435–1439.

344. Thornhill HM, Haskard DO. IL-4 regulates endothelial cell activation by IL-1, tumor necrosis factor or IFN-γ. J Immunol 1990;145:865–872.

345. Thornhill MH, Wellicome SM, Mahiouz DL, Lanchbury JSS, Kyan-Aung U, Haskard DO. Tumour necrosis factor combines with IL-4 or IFN-γ to selectively enhance endothelial cell adhesiveness for T cells. The contribution of vascular cell adhesion molecule-1-dependent and -independent binding mechanisms. J Immunol 1991;146:592–598.

346. Thornhill MH, Kyan-Aung U, Haskard DO. IL-4 increases human endothelial cell adhesiveness for T cells but not for neutrophils. J Immunol 1990;144:3060–3065.

347. Schleimer RP, Sterbinsky SA, Kaiser J, et al. IL-4 induces adherence of human eosinophils and basophils but not neutrophils to endothelium. J Immunol 1992;148:1086–1092.

348. Moser R, Fehr J, Bruijnzeel PLB. IL-4 controls the selective endothelium-driven transmigration of eosinophils from allergic individuals. J Immunol 1992;149:1432–1438.

349. Galea P, Thibault G, Lacord M, Bardos P, Lebranchu Y. IL-4, but not tumor necrosis factor-alpha, increases endothelial cell adhesiveness for lymphocytes by activating a cAMP-dependent pathway. J Immunol 1993;151:588–596.

350. Rollins BJ, Pober JS. Interleukin-4 induces the synthesis and secretion of MCP-1/JE by human endothelial cells. Am J Pathol 1991;138:1315–1319.

351. Rollins BJ, Yoshimura T, Leonard EJ, Pober JS. Cytokine-activated human endothelial cells synthesize and secrete a monocyte chemoattractant, MCP-1/JE. Am J Pathol 1990; 136:1229–1233.

352. Colotta F, Sironi M, Borre A, Luini W, Maddalena F, Mantovani A. Interleukin-4 amplifies monocyte chemotactic protein and interleukin-6 production by endothelial cells. Cytokine 1992;4:24–28.

353. Beekhuizen H, Verdegaal EM, Blokland I, van-Furth R. Contribution of ICAM-1 and VCAM-1 to the morphological changes in monocytes bound to human venous endothelial cells stimulated with recombinant interleukin-4 or rIL-1 alpha. Immunology 1992;77:469–472.

354. Howell G, Pham P, Taylor D, Foxwell B, Feldmann M. Interleukin-4 induces interleukin-6 production by endo-

thelial cells: synergy with interferon-γ. Eur J Immunol 1991;21:97–101.

355. Paleolog EM, Aluri G, Feldmann M. Interleukin-4 (IL-4) modulates the response of human vascular endothelial cells to other cytokines. J Cell Biochem 1992;16A:18.

356. Sironi M, Breviario F, Proserpio P, et al. IL-1 stimulates IL-6 production in endothelial cells. J Immunol 1989;142:549–553.

357. Joseph J, Grun JL, Lublin FD, Knobler RL. Interleukin-6 induction in vitro in mouse brain endothelial cells and astrocytes by exposure to mouse hepatitis virus (MHV-4, JHM). J Neuroimmunol 1993;42:47–52.

358. Kao J, Ryan J, Brett G, et al. Endothelial monocyte-activating polypeptide II. A novel tumor-derived polypeptide that activates host-response mechanisms. J Biol Chem 1992;267:20239–20247.

359. Tanaka Y, Albelda SM, Horgan, et al. CD31 expressed on distinctive T cell subsets is a preferential amplifier of β1 integrin-mediated adhesion. J Exp Med 1992;176:245–253.

360. Hsieh HJ, Li NQ, Frangos JA. Pulsatile and steady flow induces c-fos expression in human endothelial cells. J Cell Physiol 1993;154:143–151.

361. Grabowski EF, Zuckerman DB, Nemerson Y. The functional expression of tissue factor by fibroblasts and endothelial cells under flow conditions. Blood 1993;81:3265–3270.

362. Akira K, Ando J. Vascular endothelial cell functions and biomechanics. Endothelium 1993;1:127–130.

CHAPTER 8

ROLE OF CYTOKINES IN THE REGULATION OF HYPERSENSITIVITY RESPONSES

Angus M. Moodycliffe and Stephen E. Ullrich

Although the mechanisms of hypersensitivity responses represent important forms of adaptive immunity, these immune responses can also be harmful to individuals by producing severe pathological consequences if the response is produced in vital tissues. A conceptual advance in the study of hypersensitivity was classification of the various forms of disease into four groups, based on the immune mechanism that causes the symptoms. In type I (or immediate) hypersensitivity, an antigen combines with immunoglobulin E (IgE) bound to the surface of mast cells, causing degranulation that results in the release of vasoactive substances, which produce an acute inflammatory reaction. Type II hypersensitivity occurs when antibody binds to a cell surface antigen or to an antigen that has become attached to a cell surface, leading to cell lysis by activation of the classic complement pathway or by the action of antibody-dependent, cell-mediated cytotoxicity (ADCC). Tissue damage mediated by deposition of immune complexes (particularly soluble complexes formed in slight antigen excess) in tissues and the subsequent activation of antibody effector mechanisms is the basis of type III hypersensitivity. In contrast to types I, II, and III hypersensitivity, which are mediated by antibody, a fourth type of reaction (delayed-type hypersensitivity [DTH] or type IV) is a T-cell–dependent immune phenomenon manifested by an inflammatory response at the site of antigen deposition, usually the skin.

Cytokines are essential transmitters of intercellular communication, and they have an inherent role in the regulation of responses of the immune system. This chapter will focus on an examination of the role of cytokines in hypersensitivity. Molecular cloning of the genes encoding these factors has provided pure materials, which in turn have greatly facilitated our understanding of their biological activities. These studies have been done using in vitro model systems. On the basis of such studies, it has emerged that each cytokine has multiple functions (pleiotropy), and that more than one cytokine may mediate the same, or a very similar, function (redundancy). Therefore, instead of specific cytokines being limited to a single physiological activity, they form part of a complex cellular signaling language. Informational content therefore resides not in individual peptides, but in the pattern or set of regulatory peptide molecules to which a cell is exposed. A language based on combinations selected from a large number of peptide signaling molecules increases the amount of information that can be transmitted.

Any extrapolation of in vitro findings to the in vivo physiological effect does, however, require some degree of skepticism. The local environment in immune and inflammatory responses represents a complex milieu in which other cells and cytokines are present, raising the possibility of important synergistic or antagonistic effects, which will not be recognized when only pure cell populations are studied. Furthermore, in this situation, cytokines may exhibit very different thresholds and kinetics in terms of biological action.

Because of their plethora of activities, studies attempting to elucidate the in vivo physiological role of cytokines using recombinant/purified forms of the peptides are difficult to interpret. Making any sense of the in vivo role of a particular cytokine following its delivery into a system so finely tuned is restricted by many variables (e.g., timing, dose, site). In contrast, studies of the consequences of deleting the in vivo function of a particular cytokine have provided insight into the physiological role of these peptides in regulating immune responses. One approach undertaken by several investigators involves blocking the in vivo activity of a particular cytokine by injecting neutralizing monoclonal antibody with appropriate specificity for the molecule under investigation. Over the past several years, a number of cytokines (such as interleukins: (IL) IL-2, IL-4, and IL-10) have been subjected to the ultimate test through deletion of their genes in mice by target recombination. In simple terms, this technique involves inserting DNA into a cytokine gene with the aim of introducing a number of stop codons in all the reading frames to abolish completely the biological activity of the cytokine.

The immune mechanism involved in each class of hypersensitivity is complex, involving a coordinated interplay between cytokines and cells. Furthermore, available evidence suggests that there is more than one type of immune mechanism involved in DTH responses, depending on the type of antigen and its site of introduction or localization. As a prelude to comprehending the role of cytokines in immune reactions, a detailed analysis of the cellular mechanisms involved in these responses is necessary. Consequently, we limit the discussion to an examination of the role of cytokines in different types of DTH responses. Furthermore, although this book largely focuses on human cytokines, much of what we currently know and understand with regard to the function of cytokines in hypersensitivity responses has been based on extensive studies on the murine system, which is discussed herein.

TYPES OF DELAYED-TYPE HYPERSENSITIVITY RESPONSES

Unlike other forms of hypersensitivity, DTH reactions are T-cell–dependent responses, and they are often associated with protective immunity. However, there is not always complete correlation between DTH and protective immunity. The reaction is a biphasic phenomenon comprising an induction or afferent phase, during which sensitization is initiated, and an elicitation or efferent phase, during which the sensitized individual exhibits a delayed hypersensitivity response, following subsequent exposure to the same antigen, manifested by an inflammatory reaction at the site of antigen challenge. There are three types of DTH responses; the nature of each reaction varies according to the type of antigen and its site of administration or localization: (a) tuberculin-type (or classic DTH), (b) contact hypersensitivity (CH), and (c) granulomatous-type.

Tuberculin-type hypersensitivity

This form of hypersensitivity was originally observed by Koch. Following intradermal injection of tuberculin (a lipoprotein antigen derived from tubercle bacillus) into patients with tuberculosis, swelling developed at the site of injection after 48 hours. Typically, this form of DTH, also called classic DTH, is indurated, necrotic, and characterized by a prominent mononuclear infiltrate that is maintained at a high level for 2 to 3 days. Soluble microbial antigen, which induces a similar reaction in sensitive people when administered in the same way, is derived from *Mycobacterium leprae*. This skin reaction is now used as a clinical screening procedure to determine whether an individual has previously come into contact with these organisms. A variety of other antigens, microbial and non-microbial, are also capable of mediating this response. These antigens include herpes simplex virus, *Listeria monocytogenes, Leishmania major,* allogeneic spleen cells, haptenated spleen cells, and keyhole limpet hemocyanin (KLH). Generally, these antigens are administered intradermally, subcutaneously, or intraperitoneally in the induction and elicitation of classic DTH in animal models. In contrast to the tuberculin-type response to soluble *Mycobacterial* antigens, the DTH response exhibited at the site of antigen challenge does not normally show signs of necrosis.

Contact hypersensitivity

Contact hypersensitivity (CH) is primarily an epidermal phenomenon, in contrast to classic DTH, which is predominantly induced and elicited in the dermis or at sites proximal or distant to the skin. Furthermore, the antigen responsible for inducing this type of DTH response is usually a highly reactive chemical hapten, such as trinitrochlorobenzene (TNCB), dinitrofluorobenzene (DNFB), or dinitrochlorobenzene (DNCB). Other common haptens include nickel, chromate, urushiol (poison ivy), and certain chemicals found in rubber. Contact hypersensitivity is characterized by an infiltration of mononuclear cells and, in some instances, basophils (1), edema, and an eczematous reaction at the site of challenge. As with classic DTH, the response peaks at 24 hours following exposure, and is maintained at a high level for 2 to 3 days.

Granulomatous hypersensitivity

As previously mentioned, the immune mechanism constituting the DTH response can be protective. The tuberculin-type response is one way that this defense mechanism can appear. However, if the invading microorganism is able to evade this effector mechanism (i.e., becoming persistent), another type of DTH response can manifest: the granulomatous response. This response usually results from the persistence of microorganisms within macrophages, which the cell is unable to destroy, leading ultimately to the formation of a granuloma. Essentially, this is a localized inflammatory response composed predominantly of mononuclear cells arising during presentation of a persistent chronic antigenic stimulus. Histologically, the appearance of the granulomatous reaction is very different from that of the tuberculin-type response, which is usually a self-limiting response to antigen. Typically, a granuloma is characterized by a core of epithelioid cells, macrophages, and multinucleated giant cells. The nature of epithelioid cells and giant cells is poorly understood, although it is thought that these cells are derived from activated macrophages that no longer possess phagosomes or that have fused to form one large cell, respectively.

In contrast to tuberculin-type and CH, granulomatous reactions develop over a period of weeks. Clinically, this is the most important form of DTH; it causes many of the pathological effects in diseases that involve cell-mediated immunity. Many of the chronic diseases in humans that manifest this type of response are due to infectious agents, such as mycobacteria, fungi, and protozoa, which cause diseases such as tuberculosis, leprosy, leishmaniasis, blastomycosis, schistosomiasis, and listeriosis.

CELLULAR MECHANISM OF THE DELAYED-TYPED HYPERSENSITIVITY RESPONSE

A great deal of what we understand of the cellular mechanism of DTH has been based on studies looking at CH and classic DTH responses. Progress has been facilitated by the development of suitable animal models of CH and classic DTH, and by a greater comprehension of the molecular and cellular events that initiate and regulate immune responses in general. Although controversial, evidence generated from these studies suggests that the immune mechanism of DTH varies depending on the type of DTH reaction being expressed. Because the antigens mediating CH and classic DTH responses are very different and also delivered into distinct cellular compartments, this finding is not surprising.

Classic DTH and CH responses require the presentation of antigen in two distinct phases, termed *induction* and *elicitation phases*. During the induction phase, antigen-presenting cells (APC) pick up antigen and migrate via the afferent lymphatics to draining lymph nodes, where they present antigen in association with major histocompatibility complex (MHC) class II molecules to naive CD4+ T cells. Following activation of appropriate antigen-specific T-cell clones, they proliferate and differentiate into DTH effector T cells. The available evidence suggests that distinct populations of APC are responsible for inducing CH and classic DTH responses.

In the CH response, the processing and presentation of antigen (hapten-derivatized epidermal protein) in association with MHC class II molecules is believed to be performed by Langerhans cells (LC). These cells form a regular and almost closed network of dendrites within basal and suprabasal layers of the epidermis. They form a reticuloepithelial trap for antigen encountered at skin surfaces; they then transport it, via afferent lymphatics, to draining lymph nodes (2–4). A considerable body of evidence has been gathered to support the hypothesis that LC are important APC for the induction of CH responses. Numerous investigators have reported that the efficiency of sensitization is impaired, or actively suppressed, when hapten is applied to areas of skin naturally poor in, or depleted of, LC (5–9). Furthermore, it has been demonstrated that draining lymph node antigen-bearing dendritic cells, the majority of which are derived from LC, are potent stimulators of both primary and secondary T lymphocyte proliferative responses in vitro (10–14), and small numbers will efficiently induce CH in naive animals (12,15–17). However, there is evidence that LC are not an absolute prerequisite for the initiation of CH. Studies in the guinea pig (18) and the mouse (19) suggest that contact sensitization may proceed in the absence of epidermal LC, implying that a second pathway of cutaneous antigen presentation may exist. In support of this view is the report by Tse and Cooper (20); they showed that Ia+ DC, located in the perivascular region of the mouse dermis, when derivatized with hapten, can induce CH in naive mice.

An age-depended macrophage defeat in SJL mice that results in classic DTH unresponsiveness in young adult (≤ 8 wk old) SJL mice has been reported (21,22). Importantly, the CH response and other APC-dependent immunological effector mechanisms were normal in these mice (23), implying that different APCs are involved in inducing CH and classic DTH responses. Indeed, Matsushima and Stohlman (24) identified a unique subset of APCs in SJL mice that functions as the sole APC required for the induction of CD4+ DTH effector T cells. This cell is adherent, Mac-1+, Mac-2−, Mac-3+, and I-A+, and it does not participate in the induction of CH responses (23). As previously mentioned, available evidence suggesting that LC pick up antigen encountered in the epidermis and transport it to the draining lymph nodes is extensive. In contrast, there is no evidence that other APC populations present in different cellular compartments, such as the dermis, carry out this function, although it is considered highly likely.

It has been found that 24- to 48-hour CH and classic DTH skin swelling reactions that result from local antigen challenge of actively sensitized mice are preceded by an early skin swelling reaction, which is maximal 2 hours after challenge (24,25). Two different cells mediate the early and late components of CH and classic DTH responses: a helper cell responsible for both the early reaction and activation of the effector cell that mediates the late-phase reaction. However, although the antigen-specific, MHC-restricted Th1 (26) effector cell that mediates the late-phase reaction of CH and classic DTH is the same (i.e., Thy-1+, Lyt-1+, CD4+, CD8−, CD3+, I-A−, IL-2R+), the helper cells responsible for the early response of CH and classic DTH are different. The initiating helper cell activated in CH is a Thy-1+, Lyt-1+, CD4−, CD8−, CD3−, IL-3R+, B220+ cell and it acts in an antigen-specific but MHC-unrestricted fashion (27). In contrast, the initiating/helper cell activated in classic DTH is a Thy-1+, Lyt-1+, CD4−, CD8−, CD3−, IL-2R+, B220−, I-A− cell that also functions in an MHC-unrestricted manner, but it provides help in an antigen nonspecific manner (24). Matsushima and Stohlman (24) also identified an adherent Mac-1+, Mac-2−, Mac-3−, I-A− accessory cell that appears to be crucial in activation of the classic DTH helper cell. The interaction between these two cells is neither antigen-specific nor MHC-restricted.

In CH responses, the initiating/helper cell produces an antigen-specific DTH-initiating factor called PCL-F in picryl chloride sensitivity, or OX-F in oxazolone sensitivity (28–30). Following sensitization, these factors are produced in the lymphoid organs (28–30), and subsequently are found in the circulation (31), sensitizing the extravascular tissues (32). These antigen-specific DTH-initiating factors are analogous to Immunoglobulin E (IgE) antibodies in their ability to bind to and sensitize connective tissue mast cells for release of vasoactive amines after local antigen challenge (28–30,33,34). The antigen-specific DTH-initiating factors are, however, only functionally analogous to IgE antibodies, because extensive studies have demonstrated that these initiating factors are not IgE antibodies (28–31,33,34).

Whether DTH initiating factors are produced by initiating/helper T cells in classic DTH responses is currently not known, simply because all the investigations carried out in examining these factors focused on the CH response. It is conceivable that these helper cells do not produce these factors because they appear to be antigen-nonspecific in their function (24). It has been demon-

strated that IgE or IgG antibodies can initiate the elicitation phase of CH responses (35). Thus, antibodies may have an important role in the early phase of elicitation in classic DTH responses by negating a requirement for antigen-specific T helper cells. The early component of the elicitation phase is an immediate hypersensitivity-like reaction (36) that is due to local release of the vasoactive amine serotonin (32,37–40) from mast cells (32,40–42) and possibly other serotonin-containing cells (42,43). Released serotonin binds to serotonin receptors on the local microvasculature, creates gaps between endothelial cells (39,41), and subsequently allows local recruitment of late-acting, antigen-specific, MHC-restricted CD4+ Th1 DTH effector T cells into the tissues (26). These recruited effector DTH T cells are activated following binding of their α β T-cell receptors to antigen/MHC complexes on local APC, and they produce lymphokines that attract the 24-hour perivascular infiltrate of nonspecific inflammatory cells.

There is controversy in the literature as to whether mast cells and vasoactive amines have an imperative role in the elicitation phase of DTH responses. This discrepancy centers around studies examining the CH response. For instance, mice genetically deficient in mast cells display 24-hour challenge reactions comparable with normal animals (43,44). Also, reserpine, an agent that depletes mast-cell serotonin levels, has been demonstrated to virtually abolish expression of contact reactions in mast cell–deficient mice (42,43). It is thought that this result either is due to a direct effect of reserpine on T-lymphocyte function (44,45), or that it simply reflects the importance of other vasoactive amine-releasing cells other than mast cells in initiating the elicitation phase of DTH. Although investigations on the role of mast cells in classic DTH responses are limited, there is some evidence that this response is mast-cell–independent (46), which would further account for the antigen-nonspecific function of T initiating/helper cells involved in the early reaction of the elicitation phase of classic DTH responses.

FUNCTIONS OF Th1 AND Th2 CELLS

In 1986, two types of murine T helper clones (Th1 and Th2) were described (47) on the basis of their different cytokine secretion profiles after stimulation with either lectin or APC plus antigen. This currently remains the most clear-cut criterion for separation of mouse Th subtypes. Although both Th1 and Th2 clones secrete IL-3, tumor necrosis factor-α (TNF-α), and granulocyte-macrophage colony-stimulating factor (GM-CSF), only Th1 clones secrete interferon-γ (IFN-γ), IL-2, and TNF-β (lymphotoxin), whereas Th2 clones secrete IL-4, IL-5,

IL-6, and IL-10. Furthermore, among mouse clones, a pattern of IL-2, IL-4, IL-5, and IFN-γ (Th0) has been described (48,49); in some cases, the clones have been shown to produce all cytokines tested, including IL-3, IL-10, and GM-CSF (50). It is thought that Th0 cells represent a precursor population of Th1 and Th2 phenotypes (51,52), although it is not known whether the Th0 cell is committed to a particular phenotype before expressing the mature cytokine secretion pattern, or whether a common precursor can be induced to differentiate into either Th1 or Th2 cells.

Until recently, workers from several laboratories found no clear-cut patterns in the secretion of cytokines by panels of human T-cell clones (53–55), implying that the Th1/Th2 classification was invalid for human T cells. However, there is new evidence that supports the existence of human Th1 and Th2 CD4+ subsets. Allergen-specific CD4+ clones isolated from atopic patients (i.e., individuals expressing type 1 or immediate hypersensitivity responses) expressing high serum levels of IgE, fall into a Th2-like category and produce mainly IL-4 and IL-5, variable amounts of IL-2, and little or no IFN-γ (56). In contrast, CD4+ clones specific for the heat shock protein of *Mycobacterium leprae,* isolated from patients with tuberculoid leprosy, produce predominantly IFN-γ and IL-2 (57). Furthermore, depending on which stimulating antigen is used, Th1- and Th2-like CD4+ clones can be derived from the same healthy donors. It was found that most CD4+ clones derived from such individuals, which are specific for *Mycobacterium tuberculosis* purified protein derivative (PPD), produce IFN-γ and IL-2, but not IL-4 and IL-5 (58). In contrast, the majority of CD4+ clones specific for *Toxocara canis* excretory-secretory antigen were found to produce IL-4 and IL-5, but not IL-2 and IFN-γ (58).

The differential cytokine secretion profile of Th1 and Th2 cells correlates with different effector functions exerted by these cells: Th1 cells mediate DTH responses in adoptive hosts (26,51,59), whereas Th2 cells are more efficient at promoting B-cell responses to soluble antigen (47,60), thus stimulating IgE production (61) and enhancing the growth and differentiation of mast cells and eosinophils (62).

Because it is not yet possible to clearly assay Th1 and Th2 subsets in vivo, virtually all the evidence for involvement of specific subsets is inferred from the nature of the response and from the pattern of cytokines secreted by the stimulated cells. Thus, responses composed mainly of DTH, with very low antibody production and substantial amounts of IFN-γ mRNA but undetectable IL-4 mRNA in immune cells, may be regarded as Th1-mediated responses. Responses consisting of a large antibody response, including significant production of IgE, weak or absent DTH, and large amounts of IL-4 mRNA but no detectable IFN-γ mRNA, are regarded as being mediated by Th2 cells.

The finding that DTH is observed with adoptive transfer of Th1 and not Th2 clones and that the effector function of both these subsets is distinguished by their cytokine secretion pattern, implies that Th1-specific cytokines may be involved in mediating the effector phase of the DTH response. Furthermore, there is accumulating evidence that Th1- and Th2-specific cytokines are able to regulate the effector function of the other subset, and that a number of cytokines are important in directing the response toward a predominantly Th1 or Th2 phenotype, suggesting that these cytokines may have a significant role in initiation, elicitation, and regulation of DTH responses.

ROLE OF CYTOKINES IN THE INITIATION OF DTH RESPONSES

The possibility that Th1 and Th2 cells differentiate from a common pool of precursors leads to the question of what factors direct these differentiation pathways. A number of factors have been proposed, including the properties of the immunogen (63–65), the density of antigen presented (66), the type of APC involved (51,67–70), ongoing immune responses in the host (71,72), and cytokines (73). It is more than likely that these factors are not mutually exclusive, and that all act in concert in directing the differentiation of a precursor Th (Th0) cell toward a Th1 or Th2 phenotype.

Substantial evidence exists that certain cytokines can determine whether an antigenic challenge leads to a Th1 or a Th2 response. In particular, there is a large body of evidence from in vitro and in vivo studies that implies IFN-γ and IL-12 have significant roles in the generation of Th1 type responses.

In vitro evidence that the cytokine environment present during differentiation has an important role in determining the generation of Th1 cells was provided by Gajewski and colleagues (74). They demonstrated that Th1 cells are preferentially obtained when CD4+ cells are cloned in the presence of IFN-γ. Recently, similar findings have been obtained in humans using peripheral blood mononuclear cells cultured with allergens. The addition of both IFN-γ and anti-IL-4 antibody induced allergen-specific T cells to differentiate into Th1 cells instead of Th2 cells (75).

Clearer evidence that IFN-γ can exert decisive effects on the differentiation of virgin T cells into Th1 cells has been shown in vivo using the murine model of cutaneous leishmaniasis. Infection of different strains of mice with *Leishmaniasis major* leads to two dramatically different patterns of disease. In BALB/c mice, the immune response is unable to effectively control and eliminate the local infection; therefore, the disease disseminates to visceral organs with fatal results (nonhealer strain). In contrast, a localized lesion that heals spontaneously after a few weeks develops in most other mouse strains (healer mice), accompanied by complete resistance to reinfection. Regardless of the mouse strain, the major T-cell response is in the CD4+ population, but Th2 responses develop in nonhealer strains, as evidenced by high levels of IL-4 mRNA, but very little IFN-γ mRNA, whereas predominant Th1 responses develop in healer strains, with significant levels of IFN-γ mRNA, but no detectable IL-4 mRNA (71).

Further correlation of Th subset and disease outcome arises from studies with Th1 and Th2 *L. major*–specific lines, in which adoptive transfer of Th1 lines to BALB/c recipient mice confers almost complete resistance to infection, and transfer of a Th2 cell line exacerbates the nonhealing infection (76). Because activation by IFN-γ is clearly required for efficient parasite killing of infected macrophages (77,78), and because the combination of IL-4 and IL-3 can inhibit such activation (79,80), the principal effector function for the control of *L. major* infection is consistent with the observed correlation of disease outcome and cytokine expression. Also, the nature of the immune response varies in healer and nonhealer mice, which is consistent with a preferential activation of different subsets. Healer mice give strong DTH responses, but they produce poor antibody responses, whereas nonhealer mice express little or no DTH response (81), but they produce large antibody responses, including substantial IgE levels (71).

Studies using both susceptible and resistant strains of mice suggest that IFN-γ has a significant role in controlling early resistance to *L. major* by initiating Th1 cell differentiation. Administration of a single injection of anti-IFN-γ antibodies to healer mice at the time of *L. major* infection promotes susceptibility (82), and it inhibits the development of Th1 cells (83). Moreover, injection of IFN-γ with the parasite switches the early cytokine pattern in susceptible BALB/c mice from a Th2 to a Th1 profile (83). Importantly, alterations in the cytokine pattern following treatment with either anti-IFN-γ or IFN-γ are apparent within 3 days of infection, implying that the presence of IFN-γ at the time of antigen presentation is critical in Th1-cell subset development. Although IFN-γ inhibits the proliferation of Th2 cells, while having no inhibitory effect on Th1 cells (74), early and permanent conversion of the Th response both by anti-IFN-γ and IFN-γ suggest that alteration of the disease outcome is primarily achieved by alteration of the basic nature of the T-cell response through an influence on Th subset differentiation rather than by blocking or enhancing effector functions. Furthermore, evidence that IFN-γ stimulates differentiation of Th1 response derives from studies of its adjuvant activity (80).

Subcutaneous immunization of BALB/c mice with soluble *Leishmania* antigen (SLA) does not induce protection against challenge infection, and only limited protection is observed when SLA is used in conjunction with the adjuvant, *Corynebacterium parvum*. However, including IFN-γ with the immunization induces significant protection, which is associated with a decrease in IL-4 and an increase in IFN-γ production by cells from the immunized animals (80). Because the adjuvant activity of IFN-γ is only observed when it is mixed with the antigen, IFN-γ perhaps acts at the initial stages of T-cell activation. Indeed, conjugation of antigen to IFN-γ is extremely effective at enhancing DTH responses, but it has only marginal effects on antibody production (84).

Treatment of *L. major*–infected BALB/c mice with anti-IL-4 antibody leads to control of the infection and spontaneous healing (85,86). This effect required that the antibody be administered less than 2 weeks after infection, suggesting that the antibody acts at the beginning of the infection to alter the nature of the T-cell response, rather than to block effector or regulatory functions of IL-4. This finding is consistent with a large body of evidence implicating a role for IL-4 in the development of Th2 cells (73). More importantly, associated with the healing in anti-IL-4–treated mice was the development of a Th1 profile that required the presence of IFN-γ since coadministration of anti-IFN-γ antibody together with anti-IL-4 antibody prevented the conversion of BALB/c mice into healer mice (87).

Although there is compelling evidence that IFN-γ levels modulate Th1 development in this model, the question that arises is what the source of IFN-γ is. Two sources have been described: T lymphocytes and nature killer (NK) cells. However, it seems unlikely that T cells act as the source because IFN-γ production during the first week of infection occurs more rapidly than might be expected for a conventional primary T-cell response (88). In contrast, NK cells have been implicated in early IFN-γ production following viral (89,90), bacterial (91,92), and protozoan (93,94) infection of both conventional and T-cell–deficient mice. Indeed, evidence that NK cells have an important role in the selective development of Th1 responses has recently been provided by Scharton and Scott (88). These investigators report that NK cell activity is higher in healer C3H/HeN mice than in susceptible BALB/c mice during the first week of infection, and that removal of NK cells is associated with both an increase in susceptibility and significantly decreased IFN-γ levels and promoted IL-4 production in both the draining lymph node and the spleen.

IL-12 (also known as NK cell stimulatory factor) is a relatively newly characterized cytokine produced by monocytes, macrophages, B cells, and other accessory cells in response to bacteria, bacterial products, or parasites (95). The demonstration that it is particularly effective in inducing IFN-γ production (95,96) prompted investigators to examine the possibility that it could also induce Th1-cell generation. Following stimulation of peripheral blood lymphocytes (PBLs) from atopic patients with the allergen *Dermatophagoides pteronyssinus* group 1 (Der. p. I), the T-cell lines and the clones generated express high IL-4 and low IFN-γ production typical of Th2 cells, whereas PBL stimulation with bacterial products such as PPD generate Th1-type T-cell lines and clones that produce IFN-γ, but not IL-4. However, when PBL are stimulated with Der. p. I in the presence of IL-12, the T-cell lines generated develop a Th0 or Th1 phenotype producing either IFN-γ and IL-4 or only IFN-γ, respectively (97). Furthermore, this Th1-inducing effect of IL-12 was not inhibited by anti-IFN-γ, but it was reduced by removing NK cells from the PBL preparation, suggesting that IL-12 is able to facilitate activation and proliferation of Th1 cells in a memory response. Conversely, PPD-specific T-cell lines generated in the presence of anti-IL-12 antibodies during the initial antigen stimulation produced significant levels of IL-4, unlike cell lines generated in the absence of antibodies, and gave rise to PPD-specific CD4+ cell clones exhibiting a Th0 or Th2 phenotype, implying that endogenously produced IL-12 is an obligatory factor for Th1-cell generation (97).

Using naive T cells derived from an MHC class II–restricted, ovalbumin-specific, transgenic T-cell receptor mouse, Hsieh and associates (98) were able to demonstrate that IL-12 can initiate the development of Th1 effector cells when included during the primary stimulation with MHC-matched APC and ovalbumin in vitro. They also showed that addition of MHC class II–mismatched macrophages, in place of IL-12, conditioned with heat-killed *Listeria,* stimulated the production of CD4+ T cells of the Th1 phenotype, suggesting that the production of IL-12 by neighboring cell populations has major effects on T cells during their stimulation by cells perhaps more capable of activating naive T cells (e.g., dendritic cells). Further support for a significant role of IL-12 in generating Th1 responses is seen in vivo when administration of this cytokine into BALB/c mice protects them from *Leishmania* infection (99,100). Evidence that IL-12 induces a Th1 response to *Leishmania* in these mice is suggested by the observation that following injection of *Leishmania* antigen in the presence of IL-12, IL-4 production in the draining lymph node was inhibited, whereas IFN-γ production was boosted.

Available evidence suggests that both IFN-γ and IL-12 produced by NK cells and macrophages, respectively, have important in vivo roles in directing Th-subset differentiation toward a Th1 phenotype. Identification of IFN-γ and IL-12 as cytokines produced by components of the innate immune response that signal cognate cellular immune systems with regard to how to appropriately react to infection provides substantial clarification, although a number of fascinating questions remain concerning the roles of these cytokines and possible other cytokines in

Th1-subset development. Do these cytokines act directly on the responding Th precursors, or do they influence antigen presentation, or both? Do these cytokines act synergistically in exerting their effect, or do they act independently? Do they rely on each other for their production, and, if so, does one or both act directly in exerting their effect on Th1-cell differentiation?

Efforts to analyze the roles of other cytokines in Th1-subset differentiation in *L. major* infection have been made using antibodies to IL-2, IL-3, IL-5, IL-6, IL-10, GM-CSF, and TNF-α (73). Mice were given either a single injection of these antibodies at the time of infection, 2 days prior to infection, or multiple injections begun at the same time as the single injections and repeated at 9- to 10-day intervals for 5 weeks. Multiple injections of anti-TNF-αβ into resistant (healer) mice were found to cause a slight exacerbation of the foot pad lesion in C3H/HeN mice, but they did not prevent healing, as has been reported using a polyclonal anti-TNF-α antiserum (101). That TNF-α may have a role in Th1-subset development is perhaps not too surprising in light of the observation that this cytokine, along with IL-12, is produced in draining lymph nodes of *L. major*–infected mice (88), and that it can act synergistically with IL-12 to induce the generation of IFN-γ by NK cells (102). Also, multiple injections of anti-IL-2 into nonhealer BALB/c mice led to the development of a Th1 response and successful resolution of the infection, whereas a single injection delayed but did not prevent fatal disease. In contrast, antibodies to IL-3, IL-5, IL-6, IL-10, and GM-CSF, whether given as single or multiple injections into healer and nonhealer mice, had no effect on disease progression (73).

Although CH responses require Th1 cells to initiate a DTH response, much of what we know and understand concerning the role of cytokines in initiating this response manifests itself at the level of their influence on LC function; available evidence suggests that these cells have an imperative role in initiating the CH response. Whether Th1 development is dictated by IFN-γ and IL-12 in CH responses is currently not known, although considering the nature of the antigen, it seems less likely that the innate immune response would have an important role in the induction phase of the response.

As previously discussed, followed epicutaneous application of sensitizing chemicals, LC, many of which bear allergen, are induced to migrate from the skin, via the afferent lymphatics, to the draining lymph nodes. During this process, LC are subjected to phenotypic and functional changes, which transform them into active immunostimulatory dendritic cells (DC). Following short-term (2–3 day) culture of freshly isolated LC (fLC), these cells acquire the ability to stimulate resting T cells (103–106), and they undergo phenotypic changes, including elevated Ia (MHC class II) (107), intercellular adhesion molecule-1 (ICAM-1) (108), and B7 (109) antigen expression, as well as a gradual loss of Birbeck granules and enzyme markers, such as ATPase and nonspecific esterase (106). Similarly, compared with fLC, DC isolated from naive lymph nodes or from draining lymph nodes after skin sensitization exhibit comparable maturation. They express on average 5-fold more Ia antigen than epidermal LC from which they derive (110), which is quantitatively similar to the elevation of Ia expression observed following culture of fLC (105). Also, additional in vivo studies reveal that migration of LC from the skin is associated with a very substantial increase in the expression of ICAM-1 (111), which is consistent with the development of the ability to form stable clusters with T lymphocytes both in vivo and in vitro (112). Furthermore, a loss in the capacity of these cells to process antigen is associated with acquired potent stimulatory capacity of cultured LC for resting T cells. In contrast, fLC are able to process native protein antigens efficiently for presentation to antigen-specific T-cell clones, but they are weak in stimulating primary proliferative responses (103–106).

It is viewed that fLC and cultured LC are in vitro representatives of their in vivo counterparts: intraepidermal LC and LC that have migrated to draining lymph nodes, respectively. Therefore, it is thought that intraepidermal LC are especially programmed for efficient processing of cutaneous antigen, and that they can readily present antigen to primed or memory T cells, which possess different requirements for activation and possibly a lower stimulation threshold. In particular, the implication is that following challenge of a previously contact-sensitized animal or human, epidermal LC have an imperative role in processing and presenting the antigen to primed DTH effector T cells, which, on activation, induce the elicitation phase of the response. However, it is thought that following receipt of the stimulus to migrate and during transit from the skin (or shortly after arrival in the lymph node), LC are subjected to phenotypic and functional changes, which ultimately result in this facility being "exchanged" for increased potent immunostimulatory activity (achieved in part from the acquisition of accessory molecules) and antigen-presenting potential, thus enabling them to associate with and present chemical allergens to naive T cells.

The changes to which LC are subjected are initiated and regulated by epidermal cytokines. Although keratinocytes, the predominant cell type in the epidermis, were originally considered to be immunologically inert, it is now clear that these cells (mouse or human) are a rich source of cytokines, and they participate actively in immune and inflammatory processes (113–116). It has been found that keratinocytes produce constitutively, or can be stimulated to produce, a plethora of cytokines: IL-1α, IL-1β, IL-6, IL-8, IL-10, GM-CSF, tumor necrosis factor-alpha (TNF-α), transforming growth factor-α (TGF-α), and TGF-β. Among the cytokines of greatest relevance, with regard to their influence on LC function and the partici-

pation of LC in the induction phase of skin sensitization, are IL-1 (117), GM-CSF (118), and TNF-α (119). Using a sensitive reverse transcriptase polymerase chain reaction technique, it has been demonstrated that topical exposure of mice to the contact sensitizer picryl chloride induces the rapid appearance of epidermal cell mRNA for each of these cytokines (120). It was revealed that, in contrast to keratinocytes (the primary source of IL-1α, GM-CSF, and TNF-α), LC are the primary source of IL-1β (120).

Of the keratinocyte-derived cytokines, GM-CSF appears to have an important role in augmenting the immunostimulatory activity of fLC following culture (105,121,122). It appears that GM-CSF does more than sustain cellular integrity, because culture of LC with TNF-α maintains viability without inducing the functional maturation and enhanced stimulatory activity associated with GM-CSF (123). Furthermore, it is apparent that IL-1, which is able to enhance functional activity of lymphoid DC, can act synergistically with GM-CSF to augment further the immunostimulatory potential of cultured LC (121,124,125). Other cytokines, including IL-1, fail to maintain the viability of cultured LC (124). Thus, all three cytokines influence LC in vitro, but they exert separate or synergistic effects. GM-CSF both increases immunostimulatory function and sustains viability; TNF-α maintains LC viability, but it fails to influence functional maturation; and IL-1 does not maintain viability, but, in combination with GM-CSF, it will enhance further the function of cultured LC. Although it is inferred that the enhanced immunostimulatory activity of cultured LC is associated with augmented Ia, B7, and ICAM-1 expression, it has yet to be established whether these cytokines, alone or together, are also responsible for these changes.

Until recently, a question that remained was the nature of the signal following epicutaneous sensitization with skin allergens that provides the stimulus for LC to leave the epidermis and to transport antigen to draining lymph nodes. There is new evidence that TNF-α provides an important, and perhaps the only, signal for the movement of LC from the epidermis (126). Injection of murine recombinant TNF-α into the dermis of mice causes accumulation of DC in draining lymph nodes. In contrast, mouse recombinant GM-CSF and IL-1α were without effect, under the same conditions of exposure. A significant increase in the frequency of draining lymph node DC is observed within 4 hours of treatment. This increase contrasts with the number of DC arriving in draining lymph nodes following topical sensitization: a maximum influx of DC that occurs after 18 to 24 hours or more, with only modest changes during the first 12 hours (16,127). However, assuming that the arrival of DC in lymph nodes is secondary to the local production of TNF-α by epidermal cells following sensitization, it is perhaps not too surprising that direct administration of this cytokine accelerates this process.

Evidence substantiating the notion that TNF-α is an important migratory signal for epidermal LC is provided by the observation that there is a reduction in the density of epidermal Ia-positive LC following intradermal injection of TNF-α (128). It is conceivable that TNF-α may act indirectly on LC by inducing or up-regulating the release of another mediator that directly interacts with LC to induce their migration to draining lymph nodes. For example it has been shown that TNF-α can induce the production of IL-1 (129), which shares many biological properties with TNF-α (130,131), and that IL-1 is able to cause a reduction in the density of Ia-positive epidermal LC (132).

In contrast, precedents for a direct effect of TNF-α on LC migratory behavior exist. It has recently been found that mice possess two receptors for TNF-α, designated mTNF-R1 and mTNF-R2, which differ with respect to both extracellular nucleotide sequence and species specificity (133). Furthermore, mTNF-R1 binds human and mouse TNF-α with equivalent affinity, whereas mTNF-R2 exhibits strong species specificity for the mouse cytokine (133). Although it is not known whether both of these receptors are expressed constitutively on the surface of LC, based on the observations of Koch and associates (123) and Cumberbatch and Kimber (111), it seems reasonable to speculate that the interaction of TNF-α with mTNF-R2 expressed on the surface of LC is critical in influencing the migration of these cells. Under conditions during which murine TNF-α maintains the viability of mouse LC in culture, the same concentrations of human TNF-α are without effect (123). Also, in contrast to the increased accumulation of DC in draining lymph nodes of mice following intradermal injection of murine recombinant TNF-α, administration of human recombinant TNF-α of comparable specific activity into mice fails to have any influence on DC migration (111).

The conclusion drawn from these investigations is that after application of skin allergens, keratinocytes are induced to release cytokines such as IL-1, GM-CSF, and TNF-α, which are then responsible for initiating the migration and functional maturation of LC, which carry antigen to draining lymph nodes. Once they arrive in the lymph node, they have matured into potent immunostimulatory cells able to initiate a primary immune response.

ROLE OF Th1-DERIVED CYTOKINES IN THE ELICITATION PHASE OF DTH RESPONSES

During the course of a DTH reaction in the skin, lymphocytes (independent of their antigen specificity) (134),

mononuclear phagocytes, and granulocytes are recruited from the blood into the inflammatory site (135). Although the factors controlling this migration are poorly understood, available evidence implies that recruitment of the lymphocyte infiltrate is mediated in part by IFN-γ released by Th1 cells following their activation at the challenge site (136–141). Using radiolabeled lymphocytes injected intravenously into rats (136–138) or sheep (141), it has been found that these cells display a propensity for migrating to cutaneous DTH reactions elicited by intradermal injection of KLH (138) or PPD (141). The demonstration that approximately 50% of migration induced to skin sites injected with lymphokine containing supernatant from activated T cells can be inhibited by anti-IFN-γ monoclonal antibody suggests that a large part of this recruitment is mediated by T-cell–derived IFN-γ (137). Substantial support for this notion is provided by studies showing that lymphocytes migrate into skin sites injected intradermally with IFN-γ (136–141) and that migration into DTH reactions can be inhibited by 50% or more with polyclonal or monoclonal anti-IFN-γ antibodies.

Following adoptive transfer of Th1 clones with antigen into the footpads of naive syngeneic mice, an inflammatory reaction with the characteristics of DTH is produced (26). Treatment of these mice with anti-IFN-γ antibody at the same time as adoptive transfer was found to inhibit up to 55% of the swelling response induced by 7 of 9 Th1 clones tested, which further corroborates the notion that IFN-γ is an important mediator of Th1-induced DTH (140). Although the 24-hour DTH response was not inhibited by injection of anti-IFN-γ at 0 hours for two of the clones tested, a decrease in the swelling response at 48 hours was demonstrated when the antibody was administered at 24 hours, implying that IFN-γ released by these clones may contribute to the DTH swelling reaction during the declining phase of the response.

Although Th1-derived IFN-γ appears to be important in inducing lymphocyte migration into the DTH reaction, it is by no means the sole mediator of this migration (140,141). Thus, other cytokines released by activated Th1 cells may have an important role in inducing lymphocyte infiltration into the reaction site. Although TNF-β has been demonstrated to be very weak in stimulating lymphocyte migration into skin when administered intradermally in combination with IFN-γ, striking synergistic increases in lymphocyte migration are observed (140). IL-2, another Th1-specific cytokine, may have an indirect role in inducing cell accumulation in DTH reaction sites through its activity as a potent T cell growth and activation factor that further increases local concentrations of cytokines, such as IFN-γ and TNF-β. Indeed, it has been shown that the DTH response is enhanced when IL-2 is administered at the time of challenge (142). Conversely, anti-IL-2 receptor antibodies, if administered just prior to challenge, have been demonstrated to suppress DTH responses (143). This effect may result from abrogation of the clonal expansion of activated IL-2 receptor–positive Th1 cells, which are required to elicit the DTH response.

Although TNF-α is not uniquely synthesized by Th1 clones and would therefore not account for their unique ability to mediate DTH, it is a good stimulator of lymphocyte migration (140,141). More importantly, when TNF-α is injected intradermally with IFN-γ, there is a significant synergistic enhancement in lymphocyte migration to the skin, implicating an important in vivo physiological role for Th subset nonspecific cytokines in mediating Th subset effector functions (140). It is conceivable that the strong synergy observed when TNF-α or TNF-β is administered with IFN-γ may explain the inability of neutralizing antibodies to single cytokines to completely inhibit lymphocyte recruitment to a complex inflammatory reaction, such as DTH. Other cells, along with lymphocytes, infiltrate a DTH reaction site. In this regard, TNF-α has been shown to induce neutrophil accumulation in skin (141). Whether IFN-γ has a role in stimulating neutrophil migration is controversial (141,144,145). Two other cytokines not unique to Th1 cells that may have an important role in inducing the infiltration of cells other than lymphocytes are GM-CSF and macrophage chemotactic factor (MCF). Although GM-CSF and MCF are both chemotactic for mononuclear phagocytes, GM-CSF is also chemotactic for granulocytes (146,147).

Mobilization and targeting of the innate and adaptive defense systems to sites of antigen challenge by cytokines synthesized and released by activated Th1 cells is just one important function carried out by these mediators of the DTH response. In particular, they activate cells of the mononuclear phagocyte system following or during their migration into the site of antigen challenge for effective clearance and destruction of antigen. This effect appears to be crucial for generation of a protective DTH response to infection, and it is largely attributable to the activity of IFN-γ (148,149), which has been implicated in destruction of a number of intracellular protozoan parasites, including *Leishmania* (78,150), *Trypanosomes* (151,152), and *Toxoplasma* (77,150,153,154). It has been demonstrated that mouse or human macrophages are capable of inhibiting intracellular development of these pathogens very efficiently when cultured with IFN-γ following in vitro infection (77,78,150,151,154). These findings have been extended in studies in which murine macrophages activated in vivo by IFN-γ also display potent antimicrobial activity when infected in vitro (150,152,153). In these studies, mice treated with IFN-γ had significantly lower parasitemias and decreased morbidity compared with control mice (152,153).

Although the concept of activated macrophages was largely deduced from experimental work performed in the tuberculosis system, results on activation of tuberculocidal macrophages by IFN-γ are controversial. IFN-γ is able to enhance antimycobacterial activity of murine macrophages following in vitro culture and subsequent infection with *M. tuberculosis* (155,156). However, some strains of *M. tuberculosis* were found to be more susceptible to killing than others (155). Also, IFN-γ can enhance antimycobacterial activity of human macrophages in vitro from some donors but not others (157), whereas other studies have demonstrated that IFN-γ–activated human macrophages, although able to interfere with the replication of *Leishmania*, enhance intracellular growth of *M. tuberculosis* (158).

Similar findings have been observed with *M. avium*, in which IFN-γ inhibited intracellular growth of some strains of this organism but not others (159). Furthermore, administration of IFN-γ reduced the bacillary burden in patients with lepromatous leprosy, which was associated with an elevation in the secretion of antimicrobial products by monocytes from these patients (160). Thus, the nature of this controversy seems to reside in genetic differences of the host and the parasite that confer resistance or susceptibility to infection and destruction, respectively. Evidence that IFN-γ–activated macrophage killing of *Mycobacteria* is important in resistance to infection has recently been provided from a study using IFN-γ–deficient mice (148). Compared with wild-type mice, these mice had impaired production of macrophage antimicrobial products, reduced expression of macrophage MHC class II antigens, and were killed by a sublethal dose of the intracellular pathogen *M. bovis*.

It is inferred from these studies that resistance to infection is dependent on successful activation of macrophages for killing of intracellular microorganisms by Th1-derived IFN-γ. In support of this view is the demonstration that *T. cruzi*–specific Th1 clones (161), which confer resistance to *T. cruzi* infection in syngeneic recipients (162), can lead to dose-dependent destruction of intracellular parasites when cultured with *T. cruzi*–infected syngeneic macrophages (162).

Similar findings were obtained using two CD4+*T. cruzi*–specific T-cells lines, A10 and A28, in which trypanocidal activity of mouse macrophages was induced after culture with only the A10 line or the cell-free supernatant derived from this line. Subsequent analysis of the lymphocyte content of the supernatant from both cell lines revealed that the A10 line secreted IFN-γ and IL-2, whereas the other cell line did not. Furthermore, the trypanocidal inducing ability of the A10 line supernatant was completely abrogated by neutralizing anti-IFN-γ antibody, implying that IFN-γ secreted by *T. cruzi*–immune Th1 cells is involved in activation of the trypanocidal activity of mouse macrophages (163).

Although it is generally accepted that IFN-γ–activated macrophages represent the crucial effector cells of host resistance against intracellular parasites, little is known about the underlying mechanism. It has been suggested that reactive oxygen intermediates, such as hydrogen peroxide, are important for macrophage antimycobacterial (164–166), antitrypanosme (167), antitoxoplasma (77,150), and antileishmania (150,168) activities. In contrast, more recent evidence argues against this hypothesis, and suggests a crucial role for reactive nitrogen intermediates, such as nitric oxide, in the growth inhibition of these organisms (163,169–172). Corroboration that the generation of reactive nitrogen intermediates following activation of macrophages with IFN-γ may indeed have an imperative role in antimicrobial activity and subsequent resistance to infection has recently been reported (143).

Previously, it was demonstrated that mice infected with *M. bovis* (strain bacillus Calmette Guérin [BCG] generate macrophages with enhanced MHC class II antigen on the cell surface and enhanced capacity to kill microorganisms (173). In contrast, Dalton and colleagues (148) found that IFN-γ–deficient mice infected with a sublethal dose of BCG exhibit increased mortality and possess macrophages whose levels of MHC class II expression are significantly reduced. Furthermore, these investigators found that in response to lipopolysaccharide stimulation, macrophages from BCG-infected wild-type mice produced large quantities of nitric oxide, whereas identically treated macrophages from BCG-infected IFN-γ–deficient mice produced little detectable nitric oxide. This defect in nitric oxide production was reversed, however, if the IFN-γ mutant cells were cultured with IFN-γ for 48 hours. Thus, these findings imply an important in vivo role for IFN-γ in activating macrophages for production of reactive nitrogen intermediates and for expression of MHC class II antigen, and they further suggest that this form of activation is essential for maintaining resistance to infection by intracellular pathogens.

Although IFN-γ appears to be one of the principal cytokines that can activate macrophages for resistance to a wide variety of intracellular microbial pathogens, there are a number of other Th1-derived specific and nonspecific macrophage-activating cytokines, some of which may have a narrower spectrum of activity. In vitro studies have demonstrated that IL-3, GM-CSF, or TNF-α can activate murine or human macrophages for intracellular killing of *Leishmania* (168,174–178) and *Trypanosomes* (151,175,179–181). There is also evidence that TNF-α or GM-CSF can act synergistically with IFN-γ in activating killing of these organisms (163,176,177).

ROLE OF NON-Th1–DERIVED CYTOKINES IN THE ELICITATION PHASE OF DTH RESPONSES

It is clear that cytokines released by Th1 cells following their activation at the site of antigen challenge have a crucial role in mediating the elicitation phase of the DTH response. However, the mechanism of recruitment of the DTH effector cells into this site, which constitutes the early phase of the reaction, is not fully understood. It was mentioned earlier that the role of mast cells and their vasoactive amines in initiating the early phase of the DTH response was controversial. This controversy may be explained, however, by emerging evidence implicating a major role for epidermal and dermal cells, including mast cell–derived cytokines, in initiating and regulating this process.

An important early event following application of an antigen, either topically or intradermally, to the skin of sensitized subjects is induction of cytokine production by cells present within the epidermis and the dermis (182,183). TNF-α, produced by both epidermal keratinocytes and dermal cells (0.5 hours) following epicutaneous challenge with TNCB, appears to be a crucial mediator in facilitating expression of the elicitation phase of the CH response (182). Anti-TNF-α antibody treatment immediately prior to challenge was found to abrogate the ear swelling response (182). Furthermore, it has been demonstrated that in vivo mast cells produce and release TNF-α during cutaneous DTH reactions several hours following elicitation by challenge of sensitized subjects with DNCB (184). Other epidermal cell–derived cytokines that may exert some complementary role in initiating full expression of CH are GM-CSF and IL-3; administration of neutralizing antibodies specific for these cytokines just prior to challenge had moderate inhibitory effects on the CH response (182). Using immunohistochemical techniques, epidermal keratinocytes and dermal macrophages producing IL-1, IL-6, and TNF-α are detected at DTH reaction sites several hours after elicitation by intradermal injection of tuberculin PPD, implying that these cytokines may contribute to the early phase of a classic DTH response (183). It has been reported that DTH-initiating factors can induce macrophages to release rapidly IL-1, IL-6, and TNF-α (185). Although evidence implicating a role for these cytokines in initiating the early event of the elicitation phase of the DTH response is largely circumstantial, further evidence suggests that TNF-α may have a key role in mediating the migration of DTH effector cells into the site of challenge (184,186–189).

The vascular endothelium, which consists of a monolayer of cells lining the entire circulatory system, forms an anatomical barrier between the blood and the extravascular tissues of the body. Consequently, a mechanism must exist that signals and subsequently permits circulating skin-seeking memory CD4+ Th1 DTH effector cells to escape from the vascular tree and to enter a skin site challenged with antigen to which these cells were originally primed. It has recently been proposed that the selectin endothelial leukocyte adhesion molecule-1 (ELAM-1) may serve as the adhesion molecule directing the migration of this subset of cells into the skin (186–188). This molecule exclusively mediates adhesion of memory T cells, and its expression on inflamed endothelium is particularly prominent within skin, which has led to the suggestion that this molecule acts as an adhesion molecule, or "vascular addressin," for a specific subset of skin-homing, memory T cells (188). More importantly, induction of this molecule on the surface of endothelial cells appears to be regulated by TNF-α (184,189).

It has been demonstrated in vivo that the release of TNF-α from human dermal mast cells following their degranulation several hours after epicutaneous challenge with DNCB (184) is associated with ELAM-1 induction on dermal postcapillary venules and perivascular lymphocyte infiltration (190). Another known inducer of ELAM-1 in vitro (190) and in vivo (191) is IL-1α, a cytokine produced by epidermal keratinocytes and dermal cells immediately following challenge (182,183). Thus, it is conceivable that keratinocytes, dermal macrophages, or dermal mast cells may act as "gatekeepers" of the dermal vasculature, thus controlling initial infiltration of DTH effector cells into the site of antigen challenge through release of TNF-α or IL-1α. The subsequent induction of ELAM-1 on the surface of endothelial cells lining venules in close proximity to the site of antigen challenge would then signal and target the recruitment of antigen-specific DTH effector T cells, which, after encountering antigen, would elicit the late phase of the DTH response. The relative role of epidermal and dermal cells in initiating the DTH response may vary according to the antigen and its site of administration.

In addition to ELAM-1 induction, TNF-α can induce expression of other endothelial adhesion molecules known to have important roles in inducing migration of naive lymphocytes, neutrophils, and monocytes into skin. These molecules include the adhesion protein intercellular adhesion molecule-1 (ICAM-1), which interacts with all leukocytes, including monocytes (191–195), and vascular cell adhesion molecule-1 (VCAM-1), which binds lymphocytes (196). The coincident expression of these molecules with ELAM-1, which is also an endothelial cell adhesion molecule for neutrophils (197), is likely to collaborate in the regulation of leukocyte recruitment into extravascular tissue during both early and late phases of the DTH response.

Both IL-1 and IFN-γ are also important in inducing ICAM-1 expression on endothelial cells (192,193). Thus, following recruitment of Th1 DTH effector cells into the challenge site and their subsequent activation, Th1-derived IFN-γ may, with epidermal- or dermal-derived TNF-α and IL-1, further enhance migration of cells into the site of antigen challenge. This notion is supported by the observation that both IL-1 and TNF-α can synergize with IFN-γ to induce cell migration into a DTH reaction site (139). Also, Th1-derived TNF-α, with epidermal- or dermal-derived TNF-α, may synergize with IFN-γ to activate mononuclear phagocytes that arrive at the DTH reaction site. The local response may be amplified further following induction of ICAM-1 (198) and MHC class II (199,200) expression on the surface of keratinocytes by IFN-γ released from activated TH1 cells. Expression of MHC class II molecules may amplify the in situ potential of antigen presentation, thereby activating additional T cells, and the expression of ICAM-1 may have a role in directing T-cell migration from the dermis into the epidermis.

IMMUNOREGULATION OF DTH AND CH FOLLOWING UVB EXPOSURE

Studies of the immune suppression induced by ultraviolet-B light radiation (UVB) have added insight into how cytokines regulate DTH and CH. In addition to being carcinogenic, UVB radiation contributes to growth and pathogenesis of murine skin cancers by altering the immune system. Repeated exposure of mice to UVB radiation induces suppressor T lymphocytes that prevent immunological rejection of the developing highly antigenic skin cancers (201–203). UVB radiation suppresses certain immune responses to a variety of other antigens, other than UVB-induced tumors. For example, CH responses to chemical haptens (5,204–210) and classic DTH responses to herpes simplex virus (HSV) (211,212) and alloantigens (213–216) are suppressed. UVB-induced immunosuppression of these cell-mediated immune responses is also associated with induction of T suppressor cells, which mediate an antigen-specific unresponsive state following exposure to the same antigen.

The possible mechanisms by which UVB radiation induces the T suppressor cell pathway of the immune response have been the subject of much study and speculation for more than a decade (203,207,208,216–220). This is an important issue, because understanding how UVB radiation induces the T suppressor cell pathway may provide new insights on mechanisms of immune regulation and suggest new immunological approaches to the treatment of certain skin cancers.

Owing to the antigen-specific nature of the suppression induced and the fact that UVB radiation suppresses the induction but not the elicitation phase of CH (221), antigen presentation, specifically antigen presentation to naive T cells, is perhaps the perturbed locus for UVB-induced immunosuppression. Consequently, attention has focused on the effect of UVB radiation on antigen-presenting cells at sites of UVB exposure and in lymphoid organs, such as the spleen, where the T suppressor cells are generated. In the process of attempting to elucidate the mechanisms by which UVB radiation induces T suppressor cells, two different model systems have been employed: local and systemic immunosuppression.

Local immunosuppression is defined as the diminished immune response observed when antigen is applied at the site of irradiation, whereas systemic immunosuppression arises when the antigen is applied to a site distant from the site of UVB exposure. Because UVB radiation does not penetrate any further than the skin, it has been thought that in the local model, UVB radiation mediates its entire effect directly on APCs in the skin at the site of irradiation, whereas in the systemic model, UVB radiation exerts its effect through induction of a soluble suppressive mediator that can act on APCs at sites distant from the site of UVB exposure. In the course of examining both these models, however, evidence has emerged implicating a crucial role for keratinocyte-derived cytokines in mediating both local and systemic suppressive effects of UVB radiation.

Although TNF-α is implicated in having an important role in the induction phase of CH responses (111), there is strong evidence that it is an important and possible critical molecular mediator of the down-regulatory effect of UVB exposure on the induction of this response. In the local model of UVB-induced suppression of CH responses, administration of anti-TNF-α antibodies intraperitoneally to mice prior to UVB irradiation inhibited UVB-induced immunosuppression (222,223). Furthermore, intradermal injection of TNF-α before hapten painting at the same site suppresses the CH response (222). It is clear that UVB irradiation can stimulate the synthesis and release of TNF-α by keratinocytes (119); however, how this cytokine mediates a suppressive effect following its production at the site of UVB exposure is currently controversial. On the basis of their findings that UVB irradiation or intradermal injection of TNF-α altered the morphology of epidermal LC, Vermeer and Streilein (128) concluded that TNF-α prevents effective sensitization following UVB irradiation by immobilizing LC within the epidermis. This theory is supported by a report that no hapten-bearing APCs were present in draining lymph nodes if the skin on which the hapten was painted had been exposed previously to UVB radiation (224). Contrary to this interpretation were the findings that UVB irradiation and intradermal injection of TNF-α reduced the density of MHC class II–positive cells in the epidermis, suggesting that UVB exposure may induce LC migration through local release of TNF-α (128). Indeed, it has been demonstrated that UVB radiation increases the number of hapten-bearing DC accumulating in draining lymph nodes (225), and that this migration is mediated by UVB-induced formation of TNF-α (223).

If UVB-mediated suppression of CH is indeed attributable to changes in the behavior of LC secondary to local production of TNF-α, then it is appropriate to consider the nature of the functional deficit. It is known that migration of LC from the epidermis to the draining lymph node following skin sensitization is accompanied by changes in the membrane expression of certain molecules necessary for effective antigen presentation. Thus, compared with the epidermal LC from which they derive, the DC that accumulate in the draining nodes following skin sensitization display elevated levels of both MHC class II antigens and ICAM-1 (110,111). It is thought that this migration and functional maturation is dependent on the release of IL-1, GM-CSF, and TNF-α from keratinocytes following skin sensitization.

Because the process by which cells receive and translate messages/signals delivered by cytokines is finely tuned, any slight deviation in the timing at which a particular chemical mediator delivers its signal compared with another, or in the amount of signal delivered, will be interpreted differently by the cell. Thus, UVB-induced production of excessive local (cutaneous) amounts of TNF-α prior to sensitization may stimulate migration of LC to draining lymph nodes that are phenotypically or functionally immature but are able to pick up antigen. Consequently, these cells may be unable to activate and stimulate the proliferation of hapten-specific virgin Th1 DTH effector cells, resulting in an impaired response, or they may activate and induce proliferation of T cells capable of down-regulating Th1-mediated responses.

Within this context, it has been shown that UVB irradiation alters the selectivity of LC for Th subset cell activation. Irradiated LC were found to lose their ability to stimulate Th1 cells, while fully retaining their capacity to activate Th2 cells (226), which are capable of inhibiting activation of Th1 cells through their secretion of IL-10 (50). Moreover, they induce long-lived clonal anergy in Th1 populations (227). UVB radiation therefore may cause a changed equilibrium in the immune system and a movement away from stimulation of the Th1 cell-type response necessary for CH. Such changes may result from UVB-mediated alterations in the membrane expression by LC of determinants that govern selectivity for CD4+ subpopulations (220). This alteration may be achieved by a direct effect of UVB radiation on LC at the site of exposure, or indirectly as a consequence of UVB-induced formation of TNF-α, which may induce migration of functionally immature hapten-bearing LC lacking membrane determinants necessary for activation of Th1 DTH effector cells following their arrival in the draining lymph node. Alternatively, keratinocyte-derived IL-10 may interfere with the presentation of antigen to Th1 cells by LC, as suggested by Enk and colleagues (228).

It has been demonstrated that systemic UVB-induced suppression of classic DTH to allogeneic histocompatibility antigen can be mimicked by injecting culture supernatant from UVB-irradiated keratinocytes (214). Furthermore, injecting supernatants from UVB-irradiated keratinocytes induced formation of antigen-specific suppressor T lymphocytes in the spleens of these mice (214), and it was associated with a defect in the ability of splenic adherent cells to present antigen for a DTH reaction (229), as seen with whole body UVB irradiation (230,231). A detailed analysis of the culture supernatant revealed an essential role for IL-10 in mediating this suppressive effect (215). It was found that IL-10 mRNA expression is enhanced in UVB-irradiated keratinocytes, and that this enhancement is associated with secretion of biologically active IL-10 as measured by the ability of supernatant to suppress IFN-γ production by antigen-activated Th1 cells.

Finally, that this cytokine was indeed responsible for mediating the suppressive effect of UBV irradiation was confirmed using neutralizing anti-IL-10 antibody. Treatment of culture supernatant from UVB-irradiated keratinocytes with this antibody prior to injecting the supernatant into mice totally removed all immunosuppressive activity, and administration of anti-IL-10 antibody to mice prior to UVB exposure partially blocked the suppressive effect of UVB irradiation. Thus, the available evidence implicates an essential role for keratinocyte-derived IL-10 in the systemic suppression of DTH following UVB exposure.

Anti-TNF-α antibody treatment of mice had no effect in inhibiting systemic UVB-induced suppression of the DTH response (232), suggesting that different suppressive mechanisms may operate in CH and classic DTH responses. This finding is perhaps not too surprising considering different APCs appear to be involved in mediating these responses. Furthermore, it has been reported that IL-10 has a prominent role in modulation of splenic APC function (233). In particular, it was found that spleen cells from UVB-irradiated mice did not efficiently present antigen to Th1 clones, whereas injection of anti-IL-10 antibody after UVB exposure restored APC function. The reverse was observed when spleen cells from UVB- irradiated mice were used to present antigen to Th2 cells: UVB exposure enhanced APC function, whereas anti-IL-10 antibody treatment reversed this effect (233). Thus, IL-10 appears to be an important mediator of systemic UVB-induced immunosuppression by modulating APC function systemically in such a way that Th2 cells are preferentially activated.

Although different suppressive cytokines appear to be involved in regulating CH and DTH response, available evidence points to a common mechanism by which these cytokines may exert their effect. Thus, the long-lasting unresponsiveness induced by UVB radiation in CH and classic DTH responses may be explained by the ability of keratinocyte-derived cytokines either directly or indirectly to modify the function of APCs such that they exert a tolerogenic effect on the Th1 subset deemed to be responsible for mediating these reactions. Furthermore, because since Th2-cell activation and proliferation does not appear to be perturbed by these APCs, it is conceivable that these cells are responsible for mediating suppression of Th1-mediated responses in vivo, because Th2 cells can secrete IL-10, which has been shown to be an inhibitor of the activation of Th1 cells (50). In support of this notion is the demonstration that in both CH (233) and DTH (213) responses, T cells of the CD4+ phenotype mediate UVB-induced immunosuppression. However, that these antigen-specific CD4+ T cells are Th2 cells awaits experimental verification.

ACKNOWLEDGMENTS: This work was supported by Grant AR40824 from The National Institute of Arthritis and Musculoskeletal and Skin Diseases.

REFERENCES

1. Dvorak HF, Mihm JC Jr. Basophilic leukocytes in allergic contact dermatitis. J Exp Med 1972;135:235–242.
2. Shelley WB, Juhlin L. Langerhans' cells form a reticuloepithelial trap for external contact allergens. Nature 1976; 261:46–47.
3. Silberberg-Sinakin I, Thorbecke GJ, Baer RL, Rodenthal SA, Berezowsky V. Antigen-bearing Langerhans cells in skin, dermal lymphatics and in lymph nodes. Cell Immunol 1976;25:137–151.
4. Kripke ML, Munn CG, Jeevan A, Tang J-M, Bucana C. Evidence that cutaneous antigen-presenting cells migrate to regional lymph nodes during contact sensitization. J Immunol 1990;145:2833–2838.
5. Toews GB, Bergstresser PR, Streilein JW. Epidermal Langerhans cell density determines whether contact hypersensitivity or unresponsiveness follows skins painting with DNFB. J Immunol 1980;124:445–449.
6. Streilein JW, Toews GB, Bergstresser PR. Langerhans cells: functional aspects revealed by in vivo grafting studies. J Invest Dermatol 1980;75:17–21.
7. Semma M, Sagami S. Induction of suppressor T-cells to DNFB contact sensitivity by application of sensitizer through Langerhans cell-deficient skin. Arch Dermatol Res 1981;271:361–364.
8. Rheins LA, Nordlund JJ. Modulation of the population density of identifiable epidermal Langerhans cells associated with enhancement or suppression of cutaneous immune reactivity. J Immunol 1986;136:867–876.
9. Halliday GM, Müller HK. Sensitization through carcinogen-induced Langerhans cell-deficient skin activates specific long-lived suppressor cells for both cellular and humoral immunity. Cell Immunol 1987;109:206–221.
10. Jones DA, Morris AG, Kimber I. Assessment of the functional activity of antigen-bearing dendritic cells isolated from the lymph nodes of contact sensitized mice. Int Arch Allergy Appl Immunol 1989;90:230–236.
11. Robinson MK. Optimization of an in vitro lymphocyte blastogenesis assay for predictive assessment of immunological responsiveness to contact sensitizers. J Invest Dermatol 1989;92:860–867.
12. Knight SC, Krejci J, Malkovsky M, Colizzi V, Gautman A,

Asherson GL. The role of dendritic cells in the initiation of immune responses to contact sensitizers. I. In vivo exposure to antigen. Cell Immunol 1985;94:427–434.

13. Macatonia SE, Edwards AJ, Knight SC. Dendritic cells and the initiation of contact sensitivity to fluorescein isothiocyanate. Immunology 1986;59:509–514.

14. Macatonia SE, Knight SC, Edwards AJ, Griffiths S, Fryer P. Localization of antigen on lymph node dendritic cells after exposure to the contact sensitizer fluorescein isothiocyanate. Functional and morphological studies. J Exp Med 1987;166:1654–1667.

15. Knight SC, Bedford P, Hunt R. The role of dendritic cells in the initiation of immune responses to contact sensitizers. II. Studies in nude mice. Cell Immunol 1985;94:435–439.

16. Kinnaird A, Peters SW, Foster JR, Kimber I. Dendritic cell accumulation in draining lymph nodes during the induction phase of contact allergy in mice. Int Arch Allergy Apply Immunol 1989;89:202–210.

17. Macatonia SE, Knight SC. Dendritic cells and T cells transfer sensitization for delayed-type hypersensitivity after skin-painting with contact sensitizer. Immunology 1989;66:96–99.

18. Baker D, Parker D, Turk JL. Effect of depletion of epidermal dendritic cells on the induction of contact sensitivity in the guinea pig. Br J Dermatol 1985;113:285–294.

19. Streilein JW. Antigen-presenting cells in the induction of contact hypersensitivity in mice. Evidence that Langerhans cells are sufficient but not required. J Invest Dermatol 1989;93:443–448.

20. Tse Y, Cooper KD. Cutaneous dermal Ia+ cells are capable of initiating delayed type hypersensitivity responses. J Invest Dermatol 1990;94:267–272.

21. Stohlman SA, Matsushima GK, Casteel N, Frelinger JA. The defect in delayed-type hypersensitivity of young adult SJL mice is due to a lack of functional antigen-presenting cells. Eur J Immunol 1985;15:913–916.

22. Matsushima GK, Stohlman SA. Maturation of the delayed-type hypersensitivity response in SJL mice: absence of effector cell induction. Eur J Immunol 1988;18:1411–1416.

23. Matsushima GK, Stohlman SA. Evidence for a subpopulation of antigen-presenting cells specific for the induction of the delayed-type hypersensitivity response. Cell Immunol 1989;119:171–181.

24. Matsushima GK, Stohlman SA. Distinct subsets of accessory cells activate Thy-1+ triple negative (CD3–, CD4–, CD8–) cells and Th1 delayed-type hypersensitivity effector T cells. J Immunol 1991;146:3322–3331.

25. Van Loveren H, Kato K, Meade R. Characterization of two different Ly-1+ T-cell populations that mediate delayed-type hypersensitivity. J Immunol 1984;133:2402–2410.

26. Cher DJ, Mosmann TR. Two types of murine helper T-cell clone. II. Delayed type hypersensitivity is mediated by Th1 clones. J Immunol 1987;138:3688–3694.

27. Herzog W-R, Ferreri NR, Ptak W, Askenase PW. The DTH-initiating Thy-1+ cell is double-negative (CD4–, CD8–) and CD3–, and expresses IL-3 receptors, but no IL-2 receptors. J Immunol 1989;143:3125–3133.

28. Ptak W, Askenase PW, Rosenstein RW, Gershon PK. Transfer of an antigen specific immediate hypersensitivity-like reaction with an antigen binding factor produced by T cells. Proc Natl Acad Sci USA 1982;79:1969–1973.

29. Askenase PW, Rosenstein RW, Ptak W. T cells produce an antigen binding factor with in vivo activity analogous to IgE antibody. J Exp Med 1983;157:862–873.

30. Askenase PW, Van Loveren H, Rosenstein RW, Ptak W. Immunologic specificity of antigen-binding T cell–derived factors that transfer mast cell dependent, immediate hypersensitivity-like reactions. Monogr Allergy 1983;18:249–255.

31. Van Loveren H, Ratzlaff RE, Kato K. Immune serum from mice contact sensitized with picryl chloride contains an antigen-specific T-cell factor that transfers immediate cutaneous sensitivity. Eur J Immunol 1986;16:1203–1208.

32. Van Loveren H, Kraeuter-Kops S, Askenase PW. Different mechanisms of release of vasoactive amines by mast cells occur in T cell-dependent compared to IgE-dependent cutaneous hypersensitivity responses. Eur J Immunol 1984;14:40–47.

33. Kraeuter-Kops S, Ratzlaff RE, Meade R, Iverson GM, Askenase PW. Interaction of antigen-specific T cell factors with unique "receptors" on the surface of mast cells: demonstration in vitro by an indirect rosetting technique. J Immunol 1986;136:4515–4524.

34. Meade R, Van Loveren H, Parmentier H, Iverson GM, Askenase PW. The antigen-binding T cell factor PC1-F sensitizes mast cells for in vitro release of serotonin: comparison with monoclonal IgE antibody. J Immunol 1988;141:2704–2713.

35. Ptak W, Geba GP, Askenase PW. Initiation of delayed-type hypersensitivity by low doses of monoclonal IgE antibody. J Immunol 1991;146:3929–3936.

36. Van Loveren H, Meade R, Askenase PW. An early component of delayed-type hypersensitivity mediated by T-cells and mast cells. J Exp Med 1983;157:1604–1617.

37. Gershon RK, Askenase PW, Gershon MD. Requirement for vasoactive amines for production of delayed-type hypersensitivity skin reactions. J Exp Med 1975;142:732–747.

38. Schwartz A, Askenase PW, Gershon RK. The effect of locally injected vasoactive amines on the elicitation of delayed-type hypersensitivity. J Immunol 1977;118:159–165.

39. Askenase PW, Bursztajn S, Gershon MD, Gershon RK. T-cell–dependent mast cell degranulation and release of serotonin in murine delayed-type hypersensitivity. J Exp Med 1980;152:1358–1374.

40. Askenase PW, Metzler CM, Gershon RK. Localization of leukocytes in sites of delayed-typed hypersensitivity and in lymph nodes: dependence on vasoactive amines. Immunology 1982;47:239–246.

41. Kraeuter-Kops S, Van Loveren H, Rosenstein RW, Ptak W, Askenase PW. Mast cell activation and vascular alterations in immediate hypersensitivity-like reactions induced by a T cell-derived antigen binding factor. Lab Invest 1984;50:421–434.

42. Askenase PW, Van Loveren H, Kraeuter-Kops S, et al. Defective elicitation of delayed-type hypersensitivity in W/W^v and SI/SI^d mast cell-deficient mice. J Immunol 1983;131:2687–2694.

43. Galli SJ, Hammel I. Unequivocal delayed hypersensitivity in mast cell-deficient and Beige mice. Science 1984;226:710–713.

44. Mekori YA, Chang JCC, Wershil BK, Galli SJ. Studies on the role of mast cells in contact sensitivity responses. Pas-

sive transfer of the reaction into mast cell-deficient mice locally reconstituted with cultured mast cells: effect of reserpine on transfer of the reaction with DNP-specific cloned T-cells. Cell Immunol 1987;109:39–52.

45. Mekori YA, Weitzman GL, Galli SJ. Reevaluation of reserpine-induced suppression of contact sensitivity. Evidence that reserpine interferes with T-lymphocyte function independently of an effect on mast cells. J Exp Med 1985; 162:1935–1953.

46. Torii I, Morikawa S, Harada T, Kitamura Y. Two distinct types of cellular mechanisms in the development of delayed hypersensitivity in mice: requirement of either mast cells or macrophages for elicitation of the response. Immunology 1993;78:482–490.

47. Mosmann TR, Cherwinski H, Bond MW, Giedlin MA, Coffman RL. Two types of murine helper T-cell clone. I. Definition according to profiles of lymphokine activities and secreted proteins. J Immunol 1986;136:2348–2357.

48. Gajewski TF, Fitch FW. Anti-proliferative effect of IFN-γ in immune regulation. I. IFN-γ inhibits the proliferation of Th2 but not Th1 murine HTL clones. J Immunol 1988; 140:4245–4252.

49. Street NE, Schumacher JH, Fong TAT, et al. Heterogeneity of mouse helper T cells: Evidence from bulk cultures and limiting dilution cloning for precursors of Th1 and Th2 cells. J Immunol 1990;144:1629–1639.

50. Mosmann TR, Moore KW. The role of IL-10 in crossregulation of Th1 and Th2 responses. Immunol Today 1991;12: A49–A53.

51. Mosmann TR, Coffman RL. Heterogeneity of cytokine secretion patterns and functions of helper T cells. Adv Immunol 1989;46:111–147.

52. Firestein GS, Roeder WD, Laxer JA, et al. A new murine CD4+ T cell subset with an unrestricted cytokine profile. J Immunol 1989;143:518–525.

53. Maggi E, Del Prete GF, Macchia D, et al. Profiles of lymphokine activities and helper function for IgE in human T cell clones. Eur J Immunol 1988;18:1045–1054.

54. Paliard X, de Waal Malefyt R, Yssel H, et al. Simultaneous production of IL-2, IL-4 and IFN-γ by activated human CD4+ and CD8+ T-cell clones. J Immunol 1988;141:849–855.

55. Norma T, Nakakubo H, Sugita M, et al. Expression of different combinations of interleukins by human T cell leukemic cell lines that are clonally related. J Exp Med 1989; 169:1853–1858.

56. Wierenga EA, Snoek M, de Groot C, et al. Evidence for compartmentalization of functional subsets of CD4⁺ T lymphocytes in atopic patients. J Immunol 1990;144:4651–4656.

57. Haanen JBAG, de Waal Malefyt R, Res PCM, et al. Selection of a human T helper Type 1–like T cell subset by Mycobacteria. J Exp Med 1991;174:583–592.

58. Del Prete GF, De Carli M, Mastromauro C, et al. Purified protein derivative of Mycobacterium tuberculosis and excretory-secretory antigen(s) of Toxocara canis expand in vitro human T cells with stable and opposite (type 1 T helper or type 2 T helper) profile of cytokine production. J Clin Invest 1991;88:346–350.

59. Mosmann TR, Coffman RL. Th1 and Th2 cells: different patterns of lymphokine secretion lead to different functional properties. Ann Rev Immunol 1989;7:145–173.

60. Bottomly K. A functional dichotomy in CD4+ T-lymphocytes. Immunol Today 1988;9:268–274.

61. Lebman DA, Coffman RL. Interleukin-4 causes isotype switching to IgE in T cell-stimulated clonal B cell cultures. J Exp Med 1988;168:853–862.

62. Mosmann TR, Bond MW. Coffman RL, Ohara J, Paul WE. T cell and mast cell lines respond to B-cell stimulatory factor-1. Proc Natl Acad Sci USA 1986;83:5654–5658.

63. Finkelman FD, Katona IM, Mosmann TR, Coffman RL. IFN-γ regulates the isotypes of Ig secreted during in vivo humoral immune responses. J Immunol 1988;140:1022–1027.

64. Finkelman FC, Katona IM, Urban JF, et al. IL-4 is required to generate and sustain in vivo IgE responses. J Immunol 1988;141:2335–2341.

65. Finkelman FD, Ohara J, Goroff DK, et al. Production of BSF-1 during an in vivo, T-dependent immune response. J Immunol 1986;137:2878–2885.

66. Janeway CA, Carding S, Jones B, et al. CD4+ T cells: specificity and function. Immunol Rev 1988;101:39–80.

67. Ramila G, Sklenar I, Kennedy M, Sunshine GH, Erb P. Evaluation of accessory cell heterogeneity. II. Failure of dendritic cells to activate antigen-specific T helper cells to soluble antigens. Eur J Immunol 1985;15:189–192.

68. Gajewski TF, Schell SR, Nau G, Fitch FW. Regulation of T-cell activation: differences among T-cell subsets. Immunol Rev 1989;111:79–110.

69. Gajewski TF, Schell SR, Fitch FW. Evidence implicating utilization of different T-cell receptor associated signaling pathways by Th1 and Th2 clones. J Immunol 1990; 144:4110–4120.

70. Weaver CT, Unanue ER. The costimulatory function of antigen-presenting cells. Immunol Today 1990;11:49.

71. Heinzel FP, Sadick MD, Holaday BJ, Coffman RL, Locksley RM. Reciprocal expression of interferon gamma or IL4 during the resolution or progression of murine leishmaniasis. Evidence for expansion of distinct helper T cell subsets. J Exp Med 1989;169:59–72.

72. Sadick MD, Heinzel FP, Shigekane VM, Fisher WL, Locksley RM. Cellular and humoral immunity to Leishmania major in genetically susceptible mice after in vivo depletion of L3T4+ T cells. J Immunol 1987; 139:1303–1309.

73. Coffman RL, Varkila K, Scott P, Chatelain R. Role of cytokines in the differentiation of CD4+ T cell subsets in vivo. Immunol Rev 1991;123:189–207.

74. Gajewski TF, Joyce J, Fitch FW. Anti-proliferative effect of IFN-γ in immune regulation. III. Differential selection of TH1 and TH2 murine helper T lymphocyte clones using recombinant IL-2 and recombinant IFN-γ. J Immunol 1989; 143:15–22.

75. Maggi E, Parronchi P, Manetti R, et al. Reciprocal regulatory role of IFN-γ and IL-4 on the in vitro development of human TH1 and TH2 clones. J Immunol 1992;148:2142–2147.

76. Scott P, Natovitz P, Coffman RL, Pearce E, Sher A. Immunoregulation of cutaneous leishmaniasis. T cell lines that transfer protective immunity or exacerbation belong

to different T helper subsets and respond to distinct parasite antigens. J Exp Med 1988;168:1675–1684.

77. Nathan CF, Murray HW, Wiebe ME, Rubin BY. Identification of interferon-gamma as the lymphokine that activates human macrophage oxidative metabolism and antimicrobial activity. J Exp Med 1983;158:670–689.

78. Murray HW, Rubin BF, Rothermel CD. Killing of intracellular Leishmania donovani by lymphokine-stimulated human mononuclear phagocytes. Evidence that interferon-γ is the activating lymphokine. J Clin Invest 1983;72:1506–1510.

79. Liew FY, Millott S, Li Y, Lelchuk, R, Chan WL, Ziltener H. Macrophage activation by interferon-gamma from host-protective T cells is inhibited by interleukin (IL)3 and IL4 produced by disease-promoting T cells in leishmaniasis. Eur J Immunol 1989;19:1227–1232.

80. Scott P, Pearce E, Cheever AW, Coffman RL, Sher A. Role of cytokines and CD4+ T-cells subsets in the regulation of parasite immunity and disease. Immunol Rev 1989; 112:161–182.

81. Howard JG. Immunological regulation and control of experimental leishmaniasis. Int Rev Exp Pathol 1986;28:79–116.

82. Belosevic M, Finbloom DS, Van Der Meide PH, Slayter MV, Nacy CA. Administration of monoclonal anti-IFN-γ antibodies in vivo abrogates natural resistance of C3H/HeN mice to infection with Leishmania major. J Immunol 1989; 143:266–274.

83. Scott P. Host and parasite factors regulating the development of CD4+ T-cell subsets in experimental cutaneous leishmaniasis. Res Immunol 1991;142:32–36.

84. Health AW, Playfair JH. Conjugation of interferon-gamma to antigen enhances its adjuvanticity. Immunology 1990; 71:454–456.

85. Sadick M, Street N, Mosmann TR, Locksley RM. Cytokine regulation of murine leishmaniasis: IL-4 is not sufficient to mediate progressive disease in resistant C57BL/6 mice. Faseb J 1991;5:A1369.

86. Coffman RL, Chatelain R, Leal LMCC, Varkila K. Leishmania-major infection in mice-A model system for the study of CD4+ T-cell subset differentiation. Res Immunol 1991b;142:36–40.

87. Locksley RM, Heinzel FP, Holaday BJ, Mutha SS, Reiner SL, Sadick MD. Induction of TH1 and TH2 CD4+ subsets during murine Leishmania-major infection. Res Immunol 1991;142:28–32.

88. Scharton TM, Scott P. Natural killer cells are a source of interferon γ that drives differentiation of CD4+ T cell subsets and induces early resistance to Leishmania major in mice. J Exp Med 1993;178:567–577.

89. Welsh RM, Zinkernagel RM, Hallenbeck LA. Cytotoxic cells induced during lymphocytic virus infection of mice. II. Specificities of the natural killer cells. J Immunol 1979; 122:475–481.

90. Bukowski JF, Woda BA, Sonoku H, Okumura K, Welsh RM. Natural killer cell depletion enhances virus synthesis and virus induced hepatitis in vivo. J Immunol 1983; 131:1531–1538.

91. Wolfe SA, Tracey DE, Henney CS. Induction of 'natural killer' cells by BCG. Nature (London) 1976;262:584–586.

92. Ojo E, Haller O, Wigzell H. An analysis of conditions al-
lowing Corynebacterium parvum to cause either augmentation or inhibition of natural killer activity against tumor cells in mice. Int J Cancer 1978;21:444–452.

93. Eugui EM, Allison AC. Differences in susceptibility of various mouse strains to haemoprotozoan infections: possible correlation with natural killer activity. Parasite Immunol (Oxford) 1980;2:277–282.

94. Hatcher FM, Kuhn RE. Spontaneous lytic activity against allogeneic tumor cells and depression of specific cytotoxic responses in mice infected with Trypanosoma cruzi. J Immunol 1981;126:2436–2442.

95. D'Andrea A, Rengaraju M, Valiante NM, et al. Production of natural killer cell stimulatory factor (interleukin 12) by peripheral blood mononuclear cells. J Exp Med 1992; 176:1387–1398.

96. Chan SH, Perussia B, Gupta JW, et al. Induction of interferon γ production by natural killer cell stimulatory factor: characterization of the responder cells and synergy with other inducers. J Exp Med 1991;173:869–879.

97. Manetti R, Parronchi P, Giudizi MG. Natural killer cell stimulatory factor (interleukin 12 [IL-12]) induces T helper type (Th1)-specific immune responses and inhibits the development of IL-4 producing Th cells. J Exp Med 1993;177:1199–1204.

98. Hsieh CS, Macatonia SE, Tripp CS, Wolf SF, O'Garra A, Murphy KM. Development of Th1 CD4+ T cells through IL-12 produced by Listeria-induced macrophages. Science 1993;260:547–549.

99. Sypek JP, Chung CC, Mayor SE et al. Resolution of cutaneous leishmaniasis: interleukin 12 initiates a protective T helper type 1 immune response. J Exp Med 1993;177: 1797–1802.

100. Heinzel FP, Schoenhaut DS, Rerko RM, Rosser LE, Gately MK. Recombinant interleukin 12 cures mice infected with Leishmania major. J Exp Med 1993;177:1505–1509.

101. Titus RG, Sherry B, Cerami A. Tumor necrosis factor plays a protective role in experimental murine cutaneous leishmaniasis. J Exp Med 1989;170:2097–2104.

102. Locksley RM. Interleukin 12 in host defence against microbial pathogens. Proc Natl Acad Sci USA 1993;90:5879–5880.

103. Romani N, Koide S, Crowley M. Presentation of exogenous protein antigens by dendritic cells to T-cell clones: intact protein is presented best by immature epidermal Langerhans cells. J Exp Med 1989;169:1169–1178.

104. Streilein JW, Grammer SF. In vitro evidence that Langerhans cells can adopt two functionally distinct forms capable of antigen presentation to T lymphocytes. J Immunol 1989;143:3925–3933.

105. Witmer-Pack M, Oliver W, Valinsky J, Schuler G, Steinman RM. Granulocyte/macrophage colony-stimulating factor is essential for the viability and function of cultured murine epidermal Langerhans cells. J Exp Med 1987;166: 1484–1498.

106. Schuler G, Steinman RM. Murine epidermal Langerhans cells mature into potent immunostimulatory dendritic cells in vitro. J Exp Med 1985;161:526–546.

107. Shimada S, Caughman SW, Sharrow SO, Stephany D, Katz SI. Enhanced antigen-presenting capacity of cultured Langerhans cells is associated with markedly increased expression of Ia antigen. J Immunol 1987;139:2551–2555.

108. Tang A, Udey MC. Inhibition of epidermal Langerhans cell function by low dose ultraviolet-B radiation: ultraviolet-B radiation selectively modulates ICAM-1 (CD54) expression by murine Langerhans cells. J Immunol 1991;146: 3347–3355.

109. Young JW, Koulaova L, Soergei SA, Clark EA, Steinman RM, Dupont B. The B7/BB1 antigen provides one of several costimulatory signals for the activation of CD4 T lymphocytes by human dendritic cells in vitro. J Clin Invest 1992; 90:229–237.

110. Cumberbatch M, Gould SJ, Peters SW, Kimber I. MHC class II expression by Langerhans cells and lymph node dendritic cells: possible evidence for maturation of Langerhans cells following contact sensitization. Immunology 1991;74:414–419.

111. Cumberbatch M, Kimber I. Dermal tumour necrosis factor-α induces dendritic cell migration to draining lymph nodes, and possibly provides one stimulus for Langerhans cell migration. Immunology 1992;75:257–263.

112. Cumberbatch M, Illingworth I, Kimber I. Antigen-bearing dendritic cells in the draining lymph nodes of contact sensitized mice: cluster formation with lymphocytes. Immunology 1991;74:139–145.

113. Luger TA, Schwarz T. Evidence for an epidermal cytokine network. J Invest Dermatol 1990;95:100s–104s.

114. McKenzie RC, Sauder DN. The role of keratinocyte cytokines in inflammation and immunity. J Invest Dermatol 1990;95:105s–110s.

115. Kupper TS. Role of epidermal cytokines. In: Oppenheim JJ, Shevach EM, eds. Immunophysiology. New York: Oxford University Press, 1990:285–305.

116. Barker JNWN. Role of keratinocytes in allergic contact dermatitis. Contact Dermatitis 1992;26:145–148.

117. Kupper TS, Ballard DW, Chua AO, et al. Human keratinocytes contain mRNA indistinguishable from monocyte interleukin 1a and b mRNA: keratinocyte epidermal cell-derived thymocyte-activating factor is identical to interleukin 1. J Exp Med 1986;164:2095–2100.

118. Kupper TS, Lee F, Coleman D, Chodakewitz J, Flood P, Horowitz M. Keratinocyte derived T cell growth factor (KTGF) is identical to granulocyte macrophage colony stimulating factor (GM-CSF). J Invest Dermatol 1988;91: 185–188.

119. Kock A, Schwarz T, Kirnbauer R, et al. Human keratinocytes are a source for tumour necrosis factor: evidence for synthesis and release upon stimulation with endotoxin or ultraviolet light. J Exp Med 1990;172:1609–1614.

120. Enk AH, Katz SI. Early molecular events in the induction phase of contact sensitivity. Proc Natl Acad Sci USA 1992; 89:1398–1402.

121. Heufler C, Koch F, Schuler G. Granulocyte macrophage colony-stimulating factor and interleukin-1 mediate the maturation of murine epidermal Langerhans cells into potent immunostimulatory dendritic cells. J Exp Med 1988; 167:700–705.

122. Picut CA, Lee CS, Dougherty EP, Anderson KL, Lewis RM. Immunostimulatory capabilities of highly enriched Langerhans cells in vitro. J Invest Dermatol 1988;90:201–206.

123. Koch F, Heufler C, Kampgen E, Schneeweiss D, Bock G, Schuler G. Tumour necrosis factor α maintains the viability of murine epidermal Langerhans cells in culture, but in contrast to granulocyte/macrophage colony-stimulating factor, without inducing their functional maturation. J Exp Med 1990;171:159–171.

124. Koide SL, Inaba K, Steinman RM. Interleukin 1 enhances T-dependent immune responses by amplifying the function of dendritic cells. J Exp Med 1987;165:515–530.

125. Steinman RM. Cytokines amplify the function of accessory cells. Immunol Lett 1988;17:197–202.

126. Cumberbatch M, Peters SW, Gould SJ, Kimber I. Intercellular adhesion molecule-1 (ICAM-1) expression by lymph node dendritic cells. Comparison with epidermal Langerhans cells. Immunol Lett 1992;32:105–110.

127. Kimber I, Kinnaird A, Peters SW, Mitchell JA. Correlation between lymphocyte proliferative responses and dendritic cell migration in regional lymph nodes following skin painting with contact-sensitizing agents. Int Arch Allergy Appl Immunol 1990;93:47–53.

128. Vermeer M, Streilein JW. Ultraviolet B light-induced alterations in epidermal Langerhans cells are mediated in part by tumour necrosis factor-α. Photodermatol Photoimmunol Photomed 1990;7:258–265.

129. Dinarello CA, Cannon JG, Wolff SM, et al. Tumor necrosis factor (cachectin) is an endogenous pyrogen and induces production of interleukin 1. J Exp Med 1986;163:1433–1450.

130. Dinarello CA. Interleukin 1 and its biologically related cytokines. Adv Immunol 1989;44:153–203.

131. Le J, Vilcek J. Tumor necrosis factor and interleukin 1: cytokines with multiple overlapping biological activities. Lab Invest 1987;56:234–248.

132. Lundqvist EN, Bäck O. Interleukin-1 decreases the number of Ia+ epidermal dendritic cells but increases their expression of Ia antigen. Acta Dermatol Venereol 1990;70:391–394.

133. Lewis M, Tartaglia LA, Lee A, et al. Cloning and expression of cDNAs for two distinct murine tumor necrosis factor receptors demonstrate one receptor is species specific. Proc Natl Acad Sci USA 1991;88:2830–2834.

134. McCluskey RT, Benacerraf B, McCluskey JW. Studies on the specificity of the cellular infiltrate in delayed hypersensitivity reactions. J Immunol 1963;90:466–473.

135. Dvorak HF, Galli SJ, Dvorak AM. Expression of cell-mediated hypersensitivity in vivo—recent advances. Int Rev Exp Pathol 1980;21:119–194.

136. Issekutz TB, Stoltz JM, Van Der Meide P. Lymphocytes recruitment in delayed-type hypersensitivity. The role of IFN-γ. J Immunol 1988;140:2989–2993.

137. Issekutz TB, Stoltz JM, Van Der Meide P. The recruitment of lymphocytes into the skin by T cell lymphokines: the role of γ-interferon. Clin Exp Immunol 1988;73:70–75.

138. Issekutz TB, Stoltz JM, Webster DM. Role of interferon in lymphocyte recruitment into the skin. Cell Immunol 1986; 99:322–333.

139. Issekutz TB, Stoltz JM. Stimulation of lymphocyte migration by endotoxin, tumor necrosis factor, and interferon. Cell Immunol 1989;120:165–173.

140. Fong TAT, Mosmann TR. The role of IFN-γ in delayed-type hypersensitivity mediated by Th1 clones. J Immunol 1989;143:2887–2893.

141. Colditz IG, Watson DL. The effect of cytokines and chemotactic agonists on the migration of T lymphocytes into skin. Immunology 1992;76:272–278.

142. Zaloom Y, Walsh LP, McCulloch P, Gallagher G. Enhancement of a delayed hypersensitivity reaction to a contact allergen, by the systemic administration of interleukin-2. Immunology 1991;72:584–587.

143. Kelly VE, Nador D, Tarcic N, Gaulton GN, Strom TB. Anti-interleukin 2 receptor antibody suppresses delayed-type hypersensitivity to foreign and syngeneic antigens. J Immunol 1986;137:2122–2124.

144. Figari IS, Mori NA, Palladino MA Jr. Regulation of neutrophil migration and superoxide production by recombinant tumor necrosis factors-alpha and -beta: comparison to recombinant interferon-gamma and interleukin-1 alpha. Blood 1987;70:979–984.

145. Sayers TJ, Wiltrout TA, Bull CA, Denn AC III, Pilaro AM, Lokesh B. Effect of cytokines on polymorphonuclear neutrophil infiltration in the mouse. Prostaglandin- and leukotriene-independent induction of infiltration by IL-1 and tumor necrosis factor. J Immunol 1988;141:1670–1677.

146. Wang JM, Colella S, Allavena P, Mantovani A. Chemotactic activity of human recombinant granulocyte-macrophage colony-stimulating factor. Immunology 1987;60:439–444.

147. Tsukada H, Kawamura I, Arakawa M, Nomoto K, Mitsuyama M. Dissociated development of T cells mediating delayed-type hypersensitivity and protective T cells against Listeria monocytogenes and their functional difference in lymphokine production. Infect Immun 1991;59:3589–3595.

148. Dalton DK, Pitts-Meek S, Keshav S, Figari IS, Bradley A, Stewart TA. Multiple defects of immune cell function in mice with disrupted interferon-γ genes. Science 1993;259:1739–1742.

149. Huang S, Hendriks W, Althage A, et al. Immune response in mice that lack the interferon-γ receptor. Science 1993;259:1742–1745.

150. Murray HW, Spitalny GL, Nathan CF. Activation of mouse peritoneal macrophages in vitro and in vivo by interferon-γ. J Immunol 1985;134:1619–1622.

151. Reed SG, Nathan CF, Pihl DL, et al. Recombinant granulocyte/macrophage colony-stimulating factor activates macrophages to inhibit Trypanosoma cruzi and release hydrogen peroxide. Comparison with interferon gamma. J Exp Med 1987;166:1734–1746.

152. Reed SG. In vivo administration of recombinant IFN-γ induces macrophage activation, and prevents acute disease, immune suppression, and death in experimental Trypanosoma cruzi infections. J Immunol 1988;140:4342–4347.

153. McCabe RE, Luft BJ, Remington JS. Effect of murine interferon gamma on murine toxoplasmosis. J Infect Dis 1984;150:961–962.

154. Nathan CF, Prendergast TJ, Wiebe ME, et al. Activation of human macrophages. Comparison of other cytokines with interferon-γ. J Exp Med 1984;160:600–605.

155. Flesch IE, Kaufmann SH. Mycobacterial growth inhibition by interferon-γ–activated bone marrow macrophages and differential susceptibility among strains of Mycobacterium tuberculosis. J Immunol 1987;138:4408–4413.

156. Flesch IE, Kaufmann SH. Attempts to characterize the mechanisms involved in mycobacterial growth inhibition by gamma-interferon–activated bone marrow macrophages. Infect Immun 1988;56:1464–1469.

157. Rook GW, Steele J, Ainsworth M, Champion BR. Activation of macrophages to inhibit proliferation of Mycobacterium tuberculosis: comparison of the effects of recombinant gamma-interferon on human monocytes and murine peritoneal macrophages. Immunology 1986;59:333–338.

158. Douvas GS, Looker DL, Vatter AE, Crowle AJ. Gamma interferon activates human macrophages to become tumoricidal and leishmanicidal but enhances replication of macrophage-associated mycobacteria. Infect Immun 1985;50:1–8.

159. Shiratsuchi H, Johnson JL, Toba H, Ellner J. Strain- and donor-related differences in the interaction of Mycobacterium avium with human monocytes and its modulation by interferon-γ. J Infect Dis 1990;162:932–938.

160. Nathan CF, Kaplan G, Lewis WR, et al. Local and systemic effects of intradermal recombinant interferon-γ in patients with Lepromatous leprosy. N Engl J Med 1986;315:6–15.

161. Nickell SP, Keane M, So M. Further characterization of protective Trypanosoma cruzi-specific CD4+ T-cell clones: T helper type 1-like phenotype and reactivity with shed trypomastigote antigens. Infect Immun 1993;61:3250–3258.

162. Nickell SP, Gebremichael A, Hoff R, Boyer MH. Isolation and functional characterization of murine T cell lines and clones specific for the protozoan parasite Trypanosoma cruzi. J Immunol 1987;138:914–921.

163. Muñoz-Fernández MA, Fernández MA, Fresno M. Synergism between tumor necrosis factor-α and interferon-γ on macrophage activation for the killing of intracellular Trypanosoma cruzi through a nitric oxide-dependent mechanism. Eur J Immunol 1992;22:301–307.

164. Jackett PS, Aber VR, Mitchison DA, Lowrie DB. The contribution of hydrogen peroxide resistance to virulence of Mycobacterium tuberculosis during the first six days after intravenous infection of normal and BCG-vaccinated guinea-pigs. Br J Exp Pathol 1981;62:34–40.

165. Jackett PS, Andrew PW, Aber VR, Lowrie DB. Guinea pig alveolar macrophages probably kill M. tuberculosis H37Rv and H37Ra in vivo by producing hydrogen peroxide. Adv Exp Med Biol 1983;162:99–104.

166. Walker L, Lowrie DB. Killing of Mycobacterium microti by immunologically activated macrophages. Nature 1981;293:69–70.

167. Nathan CF, Nogueira N, Ellis J, Cohn, ZA. Activation of macrophages in vivo and in vitro. Correlation between hydrogen peroxide release and killing of Trypanosoma cruzi. J Exp Med 1979;149:1056–1068.

168. Murray HW, Cartelli DM. Killing of intracellular Leishmania donovani by human mononuclear phagocytes: evidence for oxygen-dependent and -independent leishmanicidal activity. J Clin Invest 1983;72:32–44.

169. Liew FY, Millott S, Parkinson C, Palmer RM, Moncada S. Macrophage killing of Leishmania parasite in vivo is medi-

ated by nitric oxide from L-arginine. J Immunol 1990; 144:4794–4797.

170. Green SJ, Meltzer MS, Hibbs JB Jr, Nacy CA. Activated macrophages destroy intracellular Leishmania major amastigotes by an L-arginine-dependent killing mechanism. J Immunol 1990;144:278–283.

171. Flesch IE, Kaufmann SH. Mechanisms involved in mycobacterial growth inhibition by gamma interferon-activated bone marrow macrophages: role of reactive nitrogen intermediates. Infect Immun 1991;59:3213–3218.

172. Adams LB, Hibbs JB Jr, Taintor RR, Krahenbuhl JL. Microbiostatic effect of murine-activated macrophages for Toxoplasma gondii. Role for synthesis of inorganic nitrogen oxides from L-arginine. J Immunol 1990;144:2725–2729.

173. Ezekowitz RA, Austyn J, Stahl PD, Gordon S. Surface properties of bacillus Calmette-Guérin–activated mouse macrophages. Reduced expression of mannose-specific endocytosis, Fc receptors, and antigen F4/80 accompanies induction of Ia. J Exp Med 1981;154:60–76.

174. Handman E, Burgess AW. Stimulation by granulocyte-macrophage colony-stimulating factor of Leishmania tropica killing by macrophages. J Immunol 1979;122: 1134–1137.

175. Ho JL, Reed SG, He SH, Arruda S, Wick EA, Grabstein K. Interleukin-3 (IL-3) induces antimicrobial and tumoricidal activity (abstract). Clin Res 1991;39:150.

176. Ho JL, Reed SG, Wick EA, Giordana M. Granulocyte-macrophage and macrophage colony-stimulating factors activate intramacrophage killing of Leishmania mexicana amazonensis. J Infect Dis 1990;162:224–230.

177. Weiser WY, Van Niel A, Clark SC, David JR, Remold HG. Recombinant human granulocyte-macrophage colony-stimulating factor activates intracellular killing of Leishmania donovani by human monocyte-derived macrophages. J Exp Med 1987;166:1436–1446.

178. Liew FY, Parkinson C, Millott S, Severn A, Carrier M. Tumour necrosis factor (TNF-α) in leishmaniasis. 1. TNF-α mediates host protection against cutaneous leishmaniasis. Immunology 1990;69:570–573.

179. Pihl D, Grabstein K, Reed S. Inhibition of Trypanosoma cruzi in mouse macrophages and in human monocytes and macrophages by recombinant interferon-gamma (IFN-γ) and granulocyte monocyte colony stimulating factor (GM-CSF) (abstract). Fed Proc 1987;46:1755.

180. De Titto EH, Catterall JR, Remington JS. Activity of recombinant tumor necrosis factor on Toxoplasma gondii and Trypanosoma cruzi. J Immunol 1986;137:1342–1345.

181. Wirth JJ, Kierszenbaum F. Recombinant tumor necrosis factor enhances macrophage destruction of Trypanosoma cruzi in the presence of bacterial endotoxin. J Immunol 1988;141:286–288.

182. Piguet PF, Grau GE, Hauser C, Vassalli P. Tumor necrosis factor is a critical mediator in hapten-induced irritant and contact hypersensitivity reactions. J Exp Med 1991;173: 673–679.

183. Chu CQ, Field M, Andrew E, Haskard D, Feldmann M, Maini RN. Detection of cytokines at the site of tuberculin-induced delayed-type hypersensitivity in man. Clin Exp Immunol 1992;90:522–529.

184. Walsh LJ, Trinchieri G, Waldorf HA, Whitaker D, Murphy GF. Human dermal mast cells contain and release tumor necrosis factor a, which induces endothelial leukocyte adhesion molecule 1. Proc Natl Acad Sci USA 1991;88:4220–4224.

185. Ferreri NR, Millet I, Paliwal V, et al. Induction of macrophager TNF-α, IL-1, IL-6 and PGE₂ production by DTH-initiating factor. Cell Immunol 1991;137:389–405.

186. Shimizu Y, Shaw S, Graber N, et al. Activation-independent binding of human memory T cells to adhesion molecule ELAM-1. Nature 1991;349:799–802.

187. MacKay CR. Lymphocyte homing. Skin-seeking memory T cells. Nature 1991;349:737–738.

188. Picker LJ, Kishimoto TK, Smith CW, Warnock RA, Butcher EC. ELAM-1 is an adhesion molecule for skin-homing T cells. Nature 1991;349:796–799.

189. Waldorf HA, Walsh LJ, Schechter NM, Murphy GF. Early cellular events in evolving cutaneous delayed hypersensitivity in humans. Am J Pathol 1991;138:477–486.

190. Pober JS, Lapierre LA, Stolpen AH, et al. Activation of cultured human endothelial cells by recombinant lymphotoxin: comparison with tumor necrosis factor and interleukin 1 species. J Immunol 1987;138:3319–3324.

191. Munro JM, Pober JS, Cotran RS. Tumour necrosis factor and interferon-gamma induce distinct patterns of endothelial activation and associated leukocyte accumulation in skin of Papio anubis. Am J Pathol 1989;135:121–133.

192. Dustin ML, Rothlein R, Bhan AK, Dinarello CA, Springer TA. A natural adherence molecule (ICAM-1): induction by IL-1 and interferon-gamma, tissue distribution, biochemistry and function. J Immunol 1986;137:245–254.

193. Pober JS, Gimbrone MA Jr, Lapierre LA, et al. Overlapping patterns of activation of human endothelial cells by interleukin 1, tumor necrosis factor, and immune interferon. J Immunol 1986;137:1893–1896.

194. Boyd AW, Wawryk SO, Burns GF, Fecondo JV. Intercellular adhesion molecule 1 (ICAM-1) has a central role in cell-cell contact-mediated immune mechanisms. Proc Natl Acad Sci USA 1988;85:3095–3099.

195. Dustin ML, Springer TA. Lymphocyte function-associated antigen-1 (LFA-1) interaction with intercellular adhesion molecule-1 (ICAM-1) is one of at least three mechanisms for lymphocyte adhesion to cultured endothelial cells. J Cell Biol 1988;107:321–331.

196. Osborn L, Hession C, Tizard R, et al. Direct expression cloning of vascular cell adhesion molecule 1, a cytokine-induced endothelial protein that binds to lymphocytes. Cell 1989;59:1203–1211.

197. Bevilacqua MP, Stengelin S, Gimbrone MA Jr, Seed B. Endothelial leukocyte adhesion molecule 1: an inducible receptor for neutrophils related to complement regulatory proteins and lectins. Science 1989;243:1160–1165.

198. Dustin ML, Singer KH, Tuck DT, Springer TA. Adhesion of T-lymphoblasts to epidermal keratinocytes is regulated by interferon gamma and is mediated by intercellular adhesion molecule 1 (ICAM-1). J Exp Med 1988;167:1323–1340.

199. Basham TY, Nicholoff BJ, Merigan TC, Morhenn VB. Recombinant gamma interferon differentially regulates class

II antigen expression and biosynthesis on cultured normal human keratinocytes. J Interferon Res 1985;5:23–32.

200. Aiba S, Tagami H. Functional analysis of Ia antigen bearing keratinocytes: mixed skin lymphocyte cultures between Ia bearing Pam 212 cells and allogeneic and syngeneic splenic T cells. J Invest Dermatol 1987;89:560–566.

201. Fisher MS, Kripke ML. Further studies on the tumour-specific suppressor T-cells induced by ultraviolet radiation. J Immunol 1978;121:1139–1144.

202. Fisher MS, Kripke ML. Suppressor T lymphocytes control the development of primary skin cancers in ultraviolet-irradiated mice. Science 1982;216:1133–1134.

203. Ullrich SE, Kripke ML. Mechanisms in the suppression of tumor rejection produced in mice by repeated UV irradiation. J Immunol 1984;133:2786–2790.

204. Noonan FP, Kripke ML, Pedersen JM, Greene MI. Suppression of contact hypersensitivity in mice by ultraviolet radiation is associated with defective antigen presentation. Immunology 1981;43:527–533.

205. Noonan FP, De Fabo EC, Kripke ML. Suppression of contact hypersensitivity by UV radiation and its relationship to UV-induced suppression of tumor immunity. Photochem Photobiol 1981;34:683–689.

206. Lynch DH, Gurish MF, Daynes RA. The effects of high-dose UV exposure on murine Langerhans cell function at exposed and unexposed sites as assessed using in vivo and in vitro assays. J Invest Dermatol 1983;81:336–341.

207. De Fabo EC, Noonan FP. Mechanism of immune suppression by ultraviolet irradiation in vivo. I. Evidence for the existence of a unique photoreceptor in skin and its role in photoimmunology. J Exp Med 1983;158:84–90.

208. Elmets CA, Bergstresser PR, Tigelaar RE, Wood PJ, Streilein JW. Analysis of the mechanism of unresponsiveness produced by haptens painted on skin exposed to low dose ultraviolet radiation. J Exp Med 1983;158:781–794.

209. Streilein JW, Bergstresser PR. Genetic basis of ultraviolet-B effects on contact hypersensitivity. Immunogenetics 1988; 27:252–258.

210. Vermeer M, Schmieder GJ, Yoshikawa T. Effects of ultraviolet B light on cutaneous immune responses of humans with deeply pigmented skin. J Invest Dermatol 1991;97: 729–734.

211. Howie SEM, Norval M, Maingay J. Exposure to low-dose ultraviolet-B-light suppresses delayed-type hypersensitivity to herpes simplex virus in mice. J Invest Dermatol 1986;86:125–128.

212. Yasumoto S, Hayashi Y, Aurelian L. Immunity to herpes simplex virus type 2. Suppression of virus-induced immune responses in ultraviolet-B irradiated mice. J Immunol 1987;139:2788–2793.

213. Ullrich SE. Suppression of the immune response to allogeneic histocompatibility antigens by a single exposure to ultraviolet radiation. Transplantation 1986;42:287–291.

214. Ullrich SE, McIntyre BW, Rivas JM. Suppression of the immune response to alloantigen by factors released from ultraviolet-irradiated keratinocytes. J Immunol 1990;145: 489–498.

215. Mottram PL, Mirosklavos A, Clunie GJA, Noonan FP. A single dose of UV radiation suppresses delayed type hypersensitivity responses to alloantigens and prolongs heart al-

lograft acceptance in mice. Immunol Cell Biol 1988;66: 377–385.

216. Rivas JM, Ullrich SE. Systemic suppression of DTH by supernatants from UV-irradiated keratinocytes: an essential role for interleukin 10. J Immunol 1992;149:3865–3871.

217. Kripke ML. Immunologic mechanisms in UV radiation carcinogenesis. Adv Cancer Res 1981;34:69–106.

218. Kripke ML, Morison WL. Modulation of immune function by UV radiation. J Invest Dermatol 1985;85:62s–66s.

219. Krutmann J, Elmets CA. Recent studies on mechanisms in photoimmunology (yearly review). Photochem Photobiol 1988;48:787–798.

220. Simon JC, Krutmann J, Elmets CA, Bergstresser PR, Cruz PD Jr. Ultraviolet B-irradiated antigen-presenting cells display altered accessory signaling for T-cell activation: relevance to immune responses initiated in skin. J Invest Dermatol 1992;98:66s–69s.

221. Polla L, Margolis R, Goulston C, Parrish JA, Granstein RD. Enhancement of the elicitation phase of the murine contact hypersensitivity response by prior exposure to local ultraviolet radiation. J Invest Dermatol 1986;86:13–17.

222. Yoshikawa T, Streilein JW. Genetic basis of the effects of ultraviolet light-B on cutaneous immunity. Evidence that polymorphism at the Tnfa and Lps loci governs susceptibility. Immunogenetics 1990;32:298–305.

223. Moodycliffe AM, Kimber I, Norval M. Role of tumour necrosis factor-α in ultraviolet B light induced dendritic cell migration and suppression of contact hypersensitivity. Immunology 1994;81:79–84.

224. Bigby M, Vargas R, Sy M-S. Production of hapten-specific T-cell hybridomas and their use to study the effect of ultraviolet-B irradiation on the development of contact hypersensitivity. J Immunol 1989;143:3867–3872.

225. Moodycliffe AM, Kimber I, Norval M. The effect of ultraviolet B irradiation and urocanic acid isomers on dendritic cell migration. Immunology 1992;77:394–399.

226. Simon JC, Cruz PD, Bergstresser PR, Tigelaar RE. Low dose-ultraviolet-B irradiated Langerhans cells preferentially activate CD4+ cells of the T-helper 2 subset. J Immunol 1990;145:2087–2091.

227. Simon JC, Tigelaar RE, Bergstresser PR, Edelbaum D, Cruz PD Jr. Ultraviolet B radiation converts Langerhans cells from immunogenic to tolerogenic antigen-presenting cells. Induction of specific clonal anergy in CD4+ T helper 1 cells. J Immunol 1991;146:485–491.

228. Enk AH, Angeloni VL, Udey MC, Katz SI. Inhibition of Langerhans cell antigen-presenting function by IL-10. J Immunol 1993;151:2390–2398.

229. Ullrich SE. The role of keratinocyte-derived suppressive cytokines in the systemic immunosuppression induced by ultraviolet B radiation. Trends Photochem Photobiol 1991; 2:137–154.

230. Kripke ML. Immunologic unresponsiveness induced by UV radiation. Immunol Rev 1984;80:87–102.

231. Ullrich SE, Magee M. Specific suppression of allograft rejection after treatment of recipient mice with ultraviolet radiation and allogeneic spleen cells. Transplantation 1988; 46:115–119.

232. Rivas JM, Ullrich SE. The role of IL-4, IL-10 and TNFα in the immune suppression induced by ultraviolet radiation. J Leukocyte Biology 1994 (in press).

233. Ullrich SE. Mechanism involved in the systemic suppression of antigen-presenting cell function by UV irradiation. Keratinocyte-derived IL-10 modulates antigen-presenting cell function of splenic adherent cells. J Immunol 1994;152:3410–3416.

CHAPTER 9

ROLE OF CYTOKINES IN GRAFT-VERSUS-HOST REACTION AND REJECTION FOLLOWING ALLOGENEIC BONE MARROW TRANSPLANTATION

Arnon Nagler, Vivian Barak, and Shimon Slavin

Allogeneic bone marrow transplantation (BMT) is now recognized as a conventional, occasionally even frontline mode of therapy for an increasing number of diseases not curable by other therapeutic modalities. BMT is the treatment of choice for (a) clinical syndromes associated with the life-threatening deficiency of marrow stem cells (e.g., severe aplastic anemia) or stem-cell products (e.g., T lymphocytes in severe combined immunodeficiency, osteoclasts in osteopetrosis, granulocytes in Costmann's syndrome); (b) certain genetic disorders leading to production of abnormal marrow products (e.g., β-thalassemia major) or enzyme-deficiency disorders (e.g., metachromatic leukodystrophy, Gaucher's disease); (c) malignant hematological disorders, including leukemias and lymphomas; and (d) certain solid tumors (1–3).

Despite major advances in the field and better understanding of hematopoiesis and transplantation immunobiology, graft-versus-host disease (GVHD) and graft rejection are two of the major obstacles in allogeneic BMT (4). Currently, the major goal in using allogeneic BMT for the treatment of a variety of malignant and nonmalignant disorders is to increase its success rate by preventing GVHD and graft rejection. This goal is somewhat difficult to achieve because of the inverse relationship between GVHD and graft rejection (5).

Recently, cytokines have been implicated as important mediators of infections, inflammatory reactions, and regulation of the immunohematopoietic system. Endogenously produced cytokines appear to influence multiple physiological processes affecting regulation of tumorigenicity (6,7). Identification of cytokines, a class of intermediate molecular weight, intercellular regulatory proteins, and an understanding of their function has been facilitated tremendously by the use of recombinant DNA technology. Use of specific and sensitive immunoassays using anticytokine antibodies (6) makes it possible to detect and quantify cytokines in clinical and biological samples. Measurement of cytokine levels becomes a valuable tool not just for elucidating pathophysiological mechanisms but, more importantly, for diagnosis and prognosis of a variety of diseases (7). We discuss the possible role of cytokines in GVHD and graft rejection and the potential clinical applications of cytokines following allogeneic BMT.

CYTOKINES AND GRAFT-VERSUS-HOST DISEASE

GVHD pathophysiology

GVHD is one of the major obstacles in allogeneic BMT due to its occurrence in the majority of BMT recipients; it frequently leads to morbidity and mortality within the first few weeks to the first few months after BMT. Chronic GVHD (autoimmune GVHD) may appear in subsequent months and lead to significant disability. GVHD is induced by donor-immunocompetent T lymphocytes that are reactive against alloantigens presented by the recipient tissues (8–10). However, the basic mechanisms of GVHD remain unclear. GVHD seems to be a complex multifactorial event; it is not simply determined by the reactivity of donor T cells toward disparate non-human leukocyte antigens (HLA).

GVHD is currently viewed as a three-step process: (a) up-regulation of HLA and leukocyte adhesion molecules on host target tissues; (b) activation of donor-immunocompetent T cells by host histocompatibility antigens, which then proliferate; and (c) secretion of cytokines by activated T cells, which recruit additional cells, induce the expression of histocompatibility antigens, and up-regulate the response of the donor's effector cells against recipient antigen-presenting target cells (8–10).

Cytokines have a key role in each of these steps. Recent studies indicate that mechanisms other than direct T-cell–mediated cytotoxicity may be responsible for the tissue damage associated with GVHD. An entire network of inflammatory cytokines are most probably operating as primary mediators of acute GVHD. Activation of T cells is believed to be only one event in GVHD pathophysiology. Many of the clinical manifestations of GVHD may be due in part to disequilibrium in production of inflammatory cytokines secreted by cells, such as T cells, monocytes, natural killer (NK) cells, and endothelial cells. These soluble mediators, which are released in a dysregulated fashion, may be responsible for amplification of the reactivity of the efferent arm in the immune system and the resulting tissue damage of acute GVHD.

Cytokine dysregulation during GVHD

Many cytokines are produced in an aberrant fashion during GVHD. These cytokines include interleukin-2 (IL-2), soluble IL-2 receptor (sIL-2R), tumor necrosis factor-α (TNF-α), TNF-β, interferon-γ (IFN-γ), IL-1α, Il-1β, IL-6, and IL-4 (11–13).

In the first step of GVHD, there is up-regulation of the expression of HLA and leukocyte adhesion molecules on the target tissues, such as skin, intestinal mucosa, and liver (10). It seems reasonable that this increment in expression of various cell surface molecules is influenced by cytokines released as a result of the chemical or physical insult of conditioning regimen, toxicity caused by secondary infections, and possibly the underlying disease.

It is well established that there is a direct correlation between the incidence and severity of GVHD and age; total versus selective gastrointestinal decontamination; positive serology for herpes simplex virus (HSV), Epstein Barr virus (EBV), varicella zoster virus (VZV), and cytomegalovirus (CMV); reactivation of latent infections; ad-

vanced stages of leukemia; and certain intensive conditioning regimen (8–10,14,15). These correlations may be due to epithelial and endothelial injury, which stimulate the release of inflammatory cytokines that increase expression of HLA class I and II antigens and cell surface adhesion molecules (10–13).

IL-1, TNF-α, IL-6 are inflammatory cytokines that can be produced by macrophages, epithelial cells, and endothelial cells in the gut and skin in response to inflammatory injury, and they up-regulate HLA and cell surface adhesion molecules (7,16–21). Growth of certain bacteria is enhanced by IL-1 (22), suggesting that local production of IL-1 in the gut mucosa may be associated with endotoxin injury to epithelial and endothelial cells. This finding may explain the well-known relationship between acute GVHD and infection (14).

The major role of TNF-α in the pathogenesis of GVHD is suggested by multiple authors. First, TNF is released from host tissues in the initial phases of GVHD, and it remains elevated in tissue and sera of mice and patients with acute GVHD (18,19,23–29). Moreover, Holler and colleagues (24) found a direct correlation between TNF levels and transplant-related complications and survival. Indeed, anti-TNF compounds, such as pentoxifylline and Ciprofloxacin, as well as monoclonal anti-TNF antibodies, are currently being investigated as a means for prevention and treatment of transplant-associated toxicity and GVHD (30–32). It was also shown that IL-1 receptor antagonist (IL-1RA), which inhibits IL-1, can prevent GVHD (33). It is important to note that cytokine release (e.g., TNF-α, IL-1) from host macrophages and endothelial cells in response to injury due to conditioning regimens or endotoxin is independent of alloreactivity, which may explain the occasional GVHD-like "cytokine syndromes" following syngeneic and even autologous GVHD.

Donor T-cell–mediated cytokines and GVHD

Donor-immunocompetent T cells are the key players in GVHD (8–10). Effective prevention of GVHD can therefore be accomplished by pretransplant depletion of donor-immunocompetent T lymphocytes, which can be accomplished by one of several immunological methods based on use of antibodies, although other methods based on physicochemical approaches may prove as effective (34,35). Successful T-lymphocyte depletion completely prevents GVHD, even across major histocompatibility complex (MHC) barriers, and it prevents the need for post-BMT anti-GVHD prophylaxis (34,35).

Following antigen presentation, which occurs in the first step of GVHD, there is activation of T cells. This activation involves multiple intracellular changes, which include an increase in cytoplasmic free calcium levels, activation of protein kinase C and thyrosine kinases, and secretion of cytokines (10). These events activate the transcription of genes for cytokines, such as IL-2 and their receptors.

IL-2 stimulates proliferation of both the cells that secrete it (i.e., autocrine effect) and other cells expressing the receptor (i.e., paracrine effect), and it mediates clonal expansion. Because IL-2 is critical for activation and proliferation of T lymphocytes, it may therefore have an important role in GVHD (36). IL-2 was suggested to fuel the fire of the GVHD reaction by virtue of its ability to activate and expand alloreactive T-cell clones, and also due to activation and induction of NK cell proliferation (37). However, serum IL-2 levels are not increased in GVHD, and increased mRNA for IL-2 could not be detected in both murine and human models (23,27–29). In contrast, increased levels of soluble IL-2R have been observed (37–39). Moreover, anti-IL-2R antibodies have been used successfully as a new mode of therapy in steroid-resistant GVHD (40).

Protein-toxin conjugates (e.g., diphtheria, ricin-A, and *Pseudomonas*) bound to IL-2 or to anti-IL-2R antibodies can be used for targeting IL-2–producing or IL-2–responding cells (41–43). Further attempts to treat acute GVHD were initiated in the past few years as monoclonal antibodies against selective T-lymphocyte subsets became available. The Campath-2 monoclonal antibody that can react more effectively with activated T lymphocytes, as compared with resting T cells, seems particularly promising (44).

In addition to IL-2, activated T cells can produce a variety of cytokines, such as IFN-γ, IL-4, and IL-6, which may have a direct or indirect role in GVHD (45–49). Symington and associates (50) recently evaluated serum IL-6 levels in 22 patients with GVHD, and they found direct correlation between IL-6 levels and the severity of GVHD. Moreover, IL-6 peaks tended to precede GVHD onset (50).

IFN synthesis has been implicated for a long time in GVHD (23,46,51). IFN-γ released by activated donor cells might stimulate recipient macrophages in the course of GVHD to produce IL-1, TNF, and IL-6; it thus potentiates clinical symptomatology (18,23,24,51).

IL-4 has a major role in chronic GVHD (26). However, IL-4 may down-regulate IL-2–activated NK cells (52); it therefore may also participate in the cascade of the complicated cytokine network that occurs in patients with acute GVHD (53,54).

TNF is produced by activated T cells, NK cells (55), and macrophages, and it is therefore one of the major cytokines responsible for GVHD; it has a major role in all three steps of GVHD (8–11). In a mouse model of GVHD, TNF messenger RNA (mRNA) is increased in the spleen (19,23). Moreover, subcutaneous administration of TNF produced epidermal damage characteristic of GVHD. In addition, in this mouse model (19), anti-TNF antibodies prevented systemic morbidity and mortality of GVHD, thus establishing TNF as an important mediator of GVHD. Anti-TNF in human systems was applied as well (32).

Tissue cell damage

Although acute GVHD involves primarily the cytolytic function of cytotoxic T cells, large granular lymphocytes and NK cells present in the lesions may also be directly involved in tissue damage and necrosis (9,10). Large granular lymphocytes and NK cells do not recognize HLA proteins as targets; however, they are recruited by cytokines released by T cells and macrophages. TNF is well established as a cytokine that causes direct tissue damage in experimental acute GVHD (19,56). Indeed, TNF mRNA is expressed in human blood mononuclear cells (28,29).

Using an in vitro skin explant model, the association between increased levels of TNF and IFN synthesis and the development of GVHD was recently demonstrated (57). In addition, recent experimental data demonstrate that IL-1, a central mediator of inflammation, has an important role in tissue damage secondary of GVHD (7,17,53). IL-1 can increase proliferation of fibroblasts and synoviocytes, and it can cause stimulation of collagenase secretion and prostaglandin synthesis. IL-1 mRNA increased in the skin of a murine model of GVHD and in mononuclear human cells (28,29,33). IL-1RA was able to reduce morbidity and mortality due to GVHD in mice (33).

Only certain tissues and cell types are susceptible to GVHD damage. The sites of attack are essentially the integument, the gastrointestinal mucosa and its extension into the biliary tree, and the exocrine glands. The bone marrow compartment and especially megakaryocyte production can also be affected in severe cases of GVHD, resulting in a grave prognosis (8–10).

The common features of the target structures attacked by GVHD are first, the ability to express HLA-DR (class II) antigens, and second, high cell turnover. Cytokines such as TNF and IL-1 cause a large number of endothelial cell changes that might enhance the tissue destruction associated with GVHD. TNF and IL-1 can cause cell death either by activation of phospholipase A_2 or by production of intracellular hydroxyl radicals (58,59). It is believed that TNF and IL-1 production can stimulate the release of chemotactic factors that recruit secondary cellular effector cells, such as NK cells and macrophages that may produce IFN and display enhanced cytolytic activity against host tissues. Elevated levels of IFN mRNA have recently been demonstrated in mice models of GVHD (60).

In addition, viral or other infections, or any process

that causes inflammation (e.g., ultraviolet and direct sunlight), may promote target cell damage in GVHD through activation of effector cells. Induction of IFN production enhances class II antigen expression on epidermal and endothelial cells, which further increases susceptibility to lysis and induces IL-1, TNF, and IL-6 production (61). GVHD may be activated by exciting an immune response to viral antigens expressed on dividing cells sensitive to GVHD attack. Thus, multiple inflammatory cytokines can induce tissue damage either by activating cytotoxic cells to cause direct tissue damage or as a direct mediator of tissue destruction.

Hematopoietic growth factors and GVHD

One of the concerns in using hematopoietic growth factors (HGFs) in the setting of allogeneic BMT was that treatment with the HGFs could accelerate GVHD due to activation and stimulation of donor-immunocompetent cells directly or indirectly. In several studies evaluating granulocyte-macrophage colony-stimulating factor (GM-CSF), G-CSF, and IL-3 levels, no correlation could be found between serum levels and GVHD (12,27,53). It was shown in a mouse model that neither GM-CSF nor G-CSF have a deleterious effect on the incidence or severity of GVHD (53). Moreover, Poutsiaka and colleagues (62) demonstrated the ability of GM-CSF to potentiate the production of IL-1RA, which may theoretically reduce the incidence of clinical GVHD. In the few trials already reported, GM-CSF and G-CSF enhanced neutrophil and leukocyte recovery or function following allogeneic BMT, without increasing the incidence of GVHD (63,64). Prospective evaluation in randomized comparative trials will be needed to evaluate the range of effects of all the clinically applicable biological factors.

Chronic GVHD

Chronic GVHD (cGVHD) resembles connective tissue diseases, and it is especially similar to systemic sclerosis (65). It is believed that the pathophysiological basis for cGVHD is an autoimmune one (10). In contrast to T cells in acute GVHD, which are alloreactive against host alloantigens, T cells in cGVHD are specific for a common determinant of MHC class II molecules (66). These autoreactive T cells can cause the skin abnormalities of cGVHD. cGVHD affects the musculoskeletal system, the synovia, and the exocrine glands. It can also cause lymphopenia and atrophy of lymphoid tissue, as well as a range of multiorgan (e.g., liver, gastrointestinal) symptoms and signs, which frequently resemble chronic autoimmune diseases, such as rheumatoid arthritis, systemic lupus erythematosus, and chronic active hepatitis, among

others (8–10). The autoreactive T cells in cGVHD produce cytokines, such as IL-4 and IFN-γ, which can cause modulation of fibroblasts and synoviocytes, collagen synthesis, and the skin and musculoskeletal manifestation of GVHD (54). In a mouse model of cGVHD, Umland and associates (51) were able to demonstrate the ability of anti-IL-4 therapy to delay both proteinuria and death in cGVHD mice.

In a recent study, Allen and coworkers (54) hypothesized that acute and cGVHD may be associated with differential cytokine production, in light of the recent concept that helper T cells (Th) may be divided into two types based on their cytokine secretion profile and their ability to mediate cellular (Th1) or humoral (Th2) immunity. They were able to demonstrate that IL-4, IL-10, IFN-γ, TNF-α, and macrophage inflammatory protein-1-α (MIP-1-α) are differentially expressed in acute and cGVHD (54). In another recent study, a significant difference in serum TNF-α levels was found between patients with cGVHD and patients without cGVHD. Furthermore, it was suggested that TNF release was influenced by development of cGVHD (67).

NEW MODES OF THERAPY

Traditional prophylaxis and treatment of GVHD is based on immunosuppressive agents, such as cyclosporine A, methotrexate, and steroids. A new range of immunosuppressive modalities is now being investigated, such as FK506 and deoxyspermoqualin, among others (4,8–10). However, this type of treatment is not specific: it causes additional immunosuppression in severely immunosuppressed patients, and it is associated with increased risk of fulminant infections and secondary malignancies. Moreover, methotrexate administration may lead to delayed hematopoietic reconstitution, and, together with cyclosporine A, it may be associated with an increased risk of relapse (68,69). In view of the role of immune T lymphocytes in induction of GVHD, previous attempts to prevent or treat acute GVHD were focused on depletion of T cells or well-defined T-cell subsets, such as CD3+, CD5+, and CD8+ cells (70,71). Commercial gammaglobulin may also eliminate or block subsets of active cells with Fc receptors (72,73).

In view of the possible major role of cytokine dysregulation in the pathophysiology of GVHD, blocking of cytokine bioactivity is emerging as a possible mode of therapy in GVHD. The new development of human anti-cytokine antibodies, or "cytokine antagonists," has led to development of a range of new therapeutic strategies. Herve and colleagues (40) treated patients with steroid-resistant acute GVHD with anti-IL-2R (CD25) (B-B10) monoclonal antibody with some encouraging results. Recently, clinical trials with human forms of anti-IL-2R antibodies have been started in Seattle. Antibodies directed against TNF have been demonstrated in clinical trials as being capable of temporarily abrogating steroid-resistant GVHD, and the results show promise (32).

The importance of IL-1 in GVHD has been discussed, and ongoing research focuses on evaluating different ways to block IL-1 (7,17). Antisense IL-1 prevents cultured endothelial cells from their programmed cell apoptosis (74). Intracellular IL-1RA shows similar effects on keratinocytes (75). An IL-1–specific inhibitory molecule (different than IL-1RA) (52–56 kd) secreted from the M20 human myelomonocytic cell line has been described (76).

Recently, a third member of the IL-1 gene family, known as an IL-1RA, has been purified and cloned (77). IL-1RA has been shown to prevent GVHD in a murine model without impeding immunological and hematopoietic reconstitution (33). Recently, clinical Phase I/II trials with IL-1RA for steroid-resistant GVHD have been started at the Children's Hospital and Brigham and Women's Hospital in Boston. New cytokine antagonists used as single agents or in combination should be investigated in experimental animals, pending successful results in pilot clinical trials.

CYTOKINES AND GRAFT REJECTION

Graft rejection represents a major obstacle in allogeneic BMT, especially following T-cell depletion (4,34,35). There is an inverse relationship between graft rejection and GVHD (5). Regardless of the method used for elimination of T lymphocytes, adequately depleted marrow allografts are extremely susceptible to rejection, even when no MHC disparity exists between donor and host (5). Residual host-immunocompetent cells that escape the immunosuppressive conditioning regimen are most probably responsive.

There is no agreement with regard to the optimal conditioning necessary to prevent rejection of T-cell–depleted allografts. Additional immunosuppression of residual host-immunocompetent cells (e.g., T lymphocytes, NK cells, macrophages, and perhaps other antigen-presenting cells) by more intensive radiation therapy (e.g., total body or total lymphoid irradiation; perhaps, in vivo, effective monoclonal antibodies, such as the Campath-1[15] or one of the newest immunosuppressive modalities) may be of help (44).

Biological agents may be much more effective and are far less toxic in accomplishing durable engraftment, as suggested by several studies in experimental animals and pilot clinical investigations. Monoclonal antilymphocyte

antibodies and antibodies against other lymphocyte functions (i.e., anti-lymphocyte function antigen-1 [LFA-1] antibodies, antibodies against NK cells [anti-asialo GM1 in mice]), might help overcome the rejection episodes after clinical BMT (78).

Cytokines, predominantly IL-2, are thought to have a central role in the allospecific components of the cascade of the allograft rejection reaction as a result of recruitment of other cells. The inflammatory cytokines, TNF-α, IL-1, and IL-6, may also promote induction of adhesion molecules, as well as recruitment of immunocompetent cells to the allograft; in some patients, they may directly damage the graft (79,80). A correlation between serum levels of IL-6 and engraftment was recently suggested (81).

Immunoregulatory cytokines, including IL-2, IL-4, and IFN-γ, can provide activation of growth and differentiation signals to the residual host-immunocompetent cells (T cells, NK cells, and macrophages), which are the effector cells in the allograft rejection process (52,55,82). In addition, IFN-γ may enhance MHC antigen expression on the allograft tissue, thus augmenting the immunogenicity of the graft with secondary cytotoxic attack and graft elimination (51).

Elevated levels of TNF-α, IL-1, IL-6, and IL-2 were detected in the circulation during rejection episodes (79–87). Increased levels of IL-6 mRNA were demonstrated by in situ hybridization of biopsies from kidneys undergoing acute rejection (87), whereas IL-5 gene expression was recently shown to be predominantly present in biopsies from liver allografts with histopathological evidence of acute rejection (79). Thus, rejection prevention and treatment may be achieved by targeting the cytokine network to minimize activity of cytokines that have a role in initiation or propagation of alloreactivity; by maximizing the effects of cytokines that may be involved in induction of tolerance or host immunosuppression, such as IL-10 produced by Th-2; or by activating cytokines that may enhance engraftment of donor cells.

At an early stage following BMT, IL-2 may enhance acceptance of allografts by some direct effects of T-cell subsets, as we have recently shown (88–90). Enforcement of the donor's hematopoietic cells by GM-CSF, G-CSF, IL-3, IL-6, or combinations of these agents may also enhance engraftment of T-cell–depleted marrow allografts (91), but convincing data in humans have not yet been published. Enhancement of bone marrow engraftment by infusion of in vitro cytokine-activated marrow progenitor cells may also facilitate marrow engraftment (92–95). Alternatively, using anti-IL-2 or anti-IL-2 receptor antibody, as well as anti-TNF-α, anti-IL-1, or anti-IFN-γ compounds or antibodies, produced some encouraging results in preventing graft rejection in animal models; their applicability and efficacy in clinical practice, however, has yet to be proven (30,96–100).

SUMMARY

Both graft rejection and GVHD represent major obstacles in allogeneic BMT. GVHD is induced by donor-immuno-competent T cells, whereas graft rejection is induced by residual host-immunocompetent cells. Effective prevention of GVHD can be accomplished by pretransplant depletion of donor T cells, whereas graft rejection can be prevented in the majority of transplant recipients by aggressive conditioning that eliminates host immune cells. Unfortunately, elimination of both GVHD and graft rejection is somewhat difficult to achieve, and it may be accompanied by reduction of graft-versus-leukemia effects and increased incidence of graft rejection because of the inverse relationship between the two.

Because a cascade of cytokines is actively involved in differentiation and activation of effector cells of GVHD and graft rejection, regulation of acceptance or tolerogenic signals and donor regulation of alloreactivity of host-versus-graft as well as graft-versus-host may be achieved by positive or negative feedback of cytokines, respectively.

The inflammatory cytokines (i.e., TNF-α, IL-1, IL-6) and the immunoregulatory cytokines, including IL-2, IL-4, IFN, and many more currently under investigation, have major roles in promoting the allospecific components of GVHD and graft rejection, as well as in the nonspecific secondary inflammatory response. Understanding of both processes and the ability to control them will be greatly increased with further understanding of the nature of cytokine dysregulation. Recent experiments in animal models and pilot clinical trials look promising. Systemic administration of cytokine antagonists (e.g., anti-IL2 receptor antibodies or toxin conjugates, anti-TNF, anti-IL-1 receptor antibodies, IL-1 receptor antibodies) yielded encouraging results. Combinations of these and other agents that may block cell adhesion, homing, and costimulatory signals essential for immunorectivity may permit down-regulation of production and biological reactivity of pathogenic cytokines.

A better understanding of cell interaction and cytokine biology, and further advances in down- or up-regulation of cytokine bioactivity will prove applicable to improving the outcome following allogeneic BMT and organ transplantation, as well as in naturally occurring autoimmune diseases caused by autoreactivity.

REFERENCES

1. Thomas ED. The role of marrow transplantation in the eradication of malignant disease. Cancer 1982;49:1963–1969.

2. O'Reilly RJ. Allogeneic bone marrow transplantation: current status and future directions. Blood 1983;62:941–964.

3. Slavin S, ed. Bone marrow and organ transplantation: achievements and goals. Amsterdam: Elsevier, 1984.

4. Slavin S, Nagler A. New developments in bone marrow transplantation. Curr Opin Oncol 1991;33:254–271.

5. Slavin S, Or R, Naparstek E, et al. New approaches for prevention of rejection and graft vs. host disease (GVHD) in clinical bone marrow transplantation (BMT). Isr J Med Sci 1986;22:264–267.

6. Abrams JS, Roncarolo MG, Yssel H, Andersson U, Gleich GJ, Silver JE. Strategies of anti-cytokine monoclonal antibody development: immunoassay of IL-10 and IL-5 in clinical samples. Immunol Rev 1992;127:5–24.

7. Dinarello CA. Anti-cytokine strategies. In: Ghezzi P, Mantovani A, eds. Progress in biomedical research, vol. 2. Pathophysiology and pharmacology of cytokines. Augusta: Biomedical Press, 1992:159–166.

8. Barrett AJ. Graft versus host disease—clinical features and biology. Bone Marrow Transplant 1989;4:18–22.

9. De Gast GC, Gratama JW, Ringden O, Gluckman E. The multifactorial etiology of graft versus host disease. Immunol Today 1987;8:209–212.

10. Ferrara JLM, Deeg HJD. Graft versus host disease. N Engl J Med 1991;324:667–674.

11. Antin JH, Ferrara JLM. Cytokine dysregulation and acute graft-versus-host disease. Blood 1992;80:2964–2968.

12. Rabinowitz J, Petros WP, Stuart AR, Peters WP. Characterization of endogenous cytokine concentrations after high-dose chemotherapy with autologous bone marrow support. Blood 1993;81:2452–2459.

13. Jadus MR, Wepsic HJ. The role of cytokines in graft-versus-host reactions and disease. Bone Marrow Transplant 1992;10:1–14.

14. Weisdorf D, Hakke R, Blazar B, et al. Risk factors for acute graft-versus-host disease in histocompatible donor bone marrow transplantation. Transplantation 1991;51:1197–1203.

15. Naparstek E, Or R, Nagler A, et al. Allogeneic bone marrow transplantation for leukemia using compath-1 monoclonal antibodies and post transplant alloimmunization with donor lymphocytes (abstract). Exp Hematol 1993;21:1061.

16. Peled T, Rigel M, Peritt D, et al. Effect of M20 interleukin-1 inhibitor on normal and leukemic human myeloid progenitors. Blood 1991;19:103–108.

17. Barak V, Peritt D, Flechner I, et al. The M20 IL-1 inhibitor prevents and reduces rheumatoid arthritis and IL-1 induced inflammatory response in vivo. In: Ghezzi P, Mantovani A, eds. Progress in biomedical research, vol 2. Pathophysiology and pharmacology of cytokines. Augusta: Biomedical Press, 1992:257–263.

18. Pechumer H, Leinisch E, Bender-Gotzec, Ziegler-Heitbrock HW. Recovery of monocytes after bone marrow transplantation. Rapid reappearance of tumor necrosis factor alpha and interleukin 6 production. Transplantation 1991;52:698–704.

19. Piguet PF, Grau GE, Allet B, Vassalli P. Tumor necrosis factor/cachectin is an effector of skin and gut lesions of the acute phase of graft-versus-host disease. J Exp Med 1987;166:1280–1289.

20. Norton J, Sloane JP. ICAM-1 expression of epidermal

keratinocytes in cutaneous graft-versus-host disease. Transplantation 1991;51:1203–1206.

21. Helmer ME. Adhesive protein receptors on hematopoietic cells. Immunol Today 1988;9:109–113.

22. Porat R, Clark BD, Wolf SM, Dinarello CA. Enhancement of growth of virulent Escherichia coli by interleukin-1. Science 1991;254:431.

23. Smith SR, Terminelli C, Kenworthy-Bott L, Phillips DL. A study of cytokine production in acute graft versus host disease. Cell Immunol 1991;134:336–348.

24. Holler E, Kolb HJ, Möller A, et al. Increased serum levels of tumor necrosis factor alpha precede major complications of bone marrow transplantation. Blood 1990;75:1011–1016.

25. Symington FW, Pepe MS, Chen A, Deliganis A. Serum tumor necrosis factor alpha associated with acute graft-versus-host disease in humans. Transplantation 1990;50:518–521.

26. Cohen J. Cytokines as mediators of graft-versus-host disease. Bone Marrow Transplant 1988;3:193–197.

27. Tong S, Viale M, Bacigalupo A, et al. Cytokine serum levels and acute graft versus host disease after allogeneic bone marrow transplantation. Hematologica 1992;77:365–366.

28. Parkman R, Lenarsky C, Santos R, Barrantes B, Weinberg K. Cytokines during acute graft-versus-host disease (GVHD) following matched unrelated donor (MUD) transplantation (abstract). Blood 1991;78(suppl 1): 286.

29. Weinberg K, Lawrence K, Barrantos B, Lenarsky C, Parkman R. The role of cytokines in the pathogenesis of human graft-versus-host disease (abstract). Exp Hematol 1992;20:717.

30. Bianco JA, Appelbaum FR, Nemunaitis J, et al. Phase I-II trial of pentoxifylline for the prevention of transplanted-related toxicities following bone marrow transplantation. Blood 1991;78:1205–1211.

31. Keetter Y, Singer A, Nagler A, Slavin S, Fabian I. Ciprofloxacin enhances hematopoiesis and the antibacterial activity of peritoneal polymorphonuclears in lethally irradiated bone marrow transplanted mice. Exp Hematol 1994;22:360–365.

32. Herve P, Flesch M, Tiberghien P, et al. Phase I-II trial of a monoclonal anti TNF alpha antibody (B-C7) in the treatment of refractory severe acute GVHD. Blood 1992;79: 3362–3368.

33. McCarthy PL, Abhyanhan S, Neben S, et al. Inhibition of interleukin-1 by an interleukin-1 receptor antagonist prevents graft-versus-host disease. Blood 1991;78:1915–1918.

34. Prentice HG, Blacklock HA, Janossy G, et al. Depletion of T lymphocytes in donor marrow prevents significant graft-versus-host disease in matched allogeneic leukaemic marrow transplant recipients. Lancet 1984;1:472–476.

35. Waldmann H, Polliack, A, Hale G, et al. Elimination of graft-versus-host disease by in-vitro depletion of alloreactive lymphocytes with a monoclonal anti-human lymphocyte antibody (Campath-1). Lancet 1984;2:483–486.

36. Yatsiv I, Weiss L, Ekerstein A, Slavin S. Potential role of in vivo recombinant IL-2 in allogeneic BMT. Proceedings of the XVI Meeting of International Society for Experimental Hematology 1987;15:595.

37. Nagler A, Ackerstein A, Barak V, Slavin S. Concomitant treatment of chronic myelogenous leukemia with recombinant human Interleukin-2 and Interferon-alpha 2a. Hematotherapy 1994;3:75–82.

38. Engelhard D, Nagler A, Singer R, Barak V. Soluble interleukin-2 receptor levels in cytomegalovirus disease and graft-versus-host disease after T-lymphocyte depleted bone marrow transplantation. Leuk Lymphoma 1994;12:273–280.

39. Siegert W, Josimovic-Alasevic O, Schwerdtfeger R, et al. Soluble interleukin 2 receptors in patients after bone marrow transplantation. Bone Marrow Transplant 1990;6:97–101.

40. Herve P, Wijdenes J, Bergerat JP, et al. Treatment of corticosteroid resistant acute graft-versus-host disease by in vivo administration of anti-interleukin-2 receptor monoclonal antibody (B-B10). Blood 1990;75:1017–1023.

41. LeMaistre CF, Meneghetti C, Rosenblum M, et al. Phase I trial of an interleukin-2 (IL-2) fusion toxin (DAB486IL-2) in hematologic malignancies expressing the IL-2 receptor. Blood 1992;79:2547–2554.

42. Chaudhary VK, Queen C, Junghans RP, Waldmann TA, Fitzgerald DJ, Pastan I. A recombinant immunotoxin consisting of two antibody variable domains fused Pseudomonas exotoxin. Nature 1989;339:394–397.

43. Ogata M, Lorberboum-Galski H, Fitzgerald D, Pastan I. IL-2-PE40 is cytotoxic for activated T lymphocytes expressing IL-2 receptors. J Immunol 1988;141:4224–4228.

44. Waldmann H. Immunosuppression with monoclonal antibodies: some speculation about tolerance in the context of tissue grafting. Transplant Proc 1988;20:46–52.

45. Stewart FM, Quesenberry PJ, Jones-Garrison S, Grosh W, Wheby MS. Sequential growth factor assays following bone marrow transplantation (BMT) (abstract). Exp Hematol 1993;21:1174.

46. Reyes VE, Klimpel GR. Interferon alpha/beta synthesis during acute graft-versus-host disease. Transplantation 1987;43:412–416.

47. Givon T, Slavin S, Hanan-Ghera N, Michalevicz R, Ravel M. Antitumor effects of human recombinant interleukin-6 on acute myeloid leukemia in mice and in cell cultures. Blood 1992;79:1–6.

48. Morecki S, Nagler A, Puyesky Y, et al. Effect of various cytokine combinations on induction of non-MHC-restricted cytotoxicity. Lymphokine Cytokine 1993;12:159–165.

49. Nagler A, Engelhard D, Good RA. Immunity to infection. In: Spirer Z, Rofman C, Branski D, eds. Pediatric and adolescent medicine; pediatric immunology 3. Basel: Karger, 1992:93–101.

50. Symington FW, Symington RE, Lin PY, Viguet H, Santhanam U, Shegal PB. The relationship of serum IL-6 levels to acute graft-versus-host-disease and hepatorenal disease after human bone marrow transplantation. Transplantation 1992;54:457–462.

51. Umland SP, Razac S, Nahrebne DK, Seymour BW. Effects of in vivo administration of interferon (IFN)-gamma, anti-IFN-gamma, or anti-interleukin-4 monoclonal antibodies in chronic autoimmune graft-versus-host disease. Clin Immunol Immunopathol 1992;63:66–73.

52. Nagler A, Lanier LL, Phillips JH. The effects of interleukin-4 on human natural killer cells: a potent regulator of interleukin-2 activation and proliferation. J Immunol 1988;141: 2349–2351.

53. Atkinson K, Matias C. Guiffre A, et al. In vivo administration of G-CSF, GM-CSF, IL-1 and IL-4, alone and in combination, after allogeneic murine hematopoietic stem cell transplantation. Blood 1991;77:1376–1382.

54. Allen RD, Staley TA, Sidman CL. Differential cytokine expression in acute and chronic murine graft-versus-host disease. Eur J Immunol 1993;23:333–337.

55. Nagler A, Lanier L, Cwirla S, Phillips J. Comparative studies of human FcR III-positive and negative NK cells. J Immunol 1989;143:3183–3191.

56. Piguet PF, Grau GE, Collart MA, Vassalli P, Kapauci Y. Pneumopathies of graft-versus-host reaction. Alveolitis associated with an increased level of tumor necrosis factor mRNA and chronic interstitial pneumonitis. Lab Invest 1989;61:37–45.

57. Dickinson AM, Sviland L, Dunn J, Carey P, Proctor SJ. Demonstration of direct involvement of cytokines in graft-versus-host reactions using an in vitro skin explant model. Bone Marrow Transplant 1991;7:209.

58. Neale ML, Fiera RA, Matthews N. Involvement of phospholipase A_2 in tumor cell killing by tumor necrosis factor. Immunology 1988;64:81–85.

59. Yamauchi N, Kumiyama H, Watanabe N, Neda H, Maeda M, Niitsu Y. Intracellular hydroxyl radical production induced by recombinant tumor necrosis factor and its implication in the killing of tumor cells in vitro. Cancer Res 1989;49:1671–1675.

60. Troutt AB, Kelso A. Enumeration of lymphokine mRNA containing cells in vivo in murine graft-versus-host reaction using the PCR. Proc Natl Acad Sci USA 1992;89:5276–5279.

61. Almeida GD, Pomada C, St. Jear S, Ascensao JL. Modulation of hematopoietic cytokines by human cytomegalovirus (abstract). Exp Hematol 1993;211:1183.

62. Poutsiaka DD, Clark BD, Vannier E, Dinarello CA. Production of interleukin-1 receptor antagonist and interleukin 1β by peripheral blood mononuclear cells is differentially regulated. Blood 1991;78:1275–1279.

63. Kitayama H, Ishikawa J, Yamagami T, et al. Granulocyte colony-stimulating factor in allogeneic bone marrow transplantation. Jpn J Clin Oncol 1989;19:367–372.

64. Nemunaitis J, Anasetti C, Appelbaum F, et al. Phase I/II trial of rhGM-CSF after allogeneic bone marrow transplantation (BMT). Blood 1989;74:123–127.

65. Levi-Schaffer F, Segal V, Nagler A. Mast cell and fibroblast functional activity are affected by immunocompetent cells in chronic graft versus host disease. Int Arch Allergy Appl Immunol 1992;99:238–242.

66. Parkman R. Clonal analysis of murine graft-versus-host disease: phenotypic and functional analysis of T lymphocyte clones. J Immunol 1986;46:3543–3548.

67. Fujii Y, Kaku K, Kaneko T. Tumor necrosis factor-alpha associated with chronic graft-versus-host disease in bone marrow transplantation recipients. Bone Marrow Transplant 1992;10:194–195.

68. Storb R, Deeg HJ, Whitehead J, et al. Methotrexate and cyclosporine compared with cyclosporine alone for prophylaxis of acute graft versus host disease after marrow transplantation for leukemia. N Engl J Med 1986;314:729–735.

69. Horowitz MM, Gale RP, Sondel PM, et al. Graft-versus-leu-

kemia reactions after bone marrow transplantation. Blood 1990;75:555–562.

70. Martin PJ, Hansen JA, Anasetti C, et al. Treatment of acute graft versus host disease with anti-CD3 monoclonal antibodies. Am J Kidney Dis 1989;11:149–152.

71. Pico JL, Knentz M, Herte P, et al. Efficacy of monoclonal antibodies (mAB) CD5+ CD8 for the treatment of steroid resistant graft versus host disease. Bone Marrow Transplant 1989;4:68–71.

72. Ringden O, Deeg HJ, Beschorner W, Slavin S. Effector cells of graft-versus-host disease, host resistance and the graft-versus-leukemia effect. Transplant Proc 1987;19:2758–2761.

73. Weiss L, Weigensberg M, Morecki S, Bar S, Cobbold S, Waldmann H, Slavin S. Characterization of effector cells of graft vs leukemia (GVL) following allogeneic bone marrow transplantation in mice inoculated with murine B-cell leukemia (BCL1). Cancer Immunol Immunother 1990;31:236–242.

74. Maier JAM, Voulalos P, Roeder D, Maciag J. Extension of the life span of human endothelial cells by an interleukin-1 alpha antisense oligomer. Science 1990;249:1570–1574.

75. Haskill S, Martin M, Vanle L, et al. cDNA cloning of novel form of the interleukin-1 receptor antagonist associated with epithelium. Proc Natl Acad Sci USA 1991;88:3681–3685.

76. Barak V, Treves AJ, Yanai P, et al. Interleukin-1 inhibitory activity secreted by a human myelomonocytic cell line (M20). Eur J Immunol 1986;16:1449–1452.

77. Dinarello CA, Thompson RC. Blocking IL-1: effects of IL-1 receptor antagonist in vitro and in vivo. Immunol Today 1991;12:404–410.

78. Fischer A, Blanche S, Veber F, et al. Prevention of graft failure by an anti LFA-1 monoclonal antibody in HLA-mismatched bone marrow transplantation. Lancet 4986;2:1058.

79. Martinez OM, Krans SM, Sterneck M, et al. Intragraft cytokine profile during human liver allograft rejection. Transplantation 1992;53:449–456.

80. Maury CP, Teppo AM. Raised serum levels of cachectin/tumor necrosis factor alpha in renal allograft rejection. J Exp Med 1987;166:1132–1137.

81. Ballester OF, Jannsen WJ, Perkins JB, Farmelo MJ, Smilee R. Serum interleukin-6 levels and marrow engraftment after high dose chemotherapy and autologous stem cell transplantation (abstract). Exp Hematol 1993;21:1174.

82. Nathan CF, Murray HW, Wiebe ME, Rubin BY. Identification of interferon gamma as the lymphokine that activates human macrophage oxidative metabolism and antimicrobial activity. J Exp Med 1983;158:670–689.

83. Imagawa DK, Millis JM, Olthoff KM, et al. The role of tumor necrosis factor in allograft rejection. I. Evidence that elevated levels of tumor necrosis factor-alpha predict rejection following orthotopic liver transplantation. Transplantation 1990;50:219–225.

84. Maury CP, Teppo AM. Serum immunoreactive interleukin 1 in renal transplant recipients. Transplantation 1988;45:143–147.

85. Van Oers MH, Van der Heyden AA, Aarden LA. Interleukin-6 (IL-6) in serum and urine of renal transplant recipients. Clin Exp Immunol 1988;71:314–319.

86. Simpson MA, Madras PN, Cornaby AJ, et al. Sequential determinations of urinary cytology and plasma and urinary lymphokines in the management of renal allograft recipients. Transplantation 1989;47:218–223.

87. Vandenbroecke C, Caillat-Zucman S, Legendre C, et al. Differential in situ expression of cytokines in renal allograft rejection. Transplantation 1991;51:602–609.

88. Leshem B, Tsuberi B, Lebendiker Z, Weiss L, Slavin S, Kedar E. The role of bone marrow (BM) T cells in immunological reconstitution of allogeneic BM chimeras. J Cell Biochem 1986;(suppl 10):231.

89. Nagler A, Samuel S, Or R, Slavin S. Effects of interleukin-2 on engraftment following autologous bone marrow transplantation (ABMT) in dogs. Leuk Res 1992;16:967–972.

90. Bieder A, Weiss L, Slavin S. The role of recombinant cytokines and other immunomodulators on engraftment following allogeneic bone marrow transplantation in mice. Bone Marrow Transplant 1992;9:421–426.

91. Kedar E, Tsuberi B, Landesberg A, et al. In vitro and in vivo cytokine-induced facilitation of immunohematopoietic reconstitution in mice undergoing BMT. Bone Marrow Transplant 1988;3:297–314.

92. Slavin S, Mumcuoglu M, Landesberg-Weiss A, Kedar E. The use of recombinant cytokines for enhancing immunohematopoietic reconstitution following bone marrow transplantation: I. Effects of in-vitro culturing with IL-3 and GM-CSF on human and mouse bone marrow cells purged with mafosfamide (ASTA-Z). Bone Marrow Transplant 1989;4:459–464.

93. Mumcuoglu M, Naparstek E, Slavin S. The use of recombinant cytokines for enhancing immuno-hematopoietic reconstitution following bone marrow transplantation: II. The influence of lymphokines on CFU-GM colonies from human untreated, ASTA-Z or Campath-IM treated bone marrow. Bone Marrow Transplant 1990;5:153–158.

94. Naparstek E, Hardan Y, Nagler A, et al. Enhanced marrow recovery by short preincubation of marrow allografts with human recombinant IL-3 and GM-CSF. Blood 1992;80:1673–1678.

95. Nagler A, Deutch V, Naparstek E, Mumcuoglu M, Slavin S, Eldor A. Ex-vivo treatment of marrow allografts with IL-3 and GM-CSF enhances in vitro megakaryocytopoiesis and improves thrombopoiesis in vivo (abstract). Exp Hematol 1993;21:1023.

96. Sykes M, Romick HL, Hayles KA, Sachs DH. In vivo administration of interleukin-2 plus T cell-depleted syngeneic marrow prevents graft-versus-host disease mortality and permits alloengraftment. J Exp Med 1990;171:645–658.

97. Imagawa DK, Millis JM, Olthoff KM, et al. Anti-tumor necrosis factor antibody enhances allograft survival in rats. J Surg Res 1990;48:345–348.

98. Rosenberg AS, Finbloom DS, Maniero TG, Van der Meide PH, Singer A. Specific prolongation of MHC class II disparate skin allografts by in vivo administration of anti-IFN-gamma monoclonal antibody. J Immunol 1990;144:4650.

99. Fanslow WC, Sims JE, Sassenfeld H, et al. Regulation of alloreactivity in vivo by soluble form of the interleukin-1 receptor. Science 1990;248:739–742.

100. Kupiec-Weglinski JW, Diamantstein T, Tilney NL. Interleukin-2 receptor-targeted therapy-rationale and application in organ transplantation. Transplantation 1988;46:785–792.

CHAPTER 10

ROLE OF CYTOKINES
IN ORGAN TRANSPLANT REJECTION

David K. Imagawa, Ronald W. Busuttil, and Douglas G. Farmer

Solid organ transplantation has become an established therapy for end-stage organ failure related to a number of disease processes. In Chapter 9, the role of cytokines in bone marrow transplantation is examined. Current studies are directed both at quantitation of cytokine levels to establish the diagnosis of infection or rejection, and at use of anticytokine antibodies to prevent or to treat acute rejection. In this chapter, information is presented on kidney, liver, heart, lung, pancreas, islet cell, and small bowel transplantation, with emphasis on human clinical studies.

THE REJECTION RESPONSE

The exact mechanism of allograft rejection remains undetermined, and it is beyond the scope of this discussion. Although basic immunology will be reviewed herein, for more comprehensive information, readers are directed to more detailed sources (1–4). Although antibody-mediated processes are known to be important in some forms of allograft rejection (i.e., hyperacute rejection and possibly chronic rejection), most episodes of acute rejection are mediated by a cellular, lymphocyte response. This response appears to be predominately directed against the major histocompatibility complex (MHC) antigens, which in humans are known as the human leukocyte antigen (HLA) complex, and they are located on the short arm of chromosome 6 (5). This complex encodes for four classes of genes, two of which have major roles in allograft rejection. The class I products (HLA-A, HLA-B, HLA-C) are expressed on virtually all cells except erythrocytes. Class II products (HLA-DR, HLA-DP, HLA-DQ) are found on B cells, monocytes, macrophages, and dendritic cells.

MHC restriction in the recognition of foreign antigen was first described by Zinkernagal and Doherty in 1974 (6). Foreign proteins are processed by antigen-presenting cells (APCs) into fragments that then bind to the MHC complex on the surface of APCs. These cells, known as dendritic or Langerhans cells, are derived from monocyte/macrophage lineage. This antigen-MHC complex is then recognized and bound by receptors on the surface of T cells. T-cell activation occurs when this signal is received in conjunction with an inductive molecule produced by the APC. In this situation, activation of T cells is restricted to antigen presented in association with self-MHC molecules.

Direct presentation of alloantigen also occurs. It appears that the foreign MHC complex on transplanted tissue can act as both the presenting molecule and the foreign antigen (2). If the foreign cell is of an immunological background, it may also produce the inductive molecule needed for activation (1). Foreign antigen associated with MHC class II molecules are bound by helper/inducer T cells that express the CD4 complex. Cytotoxic/suppressor T cells carry the CD8 complex, and they associate with class I MHC antigens.

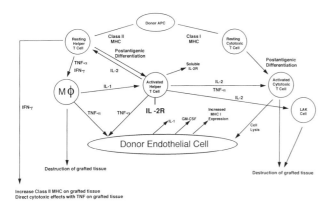

Figure 10–1. Steps involved in the development of mature T lymphocytes and in allograft rejection.

Activated T helper cells produce macrophage-activating factor (interferon-γ [IFN-γ]), which stimulates macrophages to produce interleukin-1 (IL-1) and to develop cytotoxic activity. Alternatively, the macrophage may function as the APC and be directly stimulated by foreign antigen (Fig. 10–1).

The major function of IL-1 is to trigger the proliferation of CD4+ T cells. In addition, IL-1 in association with IL-4 and IL-6, promotes B-cell growth and differentiation; increases cytotoxicity of natural killer cells; increases production of platelet-activating factor by macrophages; and has macrophage chemotactic effects (7).

Activated CD4+ T cells produce IL-2, which leads to recruitment and proliferation of new CD4+ cells. IL-2 also stimulates proliferation and differentiation of CD8+ cytotoxic T cells. A third population of non-B, non-T lymphocytes (i.e., lymphokine-activated killer cells [LAK]) are also stimulated by IL-2. Both cytotoxic T cells and LAK cells appear to actively participate in allograft destruction. (8).

In addition to IL-2 production, activated T cells begin to synthesize and express increased numbers of IL-2 receptors (IL-2R), which provides a feedback mechanism that further augments the response of these cells to increased IL-2 production (9).

A number of other cytokines are produced in increased amounts by activated T cells. IL-3 regulates proliferation and differentiation of pluripotent hematopoietic and lymphoid precursors (10). IL-4 possesses a broad spectrum of in vitro activities, which include increase in expression of MHC class II antigens on B cells; stimulate generation of cytotoxic T cells and LAK cells; and stimulate proliferation of myeloid lineage cells (11). IL-6, which appears to be the primary mediator of the acute-phase response, is induced by both tumor necrosis factor-α (TNF-α) and IL-1 (12). This mediator appears to enhance the development of cytotoxic T cells (13), and it appears to be an essential B-cell growth factor (14). IL-6, or an IL-6–induced product, has also been implicated in enhancing the expression of class I and class II MHC antigens (15,16).

IFN-γ appears to increase allograft reactivity by increasing the expression of β₂-microglobulin, which is coexpressed with HLA class I antigens (17). In addition, IFN-γ appears to stimulate expression of class II antigens on cells that do not normally express these markers (e.g., parenchymal cells, bile duct epithelial cells, vascular endothelial cells) (7). This effect is particularly augmented in the presence of TNF-α (18).

TNF-α and tumor necrosis factor-β (TNF-β; or lymphotoxin [LT]) have recently received attention as major mediators of the rejection process. The molecules share 36% identity and 51% homology in their overall amino acid sequence (19); they also share a common receptor binding domain (20). Although most studies have utilized TNF-α, it would appear that both molecules exert similar immunological effects (21).

Synthesis of TNF from monocytes is enhanced by IL-2 both in vitro and in vivo (22). In addition to possible direct cytotoxic effects on allograft tissue (23), TNF also (a) induces production of chemotactic factors (i.e., monocyte-activating factor and IL-8) for both monocytes and polymorphonuclear leukocytes (24); (b) induces IL-1 release from macrophages (25); (c) enhances expression of class I MHC antigens on vascular endothelial cells (21); (d) enhances expression of class II MHC antigens on macrophages (21); and (e) stimulates development of cytotoxic T cells (26).

In contrast to TNF, transforming growth factor-β (TGF-β) down-regulates the inflammatory response by causing (a) decreased IL-2 receptor expression; (b) decreased IL-2–induced T-cell proliferation; (c) decreased cytotoxic T-cell and LAK cell generation; and (d) decreased MHC class II antigen expression (27).

The cytokine response following foreign antigen stimulation ultimately leads to allograft destruction. This destruction is accompanied by an intense cellular infiltration of T cells, macrophages, and polymorphonuclear leukocytes. Activation of CD8+ cytotoxic T cells leads to lysis of cells through direct contact; this response is class I MHC antigen–restricted. Eicosanoids and reactive oxygen intermediates produced by activated macrophages also lead to cell death. Secondary effects (mediated by cytokines) on platelets and coagulation factors lead to graft ischemia and ultimately irreversible tissue damage. Finally, TNF and perhaps IL-1 and IFN-γ may have direct nonspecific cell necrosis capability (7,23).

IMMUNOSUPPRESSIVE AGENTS

Chemical manipulation of the immune response has become the mainstay of current clinical immunosuppression. Unfortunately, this manipulation is nonspecific, and it decreases the immune response against bacteria, virus, fungus, and malignant tumors. Therefore, continuing research is directed at developing more selective agents with fewer side effects.

Azathioprine

The immunosuppressive potential of 6-mercaptopurine, a purine analogue antimetabolite, on canine renal allografts was demonstrated by Calne and associates (28) in 1959. Subsequently, azathioprine (Imuran; Burroughs Wellcome, Research Triangle Park, NC), an analogue suitable for parenteral administration, was synthesized by Hitchings and Elion (29). The mechanism of immunosuppression is to interdict mitosis of stimulated lymphoid cells by interfering with nucleotide synthesis. The major side effect is severe leukopenia from myelosuppression.

Corticosteroids

The anti-inflammatory effects of corticosteroids were first appreciated by Glaser and colleagues (30). Subsequently, the synergistic effects of steroids with azathioprine were appreciated (31). The mechanism of immunosuppression is inhibition of antigen-driven T-cell proliferation by blocking release of IL-1 from monocytes (32).

Cyclosporine

Cyclosporine (CsA) is a metabolite of the fungal species *Tolypocladium inflatum Gams,* and it was discovered by Sandoz Ltd. in 1972. As seen in Fig. 10–2, the compound is a neutral hydrophobic cyclic peptide consisting of 11

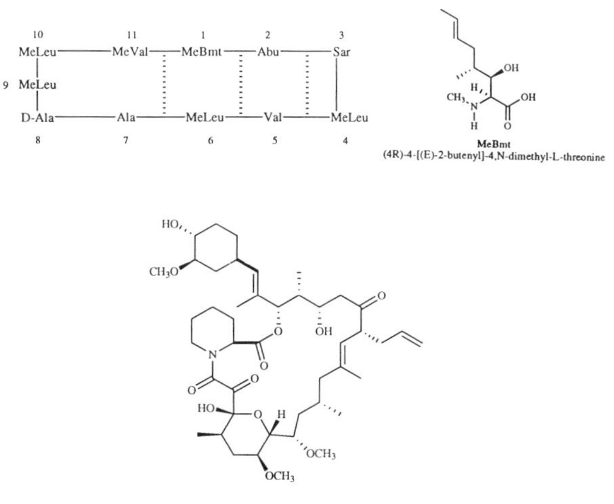

Figure 10–2. Amino acid structure of cyclosporine. The amino acid at position 1 is a novel β-hydroxy, unsaturated 9-carbon amino acid. Also shown is the structure of FK 506. Abu =- α-amino butyric acid; Sar = sarcosine; MeLeu = N-methyl-L-leucine; Val = valine; Ala = L-alanine, D-Ala, D-alanine; MeVal = N-methyl-L-valine.

amino acids. The amino acid at position 1 was previously unknown. The active immunosuppressive site is formed by the amino acids at positions 11, 1, 2, and 3 (33,34).

Although CsA interferes with both B- and T-cell activation, its major effect is interference with the function of helper T cells. This interference is accomplished by inhibiting transcription of the IL-2 gene and therefore the release of IL-2 from activated T cells (35). CsA is also reported to inhibit transcription of IL-3, Il-4, granulocyte-macrophage colony-stimulating factor (GM-CSF), TNF-α, and IFN-γ (36); however, it does not inhibit expression of IL-2R (37) or the responsiveness in vitro or in vivo of activated T cells to exogenous or endogenous cytokines (38). However, other data in mice suggest that CsA inhibits TNF-α production by blocking secretion without depressing either cell-associated TNF (translation) or TNF mRNA (transcription) (39).

Introduction of CsA into clinical practice is one of the foremost developments in organ transplantation. In initial randomized controlled multicenter studies, one-year graft survival rates of 70 to 90% were seen in cadaveric renal transplants; in contrast, standard treatment protocols yielded rates of 50 to 85% (40,41).

Despite the increased engraftment seen with CsA, side effects are common. Even with careful monitoring of serum levels, nephrotoxicity may occur (34). Concomitant rejection may also occur, often making diagnosis difficult. Other side effects include cholestasis, hirsutism, hypertension, and neuropathy. Infection with cytomegalovirus (CMV) or other opportunistic organisms can be life-threatening in immunosuppressed patients (42). Finally, there is a predilection for the development of B-cell lymphoproliferative diseases in patients receiving CsA (43). Treatment involves reduction of the immunosuppressive regimen; spontaneous regression and long-term survival occurs in many patients (44).

FK 506

Tacrolimus (FK 506) is a neutral macrolide isolated from a soil fungus, *Streptomyces tsukubaenis,* by the Fujisawa Pharmaceutical Corporation in 1984 (see Fig. 10–2). FK 506 appears to effect the same common early pathway as CsA on cytokine transcription, but it does so at 10 to 100 times lower doses than CsA (36). Early results following liver and kidney transplantation demonstrated high graft survival and apparently less toxicity than with CsA (45, 46). A randomized trial of FK 506 versus CsA as primary immunosuppression following liver transplantation conducted at the University of Pittsburgh showed that patients who received FK 506 had better graft survival and fewer side effects (47). In addition, a multicenter study recently showed FK 506 to be effective in the treatment of rejection episodes refractory to standard immunotherapy (48).

Initial reports on FK 506 for renal transplantation have also been encouraging (49). At the University of Pittsburgh, 36 patients with HLA-mismatched grafts were treated with FK 506 and low-dose prednisone. In 9 patients, transplantation was performed despite the presence of cytotoxic antibodies. Only one kidney was lost to cellular rejection; however, a total of 4 grafts were lost to irreversible humeral rejection. This finding suggests that even the use of FK 506 will not allow relaxation of classic cross-match criteria in renal transplantation.

Other agents

Rapamycin, which is structurally similar to FK 506, has also been shown to be more potent than CsA in animal models (50). Rapamycin inhibits IL-2R–induced S-phase entry and subsequent T-cell proliferation by blocking phosphorylation and activation of p70 S6 kinase. This effect can actually be competitively antagonized by FK 506, suggesting that the effects of both agents are mediated by the newly discovered FK binding protein (51).

T and B lymphocytes are uniquely dependent on a de novo pathway for purine synthesis. Mycophenolate mofetil (RS-61443), a derivative of mycophenolic acid, blocks inosine monophosphate dehydrogenases of the de novo pathway. This inhibition leads to depletion of guanosine nucleotides, thereby blocking further DNA synthesis and proliferation of activated lymphocytes (52). Animal studies have shown RS-61443 to induce tolerance and even allow xenografting, with virtually no toxicity (53). In the clinical setting, RS-61443 replaces azathioprine in standard triple therapy immunosuppression (i.e., CsA and steroids). Preliminary results from a pilot study utilizing RS-61433 for salvage of kidney, liver, and heart allograft rejection resistent to conventional immunosuppression have been encouraging (54,55).

Polyclonal antibody preparations

Polyclonal antilymphocyte serum (ALG) and polyclonal antithymocyte serum (ATG) preparations have been effectively used both for induction therapy and for treatment of acute rejection episodes. Currently, there is only one Food and Drug Administration (FDA)–licensed antithymocyte preparation available (ATGAM; Upjohn Co., Kalamazoo, Mich) (56). Many transplant centers also manufacture their own reagents; the Minnesota ALG formula, prepared by immunizing horses with a human lymphoblast cell line, is one example (57).

ALG and ATG exert their effect by combining with peripheral lymphocytes and removing them via the reticuloendothelial system. Administration of ALG or ATG is accompanied by a profound decrease in circulating lymphocytes; the lymphopenia resolves following cessation of immune sera therapy.

In addition to lymphopenia, many patients experience fever, chills, arthralgias, lumbar pain, nausea, vomiting, hypertension, tachycardia, angina, or pulmonary edema following the first administration of ATG or ALG (58). It has been suggested that these effects may be the result of cytokine release from lymphocytes. TNF levels have been shown to be significantly elevated beginning one hour after the first dose; in contrast, elevated levels of the endogenous pyrogen IL-1β were not detected (59).

During the pre-CsA era, in two large series involving cadaveric kidney transplantation, ALG was associated with a 10% increased graft survival at one and 2 years (60,61). With the introduction of CsA, protocols were developed to use ATG until renal function was established in the hopes of decreasing CsA-induced nephrotoxicity (62). ALG has also been effectively used to treat steroid-resistant rejection.

Monoclonal antibody preparations

OKT3: Currently, there is only one monoclonal antibody licensed for use in clinical organ transplantation. Orthoclone OKT3 (muromonab-CD3) is a murine monoclonal antibody directed against the human CD3 antigen, and it was developed by Kung and associates (63) in association with the Ortho Pharmaceutical Corporation. The CD3 complex is a 20,000-dalton protein located on the surface of all peripheral T cells; binding of OKT3 apparently interferes with transduction of the signal from the adjacent antigen recognition site (64). This interference prevents T-cell proliferation and activation of cytotoxic activity. The mechanism of action may be down-regulation of both the T3 and the antigen receptor structure (65). In addition, OKT3 may also interact with activated cytotoxic T cells, thereby preventing recognition or adhesion to target cells (66).

The effectiveness of OKT3 in reversing acute rejection was first demonstrated in primary cadaveric renal transplants. OKT3 reversed rejection in 94% of transplants, versus 75% with high-dose steroids (67). Subsequent studies have also demonstrated the efficacy of OKT3 in reversing renal allograft rejection in 74% of rejection episodes resistant to high-dose steroids or ATG or ALG (68).

Our initial experience with OKT3 for resistant acute hepatic allograft rejection demonstrated a graft salvage rate of 80% (69). A subsequent prospective randomized study from this institution demonstrated the superiority of OKT3 when compared with conventional triple therapy for induction therapy following hepatic transplantation (70).

Similar to ATG and ALG, the first dose of OKT3 is associated with a variety of significant adverse responses

(67). In kidney transplant patients receiving OKT3 for induction immunotherapy, significantly elevated levels of TNF-α, IFN-γ, and IL-2 were detected following the first but not subsequent doses (71); elevated levels of IL-1β, IL-1α, and GM-CSF were not detected (72). In contrast, in patients on CsA receiving OKT3 to treat acute rejection, only TNF-α levels were elevated. In addition, the severity of side effects correlated with the serum level of TNF-α (73).

Subsequent studies have attempted to modulate cytokine release and subsequent side effects following the first dose of OKT3. Administration of high-dose corticosteroids (0.5 g solumedrol) one hour prior to or at the time of OKT3 administration markedly decreased the release of TFN-α and IFN-γ; it also totally abolished the release of IL-2 (74). This premedication also significantly reduced the severity of side effects. In a mouse model, pretreatment with methylxanthine pentoxifylline (Trental; Hoechst-Roussel Pharmaceuticals Inc., Somerville, NJ) markedly attenuated release of TNF-α and IL-2 following administration of an anti-CD3 monoclonal antibody. In vitro activity of cytotoxic T cells against alloantigens was not affected by pentoxifylline treatment (75).

A recent clinical study utilized an anti-TNF monoclonal antibody (CB006; Celltech Inc., Berkshire, UK) in renal allograft patients undergoing prophylactic OKT3 induction therapy (76). Administration of either 0.4 or 2 mg/kg CB006 prevented the occurrence of life-threatening complications; however, mild symptoms did occur, and they were associated with low levels of circulating bioactive TNF-α. Administration of CB006 had no effect on the biological or clinical effectiveness of OKT3.

The adverse reactions to OKT3, however, may not be solely explained by cytokine release. Administration of the monoclonal antibody BMA031, which is directed against a public determinant of the polymorphic T-cell receptor, is associated with elevated levels of TNF-α and IFN-γ, but without any of the side effects seen with OKT3 (77).

ANTI-IL-2R: The success of OKT3 therapy, as well as its significant side effects, has led to attempts to more specifically modulate the immune response. Currently, anti-IL-2R has received the most attention. Administration of anti-IL-2R antibody was reported to prolong heterotopic cardiac allografts in mice in 1985 (78). Anti-IL-2R was also successful in prolonging renal allografts in a primate model (79).

Prophylactic use of anti-IL-2R in humans for renal allografts was first described by the group in Nantes, France, in 1987 (80). Patients in this series were treated with a 14-day course of 33B3.1, a rat monoclonal antibody directed against the Tac antigen, followed by conversion to CsA. During the first 13 postoperative days, patients treated with 5 mg/day of antibody had a rejection rate of 33%; those treated with 10 mg had a rejection rate of 6%. Patients treated with ATG had a 4% rejection rate, whereas the historical control subjects had a rejection rate of 67%. There was no "rebound" rejection following termination of monoclonal antibody therapy.

The early success of this study led to a randomized study comparing 33B3.1 with ATG for induction therapy (81). A total of 100 patients were entered into the study; there was no difference in the incidence of rejection episodes at 14, 30, 60, and 90 days after transplantation. One-year patient survival was 96%, and graft survival was 85% in both groups. Fewer total infectious episodes were noted in the 33B3.1 group (47 versus 72%), which reached statistical significance for urinary tract infections (21 versus 66%; $p < 0.001$).

Administration of 33B3.1 was well tolerated; only one patient had treatment discontinued, as opposed to 68% of ATG recipients ($p < 0.001$). As expected, immunization against 33B3.1 increased with time; by one month, 81% of patients had detectable immunoglobulin G (IgG) and IgM antibodies. Anti-idiotype antibodies were found in 34 of 46 patients with measured antirat IgG antibodies.

Soluble receptors

Recent experimental studies have examined the possibility of inhibiting a particular cytokine's action by use of its soluble receptor. In mice, a soluble IL-1 binding protein (sIL-1R) has been cloned, which binds both IL-1α and IL-1β. Administration of sIL-1R to mice increased heterotopic cardiac graft survival from 12.5 to 18.3 days. Lymph node hyperplasia in response to a localized injection of allogeneic cells was also completely blocked by sIL-1R treatment (82).

Similarly, the same investigators cloned a soluble receptor for IL-4 (sIL-4R). Although less effective than sIL-1R, sIL-4R increased cardiac survival in the mouse ear model from 10.8 to 14.9 days. The lymph node hyperplasia response was also inhibited, which was overcome by addition of recombinant IL-4 (83). These results led to the creation of a transgenic mouse that constitutively expresses elevated levels of sIL-4R. These animals developed normally, and, as expected, they had delayed rejection of heterotopic transplanted hearts (13.8 versus 9.5 days) (84).

RENAL TRANSPLANTATION

The first renal transplants in both animals and humans were performed by Ullmann in 1902. Subsequent experiments by Carrel led to the development of vascular techniques that made transplantation feasible. As the father of modern vascular surgery, Carrel was awarded the Nobel Prize in 1912. Until the early 1950s, renal transplantation was generally unsuccessful, with the exception of a series of identical twin transplantations performed by Murray (85). The first attempts at immunosuppression utilized total body irradiation, whereas Starzl's group (86) in Denver first observed that rejection could be reversed by administration of high-dose corticosteroids. As a result of the understanding of HLA typing and the introduction of CsA, one-year graft survival for HLA-A, HLA-B, HLA-DR matched kidneys approaches 85% (87). CsA also improved the survival of mismatched kidneys to 75% (88).

In 1992, in the United States, 205 centers performed 9,291 transplantations. Worldwide, 506 centers performed a total of 19,981 renal transplantations (89). Nevertheless, in the United States, 1,000 individuals are added to the waiting list for a cadaveric transplantation each month, whereas 600 undergo transplantation and 200 die or disqualifying medical problems develop. The average waiting period is now more than one year (90).

The earliest study implicating direct involvement of a cytokine in allograft rejection was by Moy and Rosenau in 1981 (91). Using a bioassay, they demonstrated the presence of cytotoxic activity, which they attributed to LT, in rejecting human renal allograft tissue. A subsequent series of studies by Lowry and colleagues (92) showed that rat kidneys could be rejected in the absence of cytotoxic T cells or specific antibody. They concluded that rejection was the result of a delayed-type hypersensitivity reaction; LT-mediated cell lysis then leads to tissue destruction (23). This hypothesis is further strengthened by the observation that TNF-α can directly cause cell death either by cytolysis and necrosis or by DNA fragmentation (apoptosis), which is enhanced in the presence of IFN-γ (93). Furthermore, TNF-α has been shown to kill endothelial cells in vitro (94). In subsequent studies utilizing systemic injections of recombinant TNF-α and LT, we were able to demonstrate accelerated rejection in an allogeneic heterotopic rat cardiac model. Histological examination of these tissues showed only a diffuse cellular infiltrate: there was no evidence of hemorrhagic or coagulative necrosis, which argues against a direct cytotoxic activity for these mediators in this setting (95).

In 1987, Maury and Teppo (96), utilizing a double-antibody radioimmunoassay, demonstrated elevated levels of TNF-α during rejection episodes following 10 cadaveric renal transplantations. Peak levels of TNF were found at the time of clinical rejection, although elevated levels were seen one to 2 days prior. These findings have been extended utilizing an enzyme-linked immunosorbent assay (ELISA) that concurrently measures serum and urine TNF-α (97). Allograft rejection was associated with significant elevations of serum TNF levels in 65% of patients; they were also elevated during episodes of systemic infection, but not during episodes of graft failure secondary to acute tubular necrosis. Elevated levels of urinary TNF were seen only in rejection (45%) and tubular necrosis (14%).

The initial observation of elevated serum and urinary IL-2 levels during episodes of renal allograft rejection was made by Cornaby and associates (98,99) in 1988. Normal control subjects had mean plasma IL-2 levels of 1.3 ng/mL, patients with stable allografts had levels of 0.9 ng/mL, and patients with acute rejection episodes had levels of 66 ng/mL. Urinary IL-2 was detected only in rejection episodes (21 ng/mL). Neither plasma nor urinary levels of IL-2 were detected in patients with CsA toxicity. Similar results were obtained by Johnson and coworkers (100) using a bioassay for IL-2. For patients with an elevated serum creatinine level, IL-2 levels greater than 5 U/mL had a sensitivity of 73%, a specificity of 86%, a positive predictive value of 78%, and a negative predictive value of 82% in diagnosing rejection.

Following an initial report in 1987 (101), a number of small studies demonstrating elevated levels of IL-2R in renal allograft rejection were presented at the 1989 International Transplant Meeting. These findings led to a multicenter retrospective study from three centers using a microparticle enzyme immunoassay (102). In patients receiving either OKT3 or ATG induction therapy, IL-2R levels increased from a mean of 3,015 U/mL to 4,815 U/mL at the time of rejection. The increased IL-2R levels were usually seen 3 days prior to clinical diagnosis of rejection. In contrast, in patients receiving standard triple immunotherapy, levels increased from a mean of 3,022 U/mL to 3,524 U/mL; elevated levels were seen only on the day of clinical diagnosis. Differences did not reach statistical significance in either group.

Increased levels of serum IL-2R appear to correlate with increased expression on helper and cytotoxic T cells. Using two-color immunofluorescence flow cytometry, increased expression of the IL-2Rβ chain was seen in CD4+ and CD8++ cells during episodes of renal allograft rejection. In contrast, a high degree of expression was seen on CD8+ and CD16+ cells, even in healthy control subjects (103).

Serial measurements of IL-6 have shown that levels of this cytokine reach peak values 2 to 3 days after transplantation, and, in uncomplicated cases, they return to normal within 3 weeks. In patients undergoing acute renal allograft rejection, IL-6 levels increase significantly in the days preceding clinical manifestations. An even more pronounced effect is seen in urine samples (104).

A subsequent larger study confirmed these findings with the following additions: (a) elevated levels of IL-6 were seen in 50% of septic episodes; (b) IL-6 levels were decreased in association with CsA-induced nephrotoxicity; (c) treatment of acute rejection episodes with a steroid pulse led to a decrease in IL-6 levels if the rejection episode was successfully treated; and (d) treatment of rejection with OKT3 or ALG was associated with a rebound increase in IL-6 levels, followed by a decrease if the episode was successfully treated (105).

A single study of 21 renal transplant patients measured an entire battery of cytokines prior to and after episodes of rejection. In contrast to other studies, TNF and IL-1 levels were not elevated at any time. Mean IL-2 and IL-3 level increases were greater prior to infectious events compared with rejection. Increases in IL-2R levels were seen prior to either infection or rejection. Of interest, GM-CSF levels greater than 5,000 pg/mL were seen in 7 of 22 patients with infection compared with none in 21 patients with rejection (p = 0.005) (106).

Detection of elevated circulating levels of cytokines appears to be related to production by graft-infiltrating cells. Using immunochemical techniques, an increased number of graft-infiltrating cells reactive to TNF-α, IFN-γ, and IL-2R were seen in renal biopsies showing acute rejection; only IL-2R–positive cells were increased in chronic rejection. Vascular smooth muscle cells within the graft stained positive for TNF, both in acute and chronic rejection (107). However, using in situ hybridization for cellular mRNA, another group was able to detect only IL-6 (not TNF-α or IFN-γ) in renal biopsies from patients with acute rejection (108).

LIVER TRANSPLANTATION

The first human orthotopic liver transplantation (OLT) was performed by Starzl and colleagues (109) in 1963. Following initial failures, a moratorium was declared until 1967. Using azathioprine, steroids, and ATG, the first successful OLT was performed by the same group in 1967 (110). Subsequent successes by other institutions ultimately led to a National Institutes of Health Consensus Conference in 1983 to declare that "liver transplantation is a therapeutic modality for end-stage liver disease that deserves broader application."

In the United States in 1992, 72 transplant centers performed 2,893 OLTs. Worldwide in 1992, a total of 157 centers performed 4,810 transplantations. The majority of mortality occurs within the first 6 months after transplantation; the cumulative mortality within the first 4 weeks is 20%. Overall 3-year survival is currently 67% in the United States (111).

Following their initial observation that IL-2 levels were elevated during episodes of renal allograft rejection (98), the New England Deaconess program extended their study to OLT patients (99). During rejection episodes, IL-2 levels increased from a mean of 2.4 ng/mL to 42 ng/mL in plasma and from 2.0 ng/mL to 76 ng/mL in bile. Urinary IL-2 levels were not detectable in either stable or rejecting allograft patients. Subsequent study measured serial IL-2 and IL-2R levels in plasma and bile from

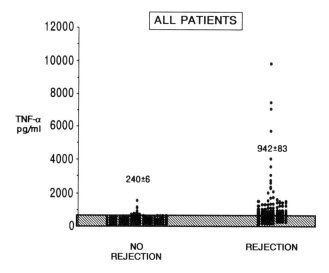

Figure 10–3. Plasma TNF-α levels from 50 patients following liver transplantation. *Shaded areas* represent mean + 2 standard deviations for the nonrejecting patients (p = 0.0001). (Reprinted by permission from Imagawa DK, Millis JM, Olthoff, et al. The role of tumor necrosis factor in allograft rejection. I. Evidence that elevated levels of tumor necrosis factor-alpha predict rejection following orthotopic liver transplantation. Transplantation 1990;50:219–225.)

46 OLT patients (112). IL-2 levels became elevated several days prior to the clinical diagnosis of rejection; higher levels were seen in bile relative to plasma. Similarly, IL-2R levels rose from a mean of 322 U/mL to 1,921 U/mL in plasma and from 386 U/mL to 2,670 U/mL in bile. In patients with CsA nephrotoxicity, neither IL-2 nor IL-2R levels were elevated.

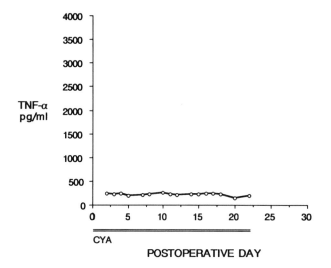

Figure 10–4. Daily plasma TNF-α levels from a liver transplant recipient experiencing no episodes of rejection. (Reprinted by permission from Imagawa DK, Millis JM, Olthoff, et al. The role of tumor necrosis factor in allograft rejection. I. Evidence that elevated levels of tumor necrosis factor-alpha predict rejection following orthotopic liver transplantation. Transplantation 1990;50:219–225.)

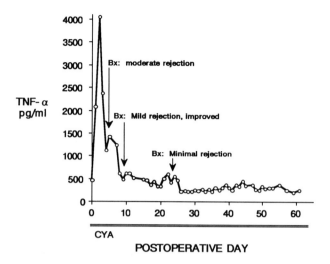

Figure 10–5. Daily plasma TNF-α levels from a liver transplant recipient with multiple episodes of rejection. (Reprinted by permission from Imagawa DK, Millis JM, Olthoff, et al. The role of tumor necrosis factor in allograft rejection. I. Evidence that elevated levels of tumor necrosis factor-alpha predict rejection following orthotopic liver transplantation. Transplantation 1990;50:219–225.)

Similar results from other institutions have been reported (113,114). The Queen Elizabeth Hospital group reported statistically elevated IL-2R levels in both serum and bile in patients undergoing acute rejection. A biliary IL-2R level of 65 U/mL or higher had a sensitivity of 94%, a specificity of 84%, a positive predictive value of 83%, and a negative predictive value of 94% in the diagnosis of acute rejection. Five patients with infectious complica-

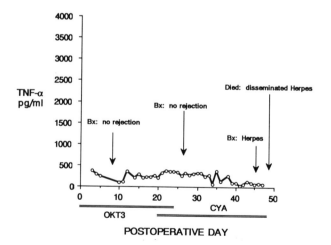

Figure 10–6. Daily plasma TNF-α levels from a liver transplant recipient who died of disseminated herpes infection. (Reprinted by permission from Imagawa DK, Millis JM, Olthoff, et al. The role of tumor necrosis factor in allograft rejection. I. Evidence that elevated levels of tumor necrosis factor-alpha predict rejection following orthotopic liver transplantation. Transplantation 1990;50:219–225.)

tions had biliary IL-2R levels in the range of acute rejection (113).

The Mayo Clinic group showed that IL-2R levels increased by a mean of 17% per day in the 10 days prior to the clinical diagnosis of rejection. Patients with CMV infections also demonstrated increased levels of IL-2R, but, overall, levels were lower than in the acute rejection group (114).

To more quickly determine IL-2R levels, the University of California San Francisco group developed a flow cytometric method (115). Using this technique, results can be obtained within 2 hours as compared with 5 hours for the ELISA, and there is a strong correlation between the two methods. They also reported that the flow cytometry results were more reproducible than the ELISA results. Once again, IL-2R levels were elevated during acute rejection episodes, as well as during infectious complications.

In 1990, we presented our initial observation that TNF-α levels were elevated during episodes of acute rejection following OLT (116). Serial plasma levels were determined in 50 consecutive adult patients. Control subjects had mean levels of 55 pg/mL; patients with stable allografts had levels of 240 pg/mL; and patients undergoing rejection had significantly elevated levels of 941 pg/mL (Fig. 10–3). Patients receiving CsA immunotherapy had overall higher TNF levels when compared with those receiving OKT3 induction therapy. In addition, elevated levels of TNF-α were seen one to 2 days prior to the clinical diagnosis. Patients with viral infections had mildly elevated levels (303 pg/mL), but levels were not statistically different from those with stable allografts (Figs. 10–4 through 10–6).

A smaller series from Heidelberg measured levels of TNF-α, in addition to IL-1, Il-2, IL-2R, and IFN-γ following OLT (117). They also showed statistically elevated levels of TNF-α during allograft rejection; however, they also found elevated levels of TNF-α associated with infectious complications. In addition, 75% of rejections and 100% of infections were associated with IL-2R levels greater than 3,700 U/mL. IL-1 and IL-2 levels were not elevated in either situation. Likewise, Tilg and colleagues (118) found elevated levels of TNF-α and IFN-γ in both acute rejection and infectious episodes. The highest levels of IL-1 were seen prior to transplantation and during episodes of rejection. IL-1 levels were depressed in patients with CMV infections.

A study from the University of Vienna examined the prognostic significance of TNF-α, endotoxin, and IL-6 levels measured during OLT (119). In contrast to our findings, there was no correlation between TNF levels on postoperative day 1 and outcome; however, all patients who experienced rejection had high plasma TNF-α levels immediately after recirculation, in contrast to low levels in recipients without complications or rejection. Detec-

TABLE 10–1 SURVIVAL OF DA LIVER GRAFTS TRANSPLANTED INTO BN RAT HOSTS

Treatment	N	Survival (d)*	P vs Control
Control	7	15.1 ± 1.5	
Preimmune sera	4	14.3 ± 0.8	NS
CyA (2 mg/kg/d, IM)	4	41.8 ± 2.0	P = .0001
Anti-LT (5,000 U/d, IV)	4	29.8 ± 2.1	P = .0003
CyA + Anti-LT	4	> 60	P = .0001

*Mean ± SEM. Reprinted by permission from Teramoto K, Baquerizo A, Imagawa DK, et al. Prolongation of hepatic allograft survival in rat recipients treated with anti-lymphotoxin antibody. Transplant Proc 1991;23:602–603.

tion of elevated IL-6 levels intraoperatively was predictive of postoperative bacterial or viral infections.

Studies attempting to demonstrate intragraft staining of cytokines have been less conclusive. Hoffmann and associates (120) found elevated levels of serum TNF-α, as well as large numbers of TNF-positive monocytes within rejecting liver allografts. In contrast, IL-1β production by macrophages and endothelial cells was restricted to episodes of severe, irreversible rejection (120).

In contrast, Bishop and coworkers (121) found no detectable difference in immunohistochemical staining of IL-1β and IFN-γ in normal versus rejecting tissues. IL-6 staining was positive in only 2 of 14 biopsies from patients with acute rejection, but it was positive in all 5 with chronic rejection (121). The San Francisco group, using the polymerase chain reaction (PCR), detected IL-1β, TNF-α, IL-4, and IL-6 with equal frequency in all biopsy specimens. IL-2 message was rarely observed in any specimens; IL-5 message was predominantly present in biopsies from patients with histopathological evidence of rejection (122).

Recently, anticytokine antibodies were developed that react with only rat/mouse or primates. Therefore, studies utilizing anticytokine antibodies in a liver transplantation model are limited. As seen in Table 10–1, rat orthotopic liver allograft survival rates were markedly increased by the administration of anti-LT for the first 10 days after transplantation. Anti-LT, in conjunction with CsA for 10 days, led to permanent engraftment (123). Using the identical model, administration of high-dose monoclonal anti-TNF-a for 10 days only modestly prolonged survival (i.e., 22 days). Histological examination of these livers showed less severe rejection, but significant liver abscesses were found in three of five animals (Table 10–2) (124).

Recently, our center began administration of granulocyte colony-stimulating factor (G-CSF) (Neupogen, Amgen Inc., Thousand Oaks, Calif) to OLT patients with persistent neutropenia. Although it was not a randomized, controlled study, all but 1 of 18 patients who received G-CSF had increases in white blood cell count, from an average nadir of 1.3×10^3 µL to a mean peak response of 12.7×10^3/µL. Despite the concern that administration of G-CSF might precipitate rejection, administration was well tolerated; only 1 episode of rejection occurred during the treatment period (125).

TABLE 10–2 SURVIVAL OF DA LIVER GRAFTS TRANSPLANTED INTO BN RAT HOSTS

Treatment	N	Survival (d)*	P vs Control	Macroscopic Findings of Liver Abscess
Control	5	12.8 ± 2.7	—	0/5
Low dose	8	12.0 ± 1.6	NS	1/8
IP	5	12.0 ± 1.6	NS	0/5
High dose	5	22.3 ± 2.7	P = 0.001	3/5

*Mean ± SD. Reprinted by permission from Shiraishi M, Shaked A, Yasunaga C, Hasuike Y, Imagawa DK, Busuttil RW. Monoclonal anit-tumor necrosis factor-α antibody suppresses rejection but enhances infectious complications in rat liver allograft recipients. Transplant Proc 1993;25:128–129.
IP = intraperitoneal

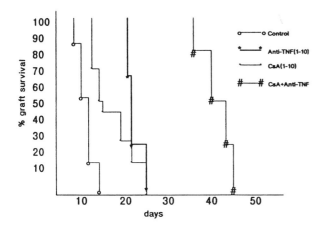

Figure 10–7. Survival curves of cardiac allografts transplanted from Buffalo donors to Lewis recipients. Control animals received no immunosuppression. Anti-TNF was administered at 2,000 U/day (IP) for days 0 to 9. CsA was administered by gastric gavage (2 mg/kg/day, days 0–9). Combination therapy consisted of anti-TNF (2,000 U) and CsA (2 mg/kg/day) for days 0 to 9 (n = 4–8 animals/group). (Reprinted by permission from Seu P, Imagawa DK, Wasef E, et al. Monoclonal anti-tumor necrosis factor-α antibody treatment of rat cardiac allografts: synergism with low-dose cyclosporine and immunohistological studies. J Surg Res 1991;50:520–528.)

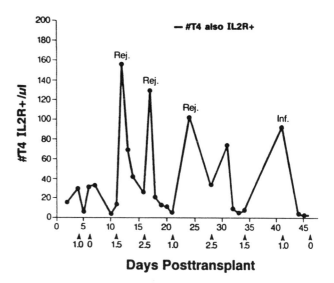

Figure 10–8. Levels of T4-IL-2R cell number in a cardiac transplantation patient with grade 2.5 rejection on days 16 and 28. Biopsy grade is given along the ordinate. An enterococcus infection (*Inf*) was detected on day 41. Peaks of T4-IL-2R associated with a rejection (*Rej*) or infection (*Inf*) are labeled as such on the graph. (Reprinted by permission from Roodman ST, Miller LW, Tsai CC. Role of interleukin 2 receptors in immunologic monitoring following cardiac transplantation. Transplantation 1988;45:1050–1056.)

CARDIAC TRANSPLANTATION

The first heterotopic heart transplantation was performed by Carrel and Guthrie (126) in 1905 when he transplanted a dog heart to the cervical vasculature of a second animal. The first attempt at human cardiac transplantation in 1964 involved a chimpanzee xenograft; the patient survived for several hours (127). The first successful human-to-human transplantation was performed by Barnard in 1967.[128]

In the United States in 1992, 132 centers performed 1,930 transplantations, whereas worldwide in 1992, 226 centers performed a total of 3,521 operations (89). In addition, 149 heart-lung transplantations were performed worldwide in 1992. Overall 5-year survival rates of 75% have been reported (129).

Implication of TNF and LT in cardiac allograft rejection was made by Lowry and associates (130) in 1986. Following their initial observation (23,92), they demonstrated the presence of both cytotoxins in rejecting rat heterotopic cardiac allografts. We have subsequently shown that antibodies to both TNF-α and LT not only prevent acute rejection but also reverse established episodes of rejection in this model (95,131). In addition, we also noted synergy when low-dose CsA was added to the anti-TNF regimen (Fig. 10–7) (132). These results have been substantiated by Bolling and colleagues (133) from the University of Michigan using a similar model. In addition, TGF-β, which opposes many of the activities of

TNF, was reported to improve graft survival in a mouse model (134).

In the clinical setting, however, there appears to be no correlation with serum TNF levels and rejection. TNF levels determined from central venous samples taken at the time of endomyocardial biopsy failed to predict either rejection or infection (135). Fyfe and coworkers (136) demonstrated that coronary sinus levels of TNF-α were elevated relative to central venous samples following heart transplantation (68 versus 17 pg/mL), but there was no correlation with rejection. There was also no correlation between peripheral or coronary sinus levels of IL-2, IL-2R, IL-4, or IL-6 and rejection (136).

Multiple studies have been reported on the utility of IL-2R levels following cardiac transplantation, with a variety of results (137–141). Using two-color flow cytometry, Roodman and associates (137) demonstrated a correlation between the presence of CD4 (T4)-positive, IL-2R–positive cells and rejection or infection. Sensitivity was 79% (73% for rejection only), and specificity was 97% during the first 5 weeks after transplantation. The utility of the test was markedly diminished after this time. Fig. 10–8 shows a representative patient in whom both rejection and infection developed (137). Serum levels of IL-2R, as measured by the same commercially available ELISA, have been reported to be significantly elevated in association with both acute rejection and severe infections by two groups (138,139). In contrast, two additional studies using the same methods failed to show elevated levels of IL-2R during acute rejection episodes in isolated (141) or serial samples (140); levels during infectious episodes were not reported.

Anti-IL-2R therapy has been utilized in the rat heterotopic cardiac transplantation model. Treatment of recipient animals with 10 days of monoclonal antibody ART 18 increased survival from 9 to 21 days; if administered in conjunction with low-dose CsA (1.5 mg/kg/day), survival was greater than 56 days (142). In addition, administration of ART 18 reversed established acute rejection in this model. The protective effect of ART 18 could also be adoptively transferred from spleen cells of antibody-treated recipients to donor-specific, but not third-party, allografts. This finding suggests that the mechanism of action of ART 18 may be via elimination of alloaggressive cytotoxic T cells, with sparing of donor-specific suppressor cells (143). Histological evidence of rejection is preceded by elevated levels of soluble IL-2R in this model, and IL-2R levels are suppressed by administration of high-dose CsA (144).

A novel approach to immunosuppression has been utilized by constructing a diphtheria toxin–related IL-2 fusion gene that produces a chimeric IL-2 toxin cytotoxic for cells carrying the high affinity IL-2 receptor (145). When administered intravenously, the toxin had a biological half-life of 20 minutes, and 95% was recovered in urine within 24 hours. A 10-day course (1 µg/day) led to permanent engraftment in four of five rats.

A recent study utilized PCR to monitor a panel of cytokines following heterotopic cardiac transplantation in cynomolgus monkeys (146). The earliest transcript was IFN-γ, which was detected 2 days after transplantation. IL-1β, IL-2, and IL-6 transcripts were noted during the early phase of rejection. With moderate and severe rejection, IL-1α, IL-1β, IL-2, IL-6, IL-8, TNF-β, and IFN-γ were all detected. The early detection of IFN-γ suggests that it may have a major and essential role in the rejection process. However, administration of monoclonal anti-IFN-γ in a rat cardiac model was unable to prolong graft survival unless given with low-dose CsA (147).

LUNG TRANSPLANTATION

The first experimental lung transplants were performed by Demikhov in 1946 (148) and clinically by Hardy in 1963 (149). Between 1963 and 1980, a total of 38 patients received lung transplants; only 2 patients survived longer than one month (149). The major limitations at that time were technical and immunological. Technically, failure of the bronchial anastomosis due to poor blood supply, high-dose corticosteroids, and rejection led to the majority of patient morbidity and mortality. In 1982, introduction of the bronchial omentopexy technique significantly improved the morbidity of bronchial anastomosis (150,151). Concomitantly, application of CsA to lung transplantation reduced both the incidence of rejection and the corticosteroid dose required. These advancements allowed the reintroduction of lung transplantation into humans.

Since 1980, several centers, including the Toronto Lung Transplant Group (152), Stanford University (153), the Washington University Lung Transplantation Group (154), as well as others (149), have reported successful single lung, double lung, and heart-lung transplantation. In 1992, 74 centers worldwide reported 674 lung transplantations (89). Most series report a one-year actuarial survival of 80 to 90%; infection and rejection are the most common problems encountered (153,154)

The role of IL-2 following lung transplantation has been investigated by Jordan and colleagues (155) in a study of 17 patients undergoing single or double lung transplantation. Serum obtained intermittently during the postoperative period was assayed for IL-2 using an ELISA, and simultaneously obtained transbronchial biopsy specimens (TBBX) were processed and graded for rejection. An increased mean serum IL-2 level in patients undergoing rejection as compared with normal control subjects (1.89 ± 3.2 ng/mL versus 0.38 ± 1.0 ng/mL; $p < 0.01$) was seen. However, a statistically significant increase in mean serum IL-2 levels was also seen in patients with CMV or bacterial/fungal pneumonia (1.97 ± 198 ng/mL, $p < 0.0006$; and 1.34 ± 1.88 ng/mL, $p < 0.01$, respectively), suggesting that elevated serum IL-2 levels after human lung transplantation are a nonspecific indicator of immune activation.

Several groups examined the relationship between soluble sIL-2R and lung rejection (156). Lawrence and associates (157) utilized ELISA to determine serum sIL-2R levels for the first 21 days after transplantation in 12 patients following lung or heart-lung transplantation. The mean serum sIL-2R level associated with rejection (3,770 U/mL) differed significantly from that associated with normal control subjects (411 U/ml; $p < 0.0001$) and nonbacterial infections (1,468 U/mL; $p < 0.05$), but not from that associated with bacterial infections (1,879 U/mL; $p =$ NS) and sepsis (5,056 U/mL; $p =$ NS). Elevations above 6,750 U/mL were associated exclusively with rejection, leading to the conclusion that marked elevations in serum sIL-2R levels correlated with lung transplant rejection, but intermediate elevations were associated with both infection and rejection.

In a similar study, Keshavjee and associates (158) examined serum sIL-2R levels in 22 lung transplant recipients, and they also found increased levels associated with both rejection and infection during the early postoperative period.

Humbert and colleagues (159) attempted to correlate serum sIL-2R levels to late rejection (4 weeks after transplantation) in 30 patients undergoing lung or heart-lung transplantation. Increased sIL-2R levels were not associated with late histological rejection; they were instead associated only with CMV pneumonia.

In contrast to renal and hepatic transplantation, the relationship between TNF-α and lung transplantation rejection has not been established. Rondeau and coworkers (160) attempted to correlate TNF-α with rejection in 10 patients after heart-lung transplantation by collecting peripheral blood and bronchoalveolar lavage (BAL) fluid on the same day at various intervals after transplantation. Peripheral blood mononuclear cells (PBMC) and BAL mononuclear cells were isolated and incubated with or without recombinant IL-2. The culture medium was subsequently assayed for TNF-α using an immunoradiometric assay. The results demonstrated that PBMC synthesized less TNF-α than BAL mononuclear cells, and rejection episodes were not associated with increased TNF-α synthesis by either PBMC or BAL cells.

In a second study, Lega and associates (161) reported 23 lung or heart-lung transplantation recipients who underwent periodic BAL, TBBX, and venopuncture for routine monitoring or clinical diagnosis after transplantation. BAL mononuclear cells or PBMC were isolated, established in culture, and incubated with or without *Escherichia coli* endotoxin lipopolysacharide [LPS]. Culture supernatant fluids were assayed for TNF-α using ELISA. Spontaneous and LPS-stimulated TNF-α production occurred in a dose-dependent manner for both alveolar and peripheral blood macrophages, and this production was identical in normal volunteers and recipients without rejection or infection. However, during episodes of rejection or infection, both BAL and PBMC demonstrated less spontaneous and LPS-stimulated production of TNF-α. The explanation for these results may be related, as the authors offered, to the timing of cell collection or to the presence of immunosuppressants. More likely, however, is the possibility that the isolation and culture process alters the immunoreactivity of the cells, and an in vivo assay would give a more accurate picture of TNF-α levels during rejection and infection episodes.

The diagnostic role of IL-6 was examined by Yoshida and coworkers (162) in a study of 17 patients undergoing lung or heart-lung transplantation. Serum samples were obtained daily for 2 to 4 weeks after transplantation, and they were assayed for the presence of IL-6 using ELISA. Sixty-eight percent of the increased IL-6 levels were associated with rejection, and conversely, 93% of the rejection episodes were associated with increased IL-6 levels. Furthermore, persistently elevated serum levels were associated with infectious states and a poor prognosis.

Neopterin, a molecule produced by activated macrophages after stimulation with INF-γ, is believed to be a marker for activated cell-mediated immunity (163). Several studies have examined its role in lung transplantation. Humbert and associates (159), as part of the study on sIL-

2R levels, assayed for serum neopterin levels in late rejection using a radioimmunoassay. Similar to the results with sIL-2R, the serum neopterin/creatinine ratio was not found to correlate with rejection, but it significantly correlated with infection. In a later prospective, blind study, the same group examined the serum neopterin/creatinine ratio in 44 patients after lung and heart-lung transplantation (164). During the first 21 days after transplantation, elevation in the neopterin/creatinine ratio was found to correlate with rejection and infection. After the third postoperative week, significant correlation was noted only in CMV pneumonia, but not rejection.

The other experimental evidence linking cytokines and lung transplantation are from animal studies. Chang and associates (165,166) assayed BAL fluid from a canine single lung transplant rejection model for TNF-α, IFN-γ, IL-2, and IL-2R using ELISA. Compared with nonrejecting allografts treated with therapeutic doses of CsA or control native lungs, rejecting allografts demonstrated marked elevations in BAL fluid TNF-α, IFN-γ, IL-2, and Il-2R levels. In two episodes of pulmonary infection, BAL fluid TNF-α, IL-2, and IL-2R levels were elevated, but to a significantly less degree than during rejection.

Using a rat model of single lung transplantation, several authors examined the correlation between cytokine levels and rejection. Jordan and colleagues (167) examined rat lung allografts for messenger RNA (mRNA) expression of IL-2, IL-2R, IL-1β, TNF-α, IFN-γ, and IL-6 by Northern blotting. Two patterns of mRNA expression were noted in the stronger rejection strain combination. In the first, IL-1β, TNF-α, IL-6, and IL-2 mRNA was detected early in rejection, and they were subsequently increased with progressing acute rejection. Alternatively, IL-2R and IFN-γ mRNA appeared early in rejection, increased in intensity 5 days after transplantation, and then decreased thereafter.

In a separate study, Francalancia and coworkers (168) examined the post-transplant day 7 intragraft expression of mRNA for IL-2 and IL-4 using quantitated reverse transcriptase PCR in rat lung isografts and allografts. A significantly elevated IL-2 mRNA level was detected in rejecting allografts as compared with isografts or allografts treated with CsA ($p < 0.05$). No significant difference was noted with IL-4.

Rolfe and associates (169) determined expression of TNF-α and IL-6 from plasma, buffy coat, BAL, and allograft tissue homogenates using a hybridoma bioassay and Northern blot analysis. BAL fluid and lung homogenate bioactivity of TNF-α and IL-6 was found to correlate with histological rejection. Lung allograft homogenate TNF-α and IL-6 mRNA expression, as detected by Northern blotting, predicted the onset of rejection by demonstrating maximal expression on post-transplant day 4, with decreasing activity thereafter. Similar results were seen with buffy coat mRNA expression of TNF-α; however, plasma levels of the cytokines did not correlate with rejection.

PANCREAS TRANSPLANTATION

Transplantation of the pancreas was developed to improve metabolic control and to prevent long-term sequela of type I diabetes mellitus. The first human pancreatic transplant was performed at the University of Minnesota in 1966 using a segmental pancreatic graft combined with a kidney graft (170). Lillehei and colleagues (171) were the first to transplant an entire pancreaticoduodenal graft, and they completed the first series of human pancreas transplantations. These early attempts were accompanied by unacceptably low patient and graft survival, as well as by high morbidity rates, leading to cessation of human pancreas transplantation.

The major technical and immunological advancements that allowed reapplication of pancreatic transplantation to humans included the introduction of CsA (33), pancreatic exocrine bladder drainage (173), duodenal segment drainage (174), and the University of Wisconsin solution for graft preservation (175). With these advancements, one-year patient and graft survival improved substantially from 41 and 5% between 1966 and 1977, respectively, to 91 and 70% between 1988 to 1990 (176), respectively. Large series on pancreatic transplantation from the University of Wisconsin (177), the University of Minnesota (178), the New England Deaconess Hospital (179), and the University of Nebraska (180) report actuarial one-year graft survival rates ranging from 68 to 100%.

Despite this improved outlook, the morbidity associated with pancreatic transplantation continues to be significant; most series report complications, such as duodenal segment leak, urinary leak, or duodenal ulceration, in as many as 20% of recipients (179,180). Furthermore, the ability of the procedure to reverse the secondary complications of diabetes mellitus, such as retinopathy, nephropathy, and neuropathy, remains controversial (181). The risk-to-benefit ratio of the requirement for exogenous insulin versus immunosuppression must also be taken into account. For these reasons, pancreatic transplantation is reserved for patients with uremia and diabetes who would benefit from concomitant kidney transplantation. More than 70% of all pancreatic transplantations are performed in conjunction with renal transplantation, and the kidney is commonly used to monitor rejection in both grafts. Isolated pancreatic transplantation is utilized only in patients with extremely poor metabolic control associated with diabetes mellitus (181).

Konigsrainer and associates (182) examined the pancreatic exocrine and urinary neopterin levels using high performance liquid chromatography in 10 recipients of combined kidney-pancreas transplantation. In the seven episodes of documented acute pancreatic rejection, pancreatic exocrine neopterin levels were elevated. Urinary neopterin levels were elevated during only four of the seven episodes. None of the seven episodes of docu-mented infection were associated with increased urinary or pancreatic exocrine neopterin levels.

Use of monoclonal antibodies as immunosuppressive agents was described. During human renal transplantation, the anti-IL-2R monoclonal antibody, 33B3.1, has been shown to be an effective immunosuppressant with few side effects (80,81) Cantarovich and associates (183) reported a randomized trial comparing 33B3.1 and rabbit ATG in 31 diabetic, uremic patients undergoing simultaneous kidney-pancreas transplantation. Immunosuppression was maintained in all patients with CsA, azathioprine, and prednisolone, and patients were randomized to receive either 10-day induction therapy with 33B3.1 (n = 14) or ATG (n = 17). The 2-year actuarial survival for the 33B3.1 and ATG groups was, respectively, 100 versus 87.4% (patient survival), 78 versus 75.5% (pancreatic graft survival), and 100 versus 81.4% (kidney graft survival). The incidence of rejection was higher in the 33B3.1 group compared with the ATG group (57 versus 29%), but side effects were less frequent. These results suggest that the anti-IL-2R monoclonal antibody 33B3.1 may be safely and effectively used in patients undergoing combined kidney-pancreas transplantation.

PANCREATIC ISLET-CELL TRANSPLANTATION

To circumvent the morbidity associated with whole organ pancreatic transplantation and to achieve euglycemia in patients with type I diabetes mellitus, human islet-cell transplantation has been attempted. The potential for islet-cell transplantation was made possible by the introduction of a procedure for successful isolation of islet cells in 1967 by Lacy and Kostianovsky (184). Islet cells were subsequently successfully transplanted experimentally in rats (185), but most early human islet-cell allotransplantations achieved only limited success (186). The first report of insulin independence after pancreatic islet-cell allotransplantation was by Scharp and colleagues in 1990 (187). Since this initial work, there have been several reports of successful islet-cell allotransplantation in humans (188–191). Two patients continue to be insulin-independent nearly 3 and 4 years, respectively, after islet allotransplantation. However, the success of the procedure is limited by islet-cell graft rejection, as well as by the potential deleterious effects of immunosuppressive agents on islet-cell function (192,193).

In contrast, islet-cell autotransplantation has been a relatively successful procedure for patients undergoing near-total or total pancreatectomy. Since the first report of successful islet-cell autotransplantation in 1980 (194), several subsequent series have been reported (193,195). The results of autotransplantation have shown that insulin independence and euglycemia can be achieved with transplantation of as few as 265,000 islet cells intraportally (193). The superior success of autotransplantation over allotransplantation is related to the absence of a rejection response and to elimination of the need for immunosuppression. This discussion on the role of cytokines in islet-cell transplantation is limited to allografts only.

In a series of experiments, Hao and associates (196) attempted to elucidate the role of Il-2, Il-3, IFN-γ, and TNF-α in rejection using a mouse model of subcapsular islet-cell allotransplantation. Cytotoxic T lymphocytes primed against donor MHC antigens were transplanted into 28-day-old subcapsular islet-cell allografts, and the effect on graft survival was analyzed using several lymphokine-depleting mechanisms. The results demonstrated that IL-2 and IL-3 were not required for rejection, whereas IFN-γ and TNF-α appeared to have a more integral role. Furthermore, induction of MHC antigens on grafted islet cells could abrogate the graft acceptance induced by CsA treatment. It can be concluded from this work that the MHC antigen expression induced by IFN-γ and TNF-α (7,17,18) are important mechanisms of mouse islet-cell allograft rejection.

The effect of TGF-β and a monoclonal anti-IFN-γ (H22) on islet-cell xenograft acceptance was examined by Carel and associates (197). Mice with streptozotocin-induced diabetes received rat islet cells transplanted under the kidney capsule. Cultured islet cells, as well as recipient mice, were treated with various combinations of TGF-β and H22 to determine the effect on islet-cell rejection. Treatment of the cultured islet cells with 7 days of TGF-β resulted in prolongation of graft survival from 27.6 ± 7.2 days in control subjects to 47.9 ± 4.4 days ($p < 0.03$). Further prolongation of graft survival to 88.9 ± 7.2 days was achieved when cultured islet cells were treated with 7 days of TGF-β and when recipients were treated with H22. No additional improvement in graft survival was noted when cultured islet cells were treated with both TGF-β and H22. These results indicate that pretreating cultured rat islet cells with TGF-β leads to decreased immunogenicity. The altered immunogenicity, with or without the monoclonal anti-IFN-γ antibody, allows significantly prolonged xenograft acceptance in this model.

SMALL INTESTINE TRANSPLANTATION

The first experimental small intestine transplantations were performed in dogs in 1901 by Carrel (198). No further studies were attempted until 1959 when Lillehei and colleagues (199) began experimentation with autotransplantation and allotransplantation of the canine small intestine. This pioneering work was followed by eight attempted human small bowel transplantations between 1964 and 1970, all of which were unsuccessful secondary to rejection, infection, or technical problems. By 1988, advancements in technique and immunosuppression provided the opportunity for the first successful human isolated small intestine transplantation (200) and combined small intestine/liver transplantation (201).

Rejection continues to be one of the major problems confronting successful human small intestine transplantation. Several centers have reported successful outcomes after small intestine transplantation using CsA as the primary immunosuppressant (202–205), but rejection has limited the success in others (206–208). With introduction of FK-506 as the primary immunosuppressant, an improved outlook in human small intestine transplantation has been seen. In 1992, Todo and coworkers (209) published the largest series of human small intestine transplantations, which included eight isolated small intestine, eight combined liver-small intestine, and one multivisceral graft. All patients were treated with FK-506, and 16 were reported alive with viable grafts from one to 23 months after surgery. The same group presented a follow-up report of 11 isolated small intestine transplant recipients that demonstrated seven patients are alive and total parenteral nutrition–independent from one month to one year after transplantation (210). Although the follow-up is short, these results represent a major advancement in the field, and they indicate a potential role for FK-506 as the primary immunosuppressant in small intestine transplantation.

The correlation between serum levels of IL-6, TNF-α, IL-2, and rejection in human small bowel allografts was investigated by Noguchi and colleagues (211). These cytokines were detected in the serum by ELISA in three patients after small intestine or liver–small intestine transplantation, and correlation with rejection was achieved with tissue biopsy. Serum IL-6 levels were elevated during rejection episodes in all patients, whereas elevations in serum IL-2 and TNF-α levels did not necessarily correlate with rejection. The results are difficult to interpret given the small number of patients, but they suggest a potential diagnostic role for serum IL-6 in small intestine transplant rejection.

The role of IL-2, IFN-γ, and IL-2R in rat small intestine transplant rejection has also been investigated (212). A heterotopic unidirectional model of rejection was established with animals killed on postoperative days 3, 5, 7, 8, 9, and 10. Tissue was blindly graded for rejection after formalin fixation and hematoxylin and eosin staining. Reverse transcriptase PCR was performed on snap frozen samples using primers specific for IL-2, IL-2R (beta chain), and IFN-γ. Intragraft IL-2R mRNA expression demonstrated constitutive expression, as did the control β-actin mRNA. However, intragraft IL-2 and IFN-γ mRNA expression in allografts increased prior to histological signs of rejection, and they demonstrated persistently higher percent expression than isografts throughout the study period. This data indicate that intragraft expression of cytokines, specifically IL-2 and IFN-γ, may be a predictor of small intestine allograft rejection in a rat model.

CONCLUSIONS

Solid organ transplantation has advanced rapidly over the past three decades. Currently, renal, hepatic, cardiac, and lung transplantation are commonly performed, whereas pancreatic, pancreatic islet cell, and small intestinal transplants have more limited application. The rapid success of solid organ transplantation is related to advancements in immunology and immunosuppression. Established immunosuppressive agents, such as azathioprine, corticosteroids, and CsA, have allowed one-year graft survival rates to approach 90% for some organ transplantations. Newer agents, such as FK-506, Rapamycin, and RS-61443, hold promise for further improvements in graft outcome.

Understanding of the mechanisms of organ transplant rejection, although still incomplete, has undergone revolutionary advancement. Cell-mediated immunity is currently believed to have the central role in acute allograft rejection; MHC antigens are a principal target in the effector cell response. Cytokines are important mediators of immune activation, proliferation, and graft destruction. The exact role of cytokines in allograft rejection is being elucidated, but it is clear that they have an integral role as intercellular and intracellular messengers in immune upregulation.

Rapid quantitation of cytokines in serum and allografts of solid organ transplant recipients using ELISA, bioassays, and molecular techniques has led to the implication of their role in the rejection process. Data currently exist to support the role of IL-2, IL-2R, TNF-α, and IL-6 in renal allograft rejection; IL-1, IL-2, IL-5, IL-2R, TNF-α, and IFN-γ in liver allograft rejection; IL-1β, IL-2, IL-2R, IL-6, TNF-α, and IFN-γ in cardiac allograft rejection; IL-1β IL-2, IL-2R, IL-6, TNF-α, IFN-γ, and neopterin in lung allograft rejection; neopterin in pancreatic allograft rejection; IFN-γ and TNF-α in islet-cell allograft rejection; and IL-2, IFN-γ, and IL-6 in small intestine allograft rejection. This experimental evidence linking cytokines to allograft rejection further elucidates the mechanisms involved, while simultaneously functioning as a diagnostic tool for its detection.

The concept of cytokines as down-regulators of the immune response, as well as use of anticytokine strategies to diminish the immune response, have been increasingly investigated. Current research supporting these concepts has demonstrated prolonged survival of heart and islet-cell allografts using TGF-β; heart and liver allografts using anti-TNF-α and anti-LT; heart, renal, and pancreas allografts using anti-IL-2R (ART 18 or 33B3.1); and islet-cell xenografts using anti-IFN-γ (H22). Development of anti-cytokine strategies and use of the so-called suppressor cytokines may be integral additions to immunosuppression and to the development of immunological unresponsiveness.

REFERENCES

1. Cerilli GJ, ed. Organ transplantation and replacement. Philadelphia: J.B. Lippincott, 1988.

2. Krensky AM, Weiss A, Crabtree G, Davis MM, Parham P. T-lymphocyte-antigen interaction in transplant rejection. N Engl J Med 1990;322:510–517.

3. Tilney NL, Kupiec-Weglinski JW. The biology of acute transplant rejection. Ann Surg 1991;214:98–106.

4. Chandler C, Passaro EP Jr. Transplant rejection: mechanisms and treatment. Arch Surg 1993;128:279–283.

5. Robinson MA, Kindt TJ. Major histocompatibility complex antigens and genes. In: Paul WE, ed. Fundamental immunology, ed 2. New York: Raven, 1989:489–539.

6. Zinkernagel RM, Doherty PC. Restriction of in vitro T cell-mediated cytotoxicity in lymphocytic choriomeningitis within a syngeneic or semi-allogenic system. Nature 1974; 248:701–702.

7. Halloran PF, Cockfield SM, Madrenas J. The mediators of inflammation (interleukin 1, interferon γ, and tumor necrosis factor) and their relevance to rejection. Transplant Proc 1989;21:26–30.

8. Kirby JA, Forsythe JLR, Proud G, Taylor RMR. Renal allograft rejection: possible involvement of lymphokine-activated killer cells. Immunology 1989;67:62–67.

9. Smith KA. The two-chain structure of high-affinity IL-2 receptors. Immunol Today 1987;8:11–13.

10. Ihle JN, Weinstein Y. Immunological regulation of hematopoietic/lymphoid stem cell differentiation by interleukin 3. Adv Immunol 1986;39:1–50.

11. Fanslow WC, Clifford KN, Park LS, et al. Regulation of alloreactivity in vivo by IL-4 and the soluble IL-4 receptor. J Immunol 1991;147:535–540.

12. Sehgal PB, Grieninger G, Tosado G. Regulation of the acute phase and immune responses: interleukin 6. Ann NY Acad Sci 1989;557:1–583.

13. Takai Y, Wong GG, Clark SC, Burakoff SJ, Hermann SH. B cell stimulatory factor-2 is involved in the differentiation of cytotoxic T lymphocytes. J Immunol 1988;140:508–512.

14. Poupart P, Vandenabeele P, Cayphas S, et al. B cell growth modulating and differentiating activity of recombinant human 26-kd protein (BSF-2, HuIFN-β2, HPGF). EMBO J 1987;6:1219–1224.

15. May LT, Helfgott DC, Sehgal PB. Anti-β-interferon antibodies inhibit the increased expression of HLA-B7 mRNA in tumor necrosis factor-treated human fibroblasts: structural studies of the β₂ interferon involved. Proc Natl Acad Sci USA 1986;83:8957–8961.

16. Lapierre LA, Fiers W, Pober JS. Three distinct classes of regulatory cytokines control endothelial cell MHC antigen expression. J Exp Med 1988;167:794–804.

17. Mantegazza R, Hughes SM, Mitchell D, Travis M, Blau HM, Steinman L. Modulation of MHC class II antigen expression in human myoblasts after treatment with IFN-γ. Neurology 1991;41:1128–1132.

18. Martin M, Schwinzer R, Schellekens H, Resch K. Glomerular mesangial cells in local inflammation: induction of the expression of MHC class II antigens by IFN-γ. J Immunol 1989;142:1887–1894.

19. Aggarwal BB, Kohr WJ, Hass PE, et al. Human tumor necrosis factor. Production, purification, and characterization. J Biol Chem 1985;260:2345–2354.

20. Aggarwal BB, Eessalu TE, Hass PE. Characterization of receptors for human tumour necrosis factor and their regulation by γ-interferon. Nature 1985;318:665–667.

21. Pober JS. Effects of tumour necrosis factor and related cytokines on vascular endothelial cells. In: Bock G, Marsh J, eds. Tumor necrosis factor and related cytotoxins. New York: Wiley, 1987:170–184.

22. Economou JS, McBride WH, Essner R, et al. Tumour necrosis factor production by IL-2 activated macrophages in vitro and in vivo. Immunology 1989;67:514–519.

23. Lowry RP, Marghesco DM, Blackburn JH. Immune mechanisms in organ allograft rejection. VI. Delayed-type hypersensitivity and lymphotoxin in experimental renal allograft rejection. Transplantation 1985;40:183–188.

24. Matsushima K, Openheim JJ. Interleukin-8 and MCAF: novel inflammatory cytokines induced by IL-1 and TNF. Cytokine 1989;1:2–13.

25. Tracey KJ, Lowry SF, Cerami A. Physiological responses to cachectin. In: Bock G, Marsh J, eds. Tumor necrosis factor and related cytotoxins. New York: Wiley, 1987:88–108.

26. Ranges GE, Figari IS, Espevik T, Palladino MA Jr. Inhibition of cytotoxic T cell development by transforming growth factor-β and reversal by recombinant tumor necrosis factor-α. J Exp Med 1987;166:991–998.

27. Fontana A, Constam DB, Frei K, Malipiero U, Pfister HW. Modulation of the immune response by transforming growth factor beta. Int Arch Allergy Immunol 1992;99:1–7.

28. Calne RY, Alexandre GPJ, Murray JE. A study of the effects of drugs in prolonging survival of homologous renal transplants in dogs. Ann NY Acad Sci 1962;99:743–761.

29. Hitchings GH, Elion GB. The role of antimetabolites in immunosuppression and transplantation. Accounts Chem Res 1969;2:202–209.

30. Glaser RJ, Berry JW, Loeb LH, Wood WB Jr. The effect of cortisone in streptococcal lymphadenitis and pneumonia. J Lab Clin Med 1951;38:363–373.

31. Goodwin WE, Kaufman JJ, Mims MM, et al. Human renal transplantation. I. Clinical experiences with six cases of renal homotransplantation. J Urol 1963;89:13–24.

32. Snyder DS, Unanue ER. Corticosteroids inhibit murine macrophage Ia expression and interleukin 1 production. J Immunol 1982;129:1803–1805.

33. Kahan BD. Drug therapy: cyclosporine. N Engl J Med 1989;321:1725–1738.

34. Tilney NL, Milford EL, Araujo J-L, et al. Experience with cyclosporine and steroids in clinical renal transplantation. Ann Surg 1984;200:605–613.

35. Krönke M, Leonard WJ, Depper JM, et al. Cyclosporine A inhibits T-cell growth factor gene expression at the level of mRNA transcription. Proc Natl Acad Sci USA 1984;81:5214–5218.

36. Tocci MJ, Matkovich DA, Collier KA, et al. The immunosuppressant FK506 selectively inhibits expression of early T cell activation genes. J Immunol 1989;143:718–726.

37. Kalman VK, Klimpel GR. Cyclosporin A inhibits the production of gamma interferon (IFN-γ) but does not inhibit production of virus-induced interferon α/β. Cell Immunol 1983;78:122–129.

38. Miyawaki T, Yachie A, Ohzeki S, et al. Cyclosporin A does not prevent expression of Tac antigen, a probable TCGF receptor molecule, on mitogen-stimulated human T cells. J Immunol 1983;130:2737–2742.

39. Remick DG, Nguyen DT, Eskandari MK, Strieter RM, Kunkel SL. Cyclosporine A inhibits TNF production without decreasing TNF mRNA levels. Biochem Biophys Res Commun 1989;161:551–555.

40. European Multicentre Trial Group. Cyclosporine in cadaveric renal transplantation: one-year follow-up of a multicentre trial. Lancet 1983;2:986–989.

41. The Canadian Multicentre Transplant Study Group. A randomized clinical trial of cyclosporine in cadaveric renal transplantation. N Engl J Med 1983;309:809–815.

42. Rubin RH. The indirect effects of cytomegalovirus infection on the outcome of organ transplantation. J Am Med Assoc 1989;261:3607–3609.

43. Penn I. Lymphomas complicating organ transplantation. Transplant Proc 1983;15:2790–2797.

44. Starzl TE, Porter KA, Iwatsuki S, et al. Reversibility of lymphomas and lymphoproliferative lesions developing under cyclosporin-steroid therapy. Lancet 1984;1:583–587.

45. Starzl TE, Todo S, Fung J, Demetris AJ, Venkataramanan R, Jain A. FK-506 for human liver, kidney and pancreas transplantation. Lancet 1989;2:1000–1004.

46. Todo S, Fung JJ, Demetris AJ, Jain A, Venkataramanan R, Starzl TE. Early trials with FK506 as primary treatment in liver transplantation. Transplant Proc 1990;22:13–16.

47. Fung J, Todo S, Abu-Elmagd K, et al. Randomized trial in primary liver transplantation under immunosuppression with FK 506 or cyclosporine. Transplant Proc 1993;25:1130.

48. US Multicenter FK 506 Liver Study Group. Use of Prograf (FK 506) as rescue therapy for refractory rejection after liver transplantation. Transplant Proc 1993;25:679–688.

49. Starzl TE, Fung J, Jordan M, et al. Kidney transplantation under FK 506. J Am Med Assoc 1990;264:63–67.

50. Morris RE, Wu J, Shorthouse R. A study of the contrasting effects of cyclosporine, FK 506, and rapamycin on suppression of allograft rejection. Transplant Proc 1990;22:1638–1641.

51. Kuo CJ, Chong J, Fiorentino DF, Flanagan WM, Blenis J, Crabtree GR. Rapamycin selectively inhibits interleukin-2 activation of p70 S6 kinase. Nature 1992;358:70–73.

52. Sweeney MJ, Hoffman DH, Esterman MA. Metabolism and biochemistry of mycophenolic acid. Cancer Res 1972;32:1803–1809.

53. Wang J, Morris RE. Effect of splenectomy and mono- or combination therapy with Rapamycin, the morpholino-ethyl ester of mycophenolic acid and deoxyspergualin on

cardiac xenograft survival. Transplant Proc 1991;23:699–702.

54. Klintmalm GB, Ascher NL, Busuttil RW, et al. RS-61443 for treatment-resistant human liver rejection. Transplant Proc 1993;25:697.

55. Sollinger HW, Belzer FO, Deierhoi MH, et al. RS-61443: rescue therapy in refractory kidney transplant rejection. Transplant Proc 1993;25:698–699.

56. Wechter WJ, Morrell RM, Bergan J, Rosenberg JC, Turcotte J, Schultz Jr. Treatment with antilymphocyte globulin (ATGAM) in renal allograft recipients. Transplantation 1979;28:365–367.

57. Najarian JS, Simmons RL, Condie R, et al. Seven years experience with antilymphoblast globulin for renal transplantation from cadaver donors. Ann Surg 1976;184:352–368.

58. Hoitsma AJ, van Lier HJJ, Reekers P, Koene RAP. Improved patient and graft survival after treatment of acute rejections of cadaveric renal allografts with rabbit antithymocyte globulin. Transplantation 1985;39:274–279.

59. Debets JMH, Leunissen KML, van Hooff HJ, van der Linden CJ, Buurman WA. Evidence of involvement of tumor necrosis factor in adverse reactions during treatment of kidney allograft rejection with antithymocyte globulin. Transplantation 1989;47:487–492.

60. Barnes BA, Olivier D. Analysis of NIAID kidney transplant histocompatibility study (KTHS): factors associated with transplant outcome. I. Transplant Proc 1981;13:65–72.

61. Spees EK, Vaughn WK, Niblack G, et al. The effect of blood transfusion on cadaver renal transplantation: a prospective study of the Southeastern Organ Procurement Foundation 1977–1980. Transplant Proc 1981;13:155–160.

62. Ferguson RM. Strategy IV—quadruple drug therapy. Transplant Immunol Lett 1985;2:3–7.

63. Kung PC, Goldstein G, Reinherz EL, Schlossman SF. Monoclonal antibodies defining distinctive human T cell surface antigens. Science 1979;206:347–349.

64. Reinherz EL, Meuer S, Fitzgerald KA, Hussey RE, Levine H, Schlossman SF. Antigen recognition by human T lymphocytes is linked to surface expression of T3 molecular complex. Cell 1982;30:735–745.

65. Goldstein G. An overview of OKT3. Transplant Proc 1986;18:927–930.

66. Landegren U, Ramstedt U, Axberg I, Ullberg M, Jondal M, Wigzell H. Selective inhibition of human T cell cytotoxicity at levels of target recognition or initiation of lysis by monoclonal OKT3 and Leu 2α antibodies. J Exp Med 1982;155:1579–1584.

67. Ortho Multicenter Transplant Study Group. A randomized clinical trial of OKT3 monoclonal antibody for acute rejection of cadaveric renal transplants. N Engl J Med 1985;313:337–342.

68. Goldstein G, Norman DJ, Shield CF III, et al. OKT3 monoclonal antibody reversal of acute renal allograft rejection unresponsive to conventional immunosuppression. Prog Clin Biol Res 1986;224:239–249.

69. Colonna JO II, Goldstein LI, Brems JJ, et al. A prospective study on the use of monoclonal anti-T3 cell antibody (OKT3) to treat steroid-resistant liver transplant rejection. Arch Surg 1987;122:1120–1123.

70. Millis JM, McDiarmid SV, Hiatt JR, et al. Randomized prospective trial of OKT3 for early prophylaxis of rejection after liver transplantation. Transplantation 1989;47:82–88.

71. Abramovicz D, Schandene L, Goldman M, et al. Release of tumor necrosis factor, interleukin-2, and gamma-interferon in serum after injectin of OKT3 monoclonal antibody in kidney transplant recipients. Transplantation 1989;47:606–608.

72. Chatenoud L, Ferran C, Legendre C, et al. In vivo cell activation following OKT3 administration. Transplantation 1990;49:697–702.

73. Gaston RS, Deierhoi MH, Patterson T, et al. OKT3 first-dose reaction: association with T cell subsets and cytokine release. Kidney Int 1991;39:141–148.

74. Chatenoud L, Legendre C, Ferran C, Bach J-F, Kreis H. Corticosteroid inhibition of the OKT3-induced cytokine-related syndrome—dosage and kinetics prerequisites. Transplantation 1991;51:334–338.

75. Alegre M-L, Gastaldello K, Abramowicz D, et al. Evidence that pentoxifylline reduces anti-CD3 monoclonal antibody-induced cytokine release syndrome. Transplantation 1991;52:674–679.

76. Ferran C, Sheehan K, Schreiber R, Bach JF, Chatenoud L. Anti-TNF abrogates the cytokine-related anti-CD3 induced syndrome. Transplant Proc 1991;23:849–850.

77. Zlabinger GJ, Pohanka E, Stuhlmeier KM, et al. Can treatment with the monoclonal antibody BMA031 induce cytokine release? Transplant Proc 1992;24:271–272.

78. Kirkman RL, Barrett LV, Gaulton GN, Kelley VE, Ythier A, Strom TB. Administration of an anti-interleukin 2 receptor monoclonal antibody prolongs cardiac allograft survival in mice. J Exp Med 1985;162:358–362.

79. Shapiro ME, Kirkman RL, Reed MH, et al. Monoclonal anti-IL-2 receptor antibody in primate renal transplantation. Transplant Proc 1987;19:594–598.

80. Soulillou JP, Le Mauff B, Olive D, et al. Prevention of rejection of kidney transplants by monoclonal antibody directed against interleukin 2. Lancet 1987;1:1339–1342.

81. Soulillou J-P, Cantarovich D, Le Mauff B, et al. Randomized controlled trial of a monoclonal antibody against the interleukin-2 receptor (33B3.1) as compared with rabbit antithymocyte globulin for prophylaxis against rejection of renal allografts. N Engl J Med 1990;322:1175–1182.

82. Fanslow WC, Sims JE, Sassenfeld H, et al. Regulation of alloreactivity in vivo by a soluble form of the interleukin-1 receptor. Science 1990;248:739–742.

83. Fanslow WC, Clifford KN, Park L, et al. Regulation of alloreactivity in vivo by IL-4 and the soluble IL-4 receptor. J Immunol 1991;147:535–540.

84. Maliszewski CR, Morrissey PJ, Fanslow WC, Sato TA, Willis C, Davison B. Delayed allograft rejection in mice transgenic for a soluble form of the IL-4 receptor. Cell Immunol 1992;143:434–448.

85. Murray JE. Reminiscences on renal transplantation. In: Chaterjee SN, ed. Organ transplantation. Littleton, MA: John Wright, 1982:1–13.

86. Starzl TE, Marchioro TL, Waddel WR. The reversal of rejection in human renal homografts with subsequent development of homograft tolerance. Surg Gynecol Obstet 1963;117:385–395.

87. Mickey MR, Carnahan B, Terasaki PI. Effectiveness of zero A, B, and DR mismatch for cadaver kidneys. Transplant Proc 1985;17:2222–2224.

88. Opelz G. Correlation of HLA matching with kidney graft survival in patients with or without cyclosporine treatment. Transplantation 1985;40:240–243.

89. Terasaki PI, Cecka JM, eds. Clinical transplants 1992. Los Angeles, CA: UCLA Tissue Typing Laboratory, 1993.

90. Randall T. Too few human organs for transplantation, too many in need . . . and the gap widens. J Am Med Assoc 1991;265:1223–1224.

91. Moy J, Rosenau W. Demonstration of α-lymphotoxin in human rejected renal allografts. Clin Immunol Immunopathol 1981;20:49–56.

92. Lowry RP, Gurley KE, Forbes RDC. Immune mechanisms in organ allograft rejection. I. Delayed type hypersensitivity and lymphocytotoxicity in heart graft rejection. Transplantation 1983;36:391–401.

93. Dealtry GB, Naylor MS, Fiers W, Balkwill FR. DNA fragmentation and cytotoxicity caused by tumor necrosis factor is enhanced by interferon-γ. Eur J Immunol 1987;17:689–693.

94. Sato N, Goto T, Haranaka K, et al. Actions of tumor necrosis factor on cultured vascular endothelial cells: morphologic modulation, growth inhibition, and cytotoxicity. J Natl Cancer Inst 1986;76:1113–1121.

95. Imagawa DK, Millis JM, Olthoff KM, et al. The role of tumor necrosis factor in allograft rejection. II. Evidence that antibody therapy against tumor necrosis factor-alpha and lymphotoxin enhances cardiac allograft survival in rats. Transplantation 1990;50:189–193.

96. Maury CPJ, Teppo A-M. Raised serum levels of cachectin/tumor necrosis factor α in renal allograft rejection. J Exp Med 1987;166:1132–1137.

97. McLaughlin PJ, Aikawa A, Davies HM, et al. Evaluation of sequential plasma and urinary tumor necrosis factor alpha levels in renal allograft recipients. Transplantation 1991;51:1225–1229.

98. Cornaby A, Simpson MA, Vann Rice R, Dempsey RA, Madras PN, Monaco AP. Interleukin-2 production in plasma and urine, plasma interleukin-2 receptor levels, and urine cytology as a means of monitoring renal allograft recipients. Transplant Proc 1988;20 (suppl 1):108–110.

99. Cornaby A, Simpson M, Vann Rice R, et al. Interleukin 2 levels and urine cytology distinguish between cyclosporine toxicity and rejection in renal and liver allograft recipients. Transplant Proc 1988;20 (suppl 3):827–830.

100. Johnson CP, Chaharmohal A, Buchmann E, Roza AM, Adams MB. Plasma IL-2 levels and diagnosis of renal transplant rejection. Transplant Proc 1990;22:1849–1851.

101. Colvin RB, Fuller C, MacKeen L, Kung PC, Ip SH, Cosimi AB. Plasma interleukin 2 receptor levels in renal allograft recipients. Clin Immunol Immunopathol 1987;43:273–276.

102. Schroeder TJ, Helling T, McKenna RM, et al. A multicenter study to evaluate a novel assay for quantitation of soluble interleukin 2 receptor in renal transplant recipients. Transplantation 1992;53:34–40.

103. Niguma T, Sakagami K, Kawamura T, et al. Expression of the interleukin 2 receptor β chain (p75) in renal transplantation—applicability of anti-interleukin-2 receptor β chain monoclonal antibody. Transplantation 1991;52:296–302.

104. Van Oers MHG, Van Der Heyden AAPAM, Aarden LA. Interleukin 6 (IL-6) in serum and urine of renal transplant recipients. Clin Exp Immunol 1988;71:314–319.

105. Yoshimura N, Oka T, Kahan BD. Sequential determinations of serum interleukin 6 levels as an immunodiagnostic tool to differentiate rejection from nephrotoxicity in renal allograft recipients. Transplantation 1991;51:172–176.

106. Daniel V, Paskar S, Reiss U, et al. Preliminary evidence that monitoring of plasma granulocyte-macrophage colony-stimulating factor may be helpful to differentiate between infection and rejection in renal transplant patients. Transplant Proc 1992;24:2770–2772.

107. Noronha IL, Eberlein-Gonska M, Hartley B, Stephens S, Cameron JS, Waldherr R. In situ expression of tumor necrosis factor-alpha, interferon-gamma, and interleukin-2 receptors in renal allograft biopsies. Transplantation 1992;54:1017–1024.

108. Vandenbroecke C, Caillat-Zucman S, Legendre C, et al. Differential in situ expression of cytokines in renal allograft rejection. Transplantation 1991;51:602–609.

109. Starzl TE, Marchiaro TL, Von Kaulla KN, Hermann G, Brittain RS, Waddell WR. Homotransplantation of the liver in humans. Surg Gynecol Obstet 1963;117:659–676.

110. Starzl TE, Groth CG, Brettschneider L, et al. Orthotopic homotransplantation of the human liver. Ann Surg 1968;168:392–415.

111. Belle SH, Beringer KC, Murphy JB, et al. Liver transplantation in the United States: 1988 to 1990. In: Terasaki PI, Cecka JM, eds. Clinical transplants 1991. Los Angeles, CA: UCLA Tissue Typing Laboratory, 1992:13–29.

112. Simpson MA, Young-Fadok TM, Madras PN, et al. Sequential interleukin 2 and interleukin 2 receptor levels distinguish rejection from cyclosporine toxicity in liver allograft recipients. Arch Surg 1991;126:717–720.

113. Adams DH, Hubscher SG, Wang L, Elias E, Neuberger JM. Soluble interleukin-2 receptors in serum and bile of liver transplant recipients. Lancet 1989;1:469–471.

114. Perkins JD, Nelson DL, Rakela J, Grambsch PM, Krom RAF. Soluble interleukin-2 receptor level as an indicator of liver allograft rejection. Transplantation 1989;47:77–81.

115. Cohen N, Gumbert M, Birnbaum J, et al. An improved method for the detection of soluble interleukin 2 receptors in liver transplant recipients by flow cytometry. Transplantation 1991;51:417–421.

116. Imagawa DK, Millis JM, Olthoff KM, et al. The role of tumor necrosis factor in allograft rejection. I. Evidence that elevated levels of tumor necrosis factor-alpha predict rejection following orthotopic liver transplantation. Transplantation 1990;50:219–225.

117. Kraus TH, Noronha IL, Manner M, Klar E, Küppers P, Otto G. Clinical value of cytokine determination for screening, differentiation, and therapy monitoring of infectious and noninfectious complications after orthotopic liver transplantation. Transplant Proc 1991;23:1509–1512.

118. Tilg H, Vogel W, Aulitzky WE, et al. Evaluation of cytokines and cytokine-induced messages in sera of patients after liver transplantation. Transplantation 1990;49:1074–1080.

119. Hamilton G, Prettenhoffer M, Zommer A, et al. Intraopera-

tive course and prognostic significance of endotoxin, tumor necrosis factor-alpha and interleukin-6 in liver transplant recipients. Immunobiology 1991;182:425–439.

120. Hoffmann MW, Wonigeit K, Steinhoff G, Herzbeck H, Flad HD, Pichlmayr R. Production of cytokines (TNF-alpha, IL-1-beta) and endothelial cell activation in human liver allograft rejection. Transplantation 1993;55:329–335.

121. Bishop GA, Matsumoto Y, McCaughan GW, Kenney JS. Identification of cytokine protein expression in human liver allograft rejection: methods development and expression of IL-1β, IL-6 IFN-γ and basic fibroblast growth factor. Transplant Proc 1992;24:2310–2312.

122. Martinez OM, Krams SM, Sterneck M, et al. Intragraft cytokine profile during human liver allograft rejection. Transplantation 1992;53:449–456.

123. Teramoto K, Baquerizo A, Imagawa DK, et al. Prolongation of hepatic allograft survival in rat recipients treated with anti-lymphotoxin antibody. Transplant Proc 1991;23:602–603.

124. Shiraishi M, Shaked A, Yasunaga C, Hasuike Y, Imagawa DK, Busuttil RW. Monoclonal anti-tumor necrosis factor-α antibody suppresses rejection but enhances infectious complications in rat liver allograft recipients. Transplant Proc 1993;25:128–129.

125. Colquhoun SD, Shaked A, Jurim O, Colonna JO, Rosove MH, Busuttil RW. Reversal of neutropenia with granulocyte colony-stimulating factor without precipitating liver allograft rejection. Transplantation 1993;56:1593–1595.

126. Carrel A, Guthrie CC. The transplantation of veins and organs. Am Med J 1905;10:1101–1102.

127. Hardy JD, Chavez CM, Kurrus FD. Heart transplantation in man: developmental studies and report of a case. JAMA 1964;188:1132–1140.

128. Barnard CN. The operation. A human cardiac transplant: an interim report of a successful operation performed at Groote Schuur Hospital, Cape Town. S Afr Med J 1967;41:1271–1274.

129. Kaye MP. Registry report: International Society for Heart and Lung Transplantation. In: Terasaki PI, Cecka JM, eds. Clnical transplants 1991. Los Angeles, CA: UCLA Tissue Typing Laboratory, 1992:39–59.

130. Lowry RP, Blais D, Marghesco D, Powell WS. Inflammatory mediators and cytotoxins in cardiac allograft rejection: current results and ongoing studies. Transplant Proc 1986; 28:116–118.

131. Imagawa DK, Millis JM, Seu P, et al. The role of tumor necrosis factor in allograft rejection. III. Evidence that anti-TNF antibody therapy prolongs allograft survival in rats with acute rejection. Transplantation 1991;51:57–62.

132. Seu P, Imagawa DK, Wasef E, et al. Monoclonal anti-tumor necrosis factor-α antibody treatment of rat cardiac allografts: synergism with low-dose cyclosporine and immunohistological studies. J Surg Res 1991;50:520–528.

133. Bolling SF, Kunkel SL, Lin H. Prolongation of cardiac allograft survival in rats by anti-TNF and cyclosporine combination therapy. Transplantation 1992;53:283–286.

134. Sporn MB, Roberts AB. Transforming growth factor-β. Multiple actions and potential clinical applications. J Am Med Assoc 1989;262:938–941.

135. Kobashigawa J, Stevenson LW, Louie H, et al. Elevated serum tumor necrosis factor is not useful for monitoring

cardiac transplant rejection (abstract). J Am Coll Cardiol 1991;17:273.

136. Fyfe A, Daly P, Galligan L, Pirc L, Feindel C, Cardella C. Coronary sinus sampling of cytokines after heart transplantation: evidence for macrophage activation and interleukin-4 production within the graft. J Am Coll Cardiol 1993;21:171–176.

137. Roodman ST, Miller LW, Tsai CC. Role of interleukin 2 receptors in immunologic monitoring following cardiac transplantation. Transplantation 1988;45:1050–1056.

138. Zucchelli GC, Clerico A, De Maria R, et al. Increased circulating concentrations of interleukin 2 receptor during rejection episodes in heart- or kidney-transplant recipients. Clin Chem 1990;36:2106–2109.

139. McNally CM, Luckhurst E, Penny R. Cell free serum interleukin-2 receptor levels after heart transplantation. J Heart Lung Transplant 1991;10:769–774.

140. Jutte NHPM, Hesse CJ, Balk AHMM, Mochtar B, Weimar W. Sequential measurements of soluble interleukin 2 receptor levels in plasma of heart transplant recipients. Transplantation 1990;50:328–330.

141. Young JB, Windsor NT, Smart FW, et al. Inability of isolated soluble interleukin-2 receptor levels to predict biopsy rejection scores after heart transplantation. Transplantation 1991;51:636–641.

142. Diamantstein T, Volk H-D, Tilney NL, Kupiec-Weglinski J. Specific immunosuppressive therapy by monoclonal anti-IL 2 receptor antibody and its synergistic action with cyclosporin. Immunobiology 1986;172:391–399.

143. Kupiec-Weglinski JW, Diamantstein T, Tilney NL, Strom TB. Therapy with monoclonal antibody to interleukin 2 receptor spares suppressor T cells and prevents or reverses acute allograft rejection in rats. Proc Natl Acad Sci USA 1986;83:2624–2627.

144. Bouchot O, Anegon I, Romaniuk A, Jacques Y, Paineau J, Soulillou JP. Interleukin 2 receptor in rat heart allograft rejection. Transplantation 1989;48:918–922.

145. Kirkman RL, Bacha P, Barrett LV, Forte S, Murphy JR, Strom TB. Prolongation of cardiac allograft survival in murine recipients treated with a diphtheria toxin-related interleukin-2 fusion protein. Transplantation 1989;47:327–330.

146. Wu CJ, Lovett M, Wong-Lee J, et al. Cytokine gene expression in rejecting cardiac allografts. Transplantation 1992; 54:326–332.

147. Didlake RH, Kim EK, Sheehan K, Schreiber RD, Kahan BD. Effect of combined anti-gamma interferon antibody and cyclosporine therapy on cardiac allograft survival in the rat. Transplantation 1988;45:222–223.

148. Demikhov VP. Some essential points of the techniques of transplantation of the heart, lungs and other organs. In: Experimental transplantation of vital organs. New York: Basil Haigh, Consultants Bureau, 1962:29–48.

149. Kamholtz SL. Current perspectives on clinical and experimental single lung transplantation. Chest 1988;94:390–396.

150. Lima O, Goldberg M, Peters WJ, Ayabe H, Townsend E, Cooper JD. Bronchial omentopexy in canine lung transplantation. J Thorac Cardiovasc Surg 1982;83:418–421.

151. Morgan E, Lima O, Goldberg M, Ferdman A, Luk SK, Cooper JD. Successful revascularization of totally ischemic

bronchial autografts with omental pedical flaps in dogs. J Thorac Cardiovasc Surg 1982;84:204–210.

152. Toronto Lung Transplant Group. Unilateral lung transplantation for pulmonary fibrosis. N Engl J Med 1986; 314:1140–1145.

153. Jamieson SW, Baldwin J, Stinson EB, et al. Clinical heart-lung transplantation. Transplantation 1984;37:81–84.

154. Trulock EP, Cooper JD, Kaiser LR, et al. The Washington University-Barnes Hospital experience with lung transplantation. JAMA 1991;266:1943–1946.

155. Jordan SC, Marchevski A, Ross D, Toyoda M, Waters PF. Serum interleukin-2 levels in lung transplant recipients: correlation with findings on transbronchial biopsy. J Heart Lung Transplant 1992;11:1001–1004.

156. Rubin LA, Nelson DL. The soluble interleukin-2 receptor: biology, function, and clinical application. Ann Intern Med 1990;113:619–627.

157. Lawrence EC, Holland VA, Young JB, et al. Dynamic changes in soluble interleukin-2 receptor levels after lung or heart-lung transplantation. Am Rev Respir Dis 1989; 140:789–796.

158. Keshavjee S, McRitchie D, Rubin L, et al. Serum interleukin-2 receptor levels in the diagnosis of rejection in lung transplant patients. Clin Invest Med 1989;12:101.

159. Humbert M, Emilie D, Cerrina J, et al. Soluble interleukin 2 receptor and neopterin serum levels after lung/heart-lung transplantation—absence of predictive value for late allograft rejection. Transplantation 1991;52:1092–1094.

160. Rondeau E, Cerrina J, Delarue F, et al. Tumor necrosis factor alpha (TNF-alpha) production by cells of bronchiolalveolar lavage (BAL) and peripheral blood mononuclear cells (PBMC) in cardiopulmonary transplants. Transplant Proc 1990;22:1855–1856.

161. Lega M, Dauber JH, Urch SE, Banas R, Whiteside TL, Griffith BP. Tumor necrosis factor-alpha production by alveolar macrophages in heart-lung transplant recipients. Am Rev Respir Dis 1992;145:1036–1041.

162. Yoshida Y, Iwaki Y, Pham S, et al. Benefits of posttransplantation monitoring of interleukin 6 in lung transplantation. Ann Thorac Surg 1993;55:89–93.

163. Woloszczuk W, Troppmair J, Leiter E, et al. Relationship of interferon-gamma and neopterin levels during stimulation with alloantigens in vivo and in vitro. Transplantation 1986;41:716–719.

164. Humbert M, Delattre RM, Cerrina J, Dartevelle P, Simonneau G, Emilie D. Serum neopterin after lung transplantation. Chest 1993;103:449–454.

165. Chang S, Hsu H, Perng R, Shiao G, Lin C. Increased expression of MHC class II antigens in rejecting canine lung allografts. Transplantation 1990;49:1158–1163.

166. Chang S, Hsu H, Perng R, Shaio G, Lin C. Significance of biochemical markers in early detection of canine lung allograft rejection. Transplantation 1991;51:579–584.

167. Jordan SC, Kondo T, Prehn J, Marchevsky A, Waters P. Cytokine gene activation in rat lung allografts: analysis by Northern blotting. Transplant Proc 1991;23:604–606.

168. Francalancia NA, Wang SC, Thai NL, et al. Graft cytokine mRNA activity in rat single lung transplants by reverse transcription-polymerase chain reaction: effect of cyclosporine. J Heart Lung Transplant 1992;11:1041–1045.

169. Rolfe MW, Kunkle S, Lincoln P, Deeb M, Lupinetti F, Strieter R. Lung allograft rejection: role of tumor necrosis factor-alpha and interleukin-6. Chest 1993;103:133.

170. Kelly WD, Lillehei RC, Merkel FK, Idezuki Y, Goetz FC. Allotransplantation of the pancreas and duodenum along with the kidney in diabetic nephropathy. Surgery 1967;61: 827–837.

171. Lillehei RC, Simmons RL, Najarian JS, et al. Pancreaticoduodenal allotransplantation: experimental and clinical experience. Ann Surg 1970;172:405–436.

172. Lillehei RC, Ruix JO, Aquino C, Goetz F. Transplantation of the pancreas. Acta Endocrinol 1976;83(suppl 205):303–318.

173. Sollinger HW, Cook K, Kamps D, Glass NR, Belzer FO. Clinical and experimental experience with pancreaticocystostomy for exocrine pancreatic drainage in pancreas transplantation. Transplant Proc 1984;16:749–751.

174. Ngheim DD, Corry RJ. Technique of simultaneous renal pancreatoduodenal transplantation with urinary drainage of pancreatic secretion. Am J Surg 1987;153:405–406.

175. Wahlberg JA, Love R, Landegaard L, Southard JH, Belzer FO. 72-hour preservation of the canine pancreas. Transplantation 1987;43:5–8.

176. Sutherland DER, Gillingham K, Moudry-Munns KC. Registry report on clinical pancreas transplantation. Transplant Proc 1991;23:55–57.

177. Sollinger HW, Knechtle SJ, Reed AR, et al. Experience with 100 consecutive simultaneous kidney-pancreas transplants with bladder drainage. Ann Surg 1991;214:703–711.

178. Sutherland DER, Dunn DL, Goetz FC, et al. A 10-year experience with 290 pancreas transplants at a single institution. Ann Surg 1989;210:274–288.

179. Shaffer D, Madras PN, Sahyoun AI, et al. Combined kidney and pancreas transplantation: a 3-year experience. Arch Surg 1992;127:574–578.

180. Stratta RJ, Taylor RJ, Zorn BH, et al. Combined pancreas-kidney transplantation: preliminary results and metabolic effects. Am J Gastroenterol 1991;86:697–703.

181. Sutherland DER. Pancreatic transplantation: state of the art. Transplant Proc 1992;24:762–766.

182. Konigsrainer A, Tilg H, Reibnegger G, et al. Pancreatic juice neopterin excretion—a reliable marker of pancreas allograft rejection. Transplant Proc 1992;24:907–908.

183. Cantarovich D, Paineau J, Le Mauff B, et al. Randomized trial of induction immunosuppression with anti-IL2-R monoclonal antibody 33B3.1 and rabbit antithymocyte globulin following simultaneous pancreas and kidney transplantation. Transplant Proc 1992;24:911–910.

184. Lacy PE, Kostianovsky M. Method for the isolation of intact islets of Langerhans from the rat pancreas. Diabetes 1967;16:35–39.

185. Ballinger WF, Lacy PE. Transplantation of intact pancreatic islets in rats. Surgery 1972;72:175–186.

186. Largiader F, Kolb E, Binswanger U. A long-term functioning human pancreatic islet allotransplant. Transplantation 1980;29:76–77.

187. Scharp, DW, Lacy PE, Santiago JV, et al. Insulin indepen-

dence after islet transplantation into type I diabetic patient. Diabetes 1990;39:515–518.

188. Tzakis AG, Ricordi C, Alejandro R, et al. Pancreatic islet transplantation after upper abdominal exenteration and liver replacement. Lancet 1990;336:402–405.

189. Scharp D, Lacy PE, Santiago JV, et al. Results of our first nine intraportal islet allografts in type I, insulin-dependent diabetic patients. Transplantation 1991;51:76–85.

190. Ricordi C, Tzakis A, Carroll P, et al. Human islet allotransplantation in 18 diabetic patients. Transplant Proc 1992; 24:961.

191. Warnock GL, Kneteman NM, Ryan EA, Rabinovitch A, Rajotte RV. Long-term follow-up after transplantation of insulin-producing pancreatic islets into patients with type I (insulin-dependent) diabetes mellitus. Diabetologia 1992;35:89–95.

192. Robertson RP. Pancreatic and islet transplantation for diabetes—cures or curiosities? N Engl J Med 1992;327:1861–1868.

193. Pyzdrowski KL, Kendall DM, Halter JB, Nakhleh RE, Sutherland DER, Robertson RP. Preserved insulin secretion and insulin independence in recipients of islet autografts. N Engl J Med 1992;327:220–226.

194. Najarian JS, Sutherland DER, Baumgartner D, et al. Total or near total pancreatectomy and islet autotransplantation for treatment of chronic pancreatitis. Ann Surg 1980; 192:526–542.

195. Farney AC, Najarian JS, Nakhleh R, et al. Long-term function of islet autotransplants. Transplant Proc 1992;24:969–971.

196. Hao L, Wang Y, Gill RG, La Rosa FG, Talmage DW, Lafferty KJ. Role of lymphokine in islet allograft rejection. Transplantation 1990;49:609–614.

197. Carel J, Schreiber RD, Falqui L, Lacy PE. Transforming growth factor β decreases the immunogenicity of rat islet xenografts (rat to mouse) and prevents rejection in association with treatment of the recipient with a monoclonal antibody to interferon-γ. Proc Natl Acad Sci USA 1990; 87:1591–1595.

198. Carrel A. La technique operatoire des anastomoses vasculaires et la transplantation des visceres. Lyon Medical 1902; 98:859–864.

199. Lillehei RC, Goott B, Miller FA. The physiological response of the small bowel of the dog to ischemia including pro-longed in vitro preservation of the bowel with successful replacement and survival. Ann Surg 1959;150:543–560.

200. Deltz E, Schroeder P, Gebhardt H. Successful clinical small bowel transplantation. Clin Transplant 1989;3:89–91.

201. Grant D, Wall W, Mimeault R, et al. Successful small-bowel/liver transplantation. Lancet 1990;335:181–184.

202. Goulet O, Revillon Y, Brousse N, et al. Successful small bowel transplantation in an infant. Transplantation 1992; 53:940–943.

203. Starzl TE, Rowe MI, Todo S, et al. Transplantation of multiple abdominal viscera. JAMA 1989;261:1449–1457.

204. Williams JW, Sankary HN, Foster PF, Lowe J, Goldman GM. Splanchnic transplantation. An approach to the infant dependent on parenteral nutrition who develops irreversible liver disease. JAMA 1989;261:1458–1462.

205. Busuttil RW, Farmer DG, Shaked A, et al. Successful combined liver and small intestine transplantation for short-gut syndrome and liver failure. West J Med 1993;158:184–188.

206. Cohen Z, Silverman R, Wassef R, et al. Small intestinal transplantation using cyclosporine: report of a case. Transplantation 1986;42:613–620.

207. Hansmann M, Deltz E, Gundlach M, Schroeder P, Radzun H. Small bowel transplantation in a child: morphologic, immunohistochemical, and clinical results. Am J Clin Pathol 1989;92:686–692.

208. Grant D, Sommerauer J, Mimeault R, et al. Treatment with continuous high-dose intravenous cyclosporine following clinical intestinal transplantation. Transplantation 1989; 48:151–152.

209. Todo S, Tzakis AG, Abu-Elmagd K, et al. Intestinal transplantation in composite visceral grafts or alone. Ann Surg 1992;216:223–234.

210. Todo S, Tzakis AG, Abu-Elmagd K, et al. Small intestinal transplantation in humans with or without the colon. Transplantation, 1994;57:840–848.

211. Noguchi K, Yoshida Y, Yagihashi A, et al. Serum levels of interleukin-6 tumor necrosis factor-α, and interleukin-2 in rejecting human small bowel allografts. Transplant Proc 1992;24:1152.

212. Farmer DG, McDiarmid SV, Kuniyoshi J, Robert ME, Shaked A, Busuttil RW. Intragraft expression of interleukin-2- and interferon-gamma-messenger RNA is a predictor of rejection in rat small intestine allografts. Surg Forum 1993;44:426–428.

CHAPTER 11

ROLE OF CYTOKINES IN AUTOIMMUNE DISEASES

Marc Feldmann, Fionula M. Brennan,
and Ravinder N. Maini

There is a group of common human diseases in which autoantibodies or autoantigen reactive T cells can be detected; the autoimmune response eventually leads to interference with various target organ functions. The most common autoimmune diseases include rheumatoid arthritis (RA), systemic lupus erythematosus, Sjögren's syndrome, insulin-dependent diabetes mellitus, and Graves' and Hashimoto's thyroiditis.

These diseases are more common in individuals of a certain human leukocyte antigen (HLA) phenotype; hence, they are termed *HLA-associated diseases*. They are most commonly associated with HLA class II antigens; for example, more than 80% of patients with RA are HLA-DR4 or HLA-DRI (1), and 90% of type I (insulin-dependent) diabetics are HLA-DR3 or HLA-DR4 (2). A smaller number of diseases are associated with HLA class I antigens; nearly all, such as ankylosing spondylitis, are associated with HLA-B27. Because the molecular function of HLA molecules is now understood to be for peptide binding and subsequent "presentation" to T-cell receptors for antigen, the observed HLA association implies a critical role for T cells at some (or several) stages in the disease process. However, it should be stressed that in no disease are the molecules responsible for HLA association completely known. As more molecules encoded in HLA are discovered, such as peptide transporters (3), proteasome (proteolytic enzymes involved in antigen processing) (4), HSP 70, and tumor necrosis factors (LT-α, LT-β, TNF-α), it is possible that several may also be involved, and much

work remains to be done in this area to elucidate the mechanisms by which HLA is associated with disease. Perhaps the most popular, and the simplest, concept is that the HLA class II molecules associated with disease are involved in the presentation of autoantigenic peptides to autoantigen-reactive T cells. However, the critical interaction could occur earlier in the pathogenesis (e.g., in the development of the T-cell repertoire) by permitting self peptides to bind in the thymus, thus influencing positive or negative selection, or at the initiation phase, thus influencing the response to a viral or a bacterial peptide.

MECHANISM OF AUTOIMMUNITY

Over the past few years, evidence has accumulated to support a conceptual framework of the pathogenesis of autoimmune diseases that was initially proposed for the endocrine autoimmune diseases (5,6). Experimentally, this hypothesis has been most extensively tested, due to readier access to the affected tissue, in patients with Graves' disease (autoimmune hyperthyroidism) (Fig. 11–1). Three stages are illustrated in our current versions of the mechanism of autoimmunity. The first stage, **initiation**, presupposes that environmental agents, in suitably genetically predisposed individuals, induce the release of cytokines, probably as a consequence of T-cell activation.

At the time the hypothesis that cytokines are involved

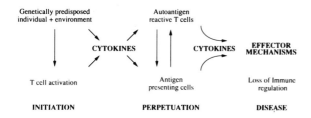

Figure 11–1 The development of autoimmunity.

in induction and maintenance of autoimmune disease was formulated, the T-cell–derived cytokine interferon-γ (IFN-γ) was the only cytokine known to induce HLA class II antigens, molecules that are critical for antigen presentation (7). It was therefore proposed that T-cell activation and relapse of IFN-γ were crucial early events leading to up-regulation of antigen-presenting capacity. In the human diseases, this concept is not directly testable because there is no indication to administer IFN-γ locally, although its administration intrathecally in patients with multiple sclerosis caused relapses (8). However, it has become apparent, as a result of therapeutic trials of the cytokines interleukin-2 (IL-2) and IFN-α in cancer patients, that autoimmunity, especially of the thyroid, is a frequent side effect (9,10). This autoimmunity is often severe enough to warrant therapy, but it resolves on cessation of therapy. Autoantibodies are usually present, and there is HLA association, suggesting that the mechanisms of cytokine-induced disease are related to the spontaneous form of the disease.

In a transgenic mouse model, the concept of whether locally acting cytokines such as IFN-γ may induce autoimmunity was tested by Sarvetnick and colleagues (11). Insulin promoter–driven IFN-γ production results in an autoimmune form of type I diabetes (11), in which T-cell tolerance has been abrogated, islet cells express class II antigens, and grafted islet cells are rejected (12). This is a direct and positive test of the hypothesis proposed. Recently, it was shown that diabetes develops in insulin promoter IFN-α transgenic mice. This finding is potentially related to the situation in humans, in whom IFN-α production by islet cells has been reported (13).

The **maintenance** phase of autoimmune disease was postulated to involve continual interactions between autoantigen-reactive T lymphocytes and tissue antigen-presenting cells. In thyroid disease, it was shown that thyroid epithelial cells can present antigen, either influenza peptides (14) or surface autoantigens (15). It was envisaged that the autoantigen-reactive cells, after stimulation by class II antigen-expressing thyrocytes acting as antigen-presenting cells (APCs), release cytokines that maintain thyrocyte class II expression and antigen-presenting function. Much evidence has been accumulated to support this concept, such as the cloning of thyrocyte-specific and stimulatable T cells from the thyroid infiltrate (15,16),

and the demonstration that cytokines such as IFN-γ and TNF-α induce thyrocyte class II antigen expression (17). Cytokines such as IFN-γ, TNF-α, IL-1, and IL-6 have been detected in the thyroid at the messenger RNA (mRNA) and protein level (18,19), and a number of the cytokines, such as IL-6, are produced by the thyrocytes. In other diseases, such as RA, in which the local cell composition is different, it is likely that the APCs are not atypical APCs, but they include conventional APCs, such as macrophages, dendritic cells, and B cells, especially CD5+ B cells (20).

There is recent evidence that there are aspects of immune regulation that are abnormal late in the autoimmune disease process. The one we uncovered during a study of the properties of T cells cloned from the thyroids of patients with Graves' disease (GD), is a relative resistance to the induction of clonal anergy. The induction of clonal anergy by antigen is a type of immunological tolerance that has been studied since 1983, and it is likely to be only one of multiple immunoregulatory mechanisms, which, if functioning optimally, may be able to switch off the autoimmune reaction. It is not clear why these T cells are refractory to anergy induction in vitro, with either the relevant peptides or with staphylococcal enterotoxins (21). The latter phenomenon excludes the possibility that the lack of anergy is due to low T-cell receptor affinity for its ligand, the peptide-class II complexes, because the enterotoxins bind the Vβ chain of the T-cell receptor, away from the peptide binding area.

Our concept for explaining the resistance to anergy is that during the development of the autoimmunity process, there is selection: T cells sensitive to anergy were probably anergized early in the autoimmunization process and, hence, are no longer detectable. Only refractory T cells would persist; hence, after the typical multiyear disease "induction" process, the T cells available for cloning are expected to be refractory to inhibitory mechanisms. T cells from the tissue sites could be refractory to immune regulation late in the autoimmunity process.

In addition to contributing to onset and maintenance of the autoimmune process, there is considerable evidence that cytokines are also involved in the **tissue-damaging or late stage** of the autoimmune process. Cytokines released by both T lymphocytes and APCs are involved in activating the effector systems of the immune response, leading to production of autoantibodies, immune complexes, complement activation, activated cytotoxic T cells, activated macrophages and natural killer (NK) cells, and activated polymorphs, among others (22).

As a consequence of tissue damage, tissue repair processes are engaged, which also involve cytokines, as does the ensuing fibrosis. Thus, cytokines are intimately involved in every stage of the autoimmune process, and therapy aimed at selectively regulating one or other cytokines may have profound clinical benefits, or it could be deleterious. One of the main goals of cytokine research in this field is to define which cytokines may be the most appropriate targets for therapy. Because of the subtle differences in mechanisms in different diseases, it is likely that optimal therapeutic targets will vary in different diseases.

THE CYTOKINE SYSTEM IN RA

Because it is clearly impossible to catalogue the extent of cytokine studies in a wide spectrum of autoimmune diseases, and partly because many diseases have not yet been extensively studied, we focus on the one disease most extensively studied (by ourselves and others) and hence most familiar. Rheumatoid arthritis (RA) also has the advantage that it is possible to biopsy the disease site at the height of the inflammatory process, which is rarely possible in other human diseases, as well as in many important diseases, such as multiple sclerosis and insulin-dependent diabetes mellitus.

In a disease such as RA, which has strong local manifestations, it would be anticipated that the cytokines produced at the site of disease would be most relevant to the disease process. Thus, we have chosen to evaluate synovial membrane cytokine expression, initially using mRNA analysis to monitor local synthesis. Because there is evidence that in some circumstances cytokine mRNA and protein levels do not correlate, cytokine protein synthesis by synovial joint cell cultures was ascertained subsequently. We did not choose to study synovial fluid cytokine levels at first because of problems associated with analysis of synovial fluids, such as high concentration of enzymes, proteins, and glycosaminoglycans, all of which render assays more difficult. Subsequently, because cytokines act locally, it became interesting to determine which cells were major cytokine producers, and which cells produced them using in situ hybridization and immunostaining.

Our studies (23–29) and those of other groups in the field have led to the realization that virtually every cytokine known and assayable can be found in the patients with synovium RA (Table 11–1). With hindsight, this finding is not surprising, because there are activated T cells, macrophages, endothelium, fibroblasts, and plasma cells in the synovium, all of which can produce cytokines actively. Therefore, the key problem was to ascertain which, if any, of the many cytokines produced were most important in the pathogenesis of the disease.

Second, the quantity of cytokines detected is not necessarily a reflection of their importance. Because macrophages are efficient secretory cells, it is expected that they produce a lot more protein, and hence cytokines, than T cells. In contrast, the physiology of T cells is to migrate to the site of the "action" and to deliver their signals

TABLE 11–1   SUMMARY OF CYTOKINES PRODUCED SPONTANEOUSLY BY RA SYNOVIAL CELLS

Cytokine	mRNA	Protein
IL-1α	Yes	Yes
IL-1β	Yes	Yes
TNF-α	Yes	Yes
LT	Yes	(+/−)*
IL-2	Yes	(+/−)
IL-3	No	No
IL-4	?	No
IFN-γ	Yes	(+/−)
IL-6	Yes	Yes
GM-CSF	Yes	Yes
IL-8/NAP-1	Yes	Yes
IL-10	Yes	Yes
RANTES	Yes	?
G-CSF	Yes	Yes
M-CSF	Yes	Yes
TGF-β	Yes	Yes
EGF	Yes	Yes
TGF-α	No	No
PDGF-A	Yes	Yes
PDGF-B	Yes	Yes

*(+/−) indicates that demonstration of protein proved difficult. IL-1 = interleukin-1; TNF-α = tumor necrosis factor; LT = lymphotoxin; IFN-γ = interferon-γ; GM-CSF = granulocyte-macrophage colony-stimulating factor; NAP-1 = neutrophil-activating peptide; RANTES = regulated on activation, normal T expressed and secreted; G-CSF = granulocyte colony-stimulating factor; M-CSF = macrophage colony-stimulating factor; TGF-β = transforming growth factor-β; EGF = epidermal growth factor; PDGF = platelet-derived growth factor.

(cytokines, or lytic granules) directly to the surface of their target. Thus, the smaller amounts of T-cell cytokines (e.g., IL-2, IL-4, IFN-γ) detected in RA synovium is not sufficient evidence to assume that T-cell–derived cytokines are not important in the disease process.

One of the observations that has permitted us to understand the regulation of cytokines in the RA joint was a result of establishing a model system to study these interactions in the diseased tissue. We found that culturing dissociated (collagenase-treated) rheumatoid synovial membrane cells in the **absence** of any extrinsic stimulus revealed that the cytokine production detected (e.g., IL-1) remained relatively stable if measured at either mRNA or protein levels for many days (24,26). Typically, we analyzed 5- or 6-day cultures, because in these cultures, the cell composition remains similar to that at the beginning of culture. In contrast, extrinsic stimulation of peripheral blood mononuclear cells (PBMCs) by mitogens, for example, induces transient cytokine mRNA production. For short-lived cytokines such as IL-1α, this cycle of synthesis can be completed within 24 hours.

These cultures of dissociated rheumatoid synovial membrane also express HLA class II antigens at high and relatively stable levels, as is found in vivo. Thus, this culture system appeared to be a useful model to study cell and molecular interactions of the rheumatoid joint in vitro, because many signs of RA activation were present. Because IL-1 was described to be important in inducing cartilage and bone destruction (30,31), we analyzed the regulation of bioactive IL-1 in these cultures. It was ascertained in parallel studies that a variety of cytokines induce IL-1. By using neutralizing antisera to TNF-α and TNF-β (potent inducers of IL-1), it was found that neutralizing TNF-α virtually abrogated IL-1 production from these cultures (26) (Fig. 11–2A). This result was surprising, because many other "signals" present in the RA joint could also induce IL-1 (e.g., IL-1, granulocyte-macrophage colony-stimulating factor [GM-CSF], IFN-γ, immune complexes). However, it was reproducible in all the RA synovial cultures, and it led to our initial awareness of the importance of TNF-α in the pathogenesis of RA. These results also prompted further experiments to investigate the role of TNF-α in RA. It was found that anti-TNF-α inhibited production of another proinflammatory cytokine, GM-CSF (Fig. 11–2B) (29), and, in studies currently in progress, diminution of IL-6 and IL-8 production (Butler DM et al., unpublished observations), as well as reducing cell adhesion and class II antigen expression. These results are summarized in Fig. 11–3. TNF-α was

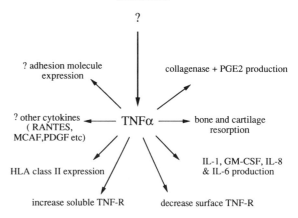

EFFECTS MEDIATED BY TNFα IN RHEUMATOID ARTHRITIS

Figure 11–3   Effects of TNF-α in RA.

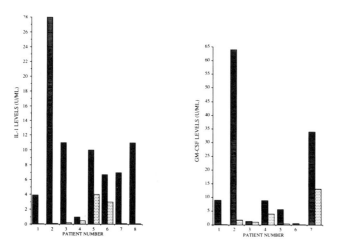

Figure 11–2   Anti-TNF-α inhibits IL-1 production in RA synovial joint cells in culture. RA synovial joint cells were cultured for 5 days with (■) or without (▦) neutralizing antibodies to TNF-α. IL-1 levels were measured using the comitogenic mouse thymocyte bioassay. (B) Anti-TNF-α inhibits GM-CSF production in RA synovial joint cells in culture. RA synovial joint cells were cultured for 5 days with (■) or without (▦) neutralizing antibodies to TNF-α. GM-CSF levels were measured using the Mo7E bioassay.

also detected by immunostaining, both in the membrane and in the cartilage pannus junction (32), which is compatible with the important role in RA pathogenesis that was emerging.

Other evidence for the importance of TNF-α has come from generation of transgenic mice. Mice with a human genomic TNF-α transgene in which the 3' untranslated UT-rich region, which yields unstable mRNA, had been replaced with the β-globin 3' UT region, have been produced (33). Asymmetrical arthritis develops in these mice from 4 weeks of age that resembles RA. It is not clear why this systemic disregulation of TNF-α should generate arthritis as virtually its only manifestation, but the finding suggests that synovial joints are highly sensitive to the effect of TNF-α. Because human TNF-α only reacts with the murine p55 TNF receptor (34), this TNF receptor is implicated as being critically involved in the arthritis process, at least in mice. One of the reasons why arthritis may develop in these mice without obviously high levels of TNF production or elevated circulating TNF is that the murine-soluble p75 receptor (the most abundant TNF inhibitor) would not be expected to act endogenously as an inhibitor of human TNF-α. We have started to investigate these mice, and it appears that they up-regulate the soluble murine p75 receptor in their serum, but not the p55 receptor (Burman WA, unpublished observations).

WHAT DOWN-REGULATES IMMUNE AND CYTOKINE RESPONSES IN RHEUMATOID JOINTS?

During a chronic disease such as RA, there is evidence of T-cell activation, as judged by cell surface markers (e.g., HLA class II, CD69), but the degree of activation by other criteria (e.g., blast morphology, proliferation, and T-cell cytokine response) is not what is seen in normal PBMC activated by mitogens. This finding strongly suggests that a homeostatic, immune regulatory effect occurs in the joint. Therefore, it was clearly of interest to attempt to evaluate what important molecular mediators may be involved. However, because it is unlikely that we know the full range of immunosuppressive cytokines, there are inherently major gaps in our knowledge of this field.

There is evidence that transforming growth factor-β (TGF-β) is capable of inhibiting the function of T lymphocytes (proliferation and cytokine release) if added to these cells prior to their activation (35,36). The effect of TGF-β on B cells is more complex, however, because it inhibits proliferation (37) and secretion of some immunoglobulin (Ig) isotypes, but at the same time, it induces IgA and IgG2b (38). On monocytes, cytokine (e.g., IL-1, TNF-α) (39) and adhesion molecule expression is downregulated if the cells are pretreated with TGF-β prior to activation. Thus, it was of considerable interest that significant quantities of TGF-β were detected in rheumatoid joint cell culture supernatants by mRNA, enzyme-linked immunosorbent assay (ELISA), and bioassay (27). Bioassay detection was important, because TFG-β requires activation to be bioactive. Experiments were performed to evaluate the effect of additional (extrinsic) TGF-β on RA joint cell cultures. However, these tests did not demonstrate any additional benefit, which is in keeping with the concept that either the maximal TGF-β effect was already manifested, or that TGF-β was ineffective because the cells were activated previously (27).

Investigations to assess the immunosuppressive potential of TGF-β in vivo have also yielded conflicting results. For example, if injected locally into the joints of normal rats, TGF-β resulted in rapid leukocyte infiltration and synovial hyperplasia leading to synovitis (40,41), whereas if injected systemically into mice "susceptible" to arthritis, it antagonized the development of polyarthritis (42,43). Furthermore, in a recent publication (44), it was found that anti-TGF-β antibody, if injected locally into the joint of rats with arthritis, diminished the ongoing inflammation. These studies indicate the multipotential properties of TGF-β, and the different effects if injected systemically or locally into the joint.

Moreover, in addition to possessing immunoregulatory properties on cytokine production, TGF-β clearly has other inflammatory effects, such as acting as a chemotactic factor for monocytes. Furthermore, TGF-β is likely to be a key cytokine involved in repair and fibrosis in the joints. For example, while inhibiting production of metalloproteinases such as collagenase, it stimulates the production of type I collagen (45) and type XI (46). Thus, TGF-β may promote local scarring and tissue repair, as well as reparative processes in arthritic synovial connective tissue by inhibiting cartilage and bone destruction. However, in chronic lesions, in which there is overproduction of TGF-β, these processes can contribute to the "ongoing" damage by recruiting inflammatory macrophages and fibroblasts with the potential for tissue destruction.

IL-4, which is produced by activated T cells, similar to other T-cell cytokines, is not found at significant levels in RA synovium (see Table 11–1). Interest has been directed toward use of IL-4 as immunomodulatory cytokine therapy in RA based on the observation that IL-4 inhibits lipopolysaccharide (LPS)-induced proinflammatory cytokine and prostaglandin E_2 production in human monocytes (47–49) and in RA synovial joint cell organ cultures (50). However, IL-4 is a multifunctional cytokine, and it also displays activities such as induction of HLA class II antigen expression on B cells and monocytes (51,52) and growth potential for T and B cells (53,54), which could be considered to be proinflammatory effects. Clearly, the overall effect of IL-4 in inflammatory tissue will depend on the target cell, the differentiation status, and the influence of other cytokines in the environment. Although the use of IL-4 as a therapeutic agent in RA has been suggested, this approach would have to be viewed in light of IL-4's T- and B-cell activation properties, as well as its effect on HLA class II antigen expression. Furthermore, we have recently shown that although IL-4 reduces TNF levels (albeit insignificantly) in RA synovial joint cell cultures (55), expression of TNF receptor on the surface of cells increased significantly, which could conceivably increase the biological effects of TNF-α. However, IL-4 production in RA joints is defective, and the incidence of allergies is lower in patients with RA (56). This finding could imply that HLA class II antigen genetic predisposition to development of autoimmunity does not predispose to development of allergies, or that there is a "Th2" defect in RA.

Interleukin-10

In the past year, we have documented that IL-10, previously known as "cytokine synthesis inhibitory factor" (57), is expressed in RA joints, and it has an important immunoregulatory role (58). The evidence for IL-10 expression is from mRNA detection by reverse transcription polymerase chain reaction and immunoassays of RA synovial joint cell culture supernatants. Furthermore, after addition of neutralizing anti-IL-10 antibodies to these cultures, augmentation in the spontaneous release of TNF and IL-1 followed. Because IL-10 was initially assayed by its inhibition of IFN-γ synthesis, it was of interest to determine the effect of neutralizing IL-10 on IFN production in the RA synovial cell cultures. In 2 of 5 cultures, there was an elevation, from undetectable (<5pg/mL) to

1,100 and 600 pg/mL. This observation needs to be confirmed with more samples, but it is conceivable that IL-10 is the major regulator of T-cell–derived cytokine production. If this result is confirmed, then the Firestein and Zvaifler (59) "hypothesis," which assumes that the late phase of RA does not involve T cells as important components, is unlikely to be valid.

We have also recently found (60) that IL-10 further modulates TNF production by inducing production of the soluble TNF receptors from monocyte cultures while down-regulating surface expression. IL-10 also up-regulates the natural inhibitor of IL-1, the IL-1 receptor antagonist protein, in monocyte cultures (61). Thus, an immunoregulatory cytokine such as IL-10 can have profound effects on the regulation of proinflammatory cytokines such as TNF and IL-1. However, it is also apparent that in chronic inflammatory tissue, such as the RA synovial membrane, IL-10 is produced, and although it has some modulatory effect on the production of proinflammatory cytokines such as TNF, it is clearly insufficient to control the disease process.

Cytokine inhibitors: soluble receptors and receptor antagonists

Over the last few years, the presence of cytokine inhibitors has also been investigated in RA. Roux-Lombard and colleagues (62) found that synovial fluid mononuclear cells secrete an IL-1 inhibitor, which was identified as the IL-1 receptor antagonist protein, IL-1 RA. A second IL-1 inhibitor was also present in synovial fluid, and it was shown to be a soluble form of the IL-1 receptor. This soluble IL-1 receptor (63), which is found in plasma, synovial fluid, and is produced by activated PBMCs, binds to IL-1β, but not to IL-1α or the IL-1 receptor antagonist. The presence of IL-1RA has been immunolocalized in RA and osteoarthritis (OA) synovial tissue (64,65), and it is found at higher levels in RA compared with OA or normal synovial tissue. Thus, in chronic inflammation, the natural antagonist of IL-1, IL-1RA, is up-regulated. However, this effect is obviously insufficient, because IL-1 bioactivity is still detected in RA joint cell cultures.

A similar observation was recently made with respect to the natural inhibitors of TNF, the soluble p55 and p75 TNF-R. We have found that both receptors are significantly elevated in RA plasma compared with normal plasma (66), and they are further increased in synovial fluid compared with other inflammatory diseases (Fig. 11–4), suggesting that the cellular source of these proteins is within the inflamed synovial joint. Indeed, soluble TNF-R are released spontaneously by RA synovial joint cells in culture, and TNF bioactivity in these culture su-

pernatants is increased after neutralization of the soluble receptors with monoclonal antibodies. However, despite increased production of the natural inhibitor, TNF bioactivity is still detectable in the synovial joint. Thus, although there is evidence that there are multiple mechanisms of cytokine regulation that occur within the RA joint, these mechanisms do not appear to be able to cope with the disease process, which can be viewed as an imbalance between the production of proinflammatory cytokines and their inhibitors. This hypothesis is summarized in Fig. 11–5.

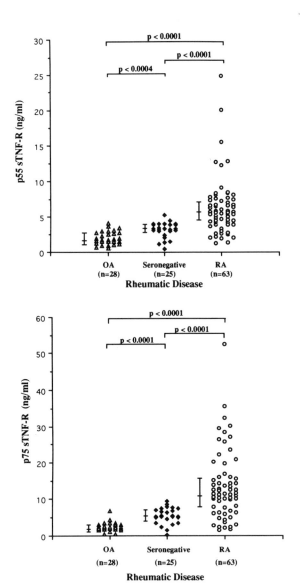

Figure 11–4 Soluble TNF receptor levels in synovial fluid. p55 sTNF receptor (above) and p75 sTNF receptor (below) in synovial fluid of osteoarthritic (▲), seronegative (◆), and rheumatoid arthritic (○) patients.

INTERACTION BETWEEN TNFα SURFACE AND SOLUBLE TNF RECEPTOR

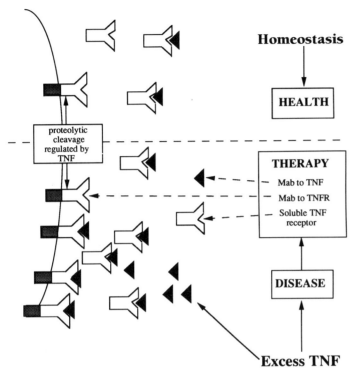

Figure 11–5 Interaction between TNF-α and the surface/soluble TNF receptors in health and disease.

WHAT CAN WE LEARN ABOUT THE CYTOKINE NETWORK FROM THERAPEUTIC CLINICAL TRIALS?

Despite that fact the cytokines are local hormones, the physiology of the cytokine system, like all other aspects of physiology, is best studied in vivo. Because animal models of autoimmune diseases such as arthritis only mimic some of the aspects of the human diseases, clinical trials may be very illuminating sources of information about cytokine physiology.

We performed a small Phase I/II clinical trial of monoclonal anti-TNF-α in patients with long-standing RA who have active disease and who have failed multiple disease-modifying treatments (67). The antibody used was a high affinity chimeric antibody (human IgG1/mouse Fv) termed cA2 (Centocor Inc., Malvern, Pa). On the basis of our studies on murine collagen-induced arthritis, during which three injections of 10 mg/kg were beneficial, but three injections of 2 mg/kg were not, the dose regimen chosen was 20 mg/kg, split over either two

or four infusions, over a 2-week period. The results were assessed both clinically and in the laboratory. The clinical measurements were of two types: subjective assessments, such as intensity of pain and duration of morning stiffness, and semiobjective assessments. Infusion of anti-TNF-α caused a rapid and marked diminution in pain scores on a 0 to 10 scale, the levels of which changed from a median of 7.4 to a median of 1.9 in 2 weeks. Similarly, morning stiffness diminished rapidly, from 180 to 5 minutes (median).

Semiobjective assessments were made by a trained nurse, and they included joint swelling and joint tenderness. There was potential for interobserver error; therefore, all patients were assessed by the same observer. Swollen joint counts decreased from a median of 18 to 5 in 6 weeks, and tender joint assessment (Ritchie Score) decreased from 23 to 6 by 6 weeks. These changes are greater than those noted for other recent attempts at biotherapy (e.g., with anti-CD4). In addition, because all patients responded, this was a good result.

However, the laboratory assessments are easiest to document objectively. There was a marked decrease in the acute-phase protein levels, such as C-reactive protein (CRP), which decreased from a pretrial median of 42 to 8 mg/L, and serum amyloid A levels decreased from 245 to 80 mg/L at week 2. The erythrocyte sedimentation rate decreased from a median of 55 to 23 mm/hour. These assays indicate that infusion of the anti-TNF-α chimeric antibody, cA2, had a marked effect on the metabolic effects of the disease. Serum IL-6 levels were measured, by two different assays, and these levels were diminished following therapy in the patients in whom they were initially elevated.

There is consensus that the dominant signal for regulation of CRP is IL-6, and the abrupt decrease in CRP levels and the decrease in serum IL-6 levels indicate that blocking TNF-α in vivo has an influence on other components of the cytokine network. These results in humans, and analogous results in mice (e.g., anti-TNF treatment of mice infected with *E. coli* resulted in reduction in IL-1 and IL-6 levels) (68), suggest that a considerable part of the cytokine network is organized in "series" and not in parallel. This finding may explain why the prediction that because inflammatory tissues, such as the RA joint, have multiple cytokines, each exerting the same action ("cytokine redundancy"), removal of a single cytokine would not have clinical benefit has proved incorrect, at least in RA.

The results obtained from both in vitro studies of RA synovial mononuclear leukocytes and clinical trials indicate that there is a "hierarchy" of cytokines, and that there is direction to the flow of information, mediated by the cytokines (Fig. 11–6). Currently, there is far too little information concerning which effects of cytokines really

How does the cytokine network operate?

-Analogy with electrical circuits

Circuit in parallel

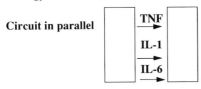

**Blocking one would have little effect.
High redundancy**

Circuit in series

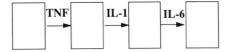

**Prediction: Blocking any one would have an
effect. Hierarchy**

Figure 11–6 The cytokine network. Evidence from RA and other diseases suggests a "circuit in series" network.

matter in vivo in immune responses and disease states. Much more information could be obtained using neutralizing antibodies in animals and in clinical trials in humans.

REFERENCES

1. Wordsworth BP, Bell JL. Polygenic susceptibility in rheumatoid arthritis. Ann Rheum Dis 1991;50:343–346.

2. Bell JI, Denney D Jr, Foster L, Belt T, Todd JA, McDevitt HO. Allelic variation in the DR subregion of the human major histocompatibility complex. Proc Natl Acad Sci USA 1987;84:6234–6238.

3. Bahram S, Arnold D, Bresnahan M, Strominger JL, Spies T. Two putative subunits of a peptide pump encoded in the human major histocompatibility complex class II region. Proc Natl Acad Sci USA 1991;88:10094–10098.

4. Kelly A, Powis SH, Glynne R, Radley E, Beck S, Trowsdale J. Second proteasome-related gene in the human MHC class II region. Nature 1991;353:667–668.

5. Bottazzo GF, Pujol-Borrell R, Hanafusa T, Feldmann M. Hypothesis: role of aberrant HLA-DR expression and antigen presentation in the induction of endocrine autoimmunity. Lancet 1983;2:1115–1119.

6. Feldmann M. Molecular mechanisms involved in human autoimmune diseases: relevance of chronic antigen presentation, class II expression and cytokine production. Immunology 1989;(suppl 2):66–71.

7. Steeg P, Moore RN, Johnson HM, Oppenheim JJ. Regulation of murine macrophage Ia antigen expression by a lymphokine with interferon activity. J Exp Med 1982;156:1780–1793.

8. Panitch HS, Hirsh RL, Haley AS, Johnson KP. Exacerbations of multiple sclerosis in patients treated with gamma interferon. Lancet 1987;1:893–894.

9. Burman P, Toterman TH, Oberg K, Karlsson FA. Thyroid autoimmunity in patients on long term therapy with leu-kocyte-derived interferon. J Clin Endocrinol Metab 1986;63:1086–1090.

10. Atkins MB, Mier JW, Parkinson DR, Gould JA, Berkman EM, Kaplan MM. Hypothyroidism after treatment with interleukin-2 and lymphokine-activated killer cells. N Engl J Med 1988;318:1557–1563.

11. Sarvetnick N, Liggitt D, Pitts SL, Hansen SE, Stewart TA. Insulin dependent diabetes mellitus induced in transgenic mice by ectopic expression of class II MHC and interferon-gamma. Cell 1988;52:773–782.

12. Sarvetnick N, Shizuru J, Liggitt D, et al. Loss of pancreatic islet tolerance induced by beta-cell expression of interferon-gamma. Nature 1990;46:844–847.

13. Foulis AK, Farquharson MA, Meager A. Immunoreactive alpha-interferon in insulin-secreting beta cells in type I diabetes mellitus. Lancet 1987;2:1423–1427.

14. Londei M, Lamb JR, Bottazzo GF, Feldmann M. Epithelial cells expressing aberrant MHC class II determinants can present antigen to cloned human T cells. Nature 1984;312:639–641.

15. Londei M, Bottazzo GF, Feldmann M. Human T-cell clones from autoimmune thyroid glands: specific recognition of autologous thyroid cells. Science 1985;228:85–89.

16. Dayan CM, Londei M, Corcoran AE, et al. Autoantigen recognition by thyroid infiltrating T cells in Graves disease. Proc Natl Acad Sci USA 1991;88:7415–7419.

17. Todd I, Pujol-Borrell R, Hammond LJ, Bottazzo GF, Feldmann M. Interferon-γ induces HLA-DR expression by thyroid epithelium. Clin Exp Immunol 1985;61:265–273.

18. Grubeck Loebenstein B, Buchan G, Chantry D, et al. Analysis of intrathyroidal cytokine production in thyroid autoimmune disease: thyroid follicular cells produce IL-1α and interleukin-6. Clin Exp Immunol 1989;77:324–330.

19. Zheng RQH, Abney E, Chu CQ, et al. Detection of IL-6 and IL-1 production in human thyroid epithelial cells by non-radioactive in situ hybridisation and immunohistochemical methods. Clin Exp Immunol 1991;83:314–319.

20. Andrew EM, Annis W, Kahan M, Maini RN. CD5 (Ly-1)-negative conventional splenic B cells make a substantial contribution to the bromelain plaque-forming cell response in CBA and BW mice. Immunology 1990;69:515–518.

21. Dayan CM, Chu NR, Londei M, Rapoport B, Feldmann M. T cells involved in human autoimmune disease are resistant to tolerance induction. J Immunol 1993;151:1606–1613.

22. Hirano T, Akira S, Taga T, Kishimoto T. Biological and clinical aspects of interleukin 6. Immunol Today 1990;11:443–449.

23. Buchan GS, Barrett K, Fujita T, Taniguchi T, Maini RN, Feldmann M. Detection of activated T cell products in the rheumatoid joint using cDNA probes to interleukin 2, IL-2 receptor and interferon γ. Clin Exp Immunol 1988;71:295–301.

24. Buchan G, Barrett K, Turner M, Chantry D, Maini RN, Feldmann M. Interleukin-1 and tumour necrosis factor mRNA expression in rheumatoid arthritis: prolonged production of IL-1α. Clin Exp Immunol 1988;73:449–455.

25. Hirano T, Matsuda T, Turner M, et al. Excessive produc-

tion of interleukin 6/B cell stimulatory factor-2 in rheumatoid arthritis. Eur J Immunol 1988;18:1797–1801.

26. Brennan FM, Chantry D, Jackson A, Maini RN, Feldmann M. Inhibitory effect of TNFα antibodies on synovial cell interleukin-1 production in rheumatoid arthritis. Lancet 1989;2:244–247.

27. Brennan FM, Chantry D, Turner M, Foxwell B, Maini RN, Feldmann M. Detection of transforming growth factor-β in rheumatoid arthritis synovial tissue: lack of effect on spontaneous cytokine production in joint cell cultures. Clin Exp Immunol 1990;81:278–285.

28. Brennan FM, Zachariae COC, Chantry D, et al. Detection of interleukin-8 biological activity in synovial fluids from patients with rheumatoid arthritis and production of IL-8 mRNA by isolated synovial cells. Eur J Immunol 1990; 20:2141–2144.

29. Haworth C, Brennan FM, Chantry D, Turner M, Maini RN, Feldmann M. Expression of granulocyte-macrophage colony stimulating factor (GM-CSF) in rheumatoid arthritis: regulation by tumour necrosis factor α. Eur J Immunol 1991;21:2575–2579.

30. Saklatavala J, Sarsfield SJ, Townsend Y. Purification of two immunologically different leukocyte proteins that cause cartilage resorption lymphocyte activation and fever. J Exp Med 1985;162:1208–1215.

31. Gowen M, Wood DD, Ihrie EJ, McGuire MKB, Russell RG. An interleukin-1 like factor stimulates bone resorption in vitro. Nature 1983;306:378–380.

32. Chu CQ, Field M, Feldmann M, Maini RN. Localization of tumor necrosis factor α in the synovial tissues and at the cartilage-pannus junction in patients with rheumatoid arthritis. Arthritis Rheum 1991;34:1125–1132.

33. Keffer J, Probert L, Cazlaris H, et al. Transgenic mice expressing human tumour necrosis factor: a predictive genetic model of arthritis. EMBO J 1991;10:4025–4031.

34. Barrett K, Taylor-Fishwick DA, Cope AP, et al. Cloning, expression and cross-linking analysis of the murine p55 tumor necrosis factor receptor. Eur J Immunol 1991;21: 1649–1656.

35. Kehrl JH, Wakefield LM, Roberts AB, et al. Production of transforming growth factor-β by human T lymphocytes. J Immunol 1986;163:1037–1050.

36. Ranges GE, Figari IS, Espevik T, Palladino MA. Inhibition of cytotoxic T cell development by transforming growth factor beta, reversal by recombinant tumour necrosis factor. J Exp Med 1987;166:991–998.

37. Kehrl JH, Roberts AB, Wakefield LM, Jakowlew S, Sporn MB, Fauci AS. Transforming growth factor β is an important immunomodulatory protein for human B lymphocytes. J Immunol 1986;137:3855–3860.

38. Coffman RL, Lebman DA, Shrader B. Transforming growth factor beta specifically enhances IgA production by lipopolysaccharide-stimulated muring B lymphocytes. J Exp Med 1989;170:1039–1044.

39. Chantry D, Turner M, Abney ER, Feldmann M. Modulation of cytokine production by transforming growth factor β. J Immunol 1989;142:4295–4300.

40. Allen JB, Manthey CL, Hand AR, Ohura K, Ellingsworth L, Wahl SM. Rapid onset synovial inflammation and hyperplasia induced by transforming growth factor β. J Exp Med 1990;171:231–247.

41. Fava RA, Olsen NJ, Postlethwaite AE, et al. Transforming growth factor β_1 (TGF-β_1) induced neutrophil recruitment to synovial tissues: implications for TFG-β-driven synovial inflammation and hyperplasia. J Exp Med 1991;173:1121–1132.

42. Brandes ME, Allen JB, Ogawa Y, Wahl SM. Transforming growth factor β_1 suppresses acute and chronic arthritis in experimental animals. J Clin Invest 1991;87:1108–1113.

43. Kuruvilla AP, Shah R, Hochwald GM, Liggitt HD, Palladino MA, Thorbecke GJ. Protective effect of transforming growth factor β_1 on experimental autoimmune diseases in mice. Proc Natl Acad Sci USA 1991;8:2918–2921.

44. Wahl SM, Allen JB, Costa GL, Wong HL, Dasch JR. Reversal of acute and chronic synovial inflammation by anti-transforming growth factor beta. J Exp Med 1993;177:225–230.

45. Lafyatis R, Thomson NL, Remmers ER, Flanders KC, Roche NS, Kim SJ. Transforming growth factor-beta production by synovial tissues from rheumatoid patients and streptococcal cell wall arthritis rats. Studies on secretion by synovial fibroblast-like cells and immunohistological localisation. J Immunol 1989;143:1142–1148.

46. Khalil N, Bereznay O, Sporn M, Greenberg AH. Macrophage production of transforming growth factor beta and fibroblast collagen synthesis in chronic pulmonary inflammation. J Exp Med 1989;170:727–737.

47. Hart PH, Vitti GF, Burgess DR, Whitty GA, Piccoli DS, Hamilton JH. Potential anti-inflammatory effects of interleukin-4: suppression of human monocyte tumour necrosis factor α, interleukin-1, and prostaglandin E_2. Proc Natl Acad Sci USA 1989;86:3803–3807.

48. Essner R, Rhoades K, McBride WH, Morton DL, Economou JS. IL-4 downregulates IL-1 and TNF gene expression in human monocytes. J Immunol 1989;142:3857–3861.

49. TeVelde AA, Huijbens K, Heije JE. Interleukin-4 (IL-4) inhibits secretion of IL-1β, tumour necrosis factor α, and IL-6 by human monocytes. Blood 1989;6:1392–1397.

50. Miossec P, Briolay J, Dechanet J, Wijdenes J, Martinez-Valdez H, Banchereau J. The inhibition of the production of proinflammatory cytokines and immunoglobulins by interleukin-4 in an ex vivo model of rheumatoid synovitis. Arthritis Rheum 1992;35:874–883.

51. Noele R, Krammer PH, Ohara J, Uhr JW, Vitetta ES. Increased expression of Ia antigens on resting B cells: an additional role for B cell growth factor. Proc Natl Acad Sci USA 1984;81:6149–6153.

52. Gerrard TL, Dyer DR, Mostowski HS. IL-4 and granulocyte-macrophage colony stimulating factor selectively increase HLA-DR and HLA-DP antigens but not HLA-DQ antigens on human monocytes. J Immunol 1990;144: 4670–4674.

53. Spits H, Yssel H, Takebe Y, et al. Recombinant interleukin-4 promotes growth of human T cells. J Immunol 1987;139: 1142–1147.

54. Defrance T, Vanbervliet B, Aubry JP, et al. B cell growth-promoting activity of recombinant human IL-4. Immunology 1987;139:1135–1141.

55. Cope AP, Gibbons DL, Aderka D, et al. Differential regulation of tumour necrosis factor receptors (TNF-Rs) by IL-4; upregulation of p55 and p75 TNF-Rs on synovial joint mononuclear cells. Cytokine 1993;5:205–212.

56. Lewis-Faning E. Report on an enquiry into the etiological factors associated with rheumatoid arthritis. Ann Rheum Dis 1950;(suppl 91):1–94.

57. Moore KW, Vieira P, Fiorentino DF, Trounstine ML, Khan TA, Mosmann TR. Homology of cytokine synthesis inhibitory factor (IL-10) to the Epstein-Barr virus gene BCRFI. Science 1990;248:1230–1234.

58. Katsikis P, Chu CQ, Brennan FM, Maini RN, Feldmann M. Immunoregulatory role at interleukin 10 [IL-10] in RA. J Exp Med 1994;179:1517–1520.

59. Firestein GS, Zvaifler NJ. How important are T cells in chronic rheumatoid synovitis? Arthritis Rheum 1990;33:768–773.

60. Joyce DA, Gibbons D, Green P, Feldmann M, Brennan FM. Two inhibitors of pro-inflammatory cytokine release, IL-10 and IL-4, have contrasting effects on release of soluble p75 TNF receptor by cultured monocytes. Eur J Immunol 1994 (in press).

61. de Waal Malefyt R, Abrams J, Bennett B, Figdor CG, de Vries JE. Interleukin-10 (IL-10) inhibits cytokine synthesis by human monocytes: an autoregulatory role of IL-10 produced by monocytes. J Exp Med 1991;174:1209–1220.

62. Roux-Lombard P, Modoux C, Vischer T, Grassi J, Dayer JM. Inhibitors of interleukin 1 activity in synovial fluids and in cultured synovial fluid mononuclear cells. J Rheumatol 1992;19:517–523.

63. Symons JA, Eastgate JA, Duff GW. Purification and characterisation of a novel soluble receptor for interleukin 1. J Exp Med 1991;174:1251–1254.

64. Firestein GS, Berger AE, Tracey DE, et al. IL-1 receptor antagonist protein production and gene expression in rheumatoid arthritis and osteoarthritis synovium. J Immunol 1992;149:1054–1062.

65. Deleuran BW, Chu CQ, Field M, et al. Localisation of interleukin 1α (IL-1α), type 1 IL-1 receptor and interleukin 1 receptor antagonist protein in the synovial membrane and cartilage/pannus junction in rheumatoid arthritis. Br J Rheumatol 1992;31:801–809.

66. Cope AP, Aderka D, Doherty M, et al. Increased levels of soluble tumor necrosis factor receptors in the sera and synovial fluid of patients with rheumatic diseases. Arthritis Rheum 1992;35:1160–1169.

67. Elliott MJ, Maini RN, Feldmann M, et al. Treatment of rheumatoid arthritis with chimeric monoclonal antibodies to TNFα, safety, clinical efficacy and regulation of the acute-phase response. Arthritis Rheum 1993;36:1681–1690.

68. Fong Y, Tracey KJ, Moldawer LL, et al. Antibodies to cachectin/tumor necrosis factor reduce interleukin-1 beta and interleukin-6 appearance during lethal bacteremia. J Exp Med 1989;170:1627–1633.

CHAPTER 12

ROLE OF CYTOKINES IN MULTIPLE SCLEROSIS, AUTOIMMUNE ENCEPHALITIS, AND OTHER NEUROLOGICAL DISORDERS

Etty N. Benveniste

In this chapter, I focus on the role of cytokines in causing or contributing to the development and progression of central nervous system (CNS) disease. Many of the cytokines discussed are products of activated lymphocytes and macrophages; however, recent work has conclusively demonstrated that glial cells of the CNS are also important sources of cytokines (1). There are two broad subgroups of glial cells: macroglia, which consist of astrocytes and oligodendrocytes, and microglia, which are considered the resident macrophage of the brain (2). In addition, neurons have been shown to secrete selected cytokines (3). All four of these CNS cell types (i.e., astrocytes, oligodendrocytes, microglia, neurons) can both respond to and produce many of the cytokines initially attributed to lymphocytes and macrophages (3,4). These cytokines include interleukin-1 (IL-1), IL-2, IL-6, IL-10, interferon-α (IFN-α), IFN-β, IFN-γ, tumor necrosis factor-α (TNF-α), TNF-β, transforming growth factor-β (TGF-β), colony-stimulating factors (CSFs), and a number of chemokines. These data indicate that within the CNS, there are local sources of cytokines, as well as cytokines produced by infiltrating cells of the peripheral immune system. The contribution of these cytokines to intracerebral immune responses and inflammation in neurological diseases that have an immunological or autoimmune component is described in detail.

MULTIPLE SCLEROSIS

Multiple sclerosis (MS) is a chronic, inflammatory, demyelinating disease of the CNS. MS most commonly affects young adults during the second or third decade of life. The clinical course is quite variable, but the most common form is characterized by relapsing neurological deficits. Early MS lesions are characterized by local accumulation of activated CD4+ and CD8+ T cells around small venules (5). Later, myelin degeneration occurs associated with perivascular inflammation consisting of T cells, B cells, plasma cells, and macrophages (6,7). T cells are also found at the leading edge of plaques, and they extend into the surrounding normal-appearing white matter. The T cells express activation molecules on their cell surface, such as IL-2 receptors and class II major histocompatibility complex (MHC) antigens (8). In addition, class II MHC expression can also be detected on infiltrating macrophages and resident CNS cells, including microglia, astrocytes, and brain capillary endothelial cells (8). Class II MHC expression in the CNS is presumably induced by IFN-γ secreted by activated T cells. These findings indicate that in early acute MS lesions, demyelination occurs in the face of an active immune response within the CNS. Gliosis is also a prominent feature of MS; this process is characterized by astrocyte proliferation, hypertrophy, and increased synthesis of glial fibrillary acidic protein (GFAP), an astrocyte-specific protein (9). This reaction eventually leads to the formation of dense glial scars in the CNS, which can contribute to motor and sensory impairment.

Different pathological findings are observed in chronic plaques: inflammatory infiltrates are less pronounced, there is evidence of abortive attempts at remyelination, and T γ/δ cells in association with heat shock proteins are detected (10). These findings indicate that the immunological reactions in chronic lesions differ from those in acute lesions, suggesting that different immunological processes take place as the disease enters a chronic phase. The primary demyelination observed in MS results from damage to the myelin sheath or to the myelin-producing cells, the oligodendrocytes. Because myelin is critical for saltatory excitation along axons, demyelination leads to loss of neurological function. Recent findings with magnetic resonance imaging (MRI) indicate that considerable subclinical disease occurs, and that there is breakdown of the blood-brain barrier (BBB) early in lesion development (11,12), which may be a crucial event in the pathogenesis of new lesions in MS.

The etiology of MS has not been defined, although a large body of experimental evidence implicates immune-mediated processes in activation and progression of MS. In addition, both genetic and environmental factors contribute to disease (13). Accumulating evidence supports the notion that MS is an autoimmune disorder mediated by T cells. This evidence includes (a) the pathology of the MS lesion; (b) immunological abnormalities in both the periphery and CNS of patients with MS; (c) immunoglobulin synthesis within the CNS; (d) exacerbation of disease after treatment with IFN-γ; (e) putative autoantigens, such as myelin basic protein (MBP) or proteolipid protein (PLP); (f) possible restricted T-cell receptor usage; and (g) involvement of cytokine networks. The first six points have been extensively reviewed elsewhere (13).

There is still little known about the pattern of cytokine production in the CNS of patients with MS, or about the cells responsible for cytokine expression within this site. More experimental data have been obtained examining cytokine levels in the serum of patients with MS or from peripheral blood mononuclear cells from these patients, but the relationship between these findings and events in the CNS are not clear. Studies on cytokine expression in the cerebrospinal fluid (CSF) of patients with MS have been inconclusive and conflicting. Currently, the number of studies examining cytokine gene expression in MS lesions have been limited, but they have generated some interesting findings. Collectively, all these studies indicate that a number of cytokines are involved in or associated with the disease of MS. These cytokines include IL-1, IL-2, IL-6, TNF-α, TNF-β, IFN-α, IFN-β, IFN-γ, and TGF-β.

Role of TNF-α and TNF-β in MS

TNF-α is a proinflammatory cytokine recognized to be an important mediator of immunological and inflammatory responses in a variety of tissues, including the CNS (14). TNF-α has a diverse range of functions in the CNS because of its direct effects on oligodendrocytes, astrocytes, and brain endothelial cells. Most relevant to CNS disease is the ability of TNF-α to mediate myelin and oligodendrocyte damage in vitro (15), and its ability to cause cell death of oligodendrocytes in vitro (16). This aspect of TNF-α activity may contribute directly to myelin damage or the demyelination process observed in MS. TNF-β, the cytokine genetically and functionally related to TNF-α (17), exerts a more potent cytotoxic effect toward oligodendrocytes than TNF-α, and it mediates its effect via apoptosis (18). Thus, both TNF-α and TNF-β can cause death of oligodendrocytes, the myelin-producing cell of the CNS.

TNF-α has multiple effects on astrocytes that are noncytotoxic in nature, and it may function in an autocrine fashion, because astrocytes express specific high affinity receptors for TNF-α (19), and they secrete TNF-α on activation (20–23). One of the pathological features of demyelinated plaques in MS is astrogliosis, during which proliferation of astrocytes and production of GFAP occurs (24). Astrocyte proliferation leads to the reactive gliosis associated with MS, and TNF-α appears to contribute to this process (25). TNF-α is also a potent inducer of cytokine production in astrocytes. Primary astrocytes and human astroglioma cell lines produce three CSFs on stimulation with TNF-α: granulocyte-macrophage CSF (GM-CSF), G-CSF, and M-CSF (26–30). These CSFs can augment inflammatory responses due to their leukocyte chemotactic properties, which would promote migration of granulocytes and macrophages to inflammatory sites within the CNS. TNF-α also induces IL-6 expression by both primary rat and human astrocytes (29,31–33). IL-6 also has proinflammatory actions (34), which in concert with TNF-α can promote inflammation within the CNS.

TNF-α may have an important role in the alteration of the BBB due to its effects on the adhesive properties of both astrocytes and brain endothelium. MS is characterized by migration of inflammatory cells from blood into the brain and subsequent invasion of the extravascular tissue (35,36). Recent studies have shown that up-regulation of adhesion molecules, such as intercellular adhesion molecule-1 (ICAM-1), on brain endothelial cells by exposure to proinflammatory cytokines such as TNF-α, IL-1β, and IFN-γ, mediates leukocyte adhesion to endothelium (37–39). Similarly, astrocytes can be induced by TNF-α, as well as by IL-1 and IFN-γ, to express ICAM-1 (40–46). Expression of ICAM-1 by CNS endothelium has been implicated in the adhesion of lymphocytes to endothelial cells in animals with experimental allergic encephalomyelitis (47,48), and studies on brain material from patients with MS have shown aberrant expression of ICAM-1 on both brain endothelium and astrocytes (49). The presence of ICAM-1 and other adhesion molecules in the vessel walls as well as on astrocytes may guide inflammatory leukocytes into and through the brain, thereby contributing to impairment of the BBB and the neuropathology of MS. The architecture of the BBB, with astrocytic end feet abutting onto cerebrovascular endothelium, suggests that astrocyte-derived TNF-α can induce ICAM-1 on neighboring endothelial cells as well as on the astrocyte, alter BBB permeability, and promote inflammatory infiltration into the CNS.

The multiple effects of TNF-α on various cell populations in the CNS suggest that TNF-α has a central role in augmenting infiltration of inflammatory cells, intracerebral immune responses, cytokine production, gliosis, and demyelination, all pathogenic events involved in immune-mediated CNS disorders such as MS. Accordingly, there has been much interest in the pattern of TNF-α expression by patients with MS. Beck and colleagues (50) performed a longitudinal study on 20 patients with MS and normal control subjects examining TNF-α production by peripheral blood mononuclear cells stimulated with phytohemagglutinin (PHA). An increase in TNF-α production was detected 2 weeks prior to disease exacerbation. In those with benign disease, or in those with fully resolved disease, the increase disappeared rapidly, often before the appearance of symptoms. When the increase in TNF-α persisted, clinical sequelae were common. In patients with chronic progressive MS, frequently intervening increases in TNF-α were observed. The authors suggested that TNF-α may trigger exacerbations, and that it may also have a role in maintaining disease in patients with chronic progressive disease. Merrill and associates (51) examined patients with acute relapsing and chronic progressive MS. TNF-α was produced in greater quantity by monocytes isolated from the peripheral blood of patients with MS, as well as by cells isolated from the CSF, which were predominantly T cells, compared with healthy control subjects. These two studies indicate that there is overproduction of TNF-α by immune cells from patients with MS, and that elevated expression of TNF-α by these cells may contribute to the neurological disease of MS.

Studies to examine TNF-α expression in the CSF of patients with MS have yielded conflicting data. Two groups did not detect TNF-α in the CSF of patients with MS (51,52). Hauser and coworkers (53) examined TNF-α production in the CSF of patients with MS and patients with other neurological diseases, and they detected higher levels of TNF-α in patients with active MS than in patients with MS in remission or patients with other neurological diseases. They suggested that the TNF-α origi-nated from cellular elements within the CNS, rather than from immune cells in the CSF, because there was no correlation between the degree of CSF pleocytosis and cytokine expression. Maimone and colleagues (54) detected TNF-α in the CSF of 23% of patients with MS and 29% of patients with other inflammatory neurological disease, which agrees with another study in which TNF-α was detected in the CSF of 13% of patients with chronic progressive MS (55). The most compelling evidence for an association of TNF-α with MS comes from Sharief and associates (56), who documented that increased TNF-α expression in the CSF of patients with MS correlated with disease progression. This same group then went on to demonstrate that a strong correlation exists between increased CSF levels of TNF-α, disruption of the BBB, CSF pleocytosis, and increased levels of circulating ICAM-1 in both the serum and the CSF of patients with active MS (57,58).

There are a number of factors that can account for the differences in the ability to detect TNF-α in the CSF of patients with MS. These factors include: (a) differences in the patients examined; (b) timing of CSF collection; and (c) instability of TNF-α in CSF if not treated with appropriate protease inhibitors. In addition, most of the TNF-α secreted within the plaques is likely to interact with TNF-α receptors on nearby cells (i.e., T cells, macrophages, microglia, astrocytes, and oligodendrocytes), thus little to any may filter to the lumbar CSF, where it may be undetectable.

The presence of TNF-α in MS brain lesions has been examined using double-labeling immunohistochemical techniques. Hofman and coworkers (59,60) demonstrated that TNF-α–positive astrocytes and macrophages are found in the plaque region of MS brains. These cells were most numerous at the lesion edge. TNF-α–positive cells were not detected in normal brain specimens, or in tissue from patients with Alzheimer's disease, but they could be identified in brain tissue from patients with subacute sclerosing panencephalitis (SSPE), a progressive, fatal form of encephalitis caused by measles virus. In SSPE brains, the TNF-α–stained cells had the morphological appearance of reactive astrocytes (60). Selmaj and associates (61) determined that both TNF-α and TNF-β are present in MS plaque regions, and that TNF-α is localized within astrocytes, whereas TNF-β is associated with microglia and T cells.

These studies, although suggestive that these cell types express TNF-α, must be verified by in situ hybridization to conclusively determine if TNF-α messenger RNA (mRNA) is localized in these cells. It is possible that the results observed with immunohistochemistry reflect the ability of astrocytes and macrophages to bind TNF-α. In vitro studies indicate that of the endogenous glial cells, both astrocytes and microglia are capable of producing TNF-α on exposure to multiple stimuli, including the

Th1 cytokine IFN-γ (20,21,23,62–65). Thus, it will be important to verify the identity of the infiltrating cells and the endogenous glial cells that are sources of TNF-α in patients with MS.

Role of IL-1 in MS

IL-1 is a 17 kd cytokine produced predominantly by activated macrophages, although other cell types, such as endothelial cells, B cells, keratinocytes, microglia, and astrocytes, can also secrete IL-1 on stimulation (66,67). IL-1 is responsible for mediating a variety of processes in the host response to microbial and inflammatory diseases, and it has a number of effects on cells of the CNS that implicate it in contributing to the pathology of MS and other neurological disease states. Purified IL-1 was shown to have a mitogenic effect on astrocyte growth in vitro (68), whereas IL-1 directly injected into the brain can stimulate astrogliosis (69). These results suggest that IL-1 may contribute to astroglial scarring.

IL-1, similar to TNF-α, is a strong inducer of cytokine production by glial cells. IL-1 can induce astrocytes, oligodendrocytes, and microglia to produce TGF-β (70), and IL-1 also stimulates astrocytes to produce a variety of cytokines, including TNF-α (20,22,71), IL-6 (29,31,32), and some of the CSFs (27,72,73). These cytokines are all involved in mediating various aspects of immune and inflammatory responses; thus, their production by resident brain cells can contribute to these processes within the CNS. IL-1 also can modulate expression of adhesion molecules on astrocytes and endothelium (41,44,74), thereby altering BBB permeability.

Similar to TNF-α, IL-1 can promote infiltration of inflammatory cells, intracerebral immune responses, cytokine production, and gliosis within the CNS. A few studies addressed the issue of IL-1 association with MS. In a study of patients with acute relapsing and chronic progressive MS, Merrill and colleagues (51) demonstrated that monocytes isolated from peripheral blood and cells isolated from CSF of patients with MS produced more IL-1 than cells from healthy control subjects. In the study by Hauser and associates (53), in which higher levels of CSF TNF-α were detected in patients with active MS, comparable findings were observed for IL-1. However, in two other studies, IL-1 could not be detected in the CSF of patients with MS (51,54).

Several studies have examined IL-1 expression in MS brain lesions. In chronic active plaques, IL-1–positive cells have been detected by immunohistochemistry (59,60). IL-1 mRNA expression was examined in acute, subacute, and chronic lesions, as well as in normal-appearing white matter by reverse transcription-polymerase chain reaction (RT-PCR) and Southern blotting. IL-1 mRNA was detected in the majority of early acute, acute,

and subacute plaques, but not in chronic lesions (75). In addition, a very low level of IL-1 mRNA was observed in some of the control brains. Thus, of the limited studies conducted, there is no correlation between IL-1 expression and type of MS plaque, and the identity of the cell types expressing IL-1 remains unknown. The cell types capable of IL-1 expression within the CNS include infiltrating macrophages, astrocytes, oligodendrocytes, and microglia (23,26,62,63,76,77).

Role of IL-6 in MS

IL-6, similar to IL-1 and TNF-α, is a pleiotropic cytokine involved in the regulation of inflammatory and immunological responses (34). IL-6, a 26 kd molecule, is secreted by a range of activated cells, including fibroblasts, monocytes, B cells, endothelial cells, T cells, microglia, and astrocytes. The two best described functions of IL-6 are on hepatocytes and B cells. IL-6 stimulates hepatocytes to synthesize several plasma proteins, such as fibrinogen and C-reactive protein, which contribute to the acute phase response. IL-6 is the principal cytokine for inducing terminal differentiation of activated B cells into immunoglobulin (Ig)-secreting plasma cells. Within the CNS, IL-6 has a mitogenic effect on bovine astrocytes (25), which may contribute to astrogliosis. Astrocytes respond to IL-6 by secreting nerve growth factor, which induces neural differentiation (32). IL-6 has been demonstrated to inhibit TNF-α production by monocytes (78). Because astrocytes can secrete TNF-α, and because TNF-α induces IL-6 production by astrocytes (31,79), IL-6 may be involved in the negative regulation of TNF-α in the CNS.

One of the hallmarks of MS is intrathecal B-cell activation, as evidenced by elevation of the CSF IgG index and by the presence of oligoclonal IgG bands in the CSF (80). Because IL-6 is involved in differentiation of B cells into Ig-secreting plasma cells (81), there has been interest in determining whether elevated IL-6 levels could be responsible for local B-cell responses within the CNS. Results have been conflicting: Three groups report that IL-6 is not detected in MS CSF (53,82,83), whereas two more recent studies suggest that IL-6 is elevated in MS CSF (54) and MS plasma (84). These latter findings suggest that there is a heightened systemic B-cell response in MS; however, in patients with MS, no relationship was observed between the incidence or the amount of intrathecal IgG synthesis or oligoclonal bands and IL-6 expression in the CSF. To date, no studies have been performed to examine IL-6 expression directly in MS lesions.

Role of IL-2 in MS

IL-2, a 14 to 17 kd glycoprotein, is the principal cytokine responsible for proliferation and maintenance of T cells

(85). IL-2 is produced primarily by CD4+ T helper cells (Th1) when they are activated, and it acts in both an autocrine and a paracrine fashion on T cells. The principal actions of IL-2 are on lymphocytes, and they include functioning as the major autocrine growth factor for T cells. Binding of IL-2 by T cells results in proliferation of these cells; enhanced secretion of other cytokines, such as IFN-γ and TNF-β; and enhanced expression of transferrin receptors. IL-2 can also stimulate the growth of natural killer (NK) cells, activated B cells, and macrophages.

IL-2 is present in the CNS only in disease states in which the BBB has been disrupted and activated T cells have infiltrated into that site. Within the CNS, IL-2 has biological effects on oligodendrocytes, the myelin-producing cell. Recombinant human IL-2 has been shown to influence proliferation and differentiation of rat oligodendrocytes (86). Oligodendrocyte numbers are increased approximately 3-fold in cultures containing IL-2, and IL-2 stimulates maturation of oligodendrocytes, assessed as the enhanced expression of myelin basic protein (MBP) in IL-2–treated oligodendrocytes. Both MBP mRNA and protein levels are increased in IL-2–stimulated oligodendrocytes (87). These findings provide evidence that an important step in oligodendrocyte differentiation, MBP mRNA and protein expression, can be amplified in part by IL-2. Two human glioblastoma cell lines with oligodendroglial phenotype proliferate in the presence of IL-2, and they also bear receptors for the IL-2 molecule, as determined by immunofluorescent staining with anti-IL-2 receptor monoclonal antibodies (88). Human oligodendroglioma cell lines expressing only IL-2 p75 receptors proliferate in response to IL-2, suggesting that the presence of p75 is sufficient to deliver the IL-2 signal to these cells (89). IL-2 appears to have an opposite effect on rat oligodendrocyte progenitor cells, because it can inhibit proliferation of these cells (90). These results suggest that IL-2 can have varying biological effects on oligodendrocytes, depending on the maturational stage of those cells. IL-2 has not been shown to modulate the function or gene expression of astrocytes or microglia; thus, it appears to have a selective effect on oligodendrocytes.

Gallo and coworkers (91) conducted a study to measure IL-2 levels in the CSF and sera from 30 patients with MS. Detectable levels of IL-2 were found in 6 sera and 9 CSF samples of 21 patients with acute relapsing MS, whereas IL-2 was not detected in either CSF or sera from 9 patients with chronic progressive MS. Trotter and associates (92) detected increased levels of IL-2 in serum from patients with chronic progressive MS. These findings suggest that systemic activation of T cells occurs in some patients with MS, most likely those with active disease. In addition, IL-2 production within the CNS could initiate and propagate immune responses within this site.

Two studies by Hofman and colleagues (8,60) demonstrated IL-2 protein expression in chronic active plaques of MS brain by immunohistochemistry, whereas normal brain specimens were negative. The source of IL-2 in MS brain is presumably activated T cells, although this source has not been formally demonstrated. Wucherpfennig and coworkers (75) examined IL-2 mRNA expression in MS brain by RT-PCR, and they demonstrated occasional expression in subacute and acute lesions.

In the animal model of MS, EAE, encephalitogenic T-cell clones are preferentially of the Th1 phenotype (i.e., they secrete IL-2, IFN-γ, and TNF-β) (93,94). Brod and associates (95) examined whether Th1- or Th2-type T cells could be identified in the peripheral blood or the CSF of patients with or without inflammatory diseases. Three patients with chronic progressive MS were part of the group with inflammatory disease, and a significant number of Th1 T-cell clones were identified in the blood and CSF of these patients with MS, as well as in patients with other inflammatory diseases. In contrast, Th1 cells were absent from the blood and CSF of patients without inflammatory disease. The authors speculate that Th1 T cells may functionally be involved in inflammatory responses within the CNS of patients with MS, as has been demonstrated for EAE.

Role of interferons in MS

The IFNs are a family of proteins related by their ability to protect cells from viral infection. On the basis of several criteria, the IFNs have been divided into three distinct classes: IFN-α, IFN-β, and IFN-γ (96). IFN-α and IFN-β (originally known as type I IFN) are the classic IFNs induced in response to viral infection. IFN-α and IFN-β display only 15 to 30% amino acid sequence homology, yet both forms bind to the same cell surface receptor. Twenty-six IFN-α genes have been identified that encode at least 22 distinct proteins (molecular weight [MW], approximately 20 kd). Recent studies suggest that the different species of IFN-α induce a distinct array of biological responses in different cell types. IFN-β exists in a single form. IFN-γ (originally known as type II IFN) is unrelated to IFN-α and IFN-β at both the genetic and the protein levels.

The single IFN-γ gene encodes a 166 amino acid polypeptide that is subsequently cleaved to give rise to a mature 143-residue protein with a predicted MW of 17 kd. Two IFN-γ proteins self-associate to form a homodimer, and only the dimer displays IFN-γ biological activity, probably because it is the only form of IFN-γ that mediates IFN-γ receptor dimerization. IFN-γ utilizes a different cellular receptor than IFN-α and IFN-β, and it functions primarily as an immunoregulatory cytokine (97). IFN-α and IFN-β can be produced by a variety of cells, whereas IFN-γ is produced only by T cells (CD4+, CD8+) and NK cells. Within the CD4+ T-cell population, IFN-γ is produced by the Th1 helper T-cell subset. IFN-α and

IFN-β are considered to be primarily antiviral agents that display some immunological activity, whereas IFN-γ is predominantly an immunomodulator that can also exert some antiviral activity. Some of the immune effects of IFN-γ include the ability to enhance the functional activity of macrophages, promotion of T- and B-cell differentiation, and modulation of both class I and class II MHC antigen expression on a variety of cells. IFN-γ is considered the most potent inducer of class II MHC antigen expression on most cell types, except B cells (98).

IFN-α, IFN-β, and IFN-γ have the capacity to modulate gene expression in astrocytes, oligodendrocytes, microglia, and neurons. These cells constitutively express very low levels of class I and II MHC antigens, which have a fundamental role in induction and regulation of immune responses (99). IFN-α, IFN-β, and IFN-γ can induce expression of class I MHC antigens on glial cells and neurons (100–103), whereas only IFN-γ induces expression of class II MHC antigens on astrocytes and microglia (103–107). The implications of class I and II MHC antigen expression on neural cells is that these cells may stimulate the development of aberrant immune responses within the CNS. IFN-β can, however, inhibit IFN-γ–induced class II MHC antigen expression in astrocytes (108,109), indicating that these two IFNs can have antagonistic effects.

Other effects of IFN-γ within the CNS include: (a) enhancement of ICAM-1 expression on astrocytes (41); (b) up-regulation of TNF-α receptors on astrocytes (19); (c) enhancement of the complement component C3 by astrocytes (110); and (d) priming of astrocytes for subsequent TNF-α and IL-6 production (20,31).

There has been much interest in the use of IFNs in clinical trials on patients with MS. The rationale for treatment of MS with IFNs was based on the hypothesis that disease activity might be related to viral persistence or latency within the CNS (111). Clinical trials of natural and recombinant IFN-α resulted in negative or equivocal clinical results (112). In 1981, an open trial of natural IFN-β administered intrathecally resulted in a decrease in frequency of exacerbations, with minimal side effects (113). A larger double-blind study followed, and patients with relapsing/remitting MS treated with IFN-β had a significantly lower exacerbation rate than the placebo group (114). A double-blind, placebo-controlled trial was recently organized at 11 centers in the United States and Canada, in which a total of 372 patients with relapsing/ remitting MS were enrolled. In this trial, IFN-β$_{ser}$ (Betaseron; Berlex Laboratories, Richmond, CA) was used. IFN-β$_{ser}$ is a nonglycosylated, recombinant form of IFN-β in which a serine residue replaced a cysteine at position 17, which greatly enhanced its stability, thus making it suitable for clinical use. This clinical trial showed that IFN-β$_{ser}$ significantly reduced the rate of exacerbations, sever-

ity of exacerbations, and accumulation of MRI abnormalities, with minimal side effects (115,116). Although the mechanisms by which IFN-β works is not known, it has been suggested that IFN-β may (a) inhibit immune activation in patients with MS, (b) lessen tissue damage by inhibiting the release of TNF within the CNS, and (c) restore T-suppressor cell function (117). In support of these suggestions, there are several reports that IFN-β downregulates TNF production by peripheral blood cells (118,119). We have also demonstrated that IFN-β is capable of inhibiting TNF-α gene expression by human astrocytes (Tang LP and Benveniste EN, unpublished observations). This clinical trial generated much excitement, and IFN-β$_{ser}$ was recently approved by the United States Food and Drug Administration. As indicated, much work needs to be performed to determine how IFN-β$_{ser}$ exerts its effect in lessening disability, and also whether IFN-β$_{ser}$ will prove to be beneficial for patients with purely progressive MS. Nonetheless, the data from this important clinical trial indicate that IFN-β$_{ser}$ can favorably and safely modulate MS disease.

Another multicenter clinical trial is currently in progress in which glycosylated recombinant IFN-β is being tested (112). Patients with relapsing/remitting MS will receive either placebo or IFN-β by intramuscular injection. The outcome measure in this trial will be differences in disability scores, rather than differences in exacerbation rates, which was used in the IFN-β$_{ser}$ trial. It is hoped that the results from both these trials will provide definitive information on the value of IFN-β in treating relapsing/remitting MS.

An entirely different outcome resulted from a pilot study to assess the effect of recombinant IFN-γ on patients with MS. It was recognized that IFN-γ induced class II MHC antigen expression on a variety of cells, including cells of the CNS and activated macrophages, which might be potentially hazardous in MS. However, a number of studies had determined that IFN-γ production was deficient in cultures from stimulated peripheral blood cells from patients with MS (120,121). Administration of IFN-γ to a group of 18 patients with relapsing/remitting MS resulted in worsening of disease in 7 (122). This trial established IFN-γ as an important mediator of MS attacks, possibly because IFN-γ or IFN-γ–activated cells (perhaps macrophages) infiltrated the CNS at sites of previous BBB damage, and then reactivated cellular responses within this site. More recent studies on the association of IFN-γ with MS demonstrated that peripheral blood lymphocytes from patients with MS produce significantly more IFN-γ than those of normal control cells (50,123). In one of the studies, increased IFN-γ production was detected prior to exacerbations, suggesting that IFN-γ contributes to exacerbation of disease (50). Examination of IFN-γ in the CSF of patients with MS indicated that IFN-γ can rarely be detected in this body fluid (124).

IFN-γ–positive cells have been detected in the CNS of patients with MS, and these cells have been identified as astrocytes (60,125). It is presumed that infiltrating activated T cells secrete IFN-γ, which can then bind to receptors on astrocytes. IFN-γ–activated astrocytes can express class II MHC antigens, thereby allowing antigen presentation, immune interactions, and activation of disease process within the CNS.

Regardless of how the IFNs work in patients with MS, it is clear that IFN-γ has a role in disease progression, whereas IFN-β has a role in suppressing exacerbations of MS. Clearly, future understanding of the immunoregulatory mechanisms by which IFN-γ and IFN-β function will provide new information on activation and regulation of the MS disease process.

Role of TGF-β in MS

Finally, there is much interest in the action of another immune system modulator, TGF-β, as a candidate for MS clinical trials. A Phase I clinical trial to assess the effect of TGF-β_2 in patients with MS was begun in April 1994 (Carlino J, Cel Trix Pharmaceutical, personal communication). The impetus for this trial comes from the very encouraging results of TGF-β in EAE. As is discussed in more detail later, TGF-β_1 and TGF-β_2 have been shown to improve the clinical course of EAE (126–129). In addition, TGF-β is detected in the CNS of animals who have recovered from EAE (130). In this regard, one article demonstrated that TGF-β–like activity can be detected from peripheral blood of patients with active MS, and within this group of patients, TGF-β activity was significantly correlated to the period of regression of symptoms (131). Although quite preliminary, these data suggest that TGF-β may contribute to regression of an exacerbation.

Summary

It is difficult to draw conclusions because some of the findings discussed are conflicting, and some of the studies are preliminary. However, what emerges is a sense that there is aberrant expression of cytokines involved in mediating immune responsiveness and inflammation, such as TNF-α, TNF-β, IL-1, IL-2, IL-6, and IFN-γ. Expression of two of these cytokines, TNF-α and IFN-γ, precedes exacerbations, suggesting a role in disease progression. In addition, all of these cytokines exert biological effects on glial cells, many of which contribute to demyelination, inflammation, and immune reactivity. These effects include lysis of oligodendrocytes, myelin damage, gliosis, expression of class I and II MHC antigens, expression of adhesion molecules, and cytokine production. IL-2, IFN-γ, and TNF-β expression is likely to come from outside the CNS by activated T cells, whereas TNF-α, IL-6, and IL-1 can be produced by both infiltrating leukocytes and endogenous glial cells. Activation of astrocytes and microglia to secrete cytokines may contribute to the propagation of intracerebral immune and inflammatory responses initiated by infiltrating T cells and macrophages.

Down-regulation of cytokine cascades, immune responses, and inflammation may be mediated by the generation of "immunosuppressive" cytokines, such as IFN-β and TGF-β. There is encouraging data that IFN-β is beneficial in reducing MS disease severity. Whether immune and inflammatory responses within the CNS are propagated or suppressed depends on a number of parameters,

TABLE 12–1   CYTOKINES ASSOCIATED WITH MULTIPLE SCLEROSIS (MS)

Cytokine	Peripheral Blood/Serum	Cerebrospinal Fluid	MS Lesions
TNF-α	Increased expression	Increased expression	TNF-α–positive astrocytes, macrophages
TNF-β	Not examined	Not examined	TNF-β–positive microglia, T cells
IL-1	Increased expression	Increased expression	IL-1 present, cell type unknown
IL-6	Conflicting results	Conflicting results	Not examined
IL-2	Increased expression	Increased expression	IL-2 present, cell type unknown
IFN-α/IFN-β	Not examined	Not examined	IFN-α present, cell type unknown
IFN-γ	Increased expression	Undetectable	IFN-γ–positive astrocytes
TGF-β	Increased expression	Not examined	Not examined

TNF = tumor necrosis factor; IL = interleukin; IFN = interferon; TGF = transforming growth factor.

including: (a) activational status of these cells, (b) cytokine receptor levels on glial and immune cells, (c) concentration and location of cytokines in the CNS, (d) timing of cytokine expression in the CNS, and (e) temporal sequence in which a particular cell is exposed to numerous cytokines. See Table 12–1 for a summary of the cytokines associated with MS.

EXPERIMENTAL ALLERGIC ENCEPHALOMYELITIS

The best-characterized experimental model for CNS autoimmune disease is EAE. This disease is induced by injection of spinal cord components such as MBP or PLP with adjuvant, injection of MBP or PLP peptides, or transfer of encephalitogenic MBP- or PLP-specific T cells to naive recipients. EAE is characterized by inflammatory infiltration of the CNS by activated T cells and macrophages; demyelination; and acute, chronic, or chronic-relapsing paralysis. The mediators of this disease are MBP- or PLP-reactive CD4+ T-helper cells that are class II MHC–restricted (132). However, not all myelin antigen–reactive CD4+ T-cell lines induce EAE; thus, there are other factors that contribute to the encephalitogenicity of these cells.

Most encephalitogenic T cells are of the Th1 subtype, which secrete IFN-γ, IL-2, TNF-α, and TNF-β (133). It has been suggested that TNF-α and TNF-β secretion by MBP-specific T-cell clones correlates with their encephalitogenic potential (134), although this correlation has not been observed for PLP-reactive T-cell clones (135). It may be that TNF production is necessary, but not always sufficient, to induce EAE.

Expression of adhesion molecules such as $\alpha4\beta1$ (or VLA4) also influences the pathogenicity of encephalitogenic T cells (93,135). Cross and associates (35) proposed that antigen-specific autoimmune T cells are responsible for initiation of disease, and that perpetuation of disease may be the result of an influx of largely non-antigen-specific inflammatory cells of the recipient animal. Susceptibility to EAE appears to be linked to MHC alleles, although non-MHC genes may have a small role in contributing to EAE (136). Cytokines have been implicated in contributing to EAE disease progression, as well as mediating recovery from disease. These cytokines include IL-1, IL-2, IL-4, IL-6, IL-10, TNF-α, IFN-γ, M-CSF, TGF-β, and chemokines.

Role of IL-1 in EAE

Because of the known inflammatory effects of IL-1 and the knowledge that glial cells can produce IL-1 within the CNS, there has been interest in the role of IL-1 in EAE.

IL-1 has been shown to enhance in vitro activation of encephalitogenic T cells, thereby enhancing the adoptive transfer of EAE (137), and guinea pigs with chronic EAE have elevated levels of IL-1 in their CSF (138). More recently, Jacobs and colleagues (139) demonstrated that in vivo administration of IL-1α enhanced severity and chronicity of clinical paralysis associated with EAE, whereas treatment of animals with soluble mouse IL-1 receptor (an IL-1 antagonist) significantly delayed the onset of EAE, reduced the severity of paralysis and weight loss, and reduced the duration of disease. These results suggest a role for IL-1 in inflammatory CNS disease states such as EAE.

There have been conflicting reports as to whether IL-1 is present in the brains of animals with EAE. In a model of chronic-relapsing EAE (CREAE) induced in Biozzi AB/H mice with autologous spinal cord homogenate, IL-1 was detected in the brains of these animals in both the acute and relapsing phases of disease (140), in addition to the cytokines TNF-α, IL-2, and IFN-γ. The cell types expressing the cytokines were not determined. Similarly, a study by Kennedy and associates (141) examining EAE induced in SJL/J mice by adoptive transfer of MBP-sensitized lymph node cells demonstrated that mRNA for IL-1 was detected in the acute phase of disease, and it remained elevated during the early chronic state. mRNA for other cytokines, such as IL-2, IL-4, IL-6, IL-10, and IFN-γ, was also detected in this model of EAE. Khoury and associates (130) examined the cytokine profiles of Lewis rats with EAE, as well as the effect of oral administration of MBP, which has been shown to suppress EAE. In this study, EAE was induced by injection of MBP in adjuvant; animals were then fed with ovalbumin (OVA) as a control, or MBP. Brains from OVA-fed animals at the peak of clinical disease showed perivascular infiltration and expression of the cytokine IL-1, as well as IL-2, IL-6, IL-8, IFN-γ, and TNF-α. In contrast, in MBP orally tolerized animals, there was marked reduction of the perivascular infiltrate, down-regulation of all the inflammatory cytokines, and an increase in expression of the inhibitory cytokines TGF-β and IL-4.

In a separate study, IL-1 protein expression was detected in the CNS of Lewis rats 10 days after immunization with spinal cord homogenate. During full-blown EAE (day 13), the number of lesions with IL-1–positive cells had increased, and in the remission phase (day 25), IL-1–positive cells could still be detected, but they were reduced in number (142). On the basis of microscopic analysis, IL-1 immunoreactivity was detected in cells with ultrastructural features of macrophages and microglia. In contrast, Merrill and colleagues (143) did not detect IL-1 protein in the brains of SJL/J and B10.PL mice immunized with MBP peptides. This finding suggests that the method of immunization by which EAE is induced may influence cytokine expression in the brain. Alternatively, the different results may be due to the sensitivity of the procedures utilized for detecting cytokine expression. Kennedy and associates (141) utilized the sensitive technique of RT-PCR to detect cytokine mRNA expression, whereas Merrill and coworkers (143) used the less sensitive method of immunohistochemistry to detect cytokine protein expression.

Role of TNF in EAE

Evidence for involvement of TNF-α and TNF-β in EAE was obtained from studies demonstrating that antibody to TNF-α and TNF-β could prevent the transfer of EAE by encephalitogenic T cells in SJL/J mice (144,145). Preincubation of MBP-sensitized T cells with anti-TNF antibody in vitro prior to injection did not diminish their ability to transfer EAE, suggesting that anti-TNF antibody inhibits the development of EAE by interfering with the effector phase of the disease (145). Another study, by Kuroda and Shimamoto (146), demonstrated that intraperitoneal injections of TNF-α resulted in significant prolongation of clinical EAE in Lewis rats. In contrast, the disease course of EAE in SJL/J mice actively immunized with spinal cord homogenate was not affected by treatment with antibody against TNF (147). These differences may be due to the route of EAE induction. These findings indicate that under certain conditions, TNF-α and TNF-β have important roles in EAE. Adding to these observations are the findings by Chung and associates (148), that astrocytes from EAE-susceptible and EAE-resistant rat strains differ in their ability to express TNF-α protein. Astrocytes from Lewis rats (EAE-susceptible) produce TNF-α in response to IFN-γ and IL-1β, whereas astrocytes from Brown Norway rats (EAE-resistant) do not. The capacity for TNF-α production by Lewis astrocytes, especially in response to disease-related cytokines such as IFN-γ and IL-1, may contribute to disease susceptibility and to the inflammation and demyelination associated with EAE.

Several studies have been conducted to examine TNF-α expression in EAE. TNF-α protein was detected by immunohistochemistry within inflammatory lesions during both the active and relapsing disease phases of CREAE (140). TNF-α was also expressed in the CNS of Lewis rats at the peak of clinical disease, whereas there was an absence of TNF-α expression in MBP orally tolerized animals (130). In SJL/J and B10.PL mice immunized with MBP peptides, cells staining positively for TNF-α and TNF-β protein were present in the brain, but not in the spinal cord of these animals (143). Expression of TNF-α and TNF-β occurred transiently (days 11 and 15 after injection), and it was not very pronounced. Again, these data illustrate that in different models of EAE using different species and modes of immunization, there is likely to be differential expression of cytokines.

Role of IFN-γ in EAE

IFN-γ appears to have a protective role in different models of EAE. Treatment with neutralizing antibody against IFN-γ caused an increase in disease severity and mortality (149,150), whereas treatment with IFN-γ resulted in enhanced survival (149). Another study examined the effect of IFN-γ on EAE in Lewis rats. Systemically administered IFN-γ did not change the disease course of EAE, whereas IFN-γ applied locally into the ventricular system of the CNS resulted in complete suppression of clinical signs (151). In addition, systemic administration of anti-IFN-γ antibody prior to the onset of clinical symptoms resulted in a more severe disease course. These results suggest that IFN-γ down-regulates the development of EAE. The findings in both murine and rat models of EAE differ from those observed in human MS trials, in which administration of IFN-γ leads to exacerbation of disease (122). These results demonstrate that IFN-γ undoubtedly can have different roles in the development of various autoimmune responses, and it may act through different molecular mechanisms. Further experimentation is needed to determine the reasons for the seemingly contradictory actions of IFN-γ in EAE compared with MS.

A number of studies have been conducted to examine IFN-γ expression in the CNS of animals with EAE. IFN-γ could be detected before the onset of clinical disease (141,143,152) and during the acute phase of disease (130,140,141); it diminished on recovery (130,140,141). By immunohistochemistry, a subpopulation of IFN-γ–positive cells were identified as T cells, and the majority were macrophages (152).

Role of TGF-β in EAE

TGF-β is a dimeric protein of approximately 28 kd that is synthesized by nearly all cell types. It is normally secreted in a latent form that must be activated by proteases (153). The TGF-β family is composed of 5 different isoforms encoded by separate genes that have high amino acid sequence homology. The actions of TGF-β are highly pleiotropic, and they include inhibiting proliferation of many cell types (e.g., epithelial, endothelial, lymphoid, and hematopoietic cells), promoting growth of new blood vessels (i.e., angiogenesis), serving as a chemotactic factor for macrophages, and inhibiting immune and inflammatory responses. TGF-β has been demonstrated to inhibit the production of numerous cytokines, and it is thought to function as a negative regulator of immune responses. TGF-β can modulate the activity of astrocytes, microglia, and oligodendrocytes. TGF-β₁ and TGF-β₂ can inhibit IFN-γ–induced class II MHC antigen expression on both human astroglioma cells and rat astrocytes (154,155), inhibit proliferation of rat astrocytes (156–158), and act as chemotactic agents for both rat astrocytes and microglia (158,159). TGF-β inhibits TNF-α production by microglia (64) and astrocytes (160), and it inhibits cytokine-induced C3 gene expression in astrocytes (161). TGF-β has also been shown to be an important mediator of oligodendrocyte differentiation (162). All three glial cells—astrocytes, microglia, and oligodendrocytes—have the capacity to produce TGF-β (70,163). Because TGF-β exerts many immunosuppressive effects, TGF-β produced by glial cells may restrict or down-regulate inflammatory processes within the CNS.

Several studies have demonstrated that TGF-β$_1$ improves the clinical course of EAE in SJL/J mice (126–128). Injection of TGF-β$_1$ delayed, but did not suppress, development of EAE; however, TGF-β$_1$ prevented relapses in these mice (128). Racke and colleagues (126) demonstrated that TGF-β$_1$ inhibited activation of MBP-specific lymph node cells in vitro, which reduced the capacity of these cells to transfer EAE. In addition, injection of TGF-β$_1$ resulted in an improved clinical course, even when administered during ongoing disease. Johns and coworkers (127) showed that in vivo injection of TGF-β$_1$ reduced the incidence of clinical disease, as well as the severity of inflammation and demyelination within the CNS. In addition, TGF-β$_1$, TGF-β$_2$, and TGF-β$_3$ were present in inflammatory lesions within the brain.

Follow-up studies have demonstrated that injections of anti-TGF-β$_1$ antibody worsen both incidence and severity of EAE (164–166). Comparable results have been obtained using TGF-β$_2$, which reduced the clinical severity of EAE and the number of relapses, and produced less inflammation and demyelination in the CNS (129,166). Of relevance to these studies are the findings that CD4+ and CD8+ T-suppressor cells that mediate recovery from EAE produce TGF-β (167,168), and that TGF-β is capable of inhibiting IFN-γ and TNF-α production by the CD4+ effector T cells that transfer disease (167,169). The implication of these studies is that TGF-β expression by T-suppressor cells is critical for recovery from EAE, and TGF-β may mediate its action by inhibiting expression of inflammatory cytokines by CD4+ effector T cells. In addition, TGF-β can inhibit TNF-α production by endogenous glial cells (64,160), thereby contributing to the control of EAE.

A recent study by Santambrogio and associates (166) examined the mechanisms by which TGF-β$_2$ protects against EAE. TGF-β$_2$ treatment on days 5 to 9 after immunization did not influence the appearance of myelin-sensitized cells in peripheral blood and lymph nodes, but it did prevent the subsequent accumulation of T cells in brain and spinal cord. These findings indicate that the protective effect of TGF-β is exerted at the level of the target organ (the CNS), or at its vascular endothelium.

TGF-β has been detected in the CNS of animals with EAE, although there are reported differences in the timing of appearance. Khoury and associates (130) detected TGF-β in MBP orally-tolerized Lewis rats, which correlated with recovery from disease, as well as in the CNS of Lewis rats that had spontaneously recovered. Expression of TGF-β was not detectable during the peak of clinical disease. The kinetics of IL-4 expression were comparable to that of TGF-β (130).

Another cytokine detected in the CNS of SJL/J mice during disease recovery is IL-10 (141). IL-4, IL-10, and TGF-β share some similar biological activities because they are all capable of inhibiting secretion of pro-inflammatory cytokines (170,171). Thus, at least in some studies, expression of IL-4, IL-10, and TGF-β within the CNS correlates with recovery from EAE. In SJL/J mice with EAE, TGF-β was detected by immunohistochemistry in areas of CNS inflammation in both acute and chronic disease, and astrocytes showed positive staining for TGF-β (165).

Expression of IL-6, IL-2, Chemokines, and M-CSFs in EAE

The studies just described investigated both the functional effects of cytokines or anticytokine antibodies on EAE disease progression, as well as cytokine expression in these animals. For IL-6, IL-2, chemokines, and M-CSF, studies have been limited to examining cytokine expression in the CNS of animals with EAE.

Increased IL-6 levels have been found in the CSF of mice suffering acute EAE, and the authors suggest that local production of IL-6 is responsible because serum levels of IL-6 were not elevated (172). IL-6 mRNA levels increase rapidly during acute EAE in SJL/J mice, and they decline when clinical symptoms resolve (141). A similar observation was made in Lewis rats with EAE (130). In contrast, IL-6 protein is not found in the CNS of SJL/J mice who acquire EAE through MBP peptide immunization (143). Again, the different methods of immunization and analysis may account for the conflicting results.

IL-2 mRNA and protein expression has been detected at the preclinical stage of disease (143) and during acute disease (130,140,141), and it diminishes on recovery (130,141). It is unknown what cell types express IL-2 within the CNS of animals with EAE.

A family consisting of at least 10 distinct 8 to 10 kd cytokines has been recently described. Collectively designated "chemokines" or "intercrines," these cytokines are the product of two related gene families, members of which exhibit sequence homology and structural similarities (173). These cytokines are expressed locally in response to inflammatory stimuli, and they act to recruit inflammatory cells via their chemoattractant properties. In mice and in humans, representative chemokines include JE/MCP-1 (monocyte chemoattractant protein 1

[MCP-1]), IP-10 (IFN-γ inducible protein; 10 kd), IL-8, and RANTES. A recent study by Ransohoff and colleagues (174) investigated chemokine production in the CNS during EAE to identify factors potentially governing inflammatory cell accumulation during immune-mediated demyelination. EAE was induced in SJL/J mice using PLP peptides, and expression of JE/MCP-1 and IP-10 mRNA was examined by RT-PCR and in situ hybridization. Astrocytes were the only cells in the CNS that expressed mRNA transcripts for JE/MCP-1 and IP-10, and expression correlated with the appearance of clinical and histological EAE. In the Lewis rat, levels of MCP-1 mRNA were elevated immediately before the onset of clinical signs, peaked with the height of disease, and declined with resolution of disease (175). The marked elevation of MCP-1 at the height of clinical disease also correlated with extensive perivascular accumulation of monocytes. The cell types producing MCP-1 were not identified in this study. Also, in the Lewis rat, IL-8 protein is expressed at the peak of disease, and it declines on recovery (130). These findings collectively indicate that expression of chemokines that specifically target cells of the immune system are an important component of the disease process in EAE.

The factors involved in development and differentiation of cells of the monocyte/macrophage series have been well characterized by their role in hematopoiesis (176). A group of four major factors have been identified; each induces lineage-specific growth of colonies from bone marrow progenitor cells. They are collectively referred to as CSFs. These factors include IL-3, GM-CSF, macrophage colony-stimulating factor M-CSF, and granulocyte-colony-stimulating factor G-CSF. IL-3, also known as multi-CSF, is produced by T-helper cells, and it acts on the most immature bone marrow progenitors to induce expansion of cells that differentiate into all known mature cell types. GM-CSF is produced by a number of activated cells, including T cells, macrophages, endothelial cells, fibroblasts, and astrocytes. GM-CSF acts on bone marrow progenitor cells already committed to differentiate to granulocytes and monocytes. GM-CSF can also interact with various mononuclear phagocytes, including microglia, to induce their activation. M-CSF, also called CSF-1, is made by macrophages, endothelial cells, fibroblasts, and astrocytes. M-CSF acts primarily on progenitor cells already committed to develop into monocytes; these progenitor cells are more mature than the targets for GM-CSF. G-CSF is made by many of the same cells that produce GM-CSF, and it acts primarily on bone marrow progenitors already committed to develop into granulocytes.

Cells of the monocyte/macrophage series are important in mediating the disease process of EAE, because in vivo depletion of these cells protects against EAE in the rat (177,178). There is only one report on the expression of CSFs in EAE, that being an examination of M-CSF and its receptor, c-fms, in Lewis rats with EAE (175). A low basal level of M-CSF mRNA was detected in non-immunized animals; in those immunized with myelin, higher levels of M-CSF mRNA were detected during the preclinical period (days 6 and 8), which peaked immediately before maximal expression of disease. Expression of M-CSF mRNA declined to baseline values when the animals recovered. Expression of the receptor for M-CSF, c-fms, was elevated immediately before disease onset, and it peaked at the height of clinical symptoms. mRNA expression of c-fms remained elevated after resolution of the acute phase of EAE.

These results indicate that production of a factor that affects monocyte growth, survival, and differentiation (i.e., M-CSF) occurs within the CNS of animals with EAE, and it correlates with disease progression and recovery. Possible cells within the CNS that could be a source of M-CSF include infiltrating T cells, as well as astrocytes. Astrocytes constitutively express M-CSF, and IL-1 and TNF-α up-regulate expression (29,62,179,180). Constitutive expression of M-CSF by astrocytes may account for the observed endogenous levels of M-CSF seen in untreated animals (175,180). The cells most likely expressing c-fms within the CNS are infiltrating macrophages or endogenous microglia (179).

Summary

I summarized studies indicating that the proinflammatory cytokines IL-1 and TNF-α contribute to initiation and/or disease progression of EAE. In contrast, the proinflammatory cytokine IFN-γ appears to impart a protective effect against EAE, which is in contrast to the effect of IFN-γ on patients with MS. In addition, TGF-β is associated with improving the clinical course of EAE, and endogenous CNS expression of TGF-β correlates with disease recovery and remission. Expression in the CNS of two other inhibitory cytokines, IL-10 and IL-4, also correlates with recovery from EAE.

These findings suggest that suppression of EAE is related to the secretion of inhibitory cytokines, such as TGF-β, IL-4, and IL-10, that actively suppress the inflammatory process in the CNS. Expression of chemokines, such as JE/MCP-1, IP-10, and IL-8, that are chemoattractants for inflammatory cells occurs in close relation to the onset of histological and clinical disease, as does expression of M-CSF, a cytokine that promotes growth, survival, and differentiation of monocytes and macrophages. The chemokines can facilitate entry of blood-borne macrophages into the CNS and then attract them to the site of injury. M-CSF can promote activation of infiltrating macrophages, as well as endogenous microglia. Collectively, the chemokines and M-CSF may have major

TABLE 12–2   CYTOKINES ASSOCIATED WITH EXPERIMENTAL
ALLERGIC ENCEPHALOMYELITIS (EAE)

Cytokine	Central Nervous System	Preclinical	Acute	Recovery	Chronic/Relapsing
IL-1	IL-1–positive macrophage/microglia	+	++	−	++
TNF-α	TNF-α–present, cell type unknown	Not examined	++	−	++
IFN-γ	IFN-γ–positive T cells/macrophages	+	++	−	Not examined
IL-6	IL-6 present, cell type unknown	Not examined	++	−	Not examined
IL-2	IL-2 present, cell type unknown	+	++	−	Not examined
Chemokines (JE/MCP-1, IP-10, IL-8)	JE/MCP-1 and IP-10–positive astrocytes	+	++	−	Not examined
M-CSF	M-CSF present, cell type unknown	+	++	−	Not examined
TGF-β	TGF-β–positive astrocytes	−	+	++	+
IL-10	IL-10 present, cell type unknown	−	+	++	Not examined
IL-4	IL-4 present, cell type unknown	−	+	++	Not examined

IL = interleukin; TNF = tumor necrosis factor; IFN = interferon; M-CSF = macrophage colony-stimulating factor; TGF = transforming growth factor; +, low expression; - = not detectable; ++ = moderate to high expression.

roles in promoting the inflammatory cascade seen within the CNS of animals with EAE. See Table 12–2 for a summary of cytokines associated with EAE.

The studies cited illustrate that multiple cytokines with both synergistic and antagonistic actions are present in the CNS of animals with EAE. As mentioned earlier for MS, it is difficult to predict the cumulative biological response to the numerous cytokine cascades ongoing in the CNS. To begin to address this issue, information on the cell types that produce or respond to the relevant cytokines must be obtained. The creation of transgenic mice to overexpress cytokines in specific brain cells will also help elucidate the role of cytokines in pathophysiological processes in the CNS. An example of this approach is a recent article by Campbell and associates (181), in which IL-6, under the regulatory control of the GFAP promoter, was overexpressed in the CNS. Severe neurological disease characterized by runting, tremor, ataxia, and seizure developed in transgenic mice with high levels of cerebral IL-6 expression. The neuropathology of the CNS included neurodegeneration, astrogliosis, angiogenesis, and induction of acute phase protein production.

These findings indicate that overexpression of IL-6 in the CNS is sufficient to induce a variety of structural and functional abnormalities, some of which are observed in autoimmune, degenerative, and trauma-induced CNS diseases in animals and humans. This strategy should provide information on the relative neuropathogenic potential of cytokines, either individually or in combination.

HUMAN IMMUNODEFICIENCY VIRUS–ASSOCIATED COGNITIVE/MOTOR COMPLEX

Human immunodeficiency virus (HIV)–associated cognitive/motor complex, or acquired immunodeficiency syndrome (AIDS) dementia complex (ADC) afflicts more than 50% of all patients infected with HIV-1 (182,183). ADC is characterized clinically by cognitive, motor, and behavioral dysfunction. Manifestations include global cognitive defects, organic psychosis, and a variety of motor abnormalities (184). Pathologically, ADC presents with cerebral atrophy and abnormalities of the white and deep gray matter structures, including the basal ganglia. These abnormalities include diffuse pallor and vacuolation of the white matter, and focal rarefaction accompanied by infiltration of macrophages, multinucleated cells, and lymphocytes. Infiltration of T lymphocytes is limited in degree, and it is primarily of the CD8+ phenotype. Discrete areas of demyelination are common, and they are associated with reactive/hypertrophied astrocytes (astrogliosis), as well as the presence of microglia, blood-derived macrophages, and multinucleated giant cells.

ADC occurs in the absence of recognized, opportunistic pathogens, and there is strong indication that direct infection of the CNS by HIV-1 is responsible for ADC. HIV-1 DNA and RNA sequences are found in the CNS tissue of individuals with ADC in an abundance greater than that of lymphoid tissues (185). HIV-1 has been directly isolated from both brain and CSF of patients with AIDS (186), and anti-HIV-1 antibodies have been detected in the CSF of patients with AIDS in levels that indicate intracerebral CNS antibody production (187).

Much attention has been directed at determining which cells in the CNS are infected by HIV-1. A number of laboratories have conclusively determined by in situ hybridization and immunohistochemistry that infiltrating monocytes and macrophages, as well as resident microglia, are infected by HIV-1 (188–191). Earlier reports suggested that brain capillary endothelial cells, astrocytes, oligodendrocytes, and neurons could occasionally be infected with HIV-1; however, these examples were quite rare (189,191). The prevailing belief is that macrophages and microglia are the principal (and probably only) cell types productively infected with HIV-1 in the CNS. In support of this finding, Watkins and colleagues (192) showed that HIV-1 infection of primary human brain explant cultures resulted in productive infection of microglial cells, whereas astrocytes remained uninfected.

Although it is clear that macrophages and microglia are the principal targets of HIV-1 infection, there is currently no satisfactory explanation for the extensive neurological impairment observed clinically in ADC. Because neurons are not directly infected with HIV-1, the severe pathophysiological manifestations of ADC are most likely mediated through indirect mechanisms. Because HIV-1–infected macrophages and microglia produce a number of different cytokines (193), it is hypothesized that cytokine production within the CNS may directly damage neurons, or alter the function of the astrocyte, thereby indirectly compromising neurons. In this regard, IFN-γ, TNF-α, and IL-1β have been shown to modulate various aspects of astrocyte ion transport systems (194–196), which are critical for maintaining a balanced ionic microenvironment for neurons. Cytokines have also been shown to modulate HIV expression in infected cells; thus, they are likely to be important in the pathogenesis of ADC (197). The role of cytokines in contributing to AIDS progression has been discussed in detail in a previous chapter, so I only briefly indicate the possible roles of some cytokines in ADC.

Role of IL-1 in ADC

Elevated levels of IL-1 are present in the CSF of patients with ADC (198,199), and IL-1–positive cells have been identified in the brains of these patients (199). The IL-1–positive cells appear to be predominantly infiltrating macrophages and resident microglia. IL-1 has been shown to enhance HIV-1 expression in cells of both T lymphocytic and monocytic lineages; thus, IL-1 expression in the CNS could propagate HIV-1 replication within this site.

Role of TNF-α in ADC

Elevated levels of TNF-α have been demonstrated in the CSF of patients with AIDS, and TNF-α staining in brains from patients with AIDS localizes with some endothelial cells and astrocytes, but primarily with macrophages and microglia (199). TNF-α has been shown to activate and enhance HIV-1 replication in macrophages (200); thus, it may contribute to the pathogenesis of ADC. Astrocytes and microglia have a direct role in this process, because TNF-α produced by these cells induces expression of HIV-1 in macrophages (201,202). Furthermore, TNF-α can act synergistically with either IL-6 or GM-CSF to induce HIV-1 expression in macrophages (203). Because astrocytes and microglia can be the source of these three cytokines (i.e., TNF-α, IL-6, GM-CSF) in the CNS, these endogenous glial cells may be involved in maintaining HIV expression in the CNS. Pentoxifylline has been shown to block TNF-α secretion in cancer patients whose symptoms were associated with elevated levels of TNF-α (204,205). With regard to HIV infection, pentoxifylline inhibits replication of HIV in T cells and peripheral blood mononuclear cells (206). Preliminary clinical trials have shown that administration of pentoxifylline to HIV-infected patients is tolerable, and it is associated with a decrease in TNF-α production by peripheral blood mononuclear cells (207). Whether pentoxifylline affects TNF- α expression or HIV replication in the CNS is currently unknown.

Role of IL-6 in ADC

Elevated CNS IL-6 levels have been demonstrated in patients with ADC (199). IL-6 has been shown to up-regulate production of HIV in infected cells of the monocytic lineage and to act synergistically with TNF-α (208). IL-6 produced by human astrocytes can stimulate HIV-1 expression in a chronically infected promonocyte clone (209); thus, local production of IL-6 by astrocytes may contribute to HIV replication within the CNS. Another possible role of CNS IL-6 may relate to B-cell differentiation. There is evidence of B-cell stimulation during ADC due to the presence of HIV-1–specific Ig in the CSF of these patients (187). Production of IL-6 by astrocytes or microglia may contribute in part to the heightened intracerebral humoral immune responses in patients with ADC.

Role of TGF-β in ADC

TGF-β₁ has been identified in the brains of patients with AIDS, but not in control brain tissue (210). TGF-β staining was localized to macrophages, microglia, and astrocytes, especially in areas of diseased brain. Moreover, HIV-1–infected monocytes secreted a factor that induced cultured astrocytes to secrete TGF-β. This factor in all likelihood is TGF-β (211).

TGF-β has bifunctional effects on HIV expression. TGF-β suppresses HIV replication in U1 cells stimulated with either phorbol ester or IL-6, but not TNF-α, as well as in primary monocytic cells (212). In contrast, treatment with TGF-β of either U937 cells or primary macrophages prior to HIV infection enhances HIV replication (212,213). Thus, HIV-1–induced TGF-β production by macrophages may act in an autocrine manner to inhibit or enhance HIV replication, or in a paracrine fashion to induce astrocytes to produce TGF-β. By either pathway, TGF-β may have an important role as a regulator of HIV expression in infected macrophages or microglia. These results indicate that TGF-β can have differential effects on HIV replication, depending on the time of exposure and the activational state of the infected cells.

Role of IFN-γ in ADC

IFN-γ staining was detected in all HIV-positive brain specimens, and endothelial cells and microglia were most frequently positive (199). Although IFN-γ levels were elevated in only one of eight CSF samples, neopterin, an indirect measure of IFN-γ–induced activation of macrophages, was elevated in all CSF and serum samples tested. In addition, class II MHC antigen–positive microglia were detected in the CNS of HIV-positive patients, presumably the result of IFN-γ stimulation. The source of IFN-γ within the CNS is likely to be infiltrating CD8+ T cells.

IFN-γ has bifunctional effects on HIV replication. In primary macrophages that were first infected, then exposed to IFN-γ, HIV production was diminished, as opposed to cells that were first stimulated with IFN-γ, then infected, in which enhancement of virus production was observed (214). Thus, IFN-γ is similar to TGF-β in that either inhibition or enhancement of HIV expression is observed on exposure.

Summary

HIV expression and replication within the CNS is governed by a number of regulatory constraints, including control by cytokine networks. The cytokines that predominantly affect HIV expression in cells of the monocyte/macrophage lineage will be the most important in the CNS because they can affect HIV expression of infected macrophages and microglia. These cytokines include IL-1, IL-4, IL-6, IL-10, IL-13, TNF-α, TNF-β, TGF-β, M-CSF, GM-CSF, IFN-α, IFN-β, and IFN-γ (197). I focused on IL-1, TNF-α, IL-6, TGF-β, and IFN-γ because these cytokines have been documented in the CNS of patients with ADC (Table 12–3). The existing literature indicates that these cytokines can either inhibit or enhance HIV expression, and the ultimate biological effect is dependent on the phase of HIV infection (i.e., acute versus chronic), presence of other regulatory factors, time of cytokine exposure, and maturational status of the infected cell. The literature on cytokine expression in ADC is still quite sparse, and more information on the repertoire of cytokines expressed in this tissue and the cells

TABLE 12–3   CYTOKINES ASSOCIATED WITH AIDS DEMENTIA COMPLEX (ADC)

Cytokine	Cerebrospinal Fluid	Brain Tissue	Effect on HIV Expression
IL-1	Increased expression	IL-1–positive macrophages, microglia	↑
TNF-α	Increased expression	TNF-α–positive endothelial cells, astrocytes, macrophages, microglia	↑
IL-6	Undetectable	IL-6–positive endothelial cells, microglia	↑
TGF-β	Not examined	TGF-β–positive macrophages, microglia, astrocytes	↑↓
IFN-γ	Undetectable	IFN-γ–positive endothelial cells, microglia	↑↓

AIDS = acquired immunodeficiency syndrome; HIV = human immunodeficiency virus; IL = interleukin; TNF = tumor necrosis factor; TGF = transforming growth factor; IFN = interferon; ↑ = increase; ↓ = decrease.

producing them will provide a foundation to start understanding the dynamics of HIV expression within the CNS.

ACKNOWLEDGMENTS: I thank Sue Wade for superb secretarial and editorial assistance in preparing this manuscript.

This work was supported in part by National Multiple Sclerosis Society Grants 2269-A-4 and 2205-B-5, and National Institutes of Health Grants NS-29719, NS-31096, and MH-50421.

REFERENCES

1. Benveniste EN. Cytokines: influence on glial cell gene expression and function. In: Blalock JE, ed. Chemical immunology: neuroimmunoendocrinology, vol 52. Basel: Karger, 1992:106–153.

2. Raff MC. Glial cell diversification in the rat optic nerve. Science 1989;243:1450–1455.

3. Patterson PH, Nawa H. Neuronal differentiation factors/cytokines and synaptic plasticity. Cell/Neuron 1993;72:123–137.

4. Benveniste EN. Inflammatory cytokines within the central nervous system: sources, function, and mechanism of action. Am J Physiol 1992;263:32:C1–C16.

5. Hauser SL, Bhan AK, Gilles FH, et al. Immunohistochemical staining of human brain with monoclonal antibodies that identify lymphocytes, monocytes and the Ia antigen. J Neuroimmunol 1983;5:197–205.

6. Prineas JW. Pathology of the early lesion in multiple sclerosis. Hum Pathol 1975;6:531–554.

7. Prineas JW, Wright RG. Macrophages, lymphocytes and plasma cells in the perivascular compartment in chronic multiple sclerosis. Lab Invest 1978;38:409–421.

8. Hofman FM, VonHanwher R, Dinarello C, Mizel S, Hinton D, Merrill JE. Immunoregulatory molecules and IL-2 receptors identified in multiple sclerosis brain. J Immunol 1986;136:3239–3245.

9. Bignami A, Eng LF, Dahl D, Uyeda CT. Localization of the glial fibrillary acidic protein in astrocytes by immunofluorescence. Brain Res 1972;43:429–435.

10. Selmaj K, Brosnan CF, Raine CS. Colocalization of lymphocytes bearing γδ T-cell receptor and heat shock protein hsp65$^+$ oligodendrocytes in multiple sclerosis. Proc Natl Acad Sci USA 1991;88:6452–6456.

11. Thompson AJ, Miller D, Youl B, et al. Serial gadolinium-enhanced MRI in relapsing/remitting multiple sclerosis of varying disease duration. Neurology 1992;42:60–63.

12. Gay D, Esiri M. Blood-brain barrier damage in acute multiple sclerosis plaques: an immunocytological study. Brain 1991;114:557–572.

13. Martin R, McFarland HF, McFarlin DE. Immunological aspects of demyelinating diseases. Annu Rev Immunol 1992;10:153–187.

14. Vilcek J, Lee TH. Tumor necrosis factor. J Biol Chem 1991;266:7313–7316.

15. Selmaj KW, Raine CS. Tumor necrosis factor mediates myelin and oligodendrocyte damage in vitro. Ann Neurol 1988;23:339–346.

16. Robbins DS, Shirazi Y, Drysdale BE, Lieberman A, Shin HS, Shin ML. Production of cytotoxic factor for oligodendrocytes by stimulated astrocytes. J Immunol 1987;139:2593–2597.

17. Paul NJ, Ruddle NH. Lymphotoxin. Annu Rev Immunol 1988;6:407–438.

18. Selmaj K, Raine CS, Farooq M, Norton WT, Brosnan CF. Cytokine cytotoxicity against oligodendrocytes: apoptosis induced by lymphotoxin. J Immunol 1991;147:1522–1529.

19. Benveniste EN, Sparacio SM, Bethea JR. Tumor necrosis factor-α enhances interferon-g mediated class II antigen expression on astrocytes. J Neuroimmunol 1989;25:209–219.

20. Chung IY, Benveniste EN. Tumor necrosis factor-α production by astrocytes: induction by lipopolysaccharide, IFN-γ and IL-1β. J Immunol 1990;144:2999–3007.

21. Lieberman AP, Pitha PM, Shin HS, Shin ML. Production of tumor necrosis factor and other cytokines by astrocytes stimulated with lipopolysaccharide or a neurotropic virus. Proc Natl Acad Sci USA 1989;86:6348–6352.

22. Bethea JR, Chung IY, Sparacio SM, Gillespie GY, Benveniste EN. Interleukin-1β induction of tumor necrosis factor-alpha gene expression in human astroglioma cells. J Neuroimmunol 1992;36:179–191.

23. Velasco S, Tarlow M, Olsen K, Shay JW, McCracken JGH, Nisen PD. Temperature-dependent modulation of lipopolysaccharide-induced interleukin-1β and tumor necrosis factor α expression in cultured human astroglial cells by dexamethasone and indomethacin. J Clin Invest 1991;87:1674–1680.

24. Raine CS. Biology of disease: analysis of autoimmune demyelination: its impact upon multiple sclerosis. Lab Invest 1984;50:608–635.

25. Selmaj KW, Farooq M, Norton WT, Raine CS, Brosnan CF. Proliferation of astrocytes in vitro in response to cytokines. A primary role for tumor necrosis factor. J Immunol 1990;144:129–135.

26. Malipiero UV, Frei K, Fontana A. Production of hemopoietic colony-stimulating factors by astrocytes. J Immunol 1990;144:3816–3821.

27. Frei K, Piani D, Malipiero UV, Van Meir E, de Tribolet N, Fontana A. Granulocyte-macrophage colony-stimulating factor (GM-CSF) production by glioblastoma cells. J Immunol 1992;148:3140–3146.

28. Tweardy DJ, Glazer EW, Mott PL, Anderson K. Modulation by tumor necrosis factor-α of human astroglial cell production of granulocyte-macrophage colony-stimulating factor (GM-CSF) and granulocyte colony-stimulating factor (G-CSF). J Neuroimmunol 1991;32:269–278.

29. Aloisi F, Care A, Borsellino G, et al. Production of hemolymphopoietic cytokines (IL-6, IL-8, colony-stimulating factors) by normal human astrocytes in response to IL-1β and tumor necrosis factor-α. J Immunol 1992;149:2358–2366.

30. Lee SC, Liu W, Roth P, Dickson DW, Berman JW, Brosnan CF. Macrophage colony-stimulating factor in human fetal astrocytes and microglia: differential regulation by cytokines and lipopolysaccharide, and modulation of class II MHC on microglia. J Immunol 1993;150:594–604.

31. Benveniste EN, Sparacio SM, Norris JG, Grenett HE, Fuller GM. Induction and regulation of interleukin-6 gene ex-

pression in rat astrocytes. J Neuroimmunol 1990;30:201–212.

32. Frei K, Malipiero UV, Leist TP, Zinkernagel RM, Schwab ME, Fontana A. On the cellular source and function of interleukin-6 produced in the central nervous system in viral diseases. Eur J Immunol 1989;19:689–694.

33. Sparacio SM, Zhang Y, Vilcek J, Benveniste EN. Cytokine regulation of interleukin-6 gene expression in astrocytes involves activation of an NF-κB-like nuclear protein. J Neuroimmunol 1992;39:231–242.

34. van Snick JV. Interleukin-6: an overview. Annu Rev Immunol 1990;8:253–278.

35. Cross AH, Cannella B, Brosnan CF, Raine CS. Homing to central nervous system vasculature by antigen-specific lymphocytes. Lab Invest 1990;63:162–170.

36. Raine CS, Lee SC, Scheinberg LC, Duijvestijn AM, Cross AH. Adhesion molecules on endothelial cells in the central nervous system: an emerging area in the neuroimmunology of multiple sclerosis. Clin Immunol Immunopathol 1990;57:173–187.

37. McCarron RM, Wang L, Racke MK, McFarlin DE, Spatz M. Cytokine-regulated adhesion between encephalitogenic T lymphocytes and cerebrovascular endothelial cells. J Neuroimmunol 1993:43:23–30.

38. Fabry Z, Waldschmidt MM, Hendrickson D, et al. Adhesion molecules on murine brain microvascular endothelial cells: expression and regulation of ICAM-1 and Lgp 55. J Neuroimmunol 1992;36:1–11.

39. Wong D, Dorovini-Zis K. Upregulation of intercellular adhesion molecule-1 (ICAM-1) expression in primary cultures of human brain microvessel endothelial cells by cytokines and lipopolysaccharide. J Neuroimmunol 1992;39:11–22.

40. Hurwitz AA, Lyman WD, Guida MP, Calderon TM, Berman JW. Tumor necrosis factor α induces adhesion molecule expression on human fetal astrocytes. J Exp Med 1992;176:1631–1636.

41. Frohman EM, Frohman TC, Dustin ML, et al. The induction of intercellular adhesion molecule-1 (ICAM-1) expression on human fetal astrocytes by interferon-γ, tumor necrosis factor-α, lymphotoxin, and interleukin-1: relevance to intracerebral antigen presentation. J Neuroimmunol 1989;23:117–124.

42. Satoh J-I, Kastrukoff LF, Kim SU. Cytokine-induced expression of intercellular adhesion molecule-1 (ICAM-1) in cultured human oligodendrocytes and astrocytes. J Neuropathol Exp Neurol 1991;50:215–226.

43. Satoh J, Kim SU, Kastrukoff LF, Takei F. Expression and induction of intercellular adhesion molecules (ICAMs) and major histocompatibility complex (MHC) antigens on cultured murine oligodendrocytes and astrocytes. J Neurosci Res 1991;29:1–12.

44. Aloisi F, Borsellino G, Samoggia P, et al. Astrocyte cultures from human embryonic brain: characterization and modulation of surface molecules by inflammatory cytokines. J Neurosci Res 1992;32:494–506.

45. Kraus E, Schneider-Schaulies S, Miyasaka M, Tamatani T, Sedgwick J. Augmentation of major histocompatibility complex class I and ICAM-1 expression on glial cells following measles virus infection: evidence for the role of type-1 interferon. Eur J Immunol 1992;22:175–182.

46. Shrikant P, Chung IY, Ballestas M, Benveniste EN. Regulation of intercellular adhesion molecule-1 gene expression by tumor necrosis factor-α, interleukin-1β, and interferon-γ in astrocytes. J Neuroimmunol 1994;51:209–220.

47. O'Neill JK, Butter C, Baker D, et al. Expression of vascular addressins and ICAM-1 by endothelial cells in the spinal cord during chronic relapsing experimental allergic encephalomyelitis in the Biozzi AB/H mouse. Immunology 1991;72:520–525.

48. Cannella B, Cross AH, Raine CS. Adhesion-related molecules in the central nervous system. Upregulation correlates with inflammatory cell influx during relapsing experimental autoimmune encephalomyelitis. Lab Invest 1991;65:23–31.

49. Sobel RA, Mitchell ME, Fondren G. Intercellular adhesion molecule-1 (ICAM-1) in cellular immune reactions in the human central nervous system. Am J Pathol 1990;136:1309–1316.

50. Beck J, Rondot P, Catinot L, Falcoff E, Kirchner H, Wietzerbin J. Increased production of interferon gamma and tumor necrosis factor precedes clinical manifestation in multiple sclerosis: do cytokines trigger off exacerbations? Acta Neurol Scand 1988;78:318–323.

51. Merrill JE, Strom SR, Ellison GW, Myers LW. In vitro study of mediators of inflammation in multiple sclerosis. J Clin Immunol 1989;9:84–96.

52. Gallo P, Piccinno MG, Krzalic L, Tavolato B. Tumor necrosis factor alpha (TNFα) and neurological diseases: failure in detecting TNFα in the cerebrospinal fluid from patients with multiple sclerosis, AIDS dementia complex, and brain tumors. J Neuroimmunol 1989;23:41–44.

53. Hauser SL, Doolittle TH, Lincoln R, Brown RH, Dinarello CA. Cytokine accumulations in CSF of multiple sclerosis patients: frequent detection of interleukin-1 and tumor necrosis factor but not interleukin-6. Neurology 1990;40:1735–1739.

54. Maimone D, Gregory S, Arnason BGW, Reder AT. Cytokine levels in the cerebrospinal fluid and serum of patients with multiple sclerosis. J Neuroimmunol 1991;32:67–74.

55. Franciotta DM, Grimaldi LME, Martino GV, et al. Tumor necrosis factor in serum and cerebrospinal fluid of patients with multiple sclerosis. Ann Neurol 1989;26:787–789.

56. Sharief MK, Phil M, Hentges R. Association between tumor necrosis factor-α and disease progression in patients with multiple sclerosis. N Engl J Med 1991;325:467–472.

57. Sharief MK, Thompson EJ. In vivo relationship of tumor necrosis factor-α to blood-brain barrier damage in patients with active multiple sclerosis. J Neuroimmunol 1992;38:27–34.

58. Sharief MK, Noori MA, Ciardi M, Cirelli A, Thompson EJ. Increased levels of circulating ICAM-1 in serum and cerebrospinal fluid of patients with active multiple sclerosis. Correlation with TNF-α and blood-brain barrier damage. J Neuroimmunol 1993;43:15–22.

59. Hofman FM, Hinton DR, Johnson K, Merrill JE. Tumor necrosis factor identified in multiple sclerosis brain. J Exp Med 1989;170:607–612.

60. Hofman FM, Hinton DR, Baemayr J, Weil M, Merrill JE. Lymphokines and immunoregulatory molecules in subacute sclerosing panencephalitis. Clin Immunol Immunopathol 1991;58:331–342.

61. Selmaj K, Raine CS, Cannella B, Brosnan CF. Identification of lymphotoxin and tumor necrosis factor in multiple sclerosis lesions. J Clin Invest 1991;87:949–954.

62. Lee SC, Liu W, Dickson DW, Brosnan CF, Berman JW. Cytokine production by human fetal microglia and astrocytes: differential induction by lipopolysaccharide and IL-1β. J Immunol 1993;150:2659–2667.

63. Chao CC, Hu S, Close K, et al. Cytokine release from microglia: differential inhibition by pentoxifylline and dexamethasone. J Infect Dis 1992;166:847–853.

64. Suzumura A, Sawada M, Yamamoto H. Marunouchi T. Transforming growth factor-β suppresses activation and proliferation of microglia in vitro. J Immunol 1993;151: 2150–2158.

65. Frei K, Siepl C, Groscurth P, Bodmer S, Schwerdel C, Fontana A. Antigen presentation and tumor cytotoxicity by interferon-γ-treated microglial cells. Eur J Immunol 1987;17: 1271–1278.

66. Arai K, Lee F, Miyajima A, Miyatake S, Arai N, Yokota T. Cytokines: coordinators of immune and inflammatory responses. Annu Rev Biochem 1990;59:783–836.

67. de Giovine FS, Duff GW. Interleukin 1: the first interleukin. Immunol Today 1990;11:13–14.

68. Giulian D, Lachman LB. Interleukin-1 stimulation of astroglial proliferation after brain injury. Science 1985;228: 497–499.

69. Giulian D, Woodward J, Young DG, Krebs JF, Lachman LB. Interleukin-1 injected into mammalian brain stimulates astrogliosis and neovascularization. J Neurosci 1988; 8:2485–2490.

70. da Cunha A, Jefferson JA, Jackson RW, Vitkovic L. Glial cell-specific mechanisms of TGF-β₁ induction by IL-1 in cerebral cortex. J Neuroimmunol 1993;42:71–86.

71. Bethea JR, Gillespie GY, Benveniste EN. Interleukin-1β induction of TNF-α gene expression: involvement of protein kinase C. J Cell Physiol 1992;152:264–273.

72. Frei K, Nohava K, Malipiero UV, Schwerdel C, Fontana A. Production of macrophage colony-stimulating factor by astrocytes and brain macrophages. J Neuroimmunol 1992; 40:189–196.

73. Tweardy DJ, Mott PL, Glazer EW. Monokine modulation of human astroglial cell production of granulocyte colony-stimulating factor and granulocyte-macrophage colony stimulating factor. I. Effects of IL-1α and IL-1β. J Immunol 1990;144:2233–2241.

74. Hong L, Imeri L, Opp MR, Postlethwaite AE, Seyer JM, Krueger JM. Intercellular adhesion molecule-1 expression induced by interleukin (IL)-1β or an IL-1β fragment is blocked by an IL-1 receptor antagonist and a soluble IL-1 receptor. J Neuroimmunol 1993;44:163–170.

75. Wucherpfennig KW, Newcombe J, Li H, Keddy C, Cuzner ML, Hafler DA. T cell receptor Vα-Vβ repertoire and cytokine gene expression in active multiple sclerosis lesions. J Exp Med 1992;175:993–1002.

76. Giulian D, Baker TJ, Shih L, Lachman LB. Interleukin-1 of the central nervous system is produced by ameboid microglia. J Exp Med 1986;164:594–604.

77. Merrill JE, Matsushima K. Production of and response to interleukin-1 by cloned human oligodendroglioma cell lines. J Biol Reg Homeost Agents 1988;2:77–86.

78. Aderka D, Le J, Vilcek J. IL-6 inhibits lipopolysaccharide-induced tumor necrosis factor production in cultured human monocytes, U937 cells, and in mice. J Immunol 1989;143:3517–3523.

79. Norris JG, Tang L-P, Sparacio SM, Benveniste EN. Signal transduction pathways mediating astrocyte interleukin-6 induction by interleukin-1β and tumor necrosis factor-α. J Immunol 1994;151:841–850.

80. Tourtellotte WW, Ma IB. Multiple sclerosis: the blood-brain barrier and the measurement of de novo central nervous system IgG synthesis. Neurology 1978;28:76–83.

81. Muraguchi A, Hirano T, Tang B, et al. The essential role of B cell stimulatory factor 2 (BSF-2/IL-6) for the terminal differentiation of B cells. J Exp Med 1988;167:332–344.

82. Frei K, Leist TP, Meager A, et al. Production of B cell stimulatory factor-2 and interferon-γ in the central nervous system during viral meningitis and encephalitis. Evaluation in a murine model infection and in patients. J Exp Med 1988; 168:449–453.

83. Houssiau FA, Bukasa K, Sindic CJM, Van Damme J, Van Snick J. Elevated levels of the 26K human hybridoma growth factor (interleukin 6) in cerebrospinal fluid of patients with acute infection of the central nervous system. Clin Exp Immunol 1988;71:320–323.

84. Frei K, Fredrikson S, Fontana A, Link H. Interleukin-6 is elevated in plasma in multiple sclerosis. J Neuroimmunol 1991;31:147–153.

85. Smith KA. Interleukin-2: inception, impact and implications. Science 1988;240:1169–1176.

86. Benveniste EN, Merrill JE. Stimulation of oligodendroglial proliferation and maturation by interleukin-2. Nature 1986;321:610–613.

87. Benveniste EN, Herman PK, Whitaker JN. Myelin basic protein-specific RNA levels in interleukin-2-stimulated oligodendrocytes. J Neurochem 1987;49:1274–1279.

88. Benveniste EN, Tozawa H, Gasson JC, Quan S, Golde DW, Merrill JE. Response of human glioblastoma cells to recombinant interleukin-2. J Neuroimmunol 1988;17:301–314.

89. Okamoto Y, Minamoto S, Shimizu K, Mogami H, Taniguchi T. Interleukin 2 receptor β chain expressed in an oligodendroglioma line binds interleukin 2 and delivers growth signal. Proc Natl Acad Sci USA 1990;87:6584–6588.

90. Saneto RP, Altman A, Knobler R, Johnson HM, de Vellis J. Interleukin 2 mediates the inhibition of oligodendrocyte progenitor cell proliferation in vitro. Proc Natl Acad Sci USA 1986;83:9221–9225.

91. Gallo P, Piccinno M. Pagni S, Tavolato B. Interleukin-2 levels in serum and cerebrospinal fluid of multiple sclerosis patients. Ann Neurol 1988;24:795–797.

92. Trotter JL, Clifford DB, Anderson CB, van der Veen RC, Hicks BC, Banks G. Elevated serum interleukin-2 levels in chronic progressive multiple sclerosis. N Engl J Med 1988; 318:1206.

93. Baron JL, Madri JA, Ruddle NH, Hashim G, Janeway CA Jr. Surface expression of α4 integrin by CD4 T cells is required for their entry into brain parenchyma. J Exp Med 1993;177:57–68.

94. Ando DG, Clayton J, Kono D, Urban JL, Sercarz EE. Encephalitogenic T cells in the B10.PL model of experimental

allergic encephalomyelitis (EAE) are of the Th-1 lymphokine subtype. Cell Immunol 1989;124:132–143.

95. Brod SA, Benjamin D, Hafler DA. Restricted T cell expression of IL-2/IFN-γ mRNA in human inflammatory disease. J Immunol 1991;147:810–815.

96. Farrar MA, Schreiber RD. The molecular cell biology of interferon-γ and its receptor. Annu Rev Immunol 1993; 11:571–611.

97. Ijzermans JNM, Marquet RL. Interferon-gamma: a review. Immunobiology 1989;179:456–473.

98. Cogswell JP, Zeleznik-Le N, Ting JP-Y. Transcriptional regulation of the HLA-DRA gene. Crit Rev Immunol 1991; 11:87–112.

99. Benacerraf B. Role of MHC gene products in immune regulation. Science 1981;212:1229–1238.

100. Hirayama M, Yokochi T, Shimokata K, Iida M, Fujuki N. Induction of human leukocyte antigen-A, -B, -C and -DR on cultured human oligodendrocytes and astrocytes by human γ-interferon. Neurosci Lett 1986;72:369–374.

101. Suzumura A, Silberberg DH, Lisak RP. The expression of MHC antigens on oligodendrocytes: induction of polymorphic H-2 expression by lymphokines. J Neuroimmunol 1986;11:179–190.

102. Suzumura A, Lavi E, Weiss SR, Silberberg DH. Coronavirus infection induces H-2 antigen expression on oligodendrocytes and astrocytes. Science 1986;232:991–993.

103. Wong GHW, Bartlett PF, Clark-Lewis I, Battye F, Schrader JW. Inducible expression of H-2 and Ia antigens on brain cells. Nature 1984;310:688–691.

104. Fierz W, Endler B, Reske K, Wekerle H, Fontana A. Astrocytes as antigen presenting cells. I. Induction of Ia antigen expression on astrocytes by T cells via immune interferon and its effect on antigen presentation. J Immunol 1985; 134:3785–3793.

105. Fontana A, Fierz W, Wederle H. Astrocytes present myelin basic protein to encephalitogenic T-cell lines. Nature 1984; 307:273–276.

106. Pulver M, Carrel S, Mach JP, de Tribolet N. Cultured human fetal astrocytes can be induced by interferon-γ to express HLA-DR. J Neuroimmunol 1987;14:123–133.

107. Suzumura A, Mezitis SGE, Gonatas NK, Silberberg DH. MHC antigen expression on bulk isolated macrophage-microglia from newborn mouse brain: induction of Ia antigen expression by γ-interferon. J Neuroimmunol 1987;15: 263–278.

108. Barna BP, Chou SM, Jacobs B, Lieberman BY, Ransohoff RM. Interferon-β impairs induction of HLA-DR antigen expression in cultured adult human astrocytes. J Neuroimmunol 1989;23:45–53.

109. Ransohoff RM, Devajyothi C, Estes ML, et al. Interferon-β specifically inhibits interferon-γ-induced class II major histocompatibility complex gene transcription in a human astrocytoma cell line. J Neuroimmunol 1991;33:103–112.

110. Barnum SR, Jones JL, Benveniste EN. Interferon-gamma regulation of C3 gene expression in human astroglioma cells. J Neuroimmunol 1992;38:275–282.

111. Johnson RT, Lazzarini RA, Waksman BH. Mechanisms of virus persistence. Ann Neurol 1981;9:616–617.

112. Panitch HS, Bever CT Jr. Clinical trials of interferons in multiple sclerosis: what have we learned? J Neuroimmunol 1993;46:155–164.

113. Jacobs L, O'Malley J, Freeman A, Ekes R. Intrathecal interferon reduces exacerbations of multiple sclerosis. Science 1981;214:1026–1028.

114. Jacobs L, Salazar AM, Herndon R, et al. Intrathecally administered natural human fibroblast interferon reduces exacerbations of multiple sclerosis. Arch Neurol 1987;44: 589–595.

115. Group TIMS. Interferon beta-1b is effective in relapsing-remitting multiple sclerosis. I. Clinical results of a multicenter, randomized, double-blind, placebo-controlled trial. Neurology 1993;43:655–661.

116. Paty DW, Li DKB, Study Group TUM, Study Group TIMS. Interferon beta-1b is effective in relapsing-remitting multiple sclerosis. II. MRI analysis results of a multicenter, randomized, double-blind, placebo-controlled trial. Neurology 1993;43:662–667.

117. Arnason BGW. Interferon beta in multiple sclerosis. Neurology 1993;43:641–643.

118. Abu-khabar KS, Armstrong JA, Ho M. Type I interferons (IFN-α and -β) suppress cytotoxin (tumor necrosis factor-α and lymphotoxin) production by mitogen-stimulated human peripheral blood mononuclear cells. J Leukocyte Biol 1992;52:165–172.

119. Noronha A, Jensen MA, Toscas A, Sihag S. IFN-beta downregulates tumor necrosis factor release. Neurology 1992;42:159.

120. Vervliet G, Claeys H, van Haver H, et al. Interferon production and natural killer (NK) activity in leukocyte cultures from multiple sclerosis patients. J Neurol Sci 1983;60:137–150.

121. Vervliet G, Carton H, Meulepas E, Billiau A. Interferon production by cultured peripheral leukocytes of MS patients. Clin Exp Immunol 1984;58:116–126.

122. Panitch HS, Hirsch RL, Schindler J, Johnson KP. Treatment of multiple sclerosis with gamma interferon: exacerbations associated with activation of the immune system. Neurology 1987;37:1097–1102.

123. Hirsch RL, Panitch HS, Johnson KP. Lymphocytes from multiple sclerosis patients produce elevated levels of gamma interferon in vitro. J Clin Immunol 1985;5:386–389.

124. Abbott RJ, Bolderson I, Gruer PJK, Peatfield RC. Immunoreactive IFN-γ in CSF in neurological disorders. J Neurol Neurosurg Psychol 1987;50:882–885.

125. Traugott U, Lebon P. Multiple sclerosis: involvement of interferons in lesion pathogenesis. Ann Neurol 1988;24:243–251.

126. Racke MK, Jalbut SD, Cannella B, Albert PS, Raine CS, McFarlin DE. Prevention and treatment of chronic relapsing experimental allergic encephalomyelitis by transforming growth factor-β₁. J Immunol 1991;146:3012–3017.

127. Johns LD, Flanders KC, Ranges GE, Sriram S. Successful treatment of experimental allergic encephalomyelitis with transforming growth factor-β₁. J Immunol 1991;147:1793–1796.

128. Kuruvilla AP, Shah R, Hochwald GM, Liggitt HD, Palladino MA, Thorbecke GJ. Protective effect of transforming growth factor β₁ on experimental autoimmune diseases in mice. Proc Natl Acad Sci USA 1991;88:2918–2921.

129. Racke MK, Sriram S, Carlino J, Cannella B, Raine CS, McFarlin DE. Long-term treatment of chronic relapsing experimental allergic encephalomyelitis by transforming growth factor-β_2. J Neuroimmunol 1993;46:175–184.

130. Khoury SJ, Hancock WW, Weiner HL. Oral tolerance to myelin basic protein and natural recovery from experimental autoimmune encephalomyelitis are associated with downregulation of inflammatory cytokines and differential upregulation of transforming growth factor β, interleukin 4, and prostaglandin E expression in the brain. J Exp Med 1992;176:1355–1364.

131. Beck J, Rondot P, Jullien P, Wietzerbin J, Lawrence DA. TGF-β-like activity produced during regression of exacerbations in multiple sclerosis. Acta Neurol Scand 1991;84:452–455.

132. Zamvil SS, Steinman L. The T lymphocyte in experimental allergic encephalomyelitis. Annu Rev Immunol 1990;8:579–621.

133. Mosmann TR, Coffman RL. TH1 and TH2 cells: different patterns of lymphokine secretion lead to different functional properties. Annu Rev Immunol 1989;7:145–173.

134. Powell MB, Mitchell D, Lederman J, et al. Lymphotoxin and tumor necrosis factor-alpha production by myelin basic protein-specific T cell clones correlates with encephalitogenicity. Intl Immunol 1990;2:539–544.

135. Kuchroo VK, Martin CA, Greer JM, Ju S-T, Sobel RA, Dorf ME. Cytokines and adhesion molecules contribute to the ability of myelin proteolipid protein-specific T cell clones to mediate experimental allergic encephalomyelitis. J Immunol 1993;151:4371–4382.

136. Gasser DL, Newlin CM, Palm J, Gonatas NK. Genetic control of susceptibility to experimental allergic encephalomyelitis in rats. Science 1973;181:872–873.

137. Mannie MD, Dinarello CA, Paterson PY. Interleukin 1 and myelin basic protein synergistically augment adoptive transfer activity of lymphocytes mediating experimental autoimmune encephalomyelitis in Lewis rats. J Immunol 1987;138:4229–4235.

138. Symons JA, Bundick RV, Suckling AJ, Rumsby MG. Cerebrospinal fluid interleukin 1-like activity during chronic relapsing experimental allergic encephalomyelitis. Clin Exp Immunol 1987;68:648–654.

139. Jacobs CA, Baker PE, Roux ER, et al. Experimental autoimmune encephalomyelitis is exacerbated by IL-1α and suppressed by soluble IL-1 receptor. J Immunol 1991;146:2983–2989.

140. Baker D, O'Neill JK, Turk JL. Cytokines in the central nervous system of mice during chronic relapsing experimental allergic encephalomyelitis. Cell Immunol 1991;134:505–510.

141. Kennedy MK, Torrance DS, Picha KS, Mohler KM. Analysis of cytokine mRNA expression in the central nervous system of mice with experimental autoimmune encephalomyelitis reveals that IL-10 mRNA expression correlates with recovery. J Immunol 1992;149:2496–2505.

142. Bauer J, Berkenbosch F, Van Dam A-M, Dijkstra CD. Demonstration of interleukin-1β in Lewis rat brain during experimental allergic encephalomyelitis by immunocytochemistry at the light and ultrastructural level. J Neuroimmunol 1993;48:13–22.

143. Merrill JE, Kong DH, Clayton J, Ando DG, Hinton DR, Hofman FM. Inflammatory leukocytes and cytokines in the peptide-induced disease of experimental allergic encephalomyelitis in SJL and B10.PL mice. Proc Natl Acad Sci USA 1992;89:574–578.

144. Ruddle NH, Bergman CM, McGrath KM, et al. An antibody to lymphotoxin and tumor necrosis factor prevents transfer of experimental allergic encephalomyelitis. J Exp Med 1990;172:1193–1200.

145. Selmaj K, Raine CS, Cross AH. Anti-tumor necrosis factor therapy abrogates autoimmune demyelination. Ann Neurol 1991;30:694–700.

146. Kuroda Y, Shimamoto Y. Human tumor necrosis factor-α augments experimental allergic encephalomyelitis in rats. J Neuroimmunol 1991;34:159–164.

147. Teuschler C, Hickey WF, Korngold R. An analysis of the role of tumor necrosis factor in the phenotypic expression of actively induced experimental allergic orchitis and experimental allergic encephalomyelitis. Clin Immunol Immunopathol 1990;54:442–453.

148. Chung IY, Norris JG, Benveniste EN. Differential tumor necrosis factor α expression by astrocytes from experimental allergic encephalomyelitis-susceptible and -resistant rat strains. J Exp Med 1991;173:801–811.

149. Billiau A, Heremans H, Vandekerckhove F, et al. Enhancement of experimental allergic encephalomyelitis in mice by antibodies against IFN-γ. J Immunol 1988;140:1506–1510.

150. Duong TT, St. Louis J, Gilbert JJ, Finkelman FD, Strejan GH. Effect of anti-interferon-γ and anti-interleukin-2 monoclonal antibody treatment on the development of actively and passively induced experimental allergic encephalomyelitis in the SJL/J mouse. J Neuroimmunol 1992;36:105–115.

151. Voorthuis JAC, Uitdehaag BMJ, De Groot CJA, Goede PH, van der Meide PH, Dijkstra CD. Suppression of experimental allergic encephalomyelitis by intraventricular administration of interferon-gamma in Lewis rats. Clin Exp Immunol 1990;81:183–188.

152. Stoll G, Müller S, Schmidt B, et al. Localization of interferon-γ and Ia-antigen in T cell line-mediated experimental autoimmune encephalomyelitis. Am J Pathol 1993;142:1866–1875.

153. Massague J. The transforming growth factor-β family. Annu Rev Cell Biol 1990;6:597–632.

154. Zuber P, Kuppner MC, de Tribolet N. Transforming growth factor-β_2 down-regulates HLA-DR antigen expression on human malignant glioma cells. Eur J Immunol 1988;18:1623–1626.

155. Schluesener HJ. Transforming growth factors type $\beta1$ and $\beta2$ suppress rat astrocyte autoantigen presentation and antagonize hyperinduction of class II major histocompatibility complex antigen expression by interferon-γ and tumor necrosis factor-α. J Neuroimmunol 1990;27:41–47.

156. Toru-Delbauffe D, Baghdassarian-Chalaye D, Gavaret JM, Courtin F, Pomerance M, Pierce M. Effects of transforming growth factor β_1 on astroglial cells in culture. J Neurochem 1990;54:1056–1061.

157. Lindholm D, Castren E, Kiefer R, Zafra F, Thoenen H. Transforming growth factor-β_1 in the rat brain: increase after injury and inhibition of astrocyte proliferation. J Cell Biol 1992;117:395–400.

158. Morganti-Kossmann MC, Kossmann T, Brandes ME,

Mergenhagen SE, Wahl SM. Autocrine and paracrine regulation of astrocyte function by transforming growth factor-β. J Neuroimmunol 1992;39:163–174.

159. Yao J, Harvath L, Gilbert DL, Colton CA. Chemotaxis by a CNS macrophage, the microglia. J Neurosci Res 1990;27:36–42.

160. Benveniste EN, Kwoon JB, Chung WJ, Sampson J, Pandya K, Tang L-P. Differential modulation of astrocyte cytokine gene expression by TGF-β. J Immunol 1994 (in press).

161. Barnum SR, Jones JL. Transforming growth factor-β₁ inhibits inflammatory cytokine-induced C3 gene expression in astrocytes. J Immunol 1994;152:765–771.

162. McKinnon RD, Piras G, Ida JA Jr, Dubois-Dalcq M. A role for TGF-β in oligodendrocyte differentiation. J Cell Biol 1993;121:1397–1407.

163. da Cunha A, Vitkovic L. Transforming growth factor-beta (TGF-β₁) expression and regulation in rat cortical astrocytes. J Neuroimmunol 1992;36:157–169.

164. Johns LD, Sriram S. Experimental allergic encephalomyelitis: neutralizing antibody to TGF-β₁ enhances the clinical severity of the disease. J Neuroimmunol 1993;47:1–8.

165. Racke MK, Cannella B, Albert P, Sporn M. Raine CS, McFarlin DE. Evidence of endogenous regulatory function of transforming growth factor-β₁ in experimental allergic encephalomyelitis. Intervent Immunol 1992;4:615–620.

166. Santambrogio L, Hochwald GM, Saxena B, et al. Studies on the mechanisms by which transforming growth factor-β (TGF-β) protects against allergic encephalomyelitis: antagonism between TGF-β and tumor necrosis factor. J Immunol 1993;151:1116–1127.

167. Karpus WJ, Swanborg RH. CD4+ suppressor cells inhibit the function of effector cells of experimental autoimmune encephalomyelitis through a mechanism involving transforming growth factor-β₁. J Immunol 1991;146:1163–1168.

168. Miller A, Lider O, Roberts AB, Sporn MB, Weiner HL. Suppressor T cells generated by oral tolerization to myelin basic protein suppress both in vitro and in vivo immune responses by the release of transforming growth factor β after antigen-specific triggering. Proc Natl Acad Sci USA 1992;89:421–425.

169. Stevens DB, Swanborg RH. Cytokine-mediated regulation of tumor necrosis factor/lymphotoxin production by effector cells of autoimmune encephalomyelitis. J Immunol 1993;150:246A.

170. Bogdan C, Paik J, Vodovotz Y, Nathan C. Contrasting mechanisms for suppression of macrophage cytokine release by transforming growth factor-β and interleukin-10. J Biol Chem 1992;267:23301–23308.

171. Chao CC, Molitor TW, Hu S. Neuroprotective role of IL-4 against activated microglia. J Immunol 1993;151:1473–1481.

172. Gijbels K, Van Damme J, Proost P, Put W, Carton H, Billiau A. Interleukin 6 production in the central nervous system during experimental autoimmune encephalomyelitis. Eur J Immunol 1990;20:233–235.

173. Oppenheim JJ, Zachariae COC, Mukaida N, Matsushima K. Properties of the novel proinflammatory supergene "intercrine" cytokine family. Annu Rev Immunol 1991;9:617–648.

174. Ransohoff RM, Hamilton TA, Tani M, et al. Astrocyte expression of mRNA encoding cytokines IP-10 and JE/MCP-1 in experimental autoimmune encephalomyelitis. FASEB J 1993;7:592–600.

175. Hulkower K, Brosnan CF, Aquino DA, et al. Expression of CSF-1, c-fms, and MCP-1 in the central nervous system of rats with experimental allergic encephalomyelitis. J Immunol 1993;150:2525–2533.

176. Golde DW, Gasson JC. Hormones that stimulate the growth of blood cells. Sci Am 1988;62–70.

177. Brosnan CF, Bornstein MB, Bloom BR. The effects of macrophage depletion on the clinical and pathologic expression of experimental allergic encephalomyelitis. J Immunol 1981;126:614–620.

178. Huitinga I, van Rooijen N, de Groot CJA, Uitdehaag BMJ, Dijkstra CD. Suppression of experimental allergic encephalomyelitis in Lewis rats after elimination of macrophages. J Exp Med 1990;172:1025–1033.

179. Hao C, Guilbert LJ, Fedoroff S. Production of colony-stimulating factor-1 (CSF-1) by mouse astroglia in vitro. J Neurosci Res 1990;27:314–323.

180. Thery C, Hetier E, Evrard C, Mallat M. Expression of macrophage colony-stimulating factor gene in the mouse brain during development. J Neurosci Res 1990;26:129–133.

181. Campbell IL, Abraham CR, Masliah E, et al. Neurologic disease induced in transgenic mice by cerebral overexpression of interleukin 6. Proc Natl Acad Sci USA 1993;90:10061–10065.

182. Levy JA. Isolation of AIDS-associated retroviruses from cerebrospinal fluid and brain of patients with neurological symptoms. Lancet 1985;9:586–588.

183. Petito CK, Cho E-S, Lemann E, Navia BA, Price RW. Neuropathology of acquired immune deficiency syndrome (AIDS): an autopsy review. J Neuropathol Exp Neurol 1986;45:635–646.

184. Navia BA, Jordan BD, Price RW. The AIDS dementia complex. Ann Neurol 1986;19:517–524.

185. Shaw GM, Harper ME, Hahn BH, et al. HTLV-III infection in brains of children and adults with AIDS encephalopathy. Science 1985;227:177–182.

186. Ho DD, Rota RR, Schooley RT, et al. Isolation of HTLV-III from the cerebrospinal fluid and neural tissues of patients with neurologic syndromes related to the acquired immune deficiency syndrome. N Engl J Med 1985;313:1493–1497.

187. Resnick L, diMarzo-Veronese F, Schupbach J, et al. Intra-blood-brain barrier synthesis of HTLV-III-specific IgG in patients with neurologic symptoms associated with AIDS or AIDS-related complex. N Engl J Med 1985;313:1498–1504.

188. Eilbott DJ, Peress N, Burger H, et al. Human immunodeficiency virus type 1 in spinal cords of acquired immunodeficiency syndrome patients with myelopathy: expression and replication in macrophages. Proc Natl Acad Sci USA 1989;86:3337–3341.

189. Gabuzda DH, Ho DD, de la Monte SM, Hirsch MS, Rota TR, Sobel RA. Immunohistochemical identification of HTLV-III antigen in brains of patients with AIDS. Ann Neurol 1986;20:289–295.

190. Koenig S, Gendelman HE, Orenstein TM, et al. Detection of AIDS virus in macrophages in brain tissue from AIDS

patients with encephalopathy. Science 1986;233:1089–1093.

191. Wiley CA, Schreier RD, Nelson JA, Lampert PW, Oldstone MBA. Cellular localization of human immunodeficiency virus infection within the brains of acquired immune deficiency syndrome patients. Proc Natl Acad Sci USA 1986; 83:7089–7093.

192. Watkins BA, Dorn HH, Kelly WB, et al. Specific tropism of HIV-1 for microglial cells in primary human brain cultures. Science 1990;249:549–553.

193. Merrill JE, Chen ISY. HIV-1, macrophages, glial cells, and cytokines in AIDS nervous system disease. FASEB J 1991; 5:2391–2397.

194. Benveniste EN, Vidovic M, Panek RB, Norris JG, Reddy AT, Benos DJ. Interferon-γ induced astrocyte class II major histocompatibility complex gene expression is associated with both protein kinase C activation and Na$^+$ entry. J Biol Chem 1991;266:18119–18126.

195. Benos DJ, Hahn BH, Bubien JK, et al. HIV-1 gp120 alters ion transport in astrocytes: Implications for AIDS dementia complex. Proc Natl Acad Sci USA 1994;91:494–498.

196. Benos DJ, McPherson S, Hahn BH, Chaikin MA, Benveniste EN. Cytokines and HIV envelope glycoprotein gp120 stimulate Na$^+$/H$^+$ exchange in astrocytes. J Biol Chem 1994;269:13811–13816.

197. Fauci AS. Multifactorial nature of human immunodeficiency virus disease: implications for therapy. Science 1993;262:1011–1018.

198. Gallo P, Frei K, Rordorf C, Lazdins J, Tavolato B, Fontana A. Human immunodeficiency virus type 1 (HIV-1) infection of the central nervous system: an evaluation of cytokines in cerebrospinal fluid. J Neuroimmunol 1989; 23:109–116.

199. Tyor WR, Glass JD, Griffin JW, et al. Cytokine expression in the brain during the acquired immunodeficiency syndrome. Ann Neurol 1992;31:349–360.

200. Poli G, Kinter A, Justement JS, et al. Tumor necrosis factor α functions in an autocrine manner in the induction of human immunodeficiency virus expression. Proc Natl Acad Sci USA 1990;87:782–785.

201. Vitkovic L, Kalebic T, da Cunha A, Fauci AS. Astrocyte-conditioned medium stimulates HIV-1 expression in a chronically infected promonocyte clone. J Neuroimmunol 1990;30:153–160.

202. Peterson PK, Gekker G, Hu S, Schoolov Y, Balfour HH Jr, Chao CC. Microglial cell upregulation of HIV-1 expression in the chronically infected promonocytic cell line U1: the role of tumor necrosis factor-α. J Neuroimmunol 1992; 41:81–87.

203. Rosenberg ZF, Fauci AS. Immunopathogenesis of HIV infection. FASEB J 1991;5:2382–2390.

204. Bianco JA, Appelbaum FR, Nemunaitis J, et al. Phase I-II trial of pentoxifylline for the prevention of transplant-related toxicities following bone marrow transplantation. Blood 1991;78:1205–1211.

205. Holler E, Kolb HJ, Möller A, et al. Increased serum levels of tumor necrosis factor α precede major complications of bone marrow transplantation. Blood 1990;75:1011–1016.

206. Fazely F, Dezube BJ, Allen-Ryan J, Pardee AB, Ruprecht RM. Pentoxifylline (trental) decreases the replication of the human immunodeficiency virus type 1 in human peripheral blood mononuclear cells and in cultured T cells. Blood 1991;77:1653–1656.

207. Dezube BJ, Pardee AB, Chapman B, et al. Pentoxifylline decreases tumor necrosis factor expression and serum triglycerides in people with AIDS. J Acquir Immune Defic Syndr 1993;6:787–794.

208. Poli G, Bressler P, Kinter A, et al. Interleukin 6 induces human immunodeficiency virus expression in infected monocytic cells alone and in synergy with tumor necrosis factor α by transcriptional and post-transcriptional mechanisms. J Exp Med 1990;172:151–158.

209. Vitkovic L. Wood GP, Major EO, Fauci AS. Human astrocytes stimulate HIV-1 expression in a chronically infected promonocyte clone via interleukin-6. AIDS Res 1991;7: 723–727.

210. Wahl SM, Allen JB, Francis NM. Macrophage- and astrocyte-derived transforming growth factor β as a mediator of central nervous system dysfunction in acquired immune deficiency syndrome. J Exp Med 1991;173:981–991.

211. Kekow J, Wachsman W, McCutchan JA, Cronin M, Carson DA, Lotz M. Transforming growth factor-β and non-cytopathic mechanisms of immunodeficiency in human immunodeficiency virus infection. Proc Natl Acad Sci USA 1990;87:8321–8325.

212. Poli G, Kinter AL, Justement JS, Bressler P, Kehrl JH, Fauci AS. Transforming growth factor β suppresses human immunodeficiency virus expression and replication in infected cells of the monocyte/macrophage lineage. J Exp Med 1991;173:589–597.

213. Lazdins JK, Klimkait T, Woods-Cook K, et al. In vitro effect of transforming growth factor-β on progression of HIV-1 infection in primary mononuclear phagocytes. J Immunol 1991;147:1201–1207.

214. Koyanagi Y, O'Brien WA, Zhao JQ, Golde DW, Gasson JC, Chen ISY. Cytokines alter production of HIV-1 from primary mononuclear phagocytes. Science 1988;241:1673–1675.

CHAPTER 13

ROLE OF CYTOKINES IN RHEUMATOID ARTHRITIS

Elaine N. Unemori and Edward P. Amento

Joint inflammation and destruction in rheumatoid arthritis is the result of inappropriate activation of resident and inflammatory cells within synovial tissue. The consequence of an initiating and as yet unknown stimulus, the cascade of inflammatory processes, unlike those in normal wound healing, are chronic and self-perpetuating. Although cell-to-cell contact undoubtedly triggers cellular activation via integrin or class II antigen binding events, the chronic nature of inflammation in the rheumatoid joint is believed to be largely mediated by aberrant cytokine production, the abnormal expression of cytokine receptors, or the absence or diminution of counter-regulatory circuits.

Normally, synovial tissue is a single layer of synoviocytes composed of macrophage-like (type A) and fibroblast-like (type B) cells. In rheumatoid arthritis, the synovial tissue is multilayered and erosive. The synovial fluid is also altered due to the changes that occur within the synovium; it becomes a reservoir of inflammatory cells and their soluble products. It is also, however, a distinct compartment within the joint that does not necessarily mirror the cellular or cytokine profiles seen within the inflamed synovial tissue. The earliest events in synovitis are not characterized in detail because they usually occur prior to the development of any overt clinical signs. However, based on a few good studies on early joint changes (1,2), as well as evidence garnered from animal models, the following events are thought to contribute to the cellular changes and self-perpetuating nature of rheumatoid arthritis: (a) influx of inflammatory cells, such as lymphocytes and macrophages, into the synovium, and neutrophils into the synovial fluid; (b) hyperplasia and activation of resident synovial and inflammatory cells; and (c) degradation of underlying cartilage and bone by the synovial pannus.

These three events, although temporally and mechanistically overlapping, are considered herein as discrete processes. Cytokines have a major role in shaping each stage, and some cytokines may contribute to more than one process. The history of studies investigating the role of cytokines in rheumatoid arthritis is a long one, and many cytokines have been detected within the synovial tissue of patients with rheumatoid arthritis (Table 13–1). Conversely, many studies have demonstrated the ability of single cytokines, such as interleukin-1 (IL-1) (3), transforming growth factor β (TGF-β) (4,5), and tumor necrosis factor-α (TNF-α) (6), to induce synovial inflammation and arthropathy when introduced into the joint in experimental animals. However, in these animal models, no single cytokine causes a progressive synovitis consistent with all the clinical signs that define rheumatoid arthritis. It is likely, therefore, that these cytokines do not act alone, but in concert and in succession, to produce this chronic, hyperplastic, and erosive disease.

TABLE 13–1 CYTOKINES DETECTED IN SYNOVIAL TISSUE OR TISSUE CELLS*

Cytokine	References
IL-1β	(102)
IL-2	(131)
IL-6	(102)
IL-8	(71)
aFGF	(28)
GM-CSF	(102)
IFN-γ	(131)
MCP-1	(94,95)
RANTES	(69)
TGF-β	(102,103)
TNF-α	(102,130)
VEGF	(18)

*See text for abbreviations.

INFLUX OF INFLAMMATORY CELLS: CHEMOATTRACTION TO AND RETENTION WITHIN THE JOINT

Judging from the example of neutrophil homing, inflammatory cell recruitment into the synovium is likely to be an active, multistep process. Initial and transient interactions, mediated by members of the selectin family, are probably common, and they are only followed by productive binding in the presence of specific activating signals. This stable binding between trafficking cells and the endothelium is regulated by members of the integrin family (7). The activation signal that triggers this firm binding can arise from the expression of specific integrin cassettes that regulate high affinity binding to other cells on the surface of endothelial cells (7). In addition, the activation state of the cells moving by the endothelium also determines the rate and affinity of stable attachment (8). Finally, the presence of chemoattractant signals, such as provided by cytokines, that promotes extravasation of cells through the endothelium provides the impetus for the tissue-specific accumulation of lymphocytes, macrophages, and neutrophils observed in inflammatory conditions. Agents that increase the permeability of the endothelium also influence the ease of cell egress.

A cytokine recently detected in the rheumatoid joint that could have a major role in increasing inflammatory cell access to the synovium is vascular endothelial growth factor (VEGF) (9), also known as vascular permeability factor (10). VEGF is a highly conserved heparin-binding molecule that shares homology with the platelet-derived growth factor (PDGF) family of proteins. It promotes protein and fluid leakage from blood vessels (11), and it is, on a molar basis, approximately 5,000 times more potent than histamine in stimulating this leak (11). It is expressed by many kinds of tumors (12,13) and in the vicinity of proliferating endothelium in neovascularizing normal tissues (14,15). Expression of VEGF and its receptor, an fms-like tyrosine kinase (16), is developmentally regulated in many tissues and organs (15,17). Recently, VEGF was localized to tissue and subsynovial macrophages in rheumatoid synovium, and it is also secreted by synovial tissue explants in culture (18). High concentrations of VEGF are also found in rheumatoid synovial fluid (386 ng/mL), in contrast to osteoarthritis synovial fluid (<0.8 ng/mL).

The vascular leakiness promoted by VEGF may increase passage of low molecular weight chemotaxins across the endothelial barrier, thus facilitating access to trafficking inflammatory cells. The existence of "leaky" vessels within the rheumatoid joint is suggested by the elevated concentration of proteins within rheumatoid synovial fluid compared with plasma (19). VEGF is also a potent mitogen for endothelial cells; it stimulates endothelial cell proliferation in the picomolar range, depending on the specific endothelial cell target. Although a number of other polypeptide factors, including fibroblast growth factor (FGF) (20), epidermal growth factor (EGF), and TGF-α (21), are also mitogenic for endothelial cells, only VEGF is believed to be specific for this cell type. EGF (22) and PDGF (23) have been shown to induce VEGF expression in certain cells. Expression of VEGF activity can confer the ability to expand (24) or a growth advantage (25) to tissues or tumors.

In the rheumatoid synovium, VEGF may contribute to the extensive neovasculature central to its pathogenesis. VEGF expression is induced in cell lines by culture under hypoxic conditions in vitro, while VEGF transcripts are detected in tumors in vivo in cells adjacent to necrotic areas, presumably where conditions are most hypoxic (26). The rheumatoid synovium contains pockets of hypoxia (27); VEGF expression in the synovium, possibly compensatory in nature, may then exacerbate inflammation by providing the means for further inflammatory cell ingress into the tissue. Acidic FGF (aFGF), another potent endothelial mitogen, is also present in stromal fibroblasts, endothelial cells, and inflammatory cells of rheumatoid synovial tissue (28).

IL-1 may also increase vascular permeability (29), although this activity may be mediated via the induction of platelet-activating factor (30), because the increase in permeability can be inhibited in part by administration of platelet-activating factor receptor antagonist (31). IL-2 also increases vascular permeability because it causes a vascular leak syndrome when administered intravenously (32). This phenomenon may be mediated, at least in part, by natural killer cells (33). The cytokine mediator of the leak, if there is one, is currently unidentified.

Lymphocyte ingress

Because the etiological agent in rheumatoid arthritis is unknown, the driving force underlying lymphocyte accumulation within the synovium is also unclear. There is indisputable evidence, however, that genetic susceptibility has a major role in predisposing individuals to the development of rheumatoid arthritis (34); therefore, it is likely that lymphocytic accumulation within the synovium is associated in some way to expression of specific human leukocyte antigen-DR (HLA-DR) sequences.

Within the synovium, T lymphocytes predominate over B lymphocytes (35), and activated lymphocytes are over-represented compared with those in the blood (36–38). Early descriptive studies demonstrate a discrete organization of lymphoid tissue within the synovial membrane (1). A large perivascular accumulation of lymphocytes is observed, adjacent to which are transitional areas composed of lymphocytes, blast cells, and macrophages. T-lymphocyte populations in the perivascular areas are composed of both activated and non-activated T cells, defined by their cell surface expression of the isoforms of the leukocyte common antigen, CD45 (37). In contrast, lymphocytes within the transitional areas are predominantly of the CD45RO+ memory phenotype (37). These studies suggest that lymphocytes may become activated once they have migrated into the deeper areas of the synovium. There is also mounting evidence that specific subsets of T lymphocytes, defined by their T-cell antigen receptor phenotype, are over-represented within the synovium (39,40). Lymphocyte immigration probably occurs by diapedesis via high endothelial venules in blood vessels within the synovium (41,42). Accumulation of these infiltrating lymphocytes is believed to be among the first events in rheumatoid synovitis (2), and it may be responsible for initiating the self-perpetuating cascade of events that eventually culminates in degenerative joint disease.

Several cytokines, when introduced in purified or recombinant form in various sites in vivo, can induce lymphocytic accumulation at the site of injection, therefore presumably having accomplished the necessary aforementioned steps. These cytokines include intra-articular TGF-β (4), intradermal IL-8 (43), intra-articular (6) or intradermal (44) TNF-α, intradermal IFN-α (44) or IFN-γ (45), and intradermal RANTES (Regulated on Activation, Normal T Expressed and Secreted) (46). However, many of these cytokines probably act through the induction of other cytokines in vivo, because only a subset can direct lymphocyte adhesion to endothelial cells or chemoattraction in vitro.

Cytokines that can increase lymphocyte-endothelial cell adhesiveness in vitro include TNF-α (47), IL-4 (48,49), IFN-γ (47,50), IL-1 (47,50), IL-8 (43), macrophage inflammatory protein-1β (MIP-1β) (51), and interferon-inducible protein-10 (IP-10) (52). Lymphocyte adhesion to endothelial cells is regulated by selectins and integrins on their cell surfaces. E and P selectins on the endothelium can bind to a subset of lymphocytes, and expression of the former is up-regulated by IL-1, TNF, and lipopolysaccharide (LPS). Their binding to the lymphocyte surface involves carbohydrate moieties, including sialyl Lewis x (sLe^x). The integrins, intercellular adhesion molecule-1 (ICAM-1) and ICAM-2 and vascular cell adhesion molecule (VCAM), on the endothelial cell surface are modulated by IL-1, TNF-α, IFN-γ, and IL-4 in specific patterns. Their ligands on the lymphocyte surface include CD11a/CD18 (LFA-1) and VLA-4. In addition, activation of T cells by stimulation with antigen in the context of class II molecules causes increased adhesiveness of CD11a/CD18. These selectins and integrins and their developmental expression on both lymphocytes and endothelial cells have been extensively reviewed (53–55). VLA-1, VLA-4 (56), and LFA-1 (57) expression by T cells, and ICAM-1, endothelial leukocyte adhesion molecule (ELAM-1), and VCAM-1 expression by endothelial and other cells are up-regulated in the rheumatoid synovium (58,59). A soluble form of the lymphocyte adhesion molecule, CD44, which may be important in lymphocyte binding to high endothelial venules, has been detected in synovial fluid (60). Moreover, it is possible that the binding of activated T cells expressing particular integrins to extracellular matrix proteins may then have a role in modulating the profile of cytokines expressed by these cells (61). For example, CD4+ peripheral blood T cells binding to fibronectin, mediated by VLA-5, results in enhanced IL-2 gene expression (62).

A number of cytokines are chemotactic for lymphocytes in vitro. Because the chemokine family of cytokines are part of an emerging cytokine literature, they and their potential roles in rheumatoid arthritis are emphasized herein. The chemokine or platelet factor 4 family is composed of small related cytokines that have a broad range of immunoregulatory activities (63–65), and they probably have important roles in many chronic inflammatory states, including rheumatoid arthritis. The family has two branches, which are defined by the relative positions of the first two of their four conserved cysteines. The "C-X-C" branch has an intervening amino acid between the first two cysteines, and it includes IL-8, melanoma growth stimulatory activity (MGSA), and IP-10 as its members. The first two cysteines in the "C-C" chemokines are directly adjacent; RANTES, monocyte chemotactic protein (MCP-1–MCP-3), and MIP-1α and MIP-1β are members of this branch of this family. RANTES (66), IL-8 (43), MIP-1α and MIP-1β (67,68), and IP-10 (52) can directly cause chemotaxis of lymphocytes in vitro, and they may therefore contribute to active lymphocyte egress from the circulation into the synovium.

RANTES can stimulate in vitro the chemotaxis of T lymphocytes of the memory phenotype, which are distinguishable from naive T cells by cell surface expression of the CD45 (66). Specifically, helper lymphocytes (CD4+) of the CD45RO+ phenotype are selectively attracted by RANTES, whereas other T cells are not. Recently, RANTES messenger RNA (mRNA) was localized by in situ hybridization to synovial lining cells in patients with rheumatoid arthritis (69). The cellular source of RANTES could be T cells; however, unlike transcripts for other members of the C-C chemokine family, mRNA for RANTES in vitro is most highly expressed in unactivated T cells with declining levels postantigen stimulation (66). It has also been shown, however, that RANTES mRNA is inducible in synovial fibroblasts by other inflammatory cytokines, such as TNF-α and IL-1β (70). These studies suggest that RANTES may participate in the recruitment of activated memory T cells into the synovium, which may be of particular significance because T cells found in the synovial lining are largely of the CD4+ phenotype with a significant CD45RO+ component (37).

Other members of the C-C branch of the chemokine family, MIP-1α and MIP-1β, are also chemoattractants for T lymphocytes, but their presence in the rheumatoid synovium has not been demonstrated. MIP-1β, although 70% identical to MIP-1α in amino acid sequence, attracts predominantly activated CD4+ lymphocytes (67,68), whereas MIP-1α is capable of stimulating migration of a broader subpopulation of cells (i.e., CD8+ T cells, B cells, and, at higher concentrations, CD4+ T cells). MIP-1β, but not RANTES or MGSA, can also stimulate T-lymphocyte binding to VCAM (51). MIP-1β is present on lymph node endothelial cell surfaces, including some with high endothelial venule morphology (51). Soluble MIP-1β is also capable of immobilization on cell surfaces via CD44, a proteoglycan. This "presentation" of MIP-1β to T cells is hypothesized to stimulate the adhesion of passing lymphocytes.

IL-8 can cause chemotaxis of T cells in vitro at picomolar concentrations 2 to 20 times less than is required to stimulate neutrophil chemoattraction (43). CD4+ and CD8+ cells exhibit equivalent chemotactic responses, but greater proportions of polyclonally activated than resting T cells are reportedly stimulated (64). IL-8 injection subcutaneously in rat ears results in a predominantly lymphocytic infiltrate at low doses (10 ng) and a neutrophil influx at higher doses (100 ng) (43). Monocytes are a minor component under both conditions. IL-8 is predominantly localized within macrophages in the synovial lining in rheumatoid arthritis (71), and it is spontaneously produced by synovial fluid mononuclear cells following isolation in vitro (72,73). It is also inducible in vitro in

fibroblasts by TNF-α and IL-1β (71,74,75) and in macrophages by LPS and IL-1 (76). IL-8 and RANTES, although both members of the chemokine family, probably bind to different cellular receptors on lymphocytes (77–80).

IP-10 is a relatively recent entrant into the C-X-C branch of the chemokine family; it also demonstrates T lymphocyte chemoattractant activity. IP-10, unlike all other known members of the C-X-C branch, is only weakly stimulatory for neutrophil movement (52). It can, however, similar to RANTES, cause directed migration of activated CD4+ T cells of the CD45RO+ memory phenotype. Both RANTES and IP-10 are also capable of stimulating the adhesion of activated T cells to IL-1–treated endothelial cell monolayers (52). The presence of IP-10 in rheumatoid synovial tissue has not yet been reported; however, it has been detected at sites of delayed–type hypersensitivity responses (81).

The biochemical basis for the incompletely overlapping properties of members of the chemokine family are currently being elucidated (82). Two receptors that bind the C-X-C chemokines exclusively with high affinity have been described (78,79). The IL-8RA receptor binds IL-8, whereas IL-8RB binds IL-8, MGSA, and neutrophil-activating protein-2 (NAP-2) (79,80). The IL-8RA receptor appears to be expressed only in neutrophils (78), whereas the IL-8RB receptor has a wider distribution; it is detectable in the Jurkat T-cell line, neutrophils, monocytes, and melanoma-cell lines (82). One C-C chemokine receptor that binds MIP-1α and RANTES has been cloned thus far (77,83). Competitive inhibition experiments using various C-C chemokines as ligands suggest the existence of several more receptors not yet discovered (84). The three chemokine receptors are G-protein–linked, and they contain seven transmembrane domains and cause an intracellular calcium flux in response to ligand binding. A fourth receptor, which binds both C-X-C and C-C chemokines with high affinity (85,86), has recently been cloned. However, unlike the other chemokine receptors, it is a nine transmembrane spanning molecule, and it is also believed to be identical to the Duffy antigen, the binding site for the malaria parasite on the red blood cell. This receptor is thought not to be present on lymphocytes (87). Its role in regulating chemokine function is currently being tested; it may function as a sink for chemokines in the circulation (87).

Recruitment of monocytes/macrophages

Cells of the monocyte/macrophage lineage are normal residents of the synovium; they constitute approximately 20 to 30% of the synoviocytes (36). In rheumatoid arthritis, an impressive increase in the number of macrophages contributes to the hypercellularity observed in the synovium. Because they are normally replaced every 20 weeks

(88), it is clear that there is a massive influx of cells of the macrophage lineage into the site.

As with other cell types, macrophage influx into the synovium is probably influenced by the expression of integrins. The Mac-1 antigen, which is expressed on mononuclear phagocytes, neutrophils, and natural killer cells, is critical to adhesion and to phagocytosis. Mac-1 exists in noncovalent association with another glycoprotein member of the integrin superfamily, the β-chain. Together the α- and β-chain heterodimer is designated CD11/CD18. The endothelial ligands for CD11/CD18 are ICAM-1 and ICAM-2, and they are inducible in endothelial cells by inflammatory cytokines, such as IL-1 and TNF-α. These molecules and their significance in immune function have been extensively reviewed (89,90).

Several cytokines, particularly those of the chemokine family, are chemotactic for monocytes. MCP-1, a member of the C-C branch of the chemokine family, is a potent chemoattractant for monocytes, but not neutrophils, in vitro (91,92). Monocytes bind MCP-1 with high affinity, and they possess approximately 1,700 binding sites per cell (93). Injection of MCP-1 into the ears of rabbits causes a monocytic infiltration into the site 6 to 16 hours later (91). In rheumatoid arthritis, MCP-1 expression has been localized to synovial lining cells by immunohistochemistry (94) and by in situ hybridization for mRNA (95). In the former study, a large percentage of rheumatoid arthritic synovial lining cells ($76 \pm 6\%$) were positive for MCP-1 staining; the tissue macrophage was identified as the major source of this chemokine. When the macrophages were isolated by enzymatic digestion of synovial tissue, they were shown to constitutively express MCP-1 protein. Peripheral blood monocytes, as well as those from synovial fluid, do not express MCP-1 basally but are inducible for its expression by IL-1 (72). Synovial fibroblasts also generally did not express MCP-1 protein or mRNA constitutively, but they were stimulated for their expression by TNF-α or IL-1β (74,94). Human articular chondrocytes also express MCP-1 mRNA in response to IL-1, TNF-α, LPS, PDGF, and TGF-β (96).

RANTES has also demonstrated monocyte chemoattractant properties (46,66), albeit at 200-fold higher concentrations than that required for lymphocyte chemotaxis (66). The biological basis for the MCP-1–RANTES similarity in monocyte chemoattraction may be due at least in part to their binding to a common cellular receptor (77), although the existence of at least one other C-C chemokine receptor on monocytes and monocyte-like cells has been suggested (46,84). Two other chemokines closely related to MCP-1, MCP-2, and MCP-3, were recently isolated from a human osteosarcoma line; they are also chemotactic for monocytes in vitro, and they cause a monocytic infiltrate in vivo (97). Their potential roles in rheumatoid arthritis have yet to be elucidated.

IL-4 can elicit a monocytic infiltrate in vivo (98), but it has no ability to cause monocyte chemotaxis in vitro. Although IL-4 inhibits the induction of IL-8 in human monocytes stimulated with IL-1, TNF, and LPS (99), it induces synthesis and secretion of MCP-1 in endothelial cells in vitro (100). Thus, MCP-1 may contribute to the monocyte chemoattractant ability of IL-4 observed in vivo.

Two isoforms of TGF-β, TGF-$β_1$ and TGF-$β_2$, have been shown to cause monocyte chemotaxis in vitro at femtomolar concentrations (4,101). TGF-β injected intraarticularly in rats can cause synovial inflammation of rapid onset, including a large activated (Ia+) monocyte component. The increase in monocyte numbers, edema, and the synovial fibroblast hyperplasia apparent 2 to 3 days after injection of TGF-β declined within several days. No erosion of cartilage is seen. The ability of TGF-β to induce these changes is likely due to its ability to stimulate expression of many other cytokines, including TNF-α, PDGF-B, TGF-α, FGF, IL-1, and TGF-β in monocytes (101). TGF-β mRNA (102), as well as TGF-β protein (103), have been detected in cells within the rheumatoid synovium. To date, five isoforms of TGF-β have been described (104,105).

TGF-β binds to cell surfaces via two high affinity receptors, type I and II receptors, as well as a type III receptor of slightly lower affinity. TGF-β signals through a heteromeric complex of the types I and II receptors (106). The type II receptor is required for TGF-β binding to the type I receptor, and its serine-threonine kinase activity is required for signaling by the complex (107). The types I and II receptors have distinct affinities for each of the TGF-β isoforms (108). The type III receptor, also called betaglycan, is also an integral membrane protein, but it is heavily modified by glycosaminoglycan groups (109). It has equal affinities for the TGF-β isoforms (108). Many potential functions have been assigned to betaglycan, including capture and presentation of TGF-β to the other signaling receptors, depletion of TGF-β from the microenvironment, and localization and presentation of basic fibroblast growth factor (bFGF) via its heparin sulfate chains (110). Betaglycan also exists in soluble form, although its function is unclear (111).

In addition to cytokines, other monocyte chemoattractants, such as activated components of complement (C5a) and neutrophil products (leukotriene B4), as well as fragments of connective tissue molecules (elastin and fibronectin), undoubtedly contribute to macrophage recruitment into synovial tissue (112).

Neutrophil influx

Neutrophils in the rheumatoid joint are found predominantly in the synovial fluid; they are relatively rare within the synovial lining (113). Their products, particularly of the icosanoid family, are responsible for the joint pain and swelling associated with the disease. Neutrophil immigration into the rheumatoid joint is probably governed by the same rules that regulate homing into other inflammatory sites. Therefore, selectin and integrin molecule expression on neutrophils and their cognate receptors of endothelium are important in determining the rate and affinity of neutrophil retention within the vasculature of the synovium. E-selectin on endothelial cells binds neutrophils, and it is induced by treatment with IL-1, TNF-α, or LPS. Like other selectins, E-selectin binds to carbohydrate moieties, including sLe^x, on the neutrophil surface. The integrin, ICAM-1, is also modulated by cell exposure to IL-1 and TNF-α on the endothelial cell surface, whereas ICAM-1 is constitutively expressed. These integrins bind to their cognate ligands, including CD11/CD18, on the neutrophil surface. These areas have been described in excellent review articles (54,55,89,90). Once at the synovium, neutrophil extravasation is driven by chemoattractants present within synovial tissue. Presumably, neutrophils then migrate into the synovial fluid by chemotaxing toward gradients of cytokines and other chemotactic agents present in that space.

IL-8 and other members of the C-X-C branch of the chemokine family can influence one of the initial phases of neutrophil accumulation in the synovial fluid (i.e., adhesion to the endothelium). IL-8, MGSA, and NAP-2 enhance the adhesiveness of neutrophils to endothelial cells by inducing expression of CD11b/CD18 on the surface of neutrophils (114). This heterodimeric integrin complex regulates not only intercellular binding, but also may be required for transendothelial migration of neutrophils, even when initial binding occurs independently (53). In this regard, IL-8 also promotes neutrophil binding to subendothelial matrix proteins (115). The endothelial ligand for CD11/CD18, ICAM-1, and ICAM-2 are up-regulated by many cytokines present at sites of inflammation, including IL-1 and TNF-α, which then strengthen neutrophil-endothelial cell adhesiveness.

IL-8 and other C-X-C chemokines are potent stimulators of neutrophil chemotaxis in vitro; they are therefore good candidates for stimulators of neutrophil accumulation within the synovial fluid. Human neutrophils bind IL-8 via both IL-8RA and IL-8RB receptors (78,79). IL-8 treatment is followed by a rapid (<2 seconds) increase in cytosolic free calcium concentrations (116), followed by down-regulation and internalization (within 10 minutes) of the IL-8 receptors (117). C5a and formylated Met-Leu-Phe (fMLP), noncytokine chemoattractants for neutrophils, also mediate the directional migration of these cells via specific G-protein–linked seven-transmembrane spanning receptors (82), suggesting a signaling pathway common among these chemoattractants. In addition to migration, IL-8 can also elicit a respiratory burst and actin polymerization within neutrophils (64). IL-8 is found at relatively high concentrations in the synovial fluid (approximately 14 ng/mL) (71), and approximately 40% of the neutrophil chemotactic activity in fluid is inhibitable with neutralizing antibody to IL-8 (71). Some studies have also found a direct correlation between IL-8 and the number of neutrophils in synovial fluid (118).

Injection of IL-8 into joint space of rabbits (≥100 ng/mL) elicits a temporary synovitis. Marked and rapid neutrophil infiltration is present even 1 hour after injection; it peaks at 4 hours and then disappears by 24 hours. Neutrophils constitute 98% of the infiltrating cells. At 24 hours, the synovial lining appears multilayered, but by 48 hours, the synovium is indistinguishable from that seen in untreated animals. No cartilage destruction is observed. These findings suggest that the continuous presence of IL-8 is necessary for maintenance of neutrophil numbers within the synovial fluid. Other members of the C-X-C chemokine family, such as MGSA and MIP-2, are also potent neutrophil chemoattractants; to date, their presence within synovial tissue or fluid has not been documented.

Granulocyte-macrophage colony-stimulatory factor (GM-CSF) is a cytokine originally identified as a factor that inhibits the migration of peripheral blood neutrophils in vitro (119). It is found in the synovial fluid (120), and it may activate neutrophils (121) and retain them at sites of inflammation. Potential sources within the rheumatoid joint are activated macrophages (122) and fibroblasts, which synthesize GM-CSF in response to IL-1 stimulation (123). IL-1 can promote the survival of neutrophils by inhibiting death by apoptosis (124). IL-1 is present in synovial fluid from patients with rheumatoid arthritis (125,126), and it may function this way. The effect of IL-1 is mediated by binding to its receptor, IL-1RI, an 80 kd transmembrane protein that is present on fibroblasts, lymphocytes, and neutrophils (127). It was recently shown that IL-4 can completely abolish the effect of IL-1 via induction of a second IL-1–binding receptor, IL-1RII (124). This receptor, which is 68 kd and has a short cytoplasmic tail, is released in soluble form and acts as a molecular decoy, or sink, for IL-1. Therefore, IL-4 can inhibit the effect of IL-1 by decreasing its bioavailability. Studies demonstrating the existence of IL-4 within synovial fluid have given conflicting results (128,129).

SYNOVIAL HYPERPLASIA

Resident as well as infiltrating cells of the rheumatoid synovium undergo cell division in the generation of a multilayered synovial pannus. Undoubtedly, the sheer increase in numbers of cells contributes to the later degradative stages of the disease. The secreted products, including cytokines, of activated lymphocytes, macrophages, and fibroblasts contribute in large part to perpetuation of the proliferative synovial pannus.

Expansion of T-lymphocyte populations in the synovial lining: proliferation and activation

Once the T lymphocytes within the synovium are activated, either by a binding event between their receptor complex and its cognate antigen in the context of class II molecules, or by a superantigen-mediated mechanism, the lymphocytes are committed to proliferating in the presence of further cytokine signals. IL-2 and IL-2 receptor expression occurs in response to signals provided by cytokines, and the autocrine action of IL-2 on the expression of newly expressed high affinity receptors leads to DNA synthesis, as well as expression of transferrin receptors on T cells. Several known T-lymphocyte mitogens, including IL-1 (102), TNF (102,130), IFN (131), IL-2 (131), and IL-6 (102), are present within the rheumatoid synovial lining.

IL-2 and IL-2 receptor mRNA are detectable within rheumatoid synovial tissue (131), and both are expressed constitutively in vitro by mononuclear cells derived from synovial membranes, as well as synovial fluid (132). This finding is in contrast to unstimulated peripheral blood mononuclear cells, which do not express IL-2 or its receptor without exogenous stimulation. Others have found IL-2 to be absent from synovial fluid (133), although this finding may be of little consequence to activated T cells within the synovial membrane. The high affinity IL-2 receptor is a heterotrimer of α, β, and γ receptor subunits (134), and it has a dissociation constant of approximately 10 pmol/L. Because of this high affinity, as well as the ability of IL-2 to synergize with other cytokines, such as IL-1, in stimulating the proliferation of T cells, relatively low molar quantities present within synovial tissue may nonetheless be biologically significant. IL-2 stimulation of T cells can induce expression of other cytokines, such as IL-3, IL-4 (135), IL-5 (136), IL-6, IL-7, GM-CSF, TNF-α, and TNF-β, TGF-β, and IFN-γ (137). Many of these cytokines have other cell types as primary targets, although IL-4, IL-6, and TGF-β will be discussed in the context of T cells here.

IL-1 has long been known as a comitogen for T lymphocytes, and it requires an additional signal provided by a growth factor or a mitogen for proliferation (138). Its presence within the synovium may therefore provide a competence factor necessary for entry into the cell cycle (139) for some T cells. IL-1 stimulation is associated with increased expression of IL-2 and high affinity IL-2 receptors in T cells and T-cell lines, and the presence of both IL-1 and IL-2 synergize to stimulate thymocyte proliferation (140). More recently, it has been suggested that only a particular subset of T-helper lymphocytes, Th2 cells, respond to IL-1 by proliferating, whereas Th1 lymphocytes are refractory (141,142). In agreement, Th2 cells bear IL-1 receptors, whereas Th1 cells do not (143). These Th1 and Th2 subsets are defined in part by their ability to synthesize and secrete IL-2 and IL-4, respectively. Th2 cells, however, are apparently not induced to express higher levels of IL-4 or IL-4 receptor in response to IL-1 (141), suggesting the existence of another mechanism for the proliferative signal.

IL-1 is detectable in the rheumatoid synovium, predominantly as the beta isoform in macrophages (102). IL-1α, the product of a separate gene, has properties largely overlapping with those of IL-1β, but it does not predominate in the synovium. Macrophages freshly isolated from the rheumatoid synovium express IL-1β (102), and many studies have demonstrated measurable levels of IL-1 in the synovial fluid (125,126). The possible existence of membrane-associated forms of IL-1 is relevant, because cell contact between T lymphocytes and other cell types undoubtedly occurs within synovial tissue. Despite the lack of a signal sequence or specific amino acid sequences consistent with the existence of a transmembrane domain in IL-1, its membrane association has been suggested via two alternative mechanisms for association. Recent studies indicating that both IL-1α and IL-1β are myristoylated in human monocytes (144) and that they can also be labeled with $D(^{14}C)$mannose (145), suggest the possibility of stimulation of T cells via membrane-bound IL-1 on monocyte cell surfaces. This mechanism could provide continuous focal stimulation of neighboring T lymphocytes by monocytes within the synovium. Stimulation of neighboring cells by a membrane-bound cytokine has recently been shown for TGF-α (146).

Although IL-6 is mainly regarded as a stimulator of B-cell differentiation, it functions as a comitogen for T cells and it enhances their proliferation in synergy with IL-1 and TNF-α (147). Some of this activity is probably due to the ability of IL-6 to induce IL-2 and its receptor in T cells (148). IL-6 is measurable in relatively high levels in synovial fluid (5,288 U/mL), compared with that measured in osteoarthritis fluid (490 U/mL), and it is also found in the serum of patients with rheumatoid arthritis (149). IL-6 is also secreted spontaneously by synoviocytes from patients with rheumatoid arthritis in culture, but the effect is also seen in normal dermal fibroblasts and it is dependent on the presence of serum during culture (150). Therefore, the significance of this finding in the context of IL-6 up-regulation in rheumatoid arthritis is unclear. However, IL-6 mRNA is present in a significant percentage (19%) of synovial tissue cells, presumably fibroblasts (a nonmacrophage, non-T-cell population) (102). Therefore, colocalization of these cytokines (i.e., IL-6, IL-1, and TNF-α) within the rheumatoid synovium may be significant in the context of T-cell stimulation within this tissue. IL-6 receptors are present on a variety of cell types, including resting normal T lymphocytes (151).

TNF-α and lymphotoxin (LT) are products of closely

related genes, and they are predominantly expressed by macrophages and lymphocytes, respectively (152). TNF-α and LT have a similar spectrum of activities and they bind the same cellular receptors. Two binding sites for these cytokines have been identified, a 55 kd (p55) and 75 kd (p75) membrane protein (153–155). Both TNF and LT exist in soluble form as homotrimers (156). Recent studies suggested that TNF-α can also exist in association with the plasma membrane (157). The effects of TNF-α on T lymphocytes include induction of TNF receptors (158), stimulation of expression of the high affinity IL-2 receptor, and increased proliferation (159). Both TNF-α and LT appear to induce proliferation of T lymphocytes by binding to p75 (160). Transcripts of TNF-α are detectable within rheumatoid synovial tissue (102); TNF-α protein is localized within the synovial lining, predominantly in monocytes (CD11b, CD14+), as well as some T cells (CD3+) (130), and it is also found in synovial fluid (161). p75 and p55 TNF receptors have been found ubiquitously (162) or localized to CD3+ lymphocytes (163) within the synovial tissue.

IL-4 can directly stimulate proliferation of some T-cell lines (164) or act as a comitogen for resting T cells (165). Conflicting data regarding the abundance of IL-4 in rheumatoid synovial fluid exist (128,129); it has not been localized in synovial tissue.

IFN-γ is a product of activated lymphocytes (137), principally of the Th1 subset of CD4+ helper cells in mice (164). Similar to other cytokine genes, transcripts for IFN-γ are unstable, and regulation of gene expression occurs principally at the level of transcription (166). IFN-γ binds as a dimer to a species-specific glycoprotein receptor that is fairly ubiquitous and that is believed to require a currently unidentified accessory protein for signal transduction (167). Genes activated by IFN-γ may share a common nucleotide consensus sequence that requires binding of an IFN-γ–activated transcriptional factor for activity (168).

IFN-γ is the major cytokine inducer of class II antigens on the surface of many cell types (169), whereas the type I interferons, IFN-α and IFN-β, are relatively weak inducers of Ia. Class II molecules are usually expressed on monocytes, B cells, and activated T cells, but they are inducible in many or all cell types. The presence of class II molecules on the cell surface allows these cells to present antigen to appropriate T cells. IFN-γ, but not IL-1β, IL-2, M-CSF, IL-6, TNF-α, GM-CSF, EGE, or bFGF (170–172), can induce HLA-DR expressed on cultured synovial fibroblasts. Class II molecules are up-regulated in synovial tissue and fluid T cells (38), indicating their activated state, but they are also present on the surface of type B or fibroblast-like synovial cells. IFN-γ is present within the rheumatoid synovial lining (131), and IFN-γ transcripts are present in synovial fluid mononuclear cells (61), although the percentage of cells expressing it at any given

time may be small (102). IFN-γ, however, causes long-lived expression of class II antigens by synovial cells, so that transient cytokine exposure may be sufficient for a significant class II molecule expression (170).

The effect of IFN-γ on class II antigen expression on synoviocytes is counteracted by IL-1 (173) and TNF-α (171) in vitro. Time course experiments demonstrate that class II expression is blocked only when IL-1 or TNF-α is added simultaneously with IFN-γ or within the first 24 hours of treatment. These data indicate the complex interplay of cytokine effects on one aspect of synoviocyte phenotype, and they may in part explain the heterogeneity in class II expression that exists within cells of the synovium.

TGF-β is an important suppressor of many lymphocyte functions, including proliferation. TGF-β_1 and TGF-β_2 have been identified in hemopoietic cells (174). Certain lymphocytes may express only types I and II receptors (175). TGF-β inhibits IL-2–dependent T-cell proliferation, and it partially inhibits IL-2–induced IL-2 and transferrin receptor expression (176). TGF-β also inhibits IL-1 receptor expression on lymphoid cell lines (177). PHA-activated T cells have a six-fold greater number of high affinity binding sites for TGF-β, they express elevated levels of TGF-β mRNA, and they secrete higher amounts of TGF-β protein than resting cells. Rheumatoid arthritis synovial fluid contains active and latent TGF-β (178,179), which suppresses CD4+ T-cell proliferation more completely than CD8+ cells, and it may be responsible for the relative reduction in CD4+ T cells in the synovial fluid (180,181).

Fibroblast mitogens

Isolated synovial tissue explants and isolated mononuclear cells from synovial tissue or fluid spontaneously secrete factors capable of stimulating fibroblast proliferation (182). Several cytokines are capable of stimulating fibroblast proliferation.

FGF, both acidic and basic, are members of the heparin-binding growth factor family, which also includes the oncogene int-2 and keratinocyte growth factor (183,184). There are five high affinity FGF receptors characterized to date; fibroblasts are likely to express at least FGF-R_1 and FGF-R_2 (185). FGF binding to its receptor is immediately followed by receptor dimerization, tyrosine kinase activity, and autophosphorylation (184). FGF can also bind to cell surfaces with low affinity through heparin sulfate proteoglycan molecules (186). These sites may function to potentiate binding to high affinity sites (187). Acidic FGF is detectable within the synovial lining in fibroblasts, endothelial cells, and inflammatory cells of patients with rheumatoid arthritis (28); the extent of anti-aFGF immunostaining correlates with the degree of mononuclear cell infiltration. Rheumatoid synovial fibroblasts constitutively express FGF after isolation in culture (188).

PDGF is a major mitogen in serum for fibroblasts and other cell types (189). PDGF is a dimer of two similar polypeptides, A and B, that can dimerize as AA, AB, and BB forms. Two cellular receptors, α and β, have been identified. The β receptor binds PDGF-BB with high affinity, the AB form with 10 times lower affinity, and it does not bind the AA form. The α receptor binds all three forms with high affinity (190). Human fibroblasts, which contain three- to four-fold more β than α receptors on their surfaces, respond to PDGF-AB and BB with proliferation, whereas PDGF-AA is only a weak mitogen (190). However, both α and β types are capable of transducing the mitogenic signal. Exposure of fibroblasts to PDGF results in rapid, transient expression of the gene encoding the PDGF-A chain and secretion of PDGF-AA (191).

PDGF is a progression factor that stimulates the movement of cells from G0 into S (139). The proto-oncogenes, cfos and cmyc, are up-regulated within 30 minutes and 8 hours of PDGF exposure, respectively (191). PDGF binding sites are present on connective tissue cells in rheumatoid synovial tissue (31). When tested for the ability to induce proliferation of cultured synovial fibroblasts, PDGF stimulated a multifold increase in thymidine incorporation (192). Rheumatoid synovial fluid was found to support cell proliferation, and 68% of this effect was blocked by the addition of neutralizing antibody to PDGF.

IL-1 can also cause fibroblast proliferation if prostaglandin synthesis is inhibited (193), although on a molar basis it is less potent than PDGF or FGF. It is also possible that IL-1 may mediate its proliferative effect via induction of PDGF-AA (194). Rheumatoid synovial fibroblasts synthesize and secrete IL-1β constitutively in culture (188).

Macrophage activation

Because of their ability to produce many inflammatory cytokines, their migratory nature, and the presence of many of their products within the joint of rheumatoid arthritis patients, macrophages are believed to have a major role in amplifying and maintaining the chronic inflammatory state of the synovial joint. Macrophages within the rheumatoid synovium are activated by cytokines within the tissue, and they in turn secrete soluble products that can influence the phenotype of neighboring cells, including fibroblasts, chondrocytes, and osteocytes.

Macrophages within tissues of the body are generally mature and activated, although they may be functionally heterogeneous due to modulating influences within a particular microenvironment. Macrophages within sites of inflammation, including the synovium, are competent antigen-presenting cells due to the abundance of surface Ia

antigen (195). A principal activator of macrophages in this regard is IFN-γ, a product of activated T cells. In addition, it also causes up-regulated expression of Fc receptors, which are necessary for antibody-dependent cellular cytotoxicity (ADCC); activation of oxidative metabolism, resulting in the generation of hydrogen peroxide and other metabolites; and induction of secretion of IL-1 and TNF-α (196). It also stimulates the release of IP-10, a T cell and monocyte chemoattractant, by monocytes (197).

IFN-γ, as well as TNF-α, also stimulates the release of prostaglandins of the E series (PGE) (198). PGE_2 is pro-inflammatory, and it is a sensitizer for evoking pain and promoting vasopermeability. PGE_2 is generally anti-inflammatory, however, in the majority of its effects on leukocytes; it inhibits neutrophil generation of superoxide anion radical in response to fMLP, it inhibits the IL-1–induced activation response of T cells, it blocks cell-mediated cytotoxicity, it inhibits immunoglobin synthesis (199), and it decreases macrophage Ia expression (200). Systemic administration of IFN-γ appears to be anti-inflammatory because it inhibits leukocyte recruitment into sites of inflammation (201,202). This inhibition may be due to induction of premature maturation of monocytes while still within the circulation, resulting in down-regulation of receptors for chemoattractants (201,203).

The pleiotropic cytokine, TGF-β, activates macrophages by increasing their expression of potent inflammatory cytokines, such as IL-1 and TNF-α (4), as well as PDGF-β, TGF-α, FGF, and TGF-β (101,174). Resting, as well as activated, monocytes express mRNA for TGF-β constitutively, but the protein is secreted only following macrophage activation (204). The protein is exported in latent form, thus requiring exogenous activation. It has been suggested that acidic microenvironments, such as those generated by macrophages (205), may cause physiologically relevant activation. Alternatively, proteinases such as plasmin or cathepsin D (206) and glycosidases (207) may participate in TGF-β activation. Coculture of cells also appears to mediate activation via a plasminogen activator-dependent mechanism (208,209), suggesting the importance of cellular cooperation and close contact in TGF-β activation. The relevance of TGF-β bioactivity may lie in such close quarters, because serum and other inactivators, such as $α_2$-macroglobulin (210), latent TGF-β binding protein (211), and matrix-associated decorin (212), are efficient inactivators of TGF-β. INF-γ and LPS, but not GM-CSF, M-CSF-1, IL-1, or TNF-α, decrease the number of TGF-β binding sites on the monocyte surface (213).

Once circulating monocytes or "resting" tissue macrophages become activated, control of this phenotype by cytokines is complex because pre-exposure of these cells to a cytokine, or to a battery of cytokines, can alter their response to others. Hence, treatment of monocytes with IFN-γ decreases their ability to respond to TGF-β due to down-regulation of the type I TGF-β receptor (213). Exposure of macrophages to IL-10, a product of Th2 lymphocytes, abrogates the LPS-induced up-regulation of IL-1 and TNF-α by promoting the degradation of their mRNA (214). TFG-β, which is proinflammatory for a certain subset of macrophages, inhibits the generation of hydrogen peroxide by macrophages once they are activated by LPS (215). GM-CSF has no effect on macrophage production of TNF-α or IL-1, but when added in the presence of IFN-γ, it specifically enhances TNF, but not IL-1, synthesis (216).

DEGRADATION OF CARTILAGE

Destruction of the underlying cartilage and neighboring bone by the synovial cells is the manifestation of massive dysregulation of function by many cell types. Degradation of connective tissue of fibroblasts, chondrocytes, and macrophages within the synovium is shaped in large part by the cytokines present within this milieu.

Proteinases of several classes are likely to be involved in cartilage degradation. Members of the matrix metalloproteinase family, including MMP-1 (interstitial collagenase), MMP-2 (the 72 kd type IV collagenase), MMP-3 (stromelysin/transin), and MMP-9 (the 92 kd type IV collagenase), are probably the principal effectors in the destruction of collagen and other extracellular matrix molecules. MMP-1 (217) and MMP-3 (218,219) have been immunolocalized in synovial lining cells in rheumatoid joints, and MMP-1 has also been found at sites of cartilage erosion in patients with rheumatoid arthritis (220). The major inhibitor of metalloproteinases, TIMP-1, is also localized to the same cells in the synovial lining, the fibroblast-like B synoviocyte (217). Fibroblasts isolated from the rheumatoid synovium demonstrate spontaneous up-regulated production of MMP-1 (221) and MMP-9 (222). Rheumatoid synovial fluid also contains MMP-1 and MMP-3 (223), as well as TIMP (217). Serine proteinases, such as plasminogen activator and plasmin, also have some degradative ability, although they can also contribute to matrix dissolution by enhancing the catalytic activity of the MMPs. Under conditions of acid pH, such as those that exist within the synovium (27) and around macrophages and osteoclasts (205), cysteine and aspartate proteinases may become relevant. These proteinases, their substrate specificities, and cell-specific regulation of expression have been extensively reviewed (224,225).

Soluble products of activated macrophages, particularly IL-1 and TNF-α, induce an aggressive matrix degradative phenotype in fibroblasts. Intra-articular injection of IL-1β causes a severe synovitis, including cartilage breakdown (3). In vitro, exposure of fibroblasts and

chondrocytes to IL-1 causes a potent induction of MMP-1 (226), MMP-3 (227), and MMP-9 (222). This battery of metalloproteinases can degrade collagen types I, II, III, IV, V, and VII, as well as fibronectin, gelatin, and laminin (225). IL-1 binds to these cells with high affinity via a small number of type I receptors (228). Following the binding event, induction of proto-oncogenes, such as cjun and cfos, is thought to mediate the activation of MMP-1 and MMP-3 transcription via binding to the TRE regions within the promoter regions 5' to the gene (229). Subsequent to extracellular activation by other proteinases, activity of the MMPs is modulated by the presence of specific inhibitors, such as tissue inhibitor of metalloproteinases (TIMP-1 or -2), or nonspecific proteinase inhibitors, such as α₂-macroglobulin.

Perhaps due to its potency, the activity of IL-1 is counterbalanced by the existence of several negative regulators. IL-1 binds to cell surfaces via two high affinity receptors, the types I and II receptors (228). The type I receptor is found on most cell types, including fibroblasts, whereas the type II receptor is expressed primarily on neutrophils, monocytes, and B cells. Although the type I receptor is believed to be important in postreceptor cell signaling, the function of the type II receptor remains unclear. It is known, however, that the type II receptor is released from the cell surface to generate a soluble receptor. Serine proteinase inhibitors can block release of this receptor into the supernatant, suggesting proteolytic cleavage. This receptor can bind IL-1β, but not IL-1α, with high affinity similar to that of the membrane-bound receptor (230). It is inducible in peripheral blood mononuclear cells by stimulation with phytohemagglutin (PHA) (230), and it is found in the synovial fluid of patients with rheumatoid arthritis (231). It is also detectable in low levels in the circulation of healthy subjects; in patients with rheumatoid arthritis, it is increased during periods of active disease (231). A soluble type I receptor produced by expression of a recombinant molecule also competitively inhibits IL-1 binding, and it demonstrates in vivo bioactivity by enhancing allograft survival in mice (232).

IL-1 receptor antagonist (IL-1RA), another negative regulator of IL-1 activity, was first described as an inhibitory activity in supernatants of human monocyte cultures (233) and simultaneously as an activity in urine of febrile patients (234). It competes for IL-1 binding sites on cells while lacking any agonist activity. IL-1RA exhibits type I receptor binding affinity equivalent to that of IL-1α or IL-1β (235). IL-1RA binds the type II receptor, which has no known intracellular signaling function, with less affinity than IL-1β. Expression of IL-1β and IL-1RA by monocytes is independently regulated, and GM-CSF (236) and TGF-β (237) induce IL-1RA production. IL-1RA is present in rheumatoid synovial tissue, both in synovial lining cells and in perivascular monocytic infiltrates, and IL-1RA protein is also expressed by isolated synoviocytes in culture (238). The addition of IL-1RA to cartilage explants can inhibit IL-1–induced proteoglycan degradation (239). IL-1RA given intravenously also partially inhibits proteoglycan degradation and neutrophil migration into the joint of rabbits given intra-articular IL-1β (240). The antagonist also inhibits collagen-induced but not antigen-induced arthritis in mice (241). However, because occupancy of only a small number of IL-1 receptors can transduce an activation signal, it has been found that IL-1RA 10- to 500-fold in excess of IL-1 levels must be given to achieve 50% inhibition of IL-1–induced responses (242).

Naturally occurring autoantibodies to IL-1 have also recently been described in 10% of healthy individuals tested (243). These immunoglobulin G (IgG) antibodies can precipitate IL-1α but not IL-1β, and they interfere with IL-1α binding to EL4 cells. The significance of this finding in the context of disease is intriguing but unclear.

TNF-α shares many of the same biological properties of IL-1. Its importance in the pathogenesis of rheumatoid arthritis is suggested by the ability of TNF-α neutralizing antibodies to ameliorate collagen-induced arthritis in the mouse model (16). Joint scores were improved, including reduction in the severity of erosions in cartilage and bone. Anti-TNF displayed the ameliorative effect even if administered after the onset of clinical disease, suggesting that TNF has a continual role in the chronic phase of the arthritis in this model. Intra-articular expression of TNF-α also causes a severe synovitis, with articular cartilage destruction (6). Addition of TNF to explant cultures causes cartilage (244) and bone (245) resorption, indicating the ability of this cytokine to stimulate the degradative ability of chondrocytes and osteoclasts, respectively. An anti-TNF antibody added to cultures of rheumatoid synoviocytes results in decreased production of IL-1, as well as GM-CSF, indicating the importance of TNF in the inflammatory cytokine circuitry of the rheumatoid joint.

TNF-α binds to cell surfaces via two high affinity receptors, p55 and p75 (153–155). Both receptors also exist in approximately 30 kd soluble forms (246,247), which are proteolytically derived cleavage products. The shed receptors retain the ability to bind TNF-α and, to a lesser extent, LT, and they can inhibit the effects of the cytokines in vitro (246). In vivo, soluble type I receptor can reduce the severity of Escherichia coli–induced shock in baboons (248). A dimeric form of the soluble receptor fused to the Fc portion of IgM (249) or IgG (250) has the ability to bind more than one TNF-α trimer with higher affinity than the membrane-bound receptor. In rheumatoid arthritis, as well as osteoarthritis, serum levels of both p55- and p75-soluble TNF receptors are elevated; soluble p75 receptor levels are 3- to 4-fold higher than p55 (161). Synovial fluid levels are 4- to 5-fold higher than serum levels, suggesting local production within the joint.

The presence of soluble IL-1 receptors, IL-1RA and

soluble TNF receptors in the rheumatoid joint may represent a frustrated attempt to down-regulate the potent inflammatory activities of IL-1 and TNF. Binding of TNF to fibroblasts induces a rapid down-modulation of both p55 and p75 TNF receptors. However, continual in vitro stimulation of fibroblasts by TNF, as well as IL-1, results in sustained up-regulation of p75 and its mRNA (251). This effect may represent the basis for the chronically activated fibroblast phenotype seen in rheumatoid arthritis, in which they are hypersensitive to the effects of TNF and IL-1 (222,229).

The role of chemokines in the degradative phase of rheumatoid arthritis is largely unexplored. It is known, however, that IL-8 and MGSA can down-regulate expression of types I and III collagens by rheumatoid synovial fibroblasts, perhaps contributing to the overall degradative phenotype of this cell (252).

TGF-β is well known as a stimulator of extracellular matrix protein synthesis (104). Expression of collagen types I, II, III, IV, V, and VII are up-regulated by TGF-β treatment of cells. Fibronectin, thrombospondin, tenascin, osteonectin, osteopontin, and proteoglycans are among other matrix components whose expression is stimulated by this cytokine. The effects of TGF-β, at least on collagen type II and fibronectin, are long-lasting, because elevated expression of their respective mRNAs is evident up to 96 hours after cytokine removal (253). Post-transcriptional, as well as transcriptional, mechanisms of regulating mRNA are involved (254,255). Chronicity is also probably contributed to by the fact that TGF-β can transcriptionally activate its own gene (256).

In addition to positively regulating matrix deposition, TGF-β also down-regulates matrix degradation in several ways. It decreases expression of matrix-degrading enzymes, such as MMP-1 (257), MMP-3 (258), and elastase (259). Although it increases expression of MMP-2 (260), production of TIMP-1 and TIMP-2 is up-regulated by TGF-β (257). The activity of serine proteinases, such as plasminogen activator (261), is also inhibited by directly decreasing their expression and by increasing production of plasminogen activator inhibitor-1 (261). TGF-β has been shown to confer protection against joint damage in collagen-induced arthritis in mice (262) and streptococcal cell wall–induced arthritis in rats (263).

Macrophages can also contribute to the matrix-degrading ability of the synovial pannus. Macrophages can express MMP-1, MMP-2, MMP-3, and MMP-9 in response to various inflammatory stimuli, including LPS (264,265). IL-4 inhibits the release of MMP-1 and MMP-9 by macrophages (266). Matrix-degrading serine proteinases, such as human leukocyte elastase, are also produced by macrophages (267).

IFN-γ can block expression of MMP-1 (268) and MMP-9 (266) by macrophages. It can also block MMP-1 collagenolytic activity in fibroblasts by inhibiting the synthesis of its activator, MMP-3 (269). However, IFN-γ also inhibits interstitial collagen synthesis by fibroblasts (172).

SUMMARY

Rheumatoid arthritis is an example of the disruption of tissue structure and function that results from inappropriate intercellular signaling involving multiple cell types. Cytokines, as mediators of intercellular communication, are contributors to every aspect of this disease. Intersecting cytokine circuits that exist in vivo are reflected even in simplified in vitro experiments conducted on isolated cell types. As modulators of almost every aspect of cellular phenotype, cytokines are powerful tools for understanding the physiology of cells, as well as the pathophysiology of disease.

REFERENCES

1. Ziff M. Relation of cellular infiltration of rheumatoid synovial membrane to its immune response. Arthritis Rheum 1974;17:313.

2. Schumacher HR, Kitridou RC. Synovitis of recent onset: a clincopathologic study during the first month of disease. Arthritis Rheum 1972;15:465.

3. Pettipher ER, Higgs GA, Henderson B. Interleukin 1 induces leukocyte infiltration and cartilage proteoglycan degradation in the synovial joint. Proc Natl Acad USA Sci 1986;83:8749–8753.

4. Allen JB, Manthey CL, Hand AR, Ohura K, Ellingsworth L,Wahl SM. Rapid onset synovial inflammation and hyperplasia induced by transforming growth factor B. J Exp Med 1990;171:2231–2247.

5. Fava RA, Olsen NJ, Postlethwaite AE, et al. Transforming growth factor β₁ (TGF-β₁) induced neutrophil recruitment to synovial tissues: implications for TGF-β-driven synovial inflammation and hyperplasia. J Exp Med 1991;173:1121–1132.

6. Keffer J, Probert L, Cazlaris H, et al. Transgenic mice expressing human tumor necrosis factor: a predictive genetic model of arthritis. EMBO J 1991;10:4025–4031.

7. Picker LJ. Mechanisms of lymphocyte homing. Curr Opin Immunol 1992;4:277–286.

8. Shimizu Y, Newman W, Gopal TV, et al. Four molecular pathways of T cell adhesion to endothelial cells: roles of LFA-1, VCAM-1, and ELAM-1, and changes in pathway hierarchy under different activation conditions. J Cell Biol 1991;113:1203–1212.

9. Leung DW, Cachianes G, Kuang WJ, Goeddel DV, Ferrara N. Vascular endothelial growth factor is a secreted angiogenic mitogen. Science 1989;246:1306–1309.

10. Keck PJ, Hauser SD, Krivi G, et al. Vascular permeability factor, an endothelial cell mitogen related to PDGF. Science 1989;246:1309–1312.

11. Connolly DT, Olander JV, Heuvelman D, et al. Human vascular permeability factor. J Biol Chem 1989;264:20017–20024.

12. Plate KH, Breier G, Weich HA, Risau W. Vascular endothelial growth factor is a potential tumour angiogenesis factor in human gliomas in vivo. Nature 1992;359:845–848.

13. Berkman RA, Merrill MJ, Reinhold WC, et al. Expression of the vascular permeability factor/vascular endothelial growth factor gene in central nervous system neoplasms. J Clin Invest 1993;91:153–159.

14. Schweiki D, Itin A, Neufeld G, Gitay-Goren H, Keshet E. Patterns of expression of vascular endothelial growth factor (VEGF) and VEGF receptors in mice suggest a role in hormonally regulated angiogenesis. J Clin Invest 1993;91:2235–2243.

15. Jakeman LB, Armanini M, Phillips HS, Ferrara N. Developmental expression of binding sites and messenger ribonucleic acid for vascular endothelial growth factor suggests a role for this protein in vasculogenesis and angiogenesis. Endocrinology 1993;133:848–859.

16. deVries C, Escobedo JA, Ueno H, Houck K, Ferrara N, Williams LT. The fms-like tyrosine kinase, a receptor for vascular endothelial growth factor. Science 1992;255:989–991.

17. Millauer B, Wizigmann-Voos S, Schnurch H, et al. High affinity VEGF binding and developmental expression suggest Flk-1 as a major regulator of vasculogenesis and angiogenesis. Cell 1993;72:835–846.

18. Koch A, Harlow LA, Haines GK, et al. Vascular endothelial growth factor: a cytokine mediating angiogenesis in rheumatoid arthritis. J Immunol 1994;152:4149–4156.

19. Wallis WJ, Simkin PA, Nelp WB. Protein traffic in human synovial effusions. Arthritis Rheum 1987;25:1307.

20. Schweigerer L, Neufeld G, Friedman J, Abraham JA, Fiddes JC, Gospodarowicz D. Capillary endothelial cells express basic fibroblast growth factor, a mitogen that promotes their own growth. Nature 1987;325:257–259.

21. Schreiber AB, Winkler ME, Derynck R. Transforming growth factor-α: a more potent angiogenic mediator than epidermal growth factor. Science 1986;232:1250–1253.

22. Goldman CK, Kim J, Wong SL, King V, Brock T, Gillespie GY. Epidermal growth factor stimulates vascular endothelial growth factor production by human malignant glioma cells: a model of glioblastoma multiforme pathophysiology. Mol Biol Cell 1993;4:121–133.

23. Finkenzeller G, Marme D, Weich HA, Hug H. Platelet-derived growth factor-induced transcription of the vascular endothelial growth factor gene is mediated by protein kinase C. Cancer Res 1992;52:4821–4823.

24. Kim KJ, Li B, Winer J, et al. Inhibition of vascular endothelial growth factor-induced angiogenesis suppresses tumor growth in vivo. Nature 1993;362:841–844.

25. Ferrara N, Winer J, Burton T, et al. Expression of vascular endothelial growth factor does not promote transformation but confers a growth advantage in vivo in Chinese hamster ovary cells. J Clin Invest 1993;91:160–170.

26. Schweiki D, Itin A, Soffer D, Keshet E. Vascular endothelial growth factor induced by hypoxia may mediate hypoxia-initiated angiogenesis. Nature 1992;359:843–845.

27. Falchuk H, Geotzl J, Kulka P. Respiratory gases of synovial fluids. Am J Med 1970;49:223.

28. Sano H, Forough R, Maier JAM, et al. Detection of high levels of heparin binding growth factor-1 (acidic fibroblast growth factor) in inflammatory arthritis joints. J Cell Biol 1990;110:1417–1426.

29. Granstein RD, Margolis R, Mizel SB, Sauder DN. In vivo inflammatory activity of epidermal cell-derived thymocyte activating factor and recombinant interleukin 1 in the mouse. J Clin Invest 1986;177:1020–1027.

30. Valone FH, Epstein LB. Biphasic platelet-activating factor synthesis by human monocytes stimulated with IL-1β, tumor necrosis factor, or IFN-γ. J Immunol 1988;141:3945–3950.

31. Rubin K, Terracio K, Ronnstrand L, Heldin C-H, Klareskog L. Expression of platelet-derived growth factor receptors is induced on connective tissue cells during chronic synovial inflammation. Scand J Immunol 1988;27:285–294.

32. Rosenstein M, Ettinghaussen SE, Rosenberg SA. Extravasation of intravascular fluid mediated by the systemic administration of recombinant IL-2. J Immunol 1986;137:1735.

33. Damle N, Doyle LV. IL-2-activated human killer lymphocytes but not their secreted products mediate increase in albumin flux across cultured endothelial monolayers. J. Immunol 1989;142:2660–2669.

34. Nepom GT, Byers P, Seyfried C, et al. HLA genes associated with rheumatoid arthritis. Arthritis Rheum 1989;32:15–21.

35. van Boxel JJ, Paget SA. A predominantly T cell infiltrate in rheumatoid synovial membranes. N Engl J Med 1975;293:517.

36. Poulter CW, Duke O, Hobbs S, Janossy G, Panayi GS. Histochemical discrimination of HLA-DR positive cell populations in the normal and arthritic synovial lining. Clin Exp Immunol 1982;48:381–388.

37. Koch AE, Robinson PG, Radosovich JA, Pope RM. Distribution of CD45RA and CD45RO T lymphocyte subsets in rheumatoid arthritis synovial tissue. J Clin Immunol 1990;10:192–199.

38. Burmester GR, Jahn B, Gramatzki M, Zacher J, Kalden J. Activated T cells in vivo and in vitro: divergence in expression of Tac and Ia antigens in the nonblastoid small T cells of inflammation and normal T cells activated in vitro. J Immunol 1984;133:1230–1234.

39. Stamenkovic I, Stegagno M, Wright RA, et al. Clonal dominance among T-lymphocyte infiltrates in arthritis. Proc Natl Acad Sci USA 1988;85:1179–1183.

40. Miltenburg AMM, Van Laar JM, Daha MR, DeVries RRP, Van Den Elsen PJ, Breedveld FC. Dominant T cell receptor-β chain gene rearrangements indicate clonal expansion in the rheumatoid joint. Scand J Immunol 1990;31:121–125.

41. Ishikawa H, Ziff M. Electron microscopic observations of immunoreactive cells in the rheumatoid synovial membrane. Arthritis Rheum 1976;19:1.

42. Rooney M, Whelan A, Feighery C, Bresnihan B. Changes in lymphocytic infiltration of the synovial membrane and the clinical course of rheumatoid arthritis. Arthritis Rheum 1989;32:361–369.

43. Larsen CG, Anderson AO, Appella E, Oppenheim JJ, Matsushima K. The neutrophil-activating protein (NAP-1) is also chemotactic for T lymphocytes. Science 1989;243:1464–1466.

44. Issekutz TB, Stoltz JM, Webster DM. Role of interferon in lymphocyte recruitment into the skin. Cell Immunol 1986;99:322–333.

45. Issekutz TB, Stoltz JM. Stimulation of lymphocyte migration by endotoxin, tumor necrosis factor, and interferon. Cell Immunol 1989;120:165–173.

46. Meuer R, van Riper G, Feeney W, et al. Formation of eosinophilic and monocytic intradermal inflammatory sites in the dog by injection of human RANTES but not human monocyte chemoattractant protein-1, human macrophage inflammatory protein 1 alpha or human interleukin 8. J Exp Med 1993;178:1913–1921.

47. Issekutz TB. Effects of six different cytokines on lymphocyte adherence to microvascular endothelium and in vivo lymphocyte migration in the rat. J Immunol 1990;144:2140–2146.

48. Masinovsky B, Urdal D, Gallatin WN. IL-4 acts synergistically with IL-1β to promote lymphocyte adhesion to microvascular endothelium by induction of vascular cell adhesion molecule-1. J Immunol 1990;145:2886–2895.

49. Thornhill MH, Kyan-Aung U, Haskard DO. IL-4 increases human endothelial cell adhesiveness for T cells but not for neutrophils. J Immunol 1990;144:3060–3065.

50. Thornhill MH, Wellcome SM, Mahiouz DL, Lanchbury JSS, Kyan-Aung U, Haskard DO. Tumor necrosis factor combines with IL-4 or IFN-gamma to selectively enhance endothelial cell adhesiveness for T cells: the contribution of vascular cell adhesion molecule-1-dependent and -independent binding mechanisms. J Immunol 1991;146:592–598.

51. Tanaka Y, Adams DH, Hubscher S, Hirano H, Siebenlist U, Shaw S. T-cell adhesion induced by proteoglycan-immobilized cytokine MIP-1β. Nature 1993;361:79–82.

52. Taub DD, Lloyd AR, Conlon K, et al. Recombinant human interferon-inducible protein 10 is a chemoattractant for human monocytes and T lymphocytes and promotes T cell adhesion to endothelial cells. J Exp Med 1993;177:1809–1814.

53. Harlan JM. Leukocyte adhesion deficiency syndrome: insights into the molecular basis of leukocyte emigration. Clin Immunol Immunopathol 1993;76:816–824.

54. Springer TA. Adhesion receptors of the immune system. Nature 1990;346:425–434.

55. Bevilacqua MP. Endothelial-leukocyte adhesion molecules. Annu Rev Immunol 1993;11:767–804.

56. Laffon A, Garcia-Vicuna R, Humbria A, et al. Upregulated expression and function of VLA-4 fibronectin receptors on human activated T cells in rheumatoid arthritis. J Clin Invest 1991;88:546–552.

57. Cush JJ, Lipsky PE. Phenotypic analysis of synovial tissue and peripheral blood lymphocytes isolated from patients with rheumatoid arthritis. Arthritis Rheum 1988;31:1230–1238.

58. Hale LP, Martin ME, McCollum DC, et al. Immunohistologic analysis of the distribution of cell adhesion molecules within the inflammatory synovial micrenvironment. Arthritis Rheum 1989;32:22–30.

59. Koch AE, Burrows JC, Hayes GK, Carlos TM, Harlan JM, Leibovich SJ. Immunolocalization of endothelial and leukocyte adhesion molecules in human rheumatoid and osteoarthritc synovial tissues. Lab Invest 1991;64:313–320.

60. Haynes BF, Liao HX, Patton KL. The transmembrane

hyaluronate receptor (CD44): multiple functions, multiple forms. Cancer Cells 1991;3:347–350.

61. Miyake S, Yagita H, Maruyama T, Hashimoto H, Miyasaka N, Okumura K. B1 integrin-mediated interactions with extracellular matrix proteins regulates cytokine gene expression in synovial fluid cells of rheumatoid arthritis patients. J Exp Med 1993;177:863–868.

62. Yamada A, Nikaido T, Nojima Y, Schlossman SF, Morimoto K. Activation of human CD4 T lymphocytes. Interaction of fibronectin with VLA-5 receptor on CD4 cells induces the AP-1 transcription factor. J Immunol 1991; 146:53.

63. Schall TJ. Biology of the RANTES/SIS cytokine family. Cytokine 1991;3:165–183.

64. Oppenheim JJ, Zachariae CCC, Mukaida N, Matsushima K. Properties of the novel proinflammatory supergene "intercrine" cytokine family. Annu Rev Immunol 1991;9:617–648.

65. Baggiolini M, Dewald B, Moser B. Interleukin-8 and related chemotactic cytokines—CXC and CC chemokines. Adv Immunol 1994; 55:97–179.

66. Schall TJ, Bacon K, Toy KJ, Goeddel DV. Selective attraction of monocytes or T lymphocytes of the memory phenotype by cytokine RANTES. Nature 1990;347:669–671.

67. Taub DD, Conlon D, Lloyd AR, Oppenheim JJ, Kelvin DJ. Preferential migration of activated CD4+ and CD8+ T cells in response to MIP-1α and MIP-1β. Science 1993;260:355–358.

68. Schall TJ, Bacon K, Camp RDR, Kaspari JW, Goeddel DV. Human macrophage inflammatory protein 1 alpha (MIP-1α) and MIP-1β chemokines attract distinct populations of lymphocytes. J Exp Med 1993;177:1821–1825.

69. Schall TJ, Lu LH, Gillett N, Amento EP. RANTES/SIS cytokine gene expression in rheumatoid synovium as analyzed by in situ hybridization. Arthritis Rheum 1991;34: S117.

70. Rathanaswami P, Hachinda M, Sadick M, Schall TJ, McColl SR. Expression of the cytokine RANTES in human synovial fibroblasts. J Biol Chem 1993;268:5834–5839.

71. Koch AE, Kunkel SL, Burrows JC, et al. Synovial tissue macrophage as a source of the chemotactic cytokine IL-8. J Immunol 1991;147:2187–2195.

72. Steitz M, Dewald B, Gerber N, Baggiolini M. Enhanced production of neutrophil-activating peptide-1/interleukin-8 in rheumatoid arthritis. J Clin Invest 1991;87:463–469.

73. Brennan FM, Zachariae COC, Chantry D, et al. Detection of interleukin 8 biological activity in synovial fluids from patients with rheumatoid arthritis and production of interleukin 8 mRNA by isolated synovial cells. Eur J Immunol 1990;20:2141–2144.

74. DeMarco D, Kunkel SL, Strieter RM, Basha M, Zurier RB. Interleukin-1 induced gene expression of neutrophil activating protein (interleukin-8) and monocyte chemotactic peptide in human synovial cells. Biochem Biophys Res Commun 1991;174:411–416.

75. Schroder JM, Sticherling M, Henneicke HH, Preissner WC, Christophers E. IL-1α or tumor necrosis factor-α stimulate release of three NAP-1/IL-8 related neutrophil chemotactic proteins in human dermal fibroblasts. J Immunol 1990; 144:2223–2232.

76. Seitz M, Dewald B, Gerber N, Baggiolini M. Enhanced pro-

duction of neutrophil-activating peptide-1/interleukin-8 in rheumatoid arthritis. J Clin Invest 1991;87:463–467.

77. Neote K, DiGregorio D, Mak JY, Horuk R, Schall TJ. Molecular cloning, functional expression, and signaling characteristics of a C-C 'chemokine' receptor. Cell 1993;72:1–20.

78. Holmes WE, Lee J, Kuang WJ, Rice GC, Wood WI. Structure and functional expression of a human interleukin-8 receptor. Science 1991;253:1278–1290.

79. Murphy PM, Tiffany HL. Cloning of complementary DNA encoding a functional human interleukin-8 receptor. Science 1991;253:1280–1283.

80. Lee J, Horuk R, Rice GC, Bennett GL, Camerato T, Wood WI. Characterization of two high affinity human interleukin 8 receptors. J Biol Chem 1992;267:16283–16287.

81. Kaplan G, Luster AD, Hancock G, Cohn ZA. The expression of a γ interferon-induced protein (IP-10) in delayed-type hypersensitivity responses in skin. J Exp Med 1987;166:1098.

82. Kelvin DJ, Michiel DF, Johnston JA, et al. Chemokines and serpentines: the molecular biology of chemokine receptors. J Leukocyte Biol 1993;54:604–612.

83. Gao J-L, Kuhns DB, Tiffany HL, et al. Structure and functional expression of the human macrophage inflammatory protein 1α/RANTES receptor. J Exp Med 1993;177:1421–1427.

84. Wang J-M, Sherry B, Firash MJ, Kelvin DJ, Oppenheim JJ. Human recombinant macrophage inflammatory protein-1α and -β and monocyte chemotactic and activating factor utilize common and unique receptors on human monocytes. J Immunol 1993;150:1–8.

85. Horuk R, Chitnis CE, Darbonne WC, et al. A receptor for the malarial parasite plasmodium vivax. The erythrocyte chemokine receptor. Science 1993;261:1182–1184.

86. Neote K, Darbonne WC, Horuk R, Schall TJ. Identification of a promiscuous inflammatory peptide receptor on the surface of red blood cells. J Biol Chem 1993;268: 12247–12249.

87. Darbonne WC, Rice GC, Mohler MA, et al. Red blood cells are a sink for interleukin 8, a leukocyte chemotaxin. J Clin Invest 1991;88:1362–1369.

88. Coulton LA, Henderson B, Bitensky L, Chayou J. DNA synthesis in human rheumatoid synovial and nonrheumatoid synovial lining. Ann Rheum Dis 1980;39:241–247.

89. Larson RS, Springer TA. Structure and function of leukocyte integrins. Immunol Rev 1990;114:179–217.

90. Arnaout MA. Structure and function of the leukocyte adhesion molecules CD11/CD18. Blood 1990;75:1037–1050.

91. Matsushima K, Oppenheim JJ. Interleukin-8 and MCAF: novel inflammatory cytokines inducible by IL-1 and TNF. Cytokine 1989;1:2–12.

92. Leonard EJ, Yoshimura T. Human monocyte chemoattractant protein-1 (MCP-1). Ummunol Today 1990;11:97–101.

93. Yoshimura T, Leonard EJ. Identification of high affinity receptors for human monocyte chemoattractant protein-1 (MCP-1) in human monocytes. J Immunol 1990;145:292–297.

94. Koch AE, Kunkel SL, Harlow LA, et al. Enhanced production of monocyte chemoattractant protein-1 in rheumatoid arthritis. J Clin Invest 1992;90:772–779.

95. Villiger PM, Terkeltaub R, Lotz M. Production of mono-

cyte chemoattractant protein-1 by inflamed synovial tissue and cultured synoviocytes. J Immunol 1992;149:722–727.

96. Villiger PM, Terkeltaub R, Lotz M. Monocyte chemo-attractant protein-1 (MCP-1) expression in human articular cartilage. J Clin Invest 1992;90:488–496.

97. Van Damme J, Proost P, Lenaerts J-P, Opdenakker G. Structural and functional identification of two human, tumor-derived monocyte chemotactic proteins (MCP-2 and MCP-3) belonging to the chemokine family. J Exp Med 1992;176:59–65.

98. Tepper RI, Pattengale PK, Leder P. Murine interleukin-4 displays potent anti-tumor activity in vivo. Cell 1989;57:503–512.

99. Standiford JJ, Strieter RM, Chensue SW, Westwick J, Kasahara K, Kunkel SL. IL-4 inhibits the expression of IL-8 from stimulated human monocytes. J Immunol 1990;145:1435.

100. Rollins BJ, Pober JS. Interleukin-4 induces the synthesis and secretion of MCP-1/JE by human endothelial cells. Am J Pathol 1991;138:1315–1319.

101. Wahl SM, Hunt DA, Wakefield LM, et al. Transforming growth factor beta (TGF-beta) induces monocyte chemotaxis and growth factor production. Proc Natl Acad Sci USA 1987;84:5788–5792.

102. Firestein GL, Alvaro-Garcia JM, Maki R. Quantitative analysis of cytokine gene expression in rheumatoid arthritis. J Immunol 1990;144:3347–3353.

103. Lafyatis R, Thomas NL, Remmers EF, et al. Transforming growth factor-β production by synovial tissues from rheumatoid aptheitns and streptococcal cell wall arthritic rats. J Immunol 1989;143:1142.

104. Roberts AB, Sporn MB. The transforming growth factor-βs. In: Sporn MB, and Roberts AB, eds. Handbook of experimental pharmacology. New York: Springer-Verlag, 1990:419–472.

105. Miyazono K, ten Dijke P, Ichijo H, Heldin C-H. Receptors for transforming growth factor-β. Adv Immunol 1994;55:181–220.

106. Wrana JL, Attisano L, Carcaom J, et al. TGF-β signals through a heteromeric protein kinase complex. Cell 1992;71:1003–1014.

107. Wieser R, Attisano L, Wrana JL, Massague J. Signalling activity of transforming growth factor β type II receptors lacking specific domains in the cytoplasmic region. Mol Cell Biol 1993;13:6239–6247.

108. Cheifetz S, Hernandez JC, Laiho M, ten Dijke P, Iwata KK, Massague J. Determinants of cellular responsiveness to the three transforming growth factor-β isoforms. J Biol Chem 1990;265:20533–20538.

109. Segarini PR, Seyedin SM. The high molecular weight receptor to transforming growth factor-β contains glycosaminoglycan chains. J Biol Chem 1988;263:8366–8370.

110. Lopez-Casillas F, Cheifetz S, Doody J, et al. Structure and expression of the membrane proteoglycan betaglycan, a component of the TGF-β receptor system. Cell 1991;67:785–795.

111. Andres JL, Stanley K, Cheifetz S, Massague J. Membrane-anchored and soluble forms of betaglycan, a polymorphic proteoglycan that binds transforming growth factor-β. J Biol Chem 1989;109:3137–3145.

112. Roska AK, Lipsky PE. Monocytes and macrophages. In: Kelley WN, DeVita VT, Dupont HL, et al. eds. Textbook of rheumatology. Philadelphia: WB Saunders, 1989:345–366.

113. Harris ED Jr. Rheumatoid arthritis: pathophysiology and implications for therapy. N Engl J Med 1990;322:1277.

114. Detmers PA, Powell DE, Walz A, Clark-Lewis I, Baggiolini M, Cohn ZA. Differential effects of neutrophil activating peptide-1/IL-8 and its homologues on leukocyte adhesion and phagocytosis. J Immunol 1991;147:4211–4217.

115. Carveth HJ, Bohnsack JF, McIntyre TM, Baggiolini M, Prescott SM, Zimmerman GA. Neutrophil activating factor (NAF) induces polymorphonuclear leukocyte adhesiveness to endothelial cells and to subendothelial matrix proteins. Biochem Biophys Res Commun 1989;162:383–393.

116. Dewald B, Thelen B, Baggiolini M. Two transduction sequences are necessary for neutrophil activation by receptor agonists. J Biol Chem 1988;263:16179–16184.

117. Samanta AK, Oppenheim JJ, Matsushima K. Interleukin 8 (MDNCF) dynamically regulates its own receptor expression on human neutrophils. J Biol Chem 1989;265:183–189.

118. Endo H, Akahoshi T, Takaggishi K, Kashiwazaki S, Matsushima K. Elevation of interleukin-8 (IL-8) levels in joint fluids of patients with rheumatoid arthritis and the induction by IL-8 of leukocyte infiltration and synovitis in rabbit joints. Lymphokine Cytokine Res 1991;10:245–252.

119. Gasson JC, Weisbart RH, Kaufman SE, et al. Purified human granulocyte-macrophage colony-stimulating factor: direct action on neutrophils. Science 1984;226:1339–1342.

120. XU W, Firestein GS, Taetle R, Kaushansky K, Zvaifler NJ. Cytokines in chronic inflammatory arthritis. II. Granulocyte-macrophage colony-stimulating factors in rheumatoid synovial effusions. J Clin Invest 1989;83:876–882.

121. Weisbart RH, Golde DW, Clark SC, Wong GG, Gasson JC. Human granulocyte-macrophage colony-stimulating factor is a neutrophil activator. Nature 1985;314:361–363.

122. Sullivan R, Gans PJ, McCarroll LA. The synthesis and secretion of granulocyte-monocyte colony stimulating activity (CSA) by isolated human monocytes: kinetics of the response to bacterial endotoxin. J Immunol 1983;130:800–807.

123. Kaushansky K, Lin N, Adamson JW. Interleukin-1 stimulates fibroblasts to synthesize granulocyte-macrophage and granulocyte-colony stimulating factors. J Clin Invest 1983;81:92–97.

124. Colotta F, Re F, Polentarutti N, et al. Interleukin-1 type II receptor: a decoy target for IL-1 that is regulated by IL-4. Science 1993;261:472–475.

125. Wood DD, Ihrie EJ, Dinarello CA, Cohen PL. Isolation of an interleukin 1-like factor from human joint effusions. Arthritis Rheum 1983;26:975–983.

126. Hopkins SJ, Humphreys M, Jayson MIV. Cytokines in synovial fluid. I. The presence of biologically immunoreactive IL-1. Clin Exp Immunol 1988;72:422–427.

127. Dower SK, Kronheim SR, March CJ. et al. Detection and characterization of high affinity plasma membrane receptors for human interleukin 1. J Exp Med 1985;162:501–515.

128. Fay AC, Trudgett A, McCrea JD, et al. Detection and partial characterization of human B cell colony stimulatory activ-

ity in synovial fluids of patients with rheumatoid arthritis. Clin Exp Immunol 1991;60:316–322.

129. Moissec P, Naviliat M, Dupuy D'Angeac A, Sany J, Banchereau J. Low levels of interleukin-4 and high levels of transforming growth factor β in rheumatoid synovitis. Arthritis Rheum 1990;33:1180–1187.

130. Chu CQ, Field M, Feldmann M, Maini RN. Localization of tumor necrosis factor α in synovial tissues and at the cartilage-pannus junction in patients with rheumatoid arthritis. Arthritis Rheum 1991;34:1125–1135.

131. Buchan G, Barrett T, Fujita T, Taniguchi T, Maini R, Feldmann M. Detection of activated T cell products in the rheumatoid joint using cDNA probes to interleukin-2 (IL-2), IL-2 receptors, and IFN-γ. Clin Exp Immunol 1988;71:295–301.

132. Lemm G, Warnatz H. Evidence for enhanced interleukin 2 (IL-2) secretion and IL-2 receptor presentation by synovial fluid lymphocytes in rheumatoid arthritis. Clin Exp Immunol 1986;64:71–79.

133. Firestein GS, Xu WD, Townsend K, et al. Cytokines in chronic inflammatory arthritis. I. Failure to detect T cell lymphokines (IL-2 and IL-3) and presence of macrophage colony-stimulating factor (CSF-1) and a novel mast cell growth factor in rheumatoid synovitis. J Exp Med 1988;168:1573–1586.

134. Takeshita T, Asao H, Ohtani K, et al. Cloning of the gamma chain of the human IL-2 receptor. Science 1992;257:379–382.

135. Howard M, Farrar J, Hilficker M, et al. Identification of a T cell-derived B cell growth factor distinct from interleukin-2. J Exp Med 1982;255:914–923.

136. Swain SC, Dennert G, Warner JF, Dutton DW. Culture supernatants of a stimulated T cell line have helper activity that acts synergistically with IL-2 in the response of B cells to antigen. Proc Natl Acad Sci USA 1981;78:2517–2521.

137. Hardy KJ, Manger B, Newton M, Stobo JD. Molecular events involved in regulating interferon-gamma gene expression during T cell activation. J Immunol 1987;138:2353–2358.

138. Gery I, Gershon RK, Waksman B. Potentiation of the T lymphocyte response to mitogens. I. The responding cell. J Exp Med 1972;136:128–142.

139. Pledger WJ, Stiles CD, Antoniades HN, Scher CD. An ordered sequence of events is required before BALB/c-3T3 cells become committed to DNA synthesis. Proc Natl Acad Sci USA 1978;75:2839–2843.

140. Mannel DN, Mizel SB, Diamantstein T, Falk W. Induction of interleukin 2 responsiveness in thymocytes by synergistic action of interleukin 1 and interleukin 2. J Immunol 1985;134:3108–3110.

141. Lichtman AH, Chin J, Schmidt JA, Abbas AK. Role of interleukin 1 in the activation of T lymphocytes. Proc Natl Acad Sci USA 1988;85:9699–9703.

142. Weaver CT, Hawrylowicz CM, Unanue ER. T helper cell subsets require the expression of distinct costimulatory signals by antigen presenting cells. Proc Natl Acad Sci USA 1988;85:8181–8185.

143. Greenbaum LA, Horowitz JB, Woods A, Pasqualami L, Reich EP, Bottomly K. Autocrine growth of CD4+ T cells. Differential effects of IL-1 helper and inflammatory T cells. J Immunol 1988;140:1555–1560.

144. Bursten SL, Locksley RM, Ryan JL, Lovett DH. Acylation of monocyte and glomerular mesangial cell proteins. Myristyl acylation of interleukin 1 precursors. J Clin Invest 1988;82:1479–1488.

145. Brody TB, Durum SK. Plasma membrane anchoring mechanism for IL-1. In: Powanda MC, et al., eds. Monokines and other non-lymphocytic cytokines. New York: Liss, 1988:101–107.

146. Massague J. Transforming growth factor-alpha. A model for membrane-anchored growth factors. J Biol Chem 1990;265:21393–21396.

147. Le J, Frederickson G, Reis LFL, et al. Interleukin 2-dependent and interleukin 2-independent pathways of regulating thymocyte function by interleukin 6. Proc Natl Acad Sci USA 1988;85:8643–8647.

148. Garman RD, Jacobs KA, Clark SC, Raulet DH. B-cell-stimulatory factor 2(β 2 interferon) functions as a second signal for interleukin 2 production by mature murine T cells. Proc Natl Acad Sci USA 1987;84:7629–7633.

149. Waage A, Kaufmann C, Espevik T, Husby G. Interleukin-6 in synovial fluid from patients with arthritis. Clin Immunol Immunopathol 1989;50:394–398.

150. Guerne P-A, Zuraw BL, Vaughan JH, Carson DA, Lotz M. Synovium as a source of interleukin 6 in vitro. J Clin Invest 1989;83:585–592.

151. Taga T, Kawanishi K, Hardy RR, Hirano T, Kishimoto T. Receptors for B cells stimulatory factor 2 (BSF-2): quantification, specificity, distribution, and regulation of expression. J Exp Med 1987;166:967–981.

152. Beutler B. Cachectin/tumor necrosis factor and lymphotoxin. In: Sporn MB, Roberts AB, eds. Peptide growth factors II. Berlin: Springer-Verlag, 1990;39–70.

153. Loetscher H, Pan YCE, Lahm HW, et al. Molecular cloning and expression of the human 55kd tumor necrosis factor receptor. Cell 1990;61:351.

154. Schall TJ, Lewis M, Koller KJ, et al. Molecular cloning and expression of a receptor for human tumor necrosis factor receptor. Cell 1990;61:361.

155. Smith CA, Davis T, Anderson D, et al. A receptor for tumor necrosis factor defines an unusual family of cellular and viral proteins. Science 1990;248:1019.

156. Smith RA, Baglioni C. The active form of tumor necrosis factor is a trimer. J Biol Chem 1987;262:6951–6954.

157. Kriegler M, Perez C, DeFay K, Albert I, Lu SD. A novel form of TNF/Cachectin is a cell surface cytotoxic transmembrane protein: ramifications for the complex physiology of TNF. Cell 1988;53:45–53.

158. Scheurich P, Thoma B, Ucer U, Pfizenmaier K. Immunoregulatory activity of recombinant human tumor necrosis factor (TNF)-alpha: induction of TNF receptors on human T cells and TNF-alpha-mediated enhancement of T cell responses. J Immunol 1987;138:1786–1790.

159. Spits H, Yssel H, Takebe Y, et al. Recombinant interleukin-4 promotes the growth of human T cells. J Immunol 1987;139:1142–1147.

160. Tartaglia LA, Goeddel DV, Reynolds C, et al. Stimulation of human T-cell proliferation by specific activation of the 75kDa tumor necrosis factor receptor. J Immunol 1993;151:4637–4641.

161. Cope AP, Aderka D, Doherty M, et al. Increased levels of

soluble tumor necrosis factor receptors in the sera and synovial fluid of patients with rheumatic diseases. Arthritis Rheum 1992;35:1160.

162. Deleuran BW, Chu C-H, Field M, et al. Localization of tumor necrosis factor receptors in the synovial tissue and cartilage-pannus junction in patients with rheumatoid arthritis. Arthritis Rheum 1992;35:1170.

163. Brennan FM, Gibbons DL, Mitchell T, Cope AP, Maini RN, Feldmann M. Enhanced expression of tumor necrosis factor receptor mRNA and protein in mononuclear cells isolated from rheumatoid arthritis synovial joints. Eur J Immunol 1992;22:1907–1912.

164. Mosmann TR, Cherwinski H, Bond MW, Giedlin MA, Coffman RI. Two types of murine helper T cell clones. I. Definition according to profiles of lymphokine activities and secreted proteins. J Immunol 1986;136:2348–2357.

165. Hu-Li J, Shevach E, Mizuguchi J, Ohara J, Mosmann T, Paul W. B cell stimulatory factor 1 (interleukin 4) is a potent costimulant for normal resting T cells. J Exp Med 1987;165:157–172.

166. Brorson KA, Beverly B, Kary SM, Lenardo M, Schwartz RH. Transcriptional regulation of cytokine genes in non-transformed T cells: apparent constitutive signals in run-on assays can be caused by repeat sequences. J Immunol 1991;147:3601–3609.

167. Gibbs VC, Williams SR, Gray PW, et al. The extracellular domain of the human interferon gamma receptor interacts with a species-specific signal transducer. Mol Cell Biol 1991;11:5860–5966.

168. DeMaeyer E, DeMaeyer-Guignard J. Interferon-γ. Curr Opin Immunol 1992;4:321–326.

169. Wong GHW, Clark-Lewis I, McKimm-Breschkin JL, Harris AW, Schrader JW. Interferon-gamma induces enhanced expression of Ia and H-2 antigens on B lymphoid, macrophage, and myeloid cell lines. J Immunol 1983;131:788–793.

170. Chin JE, Winterowd GE, Krzesicki RF, Sanders ME. Role of cytokines in inflammatory synovitis. Arthritis Rheum 1990;133:1776–1786.

171. Alvaro-Garcia JM, Zvaifler NJ, Firestein GS. Cytokines in chronic inflammatory arthritis. V. Mutual antagonism between interferon-gamma and tumor necrosis factor-alpha on HLA-DR expression, proliferation, collagenase production, and granulocyte macrophage colony-stimulatory factor production by rheumatoid arthritis synoviocytes. J Clin Invest 1990;86:1790–1798.

172. Amento EP, Bahn AK, McCullagh KG, Krane SM. Influences of gamma interferon on synovial fibroblastlike cells. Ia induction and inhibition of collagen synthesis. J Clin Invest 1985;76:837–848.

173. Johnson WJ, Kelley A, Connor JR, Dalton BJ, Meunier P. Inhibition of INF-γ-induced Ia antigen expression in synovial fibroblasts by IL-1. J Immunol 1989;143:1614–1618.

174. McCartney-Francis N, Mizel D, Wong H, Wahl L, Wahl S. Transforming growth factor-beta (TGF-β) as an immunomodulatory molecule. FASEB J 1988;2:A875.

175. Segarini PR, Rosen DM, Seyedin SM. Binding of TGF-β to cell surface proteins vary with cell type. Mol Endocrinol 1989;3:261.

176. Kerhl JH, Wakefield LM, Roberts AB, et al. Production of transforming growth factor β by human T lymphocytes and its potential role in the regulation of T cell growth. J Exp Med 1986;163:1037–1050.

177. Dubois CM, Ruscetti FW, Palaszynski EW, Falk LA, Oppenheim JJ, Keller JR. Transforming growth factor β is a potent inhibitor of interleukin 1 (IL-1) receptor expression: proposed mechanism of IL-1 action. J Exp Med 1990;172:737–744.

178. Fava R, Olsen N, Keski-Oja J, Moses H, Pincus T. Active and latent forms of transforming growth factor β activity in synovial effusions. J Exp Med 1989;169:291–296.

179. Lotz M, Kekow J, Carson DA. Transforming growth factor-β and cellular immune responses in synovial fluids. J Immunol 1990;144:4189–4194.

180. Bergroth V, Konttinen YT, Nykanen P, vonEssen R, Koota K. Proliferating cells in synovial fluid in rheumatic disease. Scand J Immunol 1985;22:383.

181. Fox RI, Fong S, Subharwal N, Carstens SA, Kung PC, Vaughan JH. Synovial fluid lymphocytes differ from peripheral blood lymphocytes in patients with rheumatoid arthritis. J. Immunol 1982;128:351.

182. Wahl SM, Malone DG, Wilder RL. Spontaneous production of fibroblast-activating factor(s) by synovial inflammatory cells. J Exp Med 1985;161:210–222.

183. Burgess WH, Maciag T. The heparin-binding (fibroblast) growth factor family of proteins. Annu Rev Biochem 1989;58:565–606.

184. Johnson DE, Williams LT. Structural and functional diversity in the FGF receptor multigene family. Adv Cancer Res 1993;60:1–42.

185. Rubin JS, Osada H, Finch PW, Taylor WG, Rudikoff S, Aaronson SA. Purification and characterization of newly identified growth factor specific for eptithelial cells. Proc Natl Acad Sci USA 1989;86:802–806.

186. Bashkin P, Doctrow S, Klagsbrun M, Svahn CM, Folkman J, Vlodavsky I. Basic fibroblast growth factor binds to subendothelial extracellular matrix and is released by heparitinase and heparin-like moleclues. Biochemistry 1989;28:1737–1743.

187. Rapraeger AC, Krufka A, Olwin BB. Requirement of heparin sulfate of bFGF-mediated fibroblast growth and myoblast differentiation. Science 1991;252:1705–1708.

188. Bucala R, Ritchlin C, Winchester R, Cerami A. Constitutive production of inflammatory and mitogenic cytokines by rheumatoid synovial fibroblasts. J Exp Med 1991;173:569–574.

189. Ross R, Raines EW, Bowen-Pope DF. The biology of platelet-derived growth factor. Cell 1986;46:155–169.

190. Ostman A, Backstrom G, Fong N, et al. Expression of three recombinant homodimeric isoforms of PDGF in Saccharomyces cerevisiae: evidence for differences in receptor binding and functional activities. Growth Factors 1989;1:271–281.

191. Paulsson Y, Bywater M, Heldin C-H, Westermark B. Effects of epidermal growth factor and platelet-derived growth factor on c-fos and c-myc mRNA levels in human fibroblasts. Exp Cell Res 1987;171:186–194.

192. Remmers EF, Lafyatis R, Kumkumian GK, et al. Cytokines and growth regulation of synoviocytes from patients with rheumatoid arthritis and rats with streptococcal cell wall arthritis. Growth Factors 1990;2:179–188.

193. Dayer JM, Goldring SR, Robinson DR, Krame SM. Effects of human mononuclear cell factor on cultured rheumatoid synovial cells. Interactions of prostaglandin E$_2$ and cyclic adenosine 3'5'-monophosphate. Biochem Biophys Acta 1979;586:87–105.

194. Raines EW, Dower SK, Ross R. Interleukin-1 mitogenic activity for fibroblasts and smooth muscle cells is due to PDGF-AA. Science 1989;243:393–396.

195. Burmester GR, Dimitriu-Bona A, Waters SJ, Winchester RJ. Identification of three major synovial lining cell populations by monoclonal antibodies directed to Ia antigens and antigens associated with monocytes/macrophages and fibroblasts. Scand J Immunol 1983;17:69.

196. Wilkinson M, Morris AG. The interaction between interferons and macrophages. In: Dean RT, Jessup W, eds. Mononuclear phagocytes: physiology and pathology. Amsterdam: Elsevier, 1985:161–174.

197. Luster AD, Unkeless JC, Ravetch JV. Gamma interferon transcriptionally regulates an early response gene containing homology to platelet proteins. Nature 1985;315:372.

198. Bachwich PR, Chensue SW, Carick JW, Kunkel SL. Tumor necrosis factor stimulates interleukin-1 and prostaglandin E$_2$ production in resting macrophages. Biochem Biophys Res Commun 1986;136:94.

199. Lewis RA. Prostaglandins and leukotrienes. In: Kelley WN, DeVita VT, Dupont HL, eds. Textbook of rheumatology. Philadelphia: WB Saunders, 1989:253–265.

200. Snyder DW, Beller DI, Unanue ER. Prostaglandins modulate macrophage Ia expression. Nature 1982;299:163–165.

201. Wahl SM, Allen JB, Ohura K, Chenoweth DE, Hand AR. IFN-γ inhibits inflammatory cell recruitment and the evolution of bacterial cell wall-induced arthritis. J Immunol 1991;146:95–100.

202. Granstein RD, Deak MR, Jacques SL, et al. The systemic administration of gamma interferon inhibits collagen synthesis and acute inflammation in a murine skin wounding model. J Invest Dermatol 1989;93:18.

203. Firestein GS, Zvaifler NJ. Down regulation of human monocyte differentiation antigens by interferon-γ and dexamethasone. Cell Immunol 1987;104:343.

204. Assoian RK, Fleurdelys BE, Steenson HC, et al. Expression and secretion of type beta transforming growth factor by activated human macrophages. Proc Natl Acad Sci USA 1987;84:6020–6024.

205. Silver IA, Murrills RJ, Etherington DJ. Microelectrode studies in the acid microenvironment beneath adherent macrophages and osteoclasts. Exp Cell Res 1988;175:266–276.

206. Lyons RM, Keski-Oja J, Moses HL. Proteolytic activation of latent transforming growth factor-β from fibroblast-conditioned medium. J Cell Biol 1988;106:1659–1665.

207. Miyazono K, Heldin C-H. Interaction between TGF-β1 and carbohydrate structures in its precursor renders TGF-β latent. Nature 1989;338:158–160.

208. Antonelli-Orledge A, Saunder KB, Smith SR, D'Amore PA. An activated form of transforming growth factor beta is produced by cocultures of endothelial cells and pericytes. Proc Natl Acad Sci USA 1989;86:4544–4548.

209. Sato Y, Rifkin DB. Inhibition of endothelial cell movement by pericytes and smooth muscle cells: activation of a latent transforming growth factor-beta a-like molecule by plasmin during co-culture. J Cell Biol 1989;109:309–315.

210. Wakefield LM, Smith DM, Broz S, Jackson M, Levinson AD. Recombinant TGF-β1 is synthesized as a two component latent complex that shares some structural features with the native platelet latent TGF-β1 complex. Growth Factors 1989;1:203–218.

211. Kanazaki T, Olofsson A, Moren A, et al. TGF-β1 binding protein: a component of the large latent complex of TGF-β, with multiple repeat sequences. Cell 1990;61:1051–1061.

212. Yamaguchi Y, Mann DM, Ruoslahti E. Negative regulation of transforming growth factor-β by the proteoglycan, decorin. Nature 1990; 346:281–283.

213. Brandes ME, Wakefield LM, Wahl SM. Modulation of monocyte type I transforming growth factor-β receptors by inflammatory stimuli. J Biol Chem 1991;266:19697–19703.

214. Bogdan C, Paik J, Vodovotz, Y, Nathan C. Contrasting mechansims for suppression of macrophage cytokine release by transforming growth factor-β and interleukin-10. J Biol Chem 1992;267:23301–23308.

215. Tsunawai S, Sporn M, Ding A, Nathan C. Deactivation of macrophages by transforming growth factor-β. Nature 1988;334:260–262.

216. Hart PH, Whitty GA, Piccoli DS, Hamilton JA. Synergistic activation of human monocytes by granulocyte-macrophage colony-stimulating factor and IFN-gamma: increased TNF-alpha but not IL-1 activity. J Immunol 1988; 141:1516–1521.

217. Okada Y, Takeuchi N, Gonoji Y, Nakanishi I, Nagase H, Hayakawa TC. Stimultaneous production of collagenase, matrix metalloproteinase-3 (stromelysin) and tissue inhibitor of metalloproteinases by rheumatoid synovial lining cells. Matrix 1992:(suppl 1)398–399.

218. Okada Y, Takeuchi N, Tomita K, Nakanishi I, Nagase H. Immunolocalization of matrix metalloproteinase 3 (stromelysin) in rheumatoid synovioblasts (B cells): correlation with rheumatoid arthritis. Ann Rheum Dis 1989; 48:645–653.

219. Case JP, Lafyatis R, Remmers EF, Kumkumian GK, Wilder RL. Transin/stromelysin expression in rheumatoid synovium. Am J Pathol 1989;135:1055–1064.

220. Woolley DE, Crossley MJ, Evanson JM. Collagenase at sites of cartilage erosion in the rheumatoid joint. Arthritis Rheum 1977;20:1231–1239.

221. Dayer JM, Krane SM, Russell RGG, Robinson DR. Production of collagenase and prostaglandins by isolated adherent rheumatoid synovial cells. Proc Natl Acad Sci USA 1976; 73:945–949.

222. Unemori EN, Hibbs MS, Amento EP. Constitutive expression of a 92-kd gelatinase (type V collagenase) by rheumatoid synovial fibroblasts and its induction in normal human fibroblasts by inflammatory cytokines. J Clin Invest 1991;88:1656–1662.

223. Walakovits LA, Moore VL, Bhardwaj N, Gallick GS, Lark MW. Detection of stromelysin and collagenase in synovial fluid from patients with rheumatoid arthritis and posttraumatic knee injury. Arthritis Rheum 1992;35:35.

224. Werb Z. Proteinases and matrix degradation. In: Kelley WN, Devita VT, Dupont HL, eds. Textbook of rheumatology. Philadelphia: W.B. Saunders, 1989:300–321.

225. Woessner JF. Matrix metalloproteinases and their inhibi-

tors in connective tissue remodeling. FASEB J 1991;5: 2145–2154.

226. Mizel SB, Dayer J-M, Krane SM, Mergenhagen SE. Stimulation of rheumatoid synovial cell collagenase and prostaglandin production by partially purified lymphocyte-activating factor (interleukin-1). Proc Natl Acad Sci USA 1981; 78:2474–2477.

227. Quinones S, Saus J, Otani Y, Harris ED, Kurkinen M. Transcriptional regulation of human stromelysin. J Biol Chem 1989;264:8339–8344.

228. Dower SK, Sims JW, Cerretti DP, Bird TA. The interleukin-1 system: receptors, ligands, and signals. In: Kishimoto T, ed. Interleukins: molecular biology and immunology. Basel: Karger, 1992:33–54.

229. Krane SN, Conca W, Stephenson ML, Amento EP, Goldring MB. Mechanisms of matrix degradation in rheumatoid arthritis. Ann NY Acad Sci 1990;580:340–354.

230. Symons JA, Eastgate JA, Duff GW. Purification and characterization of a novel soluble receptor for interleukin 1. J Exp Med 1991;174:1251–1254.

231. Symons JA, Eastgate JA, Duff GW. A soluble binding protein specific for interleukin-1β is produced by activated mononuclear cells. Cytokine 1990;2:190–198.

232. Fanslow WC, Sims JE, Sassenfeld H, et al. Regulation of alloreactivity in vivo by a soluble form of the interleukin-1 receptor. Science 1990;248:739–742.

233. Arend WP, Joslin FG, Massoni RJ. Effects of immune complexes on production by human monocytes of interleukin 1 or an interleukin 1 inhibitor. J Immunol 1985;134:3868–3875.

234. Balavoine J-F, de Rochemonteix B, Williamson P, Seckinger P, Cruchaud A, and Dayer J-M. Prostaglandin E₂ and collagenase production by fibroblasts and synovial cells is regulated by urine-derived human interleukin 1 and inhibitor(s). J Clin Invest 1986;78:1120–1124.

235. Dripps DJ, Brandhuber BJ, Thompson RC, Eisenberg SP. Interleukin-1 (IL-1) receptor antagonist binds to the 80-kDa IL-1 receptor but does not intitiate IL-1 signal transduction. J Biol Chem 1991;266:10331–10336.

236. Shields J, Bernasconi LM, Benotto W, Shaw AR, Mazzei GJ Production of a 26,000 dalton interleukin inhibitor by human monocytes is regulated by granulocyte-macrophage colony-stimulating factor. Cytokine 1990;2:122–128.

237. Turner M, Chantry D, Katsikis P, Berger A, Brennan FM, Feldmann M. Induction of the interleukin 1 receptor antagonist protein by transforming growth factor-β. Eur J Immunol 1991;21:1635–1639.

238. Firestein GS, Berger AE, Tracey DE, et al. IL-1 receptor antagonist protein production and gene expression in rheumatoid arthritis and osteoarthritis synovium. J Immunol 1992;149:1059–1062.

239. Smith RJ, En Chin J, Sam LM, Justen JM. Biologic effects of an interleukin-1 receptor antagonist protein on interleukin-1-stimulated cartilage erosion and chondrocyte responsiveness. Arthritis Rheum 1991;34:78–83.

240. Henderson B, Thompson RC, Hardingham T, Lewthwaite J. Inhibition of interleukin 1-induced synovitis and articular cartilage proteoglycan loss in the rabbit knee by recombinant human interleukin-1 receptor antagonist. Cytokine 1991;3:246–249.

241. Wooley PH, Whalen JD, Chapman DL, et al. The effect of an interleukin-1 receptor antagonist protein on type II collagen and antigen-induced arthritis in mice. Arthritis Rheum 1990;33:S20.

242. Arend WP. Interleukin 1 receptor antagonist. J Clin Invest 1991;88:1445–1451.

243. Svenson M, Poulsen K, Fornsgaard A, Bendtzen K. IgG autoantibodies against interleukin-1α in sera of normal individuals. Scand J Immunol 1989;29:489–492.

244. Saklatvala J. Tumor necrosis factor α stimulates resorption and inhibits synthesis of proteoglycan in cartilage. Nature 1986;322:547–549.

245. Bertolini DR, Nedwin GE, Bringman TS, Smith DE, Mundy GR. Stimulation of bone resorption in vitro by human tumor necrosis factor. Nature 1986;319:516–518.

246. Engelmann H, Aderka D, Rubinstein M, Rotman D, Wallach D. A tumor necrosis factor-binding protein purified to homogeneity from human urine protects cells from tumor necrosis factor toxicity. J Biol Chem 1989;264:11974–11980.

247. Engelmann H, Novick D, Wallach D. Two tumor necrosis factor-finding proteins purified from human urine: evidence for immunological cross-reactivity with cell surface tumor necrosis factor receptors. J Biol Chem 1990; 265:1531–1536.

248. van Zee KJ, Kohno T, Fischer E, Rock C, Moldawer LL, Lowry SF. Tumor necrosis factor soluble receptors circulate during experimental and clinical inflammation and can protect against excessive tumor necrosis factor-α in vitro and in vivo. Proc Natl Acad Sci USA 1992;89:4845–4849.

249. Lesslauer W, Tabuchi H, Gentz R, Brockhaus M. Recombinant soluble tumor necrosis factor receptor proteins protect mice from lipopolysaccharide-induced lethality. Eur J Immunol 1991;21:2883–2886.

250. Ashkenazi A, Marsters SA, Capon DJ, et al. Protection against endotoxic shock by a tumor necrosis factor receptor immunoadhesin. Proc Natl Acad Sci USA 1991;88: 10535–10539.

251. Winzen R, Wallach D, Kemper O, Resch K, Holtmann H. Selective upregulation of the 75kDa tumor necrosis factor (TNF) receptor and its mRNA by TNF and IL-1. J Immunol 1993;150:4346–4353.

252. Unemori EN, Amento EP, Bauer EA, Horuk R. Melanoma growth-stimulatory activity/GRO decreases collagen expression by human fibroblasts. J Biol Chem 1993;268: 1338–1342.

253. Ishikawa O, Yamakage A, LeRoy EC, Trojanowska M. Persistent effect of TGF beta 1 on extracellular matrix gene expression in human dermal fibroblasts. Biochem Biophys Res Commun 1990;169:232–238.

254. Rossi R, Karsenty G, Roberts AB, Roche NS, Sporn MB, de-Crombrugghe B. A nuclear factor 1 binding site mediates the transcriptional activation of a type I collagen promoter by transforming growth factor-beta. Cell 1988;52:405–414.

255. Raghow R, Postlethwaite AE, Keski-Oja J, Moses HL, Kang AH. Transforming growth factor-beta increases steady state levels of type I procollagen and fibronectin messenger RNAs postranscriptionally in cultured human dermal fibroblasts. J Clin Invest 1987;79:1285–1288.

256. Kim S-J, Glick A, Sporn MB, Roberts AB. Characterization of the promoter region of the human transforming growth factor-β gene responsive to GF-B1 autoinduction. J Biol Chem 1989;264:7041–7045.

257. Edwards DR, Murphy G, Reynolds JJ, Whitman SE, Docherty AJP, Angel P. Transforming growth factor beta modulates the expression of collagenase and metalloproteinase inhibitor. EMBO J 1987;6:1899–1904.

258. Kerr LD, Olashaw NE, Matrisian LM. Transforming growth factor β1 and cAMP inhibit transcription of epidermal growth factor- and oncogene-induced transin RNA. J Biol Chem 1988;263:16999–17005.

259. Redini F, Lafuma C, Pujol J-P, Robert L, Hornebecke W. Effect of cytokines and growth factors on the expression of elastase activity by human synoviocytes, dermal fibroblasts, and rabbit articular chondrocytes. Biochem Biophys Res Commun 1988;155:786–793.

260. Overall CM, Wrana JL, Sokek J. Transforming factor-beta regulation of collagenase, 72kDa-progelatinase, TIMP, and PAI-1 expression in rat bone cell populations and human fibroblasts. Connect Tissue Res 1989;20:289–294.

261. Laiho M, Saksela D, Keski-Oja J. Transforming growth factor-β induction of type 1 plasminogen activator inhibitor. J Biol Chem 1987;262:17467–17474.

262. Kuruvilla AP, Shah R, Hochwald GM, Liggitt HD, Palladino MA, Thorbecke GJ. Protective effect of transforming growth factor β1 on experimental autoimmune diseases in mice. Proc Natl Acad Sci USA 1991;88:2918–2921.

263. Brandes ME, Allen JB, Ogawa Y, Wahl SM. Transforming growth factor β1 suppresses acute and chronic arthritis in experimental animals. J Clin Invest 1991;87:1108–1113.

264. Saarialho-Kere U, Welgus HG, Parks WC. Distinct mechanisms regulate interstitial collagenase and 92-kDa gelatinase expression in human monocytic-like cells exposed to bacterial endotoxin. J Biol Chem 1993;268:17354–17361.

265. Welgus HC, Campbell EJ, Cury JD, et al. Neutral metalloproteinases produced by human mononuclear phagocytes. J Clin Invest 1990;86:1496–1502.

266. Lacraz S, Nicod L, Galve-de Rochemonteix B, Baumberger C, Dayer J-M, Welgus HG. Suppression of metalloproteinase biosynthesis in human alveolar macrophages by interleukin-4. J Clin Invest 1992;90:382–388.

267. Campbell EJ, Silverman EK, Campbell MA. Elastase and cathepsin G of human monocytes: quantification of cellular content, release in response to stimuli, and heterogeneity in elastase-mediated proteolytic activity. J Immunol 1989;143:2961–2968.

268. Shapiro SD, Campbell EJ, Kobayashi DK, Welgus HG. Immune modulation of metalloproteinase production in human macrophages. Selective pretranslational suppression of interstitial collagenase and stromelysin biosynthesis by interferon-gamma. J Clin Invest 1990;86:1204–1210.

269. Unemori EN, Bair M, Bauer EA, Amento EP. Stromelysin expression regulates collagenase activation in human fibroblasts. Dissociable control of two metalloproteinases by interferon-γ. J Biol Chem 1992;266:23477–23482.

PART 3

CYTOKINES AS MODULATORS OF PHYSIOLOGICAL FUNCTION

CHAPTER 14

ROLE OF CYTOKINES IN LIPID METABOLISM AND CACHEXIA

Riaz A. Memon, Kenneth R. Feingold, and Carl Grunfeld

The host response to infection and inflammation is usually accompanied by profound alterations in lipid metabolism, such as hypertriglyceridemia, increased lipogenesis, and decreased fatty acid (FA) oxidation and ketogenesis. Infection or endotoxin (lipopolysaccharide [LPS]) administration stimulates in many different cell types the production of a wide array of cytokines, the hormones of the immune system. Cytokines are key mediators of several physiological and pathological responses that occur during the course of infection. It is now apparent that cytokines, in addition to mediating immune and inflammatory responses, also influence lipid, glucose, and protein metabolism.

Chronic low-grade infection may also lead to cachexia, or wasting, and it has been hypothesized that cachexia associated with infection and cancer is mediated by cytokines. Because changes in lipid metabolism and cachexia may occur simultaneously during infection, it was initially proposed that a single factor, cachectin (now known as tumor necrosis factor [TNF]), caused both hypertriglyceridemia and cachexia by decreasing the clearance of triglyceride (TG)-rich lipoproteins and by decreasing the storage of fat in adipose tissue. However, many recent in vitro and in vivo studies on the metabolic effects of cytokines indicate that the pathophysiology of cachexia is much more complex than originally proposed. Multiple cytokines have overlapping effects on lipid and protein metabolism. Moreover, there are often differences between in vitro and in vivo effects of cytokines on lipid metabolism.

We summarize the changes in lipid metabolism that occur during infection and the mechanisms involved in producing these changes. We also discuss the role of cytokines in mediating these alterations. Finally, we review the role of cytokines in the pathogenesis of cachexia and its potential relationship to the changes associated with lipid metabolism.

INFECTION AND LIPID METABOLISM

Hypertriglyceridemia is a consistent finding in bacterial, viral, and protozoal infections, and it is characterized by an increase in very low density lipoprotein (VLDL) levels (1–5). Infection may increase VLDL production by stimulating de novo FA synthesis or by increasing the delivery of FA from adipose tissue (6–8). These FA are then re-esterified in the liver and secreted as VLDL. Infection may also increase VLDL levels by decreasing the activity of lipoprotein lipase (LPL), the enzyme responsible for catabolism of TG-rich lipoproteins, which results in decreased VLDL clearance (9,10). We recently showed that low doses of LPS increase serum TG levels by stimulating hepatic VLDL production, whereas high doses of LPS increase serum TG levels by decreasing LPL activity and TG clearance (11).

The effects of infection and LPS administration on cholesterol metabolism are variable between rodents and primates. These findings are in marked contrast to the effects of infection on TG metabolism, which are very similar in all species. Infection or LPS administration increase serum cholesterol levels and hepatic cholesterol synthesis in rodents (12–14), whereas infection produces hypocholesterolemia in nonhuman primates and humans (4,5,15). The mechanisms responsible for these interspecies differences during infection are not clear; however, there are marked differences in lipoprotein metabolism in rodents and primates. Rodents have low levels of LDL and high levels of high density lipoprotein (HDL), whereas primates have high LDL and low HDL levels.

In addition to the changes in TG and cholesterol metabolism, infection or endotoxin administration produce several alterations in the ketone body (KB) metabolism, which lead to significant decreases in hepatic and plasma KB levels (16). Reduction in KB levels could theoretically be caused by (a) suppression of adipose tissue lipolysis, which would decrease influx of FA substrate to the liver for KB synthesis; (b) increased hepatic levels of malonyl-CoA, the first committed intermediate in FA synthesis, and a potent inhibitor of carnitine-palmitoyltransferase-I (CPT-I), the rate-limiting enzyme in FA oxidation and ketogenesis; and (c) increased peripheral utilization of KB. Several studies have shown that all these mechanisms may be involved in the suppression of ketogenesis during infection (17–19).

The changes in lipid metabolism (i.e., enhanced lipogenesis and suppressed ketogenesis) are opposite to the expected effects that would be induced by the hormones stimulated during infection. There is a pronounced increase in plasma epinephrine, cortisol, and glucagon levels, whereas plasma insulin levels are either constant or slightly elevated during infection (17,20,21). Table 14–1 compares the typical hormonal response and the changes in lipid metabolism seen during fed and fasting states with the metabolic changes observed during infection. These hormonal changes should facilitate KB production

and suppress lipogenesis during infection. Therefore, circulating factors other than the classic hormones must be responsible for mediating changes in lipid metabolism during infection.

CYTOKINES AND LIPID METABOLISM

Availability of recombinant cytokines, such as TNF, interleukins (ILs), and interferons (IFNs), has facilitated investigation of the role of cytokines in disturbances of lipid metabolism during infection. This is a relatively new area of investigation, and the metabolic effects of several cytokines have not yet been studied in detail.

Cytokines and triglyceride metabolism

Administration of TNF rapidly increases serum TG levels in rats (22–24). This effect of TNF is acute in onset. The increase in TG levels is observed as early as 1 hour after TNF, it peaks by 2 hours, and it is sustained for at least 17 hours (22). TNF is able to increase serum TG levels under a variety of dietary conditions, ranging from a high sucrose diet, which stimulates endogenous FA synthesis, to a high fat diet, which suppresses endogenous FA synthesis (23). The increase in serum TG levels after TNF administration is due to an increase in VLDL of normal composition (24). TNF treatment has also been shown to increase serum TG levels in mice (25), nonhuman primates (26), and humans (27).

Early in vitro studies in cultured mouse adipocytes reported that TNF decreases the activity of LPL; thus, it was hypothesized that TNF produces hypertriglyceridemia by decreasing the clearance of TG-rich lipoproteins (28). However, TNF does not decrease LPL activity in

TABLE 14–1   COMPARATIVE EFFECTS OF INFECTION AND FED AND FASTING STATE ON LIPID METABOLISM AND SERUM HORMONE LEVELS

| Status | Hormone Levels | | | | Metabolic Effect | |
	Insulin*	Glucagon[†]	EPI[‡]	Cortisol[‡]	Lipogenesis	Ketogenesis
Fed	↑	↓	↓	↓	Stimulated	Inhibited
Fasting	↓	↑	↑	↑	Inhibited	Stimulated
Infection	↔/↑	↑	↑	↑	Stimulated	Inhibited

*Insulin stimulates lipogenesis and inhibits ketogenesis.
[†]Glucagon inhibits lipogenesis and stimulates ketogenesis.
[‡]EPI and cortisol enhance lipolysis and stimulate ketogenesis.
EPI = epinephrine; ↑ = increased; ↓ = decreased; ↔ = no change.

human adipocytes (29). Several in vivo studies also indicate that TNF-induced acute hypertriglyceridemia may not be mediated through the suppression of LPL activity (30–33).

Although it has been shown that TNF decreases LPL activity in epididymal fat pads in vivo, this decrease requires several hours, whereas the increase in serum TG levels occurs rapidly, and it precedes the effect of TNF on LPL activity (30). Moreover, TNF administration does not decrease LPL activity in many other adipose tissue sites or in muscle (30,31). In fact, TNF has been shown to increase total postheparin plasma lipase and hepatic lipase activity (31). Finally, TNF treatment does not decrease clearance of TG-rich lipoproteins from the circulation (32–34).

The other potential mechanism for increasing TG levels is increased VLDL production secondary to either an increase in hepatic FA synthesis or an increased mobilization of FA from the periphery (6–11). Recent studies indicate that TNF increases serum TG levels by rapidly increasing production of VLDL (32,34,35). TNF increases total hepatic TG synthesis, and the newly synthesized TGs are secreted as VLDL by the liver (35). TNF also induces a rapid increase in hepatic de novo FA synthesis that is observed within 1 to 2 hours of administration, and it is sustained for 17 hours (22). The time course of the effects of TNF on hepatic FA synthesis, hepatic TG synthesis, and VLDL secretion are consistent with the time course for TNF-induced increases in serum TG levels in vivo (22,32,35). TNF also stimulates hepatic FA synthesis in insulinopenic diabetic animals (33,34) and in adrenalectomized rats (36), suggesting that its effect on hepatic lipid synthesis is direct rather than being mediated through insulin, cortisol, or catecholamines.

In addition to stimulating hepatic FA and TG synthesis, TNF acutely stimulates lipolysis under certain dietary conditions, and these peripherally derived FA also contribute to the increase in hepatic VLDL production (37). In chow-fed animals, TNF acutely increases circulating free FA levels by inducing lipolysis. When these animals are pretreated with phenylisopropyladenosine (PIA), an inhibitor of lipolysis (38), the effect of TNF on lipolysis is abolished (37). More importantly, PIA treatment significantly blunts the effect of TNF on serum TG levels. However, TNF still stimulates hepatic FA synthesis, which results in a small but significant increase in serum TG levels. Thus, in chow-fed animals, both increased de novo FA synthesis and increased lipolysis contribute to the TNF-induced increase in serum TG levels (37). In contrast, in sucrose-fed animals, TNF does not stimulate lipolysis, and pretreatment with PIA has no effect on TNF-induced increases in serum TG levels. However, in sucrose-fed rats, TNF-stimulated FA synthesis is much higher, and it provides more FA substrate for TG synthesis. Thus, in sucrose-fed animals, TNF-induced increases

in serum TG levels are primarily due to stimulation of hepatic FA synthesis (37).

TNF does not exert any effect on the activity of hepatic enzymes involved in esterification of FA to glycerol (37), suggesting that the TNF-induced increase in hepatic TG synthesis is primarily driven by the availability of the FA substrate, which is provided by either hepatic synthesis or lipolysis. Thus, it is not surprising that prolonged starvation abolishes the effect of TNF on hepatic FA synthesis and serum TG levels (23), suggesting that nutritional status may be an important factor in modulating the mechanisms by which TNF increases serum TGs.

Recent studies indicate that several other cytokines also influence TG metabolism in vitro. In cultured adipocytes, IL-1, IL-6, lymphotoxin, IFN-α, IFN-γ, and leukemia inhibitory factor (LIF) have been shown to decrease LPL activity (39–43). In addition to TNF, lymphotoxin, IFN-α, and IFN-γ suppress de novo FA synthesis in cultured fat cells (39–43). IL-1 and LIF increase lipogenesis. Finally, TNF, IL-1, LIF and all three IFNs stimulate lipolysis in adipocytes (44). These effects of cytokines on fat cell metabolism require several hours of incubation. The in vitro effects of cytokines on TG metabolism are summarized in Table 14–2.

In contrast to these delayed in vitro effects on adipocytes, several cytokines acutely alter TG metabolism in intact animals. In vivo administration of IL-1, IL-6, lymphotoxin, and IFN-α to mice (45,46) or platelet-activating factor (PAF) to rats (47) rapidly produced an increase in hepatic FA synthesis. The ability of cytokines to induce hepatic FA synthesis is not an effect common to all cytokines, because several other cytokines, such as IL-2, and IFN-γ, do not stimulate hepatic FA synthesis under similar conditions (45). The effect of IL-1 and IFN-α on hepatic FA synthesis is sustained for several hours (45), whereas the effect of IL-6 on FA synthesis is transient (46).

IL-1 acutely increases serum TG levels in rats (48). Similar to TNF, IL-1 increases serum TG levels by stimulating hepatic FA synthesis and VLDL secretion, and not by decreasing the clearance of TG-rich lipoproteins (48). However, unlike TNF, IL-1 does not stimulate lipolysis; hence, its effect on serum TG levels is primarily due to enhanced hepatic FA synthesis and TG secretion. IFN-α and IFN-γ stimulate lipolysis in vivo (49). IFN-α and IFN-γ treatment have been shown to increase serum TG levels in humans (50–53). There is a strong correlation between hypertriglyceridemia and circulating IFN-α levels in patients with acquired immunodeficiency syndrome (AIDS) (54). Furthermore, IFN-α levels also correlate with decreases in LPL activity and TG clearance and increases in basal hepatic FA synthesis in patients with human immunodeficiency virus infection and AIDS, suggesting that several mechanisms could account for the effects of IFN-α on TG metabolism (55,56). IFN-γ

TABLE 14–2   IN VITRO EFFECTS OF CYTOKINES IN CULTURED MOUSE ADIPOCYTES

Cytokine	LPL Activity	FA Synthesis	Lipolysis
TNF	↓	↓	↑
IL-1	↓	↑	↑
IL-6	↓	?	↔
Lymphotoxin	↓	↓	↑
IFN-α	↓	↓	↑
IFN-γ	↓	↓	↑
LIF	↓	↑	↑

LPL = lipoprotein lipase; FA = fatty acid; TNF = tumor necrosis factor; IL = interleukin; IFN = interferon; LIF = leukemia inhibitory factor; ↓ = decreased; ↑ = increased; ↔ = no change; ? = not determined.

administration is also associated with inhibition of postheparin plasma lipase activity, suggesting that IFN-γ may impair the clearance of TG-rich lipoproteins (52). Table 14–3 summarizes the in vivo effects of cytokines on TG metabolism.

Studies on the mechanisms of cytokine stimulation of hepatic FA synthesis suggest that the lipogenic cytokines can be divided into two classes (57). Class I cytokines include TNF, IL-1, and IL-6. These cytokines stimulate hepatic FA synthesis by acutely increasing the hepatic levels of citrate, an allosteric activator of acetyl-CoA carboxylase, which is the rate-limiting enzyme in FA synthesis (57). Class II cytokines include IFN-α, which has no effect on hepatic citrate levels, and the mechanism by which it stimulates FA synthesis is not yet known. The stimulatory effects of TNF or IL-1 and IFN-α on hepatic FA synthesis are synergistic, whereas there is no such synergy in stimulating FA synthesis among the cytokines from the same class (57).

Finally, IL-4, which has marked inhibitory effects on the regulation of immune responses, blocks the stimulatory effects of TNF, IL-1, and IL-6 on hepatic FA synthesis by preventing the increase in hepatic citrate levels (58). In contrast, IL-4 is unable to block the stimulation of FA synthesis induced by IFN-α (58), which, as discussed, does not increase citrate levels. These results suggest that cytokines use multiple mechanisms and complex interactions to regulate hepatic lipid metabolism, and that regulation of lipid metabolism by cytokines is analogous to cytokine regulation of the immune system.

Cytokines and cholesterol metabolism

As seen with infection and LPS administration, the effects of TNF and IL-1 differ between rodents and primates. TNF and IL-1 produce a significant increase in serum cholesterol levels in mice (25). TNF also increases serum cholesterol levels in rats by increasing TG-rich VLDL and LDL levels (24). TNF and IL-1 stimulate hepatic cholesterol synthesis in mice, an effect that is delayed in onset and is observed 16 hours after cytokine treatment (45). In addition to TNF and IL-1, several other cytokines, such as lymphotoxin and IFN-γ, also stimulate hepatic cholesterol synthesis in mice (45). TNF and IL-1 increase the activity of hepatic hydroxymethylglutaryl coenzyme A (HMG-CoA) reductase (25), the rate-limiting enzyme in endogenous cholesterol synthesis, suggesting that they increase hepatic cholesterol synthesis by increasing the activity of HMG-CoA reductase. Finally, pretreatment of mice with antibodies against TNF abolishes the effect of LPS on serum cholesterol levels, hepatic cholesterol synthesis, and hepatic HMG-CoA reductase activity (25). This finding indicates that TNF is an in vivo mediator of the effect of LPS on cholesterol metabolism in mice.

In primates, TNF decreases serum cholesterol levels (26). This cholesterol-lowering effect is observed 24 hours after TNF administration. The TNF-induced decrease in serum cholesterol levels is associated with a significant decrease in cholesteryl ester content in the LDL and HDL fractions (26). TNF also decreases the concentrations of apolipoprotein B and A-1, the major apoproteins of LDL and HDL, respectively (59). TNF decreases the activity and mass of lecithin:cholesterol acyltransferase in primates, which may account for the low cholesteryl ester concentration in plasma (26). In contrast to TNF, IL-1 has no effect on cholesterol metabolism in primates (59).

Viral infections have been associated with a decrease in serum cholesterol levels in humans, and it has been postulated that this decrease may be the result of IFN induction (60). Recombinant IFNs lower serum cholesterol levels in humans (61–64). IFN-α and IFN-γ produce a significant decrease in both HDL and LDL cholesterol levels, whereas the IFN-β–induced decrease in serum cholesterol levels is primarily due to a decrease in LDL cholesterol levels (60–64). A recent study demonstrated that IFN-β decreased the synthesis of apolipoprotein B in nor-

TABLE 14–3 IN VIVO EFFECTS OF CYTOKINES ON TRIGLYCERIDE (TG) METABOLISM

Cytokine	Serum TG	Hepatic FAS	VLDL Secretion	VLDL Clearance	LPL Activity
TNF	↑	↑	↑	↔	↓
IL-1	↑	↑	↑	↔	?
IL-6	↔	↑	?	?	↓
IFN-α	↑	↑	?	?	?
IFN-γ	↑	↔	?	?	↓
Lymphotoxin	?	↑	?	?	?
PAF	↑	↑	?	?	?

FAS = fatty acid synthesis; VLDL = very low density lipoprotein; LPL = lipoprotein lipase; TNF = tumor necrosis factor; IL = interleukin; IFN = interferon; PAF = platelet-activating factor; ↓ = decreased; ↑ = increased; ↔ = no change; ? = not determined.

mal subjects, suggesting that it may lower serum cholesterol levels through reduction in the LDL production rate (65). It is not known whether the IFN-α– and IFN-γ–induced decrease in serum cholesterol levels is the result of decreased synthesis or increased clearance of lipoproteins.

Granulocyte-macrophage colony-stimulating factor (GM-CSF), a growth factor that stimulates proliferation and differentiation of hematopoietic progenitor cells, produces a significant decrease in serum cholesterol levels in humans, as well as in primates (66,67). The decrease in serum cholesterol levels is primarily due to a decrease in LDL cholesterol levels, with a variable effect on HDL cholesterol (67). It appears that the GM-CSF–induced decrease in serum cholesterol levels is due to an increase in the number of LDL receptors in spleen and bone marrow cells, which results in enhanced clearance of lipoproteins (68). The effects of cytokines on cholesterol metabolism in rodents and primates are summarized in Table 14-4 and 14–5, respectively.

Cytokines and ketone body metabolism

Similar to infection or LPS administration, low doses of TNF and IL-1 acutely decrease serum KB levels in mice in the fed state (69). However, only IL-1 is able to decrease serum KB levels in the fasting state, as is seen with LPS. Moreover, only IL-1 exerts a sustained antiketogenic effect. IL-1 also decreases hepatic KB production, whereas TNF has no such effect on hepatic KB levels (69). IL-6 has no effect on either serum or hepatic KB levels (70).

Serum KB levels are regulated by their rate of production in the liver, and also by their rate of utilization in the peripheral tissues. In contrast, the rate of KB production in the liver is dependent on the flux of FA substrate from the periphery and the ketogenic capacity of the liver, which is regulated by hepatic malonyl-CoA levels (71).

Malonyl-CoA is the first committed intermediate in FA synthesis, and it is an allosteric inhibitor of CPT-I, the rate-limiting enzyme in FA oxidation and ketogenesis. Several hormones regulate ketogenesis, either by their effects on peripheral lipolysis or through a direct action on the liver by altering the levels of malonyl-CoA or the activity of CPT-I (72).

In the fed state, IL-1 exerts its antiketogenic effect by increasing the levels of hepatic malonyl-CoA (69), a potent inhibitor of CPT-I. Inhibition of CPT-I prevents the entry of FA into the mitochondria for oxidation and KB synthesis. In the fasting state, in addition to raising hepatic malonyl-CoA levels, IL-1 also suppresses lipolysis and thereby decreases the mobilization of FA substrate to the liver (69). It is not known whether IL-1 has an effect on the peripheral utilization of KB.

Similar to IL-1, TNF also increases hepatic malonyl-CoA levels, but it has no effect on hepatic KB levels (69). The reason for this difference between TNF and IL-1 is the fact that TNF also exerts a stimulatory effect on lipolysis, resulting in an increased flux of FA substrate to the liver. The increased FA flux counterbalances the inhibitory effect of malonyl-CoA on hepatic KB production by providing additional substrate (69). This conclusion is supported by experiments in which it was demonstrated that when the lipolytic effect of TNF is blocked by pretreatment with PIA, a potent inhibitor of lipolysis, TNF produces a marked decrease in hepatic KB levels (69). Moreover, a lower dose of TNF, which does not stimulate lipolysis but does increase FA synthesis and malonyl-CoA levels, also lowers hepatic KB levels. Finally, kinetic studies in rats show that TNF decreases the rate of hepatic KB production (73). TNF may also increase peripheral utilization of KB, which may lead to a decrease in serum KB levels.

The inhibitory effect of IL-1 and TNF on hepatic ketogenesis indicates that FA substrate is directed away from oxidation; these FA are then available for re-esterification (i.e., TG synthesis), which results in increased VLDL

TABLE 14–4   IN VIVO EFFECTS OF CYTOKINES ON CHOLESTEROL METABOLISM IN RODENTS

Cytokine	Serum Cholesterol	Hepatic Cholesterol Synthesis	HMG-CoA R Activity
TNF	↑	↑	↑
IL-1	↑	↑	↑
Lymphotoxin	?	↑	?
IFN-α	↔	↔	?
IFN-γ	↔	↑	?

HMG-CoA R = hepatic hydroxymethylglutaryl coenzyme A reductase; TNF = tumor necrosis factor; IL = interleukin; IFN = interferon; ↓ = decreased; ↑ = increased; ↔ = no change; ? = not determined.

secretion. Hence, the antiketogenic effect of IL-1 and TNF is probably another mechanism by which these cytokines increase VLDL production.

In contrast to IL-1 and TNF, the effects of IFNs on KB metabolism are markedly different (49). IFN-γ exerts a dose-dependent stimulatory effect on lipolysis, resulting in an increased flux of FA to the liver. IFN-γ also increases serum and hepatic KB levels. IFN-γ has no effect on hepatic FA synthesis or malonyl-CoA levels. When the lipolytic effect of IFN-γ is blocked by prior treatment with PIA, the stimulatory effect of IFN-γ on hepatic KB production is abolished, suggesting that the ketogenic effect of IFN-γ is secondary to its effect on substrate mobilization from the periphery (49).

The effects of IFN-α on ketogenesis are more complex. IFN-α stimulates lipolysis in a dose-dependent manner, but its effect on serum and hepatic KB levels is biphasic (49). At low doses, IFN-α raises serum and hepatic KB levels, whereas at higher doses, it does not alter KB levels. At low doses, IFN-α has no effect on hepatic FA synthesis or malonyl-CoA levels; hence, it increases KB levels primarily by substrate mobilization. Thus, at low doses, the effect of IFN-α is very similar to that of IFN-γ (49).

In contrast, at higher doses, IFN-α also stimulates he-

patic FA synthesis, and it increases malonyl-CoA levels, which counteracts its lipolytic effect by inhibiting CPT-I and preventing the entry of FA into the mitochondria for oxidation and KB formation. When lipolysis induced by higher doses of IFN-α is blocked by prior treatment with PIA, IFN-α produces a decrease in hepatic KB levels, suggesting that in the absence of enhanced lipolysis, IFN-α can be antiketogenic by virtue of its effect on hepatic malonyl-CoA levels. Thus, at higher doses, the effect of IFN-α on ketogenesis resembles TNF (49).

Finally, in the fasting state, when IFN-α does not induce lipolysis, it lowers hepatic KB levels by increasing hepatic malonyl-CoA levels; thus, in the fasting state, IFN-α may act similar to IL-1 on KB metabolism. The complex interactions between the peripheral and hepatic effects of cytokines and their net effect on hepatic ketogenesis are summarized in Table 14–6.

The results of these in vivo studies reveal that unlike the effects of cytokines on lipogenesis, which are very similar, the effects of cytokines on ketogenesis are very different. The effects of cytokines on various aspects of lipid metabolism can be extremely complex in vivo, and they may depend on dose, timing of administration, and nutritional status.

TABLE 14–5   IN VIVO EFFECTS OF CYTOKINES ON CHOLESTEROL IN PRIMATES

Cytokine	Serum Cholesterol	LCAT Activity	LDL Receptors
TNF	↓	↓	?
IL-1	↔	↔	?
IFN-α	↓	?	?
IFN-β	↓	?	?
IFN-γ	↓	?	?
GM-CSF	↓	?	↑

LCAT = lecithin cholesterol acyltransferase; LDL = low density lipoprotein; TNF = tumor necrosis factor; IL = interleukin; IFN = interferon; GM-CSF = granulocyte-macrophage colony-stimulating factor; ↓ = decreased; ↑ = increased; ↔ = no change; ? = not determined.

TABLE 14–6   IN VIVO EFFECTS OF CYTOKINES ON LIPOLYSIS AND HEPATIC KETOGENESIS

Cytokine	Lipolysis	Malonyl-CoA Levels	Hepatic KB Levels
TNF (low dose)	↔	↑	↓
TNF (high dose)	↑	↑	↔
IL-1	↔	↑	↓
IFN-γ	↑	↔	↑
IFN-α (low dose)	↑	↔	↑
IFN-α (high dose)	↑	↑	↔
IL-6	↔	↔	↔

KB = ketone bodies; TNF = tumor necrosis factor; IL = interleukin; IFN = interferon; ↓ = decreased; ↑ = increased; ↔ = no change.

ROLE OF CYTOKINES IN THE PATHOGENESIS OF CACHEXIA

Cachexia, or the wasting syndrome, is characterized by persistent weight loss and abnormalities in carbohydrate, protein, and lipid metabolism. During the last several years, various investigators have postulated a role for different cytokines in the pathogenesis of cachexia. Cytokines that have been proposed to have a role in the pathophysiology of cachexia include TNF, IL-1, IL-6, IFN-γ, LIF, and TGF-β. These cytokines induce a wide spectrum of physiological and pathological effects that can be either beneficial or deleterious to the host. Whether these effects are beneficial or harmful depends on several factors, such as amount of stimulation of cytokine release; duration of cytokine release; extent of the host exposure to the cytokine; interactions among cytokines that can be antagonistic, additive, or synergistic; and, finally, nutritional status of the organism.

On the basis of early studies in cultured adipocytes, it was proposed that the TNF-induced decrease in adipose tissue LPL and de novo FA synthesis, along with an increase in lipolysis, could result in decreased TG clearance and inhibition of fat storage in adipose tissue. It was therefore proposed that by altering fat metabolism, TNF could produce both hypertriglyceridemia and cachexia (28). However, recent in vivo and in vitro studies on the effects of TNF and other cytokines indicate that the pathophysiology of cachexia is much more complex than originally proposed.

Many other cytokines, including IL-1, IL-6, IFN-α, IFN-β, IFN-γ, lymphotoxin, and LIF, exert similar catabolic effects in fat cells (38–43). Thus, if increasing fat cell catabolism is the criterion for causing cachexia, then several cytokines share this property. In addition, insulin cannot reverse the catabolic effects of these cytokines on fat cell metabolism (39). This finding is in contrast to the observations in cancer-related cachexia, in which hyperalimentation with increased insulin levels can promote the storage of fat without increasing muscle mass (74). Finally, the in vitro catabolic effects of TNF observed in adipocytes do not occur in vivo under conditions in which TNF increases plasma TG levels. In vivo, TNF administration produces hypertriglyceridemia by increasing hepatic VLDL production rather than by suppressing LPL activity or by decreasing FA synthesis in the adipose tissue (75).

Several investigators have shown that treatment with purified recombinant TNF leads to acute anorexia with weight loss, but that with repeated injections of the same dose of TNF, animals rapidly begin to gain weight (75–80). It was demonstrated in some of these studies that TNF-induced acute weight loss was the result of decreased food intake, decreased water intake, and increased urine output (79). Thus, changes in the food and fluid balance account for all the weight loss. Under these circumstances, there is little evidence for decreased muscle mass, which is the characteristic finding in true cachexia. Although repeated treatment with TNF for several days results in a state of tolerance to its anorectic and diuretic effects and the animals regain weight, the hypertriglyceridemic effect of TNF persists, suggesting that the hypertriglyceridemia of infection is not necessarily linked to cachexia (79). Similarly, there is no correlation between hypertriglyceridemia and wasting during AIDS, because patients with AIDS in whom hypertriglyceridemia develops during the course of their disease often maintain stable weight and body composition for prolonged periods (81).

TNF administration has been associated with chronic weight loss in three different experimental models. First, sequentially increasing the dose of TNF to levels that would initially be lethal produces chronic weight loss, but this loss is mainly due to anorexia because the extent of weight loss is the same in TNF-treated and pair-fed animals (82). Second, persistent anorexia and weight loss develop in chronically catheterized rats infused with TNF. In this experimental model, the muscle mass of TNF-treated rats is similar to that of pair-fed rats (83). Moreover, there could be a synergistic interaction between TNF and other inflammatory products generated at the catheterization site (84–86). Third, implantation in nude mice of a tumor that is genetically engineered to produce continuous secretion of TNF results in chronic weight loss (87). Although the circulating levels of TNF were very high in this animal model of cachexia, there is no evidence of an increase in serum TNF levels in patients with cancer-related cachexia (88,89).

Moreover, the interaction of TNF with other tumor products, cytokines, or growth factors produced by host cells in response to the tumor have not been explored in genetically engineered tumor models. There could be synergistic interactions between different cytokines in tumor-bearing animals which have been shown to be more susceptible to the toxic effects of TNF (90). Thus, the evidence suggesting that TNF is the key mediator of cachexia is inconclusive, and further studies are needed to determine its exact role in the pathogenesis of cachexia.

Unlike the tachyphylaxis to the anorectic effect of TNF, repeated injections of IL-1 induces more sustained anorexia in rodents (91,92). Administration of murine IFN-γ to experimental animals also causes a decline in food intake and weight loss (93). Treatment of cancer patients with IFN-α and IFN-γ has been associated with anorexia and weight loss (94,95). It has also been suggested that IL-6 may mediate tumor-induced anorexia in rodents (96).

Several recent studies have investigated the role of other cytokines in the pathogenesis of cachexia. Administration of monoclonal antibodies against IL-1 receptor to tumor-bearing animals results in decreased tumor growth, improved food intake, and preservation of body fat stores, suggesting that IL-1 may have a role in the progression of cancer-related cachexia (97). Treatment with TGF-β has been shown to induce cachexia and systemic fibrosis in rodents (98). Severe anorexia and profound weight loss develop in nude mice inoculated with genetically engineered Chinese hamster ovary cells, which express either a murine IL-6 gene or a murine IFN-γ gene, as compared with mice injected with cell lines that did not produce these cytokines (99,100). Moreover, hypercalcemia also develops in IL-6–secreting tumor models (99). Similarly, a fatal syndrome characterized by anorexia, abnormalities in calcium metabolism, and severe weight loss also develops in mice engrafted with a genetically engineered cell line to produce LIF (101,102). All these tumor models are similar to the genetically engineered TNF-secreting model (87), and they have the same drawbacks (i.e., interactions between different cytokines produced either by the tumor or by the host cells in response to the tumor and tumor products).

More recently, Strassmann and colleagues (103) re-ported that profound wasting of muscle and fat without anorexia develops in mice bearing the CA-26 adenocarcinoma (103). These tumors were secreting large quantities of IL-6 in vivo, and passive immunization with anti-IL-6 monoclonal antibodies prevented the weight loss associated with tumor growth (103). In another study by the same group, it was shown that the production of IL-6 was enhanced by IL-1 in vivo, because infiltrating inflammatory cells reacting to tumor margins produced IL-1 locally, which in turn stimulated the tumor cells to release IL-6 (104). These results suggest that the interactions between different cytokines are of paramount importance in mediating the syndrome of cancer-related cachexia.

Cytokines such as TNF and IL-1 may also regulate muscle protein breakdown in vivo (105). The effects of TNF and IL-1 on muscle proteolysis are dose-dependent: Very high doses of TNF and IL-1 increase the rate of total and myofibrillar protein breakdown after in vivo treatment (106–108). However, it has been difficult to demonstrate a direct effect of TNF or IL-1 on muscle proteolysis in vitro (109,110). It is not known whether other cytokines, such as IL-6, IFN-γ, and LIF, have an effect on skeletal muscle proteolysis. All these cytokines have been shown to induce the synthesis of several acute-phase proteins in the liver (111).

Although the initial hypothesis suggesting that TNF produces cachexia by altering fat cell metabolism may not be true, it is likely that the syndrome of cachexia is the result of additive or synergistic effects of multiple cytokines acting on a variety of different tissues. Anorexia may also have a key role in cytokine-induced cachexia, because the body may lose its mechanisms to compensate for decreased food intake when cytokine-induced metabolic disturbances are present (112). Continuous and sustained production of TNF, IL-1, and other unidentified cytokines can result in muscle wasting by inducing skeletal muscle protein breakdown (105–108). Similarly, TNF- and IFN-induced lipolysis (37,49,69) could deplete lipid stores, particularly in the absence of adequate food intake, resulting in reduced fat cell mass. The effect of multiple cytokines on FA synthesis (45) uses energy, and it may be a wasteful process at times when the body needs to conserve energy. Moreover, the simultaneous lipolytic and lipogenic effect of TNF and IFN-α (37,45,49,57) results in futile cycling because FAs released from adipose tissues are resynthesized into TG in the liver and resecreted as VLDL. The resultant VLDL is broken down by LPL in the periphery, and the FAs are returned to the peripheral tissues for storage as TGs. This futile cycling also wastes energy. It is likely that cytokines also induce similar futile cycles in carbohydrate and protein metabolism. Thus, a combination of cytokine-induced anorexia and additive or synergistic effects of multiple cytokines on several different metabolic pathways at a variety of sites can lead to cachexia during chronic infections and cancer.

THE METABOLIC EFFECTS OF CYTOKINES MAY BE PROTECTIVE

Low doses of cytokines that are not detrimental to the host exert several effects that can be beneficial. Animals that lack the ability to produce TNF and IL-1 are highly susceptible to the lethal effects of infection, demonstrating that these cytokines may have a physiological role in host defense mechanisms (113). Pretreatment of rodents with very low doses of TNF, IL-1, or LIF has been shown to protect against subsequent lethal endotoxemia or bacterial sepsis (114–117). Several cytokines, including TNF, IL-1, and IL-6, induce the synthesis of acute-phase proteins, which help maintain homeostasis during the course of infection and inflammation (111).

There is evidence that the increase in serum lipoprotein levels induced by endotoxin and cytokines may also be a beneficial response to the host. The half maximal dose for LPS-induced hypertriglyceridemia in the rats is 1/500,000th of the lethal dose of LPS (11). The doses required for TNF and IL-1 to stimulate hepatic FA synthesis and to increase VLDL production (22,35,45,48) are similar to those that produce fever (118,119) or that induce the synthesis of acute-phase proteins in intact animals (120). These studies suggest that the cytokine-induced increase in lipoprotein levels is not a pharmacological effect, but rather it represents a physiological response to immune stimulation.

Several studies have shown that chylomicrons, VLDL, LDL, and HDL can bind to endotoxin and prevent its ability to induce fever, hypotension, or death in rodents (121–124). A possible mechanism for this protective effect is suggested by in vitro studies, which indicate that lipoproteins can decrease the ability of endotoxin to stimulate cytokine secretion by macrophages (125,126), and it is well established that over-production of these cytokines can cause the lethal effects of endotoxin. It has also been shown that endotoxin is bound to VLDL in the circulation of normal individuals, suggesting that this detoxifying mechanism may be operative in the normal course of human activity (124).

Recent in vivo studies by our laboratory indicate that chylomicron binding of endotoxin can increase the clearance rate of endotoxin. The binding of endotoxin to chylomicrons results in its rapid clearance by hepatocytes, rather than Kupffer cells, in the liver, which results in decreased serum TNF levels (127). Hence, lipoproteins can neutralize the lethal effects of endotoxin. In addition to detoxifying endotoxin, lipoproteins can bind to a variety of viruses, which may reduce the toxic effects of these viruses (128–131). Lipoproteins have also been shown to induce lysis of the parasite *Trypanosoma brucei* (132,133). Finally, lipoproteins also bind urate crystals, and this binding can reduce the inflammatory response induced by these crystals (134). Thus, it can be postulated that the cytokine-induced increase in lipoproteins represents a nonspecific immune response that can decrease the toxicity of a variety of harmful biological and chemical agents.

REFERENCES

1. Gallin JI, Kaye D, O'Leary WM. Serum lipids in infection. N Engl J Med 1969;281:1081–1986.
2. Fiser RH, Denniston JC, Beisel WR. Infection with diplococcus pneumoniae and salmonella typhimurium in monkeys: changes in plasma lipids and lipoproteins. J Infect Dis 1972;125:54–60.
3. Kaufmann RL, Matson CF, Beisel WR. Hypertriglyceridemia produced by endotoxin: role of impaired triglyceride disposal mechanisms. J Infect Dis 1976;133:548–555.
4. Alvarez C, Ramos A. Lipids, lipoproteins and apoproteins in serum during infections. Clin Chem 1986;32:142–145.
5. Sammalkorpi K, Valtonen V, Kerttula Y, Nikkila E, Taskinen MR. Changes in serum lipoprotein pattern induced by acute infections. Metabolism 1988;37:859–865.
6. Guckian JC. Role of the metabolism in pathogenesis of bacteremia due to diplococcus pneumoniae in rabbits. J Infect Dis 1973;127:1–8.
7. Canonico PG, Ayala E, Rill WL, Little JS. Effect of pneumococcal infection on rat liver microsomal enzymes and lipogenesis by isolated hepatocytes. Am J Clin Nutr 1977; 30:1359–1363.
8. Wolfe RR, Shaw JH, Durkot MJ. Effect of sepsis on VLDL kinetics: responses in basal state and during glucose infusion. Am J Physiol 1985;248:732–740.
9. Lanza-Jacoby S, Lansey SC, Cleary MP, Rosato FE. Alterations in lipogenic enzymes and lipoprotein lipase activity during gram negative sepsis in the rat. Arch Surg 1982;117: 144–147.
10. Bagby GJ, Corll CB, Martinez RR. Triacylglycerol kinetics in endotoxic rats with suppressed lipoprotein lipase activity. Am J Physiol 1987;253:59–64.
11. Feingold KR, Staprans I, Memon RA, et al. Endotoxin rapidly induces changes in lipid metabolism that produce hypertriglyceridemia: low doses stimulate hepatic triglyceride production while high doses inhibit clearance. J Lipid Res 1992;33:1765–1776.
12. Vasconcelos PRL, Kettlewell MGW, Gibbons GF, Williamson DH. Increased rates of hepatic cholesterogenesis and fatty acid synthesis in septic rats in vivo: evidence for the possible involvement of insulin. Clin Sci 1989;76:205–211.
13. Lanza-Jacoby S, Tabares A. Triglyceride kinetics, tissue lipoprotein lipase, and liver lipogenesis in septic rats. Am J Physiol 1990;258:678–685.
14. Lanza-Jacoby S, Wong SH, Tabares A, Baer D, Schneider T. Disturbances in the composition of plasma lipoproteins during gram negative sepsis in the rat. Biochim Biophys Acta 1992;1124:233–240.
15. Auerbach BJ, Parks JS. Lipoprotein abnormalities associated with lipopolysaccharide induced lecithin-cholesteryl acyltransferase and lipase deficiency. J Biol Chem 1989; 259:10264–10270.

16. Neufeld HA, Pace JA, White FE. The effect of bacterial infections on ketone concentrations in rat liver and blood and on free fatty acid concentrations in rat blood. Metabolism 1976;25:877–884.

17. Neufeld HA, Pace JG, Kaminski MV, et al. A probable endocrine basis for the depression of ketone bodies during infectious or inflammatory state in rats. Endocrinology 1980;107:596–601.

18. Lanza-Jacoby S, Rosato E, Braccia G, Tabares A. Altered ketone body metabolism during gram-negative sepsis in the rat. Metabolism 1990;39:1151–1157.

19. Vary TC, Siegel JH, Nakatani T, Sato T, Aoyama H. A biochemical basis for depressed ketogenesis. J Trauma 1986; 26:419–425.

20. Marchuk JB, Finley RJ, Groves AC, et al. Catabolic hormones and substrate patterns in septic patients. J Surg Res 1977;23:177–182.

21. Spitzer JJ, Bagby GJ, Mesazaros K, Lang CH. Alterations in lipid and carbohydrate metabolism in sepsis. J Parenter Enter Nutr 1988;12:S53–S58.

22. Feingold KR, Grunfeld C. Tumor necrosis factor-alpha stimulates hepatic lipogenesis in the rat in vivo. J Clin Invest 1987;80:184–190.

23. Feingold KR, Soued M, Serio MK, Adi S, Moser AH, Grunfeld C. The effect of diet on tumor necrosis factor stimulation of hepatic lipogenesis. Metabolism 1990;39: 623–632.

24. Krauss RM, Grunfeld C, Doerrler WT, Feingold KR. Tumor necrosis factor acutely increases plasma levels of very low density lipoproteins of normal size and composition. Endocrinology 1990;127:1016–1021.

25. Memon RA, Grunfeld C, Moser AH, Feingold KR. Tumor necrosis factor mediates the effects of endotoxin on cholesterol and triglyceride metabolism in mice. Endocrinology 1993;132:2246–2253.

26. Ettinger WH, Miller LD, Albers JJ, Smith TK, Parks JS. Lipopolysaccharide and tumor necrosis factor cause a fall in plasma concentrations of lecithin: cholesterol acyltransferase in cynomolgus monkeys. J Lipid Res 1990; 31:1099–1107.

27. Sherman ML, Spriggs DR, Arthur KA, Imamura K, Frei E, Kufe DW. Recombinant human tumor necrosis factor administered as a five day continuous infusion in cancer patients: phase I toxicity and effects on lipid metabolism. J Clin Oncol 1988;6:344–350.

28. Beutler B, Cerami A. Cachectin and tumor necrosis factor as two sides of the same biological coin. Nature 1986;320: 584–588.

29. Kern PA. Recombinant human tumor necrosis factor does not inhibit lipoprotein lipase in primary cultures of isolated human adipocytes. J Lipid Res 1988;29:909–914.

30. Grunfeld C, Gulli R, Moser AH, Gavin LA, Feingold KR. The effect of tumor necrosis administration in vivo on lipoprotein lipase activity in various tissues of the rat. J Lipid Res 1989;30:579–585.

31. Semb H, Peterson J, Tavernier J, Olivecrona T. Multiple effects of tumor necrosis factor on lipoprotein lipase in vivo. J Biol Chem 1987;262:8390–8394.

32. Chajek-Shaul T, Friedman G, Stein O, Shiloni E, Etienne J, Stein Y. Mechanisms of the hypertriglyceridemia induced by tumor necrosis factor administration to rats. Biochim Biophys Acta 1989;1001:316–324.

33. Feingold KR, Soued M, Staprans I, et al. Effect of tumor necrosis factor on lipid metabolism in the diabetic rat: evidence that inhibition of adipose tissue lipoprotein lipase activity is not required for TNF induced hyperlipidemia. J Clin Invest 1989;83:1116–1121.

34. Feingold KR, Soued M, Adi S, et al. Tumor necrosis factor increased hepatic very low density lipoprotein production and increased serum triglyceride levels in diabetic rats. Diabetes 1990;39:1569–1574.

35. Feingold KR, Serio MK, Adi S, Moser AH, Grunfeld C. Tumor necrosis factor stimulates hepatic lipid synthesis and secretion. Endocrinology 1989;124:2336–2342.

36. Evans RD, Williamson DH. Comparison of effects of platelet activating factor and tumor necrosis factor-α on lipid metabolism in adrenalectomized in vivo. Biochim Biophys Acta 1991;1086:191–196.

37. Feingold KR, Adi S, Staprans I, et al. Diet affects the mechanisms by which TNF stimulates hepatic triglyceride production. Am J Physiol 1990;259:77–184.

38. Reaven GM, Chang H, Ho H, Jeng C, Hoffman BB. Lowering of plasma glucose in diabetic rats by antilipolytic agents. Am J Physiol 1988;254:23–30.

39. Patton JS, Shepard HM, Wilking H, et al. Interferons and tumor necrosis factor have similar catabolic effects on 3T3 L1 cells. Proc Natl Acad Sci USA 1986;83:8313–8317.

40. Beutler B, Cerami A. Recombinant interleukin-1 suppresses lipoprotein lipase activity in 3T3-L1 cells. J Immunol 1985;135:3969–3971.

41. Price SR, Mizel SB, Pekala PH. Regulation of lipoprotein lipase synthesis and 3T3-L1 adipocyte metabolism by recombinant interleukin-1. Biochim Biophys Acta 1986;889: 374–381.

42. Greenberg AS, Nordon RP, McIntosh J, Calvo JC, Scow RO, Jablons D. Interleukin-6 reduces lipoprotein lipase activity in adipose tissue of mice in vivo and in 3T3-L1 adipocytes. A possible role for interleukin-6 in cancer cachexia. Cancer Res 1992;52:4113–4116.

43. Mori M, Yamaguchi K, Abe K. Purification of a lipoprotein lipase inhibiting protein produced by a melanoma cell line associated with cancer cachexia. Biochem Biophys Res Commun 1989;160:1085–1092.

44. Feingold KR, Doerrler W, Dinarello CA, Fiers W, Grunfeld C. Stimulation of lipolysis in cultured fat cells by tumor necrosis factor, interleukin-1 and interferons is blocked by inhibition of prostaglandin synthesis. Endocrinology 1992; 130:10–16.

45. Feingold KR, Soued M, Serio MK, Moser AH, Dinarello CA, Grunfeld C. Multiple cytokines stimulate hepatic lipid synthesis in vivo. Endocrinology 1989;125:267–274.

46. Grunfeld C, Adi S, Soued M, Moser AH, Fiers W, Feingold KR. Search for mediators of the lipogenic effects of tumor necrosis factor: possible role for interleukin-6. Cancer Res 1990;50:4233–4238.

47. Evans RD, Ilic V, Williamson DH. Metabolic effects of platelet activating factor in rats in vivo: stimulation of hepatic glycogenolysis and lipogenesis. Biochem J 1990;269: 269–272.

48. Feingold KR, Soued M, Adi S, et al. Effect of interleukin-1 on lipid metabolism in the rat. Similarities to and differ-

ences from tumor necrosis factor. Arteriosclerosis Thrombosis 1991;11:495–500.

49. Memon RA, Feingold KR, Moser AH, Doerrler W, Grunfeld C. In vivo effects of interferon-α and interferon-γ on lipolysis and ketogenesis. Endocrinology 1992;131: 1695–1702.

50. Olsen EA, Lichenstein GR, Wilkinson WE. Changes in serum lipids in patients with condylomata acuminata treated with interferon alpha. J Am Acad Dermatol 1988; 19:286–289.

51. Graessle D, Bonacini M, Chen S. Alpha-interferon and reversible hypertriglyceridemia. Ann Intern Med 1993; 118:316–317.

52. Kurzrock R, Rohde MF, Quesada JR, et al. Recombinant γ-interferon induces hypertriglyceridemia and inhibits postheparin lipase activity in cancer patients. J Exp Med 1986; 164:1093–1101.

53. Kurzrock R, Feinberg B, Talpaz M, Saks S, Gutterman JU. Phase I study of a combination of recombinant tumor necrosis factor and recombinant interferon-γ in cancer patients. J Interferon Res 1989;9:435–444.

54. Grunfeld C, Kotler DP, Shigenaga JK, et al. Circulating interferon-α levels and hypertriglyceridemia in the acquired immunodeficiency syndrome. Am J Med 1991;90:154–162.

55. Grunfeld C, Pang M, Doerrler W, Shigenaga JK, Jensen P, Feingold KR. Lipids, lipoproteins, triglyceride clearance, and cytokines in human immunodeficiency virus infection and the acquired immunodeficiency syndrome. J Clin Endocrinol Metab 1992;74:1045–1052.

56. Hellerstein MK, Grunfeld C, Wu K, et al. Increased de novo hepatic lipogenesis in human immunodeficiency virus infection. J Clin Endocrinol Metab 1993;76:559–565.

57. Grunfeld C, Soued M, Adi S, Moser AH, Dinarello CA, Feingold KR. Evidence for two classes of cytokines that stimulate hepatic lipogenesis: relationships among tumor necrosis factor, interleukin-1 and interferon-alpha. Endocrinology 1990;127:46–54.

58. Grunfeld C, Soued M, Adi S, et al. Interleukin-4 inhibits stimulation of hepatic lipogenesis by tumor necrosis factor, interleukin-1, and interleukin-6 but not interferon-α. Cancer Res 1991;51:2803–2807.

59. Ettinger WH, Miller LA, Smith TK, Parks JS. Effect of interleukin-1 alpha on lipoprotein lipids in cynomolgus monkeys: comparison to tumor necrosis factor. Biochim Biophys Acta 1992;1128:186–192.

60. Cantell K, Ehnholm C, Mattila K, Kostianen E. Interferon and high density lipoproteins. N Engl J Med 1980;302: 1032–1033.

61. Ehnholm C, Aho K, Huttunen JK, et al. Effect of interferon on plasma lipoproteins and on the activity of post-heparin plasma lipases. Arteriosclerosis 1982;2:68–73.

62. Massaro ER, Borden EC, Hawkins MJ, Wiebe DA, Shrago E. Effect of recombinant interferon-α treatment upon lipid concentrations and lipoprotein composition. J Interferon Res 1986;6:655–662.

63. Rosenzweig IB, Wiebe DA, Borden EC, Storer B, Shrago ES. Plasma lipoprotein changes in humans induced by β-interferon. Atherosclerosis 1987;67:261–267.

64. Borden EC, Rosenzweig IB, Byrne GI. Interferons: from

virus inhibitor to modulator of amino acid and lipid metabolism. J Interferon Res 1987;7:591–596.

65. Schectman G, Kaul S, Mueller RA, Borden EC, Kissebah AH. The effect of interferon on the metabolism of LDLs. Arteriosclerosis Thrombosis 1992;12:1053–1062.

66. Nimer SD, Champlin RE, Golde DW. Serum cholesterol lowering activity of granulocyte macrophage colony stimulating factor. JAMA 1988;260:3297–3300.

67. Stoudemire JB, Garnick MB. Effect of recombinant human macrophage colony stimulating factor on plasma cholesterol levels. Blood 1991;77:750–755.

68. Shimano H, Yamada N, Ishibashi S, et al. Human monocyte colony stimulating factor enhances the clearance of lipoproteins containing apolipoprotein B-100 via both low density lipoprotein receptor-dependent and -independent pathways in rabbits. J Biol Chem 1990;265:12869–12875.

69. Memon RA, Feingold KR, Moser AH, et al. Differential effects of interleukin-1 and tumor necrosis factor on ketogenesis. Am J Physiol 1992;263:E301–E309.

70. Memon RA, Feingold KR, Adi S, Grunfeld C. Which cytokines mediate the metabolic effects of endotoxin? In: Fiers W, Burman W, eds. Tumor necrosis factor, vol 4. Basel: Karger, 1993:107–112.

71. McGarry JD, Woeltje KF, Kuwajima M, Foster DW. Regulation of ketogenesis and renaissance of carnitine palmitoyltransferase. Diabetes Metab Rev 1989;5:271–284.

72. Johnston DG, Alberti KGMM. Hormonal control of ketone body metabolism in the normal and diabetic state. Clin Endocrinol Metab 1982;11:329–361.

73. Beylot M, Vidal H, Mithieux G, Odeon M, Martin C. Inhibition of hepatic ketogenesis by tumor necrosis factor-α in rats. Am J Physiol 1992;263:E897–E902.

74. Popp MB, Fisher RI, Wesley R, Aamodt R, Brennan MF. A prospective randomized study of adjuvant parenteral nutrition in the treatment of advanced diffuse lymphoma: influence on survival. Surgery 1981;90:195–203.

75. Grunfeld C, Feingold KR. The metabolic effects of tumor necrosis factor and other cytokines. Biotherapy 1991;3: 143–158.

76. Patton JS, Peters PM, McCabe J, Crase D, Hansen S, Chen AB. Development of partial tolerance to the gastrointestinal effects of high doses of recombinant tumor necrosis factor alpha in rodents. J Clin Invest 1987;80:1587–1596.

77. Socher SH, Friedman A, Martinez D. Recombinant human tumor necrosis factor induces acute reductions in food intake and body weight in mice. J Exp Med 1988;167:1957–1962.

78. Stovroff MC, Fraker DL, Swedenberg JA, Norton JA. Cachectin/tumor necrosis factor, a possible mediator of cancer anorexia in the rat. Cancer Res 1988;48:920–925.

79. Grunfeld C, Wilking H, Neese R, et al. Persistence of the hypertriglyceridemic effect of tumor necrosis factor despite development of tachyphylaxis to its anorectic/cachectic effect in rats. Cancer Res 1989;49:2554–2560.

80. Mullen BJ, Harris RBS, Patton JS, Martin RJ. Recombinant tumor necrosis factor-alpha chronically administered in rats: lack of the cachectic effect. Proc Soc Exp Biol Med 1990;193:318–325.

81. Grunfeld C, Kotler DP, Hamadeh R, Tierney A, Wang J,

Pierson RN Jr. Hypertriglyceridemia in the acquired immunodeficiency syndrome. Am J Med 1989;86:27–31.

82. Tracey KJ, Wei H, Monogue KR, et al. Cachectin/tumor necrosis factor induces cachexia, anemia and inflammation. J Exp Med 1988;167:1211–1227.

83. Michi HR, Sherman ML, Spriggs DR, Rounds J, Christie M, Wilmore DW. Chronic TNF infusion causes anorexia but not accelerated nitrogen loss. Ann Surg 1989;209:19–24.

84. Rothstein JL, Schreiber H. Synergy between tumor necrosis factor and bacterial components in causing hemorrhagic necrosis and lethal shock in normal mice. Proc Natl Acad Sci USA 1988;85:607–611.

85. Oxaki Y, Oyama T, Kume S. Exacerbation of toxic effects by endotoxin contamination of recombinant human tumor necrosis factor. Cancer Chemother Pharmacol 1989;23: 231–237.

86. Williamson B, Carswell EA, Rubin BY, Prendergast JS, Old LJ. Human tumor necrosis factor produced by human B-cell lines: synergistic cytotoxic interactions with human interferon. Proc Natl Acad Sci USA 1983;80:5397–5401.

87. Oliff A, Defco-Jones D, Boyer M, et al. Tumors secreting human TNF-cachectin induce cachexia in mice. Cell 1987; 50:555–563.

88. Socher SH, Martinez D, Craig JB, Kuhn JG, Oliff A. Tumor necrosis factor not detectable in patients with clinical cancer cachexia. J Natl Cancer Inst 1988;80:595–599.

89. Waage A, Espevik T, Lamvik J. Detection of tumor necrosis factor like cytotoxicity in serum from patients with septicemia but not from untreated cancer patients. Scand J Immunol 1986;24:739–743.

90. Bartholeyns J, Freudenberg M, Galanos C. Growing tumors induce hypersensitivity to endotoxin and tumor necrosis factor. Infect Immun 1987;55:2230–2233.

91. Hellerstein MK, Meydani SN, Meydani M, Wu K, Dinarello CA. Interleukin-1 induced anorexia in the rat. J Clin Invest 1989;84:228–235.

92. Fujii T, Sato K, Ozawa M, et al. Effect of interleukin-1 on thyroid hormone metabolism in mice: stimulation by IL-1 of iodothyronine 5′- deiodinating activity (type I) in the liver. Endocrinology 1989;124:167–174.

93. Langstein HN, Doherty GM, Fraker DL, Buresh CM, Norton JA. The roles of interferon gamma and tumor necrosis factor alpha in an experimental rat model of cancer cachexia. Cancer Res 1991;51:2302–2306.

94. Sherwin SA, Knost JA, Fein S, et al. A multiple dose phase I trial of recombinant leukocyte A interferon in cancer patients. JAMA 1982;248:2461–2466.

95. Vadhan-Raj S, Al-Katib A, Bhalla R, et al. Phase I trial of recombinant interferon gamma in cancer patients. J Clin Oncol 1986;4:137–146.

96. Sehgal PB. Interleukin-6 in infection and cancer. Proc Soc Exp Biol Med 1990;193:183–191.

97. Gelin J, Moldawer LL, Lonnroth C, Sherry B, Chizzonite R, Lundholm K. Role of endogenous tumor necrosis factor-α and interleukin-1 for experimental tumor growth and the development of cancer cachexia. Cancer Res 1991;51:415–421.

98. Zugamaier G, Paik S, Wilding G, et al. Transforming growth factor β1 induces cachexia and systemic fibrosis without an antitumor effect in nude mice. Cancer Res 1991;51:3590–3594.

99. Black K, Garrett R, Mundy GR. Chinese hamster ovarian cells transfected with the murine interleukin-6 gene cause hypercalcemia as well as cachexia, leukocytosis and thrombocytosis in tumor bearing nude mice. Endocrinology 1991;128:2657–2659.

100. Matthys P, Dijkmans R, Proost P, et al. Severe cachexia in mice inoculated with interferon-γ producing tumor cells. Int J Cancer 1991;49:77–82.

101. Metcalf D, Gearing DP. Fatal syndrome in mice engrafted with cells producing high levels of leukemia inhibitory factor. Proc Natl Acad Sci USA 1989;86:5948–5952.

102. Mori M, Yamaguchi K, Honda S, et al. Cancer cachexia syndrome developed in nude mice bearing melanoma cells producing leukemia inhibitory factor. Cancer Res 1991; 51:6656–6659.

103. Strassmann G, Fong M, Kenney JS, Jacob CO. Evidence for the involvement of interleukin-6 in experimental cancer cachexia. J Clin Invest 1992;89:1681–1684.

104. Strassmann G, Jacob CO, Evans R, Beall D, Fong M. Mechanisms of experimental cancer cachexia: interaction between mononuclear phagocytes and colon-26 carcinoma and its relevance to IL-6 mediated cancer cachexia. J Immunol 1992;148:3674–3678.

105. Fischer JE, Hasselgren PO. Cytokines and glucocorticoids in the regulation of the "hepatoskeletal muscle axis" in sepsis. Am J Surg 1991;161:266–271.

106. Flores EA, Bistrian BR, Pomposelli JJ, Dinarello CA, Blackburn GL, Istfan NW. Infusion of tumor necrosis factor/cachectin promotes muscle catabolism in the rat: a synergistic effect with interleukin-1. J Clin Invest 1989;83: 1614–1622.

107. Zamir O, Hasselgren PO, Kunkel SL, Frederick J, Higashiguchi T, Fischer JE. Evidence that tumor necrosis factor participates in the regulation of muscle proteolysis during sepsis. Arch Surg 1992;127:170–174.

108. Zamir O, Hasselgren PO, Allmen D, Fischer JE. In vivo administration of interleukin-1α induces muscle proteolysis in normal and adrenalectomized rats. Metabolism 1993; 42:204–208.

109. Moldawer LL, Svaninger G, Gelin J, Lundholm KG. Interleukin-1 and tumor necrosis factor do not regulate protein balance in skeletal muscle. Am J Physiol 1987;253:766–773.

110. Rofe AM, Conyers RAJ, Bais R, Gamble JR, Vadas MA. The effects of recombinant tumor necrosis factor (cachectin) on metabolism in isolated rat adipocyte, hepatocyte and muscle preparations. Biochem J 1987;247:789–792.

111. Richards C, Gauldie J, Baumann H. Cytokine control of acute phase protein expression. Eur Cytokine Net 1991; 2:89–98.

112. Mulligan HD, Tisdale MJ. Lipogenesis in tumor and host tissues in mice bearing colonic adenocarcinomas. Br J Cancer 1991;63:719–722.

113. Cross AS, Sadoff JC, Kelly N, Bernton E, Gemski P. Pretreatment with recombinant murine tumor necrosis factor-α/cachectin and murine interleukin-1α protects mice from lethal bacterial infection. J Exp Med 1989;169:2021–2027.

114. Sheppard BC, Fraker DL, Norton JA. Prevention and treat-

ment of endotoxin and sepsis lethality with recombinant human tumor necrosis factor. Surgery 1989;106:156–162.

115. Alexander HR, Doherty GM, Fraker DL, Block MI, Swedenberg JA, Norton JA. Human recombinant interleukin-1α protection against the lethality of endotoxin and experimental sepsis in mice. J Surg Res 1991;50:421–424.

116. Alexander HR, Sheppard BC, Jensen JC, et al. Treatment with recombinant human tumor necrosis factor-alpha protects rats against the lethality, hypotension and hypothermia of gram negative sepsis. J Clin Invest 1991;88:34–39.

117. Alexander HR, Wong GGH, Doherty GM, Venzon DJ, Fraker DL, Norton JA. Differentiation factor/leukemia inhibitory factor protection against lethal endotoxemia in mice: synergistic effect with interleukin-1 and tumor necrosis factor. J Exp Med 1992;175:1139–1142.

118. Dinarello CA, Cannon JG, Mier JW, et al. Multiple biological activities of human recombinant interleukin-1. J Clin Invest 1986;77:1734–1739.

119. Dinarello CA, Cannon JG, Wolff SM, et al. Tumor necrosis factor (cachectin) is an endogenous pyrogen and induces production of interleukin-1. J Exp Med 1987;163:1433–1450.

120. Mortensin RF, Shapiro J, Lin B, Douches S, Neta R. Interaction of recombinant IL-1 and recombinant tumor necrosis factor in the induction of mouse acute phase proteins. J Immunol 1988;140:2260–2266.

121. Ulevitch RJ, Johnston AR, Weinstein DB. New function for high density lipoproteins. Their participation in intravascular reactions of bacterial lipopolysaccharides. J Clin Invest 1979;64:1516–1524.

122. VanLenten BJ, Fogelman AM, Haberland ME, Edwards PA. The role of lipoproteins and receptor mediated endocytosis in the transport of bacterial lipopolysaccharide. Proc Natl Acad Sci USA 1986;83:2704–2708.

123. Navab M, Hough GP, VanLenten BJ, Berliner JA, Fogelman AM. Low density lipoproteins transfer bacterial lipopolysaccharides across endothelial monolayers in a biologically active form. J Clin Invest 1988;81:601–605.

124. Harris HW, Grunfeld C, Feingold KR, Rapp JH. Human very low density lipoproteins and chylomicrons can protect against endotoxin induced death. J Clin Invest 1990;86:696–702.

125. Flegel WA, Wolpl A, Mannel DN, Northoff H. Inhibition of endotoxin induced activation of human monocytes by human lipoproteins. Infect Immun 1989;57:2237–2245.

126. Cavaillon JM, Fitting C, Cavaillon NH, Kirsch SJ, Warren HS. Cytokine response by monocyte and macrophage to free and lipoprotein bound lipopolysaccharide. Infect Immun 1990;58:2375–2382.

127. Harris HW, Grunfeld C, Feingold KR, et al. Chylomicrons alter the fate of endotoxin, decreasing tumor necrosis factor release and preventing death. J Clin Invest 1993;91:1028–1034.

128. Leong JC, Kane JP, Oleszko O, Levy JA. Antigen specific nonimmunoglobulin factor that neutralizes xenotropic virus is associated with mouse serum lipoproteins. Proc Natl Acad Sci USA 1977;74:276–280.

129. Seganti L, Grassi M, Matromarino P, Pana A, Superti F, Orsi N. Activity of human serum lipoproteins on the infectivity of rhabdoviruses. Mirobiology 1983;6:91–99.

130. Sernatinger J, Hoffman A, Harmon D, Kane JP, Levy JA. Neutralization of mouse xenotropic virus by lipoproteins involves binding to virons. J Gen Virol 1988;69:2651–2661.

131. Heumer HP, Menzel HJ, Potratz D, et al. Herpes simplex virus binds to human serum lipoproteins. Intervirology 1988;29:68–76.

132. Rifkin MR. Identification of the trypanocidal factor in normal human serum: high density lipoproteins. Proc Natl Acad Sci USA 1978;75:3450–3454.

133. Hajduk SL, Moore DR, Vasudevacharya J, et al. Lysis of trypanosoma bruceii by a toxic subspecies of human high density lipoprotein. J Biol Chem 1989;264:5210–5217.

134. Terkettaub R, Curtiss LK, Tenner AJ, Ginsberg MH. Lipoproteins containing apoprotein B are a major regulator of neutrophil responses to monosodium urate crystals. J Clin Invest 1984;73:1719–1730.

CHAPTER 15

ROLE OF CYTOKINES IN ACUTE-PHASE RESPONSE

Carl D. Richards and Jack Gauldie

Physiological responses to environmental stimuli are generally marked by exquisite regulation mechanisms involving multiple cell types and their interaction. In responding to tissue damage elicited by trauma or infection, the mammalian body sets in motion a complex network of molecular and cellular interactions designed to aid tissue repair and to facilitate a return to physiological homeostasis. This process is termed the *acute-phase response* (APR), and it can be initiated by inflammatory stimuli such as trauma; burns; tissue destruction due to bacterial, viral, or parasite growth; and immune-mediated events.

The APR is composed of immediate local events (at sites of inflammation), as well as activation of systemic phenomenon. In concert with other systemic features, a striking alteration in synthesis of liver-derived acute-phase proteins (APPs) by hepatocytes marks the characteristic and dramatic increases in plasma levels of APP seen in later stages (12–24 hours) of the responses. Fever, granulocytosis, and increased levels of plasma adrenocorticotrophic hormone (ACTH) and glucocorticoids accompany these changes. Cytokines have a prominent role in both local and systemic aspects of regulation, and they contribute to temporal and spatial patterns of actue inflammation.

The sequelae of these initiation events include modulation of local progression of inflammatory events and transition into resolution of inflammation. Thus, systematically induced proteins and mediators appear to slow the process of injury and aid in removal of pathogens or particles. "Shut-off" of the APR may result from clearance of initiating stimuli, as well as active suppression by certain cytokine/hormone systems. As a consequence, progression of chronic inflammation may result in part from loss of normal regulation by cytokines or other systems, as much as from the presence of ongoing stimuli.

INITIATION

Immediate local events

SMALL MEDIATORS: Signs and symptoms of local inflammation, including redness, swelling, pain, and heat, can be regulated by soluble mediators. Transection of blood vessels due to trauma can involve release of cytokines (e.g., transforming growth factor-β [TGF-β]) and eicosanoids by platelets after aggregation. Other cells, such as mast cells, can release a number of vasoactive substances (i.e., histamine and serotonin) that alter vessel permeability. Macrophages can release platelet activating factor (PAF) (another highly vasoactive substance) and products of the arachidonic acid cascade, as well as nitrous oxide and reactive oxygen radicals. These small molecular weight, "short-acting," highly unstable mediators have potent effects on vascular tone and permeability at postcapillary venules. Thus, increases in blood flow and escape of fluid and cells from the circulation into the tissues primarily accounts for redness and edema. Brady-kinin and prostaglandin also affect pain sensory nerves. Furthermore, arachidonic metabolites, such as leuko-triene B_4 (LTB_4), are chemotactic for phagocytic cells; thus, they contribute to the efflux of cells characteristic of inflammation.

INTERLEUKIN-1 AND TUMOR NECROSIS FACTOR: In addition to the small, potent, lipid-de-rived mediators, activated cells in the tissue release a se-ries of *first wave* or *proximal acting cytokines,* a term that refers to peptide hormone-like intercellular messengers possessing a spectrum of regulatory roles. The term *first wave* reflects the early and prominent release of these cytokines from cells activated by the eliciting agents. A key cell in this regard appears to be the tissue macrophage or the blood monocyte, which may be activated by bacte-rial products or recruited through chemotaxis to the af-fected locale by fragments of the complement system or by cytokines such as TGF-β. Activated macrophages re-lease a substantial amount of "first-wave" or "alarm" cytokines, such as interleukin-1 (IL-1) and tumor necro-sis factor (TNF), as well as other mediators; they are therefore thought to have the most prominent role in ini-tiation of the events that follow.

IL-1α and IL-1β interact at specific receptors on nu-merous cell types, and they produce a broad spectrum of cell responses at both the local and the systemic level. TNF-α has many similar effects, and it has been shown in certain cell types to initiate IL-1 expression (1,2), thus amplifying the "alarm cytokine" system. IL-1 and TNF are potent stimulators of cyclooxygenase activity in stromal cells, such as epithelium, endothelium, and fibroblasts, and this activation contributes to production of prosta-glandin E_2 (PGE_2) and other eicosanoids (3), which in turn affect local vascular events. Furthermore, IL-1 or TNF can potently stimulate stromal cell production of cytokines of the chemokine family, and they likely have a crucial role in orchestrating the infiltration of neutrophils and monocytes into tissues.

The chemokines (4,5) are small cytokines (5–10 kd) with similar structures that appear to control the amount and variety of cells that accumulate into inflamed tissue. The chemokines of the C-X-C group (denoting the com-mon distribution of cysteine residues), such as human IL-8, are generally chemotactic for neutrophils, whereas those of the C-C group, such as human monocyte chemo-tactic peptide (MCP-1), are generally chemotactic for mononuclear cells. The RANTES (Regulated on Activa-tion, Normal T Expressed and Secreted) gene product (also in the C-C group) also appears to attract T cells of the memory phenotype (5,6). IL-8, MCP-1, and RANTES are induced strongly in fibroblasts by IL-1 or TNF. Thus, recruitment of adjacent stromal cell populations by medi-

TABLE 15–1   CYTOKINES INVOLVED IN THE ACUTE-PHASE RESPONSE

First wave, or early-acting mediators
  IL-1 family
    IL-1α, IL-1β
  TNF family
    TNF-α
  Important cells of origin
    Macrophage/monocyte
Second wave, or distal mediators
  Chemotaxis
    IL-8
    MCP
    MIP
    RANTES
  Growth and differentiation/repair
    IL-6
    Colony-stimulating factors
    FGF
    EGF
    TGF-β
    PDGF
  Important cells of origin
    Macrophage/monocyte
    Activated stromal cells
  Immune response
    IL-2
    IL-3
    IL-4
    IL-5
    IL-7
    IL-12
    IFN-γ
  Regulatory
    IL-4
    IL-10
    IL-13
  Important cells of origin
    Activated T cells
    Monocyte/macrophage

ators released from monocytes/macrophages produces a "second wave" of cytokine release and a cascade that has an important role in the progression of inflammation (Table 15–1). In addition, monocytes and macrophages can produce their own "second wave" cytokines, such as IL-6 and IL-8 (7–9).

CELL INFILTRATION: Accumulation of neutro-phils into inflamed sites is most notable early (1–6 hours), whereas mononuclear cell infiltration is evident typically in a delayed time frame (24–48 hours). A small number of macrophages may initiate the process through the amplification pathways described. Neutrophils may respond to a variety of chemotactic agents produced at the tissue site, including those released from complement C5 or C3, mast cell degranulation products, or monocyte/macrophage- or stromal cell–derived chemokines.

IL-1 and TNF are also able to induce major changes in adhesion molecule expression on endothelial cells. Up-regulation of intercellular adhesion molecule (ICAM) and endothelial leukocyte adhesion molecule (ELAM) allows neutrophil-endothelial interaction and subsequent passage of neutrophils into tissues. More recently, it was discovered that neutrophils which cross the endothelium can be a source for both first wave (TNF) and second wave (IL-8) cytokines (10). The processes of initiation and propagation of the local response appears to involve numerous cellular mechanisms that require dynamic roles of resident macrophages, stromal cells, and infiltrating leukocytes as sources of cytokines.

Systemic events and APR of liver

Immediate local events are typically followed by systemic manifestations such as fever, neutrophilia, and alterations of plasma levels of ACTH and cortisol. The liver is also a major target; it shows marked changes in metabolic pathways and transport of ions and metabolites, as well as prominent increase in production of a series of proteins and in plasma concentrations of APPs. These proteins appear to have a crucial role in host resistance, because the APP response is conserved through phylogeny. The increase in protein concentration contributes to an increased erythrocyte sedimentation rate (ESR), which, along with fever, has long been used as a clinical indication of infection and inflammation. An example of these increases after an acute inflammatory stimulus, such as surgery, is shown in Fig. 15–1. Measurement of a typical APP, C-reactive protein (CRP), is widely used as a marker of inflammation, and, more recently, detection of increased levels of cytokines that regulate the hepatic APP response (e.g., IL-6) have also been used as measures of inflammation (11,12).

Many systemic events can be attributed to the presence of circulating cytokines derived from the site of local inflammation. Thus, IL-1 or TNF and IL-6 have been shown to modulate the temperature set point in vivo, probably by acting at the hypothalamus through induction of PGE$_2$ (13,14). IL-1 and IL-6 also act on the hypothalamus to increase corticotropin releasing hormone (15), and they subsequently effect the pituitary gland to induce ACTH production (16,17), which in turn increases cortisol production from the adrenal glands. IL-1, TNF, and IL-6 ap-

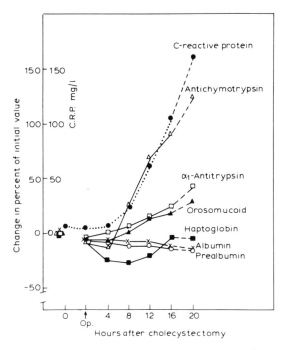

Figure 15–1 Quantitative changes in acute-phase reactants during the first day after cholecystectomy. The results are given as means for blood samples from 6 patients taken every fourth hour after the operation. C-reactive protein is given as mg/L, whereas the percentage deviation from the initial level is used for the other variables. The *broken line* between 16 and 20 hours denotes that samples were obtained from 4 of the 6 patients at 20 hours. (Reproduced by permission from Aronsen KF, Ekelund A, Kindmark CO, et al. Sequential changes of plasma protein after surgical trauma. Scand J Clin Lab Invest 1972;29:127–136.)

pear to synergistically enhance the ACTH response to lipopolysaccharide (LPS) in rodents in vivo (18).

ACUTE-PHASE PROTEINS: Typical APPs are listed in Table 15–2. They represent a heterogeneous array of molecules, some of which are markedly enhanced. CRP and serum amyloid A protein levels in humans and α_2-macroglobulin levels in rats increase by 10 to 100 times their regular concentration, whereas others, such as α_1-antichymotrypsin (α_1-ACH), α_1-acid glycoprotein (α_1-AGP), α_1-proteinase inhibitor (α_1-PI), fibrinogen, haptoglobin (HP), as well as α_1-cysteine proteinase inhibitor (α_1-CPI) (rat), and serum amyloid (SAP) levels (mouse and humans), increase to 2 to 10 times their basal levels. In reflecting the switch in liver metabolism, albumin and transferrin synthesis by the liver decreases, and these proteins are generally termed *negative APPs*. The genes for all APPs are regulated largely by transcriptional activation during an inflammatory stimulus, and protein plasma concentrations, subsequent to the increased liver synthesis, usually peaks at 24 to 48 hours. Plasma levels of APP usually return to normal by day 5 in uncomplicated acute inflammation, but each APP has its own kinetics due to its characteristic half-life ($T_{1/2}$), utilization, distribution, or other factors (19,20).

The kinetics of messenger RNA (mRNA) levels in the liver may differ between APP genes, and post-translational events, such as altered glycosylation of some APPs (21,22), may also modulate plasma levels. The APP response is relatively ubiquitous regardless of the nature of the inflammatory stimulus. Collectively, the APPs function in a homeostatic role: for removal of foreign particles, for opsonization, for replacement of utilized protein, and for demarcation of affected areas. There is evidence of extrahepatic synthesis of particular APPs (e.g., α_1-PI) (23); however, the role of this production is likely restricted to local effects.

CYTOKINE REGULATION OF APP: Historically, the investigations of Homburger (24) in 1945 were the first to show that a soluble mediator from purile exudate could enhance APP levels (fibrinogen in dogs) on injection. Studies on endogenous pyrogens and the nature of the soluble factors from leukocytes that mediate fever and leukocytosis suggested that these factors and the APP response were mediated by the same substance, termed *leukocyte endogenous mediator* (LEM) in the 1970s (25,26). In addition to the advances in technology in the early 1980s and the availability of recombinant IL-1, it became clear that IL-1 could mediate all aspects of the systemic APR when administered in vivo (13,27,28). However, during the mid-1980s, it also became clear that other factors were responsible for regulation of hepatocyte responses in vitro as part of an indirect pathway of IL-1 action in vivo. Indeed, IL-1 or TNF in vitro stimulated only a limited set of particular APPs, including α_1-AGP (in most species), SAP in mouse and humans, and the complement component C3 (29–31).

The major regulator identified thus far appears to be IL-6 because of its activity in regulating the expression of all APPs in vitro in hepatocytes and in vivo, and because of its presence in plasma during inflammation. Whereas IL-1 or TNF in conjunction with IL-6 or corticosteroids stimulate production of a set of APPs, termed *type 1 APPs*, all other APPs (type 2) are stimulated by IL-6 and steroids only. Thus, all APPs are stimulated by IL-6, but only some are stimulated by other cytokines (Table 15-2).

The plasma $T_{1/2}$ of most cytokines is relatively short (range, 7–30 minutes), and IL-6 may be found bound to various serum components, such as C4 or soluble IL-6 receptor (IL-6R) (32). Peak levels are detected prior to elevation of APP plasma concentrations (33). Administration of IL-6 causes a rapid induction of liver APP mRNA elevation and protein synthesis in vivo (34), and the association of enhanced IL-6 levels with acute and chronic inflammatory conditions is quite evident (33,35–39). Thus, regulation of IL-6 levels is closely coupled to acute inflammatory responses.

Although IL-1 and TNF have limited direct effects on hepatocyte APP synthesis, the ability of either of these first wave or alarm cytokines to initiate IL-6 production by fibroblasts, endothelial cells, and epithelial cells provides considerable enhancement of circulating IL-6 levels. Increased IL-6 plasma levels are found following intravenous administration of IL-1 or TNF (40,41).

Although this finding may suggest a causal role in inflammation, there is no evidence that IL-6 directly causes inflammation (e.g., repeated injections do not induce inflammatory sequelae other than increased APP levels). Indeed, some evidence suggests that continuous IL-6 infusion can down-regulate arthrtiic inflammation in an animal model (42), and IL-6 may inhibit release of TNF in an lipopolysacharide (LPS) model of inflammation (43). Antibodies to cytokines such as IL-6 have modulatory activity (44); however, it is not clear whether this activity is due to IL-6 clearance or prolongation of IL-6 ($T_{1/2}$) presence in the circulation (45). It therefore seems reasonable to classify IL-6 as an "inflammation-responsive" rather than a proinflammatory cytokine, such as may be said for IL-1 or TNF, which does not rule out the potential for

TABLE 15–2   ACUTE-PHASE PROTEIN GENES REGULATED BY INFLAMMATORY CYTOKINES*

Type 1—induced by IL-1/TNF and IL-6/LIF/OM/IL-11	Type 2—induced by IL-6/LIF/OM/IL-11 only
C-reactive protein (CRP)	Fibrinogen (FBG)
α_1-Acid glycoprotein (α_1-AGP)	Haptoglobin (human) (HP)
Serum amyloid A protein (SAA)	α_1-Proteinase inhibitor (α_1-PI)
Serum amyloid P (SAP)	α_1-Antichymotrypsin (α_1-ACH)
Complement C3 (C3)	Cysteine proteinase inhibitor (rat) (CPI)
Complement factor B	α_2-Macroglobulin (rat) (α_2-M)
Haptoglobin (rat) (HP)	Ceruloplasmin (CP)
Hemopexin (rat) (HX)	

*Protein expression and secretion is maximally stimulated by exposure of hepatocytes to cytokines in the presence of glucocorticosteroids.

IL-6 to be involved in the pathogenicity of certain diseases involving processes beyond acute inflammation. This finding does suggest that "IL-6–like" cytokines (in function), such as oncostatin M (OM), leukemia inhibitory factor (LIF), and IL-11, may also act as inflammation-responsive cytokines, in addition to having other important roles in hematopoiesis and differentiation.

The activity of OM on liver cells in vitro (46,47) (Fig. 15–2) and its ability to regulate APP plasma levels in vivo suggest that this regulatory cytokine has a prominent role in inflammation if sufficient plasma concentrations are reached. OM is a 28 kd monomeric protein expressed in activated T cells and monocytes (48,49), and it can be found in serum associated with as yet unidentified proteins. Whether OM is expressed at sites of inflammation is not currently clear. OM stimulates typical type 2 APP expression in human HepG2 and primary rat hepatocytes (46), and, similar to IL-6 and LIF, it acts synergistically with IL-1 in up-regulating particular APPs, such as α_1-AGP or HP. OM has at least as strong an activity as IL-6 on hepatocytes in vitro.

The sequences of complementary DNA (cDNA) and genomic clones of OM (49) and structure-based comparison to LIF predict functional similarities between these cytokines (50,51). LIF also has potent activity in regulating type 2 APP synthesis (4,52). Produced by human keratinocytes, T cells, and various cell lines (53,54), LIF, an 18-kd protein, interacts with specific receptors (55) on hepatocytes, and it induces APP stimulation that may be less than IL-6 in maximal extent.

IL-11, another 17-kd molecule, can also regulate APP expression in vitro (56). IL-11 was cloned from bone marrow cells (57), and it shares other activities with IL-6, including enhancement of hematopoietic stem-cell growth and megakaryocyte differentiation (57,58), although it utilizes a separate specific receptor complex. IL-6, OM, LIF, and IL-11 appear to be a family of cytokines that interact with separate receptors but share a common receptor complex subunit (gp130) that transduces signals intracellularly. Although this statement may oversimplify these interactions somewhat, it does provide a rationale for similar regulation of type 2 APP production by these agents.

The increase in plasma levels of corticosteroid following an inflammatory stimulus also contributes to increased levels of APPs. Figure 15–3 shows the complex interactions between cytokines, cortisol, and various cell types during an inflammatory response. Adrenalectomized animals have a markedly decreased APP response associated with inflammation (59). The ability of IL-6 or LIF to regulate various APPs is dependent on adequate corticosteroid levels. Cytokine-stimulated APPs, such as fibrinogen, α_1-ACH, α_1-AGP, and α_2-macroglobulin, are enhanced syner-

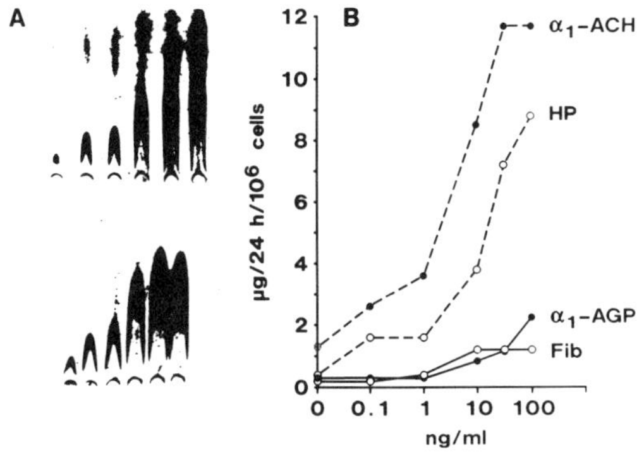

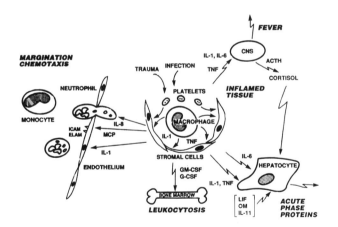

Figure 15–2 OM induces APP synthesis in HepG2 cells. HepG2 cells were cultured in the presence of OM for 72 hours (in DMEM with 10% FCS and 1 μmol/L DEX) and daily replacement with fresh medium and cytokine. Samples of supernatants collected at 72 hours (from the 48- to 72-hour incubation period) were subjected to rocket electrophoresis using antiserum to: human HP, α_1-ACH, α_1-AGP, and fibrinogen (Fib). Gels were stained with Coomassie blue to visualize precipitin lines and photographed. (A) HP (*top*) and α_1-ACH (*bottom*) content of supernatants after stimulation with (left to right) 0, 0.1, 1, 10, 50, and 100 ng/mL OM. (B) Amounts of protein secreted were calculated and graphed. Values represent the mean of two separate cultures, and determinations of protein output are given as μg secreted/24 hr/10^6 cells. (Reproduced by permission from Richards CD, Brown TJ, Shoyab M, Baumann H, Gauldie J. Recombinant oncostatin-M stimulates the production of acute phase proteins in hepatocytes in vitro. J Immunol 1992; 148:1731–1736.)

Figure 15–3 The roles of cytokines in local and systemic events are represented. Initiating cells, such as platelets and macrophages, respond to stimuli, such as trauma or infection, by releasing IL-1 or TNF, which in turn can stimulate local stromal cells. The release of chemokines, such as MCP and IL-8, regulates monocyte or neutrophil chemotaxis, whereas up-regulation of adhesion molecules, such as ICAM and ECAM, facilitates passage into tissue. Release of granulocyte-macrophage CSF (GM-CSF) and granulocyte CSF (G-CSF) modulate progenitor growth and release from bone marrow. IL-1, IL-6, and TNF can act at the CNS to mediate fever and release of ACTH. The acute-phase protein response of the liver appears to be controlled by IL-1, TNF, and IL-6 released from the site of inflammation. Leukemia-inhibiting factor (LIF) oncostatin M (OM), or IL-11 can also act on liver; however, the source of these in inflammation in vivo is not clear.

gistically by dexamethasone in culture (60–62). Plasma α_1-AGP levels can be enhanced by administration of corticosteroids alone in rodents; however, responses to cytokine/steroid combinations are much stronger.

Other cytokines may have modulatory roles by affecting hepatocyte responses to IL-6. Interferon-γ (IFN-γ) inhibits IL-6–induced α_1-ACH, fibrinogen, and HP expression (63), whereas epidermal growth factor (EGF) modulates IL-6–induced albumin synthesis (64). TGF-β causes a small enhancement of α_1-ACH, α_1-PI, and fibrinogen production in hepatoma cells (64). These factors could contribute to the profile of cytokines the liver is exposed to, which presumably is continually altered in a temporal fashion and in different disease states, thus accounting for variation of APP levels in vivo (65,66).

RECEPTORS/SIGNAL TRANSDUCTION: Hepatocytes possess different surface receptors (α-subunit) for IL-6, OM, LIF, and IL-11 that share a common β-subunit, gp130 (67). IL-6R and LIF-R are present at relatively low numbers per cell (400–600) (55,68–70). It has been shown in elegant transfection studies that although an 80 kd IL-6 α-subunit can bind the IL-6 ligand, coexpression of gp130 (β-subunit) is necessary for mediation of biological effects (71,72). The unique LIF-R α-subunit shows homology to gp130 (73), whereas the putative α-subunits of the OM and IL-11R complexes are not yet characterized at the molecular level. Similar to the IL-6Rα, presence of gp130 is necessary for formation of a high affinity receptor complex and signal transduction by OM, LIF, or IL-11 (55,67,73,74). Differences in tissue expression of the α-subunits may impart differences in cellular responses to these cytokines. A fifth member of the IL-6–like family of cytokines is ciliary neurotrophic factor (CNTF), which also utilizes gp130 for signal transduction. CNTF is apparently limited in activity to the nervous system due to the necessity of a unique receptor subunit, in addition to LIF-R and gp130, to make up the receptor complex (75,76). Antibodies to gp130 can suppress signaling by all these receptors (77).

The gp130 serves as an affinity converter molecule, and it is rapidly phosphorylated at various residues in its cytoplasmic domain after ligand binding (76,78). The receptor complexes or α-subunits do not have intrinsic kinase activity; therefore, activation of local kinases is likely. The nature of these steps is not known in hepatocytes; however, OM is capable of activating tyrosine kinases, such as p62 and p56, in endothelial cells (79).

Tyrosine phosphorylation may also be involved in IL-6 receptor activation of B cells (80). Tyrosine phosphorylation inhibitors can inhibit OM-induced low density lipoprotein (LDL) responses in HepG2 cells, although whether APP protein responses are also inhibited is not clear. Thus, tyrosine phosphorylation is a likely critical step in signal transduction by these cytokines; however,

the nature of the specific enzymes involved is not clear. Subsequent signaling steps are not known, but there is evidence that a serine/threonine kinase is also part of the pathway, because inhibitors are capable of modulating responses even in the presence of the initial tyrosine phosphorylation of gp130 (67). More recently, it was shown that CNTF stimulation of a neuroblastoma cell line (SK-N-MC) resulted in tyrosine phosphorylation of p91 and related proteins implicated in IFN signal pathways (81). These proteins then translocate to the nucleus, where they bind to DNA sequences that are found in CNTF-responsive genes. Whether a similar mechanism is involved in other cell types and the IL-6–related cytokines awaits future studies.

IL-1 interacts at either type 1 or 2 IL-1Rs, although the type 1 IL-1R appears to be responsible for signal transduction (82). The type 2 IL-1R has a very short cytoplasmic tail, and although it is expressed on HepG2 cells (83), whether it induces signal transduction is not clear. The type 1 IL-1R is an 80 kd single-chain protein expressed on fibroblasts, connective tissue cells, and a variety of other cells, including low numbers expressed on hepatocytes. TNF interacts with two receptors, a high affinity type 1 receptor, TNF-R1, and a lower affinity type 1 receptor, TNF-R2 (84). TNF-R1 may dimerize in signaling hepatoma cells to express APPs (85).

IL-1 and TNF share many biological activities (86,87), and they may activate several signal pathways in regulating nuclear events. IL-1–induced phosphorylation of the small molecular weight heat shock protein, HSP-27, occurs due to activation of a serine/threonine kinase (88,89). In an epidermal cell line, inhibitors of map kinase (MAPK) activity can cause a profound decrease in IL-1–stimulated IL-6 or PGE$_2$ production, but not IL-1–induced nuclear factor kappa β (NF-$k\beta$) activation (90). MAPK is activated by IL-1, but it is also activated by other ligands, such as IL-6 and insulin, and whether such kinases are regulated similarly in hepatocytes is not clearly defined. Involvement of separate enzymes and their activation is possible in the regulation of expression of many APPs.

RECEPTOR MODULATION IN INFLAMMATION: The APR of hepatocytes to cytokines also depends on the level of expression or activation of cell receptors. In vitro, the mRNA for IL-6R α-subunit (IL-6Rα) can be up-regulated in hepatocytes on HepG2 cells by various combinations of glucocorticoid, IL-1, and IL-6 (91–95) in a time-dependent fashion. The mRNA for gp130 is up-regulated in HepG2 cells by the combination of IL-6 and glucocorticoid (96) (Richards CD, Gauldie J, unpublished observations). Epithelial cell types have also shown up-regulation of gp130 mRNA by treatment with IL-1, TNF, and IL-6 in vitro (97). Treatment of rat hepatocytes in vitro with IL-1 or IL-6 resulted in down-regula-

tion of surface receptors and mRNA for IL-6R and gp130 (93). Whether these changes in mRNA expression and surface expression of receptors alter responsiveness of these cells to IL-6 is not yet clear.

Models of inflammation in vivo also show that IL-6R is regulated at the mRNA level in liver. This regulation occurs as early as 3 hours, and it peaks 3 to 6 hours after rats were treated with LPS (IV), Freund's adjuvant (IP), or turpentine (SC) (Fig. 15–4) (91). Animals injected with recombinant IL-6 showed a similar increase in liver mRNA levels for the α-subunit of the receptor. Thus, dur-

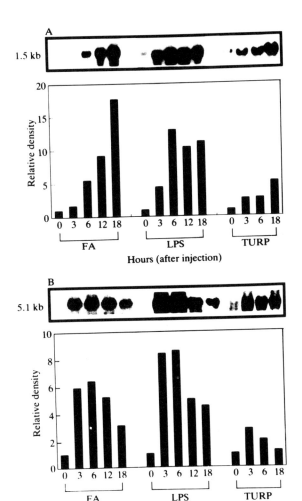

Figure 15–4 Regulation of IL-6 receptor mRNA in vivo. Sprague-Dawley rats (200 gm) were treated intraperitoneally with 0.5 mL Freund's complete adjuvant, intravenously with 200 μg CPS, or subcutaneously with 0.2 mL turpentine. Rats were killed at the various time points indicated, and RNA was extracted from liver tissue samples. PolyA+ RNA was prepared by oligo dT chromatography, and 30 μg was loaded per lane for Northern analysis. The blots were probed for (A) α₁-cysteine proteinase inhibitor (CPI) and (B) IL-6R using labeled rat cDNA probes. Changes in levels were quantitated using densitometry scans (*black bars*). (Reproduced by permission from (Geisterfer M, Richards CD, Baumann M, Fey G, Gwynne D, Gauldie J. Regulation of IL-6 and hepatic IL-6 receptor in acute inflammation in vivo. Cytokine 1993;5:1–7.)

ing inflammation, there is a rapid increase in serum IL-6 content as well as in IL-6Rα component expression by liver, and both factors govern the nature of the hepatic response to IL-6. In vivo regulation of other cytokine receptors and their components on hepatocytes may also be modified in a time-dependent fashion, although this hypothesis has not been proved.

The existence of soluble forms of receptors for IL-1, TNF, and IL-6 represents an additional mechanism by which responses to ligand presence during the APR may be regulated. Soluble binding proteins for these cytokines have been found in body fluids such as urine and serum (98–100). Proteins that bind IL-1 or TNF have been shown to be forms of the cell surface receptors, and, when bound to ligand, they inhibit biological activity. In contrast, in vitro evidence suggests that the α-chain of IL-6R can bind IL-6 in soluble form, but they then cause signal transduction in cells that express gp130 (72,101). Narazaki and associates (102) showed that high levels of soluble gp130 are present in serum, and the authors suggested that soluble gp130 could compete for the IL-6R/IL-6 complex with cell-associated gp130. Whether this competition may occur in vivo is not clear; however, altered levels of soluble IL-6R are evident in diseases such as human immunodeficiency virus (100), which suggests that elevation of soluble IL-6R could have a role in modulation of cell responses. Soluble IL-6R produced by genetic engineering can bind IL-6 and enhance APP synthesis by HepG2 cells (101). One report suggests that soluble IL-6R can be generated by shedding of the surface protein (103), and another suggests that a second alternately spliced mRNA exists for IL-6R on various cell types that lacks the entire transmembrane region, but is otherwise similar (104). The role of these receptor components, as well as soluble IL-1R and TNF-R, in liver responses in vivo awaits further investigation.

GENE REGULATION: Study of the regulation of APP gene transcription has revealed, as in other genes, that multiple nuclear factors (NF) appear to be involved in the expression of any single APP gene, and that cooperation or repression can result from the interaction of different nuclear factors either at the protein–protein level, or by protein–DNA interaction. A number of transcriptional regulating proteins have been defined that can bind to specific sequences or regulatory elements found in APP promoter and enhancer gene regions. Glucocorticoid receptor can modulate genes containing recognizable response elements (GRE), and it probably accounts for the synergistic activity in enhanced expression of α₁-AGP, HP, and fibrinogen by glucocorticoid (105–107).

A second set of nuclear factors involved are those of the C/EBP group. These factors include C/EBP-β, which has also been termed *NFIL-6α* in human, *LAP* and *IL-6*

DBP in rats, or *AGP/EBP* in mouse; and C/EBP-δ, which is analogous to NFIL-6β in humans (108–110). It appears that the C/EBP-β group can interact with the C/EBP-δ group, and cotransfection of NFIL-6α and NFIL-6β can synergize in transcriptional activation of sequences containing responsive elements (111). These elements bind to a consensus sequence, ACATTGCACAATCT, present in type 1 APP genes, such as α_1-AGP, C3, and CRP, as well as the IL-6 promoter. IL-6 has been shown to induce NFIL-6α/IL-6 DBP activity by post-translational modification, whereas NFIL-6β/CEBP-δ is transcriptionally induced by IL-6, implicating both mechanisms in the regulation of APP genes possessing the ACATTGCACAATCT motif.

Protein-protein interaction of the glucocorticoid receptor and NFIL-6 synergistically enhances transcription of sequences of the rat α_1-AGP gene (112). Other experiments have shown that interaction of the glucocorticoid receptor with the AP-1 complex causes inhibition of AP-1–driven transcription (113). In addition, the distinct nuclear factor NF-kβ may also interact with NFIL-6 to mod-

ulate transcription (114). NF-kβ can bind sequences and activate transcription of the SAA, angiotensinogen, and α_1-AGP genes (115), in addition to having a role in IL-6 expression (116,117).

Separate nuclear factors have been implicated further in type 2 APP genes, such as α_2-macroglobulin, fibrinogen, HP, α_1-CPI, and CRP (118–120), which contain a consensus sequence (*CTGGGAA*) termed *IL-6RE*. These factors, termed *IL-6 response element binding protein (IL-6REBP)* in human cells and *APR factor (APRF)* in rat cells, appear specifically to bind IL-6RE (118,121,122) and to activate transcription after cellular responses to IL-6. We have shown that OM, LIF, and IL-6 can strongly regulate CAT genes downstream of IL-6RE (46) (Fig. 15–5). The nature and function of these factors have been elusive thus far, although IL-6 stimulation of hepatocytes apparently alters activity through post-translational modification (122). Other transcription factors, including hepatocyte nuclear factor-1 (HNF-1), contribute to the tissue specificity of APP gene regulation (120); others, such as the ets oncogene family, may also have a role in regulating APP with ets-binding sequences in their genes. Furthermore, cytokine stimulation of hepatoma cells results in elevated levels of early-response genes, such as c-jun in IL-1–stimulated cells and jun B in IL-6–stimulated cells (123). The role these early responses have in APP gene regulation is not known.

Other local events

Production of cytokines and cell infiltration caused by immediate local events are associated with additional sequelae at the site of inflammation. Recruitment of phagocytic cells can result in release of catabolic enzymes, such as elastases, cathepsin G, metalloproteinases, and superoxide radicals from granulocytes and macrophages. These products aid in destruction of foreign particles, but they can also damage nearby host tissue, resulting in cytopathology. The proinflammatory cytokines IL-1 and TNF can prime phagocytes for release of these agents. In addition, IL-1 and TNF are powerful inducers of matrix metalloproteinase (MMP) expression by local connective tissue cells (124,125).

Enhanced expression of collagenase (MMP-1) or stromelysin (MMP-3) is evident in vivo in both acute and chronically inflamed tissue (126,127). These enzymes contribute to the tissue remodeling process; if they are not regulated appropriately, they are thought to have a central role in chronic destructive tissue diseases (128,129). The metalloproteinases are activated by cleavage of propeptide to yield active enzyme. These enzymes are then inhibited by the natural tissue inhibitors of metalloproteinases, TIMP-1 and TIMP-2, which are also expressed by connective tissue cells, among others (130,131). The balance of MMP and

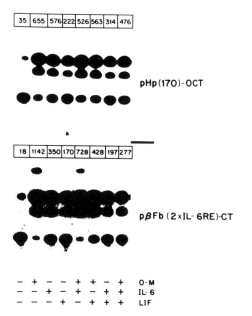

Figure 15–5 OM controls transcription via IL-6 regulatory elements. HepG2 cells were transfected with either pHp(170)-OCT or pβFb(2xIL-6RE)-CT constructs containing CAT expression genes. Each transfection mixture included the reference plasmid, pIE MUP, whose level of expression allowed normalization of transfection efficiency. Twenty-four hours after subdividing the transfected cells, OM (O-M; 100 ng/mL), IL-6 (100 ng/mL), or LIF (10 U/mL) and the various combinations were used to stimulate the cells. CAT activity was determined and calculated relative to the expression of major urinary protein, and it is expressed as percent conversion of substrated to product per hour and per pg major urinary protein. (Reproduced by permission from Richards CD, Brown TJ, Shoyab M, Baumann H, Gauldie J. Recombinant oncostatin-M stimulates the production of acute phase proteins in hepatocytes in vitro. J Immunol 1992;148:1731–1736.)

TIMPs provides a net enzymatic activity, and they can also be regulated at other stages, such as during proenzyme gene expression or inhibition of activation.

Although IL-1/TNF can elevate MMP expression, cytokines such as IL-6 and OM can specifically up-regulate TIMP-1 expression in fibroblasts and certain tumor cells in vitro (Fig. 15–6) (132–134). Other evidence suggests that IL-6 can enhance IL-1–induced MMP expression in human synovial fibroblasts (135). Furthermore, PGE$_2$ has been shown to inhibit stromelysin expression (136) and to enhance TIMP-1 expression (137) in human fibroblast cell cultures. Thus, IL-6 and PGE$_2$ released by local cells may have a paracrine/autocrine effect on the production of active enzymes and their inhibitors. Whether such an effect occurs in phagocytic cells is not clear. Furthermore, in vitro data suggest that IL-1–induced PGE$_2$ has modulatory effects on connective tissue cytokine production: PGE$_2$ can inhibit granulocyte-macrophage colony-stimulating factor (GM-CSF) production and simultaneously enhance G-CSF production by fibroblasts (138). We have shown that OM can also act on fibroblasts to further enhance IL-1–induced IL-6 expression (137). Thus, the cytokines produced by proinflammatory or first wave cytokines may be further modulated by locally produced mediators. OM up-regulates the production of IL-6 by endothelial cells (139), which may further contribute to systemic IL-6 levels in vivo.

ROLE OF ACUTE-PHASE PROTEINS

Initiation of the liver APP response results in increased systemic levels of positive APP that peak at 24 to 48 hours in vivo after inflammatory stimuli. These increased levels may thus modify activity of cells or proteins in the blood, or, after entering extravascular tissue, they may modify activity of cells or molecular interactions at sites of inflammation. Collectively, APPs provide a number of activities that appear to function in a homeostatic nature: they replace proteins utilized in coagulation; they provide proteins that inhibit protease activity, thereby curbing excessive proteolysis; and they provide opsonization of certain agents, thus modulating local inflammation.

Hemostasis and transport proteins

Tissue damage, including bleeding and blood coagulation, results in the rapid utilization of fibrinogen, which also serves to demarcate the affected tissue site. The liver response (i.e., elevating fibrinogen output 4- to 10-fold) replaces the fibrinogen used and prepares for the possibility of further blood vessel damage. In addition, the elevation of α$_2$-plasmin inhibitor during the acute phase inhibits fibrinolysis and thus aids coagulation. Deficiency of this protein is associated with severe bleeding disorders that can be managed with replacement therapy. Fibrinogen and α$_2$-plasmin inhibitor both aid in homeostasis after transection of blood vessels. Ritchie and Fuller (140) suggested that peptides D and E, derived from the cleavage of fibrin, enhance macrophage production of IL-6, which acts as a positive feedback to enhance fibrinogen output by the liver.

In addition, APPs also transport and remove molecules during inflammation. Haptoglobin binds hemoglobin released during tissue damage involving hemolysis, whereas hemopexin binds heme released during such processes. Ceruloplasmin is a transport protein for copper, but it can also inhibit superoxide anion–dependent enzyme reactions, and it possibly has a role in neutralizing oxygen-derived reactive metabolites.

Antiprotease action

Proteinase inhibitors that are elevated during the acute phase include members of the serpins (inhibitors of serine proteases), cystatin (inhibitors of cysteine proteinases), and α-macroglobulin (inhibitor of a broad range of pro-

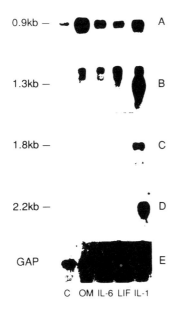

Figure 15–6 OM, IL-6, LIF, and IL-1α induce TIMP-1 mRNA in fibroblasts. Confluent human lung fibroblasts were cultured for 18 hours in 2% FCS/DMEM with: no addition (C), OM (50 ng/mL), IL-6 (50 ng/mL), LIF (5,000 U/mL), or IL-1α (5 ng/mL). RNA was extracted and 10-μg aliquots were run in formaldehyde-denaturing 1% agarose gels. RNA was sequentially probed (then stripped and reprobed) for (A) TIMP-1, (B) IL-6, (C) stromelysin, (D) collagenase, and (E) glyceraldehyde-3-p-dehydrogenase (GAP). The size of each RNA species signal is indicated in kb. (Reproduced by permission from Richards CD, Shoyab M, Brown TJ, Gauldie J. Selective regulation of tissue inhibitor of metalloproteinases (TIMP-1) by oncostatin M in fibroblasts in culture. J Immunol 1993;150:5596–5603.)

teinases) superfamilies. α_1-Proteinase inhibitor, which inhibits neutrophil elastase, and α_1-ACH, which inhibits neutrophil cathepsin G and mast-cell chymase (141), are the most prominent serpins evident during the APR in humans. Elevated levels would gain control of proteinases released by invading organisms or by host cells in response to inflammatory stimuli, such as the neutrophil products noted. This process would help protect the integrity of normal host tissue in a time frame that would allow a burst of enzyme activity early in the process; however, if sustained, this burst would cause unnecessary destruction of nearby tissue. Although this is the simplest explanation of why such a liver response has been so well conserved through evolution, it is difficult to determine if such a purpose is critical in vivo. Because no reports exist of individuals with defects in this system (other than an α_1-PI deficiency), such defects may be incompatible with life.

In the APP response in rats, the major increases in serum levels are seen in a cystatin member called thiostatin (also called α_1-CPI, α_1-MAP, t-kininogen), as well as in α_2-macroglobulin. The targets for thiostatin are not known, but it presumably endows rats with a defense in inflammation for an unknown function. α_2-Macroglobulin has the broadest activity in vitro: It inhibits serine-, cysteine- and metalloproteinases, but due to its size (725 kd), it is restricted mainly to the plasma compartment. It has been suggested that α_2-macroglobulin is a support inhibitor to back up more specific ones if they are saturated by substrates (141,142). Evidence shows that transfer of proteases from one inhibitor (e.g., TIMP [143]) to α_2-macroglobulin does occur, which provides another sink for disposal of excess proteases. Recent evidence suggests that serpin-protease complexes enhance IL-6 release by monocytes in vitro (144) and that proteolytically modified α_1-PI can also enhance IL-6 production. This effect raises the possibility that other inhibitors may release cytokine-inducing fragments after binding to their substrate, thus contributing to cytokine modulation.

Opsonization

CRP is a major APP in humans (i.e., it increases 100-fold in serum levels) to which a number of functions have been ascribed, including binding activity of phosphocholine moieties, such as those on the C-polysaccharide of pneumococci cell wall (thus originally termed *C-reactive protein*) that appear to require Ca^{2+}; and binding of chromatin, probably through binding of histones (145). CRP has also been reported to bind to fibronectin and various galactans (146). CRP clearly enhances phagocytosis of gram-positive and gram-negative bacteria by blood leukocytes. Binding of CRP can activate complement through the classic pathway, resulting in C3 convertase and re-

lease of C3a; however, an efficient C5 convertase is apparently not formed so that the complement lytic complex C5-C9 may not proceed (147). CRP is found deposited at local sites of inflammation, and it can bind to neutrophils and enhance tumoricidal activity of monocytes through what appear to be specific receptors (145). In addition to CRP, complement component C3 is a minor APP, and it presumably functions at least in part to replace complement utilized at sites of inflammation. The role of complement in opsonization is well established.

Immunomodulation and proliferation

Several acute phase proteinase inhibitors exhibit effects on immune function and cell proliferation in vitro, and thus may provide a dampening action on immune responses in vivo, thereby contributing to control of specific immunity. α_1-PI inhibits proliferative responses of mononuclear cells to lectins (148), and purified antiproteinases have been reported to modulate natural killer (NK) cell activity and antibody-dependent cellular cytotoxicity (ADCC) cell function (149–151), as well as endotoxin shock (152,153). SAA and α_1-PI inhibit plaque-forming cell responses, whereas CRP also inhibits T-cell proliferation and production of cytokines in vitro. These functions could serve as a fine-tuning mechanism whereby events at local sites of immune-mediated tissue destruction are modulated.

Cytokine/cytokine inhibitor production

More recent studies have suggested that APPs also modulate production of certain cytokines by some cell types. Treatment of monocytes, for example, with complexes of α_1-ACH/chymotrypsin will enhance IL-6 production and APP stimulating activity of the monocyte supernatants (144). Recent findings suggest a more defined feedback anti-inflammatory role for IL-6–induced APP. In cancer patients receiving IL-6 infusion as part of their therapy regimen, increased levels of IL-1RA (i.e., the IL-1R antagonist that blocks IL-1 function [154–156]), are found (157). Moreover, the APPs induced by IL-6, including CRP, α_1-PI, and α_1-AGP all induce IL-1RA synthesis by peripheral blood mononuclear cells in vitro (157,158), thus demonstrating a link between IL-6 release, IL-6 function, and APP function in regulation and resolution of the APR.

RESOLUTION

Enhanced liver expression of APPs returns to normal by day 2 to 3 after an acute stimulus, accompanied by a decrease to normal APP plasma levels by day 5 to 10. In cultured hepatocytes/hepatoma cells, this up-regulation and down-regulation in response to an IL-6 stimulus is more rapid, presumably due to the nature of "one-shot" stimulation versus a continuous and evolving mixture of cytokines the liver is exposed to in vivo. The natural decay of the response is presumably due in large part to removal or inactivation of the initial inflammatory agent and the resultant lack of generation of cytokines and mediators. Because the plasma $T_{1/2}$ of cytokines such as IL-1, TNF, and IL-6 is relatively short, there is a reduction of active circulating cytokines able to regulate hepatocyte APP synthesis. In turn, because the up-regulation of acute phase gene expression is transient, hepatocyte synthesis returns to a normal profile of proteins produced.

In addition to this mechanism, processes may also exist that actively turn the liver response down by directly acting on hepatocytes, although no evidence for this effect has been shown. However, it is apparent that specific mediators (including corticosteroid and certain cytokines) can actively down-regulate the production of first and second wave cytokines and thus may indirectly regulate the hepatic response.

Corticosteroid

Enhanced levels of cortisol due to inflammatory stimuli can aid in the expression of certain APPs in which synergistic action is evident in combination with IL-1 or IL-6 (18). In addition, corticosteroid may enhance expression of IL-6R mRNA and thus the potential response of hepatocytes to IL-6. The effects of glucocorticoids on other cell types is wide-ranging; however, a critical effect is their ability to markedly inhibit production of cytokines such as IL-1, TNF, IL-6, IL-8, GM-CSF (159–163), matrix metalloproteinases (164–166), and prostaglandins (167). These effects occur at physiologically relevant levels of steroid; thus, they contribute to regulation of mediators released by monocytes, macrophages, and stromal cells, such as fibroblasts or endothelium.

The mechanism by which this regulation occurs has been examined closely in several systems. The glucocorticoid receptor/glucocorticoid complex (GR) may interact by protein–protein interaction with AP-1 nuclear complex to inhibit transcription of metalloproteinase (168, 169). This GR complex may also interact with other nuclear factors in a similar fashion to regulation transcription of IL-6 as noted. Corticosteroid also appears to decrease stability of mRNA for IL-1α, IL-1β, and IL-6 in monocytes (159), as well as the stability of mRNA for IL-8, IL-6, and GM-CSF in fibroblasts (162). The mechanism by which these effects occur is not clear. Many cytokines, including the ones mentioned, possess the AUUUA motif in the 3' untranslated region of the mRNA transcript, which confers instability to the molecule (170,171). This

instability provides a transience to the cytokine system that allows natural decay of induced responses.

Cytokines

A number of cytokines exhibit in vitro activities that result in down-regulation of proinflammatory molecules and mediators. IL-1RA is thought to provide a mechanism for IL-1 shutoff, which could inhibit the cytokine cascade. IL-1RA is found in body fluids from inflammatory sites and thus may contribute to control of inflammation in vivo. Pharmacological administration of IL-1RA had marked effects in animal models (172); however, the physiological concentrations generated naturally are low in comparison to those needed for significant responses in the animals. The effects of IL-1RA could be broad because IL-1 acts on many cell types.

Several other cytokines have been shown to modulate monocyte production of proinflammatory molecules, including IL-6, which inhibits IL-1 and TNF production by monocytes and monocytic cell lines in vitro (173,174). The T-cell–derived cytokines IL-4 and IL-10 (175–177) have been shown to inhibit expression of TNF, IL-1, IL-8 (178–180), and MIP-1α (181) by monocytes, whereas IL-4 simultaneously enhances expression of IL-1RA (182,183). In addition, IL-4 has been shown to up-regulate soluble IL-1R type 2, which does not transduce signals, thus inhibiting IL-1 activity due to extracellular binding (184). IL-13, a recently characterized molecule, has activities very similar to IL-4. The roles of IL-4, IL-10, and IL-13 in inflammation are not clear because expression of these molecules in tissues has not been extensively studied; however, administration of IL-10 to mice protected the animals from the lethal effects of LPS challenge (185). Down-regulation of the macrophage and its production of IL-6 and IL-6–inducing cytokines (i.e., IL-1, TNF) may indeed be central in shaping the APR in certain conditions.

Thus, there appears to be various mechanisms by which the acute inflammatory cascade and the liver response may be turned off. This redundancy may mirror that which characterizes the mechanisms by which the liver response is initiated, thereby providing a variety of ways to allow a normal course of events to occur, followed by a return to homeostasis. After further investigation, however, it may become clear that certain subtle alterations in one or more of these processes may contribute to aspects of chronic inflammation, because the return to homeostasis is avoided and the cascade of cytokine and cellular events continues.

REFERENCES

1. Feldman M, Brennan FM, Chantry D, et al. Cytokine production in the rheumatoid joint: implications for treatment. Ann Rheum Dis 1990;49:480–486.

2. Feldmann M, Brennan FM, Williams RO, et al. Evaluation of the role of cytokines in autoimmune disease: the importance of TNFα in rheumatoid arthritis. Prog Growth Factor Res 1992;4:247–255.

3. DeWitt DL. Prostaglandin endoperoxide synthase: regulation of enzyme expression. Biochim Biophys Acta 1991; 1083:121–134.

4. Baumann H, Won K-A, Jahreis GP. Human hepatocyte-stimulating factor-III and intrleukin-6 are structurally and immunologically distinct but regulate the production of the same acute phase plasma proteins. J Biol Chem 1989; 264:8046–8051.

5. Schall TJ. Biology of the RANTES/SIS cytokine family. Cytokine 1991;3:1–18.

6. Schall T, Bacon K, Toy K, Goeddel D. Selective attraction of monocytes and T lymphocytes of the memory phenotype by cytokine RANTES. Nature 1990;347:669–671.

7. Matsushima K, Oppenheim JJ. Interleukin 8 and MCAF: novel inflammatory cytokines inducible by IL 1 and TNF. Cytokine 1989;1:2–13.

8. Gauldie J, Richards C, Harnish D, Lansdorp P, Baumann H. Interferon-beta2/B-cell stimulatory factor type 2 shares identity with monocyte hepatocyte-stimulating factor and regulates the major acute phase protein response in liver cells. Proc Natl Acad Sci USA 1987;84:7251–7255.

9. Baumann H, Gauldie J. Regulation of hepatic acute phase plasma protein genes by hepatocyte stimulating factors and other mediators of inflammation. Mol Biol Med 1990;7: 147–159.

10. Xing Z, Jordana M, Kirpalani H, Driscoll KE, Schall TJ, Gauldie J. Cytokine expression by neutrophils and macrophages in vivo: endotoxin induces tumor necrosis factor α, macrophage inflammatory protein-2, interleukin-1β and interleukin-6, but not RANTES or transforming growth factor β1 mRNAs expression in acute lung inflammation. Am J Respir Cell Mol Biol 1994;10:148–153.

11. Whicher JT, Gauldie J, Baumann H, Westacott C. Acute phase proteins. In: Bomford R, Henderson B, eds. Interleukin-1, inflammation and disease, research monographs in cell and tissue physiology, vol 16. Amsterdam: Elsevier, 1989:191–216.

12. Ohzato H, Yoshizaki K, Nishimoto N, et al. Interleukin-6 as a new indicator of inflammatory status: detection of serum levels of interleukin-6 and C-reactive protein after surgery. Surgery 1992;111:201–209.

13. Dinarello CA. Biology of interleukin-1. FASEB J 1988;2: 108.

14. Navarra P, Pozzoli G, Brunetti L, Ragazzoni E, Besser M, Grossman A. Interleukin-1beta and interleukin-6 specifically increase the release of prostaglandin E$_2$ from rat hypothalamic explants in vitro. Neuroendocrinology 1992;56: 61–68.

15. Navarra P, Tsagarakis S, Faria MS, Rees LH, Besser M, Grossman AB. Interleukins-1 and -6 stimulate the release of corticotropin-releasing hormone-41 from rat hypothalamus in vitro via the Eicosanoid cyclooxygenase pathway. Endocrinology 1991;128:37–44.

16. Woloski BMRNJ, Smith EM, Meyer WJ III, Fuller GM, Blalock JE. Corticotropin-releasing activity of monokines. Science 1985;230:1035–1037.

17. Naitoh Y, Fukata J, Tominaga T, et al. Interleukin-6 stimu-

lates the secretion of adrenocorticotropic hormone in conscious, freely-moving rats. Biochem Biophys Res Commun 1988;155:1459–1463.

18. Perlstein R, Whitnall M, Abrams J, Mougey E, Neta R. Synergistic roles of interleukin-6, interleukin-1 and tumor necrosis factor in the adrenocorticotropin response to bacterial lipopolysaccharide in vivo. Endocrinology 1993;132: 946–952.

19. Schreiber G. Synthesis, processing and secretion of plasma proteins by the liver (and other organs) and their regulation. Plasma Proteins 1987;5:293–363.

20. Schreiber G, Tsykin A, Aldred AR, et al. The acute phase response in the rodent. Ann NY Acad Sci 1989;557:61–86.

21. Mackiewicz A, Ganapathi MK, Schultz D. Monokines regulate glycosylation of acute phase proteins. J Exp Med 1987;166:253–258.

22. Mackiewicz A, Kushner I. Role of IL-6 in acute phase protein glycosylation. Ann NY Acad Sci 1989;557:515–517.

23. Lamontagne LR, Stadynk AW, Gauldie J. Synthesis of alpha-1-protease inhibitor by resident and activated mouse alveolar macrophages. Am Rev Respir Dis 1985;131:321–325.

24. Homburger F. A plasma fibrinogen-increasing factor obtained from sterile abscesses in dogs. J Clin Invest 1945;24: 43–45.

25. Kampschmidt R, Upchurch HF. Effect of leukocytic endogenous mediator on plasma fibrinogen and haptoglobin. Proc Soc Exp Biol Med 1974;146:904–907.

26. Kampschmidt RF, Upchurch HP, Pulliam LA. Characterization of a leukocyte-derived endogenous mediator responsible for increased plasma fibrinogen. Ann NY Acad Sci 1982;389:338–353.

27. Bornstein DL. Leukocytic pyrogen: a major mediator of the acute phase reaction. Ann NY Acad Sci 1982;389:323–337.

28. Kampschmidt RF, Mesecher M. Interleukin-1 from P388D: effects upon neutrophils plasma iron, and fibrinogen in rats, mice, and rabbits. Proc Soc Exp Biol Med 1985;179: 197–200.

29. Ramadori G, Sipe JD, Dinarello CS, Mizel SB, Colten HR. Pretranslational modulation of acute phase hepatic protein synthesis by murine recombinant interleukin-1 (IL-1) and purified human IL-1. J Exp Med 1985;162:930–942.

30. Perlmutter DH, Dinarello CA, Punsal PI, Coltent HR. Cachectin/tumor necrosis factor regulates hepatic acute phase gene expression. J Clin Invest 1986;78:1349–1354.

31. Le PT, Mortensen RF. In vitro induction of hepatocyte synthesis of the acute phase reaction mouse serum amyloid P-component by macrophages and IL-1. J Leuk Biol 1984;35:587–603.

32. May L, Viguet H, Kenney J, Ida N, Allison A, Sehgal P. High levels of "complexed" interleukin-6 in human blood. J Biol Chem 1992;267:19698–19704.

33. Nijsten M, deGroot E, TenDuuis H, Klensen H, Hack C, Aarden L. Serum levels of interleukin-6 and acute phase responses. Lancet 1987;2:921.

34. Geiger T, Andus T, Klapproth J, Hirano T, Kishimoto T, Heinrich PC. Induction of rat acute-phase proteins by interleukin 6 in vivo. Eur J Immunol 1988;18:717–721.

35. Ulich T, Guo K, Remick D, Castillo J, Yin S. Endotoxin-induced cytokine gene expression in vivo. IL-6 mRNA and

serum protein expression and the in vivo hematologic effect of IL-6. J Immunol 1991;146:2316–2323.

36. Hirano T, Akira S, Taga T, Kishimoto T. Biological and clinical aspects of interleukin 6. Immunol Today 1990;11:443–449.

37. Hirohata S, Tanimoto K, Ito K. Elevation of cerebrospinal fluid interleukin-6 activity in patients with vasculitides and central nervous system involvement. Clin Immunol Immunopathol 1993;66:225–229.

38. Honssiau F. Bukasa K, Sindic C, Van Damme J, Van Snick J. Interleukin-6 in synovial fluid and serum of patients with rheumatoid arthritis and other inflammatory arthritides. Arthritis Rheum 1988;31:784–788.

39. Eastgate JA, Symons JA, Wood NC, Grinlinton FM, di Giovine FS, Duff GW. Correlation of plasma interleukin 1 levels with disease activity in rheumatoid arthritis. Lancet 1988;2:706–709.

40. Libert C, Brouckaert P, Shaw A, Fiers W. Induction of interleukin 6 by human and murine recombinant interleukin 1 in mice. Eur J Immunol 1990;20:691–694.

41. Jablons DM, Mule JJ, McIntosh JK, et al. IL-6/IFN-beta2 as a circulating hormone. Induction by cytokine administration in humans. J Immunol 1989;142:1542–1547.

42. Mihara M, Ikuta M, Koishihara Y, Ohsugi Y. Interleukin 6 inhibits delayed-type hypersensitivity and the development of adjuvant arthritis. Eur J Immunol 1991;21:2327–2331.

43. Ulich TR, Yin S, Guo K, Yi ES, Remick D, del Castillo J. Intratracheal injection of endotoxin and cytokines. Am J Pathol 1991;138:1097–1101.

44. Starnes HF Jr, Pearce MK, Tewari A, Yim JH, Zou J-C, Abrams JS. Anti-IL-6 monoclonal antibodies protect against lethal Escherichia coli infection and letal tumor necrosis factor-alpha challenge in mice. J Immunol 1990;145:4185–4191.

45. Finkelman FD, Madden KB, Morris SC, et al. Anti-cytokine antibodies as carrier proteins. Prolongation of in vivo effects of exogenous cytokines by injection of cytokine–anti-cytokine antibody complexes. J Immunol 1993;151:1235–1244.

46. Richards CD, Brown TJ, Shoyab M, Baumann H, Gauldie J. Recombinant oncostatin-M stimulates the production of acute phase proteins in hepatocytes in vitro. J Immunol 1992;148:1731–1736.

47. Grove RI, Mazzucco CE, Radka SF, Shoyab M, Keiner PA. Oncostatin M upregulates low density lipoprotein receptors in HepG2 cells by a novel mechanism. J Biol Chem 1991;266:18194–18199.

48. Brown TJ, Lioubin MN, Marquardt H. Purification and characterization of cytostatic lymphokines produced by activated human T lymphocytes. J Immunol 1987;139:2977–2983.

49. Malik N, Kallestad JC, Gunderson NL, et al. Molecular cloning, sequence analysis, and functional expression of a novel growth regulator, oncostatin M. Mol Cell Biol 1989;9:2847–2853.

50. Rose TM, Bruce AG. Oncostatin M is a member of the cytokine family which includes LIF, GM-CSF and IL-6. Proc Natl Acad Sci USA 1991;88:8641–8645.

51. Bazan F. Neuropeptide cytokines in the hematopoietic fold. Neuron 1991;7:197–208.

52. Baumann H, Wong GG. Hepatocyte-stimulating factor III shares structural and function identity with leukemia inhibitory factor. J Immunol 1989;143:1163–1167.

53. Northemann W, Hattori M, Baffet G, et al. Production of interleukin 6 by hepatoma cells. Mol Biol Med 1990;7:273–285.

54. Fey GH, Hattori M, Northemann W, et al. Regulation of rat liver acute phase genes by interleukin-6 and production of hepatocyte stimulating factors by rat hepatoma cells. Ann NY Acad Sci 1989;557:317–331.

55. Gearing DP, Bruce AG. Oncostatin M binds the high-affinity leukemia inhibitory factor receptor. New Biologist 1991;4:61–65.

56. Baumann H, Schendel P. Interleukin-11 regulates the hepatic expression of the same plasma protein genes as interleukin-6. J Biol Chem 1991;266:1–4.

57. Megidish T, Mazurek N. A mutant protein kinase C that can transform fibroblasts. Nature 1989;342:807–811.

58. Kishimoto T. The biology of interleukin-6. Blood 1989;74:1–10.

59. Baumann H, Gauldie J. Regulation of hepatic acute phase plasma protein genes by hepatocyte stimulating factors and other mediators of inflammation. Mol Biol Med 1990;7:147–159.

60. Koj A, Gauldie J, Regoeczi E, Sauder DN, Sweeney GD. The acute-phase response of cultured rat hepatocytes. System characterization and the effect of human cytokines. Biochem J 1984;224:505–514.

61. Baumann H. Hepatic acute phase reaction in vivo and in vitro. In Vitro Cell Dev Biol 1989;25:115–126.

62. Baumann H, Firestone GL, Burgess TL, Gross KW, Yamamoto KR, Held WA. Dexamethasone regulaton of alpha-1-acid glycoprotein and other acute phase reactants in rat liver and hepatoma cells. J Biol Chem 1983;258:563–570.

63. Magielska-Zero D, Bereta J, Czuba-Pelech B, Pajdak W, Gauldie J, Koj A. Inhibitory effect of human recombinant interferon gamma on synthesis of acute phase proteins in human hepatoma Hep G2 cells stimulated by leukocyte cytokines, TNFα and IFN-β2/BSF-2/IL-6. Biochem Int 1988;17:17–23.

64. Rokita H, Bereta J, Koj A, Gordon AH, Gauldie J. Epidermal growth factor and transforming growth factor-beta differently modulate the acute phase response elicited by interleukin-6 in cultured liver cells from man, rat and mouse. Comp Biochem Physiol [A] 1990;95:41–45.

65. Gauldie J, Lamontagne L, Stadnyk A. Acute phase response in infectious disease. Surv Synth Pathol Res 1985;4:126–151.

66. Whicher JT, Banks RE, Thompson D, Evans SW. The measurement of acute phase proteins as disease markers. In: Mackiewicz A, Kushner I, Baumann H, eds. Acute phase proteins. Boca Raton, FL: CRC Press, 1993:633–650.

67. Taga T, Kishimoto T. Cytokine receptors and signal transduction. FASEB J 1992;6:3387–3396.

68. Yamasaki K, Taga T, Hirato Y, et al. Cloning and expression of the human interleukin-6 (BSF-2/IFNbeta 2) receptor. Science 1988;241:825–828.

69. Hirano T, Taga T, Yamasaki F, et al. Molecular cloning of the cDNAs for IL-6/B cell stimulatory factor 2 and its receptor. Ann NY Acad Sci 1989;557:167–180.

70. Baumann H, Isseroff H, Latimer J, Jahreis G. Phorbol ester modulates interleukin 6- and interleukin 1-regulated expression of acute phase plasma proteins in hepatoma cells. J Biol Chem 1988;263:17390–17396.

71. May L, Ghrayeb J, Santhanam U, et al. Synthesis and secretion of multiple forms of beta2-interferon/B-cell differentiation factor-2/hepatocyte stimulating factor by human fibroblasts and monocytes. J Biol Chem 1988;263:7760–7766.

72. Hibi M, Murakami M, Saito M, Hirano T, Taga T, Kishimoto T. Molecular cloning and expression of an IL-6 signal transducer, gp130. Cell 1990;63:1149–1157.

73. Gearing DP, Thut CJ, VandenBos T, et al. Leukemia inhibitory factor receptor is structurally related to the IL-6 signal transducer, gp130. EMBO J 1991;10:2839–2848.

74. Liu J, Modrell B, Aruffo A, et al. Interleukin-6 signal transducer, gp130 mediates oncostatin M signaling. J Biol Chem 1993;267:16763–16766.

75. Miyajima A, Hara T, Kitamura T. Common subunits of cytokine receptors and the functional redundancy of cytokines. TIBS 1992;17:378–382.

76. Ip N, Nye S, Boulton T, et al. CNTF and LIF act on neural cells via shared signalling pathways that involve the IL-6 signal transducing receptor component gp130. Cell 1992;69:1121–1132.

77. Taga T, Narazaki M, Yasukawa K, et al. Functional inhibition of hematopoietic and neutrophic cytokines by blocking the interleukin 6 transducer gp130. Proc Natl Acad Sci USA 1992;89:10998–11001.

78. Murakami M, Narazaki M, Hibi M, et al. Critical cytoplasmic region of the interleukin 6 signal transducer gp130 is conserved in the cytokine receptor family. Proc Natl Acad Sci USA 1991;88:11349–11353.

79. Schieven G, Kallestad J, Brown J, Ledbetter J, Linsley P. Oncostatin M induces tyrosine phosphorylation in endothelial cells and activation of p62 yes tyrosine kinase. J Immunol 1992;149:1676–1682.

80. Nakajima K, Wall R. Interleukin-6 signals activating junB and TIS11 gene transcription in a B-cell hybridoma. Mol Cell Biol 1991;11:1409–1418.

81. Bonni A, Frank DA, Schindler C, Greenberg ME. Characterization of a pathway for ciliary neurotrophic factor signaling to the nucleus. Science 1993;262:1575–1579.

82. Sims JE, March CJ, Cosman D, et al. cDNA expression cloning of the IL-1 receptor, a member of the immunoglobulin superfamily. Science 1988;241:585–588.

83. Giri JG, Robb R, Wong WL, Horuk R. HepG2 cells predominantly express the type II interleukin 1 receptor (biochemical and molecular characterization of the IL-1 receptor). Cytokine 1992;4:18–23.

84. Tartaglia LA, Goeddel DV. Two TNF receptors. Immunol Today 1992;13:151–153.

85. Baumann H, Morella KK, Wong GHW. Interferon α1, IL-β and hepatocyte growth factor cooperate in stimulating specific acute phase protein genes in red hepatoma cells. J Immunol 1993;151:4248–4257.

86. Dinarello CA. Interleukin-1. Rev Infect Dis 1984;6:51–95.

87. Le J, Vilcek J. Biology of disease. Tumor necrosis factor and interleukin I: cytokines with multiple overlapping biological activities. Lab Invest 1987;56:234–248.

88. Kaur P, Welch WJ, Saklatvala J. Interleukin 1 and tumour necrosis factor increase phosphorylation of the small heat shock protein. FEBS Lett 1989;258:269–273.

89. Kaur P, Saklatvala J. Interleukin 1 and tumour necrosis factor increase phosphorylation of fibroblast proteins. FEBS Lett 1988;241:6–10.

90. Bird TA, Schule HD, Delaney PB, Sims JE, Thoma B, Dower SK. Evidence that MAP (mitogen-activated protein) kinase activation may be a necessary but not sufficient signal for a restricted subset of responses in IL-1-treated epidermoid cells. Cytokine 1992;4:429–440.

91. Geisterfer M, Richards CD, Baumann M, Fey G, Gwynne D, Gauldie J. Regulation of IL-6 and hepatic IL-6 receptor in acute inflammation in vivo. Cytokine 1993;5:1–7.

92. Rose-John S, Schooltink H, Lenz D, et al. Studies on the structure and regulation of the human hepatic interleukin-6 receptor. Eur J Biochem 1990;190:79–83.

93. Nesbitt JE, Fuller GM. Differential regulation of interleukin-6 receptor and gp130 gene expression in rat hepatocytes. Mol Biol Cell 1992;3:103–112.

94. Bauer J, Lengyel G, Bauer TM, Acs G, Gerok W. Regulation of interleukin-6 receptor expression in human monocytes and hepatocytes. FEBS Lett 1989;249:27–30.

95. Gauldie J, Geisterfer M, Richards C, Baumann H. IL-6 regulation of the hepatic acute phase response. In: Revel M, ed. IL-6 physiopathology and clinical potentials. Serono Symposia Publ, vol 88. New York: Raven, 1992:151–162.

96. Schooltink H, Schmitz-Van de Leur H, Heinrich PC, Rose-John S. Up-regulation of the interleukin-6-signal transducing protein (gp130) by interleukin-6 and dexamethasone in HepG2 cells. FEBS Lett 1992;297:263–265.

97. Snyers L, Content J. Enhancement of IL-6 receptor beta chain (gp130) expression by IL-6, IL-1 and TNF in human epithelial cells. Biochem Biophys Res Commun 1992;185:902–908.

98. Fernandez-Botran R. Soluble cytokine receptors: their role in immunoregulation. FASEB J 1991;5:2567–2574.

99. Novick D, Engelmann H, Wallach D, Rubinstein M. Soluble cytokine receptors are present in normal human urine. J Exp Med 1989;170:1409–1414.

100. Honda M, Yamamoto S, Cheng M, et al. Human soluble IL-6 receptor: its detection and enhanced release by HIV infection. J Immunol 1992;148:2175–2180.

101. Mackiewicz A, Schooltink H, Heinrich P, Rose-John S. Complex of soluble human IL-6 receptor/IL-6 up-regulates expression of acute-phase proteins. J Immunol 1992; 149:2021–2027.

102. Narazaki M, Yasukawa K, Saito T, et al. Soluble forms of the interleukin-6 signal-transducing receptor component gp130 in human serum possessing a potential to inhibit signals through membrane-anchored gp130. Blood 1993; 82:1120–1126.

103. Mullberg J, Schooltink H, Stoyan T, et al. The soluble interleukin-6 receptor is generated by shedding. Eur J Immunol 1993;23:473–480.

104. Lust JA, Donovan KA, Kline MP, Greipp PR, Kyle RA, Maihle NJ. Isolation of an mRNA encoding a soluble form of the human interleukin-6 receptor. Cytokine 1992;4:96–100.

105. Baumann H, Maquat LE. Localization of DNA sequences

involved in dexamethasone-dependent expression of the rat alpha1-acid glycoprotein gene. Mol Cell Biol 1986;6: 2551–2561.

106. Baumann H, Prowse KR, Marinkovic S, Won K-A, Jahreis GP. Stimulation of hepatic acute phase response by cytokines and glucocorticoids. Ann NY Acad Sci 1989; 557:280–296.

107. Prowse KR, Baumann H. Molecular characterization and acute phase expression of the multiple Mus caroli alpha1-acid glycoprotein (AGP) genes. J Biol Chem 1990;265: 10201–10209.

108. Akira S, Isshiki H, Sugita T, et al. A nuclear factor for IL-6 expression (NF-IL6) is a member of a C/EBP family. EMBO J 1990;9:1897–1906.

109. Ramji DP, Vitelli A, Tronche F, Cortese R, Ciliberto G. The two C/EBP isoforms, IL-6DBP/NF-IL6 and C/EBPdelta/NF-IL6beta, are induced by IL-6 to promote acute phase gene transcription via different mechanisms. Nucleic Acids Res 1993;21:289–294.

110. Poli G, Mancini FP, Cortese R. IL-6DBP, a nuclear protein involved in interleukin-6 signal transduction, defines a new family of leucine zipper proteins related to C/EBP. Cell 1990;63:643–653.

111. Kinoshita S, Akira S, Kishimoto T. A member of the C/EBP family, NF-IL6B, forms a heterodimer and transcriptionally synergizes with NF-IL6. Proc Natl Acad Sci USA 1992; 89:1473–1476.

112. Nishio Y, Isshiki H, Kishimoto T, Akira S. A nuclear factor for interleukin-6 expression (NF-IL6) and the glucocorticoid receptor synergistically activate transcription of the rat alpha1-acid glycoprotein gene via direct protein-protein interaction. Mol Cell Biol 1993;13:1854–1862.

113. Jonat C, Rahmsdorf HJ, Park K-K, et al. Antitumor production and antiinflammation: down-modulation of AP-1 (fos/jun) activity by glucocorticoid hormone. Cell 1990;62: 1189–1204.

114. LeClair K, Blanar M, Sharp P. The p50 subunit of NF-kB associates with the NF-IL6 transcription factor. Proc Natl Acad Sci USA 1992;89:8145–8149.

115. Baumann H, Gauldie J. The acute phase response. Immunol Today 1994;15:74–80.

116. Zhang Y, Lin J-X, Vilcek J. Interleukin-6 induction by tumor necrosis factor and interleukin-1 in human fibroblasts involves activation of a nuclear factor binding to a kB-like sequence. Mol Cell Biol 1990;10:3818–3823.

117. Libermann TA, Baltimore D. Activation of interleukin-6 gene expression through the NF-kB transcription factor. Mol Cell Biol 1990;10:2327–2334.

118. Hattori M, Abraham LJ, Northemann W, Fey GH. Acute-phase reaction induces a specific complex between hepatic nuclear proteins and the interleukin 6 response element of the rat alpha2-macroglobulin gene. Proc Natl Acad Sci USA 1990;87:2364–2368.

119. Marinkovic S, Baumann H. Structure, hormonal regulation, and identification of the interleukin-6- and dexamethasone-responsive element of the rat haptoglobin gene. Mol Cell Biol 1990;10:1573–1583.

120. Dalmon J, Laurent M, Courtois G. The human B fibrinogen promoter contains a hepatocyte nuclear factor 1-dependent Interleukin-6 responsive element. Mol Cell Biol 1993; 13:1183–1193.

121. Stetler-Stevenson WG, Brown PD, Onisto M, Levy AT, Liotta LA. Tissue inhibitor of metalloproteinases-2 (TIMP-2) mRNA expression in tumor cell lines and human tumor tissues. J Biol Chem 1990;265:13933–13938.

122. Wegenka U, Buschmann J, Lutticken C, Heinrich P, Horn F. Acute-phase response factor, a nuclear factor binding to acute-phase response elements, is rapidly activated by Interleukin-6 at the posttranslational level. Mol Cell Biol 1993;13:276–288.

123. Won K-A, Campos SP, Baumann H. Experimental systems for studying hepatic acute phase response. In: Mackiewicz A, Kushner I, Baumann H, eds. Acute phase proteins. Boca Raton, FL: CRC Press, 1993:255–267.

124. Woessner JF Jr. Matrix metalloproteinases and their inhibitors in connective tissue remodelling. FASEB J 1991;5: 2145–2154.

125. Matrisian LM. The matrix-degrading metalloproteinases. BioEssays 1992;14:455–463.

126. Walakovitis L, Moore V, Bhardwaj N, Gallick G, Lark M. Detection of stromelysin and collagenase in synovial fluid from patients with rheumatoid arthritis and post-traumatic knee injury. Arthritis Rheum 1992;35:35–42.

127. McDonnell J, Hoerrner L, Lark M, et al. Recombinant human interleukin-1B-induced increase in levels in stromelysin, and leukocytes in rabbit synovial fluid. Arthritis Rheum 1992;35:799–805.

128. Docherty AJP, Murphy G. The tissue metalloproteinase family and the inhibitor TIMP: a study using cDNAs and recombinant proteins. Ann Rheum Dis 1990;49:469–479.

129. Opdenakker G, Van Damme J. Cytokines and proteases in invasive processes: molecular similarities between inflammation and cancer. Cytokine 1992;4:251–258.

130. Khokha R, Denhardt DT. Matrix metalloproteinases and tissue inhibitor of metalloproteinases: a review of their role in tumorigenesis and tissue invasion. Invasion Metastasis 1989;9:391–405.

131. Liotta LA, Steeg PS, Stetler-Stevenson WG. Cancer metastasis and angiogenesis: an imbalance of positive and negative regulation. Cell 1991;64:327–336.

132. Lotz M, Guerne P-A. Interleukin-6 induces the synthesis of tissue inhibitor of metalloproteinases-1/erythroid potentiating activity (TIMP-1/EPA). J Biol Chem 1991;266:2017–2020.

133. Sato T, Ito A, Mori Y. Interleukin 6 enhances the production of tissue inhibitor of metalloproteinases (TIMP) but not that of matrix metalloproteinases by human fibroblasts. Biochem Biophys Res Commun 1990;170:824–829.

134. Richards CD, Shoyab M, Brown TJ, Gauldie J. Selective regulation of tissue inhibitor of metalloproteinases (TIMP-1) by oncostatin M in fibroblasts in culture. J Immunol 1993; 150:5596–5603.

135. Ito A, Itoh Y, Sasaguri Y, Morimatsu M, Mori Y. Effects of Interleukin-6 on the metabolism of connective tissue components in rheumatoid synovial fibroblasts. Arthritis Rheum 1992;35:1197–1201.

136. Hamilton JA. Hypothesis: in vitro evidence for the invasive and tumor-like properties of the rheumatoid pannus. J Rheumatol 1983;10:845–851.

137. Richards CD, Agro A. Interaction between oncostatin-M, interleukin 1 and prostaglandin E$_2$ in induction of IL-6 expression in human fibroblasts. Cytokine 1994;6:40–47.

138. Hamilton JA, Piccoli DS, Cebon J, et al. Cytokine regulation of colony-stimulating factor (CSF) production in cultured human synovial fibroblasts. II. Similarities and differences in the control of interleukin-1 induction of granulocyte-macrophage CSF and granulocyte-CSF production. Blood 1992;79:1413–1419.

139. Brown TJ, Rowe JM, Lui J, Shoyab M. Regulation of interleukin-6 expression by oncostatin M. J Immunol 1991;147:2175–2180.

140. Ritchie DG, Fuller GM. Hepatocyte-stimulating factor: a monocyte-derived acute-phase regulatory protein. Ann NY Acad Sci 1983;408:409–502.

141. Travis J, Salvesen GS. Human plasma proteinase inhibitors. Annu Rev Biochem 1983;52:665–709.

142. Salvesen G, Enghild JJ. Proteinase inhibitors: an overview of their structure and possible function in the acute phase. In: Mackiewicz A, Kushner I, Baumann H, eds. Acute phase proteins. Boca Raton, FL: CRC Press, 1993:117–147.

143. Murphy G, Koklitis P, Carne AF. Dissociation of tissue inhibitor of metalloproteinases (TIMP) from enzyme complexes yields fully active inhibitor. Biochem J 1989;261:1031–1034.

144. Kurdowska A, Travis J. Acute phase protein stimulation by alpha1-antichymotrypsin-cathepsin G complexes. J Biol Chem 1990;265:21023–21026.

145. Agrawal A, Kilpatrick JM, Volanakis JE. Structure and function of human C-reactive protein. In: Mackiewicz A, Kushner I, Baumann H, eds. Acute phase proteins. Boca Raton, FL: CRC Press, 1993:79–92.

146. Kottgen E, Hell B, Kage A, Tauber R. Lectin specificity and binding characteristics of human C-reactive protein. J Immunol 1992;149:445–453.

147. Berman S, Gewurz H, Mold C. Binding of C-reactive protein to nucleated cells leads to complement activation without cytolysis. J Immunol 1986;136:1354–1359.

148. Simon PL, Willoughby JB, Willoughby WF. Inhibition of T-cell activation by alpha1-antiprotease is reversed by purified rabbit interleukin-1. In: Oppenheim JJ, Cohen S, eds. Interleukins, lymphokines and cytokines. New York: Academic Press, 1983:487–493.

149. Hudig D, Haverty T, Fulcher C, Redelman D, Mendelsohn J. Inhibition of human natural cytotoxicity by macromolecular antiproteases. J Immunol 1981;126:1569–1574.

150. Ades EW, Hinson A, Chapuis-Cellier C, Arnaud P. Modulation of the immune response by plasma protease inhibitors. I. Alpha$_2$-macroglobulin and alpha1-antitrypsin inhibit natural killing and antibody-dependent cell-mediated cytotoxicity. Scand J Immunol 1982;15:109–113.

151. Hooper DC, Steer CJ, Dinarello CA, Peacock AC. Haptoglobin and albumin synthesis in isolated rat hepatocytes. Response to potential mediators of the acute-phase reaction. Biochim Biophys Acta 1981;653:118–129.

152. Van Vugt H, van Gool J, de Ridder L. Alpha$_2$-macroglobulin of the rat, an acute phase protein, mitigates the early course of endotoxin shock. Br J Exp Pathol 1986;67:313–319.

153. Hoffman M, Feldman SR, Pizzo SV. Alpha$_2$-macroglobulin "fast" forms inhibit superoxide production by activated macrophages. Biochim Biophys Acta 1983;760:421–423.

154. Hannum CH, Wilcox CJ, Arend WP, et al. Interleukin-1 receptor antagonist activity of a human interleukin-1 inhibitor. Nature 1990;343:336–340.

155. Eisenberg SP, Evans RJ, Arend WP, et al. Primary structure and functional expression from complementary DNA of a human interleukin-1 receptor antagonist. Nature 1990;343:341–346.

156. Seckinger P, Kaufmann M-T, Dayer J-M. An interleukin 1 inhibitor affects both cell-associated interleukin 1-induced T cell proliferation and PGE2/collagenase production by human dermal fibroblasts and synovial cells. Immunobiology 1990;180:316–327.

157. Tilg H, Trehu E, Atkins MB, Dinarello CA, Mier JW. Interleukin-6 as an anti-inflammatory cytokine: induction of circulating interleukin-1 receptor antagonist and soluble tumor necrosis factor receptor p55. Blood 1994;83:113–118.

158. Tilg H, Vannier E, Vachino G, Dinarello CA, Mier JW. Anti-inflammatory properties of hepatic acute phase proteins: preferential induction of interleukin-1 receptor antagonist over interleukin-1β synthesis by human PBMC. J Exp Med 1993;178:1629–1636.

159. Amano Y, Lee S, Allison A. Inhibition of glucocorticoids of the formation of interleukin-1a, interleukin-1B and interleukin-6: mediation by decreased mRNA stability. Mol Pharmacol 1992;43:176–182.

160. Seitz M, Dewald B, Gerber N, Baggiolini M. Enhanced production of neutrophil-activating peptide-1/Interleukin-8 in rheumatoid arthritis. J Clin Invest 1991;87:463–469.

161. Waage A, Slupphaug G, Shalaby R. Glucocorticoids inhibit the production of IL6 from monocytes, endothelial cells and fibroblasts. Eur J Immunol 1990;20:2439–2443.

162. Tobler A, Meier R, Seitz M, Dewald B, Baggiolini M, Fey M. Glucocorticoids downregulate gene expression of GM-CSF, NAP-1/IL-8, and IL-6, but not of M-CSF in human fibroblasts. Blood 1992;79:45–51.

163. Ray A, Prefontaine KE. Physical association and functional antagonism between the p65 subunit of NF-kB and the glucocorticoid receptor. Proc Natl Acad Sci USA 1994;91:752–756.

164. Clark SD, Kobayashi DK, Welgus HG. Regulation of the expression of tissue inhibitor of metalloproteinases and collagenase by retinoids and glucocorticoids in human fibroblasts. J Clin Invest 1987;80:1280–1288.

165. Frisch SM, Ruley HE. Transcription from the stromelysin promoter is induced by interleukin-1 and repressed by dexamethasone. J Biol Chem 1987;262:16300–16304.

166. Munck A, Mendel DB, Smith LI, Orti E. Glucocorticoid receptors and actions. Am Rev Respir Dis 1990;141:2–10.

167. Duval D, Freyss-Beguin M. Glucocorticoids and prostaglandin synthesis: we cannot see the wood for the trees. Prostaglandins Leukotrienes Essential Fatty Acids 1992;45:85–112.

168. Auble DT, Brinckerhoff CE. The AP-1 sequence is necessary but not sufficient for phorbol induction of collagenase in fibroblasts. Biochemistry 1991;30:4629–4635.

169. Grassi J, Roberge C, Frobert Y, Pradelles P, Poubelle P. Determination of IL-1a, IL-1B and IL-2 in biological media using specific enzyme immunometric assays. Immunol Rev 1991;119:125–145.

170. Shaw G, Kamen RA. Conserved AU sequence from the 3′

untranslated region of GM-CSF mRNA mediates selective mRNA degradation. Cell 1986;46:659–667.

171. Bagby GC, Shaw G, Heinrich MC, et al. Interleukin-1 stimulation stabilizes GM-CSF mRNA in human vascular endothelial cells: preliminary studies on the role of the 3′ au rich motif. Progress in Clinical and Biological Research 1990; 352:233–239.

172. Henderson B, Thompson RC, Hardingham T, Lewthwaite J. Inhibition of interleukin-1-induced synovitis and articular cartilage proteoglycan loss in the rabbit knee by recombinant human interleukin-1 receptor antagonist. Cytokine 1991;3:246–249.

173. Schindler R, Mancilla J, Endres S, Ghorbani R, Clark SC, Dinarello CA. Correlations and interactions in the production of interleukin-6 (IL-6), IL-1, and tumor necrosis factor (TNF) in human blood mononuclear cells: IL-6 suppresses IL-1 and TNF. Blood 1990;75:40–47.

174. Aderka D, Le J, Vilcek J. IL-6 Inhibits lipopolysaccharide-induced tumor necrosis factor production in cultured human monocytes, U937 cells, and in mice. J Immunol 1989;143:3517–3523.

175. Boulay J-L, Paul WE. The interleukin-4 family of lymphokines. Curr Opin Immunol 1992;4:294–298.

176. de Waal Malefyt R, Yssel H, Roncarolo M-G, Spits H, de Vries JE. Interleukin-10. Curr Opin Immunol 1992;4:314–320.

177. Howard M, O'Garra A. Biological properties of interleukin 10. Immunol Today 1992;13:198–200.

178. Hart PH, Vitti GF, Burgess DR, Whitty GA, Piccoli DS, Hamilton JA. Potential anti-inflammatory effects of interleukin 4: suppression of human monocyte tumor necrosis factor α, interleukin 1 and prostaglandin E_2. Proc Natl Acad Sci USA 1989;86:3803–3807.

179. Donnelly R, Fenton M, Kaufman J, Gerrard T. IL-1 expression in human monocytes is transcriptionally and post-transcriptionally regulated by IL-4. J Immunol 1991;146: 3431–3436.

180. Standiford TJ, Strieter RM, Chensue SW, Westwick J, Kasahara K, Kunkel SL. IL-4 inhibits the expression of IL-8 from stimulated human monocytes. J Immunol 1990;145: 1435–1439.

181. Standiford TJ, Kunkel SL, Liebler JM, Burdick MD, Gilbert AR, Strieter RM. Gene expression of macrophage inflammatory protein-1alpha from human blood monocytes and alveolar macrophages is inhibited by interleukin-4. Am J Respir Cell Mol Biol 1993;9:192–198.

182. Fenton M, Buras J, Donnelly R. IL-4 reciprocally regulates IL-1 receptor antagonist expression in human monocytes. J Immunol 1992;149:1283–1288.

183. Orino E, Sone S, Nii A, Ogura T. IL-4 up-regulates IL-1 receptor antagonist gene expression and its production in human blood monocytes. J Immunol 1992;149:925–931.

184. Colotta F, Re F, Muzio M, et al. Interleukin-1 type II receptor: a decoy target for IL-1 that is regulated by IL-4. Science 1993;261:472–475.

185. Howard M, Muchamuel T, Andrade S, Menon S. Interleukin 10 protects mice from lethal endotoxemia. J Exp Med 1993;177:1205–1208.

CHAPTER 16

ROLE OF CYTOKINES IN GLUCOSE METABOLISM

Charles H. Lang

The purpose of this chapter is to present a concise review of the literature specifically related to the effects of different cytokines on carbohydrate metabolism. For the most part, only studies dealing with the injection of either highly purified or recombinant cytokines are discussed. However, readers are encouraged to review the early work by Berry (1) and Filkins (2) and their colleagues, who pioneered the concept that soluble mediators from reticuloendothelial cells could influence glucose homeostasis by altering glucose production and glucose utilization.

For convenience, this chapter is divided into sections describing the particular actions of a given cytokine. Although this format aids in the enumeration of the various metabolic actions of each cytokine, it is important to remember that cytokines are rarely, if ever, secreted individually in the body. Moreover, they are likely to modulate metabolism in an autocrine or a paracrine manner, or both. Thus, large bolus injections of these biological response modifiers, which constitutes the method most commonly employed in in vivo studies, may not necessarily produce physiologically relevant findings.

Despite these caveats, evidence is presented that multiple cytokines have the potential to alter whole body glucose metabolism either directly or by secondary stimulation of more classic neuroendocrine pathways. The ability of cytokines working alone and in combination with glucoregulatory hormones to mediate metabolism must be considered an important aspect of their biological function.

TUMOR NECROSIS FACTOR

In vivo effects on metabolism

Tracey and colleagues (3) were the first to inject recombinant human (rh) tumor necrosis factor (TNF) into rats and to demonstrate that this cytokine could produce circulatory shock and elicit many of the deleterious effects of endotoxin (Table 16–1). Among the effects reported were an initial hyperglycemia that appeared to be dose-dependent, and a later hypoglycemic phase that occurred preterminally when TNF was injected in relatively high doses. Early studies concerning the mechanism for the TNF-induced hyperglycemia were performed by Bagby and associates (4). Their data show that when either rh TNF-α or a monokine mixture from macrophages (i.e., RAW 264.7 cells) was infused into overnight fasted rats, glucose levels were increased by stimulating hepatic glucose production (HGP) to a greater extent than peripheral glucose uptake.

Although TNF decreases hepatic glycogen content (5,6), liver reserves are already low because of the overnight fast. Thus, in overnight fasted rats that received TNF, glycogenolysis initially supports the enhanced HGP production, but the relatively sustained increase in glucose output must result from de novo glucose synthesis. Comparable increases in glucose production after TNF have subsequently been confirmed in rats (7,8), and they have been reported to occur in dogs, rabbits, sheep, and humans (9–12). In studies in which TNF fails to stimulate HGP, the cytokine was administered in too small a dose (13).

There is little evidence to support a direct effect of TNF on hepatic gluconeogenesis or glycogenolysis. The TNF-induced increase in HGP is undoubtedly partially due to an increased precursor delivery. Hyperlactacidemia is a common manifestation of TNF administration (4,7,14,15), and it is associated with an elevated lactate efflux from skeletal muscle (14). Moreover, net flux of alanine and glutamine from muscle also increases after TNF (16).

Thus, TNF results in an interorgan transfer of 3-carbon units from peripheral tissues to the liver to support gluconeogenesis. Furthermore, although TNF has no direct effect on hepatic amino acid uptake, it does enhance uptake stimulated by glucagon (17). Low doses of TNF, however, do not appear to produce physiologically significant changes in the activity of key hepatic gluconeogenic enzymes (18). In general, the increased HGP is associated with dose-dependent increases in catecholamines, glucagon, adrenocorticotrophic hormone (ACTH), and glucocorticoids (14,15,19). These hormones, individually or together, have the ability to stimulate HGP.

The role of the adrenergic nervous system in mediating the in vivo effects of TNF has been investigated by Lang (20) and Bagby and colleagues (8). In one study, rats were infused with TNF for 30 minutes (150 µg/kg), and enhancement of HGP was found to be prevented by the concomitant infusion of α-adrenergic and β-adrenergic antagonists (i.e., phentolamine and propranolol) (8). Because these antagonists block catecholamine actions and do not influence the TNF-induced increases in glucagon and glucocorticoids, adrenergic activation appears to have a major role in mediating the effect of TNF-α on HGP. This mediating role is consistent with the known stimulatory effect of epinephrine, and to a lesser extent norepinephrine, on hepatic glycogenolysis and gluconeogenesis.

In contrast, in another study, rats were infused with a low dose of TNF for 18 hours (1 µg/h/kg), and adrenergic blockade was found to be unable to prevent the increased basal glucose output by the liver (20). The apparent disparity between the findings of these two studies may be explained if catecholamines are more important in the control of metabolism following a TNF challenge that has a relatively rapid onset or is of greater severity. Under more protracted conditions, TNF may possibly enhance HGP by mechanisms that are largely independent of control by catecholamines (and maybe other counter-regulatory hormones), which may indicate a direct effect of the cytokine on liver and muscle metabolism.

As indicated, the plasma glucose response to TNF is dose-dependent; large doses invariably produce severe and protracted hypoglycemia (3,9,21,22). Detailed studies on whole body glucose flux and tissue glucose uptake under hypoglycemic conditions have not been conducted. However, if data from endotoxic shock can be extrapolated (23), the primary cause of the TNF-induced hypoglycemia is perhaps failure of the hepatic glucose

TABLE 16-1   EFFECTS OF TNF ON CARBOHYDRATE METABOLISM

Blood glucose (variable)	Rat, rabbit, dog, human
Initial hyperglycemia/late hypoglycemia with high dose; no change or slight increase in glucose with low doses	
Increased hepatic glucose production	
Increased glycogenolysis	
Increased gluconeogenesis	
Increased peripheral glucose uptake	
Primarily macrophage-rich tissues	
Chronic exposure increases uptake by skeletal muscle	
Increases stress hormone levels in blood	
Produces insulin resistance mediated in part by β-adrenergic stimulation	
Hepatic	
Peripheral	
No change in glucose oxidation	Adipocytes, rat
No change in glycogenolysis or gluconeogenesis	Hepatocytes, rat
No change in glycolysis	Diaphragm, rat
Increased glucose uptake and lactate production	L6 myotubes
Increased glucose uptake	3T3-L1 preadipocytes
Increased glucose uptake and decreased IMGU	3T3-L1 adipocytes

output to meet the increased demands of peripheral tissues. This hepatic failure is obviously multifactorial, including decreased gluconeogenic substrate availability resulting from a decrease in hepatic blood flow, and metabolic changes related to regional or global hepatic ischemia or hypoxia.

The TNF-induced increase in HGP is a compensatory response that benefits the host by supplying the increased glucose demands of various peripheral tissues. In vivo tracer studies, using [6-³H]-glucose or [3-³H]-glucose and conducted in numerous species, clearly indicate that TNF enhances the rate of whole body glucose disappearance or uptake (7–12). Meszaros and coworkers (24) reported that 3 hours after TNF challenge in rats, in vivo glucose uptake was increased in spleen, liver, lung, ileum, skin, and kidney (30–100%) (Fig. 16–1). Increased glucose uptake by these macrophage-rich tissues was reported after a bolus injection of TNF to mice and after more prolonged infusions of TNF into rats (7,8,20,25,26). The major difference in these studies is the involvement of skeletal muscle. Glucose uptake by muscle has been shown to be unaltered following short-term (30 minutes) infusion of TNF (8,24,26), increased after overnight infusion of TNF (7,20), or decreased after intraperitoneal (IP) injection of TNF into mice (25). Evans and associates (9) also reported an increased uptake of glucose across the hindlimb in dogs after 6 hours (but not 3 hours) of TNF infusion. It seems likely that the ability of TNF to enhance glucose uptake by skeletal muscle may require prolonged tissue exposure to the cytokine, and therefore is only seen under relatively long term experimental conditions. This speculation is supported by the in vitro findings of Lee and colleagues (27), in which the ability of TNF to stimulate maximal glucose uptake in L6 myotubes is evident only after prolonged exposure (approximately 16 hours). Glucose uptake by muscle appears to be reduced only in hypoglycemic animals (25).

In general, glucose uptake by peripheral tissues occurs by one of two mechanisms. The first is insulin-mediated glucose uptake (IMGU); by definition, it only occurs in insulin-sensitive tissues, such as adipose tissue and muscle. The second mechanism, known as noninsulin-mediated glucose uptake (NIMGU), can occur in both insulin-sensitive and insulin-nonsensitive tissues. Under basal postabsorptive conditions, NIMGU is responsible for approximately 75% of the total rate of whole body glucose disposal in humans and rats (28). Although the glucose counter-regulatory hormones, such as epinephrine, glucagon, and glucocorticoids impair IMGU, they do not appear to modulate NIMGU. Therefore, based on this evidence, these two pathways for glucose uptake appear to be regulated independently. In the studies reviewed, plasma insulin levels are either unchanged or depressed after in vivo injection of TNF-α. In addition, TNF also impairs IMGU. The increment in peripheral glucose dis-

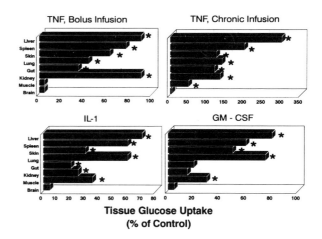

Figure 16–1 In vivo glucose uptake by selected tissues in animals infused with various cytokines. Animals received TNF-acute (50 µg/kg for 3 hours), TNF-chronic (1 µg/hr/kg for 18 hours), IL-1 (50 U; tissues sampled at 30 minutes), or GM-CSF (30 µg/kg; tissues sampled at 30 minutes). Values are represented as percent of time-matched values from saline-treated control animals. $^*p < 0.05$ compared with control values.

posal observed after TNF therefore appears to occur primarily by noninsulin-mediated pathways.

One of the consistent findings of all of the studies mentioned is TNF-induced increase in glucose uptake by the liver. Enhanced uptake of glucose occurs concomitantly with an increased rate of glucose production. Because the liver is composed of a heterogenous population of cells, TNF might stimulate glucose consumption by one cell type and enhance glucose production by another. This possibility was investigated by Spolarics and associates (26). By combining the tracer [¹⁴C]-2-deoxyglucose technique and centrifugal elutriation, they determined that in vivo injection of TNF increased glucose uptake in only the Kupffer cells (i.e., hepatic macrophages) and the endothelial cells of the liver. Therefore, after TNF administration, the parenchymal cells are stimulated to produce more glucose, whereas the nonparenchymal cells are one of the cell populations that have an increased demand for this substrate. In this situation, however, there is still a net output of glucose by the liver. In subsequent studies, the TNF-induced increase in glucose uptake by Kupffer cells was shown to support enhanced rates of glucose oxidation, as well as increased hexose monophosphate shunt activity (29).

Insulin resistance

In several studies by Lang and coworkers (7,20), the euglycemic hyperinsulinemic clamp methodology was used to determine whether TNF impairs in vivo insulin action and produces insulin resistance. Insulin resistance can be defined as a smaller than expected response to a given

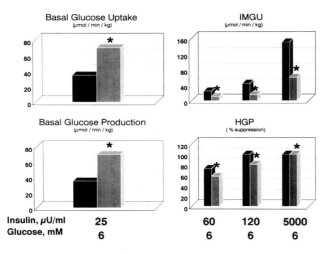

Figure 16–2 In vivo glucose metabolism under basal and hyperinsulinemic conditions in control (*dark bars*) and TNF-infused (*light bars*) rats. Basal rates of glucose production and utilization were determined after 18 hours of TNF infusion (1 μg/hr/kg); thereafter, a euglycemic hyperinsulinemic clamp was performed to determine insulin-mediated glucose uptake (IMGU) and the degree of suppression of hepatic glucose production (HGP). $^*p < 0.05$ compared with control values at the same insulin level.

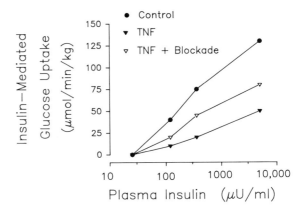

Figure 16–3 Dose-response relationship between arterial insulin concentrations and peripheral glucose uptake in control (*squares*) and TNF-infused (*open circles*) rats. In addition, a separate group of TNF-treated rats were concomitantly infused with propranolol, a nonselective β-adrenergic antagonist (*triangles*). All values for the TNF-infused rats are significantly lower ($p < 0.05$) than control values at the same plasma insulin level. All values for the propranolol + TNF group are significantly greater ($p < 0.05$) than values for the TNF group.

dose of insulin. In these experiments, rats received a constant intravenous (IV) infusion of rhTNF-α for 18 to 24 hours, as described. Under hyperinsulinemic conditions, the glucose infusion rate necessary to maintain euglycemia was 30% lower in TNF-treated rats. This insulin-resistant state results from an impaired ability of insulin both to suppress HGP and to stimulate peripheral glucose uptake in TNF-treated rats (Fig. 16–2). Importantly, decreased IMGU by peripheral tissues occurs at both physiological and pharmacological plasma insulin concentrations. Although an entire insulin dose-response curve was not generated, these data are consistent with a decrease in both insulin sensitivity (i.e., an increased ED_{50}) and maximal responsiveness.

These alterations suggest that TNF produces both a receptor and a postreceptor defect. Infusion of propranolol (a nonselective β-adrenergic antagonist), but not atenolol (a $β_1$-antagonist) or phentolamine (an α-adrenergic antagonist), partially prevents the TNF-induced impairment in whole body insulin-stimulated glucose uptake (Fig. 16–3).

Subsequent studies using [^{14}C]-2-deoxyglucose indicated that the increment in glucose uptake by skeletal muscle and skin accounts for the majority (85%) of glucose disposal under hyperinsulinemic conditions in control rats. However, in TNF-infused animals, hyperinsulinemia failed to increase glucose uptake by skin, and it greatly blunted IMGU by skeletal muscle. The TNF-induced impairment in IMGU was not found in all muscle types, because glucose uptake by diaphragm and heart ("working muscles") was comparable in control rats and

TNF-treated rats under hyperinsulinemic conditions. Continuous infusion of propranolol selectively prevented the decreased glucose disposal by skeletal muscle, but it did not attenuate the inhibition of IMGU by skin. Because atenolol, a selective $β_1$-adrenergic antagonist, did not reverse the insulin resistance, these data suggest that β-adrenergic stimulation, probably mediated by a $β_2$-adrenergic mechanism, is partially responsible for the development of the peripheral insulin resistance in animals infused with TNF. A large portion of the TNF-induced insulin resistance is therefore mediated by mechanisms other than sympathetic stimulation.

The exact location and the nature of the biochemical lesion responsible for the TNF-induced impairment in insulin action remain to be determined (Fig. 16–4). It is well established that the biological actions of insulin are initiated by hormone binding to insulin's high-affinity membrane-bound receptor. No studies have been done to examine alterations in insulin binding or affinity by TNF. Likewise, tyrosine kinase activity, which is known to be reduced in other insulin-resistant conditions, has not been assessed. However, some studies have implicated enhanced adrenergic activity in TNF-induced insulin resistance, and catecholamines are known to alter both insulin binding and tyrosine kinase activity. It also seems likely that at least part of the insulin resistance is due to a postreceptor defect. Such alterations might include depletion or decreased translocation of the insulin-sensitive glucose transporter (GLUT 4), or an impaired intracellular disposition of glucose. The first possibility is consistent with the in vitro findings of Stephens and Pekala (30). In their experiments, chronic incubation of 3T3-L1

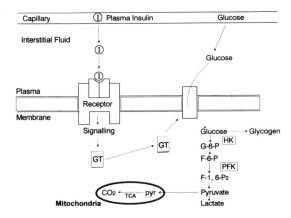

Figure 16–4 Potential cellular sites for cytokine-induced impairment of insulin action of peripheral glucose uptake.

cells with TNF-α resulted in a marked reduction of IMGU, which resulted primarily from a severe reduction in GLUT 4 transporter protein content.

In vitro effects on metabolism

In 1987, Lee and colleagues (27) reported that a crude monokine preparation from endotoxin-stimulated macrophages rapidly depletes glycogen reserves within 3 hours in fully differentiated L6 myotubes. Thereafter, gradual stimulation of glucose uptake and lactate production occurs to maintain intracellular high energy reserves. The investigators found that when the monokine mixture was treated with a neutralizing antibody to TNF, most, but not all, of the enhanced glucose metabolism was prevented. Incubation of L6 myotubes with TNF-α mimicked the changes in glucose uptake seen with the monokine mixture. The enhanced glucose uptake was due to an increase in membrane-bound glucose transporters, based on data from photoaffinity and equilibrium binding studies with [^{3}H]-cytochalasin B. Subsequent Northern blot analysis indicated an increased level of glucose transporter messenger RNA (mRNA) (31). In contrast, no increase in glucose uptake was observed after short-term exposure (30–120 minutes) of hemidiaphragms (or adipocytes or hepatocytes) to TNF (32).

Studies by Cornelius and associates (33) demonstrate that TNF-α also enhances glucose uptake by 3T3-L1 fibroblasts (preadipocytes) in a time- and dose-dependent manner. In these experiments, glucose uptake was increased as early as 30 minutes, but the maximal effect required approximately 16 hours of exposure. This increased hexose transport appears to be caused by an increased number of GLUT 1 transporters, as well as activation of their intrinsic activity. Although TNF's influence on glucose uptake in 3T3-L1 cells appears related to its ability to stimulate mitogenesis, this cytokine is also capable of enhancing hexose uptake by fully differenti-

ated 3T3-L1 adipocytes (30). Prolonged treatment (12 days) of these cells with TNF decreases the GLUT 1 protein content of the intracellular membranes, as well as decreases GLUT 4 (insulin-responsive glucose transporter) protein levels in both plasma and inner-membrane pools.

INTERLEUKIN-1

In vivo effects on metabolism

One of the earliest studies, if not the first, to examine the impact of interleukin-1 (IL-1) on glucose homeostasis was performed by George and colleagues (34). In this study, a relatively crude supernatant from stimulated rabbit peritoneal macrophages was used (i.e., leukocyte endogenous mediator [LEM]). After a single IP injection of LEM into rats, glucose concentrations were gradually reduced, and they reached a nadir 5 hours after injection (Table 16–2). This hypoglycemia was associated with depletion of hepatic glycogen and elevated circulating levels of glucagon. Similarly, Del Ray and Besedovsky (35) showed that purified human IL-1 produces transient hypoglycemia in mice that reaches a nadir 2 hours after injection. This decrease in glucose was associated with relatively more sustained elevations in insulin, glucagon, and corticosterone levels, as well as more transient changes in catecholamine levels (36). Both the maximal response of glucose and the glucoregulatory hormones appear to be directly proportional to the amount of IL-1 injected. Furthermore, IL-1 normalizes blood glucose levels in various types of insulin-resistant diabetic mice (37,38). These authors suggest that the hypoglycemic effect of IL-1 is direct and not due to the insulin secretagogue actions of this cytokine. However, their conclusions are based exclusively on blood glucose measurements, and they did not determine glucose uptake by peripheral tissues or HGP.

In contrast, there are a comparable number of studies using recombinant or highly purified IL-1 that indicate injection of IL-1 fails to alter or produces only minor changes in circulating levels of glucose when injected into rats (39–42). When present, this hyperglycemia appears to result from both an increased rate of glycogenolysis (34) and enhanced gluconeogenesis. This latter facet of IL-1 action is based on the observation that hepatocytes isolated from rats injected in vivo with purified IL-1 had an enhanced rate of ^{14}C-alanine conversion to glucose (43). However, no stimulatory effect was observed when hepatocytes from control rats were incubated in vitro with different doses of IL-1. Fischer and coworkers (44) also demonstrated a dose-dependent increase in glucose concentrations following IV injection of IL-1α into baboons. It appears that the IL-1–induced changes in blood

TABLE 16–2 EFFECTS OF IL-1 ON CARBOHYDRATE METABOLISM

IL-1α and IL-1β	
Blood glucose levels (variable)	Rat, whole body
Initial hyperglycemia/late hypoglycemia with high doses; no change or slight increase in blood glucose with low doses	
Increased hepatic glucose production	
Increased peripheral glucose uptake, primarily in macrophage-rich tissues	
Increases insulin secretion	
Peripheral insulin resistance (no consistent change)	
IL-1α	
ICV administration enhances glucose flux and stress hormone release	
IL-1β	
Increased glucose uptake	Synoviocytes, human
IL-1α	
Increased glucose uptake	Fibroblasts, human
Increased glycolysis	
Decreased glucose oxidation	
Increased Fru, 2,6-bisphosphate	
IL-1α	
Increased glucose transport	Renal tubular epithelium, rat
IL-1β	
Increased glucose uptake	Adipocytes, rat
IL-1α	
No change in glucose uptake	Adipocytes, rat
IL-1β	
No change in glucose uptake	Islet, rat
Decreased glucose oxidation	
IL-1	
No effect on glycolysis	Hepatocytes, rat
IL-1β	
Decreased glycogen content	Hepatocytes, rat
Increased glycogen phosphorylase	
Decreased glycogen synthetase	

glucose, either increases or decreases, are relatively short-lived. Therefore, transient periods of hypoglycemia and hyperglycemia will likely be missed unless multiple blood samples are taken over several hours after injection of IL-1 (44).

One cytokine synergistic with IL-1 is TNF. When a combined infusion of rhIL-1 and rhTNF was administered to rabbits (in doses at which neither cytokine alone had any effect), whole body glucose turnover was elevated 33% above time-matched control values (12). Because these animals were fasted prior to IL-1/TNF infusion, most of the increment in HGP under these conditions was due to enhanced gluconeogenesis. The calculated metabolic clearance rate (MCR) for glucose (which estimates the body's avidity for glucose) was unchanged, suggesting that the elevated rate of glucose uptake was primarily due to a mass action effect resulting from the hyperglycemia. Glucose recycling was also dramatically increased 600%, indicating enhanced Cori cycle activity and further supporting the concept that IL-1 enhances gluconeogenesis.

One possible mechanism by which IL-1 can induce hypoglycemia is by impairing gluconeogenesis. Data from Hill and colleagues (45) indicate that IL-1 down-regulates intracellular glucocorticoid receptors, which impair the induction of phosphoenolpyruvate carboxykinase (PEPCK). Because PEPCK is a primary rate-controlling enzyme of gluconeogenesis, this alteration might be expected to decrease the rate of gluconeogenesis and to produce a decrease in circulating glucose levels. Alternatively, or in addition, IL-1 can influence glucose levels by altering plasma insulin levels.

One of the most consistent hormonal disturbances produced by IL-1 is increased insulin secretion. Hyperinsulinemia has been reported following IV, intracerebroventricular (ICV), or preoptic injection of various types and doses of IL-1 (34,35,40–42,46,47). When the pancreas is removed 30 minutes after an in vivo injection of IL-1, both first-phase and second-phase glucose-stimulated insulin secretion is enhanced (48). IL-1β has a similar effect when perfused directly into the pancreas (49). In contrast to these immediate effects, relatively long-term exposure of islet cells to IL-1 is often cytotoxic, and it impairs insulin secretion (50).

Injection of rhIL-1β into rats increases whole body glucose turnover, as assessed by continuous infusion of [6-³H]- glucose, for up to 4 hours (13). This elevation was found to be accomplished with only a small elevation in glucose concentration; thus, the MCR for glucose was unchanged. Glucose recycling was unaltered by IL-1. Work by Lang and Dobrescu (40) specifically determined whether IL-1 could enhance glucose uptake by peripheral tissues, and whether that increase was insulin-dependent. When human purified IL-1 was given IV to catheterized conscious rats, plasma insulin levels increased, and glucose uptake was enhanced by lung, spleen, liver, skin, skeletal muscle, and diaphragm (see Fig. 16–1). To minimize IMGU, somatostatin was infused for 1 hour prior to administration of IL-1. Somatostatin prevented IL-1–induced hyperinsulinemia and the increased glucose uptake by peripheral tissues. Furthermore, IL-1 injected into streptozotocin-induced diabetic rats failed to increase tissue glucose uptake. These data suggest that in vivo administration of IL-1 to rats increases organ glucose uptake by insulin-dependent mechanisms. Although IL-1 is known to have many effects on the central nervous system (CNS) (51), when injected IV into rats, this cytokine fails to alter either total or regional cerebral glucose uptake (40,52).

There have been several in vivo studies in which the ability of IL-1 to modulate insulin-stimulated glucose disposal has been investigated. Unfortunately, there is no consensus among these studies. In early work by Watters and colleagues (53), normal patients received etiocholanolone, an inflammatory agent whose mode of action is believed to be mediated principally by induction of IL-1. Although this agent was biologically active and produced an intense acute-phase response, it failed to affect IMGU by the forearm under well controlled euglycemic hyperinsulinemic conditions. In contrast, when a single injection of rIL-1β was given to rats, it slightly improved glucose tolerance, as determined by an IP glucose tolerance test (GTT) (54). An improvement in the half-life ($T_{1/2}$) value for an IV GTT was also reported for rats 30 minutes after injection of purified IL-1 (41). However, glucose tolerance was moderately impaired after five daily injections of IL-1 (54). Although the standard GTT is a valuable screening aid in the detection of diabetes mellitus, it must be emphasized that results from these tests provide little insight into the mechanisms responsible for the glucose dyshomeostasis observed following cytokine administration (55).

Central nervous system effects on metabolism

It is recognized that there is extensive intercommunication between the neuroendocrine and the immune systems. On the basis of its diverse biological activities, IL-1 appears to coordinate many aspects of this cross-talk between the hypothalamus, the pituitary, and the immune network. As described, systemic injection of this cytokine has been shown to affect different facets of glucose homeostasis. However, various cell types within the brain can also elaborate IL-1 after appropriate stimulation, and IL-1 produced by peripheral tissues may gain access to the CNS via areas not protected by the blood-brain barrier (56,57).

There are numerous reports that CNS administration of IL-1 alters hormone secretion by the hypothalamic-pituitary-adrenal axis (58). However, few studies in which the accompanying changes in carbohydrate metabolism following CNS administration of IL-1 have been described. Initially, Cornell (59) reported that ICV injection of human purified IL-1 did not alter the plasma glucose concentration in conscious rats, although it did produce

hyperinsulinemia. However, in a recent study by Lang and colleagues (46), ICV injection of 100 ng rhIL-1α increased glucose levels within 20 minutes, and they remained elevated for up to 3 hours (Fig. 16–5). The hyperglycemia resulted from an approximately 50% increase in HGP, which preceded a proportional increase in peripheral glucose utilization. No increase in MCR for glucose was observed, suggesting that the increased glucose uptake by peripheral tissues was the result of mass action. Moreover, no change in glucose metabolism occurred when the same dose of IL-1α was injected IV, indicating that the observed glucose metabolic response to ICV administered IL-1 is not due to a spillover of cytokine into the peripheral circulation.

The glucoregulatory action of IL-1 appears to be mediated by prostaglandins, because pretreating rats with indomethacin prior to IL-1 injection completely prevents the enhanced glucose metabolic response. In addition, ICV injection of prostaglandin E_2 (PGE_2) also produces comparable increases in glucose flux. These results indicate that IL-1α can act centrally to enhance whole body glucose metabolism, and that this response is mediated within the CNS by prostaglandins. In contrast to these findings, ICV injection of rh TNF-α (1–1000 ng/rat) failed to alter whole body carbohydrate metabolism (Lang CH, unpublished observations).

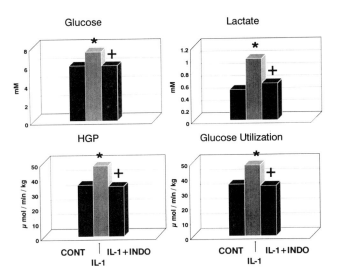

Figure 16–5 In vivo glucose metabolic response 3 hours after an intracerebroventricular (ICV) injection of IL-1α (100 ng), IL-1α + indomethacin (INDO), or water (control). Data are expressed as means ± SEM. $^*p < 0.05$ compared with time-matched control rats injected (ICV) with water; $^+p < 0.05$ compared with time-matched values of animals injected (ICV) with IL-1. Animals injected intravenously (IV) with 100 ng IL-1 showed no change in glucose metabolism.

In vitro effects on metabolism

There are a number of studies in which various cell types have been incubated with IL-1. In general, the findings are remarkably consistent. Incubation of either rheumatoid or nonrheumatoid synovial cells with rhIL-1β increases glucose uptake in a time-dependent and dose-dependent manner (60). Significant stimulation of uptake first occurs at approximately 3 hours, and it continues to increase for up to 24 hours. Prostaglandins are well-known mediators of many IL-1 effects; however, under these conditions, coincubation of synovial cells with indomethacin does not alter the IL-1β–induced increase in glucose uptake. Because kinetic measurements indicate that IL-1 increases V_{max}, but not Km, it appears that IL-1 increases the synthesis of new hexose transporters in these cells. Comparable enhancement of glucose uptake and glycolysis (as measured by lactate production) is also observed in porcine synovial cells incubated for 30 hours with IL-1 (61). IL-1α and IL-1β produce similar effects in these cells (62). In addition, Taylor and associates (62,63) demonstrated that IL-1 increases cellular levels of fructose 2,6-bisphosphate, a potent stimulator of phosphofructokinase (PFK), which is a rate-controlling enzyme of glycolysis.

These studies indicate that cyclo-oxygenase inhibition, although able to decrease PGE$_2$ production, does not block enhanced glucose metabolism. Inhibition of the IL-1–induced increase in glycolysis was only possible when cycloheximide was used to inhibit de novo protein synthesis. Human gingival fibroblasts are also responsive to IL-1. After incubation, IL-1 enhanced glucose uptake and glycolysis, but it inhibited glucose oxidation (61–63). Pulse-labeling experiments showed a net synthesis of glucose transporters (probably GLUT 1) that is proportional to the enhanced rate of glucose uptake (62). It has been suggested that IL-1 functions as a mitogen for synovial cells and fibroblasts, and that the subsequent increase in glucose uptake and glycolysis by these cells after relatively long-term exposure to IL-1 is an essential part of the differentiation process.

IL-1β, but not IL-1α, also produces time-dependent and dose-dependent increases in glucose uptake by isolated rat adipocytes (64). In this cell system, the maximal effect occurs after 3 hours of incubation, and the IL-1β effect is partially blocked by cycloheximide. IL-1 also enhances glucose uptake into proximal renal tubular cells (65). In addition, work by Eizirik (66) showed that after 48 hours of incubation with IL-1, glucose utilization was unaltered, but glucose oxidation was suppressed, in pancreatic islet cells. Furthermore, IL-1–induced inhibition of mitochondrial oxidation in islet cells appears mediated, at least in part, by nitric oxide, which inhibits the Krebs' cycle enzyme aconitase (67,68). Exposure of fully differentiated L6 myotubes to IL-1α does not alter hexose uptake (19). Finally, IL-1 fails to alter glucose utilization in hepatic parenchymal cells (69); however, this cytokine has been shown to enhance glycogenolysis in cultured rat hepatocytes (70). This effect results from both decreased glycogen synthase and increased glycogen phosphorylase-α activity, which is seen in hepatocytes incubated with IL-1β for 15 hours.

INTERLEUKIN-6

Most of the work on IL-6 relates to this ability to influence the acute phase protein response of the liver. In addition, however, IL-6 has been shown to alter hepatic carbohydrate metabolism under specific experimental conditions (Table 16–3). The ability of IL-6 to enhance hepatic glycogenolysis has been examined by Ritchie (71). In this study, ^{14}C-glucose was used to prelabel the glycogen pool in cultured rat hepatocytes. Concentrated conditioned medium from cultured human monocytes produced a dose-dependent release of ^{14}C-labeled glucose; the maximal response was comparable to that obtained using a maximally stimulating dose of glucagon. Partial purification of the monocyte-conditioned medium indicated a biologically active glycogenolytic factor with a relative molecular weight of 20 kd, which was heat-labile. Preincubation of conditioned medium with antisera

TABLE 16–3 EFFECTS OF IL-6 AND INF-α ON CARBOHYDRATE METABOLISM

IL-6	
Increased hepatic glycogenolysis	Hepatocytes, rat
Increased insulin secretion	Islets, rat
Decreased glucose-stimulated insulin release	
No change in glucose uptake	
Increased glucose oxidation	
Decreased hormonal stimulation of PEPCK	Hepatoma
Increased secretion of anterior pituitary hormones	In vivo, rat
INF-α	
Decreased glucose tolerance	In vivo, human
Decreased IMGU	
Increased catabolic hormones, insulin	
Increased insulin binding	Adipocytes, human
Increased glucose transport	

against human IL-6 produced a marked reduction in ^{14}C-glucose release. Subsequent experiments indicated that rhIL-6, but not rhTNF, rhIFN, or human IL-1, is also able to enhance hepatic glycogenolysis in this system.

Purified IL-6 has also been reported to produce dose-dependent inhibition of the hormonal induction of PEPCK mRNA in Reuber hepatoma cells (72). It has been suggested that by inhibiting PEPCK activity, this cytokine and others should attenuate stimulation of gluconeogenesis mediated by various endocrine hormones in stress states, thereby potentially leading to the development of hypoglycemia.

IL-6 has also been demonstrated to alter insulin secretion under in vitro conditions, an outcome that would be expected to influence glucose homeostasis (73). Incubation of rhIL-6 with cultured rat islet cells for 48 hours results in a 40 to 50% increase in insulin accumulation in the incubation medium. In addition, IL-6 blunts normal glucose-induced insulin release (73,74). Although IL-6 does not alter the rate of glucose utilization, as determined by the formation of ^3H_2O from $[5\text{-}^3H]$-glucose, it does increase glucose oxidation. However, these changes in insulin secretion and glucose metabolism do not appear to be immediate effects because they are not observed after short-term (1–2 hours) exposure of islet cells to IL-6.

IL-6 stimulates secretion of a number of anterior pituitary hormones under both in vitro and in vivo conditions, including ACTH, growth hormone, and β-endorphins (75), all of which can potentially influence glucose metabolism. Information regarding the ability of IL-6 to alter in vivo production of glucoregulatory hormones (i.e., insulin, glucagon, and catecholamines) is lacking. It remains to be shown whether any of these described effects of IL-6 are physiologically relevant.

INTERFERON

Overnight intramuscular administration of natural human leukocyte interferon-α (IFN-α) to healthy humans was found to produce a mild increase in plasma glucose concentrations (76). This hyperglycemia was associated with increases in circulating levels of insulin, cortisol, glucagon, and growth hormone. IFN-α impaired glucose tolerance in these subjects as manifested by a slower rate of glucose disappearance and a larger area under the curve following either oral or IV GTTs. However, subsequent studies found that basal HGP and peripheral glucose uptake are unchanged by IFN-α. This cytokine markedly impairs IMGU by peripheral tissues when assessed under euglycemic hyperinsulinemic conditions. This peripheral insulin resistance appears to result from overproduction of various counter-regulatory

hormones or subsequent release of other mediators, because INF-α fails to impair either insulin binding or glucose uptake by isolated human adipocytes (77). In fact, 5- and 24-hour incubation of adipocytes with IFN-α increased high-affinity insulin binding and enhanced insulin-stimulated glucose transport.

COLONY-STIMULATING FACTORS

Colony-stimulating factors (CSFs) promote proliferation and differentiation of hemopoietic progenitor cells. Prolonged exposure to these factors results in increased numbers of circulating leukocytes. In addition, these factors also enhance many effector functions of mature white blood cells. There are four colony-stimulating factors (multi-CSF [IL-3], granulocyte-macrophage CSF [GM-CSF], macrophage CSF [M-CSF or CSF-1], and granulocyte-CSF [G-CSF]), which were originally categorized based on the major cell types they affected.

Granulocyte-macrophage colony-stimulating factor

In an early study, Heidenreich and colleagues (78) demonstrated that elicited peritoneal macrophages treated with GM-CSF for 20 hours had an increased rate of lactate production (Table 16–4). However, it was not determined whether this increase resulted from a change in the rate of glucose uptake, glycolysis, or the Krebs' cycle.

GM-CSF has also been shown to rapidly alter in vivo glucose metabolism in conscious unrestrained rats (79). A single intra-arterial injection of recombinant murine GM-CSF produced transient mild hyperglycemia and increased whole body glucose turnover for up to 3 hours. The resultant elevation in HGP is not associated with an increase in circulating glucagon levels, and the enhanced peripheral uptake of glucose occurs concomitantly with unchanging arterial insulin levels. Using the in vivo tracer 2-deoxyglucose technique, glucose uptake by lung, liver, spleen, and skin was shown to be increased 0.5 hour after administration of GM-CSF. In addition to its transient effect on glucose uptake by these macrophage-rich tissues, GM-CSF also increases glucose uptake by skeletal muscle for up to 6 hours (Fig. 16-1). GM-CSF fails to elevate circulating levels of TNF; therefore, the glucose metabolic response appears to occur independently of this cytokine.

Subsequent studies by the same group investigated in vivo glucose uptake by circulation neutrophils and mononuclear cells, as well as by various liver cell types (80). A single injection of GM-CSF was found to increase glucose uptake several-fold by circulating neutrophils and mononuclear cells. In addition, the cells responsible for the

TABLE 16–4   EFFECTS OF COLONY-STIMULATING FACTORS ON CARBOHYDRATE METABOLISM

GM-CSF	
Increased glucose production	In vivo, rat
Increased peripheral glucose uptake in macrophage-rich tissues and muscle	
Increased glucose uptake by blood neutrophils	
Increased glucose uptake by parenchymal, Kupffer, and endothelial cells in liver	
Increased lactate production	Macrophages
G-CSF	
No change in basal glucose production or uptake	In vivo, rat
Enhanced uptake of glucose by macrophage-rich tissues in response to a secondary stimulus (endotoxin)	
M-CSF	
Increased glucose uptake	Macrophages
Increased hexokinase activity	
Primes macrophages for secondary stimulus and enhances HMP shunt	
Multi-CSF	
Increases glucose uptake	IL-3–dependent cell line

increased hepatic glucose uptake were assessed. Using centrifugal elutriation, GM-CSF was found to stimulate uptake in both parenchymal and nonparenchymal cells (both hepatic endothelial and Kupffer cells). Enhanced glucose uptake was also observed in neutrophils that had infiltrated the liver. These changes appear to be independent of prostanoid production because pretreatment of rats with indomethacin failed to attenuate the GM-CSF–induced increment in glucose uptake by these various hepatic and circulating cells. These observations are in accord with earlier findings that GM-CSF elevates glucose transport in bone marrow–derived and peritoneal macrophages (81). The increased glucose uptake seen after GM-CSF is insulin-independent, and it is not dependent on a mass action effect.

Granulocyte colony-stimulating factor

Lang and associates (82,83) conducted two studies to examine whether in vivo administration of G-CSF alters whole body and tissue glucose metabolism under basal conditions, or if it modifies either endotoxin-induced or sepsis-induced changes in glucose flux. In these studies, rats were injected twice daily subcutaneously with rhG-CSF, and glucose metabolism was studied approximately 12 hours after the final injection. This dosage regimen resulted in a greater than 8-fold elevation in the number of circulating granulocytes, but no detectable changes in hemodynamics or whole body or tissue glucose metabolism were seen (82,83). However, G-CSF was a potent immunomodulatory agent, and it altered glucose flux in response to a secondary challenge (i.e., endotoxin). Rates of HGP and peripheral glucose uptake in both control and G-CSF–treated rats were rapidly increased by endotoxin; however, the increment in glucose flux was 50 to 100% greater in the G-CSF–treated group (82). The enhanced HGP in this group occurred despite lower plasma lactate and glucagon levels, suggesting an increased hepatic gluconeogenic efficiency.

The elevated rate of whole body glucose uptake was attributed to G-CSF–enhanced, endotoxin-induced increase in uptake by intestine, spleen, liver, and lung. Furthermore, endotoxin increased glucose uptake by skeletal muscle in G-CSF–treated rats, but not in control animals. Importantly, enhanced glucose disposal in G-CSF–treated rats was not mediated by increases in plasma glucose or insulin concentrations. The mechanism for direct or indirect increase in tissue avidity for glucose remains unknown. In contrast, when gram-negative hypermetabolic sepsis was induced in rats, the resultant elevation in whole body glucose production, utilization, and MCR were unaffected by prior treatment with G-CSF (83). This cytokine was able, however, to modify enhanced glucose uptake by tissues at the site of inflammation.

These studies demonstrate that G-CSF, in the absence of a secondary stimulus, results in no detectable changes in whole body or tissue glucose metabolism, whereas G-CSF appears to prime cells so that subsequent administration of immunomodulators (e.g., endotoxin) produces a greater increase in glucose uptake than in control animals. Under these conditions, euglycemia is maintained by a proportional increase in the HGP.

Macrophage colony-stimulation factor (or CSF-1)

Purified M-CSF produces a dose-dependent increase in glucose uptake and phosphorylation in murine bone marrow–derived macrophages (84) and resident peritoneal macrophages (81). It has been suggested by a number of investigators that cytokine-induced changes in glucose uptake represent an increased hexose monophosphate shunt activity. Rist and coworkers (85), using C-1-^{3}H-labeled and C-2,6-^{3}H-labeled 2-deoxyglucose, examined this possibility in a series of elegant experiments. Their results indicate that 1-hour incubation of rat or mouse macrophages with rhM-CSF results in an equal accumulation of both 2-deoxyglucose labels within the cells, suggesting that this cytokine stimulates hexokinase activity without altering metabolism through the hexose monophosphate shunt or superoxide production. In contrast, there was a disparity between uptake of the two labels in macrophages treated with phorbol 12-myristate 13-acetate (PMA), indicating enhanced activity of the shunt pathway. Moreover, when cells were incubated simultaneously with M-CSF and PMA, there was a synergistic effect, with dual activation of both hexokinase and the pentose shunt. Additional studies by this same group (86) suggest that the M-CSF–induced increase in glucose uptake is most likely due to enhanced hexokinase activity and not an increased number of glucose transporters.

These results confirm the observations described by Hamilton and associates (84), but they also indicate that enhanced glucose uptake alone is not an accurate index of shunt activity. In addition, these results are consistent with those of Lang and colleagues (82,83), which showed that G-CSF was able to prime cells in macrophage-rich tissues to increase glucose uptake in response to endotoxin, a known activator of the pentose shunt.

Multi-colony-stimulating factor/interleukin-3

Whetton and coworkers (87) performed experiments using a multipotent hemopoietic stem-cell line, FDC-Mix 1. A 4-hour incubation of these cells with IL-3 increased 2-deoxyglucose uptake. The enhanced glucose transport appears to be attributable to improved glucose transporter function (i.e., activation) and not to increased transport number (88).

ROLE OF CYTOKINES IN THE GLUCOSE METABOLIC RESPONSE TO DISEASE

Numerous cytokines can modulate carbohydrate metabolism under in vivo and in vitro conditions. However, a cytokine's ability to influence metabolism under controlled experimental conditions only indicates its potential actions. The actual role of these cytokines in regulating metabolism in disease states associated with their increased production remains unclear. These cytokines have most often been suggested to be key regulators of the protein, lipid, and carbohydrate changes that occur in chronic disease states, such as infection, neoplasia, and inflammation.

There is little doubt that passive immunoneutralization of circulating TNF protects animals from the lethal

consequences of bacteremia or endotoxic shock (89,90); however, its ability to reverse metabolic sequelae is controversial. Work by Hinshaw and associates (90) showed that anti-TNF antibodies administered to baboons prior to IV injection of live *Escherichia coli* attenuated the early hyperglycemic response. In contrast, Bagby and colleagues (91,92) and Lang and associates (93) reported that the antibodies against TNF were unable to prevent the endotoxin-induced increase in plasma glucose, HGP, or tissue glucose uptake in rats, although it did blunt hyperlactacidemia and hyperglucagonemia. Likewise, injection of a polyclonal antibody against recombinant murine TNF into rats prior to the induction of gram-negative hypermetabolic sepsis was unable to prevent either enhanced peripheral glucose uptake observed under basal conditions or impairment of IMGU under hyperinsulinemic conditions (94). On the positive side, however, neutralization of TNF-α in obese *fa/fa* rats was found to achieve significant improvement in glucose uptake by peripheral tissues under hyperinsulinemic conditions (95).

Substances that block IL-1 binding to its receptor have also been employed as possible therapeutic agents in shock. Administration of the IL-1 receptor antagonist (RA) improves survival and the hemodynamic performance of shocked animals (96). However, in a study by Fischer and colleagues (97), IL-1RA was unable to block the plasma glucose and lactate changes produced by either a sublethal dose of endotoxin or an LD_{100} dose of live *E. coli* in baboons. The relevancy of TNF, IL-1, and other cytokines as modulators of the glucose dyshomeostasis observed in various disease states remains unresolved. As a result of widening availability of neutralizing antibodies and receptor blocking agents, a better understanding of the role of cytokines in infection, cancer, autoimmune disease, and other chronic catabolic illnesses should be forthcoming.

ACKNOWLEDGMENTS: This work was supported by National Institute of General Medical Science grant GM38032.

I would also like to thank my collaborators and colleagues, Drs. John Spitzer, Gregory Bagby, Zoltan Spolarics, and Karoly Meszaros, Department of Physiology, Louisiana State University Medical Center, New Orleans, LA, for their assistance and advice throughout my stay at that institution.

REFERENCES

1. Berry LJ. Bacterial toxins. Crit Rev Toxicol 1977;5:239–318.
2. Filkins JP. Insulin-like activity (ILA) of a macrophage mediator on adipose tissue glucose oxidation. J Reticuloendothel Soc 1979;25:591–594.
3. Tracey KJ, Beutler B, Lowry SF, et al. Shock and tissue in-

jury by recombinant human cachectin. Science 1986;234: 470–474.

4. Bagby GJ, Lang CH, Hargrove DM, Thompson JJ, Wilson LA, Spitzer JJ. Glucose kinetics in rats infused with endotoxin-induced monokines or tumor necrosis factor. Circ Shock 1988;24:111–121.

5. Arbos J, Lopez-Soriano FJ, Carbo N, Argiles JM. Effects of tumour necrosis factor-α (cachectin) on glucose metabolism in the rat: intestinal absorption and isolated enterocyte metabolism. Mol Cell Biochem 1992;112:53–59.

6. Chajek-Shaul T, Barash V, Wiedenfed J, et al. Lethal hypoglycemia and hypothermia induced by administration of low doses of tumor necrosis factor to adrenalectomized rats. Metabolism 1990;39:242–250.

7. Lang CH, Dobrescu C, Bagby GJ. Tumor necrosis factor impairs insulin action on peripheral glucose disposal and hepatic glucose output. Endocrinology 1992;130:43–52.

8. Bagby GJ, Lang CH, Skrepnik N, Spitzer JJ. Attenuation of glucose metabolic changes resulting from TNFα administration by adrenergic blockade. Am J Physiol 1992;262: R628–R635.

9. Evans DH, Jacobs DO, Wilmore DW. Tumor necrosis factor enhances glucose uptake by peripheral tissues. Am J Physiol 1989;257:R1182–R1189.

10. Douglas RG, Gluckman PD, Breier BH, McCall JL, Parry B, Shaw JHF. Effects of recombinant IGF-1 on protein and glucose metabolism in rTNF-infused lambs. Am J Physiol 1991;261:E606–E612.

11. Van Der Poll T, Romijn JA, Endert E, et al. Tumor necrosis factor mimics the metabolic response to acute infection in healthy humans. Am J Physiol 1991;261:E457–E465.

12. Tredget EE, Yu YM, Zhong S, et al. Role of Interleukin-1 and tumor necrosis factor on energy metabolism in rabbits. Am J Physiol 1988;255:E760–E768.

13. Flores EA, Istfan N, Pomposelli J, Blackburn GL, Bistrian BR. Effect of interleukin-1 and tumor necrosis factor/cachectin in glucose turnover in the rat. Metabolism 1990; 39:738–743.

14. Tracey KJ, Lowry SF, Fahey TJ, et al. Cachectin/tumor necrosis factor induces lethal shock and stress hormone responses in the dog. Surg Gynecol Obstet 1987;164:415–422.

15. Darling G, Goldstein DS, Stull R, Gorschboth CM, Norton JA. Tumor necrosis factor: immune endocrine interaction. Surgery 1989;106:1155–1160.

16. Warren RS, Starnes F, Gabrilove JL, Oettgen HF, Brennan MF. The acute metabolic effects of tumor necrosis factor administration in humans. Arch Surg 1987;122:1396–1400.

17. Warren RS, Donner DB, Starnes HF, Brennan MF. Modulation of endogenous hormone action by recombinant human tumor necrosis factor. Proc Natl Acad Sci USA 1987; 84:8619–8622.

18. Yasmineh WG, Theologides A. Effect of tumor necrosis factor on enzymes of gluconeogenesis in the rat. Proc Soc Exp Biol Med 1992;199:97–103.

19. Warren RS, Starnes HF, Alcock N, Calvano S, Brennan MF. Hormonal and metabolic response to recombinant human tumor necrosis factor in rat: in vitro and in vivo. Am J Physiol 1988;255:E206–E212.

20. Lang CH. β-adrenergic blockade attenuates insulin resistance induced by tumor necrosis factor. Am J Physiol 1993; 264:R984–R991.

21. Cianco MJ, Hunt J, Jones SB, Filkins JP. Comparative and interactive in vivo effects of tumor necrosis factor-α and endotoxin. Circ Shock 1991;33:108–120.

22. Kettelhut IC, Fiers W, Goldberg AL. The toxic effects of tumor necrosis factor in vivo and their prevention by cyclooxygenase inhibitors. Proc Natl Acad Sci USA 1987; 84:4273–4277.

23. Lang CH, Spolarics Z, Ottlakan A, Spitzer JJ. Effect of high-dose endotoxin on glucose production and utilization. Metabolism 1994;442:1351–1358.

24. Meszaros K, Lang CH, Bagby GJ, Spitzer JJ. Tumor necrosis factor increases in vivo glucose utilization of macrophage-rich tissues. Biochem Biophys Res Commun 1987;149:1–6.

25. Mahony SM, Tisdale MJ. Metabolic effects of TNF-α in NMRI mice. Br J Cancer 1990;61:514–519.

26. Spolarics Z, Schuler A, Bagby GJ, Lang CH, Meszaros K, Spitzer JJ. Tumor necrosis factor increases in vivo glucose uptake in hepatic nonparenchymal cells. J Leukocyte Biol 1991;49:309–312.

27. Lee MD, Zentella A, Pekala PH, Cerami A. Effect of endotoxin-induced monokines on glucose metabolism in the muscle cell line L6. Proc Natl Acad Sci USA 1987;84:2590–2594.

28. Lang CH, Dobrescu C. Gram-negative infection increases noninsulin-mediated glucose disposal. Endocrinology 1991; 128:645–653.

29. Spolarics Z, Bagby GJ, Lang CH, Spitzer JJ. Up-regulation of glucose metabolism in Kupffer cells following infusion of tumour necrosis factor. Biochem J 1991;278:515–519.

30. Stephens JM, Pekala PH. Transcriptional repression of the GLUT 4 and c/ebp genes in 3T3-L1 adipocytes by tumor necrosis factor-α. J Biol Chem 1991;266:21839–21845.

31. Cornelius P, Lee MD, Marlowe M, Pekala PH. Monokine regulation of glucose transporter mRNA in L6 myotubes. Biochem Biophys Res Commun 1989;165:429–436.

32. Rofe AM, Conyers AJ, Bais R, Gamble JR, Vadas MA. The effects of recombinant tumor necrosis factor (cachectin) on metabolism in isolated rat adipocyte, hepatocyte and muscle preparations. Biochem J 1987;247:789–792.

33. Cornelius P, Marlowe M, Lee MD, Pekala PH. The growth factor-like effects of tumor necrosis factor-α. J Biol Chem 1990;265:20506–20516.

34. George DT, Abeles FB, Mapes CA, Sobocinski PZ, Zenser TV, Powanda MC. Effect of leukocytic endogenous mediators on endocrine pancreas secretory responses. Am J Physiol 1977;233:E240–E245.

35. Del Ray A, Besedovsky H. Interleukin 1 affects glucose homeostasis. Am J Physiol 1987;253:R794–R798.

36. Berkenbosch F, de Goeij DEC, Del Ray A, Besedovsky HO. Neuroendocrine, sympathetic and metabolic responses induced by interleukin-1. Neuroendocrinology 1989;50: 570–576.

37. Besedovsky HO, Del Ray A. Interleukin-1 and glucose homeostasis: an example of the biological relevance of immune-neuroendocrine interactions. Horm Res 1989;31: 94–99.

38. Del Ray A, Besedovsky H. Antidiabetic effects of interleukin 1. Proc Natl Acad Sci USA 1989;86:5943–5947.

39. Keenan RA, Moldawer LL, Sakamoto A, Blackburn GL, Bistrian BR. Effect of leukocyte endogenous mediator(s) on insulin and substrate profiles in the fasted rat. J Surg Res 1982:33:151–157.

40. Lang CH, Dobrescu C. Interleukin-1 induced increases in glucose utilization are insulin mediated. Life Sci 1989;45: 2127–2134.

41. Sacco-Gibson N, Filkins JP. Glucoregulatory effects of interleukin-1: implications to the carbohydrate dyshomeostasis of septic shock. In: Bond RF. Perspectives in shock research. New York: Liss, 1988:355–360.

42. Cornell RP, Schwartz DB. Central administration of interleukin 1 elicits hyperinsulinemia in rats. Am J Physiol 1989;256:R772–R777.

43. Roh MS, Moldawer LL, Ekman LG, et al. Stimulatory effect of interleukin-1 upon hepatic metabolism. Metabolism 1986; 35:419–424.

44. Fischer E, Marano MA, Barber AE, et al. Comparison between effects of interleukin-1α administration and sublethal endotoxemia in primates. Am J Physiol 1991;261: R442–R452.

45. Hill MR, Stith RD, McCallum RE. Interleukin 1: a regulatory role in glucocorticoid-regulated hepatic metabolism. J Immunol 1986;137:858–862.

46. Lang CM, Molina PE, Yousef KA, Tepper PG, Abumrad NN. Role of IL-1α in central nervous system immunomodulation of glucoregulation. Brain Res 1993;624: 53–60.

47. Cornell RP. Central interleukin 1-elicited hyperinsulinemia is mediated by prostaglandins but not autonomics. Am J Physiol 1989;257:R839–R846.

48. Yelich MR. In vivo endotoxin and IL-1 potentiates insulin secretion in pancreatic islets. Am J Physiol 1990;258: R1070–R1077.

49. Wogensen LD, Kolb-Bachofen V, Christensen P, et al. Functional and morphological effects of interleukin-1β on the perfused rat pancreas. Diabetologia 1990;33:15–23.

50. Argiles JM, Lopez-Soriano J, Ortiz MA, Pou JM, Lopez-Soriano FJ. Interleukin-1 and β-cell function: more than one second messenger? Endocr Rev 1992;13:515–524.

51. Rothwell NJ. Functions and mechanisms of interleukin 1 in the brain. TIPS 1991;12:430–435.

52. Donner FR, Mori K, Dinarello CA, Sokoloff L. Effects of leukocytic pyrogen (interleukin-1) on local cerebral glucose utilization in rats with and without premedication with indomethacin or dexamethasone. J Cereb Blood Flow Metab 1988;8:173–178.

53. Watters JM, Bessey PQ, Dinarello CA, Wolff SM, Wilmore DW. The induction of interleukin-1 in humans and its metabolic effects. Surgery 1985;98:298–306.

54. Wogensen L, Reimers J, Mandrup-Poulsen T, Nerup J. Repeated intraperitoneal injections of interleukin 1β induce glucose intolerance in normal rats. Acta Endocrinol 1991; 124:470–478.

55. Bergman RN, Finegood DT, Ader M. Assessment of insulin sensitivity in vivo. Endocr Rev 1985;6:45–86.

56. Banks WA, Ortiz L, Plotkin SR, Kastin AJ. Human interleukin (IL)-1α, murine IL-1α and murine IL-1β are transported from blood to brain in the mouse by a shared saturable mechanism. J Pharmacol Exp Ther 1991;259: 988–996.

57. Benveniste EN. Inflammatory cytokines within the central nervous system: sources, function, and mechanism of action. Am J Physiol 1992;263:C1–C16.

58. Bateman A, Sungh A, Kral T, Soloman S. The immune-hypothalamic-pituitary-adrenal axis. Endocr Rev 1989;10: 92–112.

59. Cornell RP. Central administration of interleukin 1 elicits hyperinsulinemia in rats. Am J Physiol 1989;265:R772–R777.

60. Hernvann A, Aussel C, Cynober L, Moatti N, Ekindjian OG. IL-1β, a strong mediator for glucose uptake by rheumatoid and non-rheumatoid cultured human synoviocytes. FEBS Lett 1992;303:77–80.

61. Bird TA, Davies A, Baldwin SA, Saklatvala J. Interleukin 1 stimulates hexose transport in fibroblasts by increasing the expression of glucose transporters. J Biol Chem 1990;265: 13578–13583.

62. Taylor DJ, Whitehead RJ, Evanson JM, et al. Effect of recombinant cytokines on glycolysis and fructose 2,6-bisphosphate in rheumatoid synovial cells in vitro. Biochem J 1988;250:111–115.

63. Taylor DJ, Faragher EB, Evanson JM. Inflammatory cytokines stimulate glucose uptake and glycolysis but reduce glucose oxidation in human dermal fibroblasts in vitro. Circ Shock 1992;37:105–110.

64. Garcia-Welsh A, Schneiderman JS, Baly DL. Interleukin-1 stimulates glucose transport in rat adipose cells. Evidence for receptor discrimination between IL-1β and IL-1α. FEBS Lett 1990;269:421–424.

65. Kohan DE, Schreiner GF. Interleukin 1 modulation of renal epithelial glucose and amino acid transport. Am J Physiol 1988;254:F879–F886.

66. Eizirik DL. Interleukin-1 induced impairment in pancreatic islet oxidative metabolism of glucose is potentiated by tumor necrosis factor. Acta Endocrinol 1988;119:321–325.

67. Corbett JA, Wang JL, Hughes JH, et al. Nitric oxide and cyclic GMP formation induced by interleukin 1β in islets of Langerhans. Biochem J 1992;287:229–235.

68. Welsh N, Eizirik DL, Bendtzen K, Sandler S. Interleukin-1β-induced nitric oxide production in isolated rat pancreatic islets requires gene transcription and may lead to inhibition of the krebs cycle enzyme aconitase. Endocrinology 1991;129:3167–3173.

69. Miller BC, Uyeda K, Cottam GL. Endotoxin stimulation of liver parenchymal cell phosphofructokinase activity requires nonparenchymal cells. Eur J Biochem 1992;203: 593–598.

70. Lee JD, Cho S-W, Hwang O. Interleukin 1β regulates glycogen metabolism in primary cultured rat hepatocytes. Biochem Biophys Res Commun 1993;191:515–522.

71. Ritchie DG. Interleukin 6 stimulates hepatic glucose release from prelabeled glycogen pools. Am J Physiol 1990; 258:E57–E64.

72. Hill MR, Stith RD, McCallum RE. Mechanism of action of interferon-β2/Interleukin-6 on induction of hepatic liver enzymes. Ann NY Acad Sci 1989;57:502–504.

73. Sandler S, Bendtzen K, Eizirik DL, Welsh M. Interleukin-6

affects insulin secretion and glucose metabolism of rat pancreatic islets in vitro. Endocrinology 1990;126:1288–1294.

74. Southern C, Schulster D, Green IC. Inhibition of insulin secretion from rat islets of Langerhans by interleukin-6. Biochem J 1990;272:243–245.

75. Lyson K, McCann SM. The effect of interleukin-6 on pituitary hormone release in vivo and in vitro. Neuroendocrinology 1991;54:262–266.

76. Koivisto VA, Pelkonen R, Cantell K. Effect of interferon on glucose tolerance and insulin sensitivity. Diabetes 1989;38: 641–647.

77. Kolaczynski JW, Taskinen M-R, Hilden H, Kiviluoto T, Cantell K, Koivisto VA. Effects of interferon alpha on insulin binding and glucose transport in human adipocytes. Eur J Clin Invest 1992;22:292–299.

78. Heidenreich S, Gong J-H, Schmidt A, Nain M, Gemsa D. Macrophage activation by granulocyte/macrophage colony-stimulating factor. J Immunol 1989;143:1198–1205.

79. Schuler A, Spolarics Z, Lang CH, Bagby GJ, Nelson S, Spitzer JJ. Upregulation of glucose metabolism by granulocyte-macrophage colony-stimulating factor. Life Sci 1991; 49:899–906.

80. Spolarics Z, Schuler A, Bagby GJ, Lang CH, Nelson S, Spitzer JJ. In vivo metabolic response of hepatic non-parenchymal cells and leukocytes to granulocyte-macrophage-stimulating factor. J Leukocyte Biol 1992;51:360–365.

81. Hamilton JA, Vairo G, Lingelbach SR. Activation and proliferation signals in murine macrophages: stimulation of glucose uptake by hemopoietic growth factors and other agents. J Cell Physiol 1988;134:405–412.

82. Lang CH, Bagby GJ, Dobrescu C, Nelson S, Spitzer JJ. Modulation of glucose metabolic response to endotoxin by granulocyte colony-stimulating factor. Am J Physiol 1992; 263:R1122–R1129.

83. Lang CH, Bagby GJ, Dobrescu C, Nelson S, Spitzer JJ. Effect of granulocyte colony-stimulating factor on sepsis-induced changes in neutrophil accumulation and organ glucose uptake. J Infect Dis 192:166:336–343.

84. Hamilton JA, Vairo G, Lingelbach SR. CSF-1 stimulates glucose uptake in murine bone marrow-derived macrophages. Biochem Biophys Res Commun 1986;138:445–454.

85. Rist RJ, Jones GE, Naftalin RJ. Synergistic activation of 2-deoxy-D-glucose uptake in rat and murine peritoneal macrophages by human macrophage colony-stimulating factor-stimulated coupling between transport and hexokinase activity and phorbol-dependent stimulation of pentose phosphate-shunt activity. Biochem J 1990;265:243–249.

86. Rist RJ, Jones GE, Naftalin RJ. Effects of macrophage colony-stimulating factor and phorbol myristate acetate on 2-D-deoxyglucose transport and superoxide production in rat peritoneal macrophages. Biochem J 1991;278:119–128.

87. Whetton AD, Heyworth CM, Dexter TM. Phorbol esters activate protein kinase C and glucose transport and can replace the requirement for growth factor in interleukin-3-dependent multipotent stem cells. J Cell Sci 1986;84:93–104.

88. Nefesh I, Bauskin AR, Alkalay I, Golembo M, Ben-Neriah Y. IL-3 facilitates lymphocyte hexose transport by enhancing the intrinsic activity of the transport system. Int Immunol 1991;3:827–831.

89. Mathison JC, Wolfson E, Ulevitch RJ. Participation of tumor necrosis factor in the mediation of gram negative bacterial lipopolysaccharide-induced injury in rabbits. J Clin Invest 1988;81:1925–1937.

90. Hinshaw LB, Tekamp-Olson P, Chang A, et al. Survival of primates in LD100 septic shock following therapy with antibody to tumor necrosis factor (TNFα). Circ Shock 1990; 30:279–292.

91. Bagby GJ, Plessala KJ, Wilson LA, Thompson JJ, Nelson S. Divergent efficacy of anti-TNFα antibody in intravascular and peritonitis models of sepsis. J Infect Dis 1991;163:83–88.

92. Bagby GJ, Lang CH, Skrepnik N, Golightly G, Spitzer JJ. Regulation of glucose metabolism is largely independent of endogenous tumor necrosis factor. Circ Shock 1993;39: 211–219.

93. Lang CH, Obih J-C A, Bagby GJ, Bagwell JN, Spitzer JJ. Endotoxin-induced increases in regional glucose utilization by small effect. Am J Physiol 1991;260:G548–G555.

94. Lang CH. Mechanism of insulin resistance in infection. In: Schlag G, Redl H, eds. Pathophysiology of shock, sepsis and organ failure. Heidelberg: Springer-Verlag, 1993:609–625.

95. Hotamisligil GS, Shargill NS, Spiegelman BM. Adipose expression of tumor necrosis factor α: direct role in obesity-linked insulin resistance. Science 1993;259:87–91.

96. Arend WP. Interleukin 1 receptor antagonist: a new member of the interleukin 1 family. J Clin Invest 1991;88:1445–1451.

97. Fischer E, Marano MA, VanZee KJ, et al. Interleukin-1 receptor blockade improves survival and hemodynamic performance in Escherichia coli septic shock, but fails to alter host responses to sublethal endotoxemia. J Clin Invest 1992;89:1551–1557.

CHAPTER 17

ROLE OF CYTOKINES IN REGULATION OF BONE REMODELING AND OSTEOPOROSIS

Gregory R. Mundy, G. David Roodman, and Toshiyuki Yoneda

All diseases of bone are superimposed on the normal bone remodeling sequence. Bone remodeling is carried out in discrete, geographically distinct packets throughout the skeleton. The cellular events responsible for bone remodeling are the same both in Haversian bone and on the endosteal surfaces of cancellous bone, but they are clearly controlled locally, because the stage of remodeling in one bone remodeling packet may be different from that of other bone remodeling packets. For these reasons, there has been intense interest over the past 20 years in identifying local factors or cytokines responsible for control of the normal bone remodeling sequence, as well as what happens to these factors in disease states, such as osteoporosis.

NORMAL BONE REMODELING

The sequence of cellular events that occurs in Haversian systems of cortical bone and on the surface of cancellous bone always involves osteoclastic bone resorption followed by bone formation by osteoblasts (1). This is a complex and prolonged sequence that takes several months on human bone surfaces. The process of osteoclastic bone resorption usually takes approximately 10 days, and the period of bone formation lasts several months. Although the sequence is the same in both cortical and cancellous bone, it is likely that the factors re-

sponsible for modulating the cellular events in cancellous bone are different from those in cortical bone, because the surfaces of cancellous bone are much more closely in contact with the mononuclear cells of the marrow cavity.

The initial event in the remodeling sequence is osteoclastic bone resorption. The osteoclast is a large multinucleated cell unique to bone. It is the only cell in the body that has the capacity to resorb bone. It does so across a specialized area of the cell membrane known as the ruffled border. The osteoclast becomes highly polarized with respect to intracellular organelles, and it mediates bone resorption by production of protons through a novel vacuolar adenosine triphosphatase (ATPase) located at the ruffled border and by secretion of proteolytic enzymes (2). Osteoclast formation is under the control of cytokines generated in the microenvironment of the osteoclast, as well as systemic factors, such as parathyroid hormone, calcitonin, and 1,25-dihydroxyvitamin D. Because these latter factors are primarily responsible for controlling calcium homeostasis, it appears more likely that the cytokines generated in the microenvironment of resorbing osteoclasts are responsible for regulating osteoclast activity.

Recent data suggest that attachment of osteoclasts to the mineralized matrix is essential for bone resorption to occur. This attachment may be mediated by integral membrane proteins or integrins. One integrin implicated in bone resorption is the vitronectin receptor (3). Antibodies to the vitronectin receptor have been shown to block bone resorption. Moreover, recent data suggest that interaction of the vitronectin receptor with arginine-glycine-aspartic acid (RGD) sequences in matrix proteins, such as osteopontin, leads to changes in intracellular calcium that may be responsible for osteoclast activation. A series of proto-oncogenes may be expressed in osteoclasts, and they are essential for osteoclast function. These proto-oncogenes include the nonreceptor tyrosine kinase, c-src, the receptor tyrosine kinase, c-fms, and the c-fos proto-oncogenes (4,5). Whether these proto-oncogenes are linked or independent in their action is unknown. It is certainly likely that c-src and c-fms are linked, because there is ample precedent for associations of nonreceptor and receptor tyrosine kinases in other systems. Gene knockout experiments have shown that c-fos and c-src are required for normal osteoclastic bone resorption: osteopetrosis develops in mice with deficient expression of c-fos and c-src. In the case of c-fms, although gene knockout experiments have not been reported as yet, deficient expression of the ligand for c-fms, namely monocyte-macrophage colony-stimulating factor (M-CSF), causes a neonatal form of osteopetrosis in the mouse (6–9).

The process of bone formation during which a previous packet of bone removed by osteoclasts is replaced is much more prolonged than that of bone resorption. The cellular sequence of events is highly integrated, and it is clearly stimulated by the process of resorption. Although the precise mechanism by which bone formation is initiated at previous sites of resorption is unknown, it appears likely that local factors generated as a consequence of resorption are responsible. These factors may be released from the bone matrix, by bone cells, or even by osteoclasts. The bone matrix is an abundant source of growth regulatory factors for osteoblasts (10), including insulin-like growth factors I and II, heparin-binding fibroblast growth factors, transforming growth factor-β (TGF-β), bone morphogenetic proteins, and platelet-derived growth factor.

The cellular events involved in bone formation are multiple. These events include migration of osteoblast precursors to the sites of resorption defects (chemotaxis), stimulation of proliferation of osteoblast precursors, differentiation of osteoblast precursors to form mature osteoblasts, secretion of proteins such as type I collagen and the other proteins of the mature bone matrix, and, finally, mineralization of the bone matrix to form normal mineralized bone. These events are obviously highly complex, but they must be very tightly coordinated to produce a packet of bone that replaces exactly the packet of bone removed by previous osteoclastic bone resorption. In an attempt to devise an in vitro model to study these complex events, Bellows and colleagues (11) and Stein and associates (12) used prolonged cultures of fetal rat calvarial osteoblasts. In

this system, it is possible to study all the events involved in osteoblast proliferation and differentiation, including formation of mineralized bone nodules. It is also possible to study the expression of specific gene products associated with bone formation and to study the regulation of this process by growth regulatory factors.

Interleukin-1

Interleukin-1 (IL-1) is the cytokine most extensively studied for its effects on bone. It is a powerful bone-resorbing factor. It is a systemic mediator of osteoclastic bone resorption, and it rapidly promotes hypercalcemia because of its powerful effects on osteoclasts (13,14). It causes hypercalcemia and increased osteoclastic bone resorption whether it is injected intermittently or delivered in a bolus form, or whether it is infused via an osmotic mini-pump into the subcutaneous tissue. The osteoclasts formed are very large and hyperactive. The effects of IL-1 on osteoclastic bone resorption can be partially impaired by inhibition of prostaglandin synthesis, indicating that they are at least in part mediated by local generation of prostaglandins in bone tissue (15). IL-1 increases the formation of osteoclasts from precursors, which may be its major effect (16). However, it also enhances differentiation of committed precursors in the osteoclast lineage. Although effects of IL-1 have also been described on mature osteoclasts, these findings are controversial. In the hands of some people, IL-1 works indirectly on osteoclasts through intermediate cells to stimulate osteoclast activation (17), but in the hands of others, IL-1 may in fact have inhibitory effects on mature cells (18). Whether the effects on the mature cell are stimulatory or inhibitory, there is no question about the overall powerful stimulatory effects of IL-1 on bone resorption.

IL-1 may also cause enhanced bone formation, but this process does not happen unless there is preceding osteoclastic bone resorption initiated by intermittent IL-1. It stimulates osteoblast proliferation (19), but it inhibits differentiated function in osteoclasts exposed to its continued presence (20). It has an inhibitory effect on markers of differentiated function, such as alkaline phosphatase content and type I collagen synthesis. We have found that intermittent exposure to IL-1 in vivo enhances coupling (13), presumably because of secondary factors produced as a consequence of the coupling phenomenon.

Although the effects of IL-1 in vivo are to enhance bone resorption and to cause hypercalcemia, there is a transient initial decrease in serum calcium levels following exposure to IL-1 (15). This decrease appears to be related to prostaglandin synthesis, and the mechanism is unknown.

IL-1 may be involved in chronic inflammatory diseases, certain malignancies associated with bone resorption and hypercalcemia, and osteoporosis. Its potential role in osteoporosis is discussed in more detail in another section.

Tumor necrosis factor

Tumor necrosis factor (TNF) is an interesting bone resorbing cytokine with many biological effects on bone that overlap with those of IL-1. Like IL-1, it is a powerful stimulator of osteoclastic bone resorption in vivo, and it causes hypercalcemia (21). Its effects on bone have not been studied in as much detail as those of IL-1, although it seems to have very similar effects in all the in vitro systems in which it has been tested. For example, it is known that TNF stimulates proliferation of osteoclast precursors and enhances differentiation of committed precursors to form mature cells (16). Moreover, there is information to suggest that, like IL-1, it can stimulate isolated osteoclasts to form resorption pits on calcified matrices (22). Its major effects on osteoclasts still have to be clarified.

TNF seems to also have identical effects as those of IL-1 on cells in the osteoblast lineage (19). It stimulates proliferation of normal osteoblast precursors, but it probably inhibits proliferation. In some osteosarcoma cell lines, it seems to have different types of effects, and it can actually enhance differentiated function. The relevance of these observations to normal osteoblastic bone formation remains unclear.

TNF is produced by activated macrophages, but it is also produced by bone cells. It is not known to be produced by solid tumors, unlike IL-1α. However, lymphotoxin (also known as TNF-β) stimulates osteoclastic bone resorption (23), and hypercalcemia has been implicated in the bone resorption associated with myeloma (24). Certainly, established cell lines from human and animal myeloma cells express lymphotoxin, and part of the bone resorbing activity produced by these cells can be accounted for by lymphotoxin. However, whether this is the sole mediator responsible for bone destruction in myeloma, and whether myeloma cells in situ behave identically to myeloma cells in long-term culture remains obscure.

TNF may be responsible for other paraneoplastic syndromes associated with malignancy. Chinese hamster ovarian cells transfected with TNF cause a number of paraneoplastic syndromes when carried in tumor-bearing nude mice (21,25). For example, such tumors can cause hypercalcemia, cachexia, leukocytosis, hypertriglyceridemia, and anemia. In situations in which TNF is overproduced, all these syndromes seem likely to be important. Although this correlation is unlikely to be true very often in patients with solid tumors because of direct production of TNF by the solid tumor cells, it nevertheless appears likely that TNF is often produced by normal host cells in some patients with cancer. This effect has been clearly demonstrated in a number of human and animal tumors. In the best documented case, a human squamous-cell carcinoma was shown to stimulate normal host immune cells to produce TNF (26,27). In tumor-bearing nude mice, hypercalcemia and other paraneoplastic syndromes are relieved when the tumor is removed, but they are also relieved when the spleen is removed. The mechanisms with which solid tumor cells may stimulate TNF production are probably multiple, and they may include production of mediators such as granulocyte-macrophage colony-stimulating factor (GM-CSF), as has been shown in some human tumor models (28,29), as well as other unidentified soluble factors. Cell-to-cell contact may also be important.

TNF may have a role in the bone loss associated with estrogen withdrawal or the aging state. It has been shown that cytokines, such as IL-1 and TNF, are overproduced by monocytic cells following estrogen withdrawal in vivo (30). The importance of these observations has yet to be confirmed.

Interleukin-6

IL-6 is a novel cytokine that has very unusual effects on bone resorption. Its effects in bone have been controversial because in many of the traditional models for studying bone resorption, IL-6 seems to have no effect. However, it is clear that IL-6 causes hypercalcemia in vivo (31), and that it stimulates osteoclastic bone resorption in some systems. It also probably stimulates osteoclastic bone resorption in vivo. Most of the information comes from specialized in vitro systems, including isolated osteoclasts (32), isolated osteoclast-like cells derived from giant-cell tumors of bone (33,34), human marrow cell culture systems (35), and several murine fetal organ culture systems in which cells that are clearly precursors of osteoclasts are assessed (32).

IL-6 has received a lot of attention for its potential role in osteoporosis by the observations of Manolagas and colleagues over the last 2 years (36,37). These workers showed that human bone cells express IL-6, and that IL-6 production by these bone cells can be modulated by estrogens. Moreover, they showed that there was overproduction of IL-6 in rats undergoing ovariectomy, and that the rapid bone loss associated with the estrogen withdrawal state could be ablated by neutralizing antibodies to estrogen, as well as by sex steroids, such as estrogen and, in male rats, testosterone. These data have received a lot of attention, and they may have considerable significance as far as the estrogen withdrawal state is concerned.

IL-6 is also likely to be important in bone loss associated with several other pathological situations. Many solid tumors express IL-6, and some of the paraneoplastic syndromes associated with IL-6 in these tumors can be ablated by neutralizing IL-6 passively in neutralizing antibodies, by inoculation of the neutralizing antibodies (38). Similarly, IL-6 has been implicated in the bone loss associated with myeloma (39). Patients with severe myeloma, such as plasma-cell leukemia, have increased circulating concentrations of IL-6, and, in several patients, neutralization of IL-6 resulted in a change not only in the disease state but also in the treatment of the hypercalcemia.

Monocyte-macrophage colony-stimulating factor

M-CSF is clearly important for osteoclast formation, particularly during the neonatal period. This relationship has been demonstrated in an experiment of nature, the op/op form of murine osteopetrosis. In this type of osteopetrosis, there is defective formation of normal osteoclasts during the mouse neonatal period, and osteopetrosis develops (40). The disease can be cured by injections with recombinant M-CSF. There is deficient production of M-CSF by stromal cells due to a defect in the coding region for the M-CSF gene (40,41). As a result, precursors for the osteoclast lineage cannot respond to M-CSF, and there is impaired osteoclast formation. In vitro findings are consistent with these in vivo findings (42). M-CSF enhances the formation of cells with the osteoclast phenotype from precursors present in the human bone marrow (43).

M-CSF exerts its effects on a receptor tyrosine kinase, the normal counterpart of the fms proto-oncogene (44). This receptor is expressed on cells in the osteoclast lineage. The associations between this tyrosine kinase and other tyrosine kinases important in osteoclastic bone resorption, such as src tyrosine kinase, remain unknown.

Interferon-γ

Interferon-γ (IFN-γ) inhibits osteoclastic bone resorption in vitro (20). It also inhibits the formation of osteoclasts from their precursors (45). It probably exerts effects both on proliferation and on differentiation, but its major effects may be on differentiation. This is a different response to IFN-γ than that seen in other systems. In most other systems, IFN-γ seems to synergize with the effects of cytokines such as IL-1 and TNFs and it exerts its major effects on proliferation. With respect to osteoclasts, IFN-γ appears to oppose the effects of IL-1 and TNF, and it has its major effects on differentiation rather than on cell proliferation.

Whether IFN-γ exerts important effects in vivo on osteoclast formation remains unknown. In our hands, it appears to have effects in vivo only at toxic doses.

Interleukin-4

Another cytokine that appears to be an inhibitor of osteoclast formation and osteoclastic bone resorption is IL-4 (46). This is also a pleiotropic cytokine that has multiple effects on many systems. A recent report suggests that IL-4 may also stimulate cells with the osteoblast phenotype to form bone nodules (47). A form of bone loss or osteopenia likened to postmenopausal osteoporosis (48) has been shown to develop in transgenic mice over-expressing IL-4. As with IFN-γ, the precise role of IL-4 and the control of normal bone resorption remains to be determined.

Leukemia inhibitory factor

Leukemia inhibitory factor (LIF) is expressed by osteoblasts, and it stimulates osteoclastic bone resorption in organ culture (49,50). It has characteristics in common with those of IL-6, including some homology at the amino acid level. However, its effects on bone resorption appear to be different from those of IL-6. Its precise role in the control of normal osteoclastic bone resorption remains to be determined.

IMPLICATION FOR THE ROLE OF CYTOKINES IN DISEASE STATES

The expanding list of cytokines has led to these factors being implicated in a number of disease states, particularly in those diseases associated with localized bone loss. In most cases, evidence is based on knowledge of their effects on target cells, as well as the discovery that they are produced in sufficient amounts in those diseases to account for the localized osteolysis. For example, in patients with rheumatoid arthritis and in periodontal disease, collections of chronic inflammatory cells occur in inflamed synovia or gingiva, respectively, and osteoclasts are stimulated in adjacent bone and bone destruction occurs. In these circumstances, it appears very likely that peptide cytokines, such as IL-1, TNF, lymphotoxin, and IL-6, as well as arachidonic acid metabolites, such as prostaglandins of the E series and the leukotrienes, are responsible. There is now a body of literature that indicates all of these factors are produced by these chronic inflammatory infiltrates.

Cytokines have also been associated with bone destruction associated with neoplastic cells. There have been two different types of phenomena demonstrated. Some tumor cells have been shown to express bone-resorbing cytokines directly (24,38). This effect is true for both hematological malignancies as well as for solid tumors. Among the hematological malignancies, human and animal myeloma cells have been shown to express the cytokines lymphotoxin and IL-6, and there is evidence to suggest that both cytokines may be important in the bone destruction and hypercalcemia common in this disease.

Established cell lines derived from patients with myeloma express lymphotoxin, and the bone-resorbing activity produced by these cell lines in vitro can be inhibited by neutralizing antibodies to lymphotoxin (24). Patients with myeloma have increased circulating levels of IL-6, and antibodies to IL-6 have been shown to reduce serum calcium levels in these patients (24,39). In solid tumors, cytokines such as IL-1α and IL-6 may be produced by the tumor cells directly. This process has been demonstrated for a number of human squamous-cell carcinomas (51–53). These factors may act alone or in conjunction with other cytokines or circulating factors, such as the parathyroid hormone-related protein, to cause hypercalcemia (53). However, there is another important mechanism by which cytokines may influence bone cell behavior and calcium homeostasis in patients with solid tumors.

The cytokines may be produced not by the tumor cells, but rather by normal host cells stimulated by the presence of the tumor. This effect has been clearly documented in several animal and human tumors (26–29). The most convincing demonstration is a human squamous-cell carcinoma of the maxilla associated with hypercalcemia, in which TNF was shown to be produced by immune cells in response to tumor products (26,27). In this particular tumor, hypercalcemia developed in nude mice carrying the human tumor, and hypercalcemia was reduced following splenectomy. (The spleen contains the majority of immune cells in nude mice.) There were no neoplastic cells in the spleen. These animals had high circulating levels of TNF, which were reduced when the spleen was removed, and the hypercalcemia was reduced by treatment of the animals with neutralizing antibodies to TNF. The tumor cells did not express TNF. In these studies, one of the interesting facets is the mechanism by which the tumor cells stimulate host cells to release bone-resorbing cytokines, such as TNF. Cell-to-cell contact may be involved, but there is also clearly evidence for the production of soluble mediators by the tumor cells. These mediators include GM-CSF (28,29), as well as other peptide growth factors (26,27).

The potential role of cytokines in the bone loss associated with estrogen withdrawal is discussed. It has recently been shown that TGF-β expression by bone cells is decreased following ovariectomy in rats (54).

IMPLICATIONS FOR THE ROLE OF CYTOKINES IN OSTEOPOROSIS

There are several distinct types of abnormalities in bone remodeling that occur in elderly patients with osteoporosis. These abnormalities are in part related to the estrogen withdrawal state that occurs during the decade or so after onset of menopause in women, as well as the aging state. During the postmenopausal period, there is an increase in osteoclastic bone resorption on cancellous bone surfaces that is not balanced by adequate new bone formation. This defect in balance between bone resorption and bone formation can be reversed by therapy with estrogens. The mechanism for the increased osteoclastic bone resorption associated with estrogen withdrawal is highly controversial. Estrogen deficiency leads predominantly to increased thinning and fragmentation of cancellous bone plates, and decreased with the cortical bone due to increased endosteal osteoclastic bone resorption.

The second abnormality in bone remodeling that occurs in osteoporosis has been linked with aging. It is characterized by bone histomorphometrists as a decrease in mean wall thickness, and it is seen predominantly in the Haversian systems of cortical or compact bone. The cellular abnormality is a defect in the capacity of the osteoblasts to repair defects made by previously resorbing osteoclasts. As a consequence, resorption cavities are incompletely filled, and bone is progressively lost. The cortical or compact bone becomes progressively more porous, which is likely to lead to fractures of long bones and particularly fractures of the neck or the femur, which are particularly common following falls in elderly people.

The mechanisms responsible for the abnormalities in bone remodeling that cause these changes remain unknown. Most attention has been given to the estrogen withdrawal status associated with menopause. Recently, estrogen receptors have been detected in osteoclasts, and they have been linked to functional characteristics (55). Thus, it has been shown in vitro that avian osteoclasts have estrogen receptors and that estrogen prevents these osteoclasts from releasing previously incorporated mineral from bone chips.

More attention, however, has been focused on indirect effects of estrogens to regulate bone resorption via regulation of cytokines. In a series of studies, Pacifici and colleagues (30,56) showed that in patients with postmenopausal osteoporosis, circulating monocytes produce increased amounts of the cytokine IL-1 in vitro. The presumption is that these cells represent similar cells adjacent to bone surfaces in these patients, and that increased IL-1 production in the absence of estrogen in these patients leads to the high bone turnover state associated with bone loss. When patients are treated with estrogen, IL-1 production by peripheral blood monocytes in vitro is decreased.

Not all workers have been able to confirm these findings (57). Other cytokines have also been shown to be produced by peripheral blood monocytes under these circumstances. These workers claim that these defects can be inhibited in vivo by the IL-1 receptor antagonist, a cytokine that specifically blocks the effects of IL-1α and IL-1β on bone.

An alternative possibility recently raised by Manolagas and coworkers (58,59) is that the critical cytokine for the bone loss associated with the postmenopausal state may be IL-6. These workers showed that cells of the osteoblast lineage express IL-6, a finding that had been made earlier by a number of workers, including most notably Feyen and associates (60). However, Girasole and colleagues (58) showed that normal and transformed cells with the osteoblast phenotype could be inhibited in vitro by treatment with estrogens. More convincingly, this group performed in vivo experiments in ovariectomized rats (37). In this model, they showed that ovariectomy led to increased production of IL-6, and that the changes in bone resorption that could be demonstrated by bone histomorphometry in ovariectomized rats could be inhibited by treatment of the rats both with estrogens and neutralizing antibodies to IL-6.

It is possible that these mechanisms are not mutually exclusive. For example, a cascade of cytokines associated with bone loss may be released during the estrogen withdrawal state. For example, it is possible that IL-1 is released earlier and IL-6 later, and that they work in concert to stimulate bone resorption.

These findings address the loss of bone associated with the estrogen withdrawal state, but not the loss of bone associated with aging, during which the changes may be much more complex. One possibility recently suggested is that the defect in osteoblast function seen in all elderly individuals, whether male or female, may be related to either decreased production of growth regulatory factors in the bone microenvironment or decreased responsivity of these cells to growth regulatory factors. The latter hypothesis seems less likely. However, it is well known that a number of powerful osteoblast growth regulatory factors are stored in the bone matrix. These factors are released in active form during the bone resorption process, and if aging is associated with either increased storage of these factors in the matrix or decreased storage and release in active form, then this process could account for changes seen during aging. This is obviously an area of potentially fruitful investigation.

REFERENCES

1. Mundy GR, Roodman GD. Osteoclast ontogeny and function. In: Peck WA, ed. Bone and mineral research V. Amsterdam: Elsevier, 1987:209–280.

2. Blair HC, Teitelbaum SL, Ghiselli R, Gluck S. Osteoclastic bone resorption by a polarized vacuolar proton pump. Science 1989;245:855–857.

3. Horton MA, Davies J. Perspectives—adhesion receptors in bone. J Bone Miner Res 1989;4:803–808.

4. Soriano P, Montgomery C, Geske R, Bradley A. Targeted disruption of the c-src proto-oncogene leads to osteopetrosis in mice. Cell 1991;64:693–702.

5. Johnson RS, Spiegelman BM, Papaioannou V. Pleiotropic effects of a null mutation in the c-fos proto-oncogene. Cell 1992;71:577–586.

6. Wiktor-Jedzrejzcak W, Ahmed A, Szczylik C, et al. Hematological characterization of congenital osteopetrosis in op/op mouse. J Exp Med 1982;156:1516–1527.

7. Felix R, Cecchini MG, Fleisch H. Macrophage colony stimulating factor restores in vivo bone resorption in the op/op osteopetrotic mouse. Endocrinology 1990;127:2592–2594.

8. Kodama H, Nose M, Niida S, Yamasaki A. Essential role of macrophage colony-stimulating factor in the osteoclast differentiation supported by stromal cells. J Exp Med 1991;173:1291–1294.

9. Kodama H, Yamasaki A, Nose M, et al. Congenital osteoclast deficiency in osteopetrotic (op/op) mice is cured by injections of macrophage colony stimulating factor. J Exp Med 1991;173:269–272.

10. Hauschka PV, Mavrakos AE, Lafrati MD, Doleman SE, Klagsbrun M. Growth factors in bone matrix. J Biol Chem 1986:261;12665–12674.

11. Bellows CG, Aubin JE, Heersche JN, Antosz ME. Mineralized bone nodules formed in vitro from enzymatically released rat calvaria cell populations. Calcif Tissue Int 1986;38:143–154.

12. Stein GS, Lian JB, Owen TA. Relationship of cell growth to the regulation of tissue-specific gene expression during osteoblast differentiation. FASEB J 1990;4:3111–3123.

13. Boyce BF, Aufdemorte TB, Garrett IR, Yates AJP, Mundy GR. Effects of interleukin-1 on bone turnover in normal mice. Endocrinology 1989;125:1142–1150.

14. Sabatini M, Boyce B, Aufdemorte T, Bonewald L, Mundy GR. Infusions of recombinant human interleukin-1 α and β cause hypercalcemia in normal mice. Proc Natl Acad Sci USA 1988;85:5235–5239.

15. Boyce BF, Yates AJP, Mundy GR. Bolus injections of recombinant human interleukin-1 cause transient hypocalcemia in normal mice. Endocrinology 1989;125:2780–2783.

16. Pfeilschifter J, Chenu C, Bird A, Mundy GR, Roodman GD. Interleukin-1 and tumor necrosis factor stimulate the formation of human osteoclast-like cells in vitro. J Bone Miner Res 1989;4:113–118.

17. Thomson BM, Atkinson SJ, McGarrity AM, Hembry RM, Reynolds JJ, Meikle MC. Type-I collagen degradation by mouse calvarial osteoblasts stimulated with 1,25-dihydroxyvitamin D₃. Evidence for a plasminogen-plasmin-metalloproteinase activation cascade. Biochim Biophys Acta 1989;1014:125–132.

18. Murrills RJ, Stein LS, Dempster DW. Inhibition of bone resorption by interleukin-1 alpha in the bone slice assay. J Bone Miner Res 1991;7(suppl 1):888.

19. Smith D, Gowen M, Mundy GR. Effects of interferon

gamma and other cytokines on collagen synthesis in fetal rat bone cultures. Endocrinology 1987;120:2494–2499.

20. Gowen M, Nedwin G, Mundy GR. Preferential inhibition of cytokine stimulated bone resorption by recombinant interferon gamma. J Bone Miner Res 1986;1:469–474.

21. Johnson RA, Boyce BF, Mundy GR, Roodman GD. Tumors producing human TNF induce hypercalcemia and osteoclastic bone resorption in nude mice. Endocrinology 1989;124:1424–1427.

22. Thomson BM, Mundy GR, Chambers TJ. Tumor necrosis factors alpha and beta induce osteoblastic cells to stimulate osteoclastic bone resorption. J Immunol 1987;138:775–779.

23. Bertolini DR, Nedwin GE, Bringman TS, Smith DD, Mundy GR. Stimulation of bone resorption and inhibition of bone formation in vitro by human tumour necrosis factors. Nature 1986;319:516–518.

24. Garrett IR, Durie BGM, Nedwin GE, et al. Production of the bone resorbing cytokine lymphotoxin by cultured human myeloma cells. N Engl J Med 1987;317:526–532.

25. Oliff A, Defea-Jones D, Boyer M, et al. Tumors secreting human TNF/cachectin induce cachexia in mice. Cell 1987; 50:555–563.

26. Yoneda T, Alsina MM, Chavez JB, Bonewald L, Nishimura R, Mundy GR. Evidence that tumor necrosis factor plays a pathogenetic role in the paraneoplastic syndromes of cachexia, hypercalcemia, and leukocytosis in a human tumor in nude mice. J Clin Invest 1991;87:977–985.

27. Yoneda Y, Aufdemorte TB, Nishimura R, et al. Occurrence of hypercalcemia and leukocytosis with cachexia in a human squamous cell carcinoma of the maxilla in athymic nude mice. A novel experimental model of three concomitant paraneoplastic syndromes. J Clin Oncol 1991;9:468–477.

28. Sabatini M, Chavez J, Mundy GR, Bonewald LF. Stimulation of tumor necrosis factor release from monocytic cells by the A375 human melanoma via granulocyte-macrophage colony stimulating factor. Cancer Res 1990;50: 2673–2678.

29. Sabatini M, Yates AJ, Garrett R, et al. Increased production of tumor necrosis factor by normal immune cells in a model of the humoral hypercalcemia of malignancy. Lab Invest 1990;63:676–681.

30. Pacifici R, Rifas L, McCracken R, et al. Ovarian steroid treatment blocks a postmenopausal increase in blood monocyte interleukin-1 release. Proc Natl Acad Sci USA 1989;86:2398–2402.

31. Black K, Garret IR, Mundy GR. Chinese hamster ovarian cells transfected with the murine interleukin-6 gene cause hypercalcemia as well as cachexia, leukocytosis and thrombocytosis in tumor-bearing nude mice. Endocrinology 1991;128:2657–2659.

32. Ishimi Y, Miyaura C, Jin CH, et al. IL-6 is produced by osteoblasts and induces bone resorption. J Immunol 1990; 145:3297.

33. Ohsaki Y, Scarcez T, Demulder A, Nishihara T, Williams R, Roodman GD. Evidence for an autocrine/paracrine role for IL-6 in bone resorption by giant cell tumors of bone. Endocrinology 1992;131:2229–2234.

34. Reddy SK, Takahashi S, Dallas M, Williams RE, Neckers L, Roodman GD. Interleukin-6 antisense deoxyoligo-

nucleotides inhibit bone resorption by giant cells from human giant cell tumors of bone, J Bone Miner Res 1994; 9:753–757.

35. Kurihara N, Bertolini D, Suda T, Akiyama Y, Roodman GD. Interleukin-6 stimulates osteoclast-like multinucleated cell formation in long-term human marrow cultures by inducing IL-1 release. J Immunol 1990;144:426–430.

36. Girasole G, Jilka RL, Passeri G, et al. 17β-estradiol inhibits interleukin-6 production by bone marrow derived stromal cells and osteoblasts in vitro. A potential mechanism for the antiosteoporotic effect of estrogens. J Clin Invest 1992; 89:883–891.

37. Jilka RL, Hangoc G, Girasole G, et al. Increased osteoclast development after estrogen loss-mediation by interleukin-6. Science 1992;257:88–91.

38. Yoneda T, Nakai M, Moriyama K, et al. Neutralizing antibodies to human interleukin-6 reverse hypercalcemia associated with a human squamous carcinoma. Cancer Res 1993;53:737–740.

39. Klein B, Bataille R. Recent advantages in the biology of IL-6 in multiple myeloma. Cancer J 1991;4:81–82.

40. Wiktor-Jedrzejczak W, Bartocci A, Ferrante AWJ, et al. Total absence of colony-stimulating factor 1 in the macrophage-deficient osteopetrotic (op/op) mouse. Proc Natl Acad Sci USA 1990;87:4828–4832.

41. Yoshida H, Hayashi SI, Kunisada T, et al. The murine mutation osteopetrosis is in the coding region of the macrophage colony stimulating factor gene. Nature 1990;345: 442–444.

42. Takahashi N, Udagawa N, Akatsu T, Tanaka H, Isogai Y, Suda T. Deficiency of osteoclasts in osteopetrotic mice is due to a defect in the local micro-environment provided by osteoblastic cells. Endocrinology 1991;128:1792–1796.

43. MacDonald BR, Mundy GR, Clark S, et al. Effects of human recombinant CSF-GM and highly purified CSF-1 on the formation of multinucleated cells with osteoclast characteristics in long term bone marrow cultures. J Bone Miner Res 1986;1:227–233.

44. Sherr CJ, Rettenmier W, Sacca R, Roussel MF, Look AT, Stanley ER. The c-fms proto-oncogene product is related to the receptor for the mononuclear phagocyte growth factor, CSF-1. Cell 1985;41:665–676.

45. Takahashi N, Mundy GR, Kuehl TJ, Roodman GD. Osteoclast like formation in fetal and newborn long term baboon marrow cultures is more sensitive to 1,25-dihydroxyvitamin D$_3$ than adult long term marrow cultures. J. Bone Miner Res 1987;2:311–317.

46. Lewis DB, Liggitt HD, Effmann EL, et al. Osteoporosis induced in mice by overproduction of interleukin 4. Proc Natl Acad Sci USA 1993;90:11618–11622.

47. Ueno K, Katayama T, Miyamoto T, Koshihara Y. Interleukin-4 enhances in vitro mineralization in human osteoblast-like cells. Biochem Biophys Res Commun 1992;189: 1521–1526.

48. Lewis DB, Liggit D, Teitelbaum S, Perlmutter R. Mechanism of osteoporosis in IL-4 transgenic mice. J Bone Miner Res 1992;7(suppl 1):20.

49. Abe E, Tanaka H, Ishimi Y, et al. Differentiation-inducing factor purified from conditioned medium of nitrogen-treated spleen cell cultures stimulates bone resorption. Proc Natl Acad Sci USA 1986;83:5958–5962.

50. Lowe C, Cornish J, Martin TJ, Reid IR. Effects of leukemia inhibitory factor on bone resorption and DNA synthesis in neonatal mouse calvaria. Calcif Tissue Int 1991;49:394–397.

51. Fried RM, Voelkel EF, Rich RH, Levine L, Tashjian AH. Evidence for multiple bone resorption-stimulating factors produced by normal human keratinocytes in culture. Endocrinology 1988;122:2467–2475.

52. Fried RM, Voelkel EF, Rice RH, Levine L, Gaffney EV, Tashjian AH. Two squamous cell carcinomas not associated with humoral hypercalcemia produce a potent bone resorption-stimulating factor which is interleukin-1 alpha. Endocrinology 1989;125:742–751.

53. Sato K, Fujii Y, Kasono K, et al. Parathyroid hormone related protein and interleukin-1 alpha synergistically stimulate bone resorption in vitro and increase the serum calcium concentration in mice in vivo. Endocrinology 1989;124:2172–2178.

54. Finkelman RD, Bell NH, Strong DD, Demers LM, Baylink DJ. Ovariectomy selectively reduces the concentration of transforming growth factor β in rat bone: implications for estrogen deficiency-associated bone loss. Proc Natl Acad Sci USA 1992;89:12190–12193.

55. Oursler MJ, Osdoby P, Pyfferoen J, Riggs BL, Spelsberg TC. Avian osteoclasts as estrogen target cells. Proc Natl Acad Sci USA 1991;88:6613–6617.

56. Pacifici R, Rifas L, Teitelbaum S, et al. Spontaneous release of interleukin-1 from human blood monocytes reflects bone formation in idiopathic osteoporosis. Proc Natl Acad Sci USA 1987;84:4616–4620.

57. Zarrabeitia MT, Riancho JA, Amado JA, Napal J, Gonzalez-Macias J. Cytokine production by peripheral blood cells in postmenopausal osteoporosis. Bone Miner 1991;14:161–167.

58. Girasole G, Jilka RL, Passeri G, et al. 17β estradiol inhibits interleukin-6 production by bone marrow derived stromal cells and osteoblasts in vitro—a potential mechanism for the antiosteoporotic effect of estrogens. J Clin Invest 1992;89:883–891.

59. Manolagas SC, Jilka RL. Cytokines, hematopoiesis, osteoclastogenesis, and estrogens. Calcif Tissue Int 1992;50:199–202.

60. Feyen JHM, Elford P, Dipadova FE, Trechsel U. Interleukin-6 is produced by bone and modulated by parathyroid hormone. J Bone Miner Res 1989;4:633–638.

CHAPTER 18

ROLE OF CYTOKINES
IN HYPOTHALAMIC-PITUITARY FUNCTIONS

Samuel M. McCann, Sharada Karanth, Amrita Kamat, W. Les Dees,
Krzysztof Lyson, Martha Gimeno, and Valeria Rettori

The pattern of release of pituitary hormones in infection is probably brought about by cytokine-induced release of hypothalamic peptides that alter the release of pituitary hormones. Furthermore, direct actions of these cytokines on the pituitary gland can alter pituitary hormone release and responsiveness of the gland to hypothalamic peptides (1).

In this brief review, the means by which cytokines reach the hypothalamus is considered first. Then, the responses to various cytokines are characterized and compared. Their mechanisms of action at both the hypothalamic and the pituitary level are discussed. Finally, the means by which the action of the cytokines can be suppressed is described. Evidence is mounting that excessive production of cytokines can be very harmful, for example, in toxic shock, during which secretion of cachectin is principally involved, and also in central nervous system (CNS) infections, such as acquired immunodeficiency syndrome (AIDS), during which production of cytokines within the brain may be responsible for the neuropathological changes that bring about the signs and symptoms of CNS AIDS.

PENETRATION OF CYTOKINES
TO THE HYPOTHALAMUS
AND THE PITUITARY GLAND

Introduction of bacteria into the body causes liberation of toxic soluble products of the bacterial cell wall, for example, bacterial lipopolysaccharide (LPS), which circulates in the blood and acts on immune cells, particularly monocytes and macrophages. LPS combines with its receptors on these cells and induces synthesis and release of various cytokines, such as interleukin-1 (IL-1), cachectin, IL-6, IL-2, interferon-γ (IFN-γ), and others. The pattern of release probably depends on the infective agent and the severity of the infection (2).

Because there is no arterial blood supply to the anterior pituitary gland, cytokines released into the circulation reach the hypophyseal portal capillaries in the median eminence (ME) of the tuber cinereum only via the anterior hypophysial arteries (3). Cytokines (molecular weight, 15 kd) diffuse into the ME because there is little or no blood-brain barrier there. Therefore, the concentration of cytokines delivered to the anterior lobe sinusoids by the hypophyseal portal veins will be less than in arterial blood. The concentration of cytokines in blood reaching the anterior lobe via the short portal vessels is similarly reduced by their diffusion into neural lobe tissue. One third the blood supply of the anterior lobe is provided by these vessels (3).

Transport of cytokines to the hypothalamus presents a more difficult problem except in regions where the blood-brain barrier is defective, in the ME, and in other circumventricular organs: the organum vasculosum lamina terminalis, the subfornical organ, the subcommisural organ, the area postrema, and the pineal gland (4–7). Also, permeability is probably enhanced in the choroid plexus. Banks and Kastin (8) even reported a transport system that carries IL-1 into the brain. Clearly, peripherally injected cytokines effectively reach the brain, because IL-1 injected intravenously can induce fever and increase adrenocorticotrophic hormone (ACTH) secretion by hypothalamic action.

Evidence is mounting for the production of various cytokines also by glial elements within the brain, particularly IL-1, IL-2, and IL-6, and perhaps others (9). Bacterial LPS appears to be capable of increasing the production of cytokines, such as IL-6, within glial elements (10).

In addition, a neuronal system that produces IL-1β has been described in humans (11). The cell bodies of these neurons are located particularly in the paraventricular nucleus, with axons projecting to the ME; therefore, IL-1β released from these neurons could reach the anterior lobe and even the peripheral circulation after uptake by portal vessels.

We discovered an IL-1α–immunoreactive neuronal system with cell bodies in the dorsolateral preoptic area and the anterior hypothalamus and relatively short axons that could not be traced to the ME. Intravenous injection of LPS led to a dramatic increase in the number of these immunostained neurons, suggesting that LPS induced the synthesis of IL-1α in these neurons (12). Therefore, it is apparent that cytokines can act on the hypothalamus following their delivery via the vascular system or after local production by glial and neuronal elements, and that cytokine production in these cells may be enhanced by LPS.

IL-1 RECEPTORS IN THE BRAIN

Several groups have found IL-1 receptors in the brain and the pituitary gland; however, the number of receptors in the hypothalamus appears to be low (13,14). Possibly, this finding is another example of the so called receptor mismatch, in which receptor numbers are higher in areas where the transmitter is not produced and lower near the areas of production. This process may represent downregulation of receptors in response to release of the endogenous transmitter. It appears that IL-1α and IL-1β utilize the same receptors (13,14). However, there have been reports of differences in potency of the two forms of IL-1 (15); whether these differences are real or are related to the purity and the species from which the cytokine tested was derived has not yet been determined.

PRODUCTION OF CYTOKINES IN THE ANTERIOR PITUITARY GLAND

Evidence that IL-6 is produced in the anterior pituitary gland is quite convincing. Production of the cytokine is increased by in vitro exposure of the gland to LPS (10). The site of origin appears to be folliculostellate cells (16), a cell type known for a long time, but its function is obscure. These cells appear to be modified macrophages; it would therefore not be surprising if they also produced other cytokines.

CHARACTERIZATION OF THE EFFECTS OF CYTOKINES ON THE HYPOTHALAMUS

IL-1

IL-1 was the first cytokine synthesized (17). Recombinant human IL-1α and IL-1β are available. Intravenous (IV) or intraperitoneal (IP) administration of IL-1 increases plasma ACTH levels in the rat (18,19). This release is at least in part caused by secretion of corticotropin-releasing hormone (CRH) into the hypophyseal portal vessels, because there is an increase of CRH levels in portal blood following injection of IL-1 (19). It is apparent that vasopressin is also released by IL-1 (19), and it is at least partially responsible for the ensuing ACTH release. Both peptides can directly stimulate release of ACTH from the pituitary gland, and vasopressin potentiates CRH-induced ACTH release (20). Antisera directed against CRH block the response to systemic administration of IL-1, again indicating the importance of CRH to the response (21). Not only does IL-1β stimulate release of CRH, but it also increases the messenger RNA for CRH in the paraventricular nucleus, as determined from in situ hybridization studies (15), which suggests that IL-1β increases synthesis as well as release of CRH.

In conscious rats, an increase in plasma growth hormone (GH) and prolactin (PRL), an elevation in body temperature, and a decrease in plasma thyrotropin-secreting hormone (TSH) concentrations occurred within 15 minutes after third ventricular (3V) administration of 0.3 pmol IL-1. However, the responses were not observed when a higher dose (1.5 pmol) was given (22), although a higher fever was observed. This was the first example of a bell-shaped dose-response curve frequently seen following in vivo administration of cytokines. IL-1β stimulated CRH release in vitro from medial hypothalamic fragments with a minimal effective concentration of 10^{-14}mol/L, but, as in the in vivo experiments cited, there was a bell-shaped dose-response relationship (23). Because IL-1 incubated with hypothalami in vitro releases prostaglandin E_2 (PGE$_2$), but not PGF$_{1\alpha}$, at a lower (10^{-14}mol/L) but not a higher concentration (10^{-11}mol/L) (Rettori V, et al., unpublished observations), we hypothesize that this decreased effect of higher doses on prostaglandin release may be involved in the bell-shaped dose-response curve because PGE$_2$ stimulates CRH release in vitro (23).

The 3V injection of as little as 0.06 pmol recombinant human IL-1α suppressed pulsatile luteinizing hormone (LH) but not follicle-stimulating hormone (FSH) release in conscious, castrate male rats. LH pulses ceased completely, but with a different latency among the rats; all animals had stopped pulsing by 1 hour, and there were no pulses during the second hour after 3V injection (24). IL-1β was also active in this regard following lateral cerebroventricular administration of the monokine (15).

In sharp contrast, pulsatile release of FSH was barely altered; the only change was a borderline significant increase in the height of the FSH pulses (24). We postulated that IL-1 selectively blocked pulsatile release of LH but not FSH. This hypothesis supports our previous observations indicating separate hypothalamic control of LH and FSH (i.e., LH is controlled by LH-releasing hormone and FSH is controlled by FSH-releasing factor) (24). Intraventricular injection of IL-1 has also been found to block the proestrous release of LH (25).

Tumor necrosis factor (cachectin)

The pattern of change in pituitary hormone secretion after 3V injection of tumor necrosis factor-α (TNF-α) into conscious male rats was similar to that observed with IL-1: It stimulated ACTH, PRL, and GH secretion, and it inhibited secretion of TSH, the latter only after a 2-hour delay (26). Although the minimal effective dose (MED) of TNF that elevated body temperature was less than that of IL-1, the maximal increase (1–1.5°C) was much less than that obtained with IL-1 (3.4°C). The cytokine was also much less potent than IL-1 with respect to effects on hormone secretion, because ACTH and GH release were only increased with the largest dose evaluated (6 pmol), whereas in the prior experiments, IL-1 (0.3 pmol) stimulated PRL and GH release. However, in the case of TNF-α, we did not observe the absence of the response with higher doses observed with IL-1, perhaps because we did not administer an adequate amount of the cytokine. Thus, cachectin can produce the same pattern of pituitary hormone release, but, unlike IL-1, it is much less potent on a molar basis.

Interleukin-6

Following 3V injection into conscious, castrate male rats, IL-6 elevated body temperature accompanied by an increase in plasma ACTH levels within 15 minutes; TSH levels were significantly reduced, but PRL and GH levels were not changed. Plasma gonadotropin levels were also unaltered by these doses of IL-6 in castrate males, a result dissimilar from that obtained with IL-1. The effects on

rectal temperature and hormone release were directly related to the doses of monokine injected with an MED of 1.5 pmol, which is essentially five times the MED for IL-1α. The pattern of hormonal responses was similar, in part, to those obtained with IL-1 and cachectin, except that there was no effect on PRL or GH levels. There was also no effect on LH levels, which was not evaluated with regard to cachectin (27).

IL-6 increased CRH release from medial hypothalamic tissue, including the ME, with an MED of 10^{-13}mol/L (23). As with IL-1, the effect was not observed with higher concentrations of IL-6 (10^{-12}mol/L). Therefore, it is likely that the increase in plasma ACTH levels observed following 3V injection of IL-6 was caused by CRH release, which in turn stimulated the release of ACTH by the corticotrophs. Navarra and associates (28) also observed the stimulatory effect of 10^{-13}mol/L IL-6; however, they did not increase the dose further, so it is not clear whether they would have also observed a bell-shaped dose-response curve.

IL-2

IL-2 is secreted by T lymphocytes. Following 3V injection into conscious rats, it stimulated ACTH, PRL, and TSH release, but it inhibited FSH, LH, and GH release (Karanth S, McCann SM, unpublished observations). That these actions were mediated at least in part by direct effects on the hypothalamus is supported by the fact that IL-2 stimulated CRH release from medial hypothalamic fragments incubated in vitro at doses of 10^{-13}mol/L (29). At the same concentration, it inhibited the release of luteinizing hormone-releasing hormone (LHRH) (Karanth S, et al., unpublished observations). Furthermore, it stimulated the release of somatostatin, and it blocked dopamine-induced growth releasing hormone (GRH) release, which might account for its ability to inhibit GH release (30). Thus, IL-2 administered centrally induced a somewhat different pattern of response than the other cytokines because it stimulated instead of inhibited TSH release, and it also inhibited GH release, which was stimulated by low doses of IL-1 and cachectin. As with IL-1, IL-2 inhibited LH release, but it also inhibited FSH release. Thus, this cytokine has powerful actions at the hypothalamic level to alter pituitary hormone release.

Interferon-γ

The 3V injection of 0.3 pmol IFN-γ stimulated ACTH release, accompanied by delayed inhibition of GH and TSH release; it had no effect on PRL release. Similar to IL-1, there was no effect when the dose was increased to 1.5 pmol. Thus, like IL-1, IFN-γ exhibited a bell-shaped dose-response relationship following in vivo injection.

However, this cytokine had little effect on body temperature, which rules out the argument that the lack of response of pituitary hormones at high doses of cytokines in vivo could be due to further elevation of body temperature (31). In fact, because we have found similar bell-shaped dose-response curves from incubation with hypothalamic fragments in vitro, it appears that the mechanism is probably related to the ability of low but not high doses of cytokines to stimulate the release of prostaglandins, as mentioned earlier.

IFN-γ also stimulated the release of somatostatin from medial basal hypothalami (MBH) incubated in vitro at concentrations of 10^{-8} and 10^{-9}mol/L, supporting its ability to inhibit GH release in vivo, presumably by stimulating the release of somatostatin. Higher concentrations resulted in loss of the stimulatory action on somatostatin release, again reproducing the bell-shaped dose-response curve (32).

Thymosin-α₁

Central administration of thymosin-α_1 (Tα_1), the first thymic peptide synthesized, produced a dose-related decrease in plasma TSH and ACTH levels, a decrease in PRL levels, but no significant change in plasma GH concentrations (33). The decreases in ACTH and TSH levels were caused by decreased release of CRH and TRH because in vitro incubation of MBH revealed that Tα_1 suppressed release of these neuropeptides (34).

In many previous instances, we have found that a peptide will influence the release of another hypothalamic peptide, but in most instances, these actions are mediated via interneurons. To test this hypothesis, we incubated hypothalami in the presence of metergoline, a blocker of serotonin receptors. Metergoline blocked the decrease of TSH release induced by serotonin, and it reversed the Tα_1-induced inhibition of TRH release, indicating that a serotoninergic receptor was probably involved in the pathway of inhibition of TRH by Tα_1 (34). The hypotha-

lamic actions of these various cytokines are summarized in Table 18–1.

ACTIONS OF CYTOKINES DIRECTLY ON THE ANTERIOR PITUITARY GLAND

IL-1

The possible direct action of IL-1 on the pituitary gland is controversial. It was first reported that IL-1 releases ACTH from AT-10 tumor cells, which consist of modified corticotrophs (35). It was then reported that IL-1 releases ACTH and other pituitary hormones from perfused pieces of pituitary glands (36); however, it was found to be ineffective in altering ACTH release from 4-day monolayer, cultured pituitary cells (18,37,38).

We found actions on the pituitary gland for the other cytokines; however, it required a period of 1 to 2 hours for these actions to become manifest, and they have been much easier to observe in hemipituitaries than in overnight-cultured, dispersed cells (39). Therefore, we believe that the actions of IL-1 directly on the pituitary will ultimately be clearly established. The failure to find these actions in monolayer-cultured, dispersed cells may be due to the loss of paracrine actions on adjacent pituitary cells of different cell type from that of the hormones released, or it may be related to down-regulation of IL-1 receptors on pituitary cells during long-term (4 days) culture in the absence of the ligand.

Cachectin

After at least 1 hour of incubation, cachectin was capable of stimulating the release of ACTH, GH, TSH and PRL (minimally) from either overnight-cultured, dispersed pi-

TABLE 18–1   ACTIONS OF CYTOKINES ON THE HYPOTHALAMIC-PITUITARY UNIT

Cytokine	Fever	ACTH	PRL	LH	FSH	GH	TSH
IL-1	+	+	+	−	0	+	−
TNF*	+	+	+	?	?	+	−
INF-γ	+	+	0	?	?	−	−
IL-6	+	+	0	0	0	−	−
IL-2	?	+	+	−	−	−	+
Tα₁	+	−	−	+†	0	0	−

*TNF = cachectin.
† In vitro on hemipituitaries.

tuitary cells or hemipituitaries (39); however, the MED for these actions of cachectin was 100-fold greater with dispersed cells than with hemipituitaries. As indicated, we speculate that this decreased sensitivity in the dispersed cell preparation is due either to loss of receptors or to some paracrine actions of various pituitary cells to augment the effects on other pituitary cells in the hemipituitary preparation. There was a bell-shaped dose-response curve of the pituitaries, and the MED (10^{-12}mol/L) for the hemipituitaries is within the concentrations that might be encountered in vivo in infection. Consequently, we concluded that cachectin may have an important role in altering pituitary hormone release by direct actions on the gland in infection; however, because of the relatively slow onset of these actions, it is likely that the acute response to infection is brought about by alterations in the release of hypothalamic releasing and inhibiting hormones, which then affect the gland. During more chronic infection, the actions at the pituitary would modulate effects on release of the hypothalamic peptides.

IL-6

Incubation of IL-6 with hemipituitaries in vitro for at least 2 hours increased the release of ACTH and GH into the culture medium at the single concentration of 10^{-13}mol/L. Concentrations of 10^{-14} or 10^{-12}mol/L were ineffective. Again, there was a bell-shaped dose-response curve; abolition of the actions occurred at higher doses (23). Using 4-day monolayer cultured cells, Spangelo and colleagues (10) found not only an IL-6–induced increase in GH release, but also an increase in PRL release. These differences from our results may be accounted for by the different preparations of IL-6 used, or, perhaps more likely, by their use of the dispersed cell system. This system may result in up-regulation or down-regulation of receptors for IL-6 in the relative absence of endogenous ligand, as well as loss of paracrine actions because of separation of the cells.

Because IL-6 is clearly produced by the pituitary gland, and because IL-6 is increased by LPS (40), it is quite likely that IL-6 has important direct actions on the pituitary to modify pituitary hormone release. These actions probably modulate the effects of hypothalamic hormones on the release of pituitary hormones, as mentioned.

Therefore, the effect of IL-6 released from the hypothalamus and the pituitary, as well as IL-6 reaching the gland after release in the periphery during infection, would be the result of its actions at both the hypothalamic and the pituitary levels: induction of stimulation of ACTH and GH, and a decrease in TSH release in acute situations in vivo.

We have not investigated chronic exposure to IL-6. It is quite likely that there might be other effects, perhaps similar to those that occur in infection, with chronic exposure to this interleukin. Indeed, we can characterize the acute effects of most of the cytokines at hypothalamic and pituitary sites over a short period of 1 or 2 hours; however, much more research should be done to characterize the effects of more prolonged exposure of both the hypothalamus and the pituitary gland to these substances.

IL-2

IL-2 is the most potent agent known to act directly on the pituitary gland to alter pituitary hormone release. At concentrations of 10^{-15}mol/L, it elevated PRL and TSH release and inhibited release of FSH, LH, and GH from hemipituitaries in vitro. ACTH release was induced with a higher concentration (10^{-12}mol/L). After reaching the minimal effective stimulatory or inhibitory concentration, the dose-response curve was flat, but at much higher concentrations (10^{-9} or 10^{-8}mol/L), responses tended to diminish to insignificant values. Again, bell-shaped dose-response curves were obtained, similar to those observed with other cytokines (41).

IFN-γ

Incubation of IFN-γ with hemipituitaries in vitro revealed no effect on the release of PRL, TSH, and GH, but there was stimulation of ACTH release only at the relatively high concentration of 10^{-8}mol/L. Later studies revealed that at a concentration of 10^{-12}mol/L, IFN-γ also decreased release of GH from pituitaries incubated in vitro (42). At much higher concentrations (10^{-8}mol/L), INF-γ potentiated GH release induced by GRH, but it had no direct effect by itself. Because this is a 10,000-fold increase in dose over that which produced inhibition of release, we question whether it is of pathophysiological significance. This inhibitory action on GH release vanished with higher doses, again producing the bell-shaped dose-response curve.

Tα₁

Tα₁ evoked a dose-dependent release of TSH and ACTH, although there was no effect on the release of PRL and GH from hemipituitaries incubated in vitro (33). There was a remarkable ability of the peptide to stimulate LH release in a dose-related manner at doses as low as 10^{-12}mol/L, whereas FSH release was unaltered (33). Because Tα₁ has been localized to both the hypothalamus and the pituitary, it may have physiological significance in neuroendocrine immunology. As with the other cytokines, both hypothalamic and pituitary sites of action may be important for induction of the changes in pituitary hormone release.

MECHANISM OF ACTION OF CYTOKINES TO ALTER RELEASE OF HYPOTHALAMIC PEPTIDES

It is axiomatic that the actions of the cytokines at hypothalamic and pituitary levels must be mediated after combination with their receptors on particular cell types. We suspect that the mechanism of action may be quite similar for the various cytokines when they evoke a similar action on hypothalamic neurons.

Mechanism of CRH-releasing action of cytokines

The most uniform action of the cytokines is to stimulate CRH release. The exception to this rule is the thymic peptide, $T\alpha_1$, which inhibits CRH release. The mechanism by which IL-2 stimulates CRH release has been studied most extensively. We and others have demonstrated that acetylcholine or carbachol, a cholinergic agonist, stimulates CRH release from hypothalami incubated in vitro (29). The action occurs via muscarinic cholinergic receptors because it can be blocked by atropine. Because the release of CRH induced by IL-2 can be blocked by atropine, it appears that IL-2 acts on its receptors on cholinergic interneurons near the perykaria of CRH neurons in the paraventricular nucleus. The acetylcholine released stimulates a muscarinic-type receptor, which in turn stimulates CRH release from the CRH neuron.

In the periphery, cytokines induce synthesis of nitric oxide synthase (NOS), an enzyme that converts L-arginine into L-citrulline and nitric oxide (NO) (43,44). NO is believed to be responsible for the cytotoxic action of these agents. In addition to this inducible form of NOS, a constitutive form of NOS has been found in vascular endothelium, and its release is stimulated by cholinergic terminals ending on the endothelial cells (43,44). The released NO then acts on vascular smooth muscle to induce vasodilation. Recently, a very similar constitutive form of NOS was located in neurons in the CNS, and it has been shown to have a neurotransmitter role in cerebellum and hippocampal function (45).

We therefore explored the probability that IL-2 and synaptic transmitters might release CRH in vitro via NO (29). L-arginine, the substrate for NOS, was added in varying concentrations to determine whether it would alter basal CRH release or the CRH release induced by IL-2. During a short incubation period (30 minutes) in

Krebs-Ringer bicarbonate glucose buffer, L-arginine had no effect on either basal or IL-2–induced CRH release. However, when the incubation was continued for an additional 30 minutes after changing the medium, arginine significantly elevated both basal and IL-2–induced CRH release, presumably because the endogenous substrate had been depleted during the initial 30 minute incubation period.

N^G-monomethyl-L-arginine (NMMA) is a competitive inhibitor of NOS. It had no effect on basal release of CRH; however, 100 or 300 μmol/L NMMA completely blocked the IL-2–induced release of CRH, as well as that caused by IL-2 plus acetylcholine or carbachol. IL-2 plus carbachol produced an additive effect on CRH release. Thus, the results indicate that IL-2 activates constitutive NOS, leading to increased NO release, which activates CRH release. It appears that NO is also involved in the release of CRH induced by acetylcholine.

In nearly all systems studied, the NO pathway involves several cells. We speculate that IL-2 acts on its receptors on cholinergic neurons to cause the release of acetylcholine because IL-2–induced CRH release is blocked by atropine (Fig. 18–1). The acetylcholine released activates

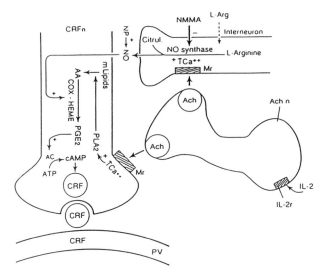

Figure 18–1 The possible interaction of a cholinergic neuron (Achn) with an interneuron and CRF neuronal terminals (CRFn) to generate NO, prostaglandin E_2 (PGE$_2$), cyclic AMP (cAMP), and CRF release. n = neuron; m lipids = membrane phospholipids; AA = arachidonic acid; COX-HEME = cyclo-oxygenase; AC = adenylate cyclase; L-arg = L-arginine; NMMA = N^G-monomethyl L-arginine; ATP = adenosine triphosphate; NP = nitroprusside; citrul = citrulline; Ca^{++} = internal Ca concentration; IL-2R = IL-2 receptor; Mr = muscarinic receptor; PLA$_2$ = phospholipase A$_2$; PV = portal vessel; + = stimulation or increase; − = inhibition or decrease. (Reproduced by permission from Karanth S, Lyson K, McCann SM. Role of nitric oxide in interleukin 2induced corticotropin-releasing factor release from incubated hypothalami. Proc Natl Acad Sci USA 1993;90:3383–3387.)

muscarinic receptors on interneurons, termed *NOergic neurons,* to activate NOS, which causes the release of NO. This NO diffuses to the CRH neuron, and it activates CRH release by its ability to activate the cyclo-oxygenase enzyme (29), leading to the generation of PGE_2. PGE_2 activates CRH via activation of adenylate cyclase and generation of cyclic adenosine monophosphate (AMP). Cyclic AMP activates protein kinase A, which induces exocytosis of CRH secretory granules.

We recently reported that NO activates cyclo-oxygenase in vitro in similar hypothalamic fragments (24). Activation of the constitutive NOS requires an elevation in intracellular calcium levels, which interacts with calmodulin to activate the enzyme. We showed that high potassium concentrations in the medium increases CRH release (Karanth S, et al., unpublished observations), presumably by opening voltage-dependent calcium channels in the NOergic neurons to elevate intracellular calcium levels, thereby leading to activation of NOS and generation of NO. The NO diffuses into the CRH neuron, and it activates cyclo-oxygenase by interaction with the heme group of the enzyme (24). The cholinergic neuron is also believed to act on the CRH neuron via muscarinic receptors to increase free calcium levels in the CRF neuron, thereby leading to activation of phospholipase A_2 (29). This process would cause breakdown of membrane phospholipids to arachidonate to provide substrate for the activated cyclo-oxygenase enzyme, which results in production of PGE_2. It is also possible that there may be activation of other Fe^{2+}-containing enzymes involved in arachidonic acid metabolism, such as lipoxygenase and epoxygenase, because NO possibly activates cyclo-oxygenase via the Fe^{2+} in the heme group present in this enzyme. Our previous studies have shown that indomethacin can block the response to IL-2 (Karanth S, et al., unpublished observations). Indomethacin is an inhibitor of the cyclo-oxygenase enzyme; therefore, this result fits the concept outlined. It is likely that other cytokines that stimulate CRF release, such as IL-1, IL-6, INF-γ, and cachectin, also act via the NO pathway.

Recently, we studied the mechanism by which IL-6 stimulates the release of CRH in vitro. We believe that arachidonic acid metabolites are also involved. Dexamethasone, the synthetic glucocorticoid, may act after combination with the glucocorticoid receptors to inhibit ACTH release by blockade of phospholipase A_2, the enzyme that stimulates synthesis of arachidonic acid. Dexamethasone was capable of blocking the action of IL-6 to increase CRH release from medial basal hypothalamic fragments incubated in vitro at the very low concentration of 10^{-11}mol/L (23).

We then studied the effect of inhibitors of the three pathways of arachidonic acid metabolism, and we found that the most effective inhibitor was clotrimazole, which blocks the epoxygenase enzyme involved in synthesis of epoxides. This agent was effective at a dose of 10^{-9}mol/L, whereas blockade of cyclo-oxygenase by indomethacin (to inhibit prostaglandin synthesis) or lipoxygenase (to inhibit leukotriene synthesis) by 5,8,11-eicosatriynoic acid was much less effective. Therefore, the results suggest that IL-6 stimulates CRH release by activation of the arachidonic acid cascade, and that the most effective compounds activating CRH release are the epoxides (23). Glucocorticoids may inhibit IL-6–induced CRH release by blocking arachidonic acid synthesis.

α-Melanocyte-stimulating hormone (α-MSH), which has important antipyretic (46) and anti-inflammatory actions (47), blocks the release of CRH induced by IL-6 at a concentration of 10^{-13}mol/L, an action shared by ACTH (48). Because the MED for the inhibitory effect of ACTH is 10 to 100 times less than that of α-MSH and α-MSH is ACTH 1–13, the action of α-MSH may be the result of its ability to combine with ACTH receptors.

These actions of ACTH and α-MSH might have therapeutic value by reducing the release of CRH, which has the ability to inhibit immune responses via its stimulation of ACTH release and consequent adrenal cortical steroid release. In this respect, because of the lack of action on the adrenal cortex, α-MSH could be more valuable in suppressing release of cytokines and preventing their peripheral action.

We speculate that the actions of the other cytokines that cause release of CRH are mediated similarly; however, much more work needs to be done to determine whether they all have common mechanisms of action.

Mechanism of action of cytokines to alter LHRH release

We studied the mechanism of the inhibitory action of IL-1α on LHRH release in detail. In vivo, 3V injection of a minute dose of recombinant human IL-1α (0.06 pmol) induced suppression of pulsatile LH release, but not FSH release, suggesting that it blocked the release of LHRH without affecting the release of a putative FSH releasing factor that controls pulsatile FSH release. IL-1α slightly lowered basal release of LHRH when MBH were incubated in vitro, and it completely blocked the norepinephrine (NE) (5×10^{-5}mol/L)-induced release of LHRH. We had previously shown that PGE_2 is critical for LHRH release and that NE releases PGE_2. The action of NE to release PGE_2 was completely blocked by 10^{-11}mol/L IL-1α, whereas the basal release of PGE_2 was unaffected. Therefore, we postulated that IL-1 reacts with its newly discovered receptors in the basal hypothalamus to inhibit the NE-induced release of PGE_2, thereby blocking the release of LHRH (24).

Because constitutive NOS has been located in a large number of neurons in the brain, including neurons in the hypothalamus, we investigated the possible role of NO in the control of LHRH release. Indeed, sodium nitroprusside, which spontaneously releases NO, increased LHRH release by medial basal hypothalamic explants incubated in vitro, and this release was prevented by hemoglobin, which combines with the NO released. The inhibitor of NOS, NMMA, blocked the release of LHRH induced by NE. Neither NMMA nor hemoglobin altered "basal" release of LHRH, indicating that NO had no role in this release (49).

PGE$_2$ release has been shown to be required for LHRH release, and we demonstrated that NO releases PGE$_2$ and that its removal by NMMA or hemoglobin inhibits PGE$_2$ release (24).

The mechanism by which NE operates to control LHRH release is conceptualized to involve three neurons (Fig. 18–2). A NE terminal synapses with a NOergic neuron, and it also makes an axoaxonal synapse on an axon of the LHRH neuron that terminates on a portal capillary. The NE neuron perhaps arises from the locus ceruleus; lesions of the locus ceruleus can block preovulatory and pulsatile release of LH (Franci J, McCann SM, unpublished data). We hypothesize that the NE terminal synapses on the NOergic neuron, and on adjacent LHRH terminals, via α_1-adrenergic receptors. Activation of each of these receptors leads to conversion of inositol phosphates (IPs) into IP3. IP3 activates protein kinase C, which liberates calcium from intracellular stores. In the NOergic neuron, the increased intracellular calcium interacts with calmodulin, and it activates the constitutive NO synthase in this cell, which leads to generation of NO plus citrulline. The NO diffuses across to the axon of the LHRH neuron, and it activates cyclo-oxygenase by interaction with the heme group on the enzyme. We demonstrated the presence of NOergic neurons in proximity to the LHRH neuronal axons (49). The increased calcium levels generated by the α_1 receptor combination with NE on the LHRH axon activates phospholipase A$_2$ to provide arachidonate from hydrolysis of membrane phospholipids. Arachidonate is then converted by activated cyclo-oxygenase to PGE$_2$, which activates adenyl cyclase, leading to an increase in cyclic AMP and activation of protein kinase A, which induces exocytosis of LHRH secretory granules.

We believe that NO acts on the cyclo-oxygenase enzyme rather than by its conventional mechanism (i.e., activation of the soluble guanylate cyclase) (45), because the postulated increase in intracellular calcium levels in the LHRH terminal should inhibit guanylate cyclase. That the cyclo-oxygenase enzyme is activated is indicated by the ability of indomethacin, an inhibitor of cyclo-oxygenase, to block the PGE$_2$ and LHRH release induced by NE (24).

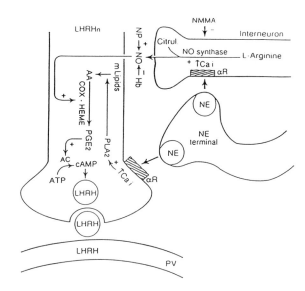

Figure 18–2   Hypothetical interactions of NE terminals with nitric oxidergic interneuron and LHRH terminals to generate nitric oxide, PGE$_2$, cyclic AMP, and LHRH release. n = neuron; m lipids = membrane phospholipids; AA = arachidonic acid; COX-HEME = cyclo-oxygenase; AC = adenylate cyclase; ATP = adenosine triphosphate; NP = nitroprusside; Hb = hemoglobin; citrul = citrulline; Cai = internal calcium ion concentration; alpha R = α_1 adrenergic receptor; PLA$_2$ = phospholipase A$_2$; PV = portal vessel; + = stimulation or increase; – = inhibition or decrease. (Reproduced by permission from Rettori V, Gimeno MF, Karara A, Gonzalez MC, McCann SM. Interleukin 1α inhibits prostaglandin E$_2$ release to suppress pulsatile release of luteinizing hormone but not follicle-stimulating hormone. Proc Natl Acad Sci USA 1991;88:2763–2767.)

We hypothesized that IL-1α blocks release of LHRH in vivo and in vitro by interfering with this pathway of activation of LHRH involving NO (50). Indeed, in vivo experiments showed that intraventricular injection of IL-1 inhibited pulsatile LH but not FSH release in a manner exactly similar to that of the inhibitor of NOS (NMMA), except that blockade was delayed. When the two substances were microinjected into the 3V, they had an additive effect to suppress LH but not FSH release. These results suggest that IL-1 blocks the pathway of LHRH release that involves NO. As indicated, previous in vitro experiments with medial basal hypothalami had shown that IL-1 action was identical to that of NMMA, because it blocked NE-induced PGE$_2$ and LHRH release. Therefore, IL-1α presumably acts on its receptors on either the NOergic neurons or the LHRH terminals to block either the release of NO from the former or the response to NO by the latter neurons.

To test the hypothesis that IL-1α directly inhibits the response of the LHRH terminals to NO, we incubated hypothalamic explants with sodium nitroprusside (NP; 500 μmol/L), which spontaneously releases NO. NP-induced

LHRH release was blocked by IL-1α (10 pmol/L). Therefore, we conclude that IL-1α directly suppresses the response of LHRH terminals to NO. This is one mechanism by which it suppresses LHRH release; however, this finding does not exclude the possibility that it may also suppress other neurons in this pathway. Further experiments are needed to determine this action.

MECHANISM OF ACTION OF CYTOKINES AT THE PITUITARY LEVEL

Little work has been done on the mechanism of action of the various cytokines at the pituitary level. We studied the mechanism by which cachectin (TNF) can alter secretion of pituitary hormones in extenso (39). The data indicate a role of prostaglandins in these effects because indomethacin, an inhibitor of cyclo-oxygenase, completely or partially blocked the effects. Cachectin produced dose-related suppression of cyclic AMP levels in the pituitary gland, and this effect was blocked by somatostatin, which produced a remarkable stimulation of PRL release by TNF (39). This stimulation was possibly caused by the elevation of cyclic AMP levels, which occurred in the presence of both cachectin and somatostatin, because cyclic AMP is a known stimulator of PRL release from the lactotrophs. Much more work needs to be done to characterize the mechanism of these actions, which have a longer latency than those at the hypothalamic level. It will be of interest to see if there is any role for NO in the actions of the cytokines at the pituitary level.

CONCLUSIONS

It is apparent that the stress-response is mimicked by infections and by most immunization procedures that lead to an altered pattern of pituitary hormone secretion. There is increased ACTH secretion, leading to immunosuppressive actions, and there is increased release of PRL and GH, which tends to augment immune responses. The effects of infection are brought about by a complex interplay of monokines and cytokines on hypothalamic neurons that results in altered release of hypothalamic peptides, which in turn alters release of the peptides into the hypophyseal portal vessels to bring about the expected pituitary response.

It appears that all these cytokines have actions at both hypothalamic and pituitary levels; the rapid effects produced by hypothalamic action alter releasing hormone discharge, and the pituitary actions are slower and probably important in responses to more prolonged release of the monokines, as occurs in infection. The pattern of modification of pituitary hormone release varies depending on the cytokine studied, and we are still not sure of the relative importance of the various cytokines.

Following combination with their receptors, it appears cytokine actions are mediated by activation or inhibition of particular hypothalamic neurons. For example, IL-2 stimulation of CRH release is mediated by a cholinergic interneuron that releases acetylcholine to combine with muscarinic receptors on a NOergic neuron and on the CRH neuron to increase internal calcium ion concentrations in each of these neurons. In the NOergic neuron, the increased internal calcium levels combine with calmodulin to activate the constitutive NOS, which causes the release of NO. This NO diffuses to the CRH neuron and activates it. The muscarinic synapse also has elevated internal calcium levels in the CRH neuron, leading to activation of phospholipase A_2 (PLA$_2$), which converts membrane phospholipids to arachidonate. Arachidonate is converted to PGE$_2$ via activation of cyclo-oxygenase by NO, leading to generation of cyclic AMP, activation of protein kinase A, and release of CRH from the CRH terminal. In contrast, the action of IL-1 is opposite on the LHRH neuron: It blocks the NOergic activation of the LHRH terminal by combining with its receptors on the terminal and inhibiting its response to NO.

Arachidonic acid metabolites appear to be involved in the mechanism of action to stimulate hypothalamic hormone release, and, in patients in whom this action is inhibited, the cytokine causes inhibition of the release of these metabolites. The cyclo-oxygenase enzyme is certainly important via PGE$_2$; however, in the case of IL-6, it may be that the epoxygenase enzyme and its products, the epoxides, are more important.

The stimulatory action of IL-1, IL-6, and IL-2 to release CRH can be blocked by the glucocorticoid, dexamethasone, which presumably combines with glucocorticoid receptors on the CRH neuron or other neurons in the pathway of activation to prevent the increase in intracellular free calcium levels necessary for activation of PLA$_2$, generation of arachidonic acid metabolites, and consequent CRH release.

ACTH and α-MSH can also block the action of cytokines to release CRH; ACTH is more potent, presumably because these peptides interact with ACTH rather than α-MSH receptors on the surface of cells in the pathway of activation of CRH, perhaps on the CRH neuron itself. Activation of this receptor prevents elevation of intracellular free calcium levels by the cytokine, thereby preventing, as in the case of dexamethasone, the activation of PLA$_2$ required for conversion of membrane phospholipids into arachidonic acid and subsequent conversion to PGE$_2$ via NO, as well as activation of CRH release. Further studies are needed to determine the precise mechanism of both these inhibitory effects. They may be therapeutically useful in situations of excessive production of cytokines.

ACKNOWLEDGMENTS: This work was supported by National Institutes of Health grants DK10073[(S.M.McC.)], DK43900[(S.M.McC.)], and AA00104[(W.L.D.)]

REFERENCES

1. McCann SM, Rettori V, Milenkovic L, Jurcovicova J, Gonzalez MC. Role of monokines in control of anterior pituitary hormone release. In: Porter JC, Jezova D, eds. Circulating regulatory factors and neuroendocrine function, vol 274. New York: Plenum Press, 1990:315–329.

2. McCann SM, Milenkovic L, Gonzalez MC, Lyson K, Karanth S, Retorri V. Endocrine aspects of neuroimmunomodulation: methods and overview. In: De Souza EB, ed. Neurobiology of cytokines, Part A. Methods in neurosciences. San Diego: Academic Press, 1993:87–210.

3. Porter JC, Sissom JF, Arita J, Reymond MJ. The hypothalamic-hypophysial vasculature and its relationship to secretory cells of the hypothalamus and pituitary gland. Vitam Horm 1983;40:145–174.

4. Hetier E, Ayala J, Denèfle P, Bousseau A, Rouget P, Mallat M, Prochiantz A. Brain macrophages synthesize interleukin-1 and interleukin-1 mRNAs in vitro. J Neurosci Res 1988;21:391–397.

5. Fontana A, McAdam KPWJ, Kristensen F, Weber E. Biological and biochemical characterization of an interleukin 1-like factor from rat C_6 glioma cells. Eur J Immunol 1983; 13:685–689.

6. Stitt JT. Prostaglandin E as the neural mediator of the febrile response. Yale J Biol Med 1986;59:137–149.

7. Katsuura G, Gottschall PE, Dahl RR, Arimura A. Adrenocorticotropin release induced by intracerebroventricular injection of recombinant human interleukin-1 in rats: possible involvement of prostaglandin. Endocrinology 1988; 122:1773–1779.

8. Banks WA, Kastin AJ. Measurement of transport of cytokines across the blood-brain barrier. In: De Souza EB, ed. Neurobiology of cytokines, Part A. Methods in neurosciences. San Diego: Academic Press, 1993:67–77.

9. Koenig JI. Presence of cytokines in the hypothalamo-pituitary axis. Prog Neuroendocrinol Immunol 1991;4:143–153.

10. Spangelo BL, MacLeod RM, Isakson PC. Production of interleukin-6 by anterior pituitary cells in vitro. Endocrinology 1990;126:582–586.

11. Breder CD, Dinarello CA, Saper CB. Interleukin-1 immunoreactive innervation of the human hypothalamus. Science 1988;240:321–324.

12. Rettori V, Dees WL, Hiney JK, Milenkovic L, McCann SM. Interleukin-1 alpha (IL-1α)-immunoreactive neurons in the hypothalamus of the rat are increased after lipopolysaccharide (LPS) injection. Abstracts of the 74th Annual Meeting of the Endocrine Society 1992;534:185.

13. Takao T, Tracey DE, Mitchell WM, De Souza EB. Interleukin-1 receptors in mouse brain: characterization and neuronal localization. Endocrinology 1990;127:3070–3078.

14. Cunningham ET Jr, De Souza EB. Localization of type I interleukin-1 receptor mRNA in brain and endocrine tissues using in situ hybridization histochemistry. In: De Souza EB, ed. Neurobiology of cytokines, Part A. Methods in neurosciences. San Diego: Academic Press, 1993:112–127.

15. Rivier C. Role of endotoxin and interleukin-1 in modulating ACTH, LH and sex steroid secretion. In: Porter JC, Jezova D, eds. Circulating regulatory factors and neuroendocrine function, vol 274. New York: Plenum Press, 1990: 295–301.

16. Vankelecom H, Carmeliet P, Van Damme J, Billiau A, Denef C. Production of interleukin-6 by folliculo-stellate cells of the anterior pituitary gland in a histiotypic cell aggregate culture system. Neuroendocrinology 1989;49:102–106.

17. Duff GW, Durum SK. Fever and immunoregulation: hyperthermia, interleukins 1 and 2, and T-cell proliferation. Yale J Biol Med 1982;55:437–442.

18. Berkenbosch F, Van Oers J, Del Rey A, Tilders F, Besedovsky H. Corticotropin-releasing factor-producing neurons in the rat activated by interleukin-1. Science 1987; 238:524–526.

19. Rivier C, Vale W. In the rat, interleukin-1α acts at the level of the brain and the gonads to interfere with gonadotropin and sex steroid secretion. Endocrinology 1989;124:2105–2109.

20. McCann SM, Lumpkin MD, Samson WK. The role of vasopressin and oxytocin in control of anterior pituitary hormone secretion. In: Baertsche AJ, Dreifuss JJ, eds. Neuroendocrinology of vasopressin, corticoliberin and opiomelanocortins. London: Academic Press, 1982:319–329.

21. Sapolsky R, Rivier C, Yamamoto G, Plotsky P, Vale W. Interleukin-1 stimulates the secretion of hypothalamic corticotropin-releasing factor. Science 1987;238:522–524.

22. Rettori V, Jurcovicova J, McCann SM. Central action of interleukin-1 in altering the release of TSH, growth hormone and prolactin in the male rat. J Neurosci 1987; 18:179–183.

23. Lyson K, McCann SM. Involvement of arachidonic acid cascade pathways in interleukin-6-stimulated corticotropin-releasing factor release in vitro. Neuroendocrinology 1992; 55:708–713.

24. Rettori V, Gimeno MF, Karara A, Gonzalez MC, McCann SM. Interleukin 1α inhibits prostaglandin E_2 release to suppress pulsatile release of luteinizing hormone but not follicle-stimulating hormone. Proc Natl Acad Sci USA 1991;88:2763–2767.

25. Kalra PS, Sahu A, Kalra SP. Interleukin-1 inhibits the ovarian steroid-induced luteinizing hormone surge and release of hypothalamic luteinizing hormone-releasing hormone in rats. Endocrinology 1990;126:2145–2152.

26. Rettori V, Mikenkovic L, Beutler BA, McCann SM. Hypothalamic action of cachectin to alter pituitary hormone release. Brain Res Bull 1989;23:471–475.

27. Lyson K, McCann SM. The effect of interleukin-6 on pituitary hormone release in vivo and in vitro. Neuroendocrinology 1991;54:262–266.

28. Navarra P, Tsagarakis S, Faria MS, Rees LH, Besser GM, Grossman AB. Interleukins-1 and -6 stimulate the release of corticotropin-releasing hormone-41 from rat hypothalamus in vitro via the eicosanoid cyclooxygenase pathway. Endocrinology 1991;128:37–44.

29. Karanth S, Lyson K, McCann SM. Role of nitric oxide in interleukin 2-induced corticotropin-releasing factor release from incubated hypothalami. Proc Natl Acad Sci USA 1993;90:3383–3387.

30. Karanth S, Aguila MC, McCann SM. The influence of interleukin-2 on the release of somatostatin and growth hormone-releasing factor by mediobasal hypothalamus. Neuroendocrinology 1993;58:185–190.

31. Gonzalez MC, Riedel M, Rettori V, Yu WH, McCann SM. Effect of recombinant human γ-interferon on the release of anterior pituitary hormones. Prog Neuroendocrinol Immunol 1990;3:49–54.

32. Gonzalez MC, Aguila MC, McCann SM. In vitro effects of recombinant human gamma-interferon on growth hormone release. Prog Neuroendocrinol Immunol 1991;4:222–227.

33. Milenkovic L, McCann SM. Effects of thymosin alpha-1 on pituitary hormone release. Neuroendocrinology 1992;55:14–19.

34. Milenkovic L, Lyson K, Aguila MC, McCann SM. Effect of thymosin alpha-1 on hypothalamic hormone release. Neuroendocrinology 1992;56:674–679.

35. Woloski BMRNJ, Smith EM, Meyer WJ III, Fuller GM, Blalock JE. Corticotropin-releasing activity of monokines. Science 1985;230:1035–1037.

36. Bernton EW, Beach JE, Holaday JW, Smallridge RC, Fein HG. Release of multiple hormones by a direct action of interleukin-1 on pituitary cells. Science 1987;238:519–522.

37. Sapolsky R, Rivier C, Yamamoto G, Plotsky P, Vale W. Interleukin-1 stimulates the secretion of hypothalamic corticotropin-releasing factor. Science 1987;238:522–524.

38. Uehara A, Gillis S, Arimura A. Effects of interleukin-1 on hormone release from normal rat pituitary cells in primary culture. Neuroendocrinology 1987;45:343–347.

39. Milenkovic L, Rettori V, Snyder GD, Beutler B, McCann SM. Cachectin alters anterior pituitary hormone release by a direct action in vitro. Proc Natl Acad Sci USA 1989;86:2418–2422.

40. Spangelo BL, Jarvis WD, Judd AM, MacLeod RM. Induction of interleukin-6 release by interleukin-1 rat anterior pituitary cells in vitro through an eicosanoid-dependent mechanism. Abstracts of the 73rd Annual Meeting of the Endoctrine Society 1991;1605:432.

41. Karanth S, McCann SM. Anterior pituitary hormone control by interleukin-2. Proc Natl Acad Sci USA 1991;88:2961–2965.

42. Gonzalez MC, Aguila MC, McCann SM. In vitro effects of recombinant human gamma-interferon on growth hormone release. Prog Neuroendocrinol Immunol 1991;4:222–227.

43. Lancaster JR Jr. Nitric oxide in cells. Am Sci 1992;80:248–259.

44. Moncada S, Palmer RMJ, Higgs EA. Nitric oxide: physiology, pathophysiology, and pharmacology. Pharmacol Rev 1991;43:109–142.

45. Bredt DS, Snyder SH. Nitric oxide, a novel neuronal messenger. Neuron 1992;8:3–11.

46. Glyn JR, Lipton JM. Hypothalamic and antipyretic effects of centrally administered ACTH (1–24) and α-melanotropin. Peptides 1981;2:177–187.

47. Lipton JM. Modulation of host defense by the neuropeptide α-MSH. Yale J Biol Med 1990;63:173–182.

48. Lyson K, McCann SM. Alpha-melanocyte-stimulating hormone abolishes IL-1- and IL-6-induced corticotropin-releasing factor release from the hypothalamus in vitro. Neuroendocrinology 1993;58:191–195.

49. Rettori V, Belova N, Dees WL, Nyberg CL, Gimeno M, McCann SM. Role of nitric oxide in the control of luteinizing hormone-releasing hormone release in vivo and in vitro. Proc Natl Acad Sci USA 1993;90:10130–10134.

50. Rettori V, Belova N, Kamat A, Lyson K, McCann SM. Blockade by interleukin-1 alpha of the nitricoxidergic control of luteinizing hormone-releasing hormone release in vivo and in vitro. Neuroimmunomodulation 1993;1:82–85.

CHAPTER 19

ROLE OF CYTOKINES IN SLEEP, FEVER, AND ANOREXIA

Levente Kapás, Masaaki Shibata, and James M. Krueger

Sleepiness, loss of appetite, and fever are constitutional symptoms of almost all infectious diseases. These responses represent facets of the acute-phase response regulated by the central nervous system (CNS). These symptoms have been recognized throughout history as being hallmarks of infection, and physicians have spent considerable effort to treat fevers despite evidence that febrile responses are adaptive. Conversely, physicians seldom fail to prescribe bed rest, although there is no direct evidence that sleep aids the recuperative processes. It is likely, however, that sleep and loss of appetite, like fever and other host responses to infection, are in toto adaptive.

A variety of microbial products (e.g., muramyl peptides, endotoxin, viral double-stranded RNA) are effective stimulants of inflammatory mediators (1). One class of these mediators, the cytokines, are involved in triggering CNS responses to acute illness. Much evidence has accumulated in the past few years to indicate that most aspects of the acute-phase response are driven by a complex array of cytokines in association with classic stress hormones. The hypothesis that cytokines are involved in physiological processes is currently debated. The central idea invoked by this hypothesis is that, under normal conditions, low basal levels of cytokine production and effects vary in subtle ways with one or more physiological processes. Specificity of response for any one physiological function (e.g., sleep) would arise from a network of interactions of several cytokines and hormones with multiple neuronal groups, each having a different array of sensitivities to different cytokines and hormones (2). After pathological disturbances, production of one or more cytokines would be greatly amplified via microbial (or other pathological) stimuli in a site-specific manner. Such amplified cytokine production would then produce pathology analogous to the pathologies produced by excessive hormone production. The fact that cytokines such as tumor necrosis factor-α (TNF-α) induce and act in synergy with other cytokines such as interleukin-1 (IL-1), which in turn also affect CNS functions, has greatly complicated interpretation of physiological responses to individual cytokines.

In this review, we focus on the role that cytokines have in regulating CNS responses to infection, although the evidence that IL-1 is involved in physiological sleep regulation is also briefly reviewed. Fever has been investigated for more than 100 years, and there is thus an extensive body of literature (3); our focus is on central mechanisms of cytokine-induced fevers. In contrast, sleep and food intake response to infection have only recently been studied. As a consequence, a discussion involving citation of most of the literature relating cytokines to sleep and appetite is possible.

SLEEP

Almost everyone is aware of the subjective feelings of sleepiness and fatigue associated with the onset of infectious illness. This knowledge, coupled with the discovery that some sleep-promoting substances also serve as immune response modifiers, led to the first systematic investigations of sleep over the course of infectious disease (4). The following findings were demonstrated: (a) the time course of sleep responses depends on the infectious agent used (4); (b) the temporal patterns of bacteria-induced sleep varied with the route of administration (5); and (c) dead bacteria (4) or bacterial cell walls (6) elicited sleep effects similar to those of viable bacteria. These results are consistent with previous studies showing that sleep responses are elicited by muramyl peptides tailored from bacterial cell wall peptidoglycan by mammalian macrophages (7).

It is hypothesized that viral infections are linked to a variety of sleep disorders (e.g., chronic fatigue syndrome) (8). Indeed, human immunodeficiency virus–seropositive individuals who are otherwise healthy have an excess of nonrapid-eye-movement sleep (NREMS) (9), although, after acquired immunodeficiency syndrome (AIDS) develops, sleep is greatly disrupted (10). Rabbits inoculated with influenza virus (an abortive infection) respond by enhancing NREMS (11). Furthermore, mice inoculated with influenza virus (a productive infection) exhibit prolonged (4–7 days) NREMS enhancement (Toth LA, unpublished observations; Fang J, Krueger JM, unpublished observations).

After either bacterial or fungal challenge, the specific sleep pattern that develops is related to the clinical response of the animal; a more favorable prognosis is associated with prolonged duration and intensity of NREMS after infectious challenge (12). It is therefore possible that excess sleep, like fever, may be beneficial during infection. This notion is indirectly supported by the finding that mice immunized against influenza virus failed to clear the virus from their lungs after a second exposure to the virus if they were sleep-deprived (13). Similarly, it has been reported that rats became septicemic during prolonged sleep deprivation (14). Regardless of whether sleep aids recuperation, it is currently clear that infectious diseases affect sleep and cytokine production.

Much of our information concerning the somnogenic actions of cytokines is derived from studies in which IL-1 was used. The first indication that IL-1 was somnogenic came from experiments in which an extract of stimulated rabbit peritoneal exudate cells or human mononuclear cells was injected into rabbits (15). This preparation was called "endogenous pyrogen," and it most likely contained not only IL-1 but several other cytokines. Nevertheless, both intravenous (IV) and intracerebroventricular (ICV) injections of that preparation resulted in dose-dependent increase in NREMS and fever. Sleep intensity, as indicated by increased electroencephalographic (EEG) slow-wave amplitudes during NREMS, was also stimulated. In subsequent studies, similar somnogenic actions of recombinant human (rhu)-IL-1β and rhu-IL-1α were

demonstrated in rabbits (16,17). ICV bolus injection of 1 to 20 ng rhu-IL-1β or rhu-IL-1α induces dose-dependent increases in NREMS and suppression of rapid-eye-movement sleep (REMS) during a 6 hour postinjection period. Both the pyrogenic and the somnogenic actions of IL-1 are prevented by heat treatment of the preparation (17). The 208 to 240 amino acid region of the parent molecule, a sequence necessary for the IL-1-to-IL-1 receptor complex translocation to the cell nucleus (18), showed similar, but approximately 5,000 times less potent, somnogenic activities (17). The somnogenic activities of this fragment are blocked by the IL-1 receptor antagonist (IL-1RA) (19).

The somnogenic effects of IL-1β have been demonstrated in rats (20,21), cats (22), and monkeys (23). In rats, the effects of IL-1 are biphasic; initial sleep enhancement is followed by a secondary suppression in sleep (24), and the effect is strongly influenced by circadian factors (21). If injected at dark onset (the period when nocturnal rats are the most active), 0.5 to 10 ng IL-1 promotes NREMS. If injected during the light period, however, when rats sleep the most spontaneously, low doses of IL-1 (0.5–2.5 ng) do not increase the time spent in sleep, but they do increase EEG slow-wave amplitudes ("sleep intensity"), whereas higher doses (10–25 ng) decrease NREMS duration but stimulate sleep intensity. The specificity of the somnogenic effects of IL-1 is supported by the findings that IL-1–induced sleep can be reversed by administration of IL-1RA (25) or another endogenous antagonist of IL-1, α-melanocyte stimulating hormone (α-MSH) (26).

It is likely that the somnogenic effects of IL-1 after ICV administration are mediated through central mechanisms. Systemic injections of centrally active doses of IL-1 do not affect sleep, and the exact site of the somnogenic action is not known. IL-1 was not effective in inducing sleep, but it elicited fever when injected into the basal forebrain, the posterior hypothalamus, and the brainstem areas in rabbits (27).

Current models of sleep regulation are based on the hypothesis that sleep is not regulated by a single humoral agent or by a single "sleep center" in the brain; rather, a complex network of sleep factors interacts with various neuronal groups to elicit sleep (2,28). It is likely that IL-1, as a crucial part of the sleep regulatory network, exerts its effects on sleep through other substances that affect sleep. Prostaglandins (PGs) are implicated in sleep regulation; PGD$_2$ induces sleep in several species (29), and IL-1 stimulates PG production. The somnogenic actions of IL-1, however, are not attenuated by the cyclo-oxygenase inhibitor, indomethacin, indicating that the sleep effects are independent from cyclo-oxygenase products (30). Pancreatic insulin, another sleep-promoting hormone regulated in part by IL-1, also does not contribute to the effects of IL-1 because the somnogenic actions of IL-1 are preserved in diabetic rats (24). The inability of naloxone to suppress IL-1–induced sleep indicates that opioids probably are also not crucial for this effect of IL-1 (31). In contrast, IL-1 stimulates production of nitric oxide (NO), a recently identified transmitter in the nervous system. NO may be a part of sleep regulatory mechanisms because inhibition of NO production in rabbits (32) and rats (33) results in profound sleep loss. When rabbits were pretreated with an NO synthase inhibitor prior to IL-1 injection, the expected IL-1–enhanced NREMS was suppressed for several hours. Because the NO inhibitor suppressed normal sleep, unequivocal conclusions cannot be drawn; it is either an additive interaction between independent opposite effects, or specific interactions took place between IL-1 and NO (32).

IL-1 stimulates production of growth hormone (GH) via growth hormone-releasing hormone (GHRH) (34), another peptide hormone with strong somnogenic activities. GHRH is likely to contribute to IL-1–induced sleep because anti-GHRH antibodies attenuate IL-1–induced GH release and NREMS in rats (35). Cytokines are organized in regulatory networks, and it is possible that other somnogenic cytokines, such as TNF or interferons (IFNs), contribute to the sleep effects of IL-1. It is unlikely, however, that IL-2 (36) or IL-6 (37) mediates IL-1 sleep because these cytokines lack somnogenic activity in rabbits. The suppression of NREMS after high doses of IL-1 and the secondary sleep decrease that follows the somnogenic effects of IL-1 are assumed to be mediated by corticotrophin-releasing hormone (CRH). IL-1 stimulates CRH secretion, and exogenously administered CRH attenuates the somnogenic actions of IL-1 (38).

It is hypothesized that IL-1 is involved not only in sleep responses to generalized infections but also in regulation of normal sleep. Much evidence supports this hypothesis: (a) IL-1β, IL-1RA, and IL-1 receptors are present in normal brain; (b) IL-1 affects neural activity in the CNS; (c) IL-1 levels in cerebrospinal fluid (CSF) vary with the sleep-wake cycle, and they are highest at sleep onset (39,40); (d) spontaneous sleep is suppressed by administering anti-IL-1 antibodies in rats or rabbits, or IL-1RA in rabbits (41,42); and (e) the rebound sleep after sleep deprivation is attenuated by IL-1RA or anti-IL-1β antibodies (42).

The effects of TNF on sleep are very similar to that of IL-1. IV injection of 10 μg/kg rhu-TNF-α induces robust increases in NREMS, enhanced EEG slow-wave activity, and suppression of REMS in rabbits. The sleep effects last for at least 6 hours. The effects of ICV injection of 5 μg TNF-α (approximately 1 μg/kg) were similar in magnitude and duration (16,43). Enhanced sleep is accompanied by biphasic febrile responses. The effects of TNF-β are identical to that of TNF-α (44). Fragments of TNF-α are capable of inducing sleep, as well as febrile and anorectic responses (43). All the somnogenic fragments shared the amino acid sequence 31–36. This segment is located close to the region assumed to be involved in the binding of TNF-α to its receptor (45). The somnogenic sequences were different from the sequence active in food intake suppression, but they partially overlapped with regions that showed pyrogenic activities.

Blocking endogenous TNF-α results in decrease of spontaneous sleep, indicating that TNF-α may contribute to initiation and maintenance of normal sleep. In rats, ICV injection of 10 μg anti-TNF-α antibodies during the light period significantly suppressed NREMS for 3 hours; thereafter, NREMS tended to be below the baseline level (Kapás L, Krueger JM, unpublished observations). Similarly, ICV injection of TNF binding protein I suppressed normal sleep in rabbits (Tooley DD, et al., unpublished observations). Furthermore, TNF-α and its receptors are found in normal brain (46).

IFNs were originally defined by their ability to suppress virus proliferation. They are widespread in the body; almost all nucleated cells can produce IFN-α after appropriate stimulation. The first indications suggesting that IFNs may be involved in sleep regulation came when sleepiness and fatigue were reported as side effects during IFN therapy. The first experimental evidence for the somnogenic actions of IFN came from experiments in rabbits: Animals injected with rhu-IFN-α$_2$ had increased NREMS and EEG slow-wave activity (47,48). Subsequently, the somnogenic activity of rhu-IFN-α and rabbit IFN-α were reproduced in rabbits (49); this study also demonstrated that the somnogenic activity of IFNs, but not antiviral activity, is relatively species-specific in that the effective dose of rhu-IFN-α in rabbits was approximately 10^3-fold greater than the effective dose of rabbit IFN. Rhu-IFN-α also enhances cortical EEG synchronization in rats (50,51), and it reduces the latency to REM sleep in monkeys (52). The observation that increases in plasma antiviral activities (IFN) parallel somnogenic responses after viral challenge support the hypothesis that IFN may contribute to increased sleep during viral infections (11). The role that IFNs may have in physiological sleep regulation has not been investigated.

ANOREXIA

Anorexia and cachexia are commonly associated with malignant tumors and chronic infections. In the search for an endogenous, blood-born anorectic factor, a peptide, cachectin, was isolated from cachectic, *Trypanosoma* infected rabbits. This factor later proved to be identical to TNF. Injection of dialyzed conditioned medium obtained from lipopolysaccharide (LPS)-stimulated peritoneal macrophages, which contains TNF, causes anorexia and weight loss in mice (53). The anorectic effects of recombinant

TNF-α were demonstrated subsequently in several species, including rat (54,55), mouse (54,56,57), goat (58), and human (59). TNF endogenously produced by TNF-secreting tumors in nude mice causes anorexia and weight loss (60). TNF$_{69-100}$ induces reduced food intake; other TNF fragments, although they possess somnogenic or pyrogenic activities, did not affect food intake (43). TNF-β, which has approximately 30% homology with TNF-α at the amino acid level and binds to the same receptors, has similar anorectic activities to that of TNF-α when injected into rats ICV (44).

Tolerance to the anorectic effects of TNF develops rapidly after systemic administration (54–57,61–63). This tolerance to the anorectic effects of TNF may be due to the use of very high, sublethal doses of nonspecies-specific (human) TNF preparations, and it does not necessarily change the role of endogenously produced TNF in tumor-associated cachexia. The metabolic changes after TNF-α (and IL-1α) administration are similar to those that occur after endotoxin administration or during chronic diseases. These changes do not simply mimic the changes seen after starvation (64). Animals that show tolerance to TNF after repeated injections also show decreased sensitivity to tumor-associated anorexia and cachexia, indicating a role for endogenous TNF in tumor-associated cachexia (65).

CNS mechanisms likely mediate TNF-induced anorexia. Centrally active doses of TNF do not affect feeding when injected systemically (66–68). Furthermore, cachexia develops rapidly if TNF-secreting tumor is implanted in the brain, but not if it is implanted in muscle, although plasma TNF levels were similar in both scenarios (69). TNF also mimics the effects of glucose on the activity of ventromedial hypothalamic neurons (66). PGs are not involved in the anorectic effects of TNF (69,70) or the anorexia accompanied with tumor growth (71). In addition to the central effects, peripheral mechanisms (e.g., decreased gastric emptying, gastrointestinal inflammation) (54) may also contribute to the anorectic effects of systemically injected or produced TNF.

The first data indicating that IL-1 suppresses food intake are from the experiments of McCarthy and co-workers (72): Systemic injection of monocyte supernatant or recombinant murine IL-1β suppressed short-term feeding in rats. These results were later confirmed in rats using rhu-IL-1 (73), as well as in mice (74–76) and goats (77). The effective systemic doses are in the pyrogenic dose range of 6 to 10 μg/kg. Similar to TNF, continuous systemic intraperitoneal (IP) or subcutaneous infusion of IL-1 results in loss of its anorectic potency (78–81). Because IL-1 is a potent proinflammatory substance, the decreased biological activity may be the consequence of a local inflammatory reaction, such as the appearance of scar tissue around the tip of the cannula. If these tolerant animals are challenged with a single bolus injection of IL-1, anorectic

responses can be elicited (82). Furthermore, repeated systemic bolus injections do not elicit tolerance (75,82–84).

Central injection of IL-1 requires much lower doses to elicit anorexia (66,76). The first attempt to elicit anorexia by ICV injection of a crude IL-1 preparation failed (85), but subsequent experiments revealed that ICV injection of 1 to 20 ng rIL-1 suppresses food intake in rats (66,85–91) and mice (76). It is assumed that IL-1 acts directly on CNS sites, most probably on the hypothalamus, to decrease food intake. Microinjections of rhu-IL-1α into the hypothalamus suppress feeding in rats (92). IL-1β mimics the effects of glucose on neural activity in the lateral (66) and the ventromedial hypothalamus (93).

CRH (but not corticosteroids [85]), PGs, lipoxigenase enzyme products (94), and IL-6 (95) may be involved in mediating IL-1–induced anorexia. Anti-CRH antibodies (96) or dexamethasone (91) suppress the anorectic effects of IL-1. The cyclo-oxygenase inhibitor, indomethacin, also prevents the anorectic effects of IL-1 in rats (94) and mice (74). The role of peripherally produced PGs seems relatively important (84,87), although the effects of IL-1 on the activities of glucose-sensitive hypothalamic neurons are also prostaglandin-dependent (92). Endogenous antagonists of IL-1, such as IL-1RA (88), α-MSH (90), C-terminal α-MSH tripeptide (90), and the Lys-Pro dipeptide portion of the tripeptide (89), block the food intake suppressive effects of exogenous IL-1. IL-1α (64,75,78, 86) also has anorectic activities. IL-2 does not suppress food intake in rat (86), mouse (75), or goat (77). ICV, but not IP, injection of IL-8 elicits similar effects to that of IL-1: it suppresses short-term food intake, decreases locomotor activity, and elicits moderate fever in rats (97).

Early clinical observations indicated that patients undergoing IFN therapy experienced fever, fatigue, and anorexia. Systemic injection of IFN-α (98) and IFN-γ (77,99,100) reduces food intake in mice, rats, and goats. The effects are independent from the PG system (101). ICV injection of IFN also suppresses feeding in rats (102). The food intake suppressive effects of IFN, similar to the somnogenic actions of IFN, show relative species specificity (98,102). IFN-α modulates neuronal activity in the ventromedial hypothalamus in a manner similar to glucose and IL-1 (93). Finally, in tumor-bearing rats (100) and mice (103), food intake can be stimulated by anti-IFN-γ antibodies, suggesting a role for IFN-γ in tumor-associated anorexia.

FEVER

One of the most studied host defense responses induced by cytokines is fever, perhaps because fever is the most manifest and often the earliest sign of infection. It is generally believed that in response to pathogens, endogenously released cytokines from diverse cell types are transported by the blood to the brain, where they somehow penetrate. These pyrogenic cytokines include IL-1α, IL-1β, IL-6, TNF-α, TNF-β, and IFN-α_2. The most critical regions of the brain for fever induction are the preoptic area and the anterior hypothalamus (PO/AH), where blood-borne cytokines directly or indirectly affect thermosensitive neurons (104).

The importance of the CNS in regulation of body temperature was noted in the late 1930s. The hypothalamus was identified as a critical brain area for temperature regulation: Animals with hypothalamic lesions were unable to maintain their body temperature at varying room temperatures (105). These findings were later confirmed by the fact that local cooling or heating of the hypothalamus through an implanted device evoked dramatic thermoregulatory responses (106–109). In the early 1960s, two types of PO/AH neurons that show distinctly different activity to local temperature changes were described (109–113): Warm-sensitive neurons increase their firing rate when the PO/AH temperature is raised higher than normal (approximately 37°C), and cold-sensitive neurons increase their firing rate below normal PO/AH temperature. The activity of PO/AH warm-sensitive and cold-sensitive neurons decrease and increase, respectively, in conjunction with fever with IV bacterial or endogenous pyrogens (114,115). These neurons also similarly changed their activity when endogenous pyrogens were microinjected or when small amounts of purified IL-1 were iontophoretically injected in the immediate vicinity of the neurons in anesthetized animals (116,117). Coinjection of sodium acetyl salicylate blocked the IL-1 effect. The thermosensitivity of PO/AH neurons can be maintained in isolated incubated brain slices, and they respond to TNF-α and IFN-α_2 in the same manner as those in vivo preparations (118). It is assumed that increased activity of warm-sensitive neurons would induce panting, cutaneous vasodilation, sweating, and a decrease in body temperature (i.e., mimics fever lysis) (106,107). Conversely, enhanced activity of cold-sensitive neurons would provoke shivering, cutaneous vasoconstriction, and an increase in body temperature (i.e., mimics fever production) (108,109). Although there is no direct anatomical evidence for efferent connections of PO/AH thermosensitive neurons to thermoeffectors, it is generally presumed that these neurons are in fact the most critical element of central thermoregulatory/fever mechanisms.

Two fundamental questions regarding central mechanism of fever induction by blood-borne pyrogenic cytokines still remain unanswered. First, where do blood-borne pyrogenic cytokines affect the brain? Second, how are cytokine signals transduced into neuronal signals? It has been hypothesized that blood-borne cytokines may act on circumventricular organs (CVOs), which lack blood-brain barrier (BBB). The hypothesis is based on a number of observations. Circulating cytokines do not readily cross the BBB (119,120), and they do not appear to enter the brain at a rate which may explain the relatively rapid onset of fever (10–15 min) after IV injection (121), although there may be a transport system for IL-1 from blood to brain (122). Lesions and sensitization of the organum vasculosum laminae terminalis (OVLT), one of the CVOs closely located to the PO/AH, abolish and enhance fever, respectively, to systemic pyrogens (123,124).

The CVOs are very rich in vasculature, and fenestration of the vascular endothelium may allow large molecules such as cytokines to directly enter into the OVLT (125). Neurons in the OVLT are sensitive to TNF-α and IFN-α_2 (126). It is therefore likely that the OVLT may be where the chemical signals of blood-borne cytokines are transduced into neuronal signals, and that the OVLT may affect the activity of the PO/AH-thermosensitive neurons trans-synaptically involving neurotransmitters, such as serotonin or PGE$_2$ (127,128). It is, however, currently not known whether blood-borne cytokines bind to the cellular elements of the OVLT or actually enter the OVLT. It is also not known whether the OVLT has an efferent connection to the PO/AH-thermosensitive neurons. Nevertheless, it has been suggested that PGE$_1$ and PGE$_2$ act as central mediators of fever. PGEs induce hyperthermia after ICV or intrahypothalamic injection, and PG synthase inhibitors reduce both cytokine-induced fever and increased PGE levels in ventricular or cisternal CSF (129–132). Intrahypothalamic or ICV injection of PGEs cause activity changes of the PO/AH-thermosensitive neurons that are consistent with fever induction (133,134). Brain, as well as peripheral vascular endothelial cells, are able to synthesize PGE$_2$ in response to cytokines (135,136). Plasma PGE$_2$ levels increase concomitantly with fever following IV IL-1 injection (137). Finally, IV injected PGE$_2$ induces fever (138).

Despite the evidence supporting PGE$_2$ as a major mediator of fever, very little is known about where and how it acts in the brain. Two hypotheses have been proposed with regard to PGE$_2$: (a) PGE$_2$ may be produced within the region of the OVLT, and it may diffuse toward the PO/AH (139); or (b) PGE$_2$ is synthesized peripherally in response to blood-borne pyrogens, and it is carried to the brain, where it may diffuse into the PO/AH (137). Both hypotheses assume that PGE$_2$ diffuses toward thermosensitive neurons in the PO/AH; it is not clear whether such diffusion of PGE$_2$ requires a specific transport mechanism.

NO may also be considered as one of the fever mediators released by cytokines. NO production is stimulated by cytokines and bacterial endotoxins (140,141). Once the inducible form of NO synthase is activated by cytokines or endotoxin, the enzyme continues to produce NO for lengthy periods (142,143). This characteristic may explain why bolus injection of cytokines induces long-lasting fevers. Following bacterial endotoxin injection, levels of the stable metabolite of NO, nitrate, increase in urine as well as in plasma in conjunction with fever (144,145). Hyperthermia induced by hypothalamic microinjection of PGE_2 is attenuated by a NO inhibitor, N^G-monomethyl-L-arginine (146). Finally, cytokines increase cyclic guanosine monophosphate (cGMP) in glial cells through the L-arginine NO pathway (147–149), and ICV injection of cGMP induces hyperthermia (150). Such evidence may suggest that the cytokine-NO-cGMP pathway is a possible mechanism of fever. However, because another NO synthase inhibitor, N^ω-nitro-L-arginine methyl ester, only slightly attenuated IL-1β–induced fever (32), and because the PG inhibitor, indomethacin, does not block IL-1β–induced increase in cGMP in vitro (Shibata M, unpublished data), the involvement of NO and cGMP in cytokine-induced fever needs further evaluation.

CONCLUSIONS

Cytokines, such as IL-1, TNF-α, and TNF-β, and IFNs, elicit behavioral changes characteristic of infections: increased NREMS, suppressed food intake, and fever. It is likely that these symptoms are part of host defense mechanisms rather than undesirable side effects of infections or chronic diseases. There is a positive correlation, for example, between the amount and intensity of slow-wave sleep occurring during the initial responses to infectious challenge and a favorable clinical process in rabbits (12). Whether such a correlation is indicative of causative relationships between increased sleep and survival is currently unknown. It may seem naive to assume that suppressed eating helps recuperation during wasting diseases, especially in the light of the common and successful practice of roborative (and, if needed, parenteral) therapies for acute or chronic diseases. Nevertheless, it is posited that anorexia is a part of the host defense response by reducing the availability of nutrients for the microbial agents. This idea is supported by experiments in which the survival rate of force-fed infected mice was below that of nonforce-fed infected control mice (151). Mild elevations in body temperature also likely help recuperation (3).

There are well described general interactions between thermoregulation and sleep, feeding and sleep, and feeding and thermoregulation. It seems likely, however, that sleep, fever, and anorexia, which occur in response to cytokines, are not the consequences of each other; rather they represent independent, parallel behavioral and, autonomic output of a common (cytokine) trigger. For example, passive increase in body temperature promotes sleep, but the sleep effects of cytokines are unlikely due to the fever because the somnogenic effects of IL-1 are not affected by antipyretics, whereas the fever is blocked (15,30). Furthermore, fever does not necessarily induce sleep, as evidenced by the lack of somnogenic effects of the otherwise pyrogenic IL-6 (37) and pyrogenic fragments of TNF-α (43). Finally, subpyrogenic doses of IL-1 elicit sleep (24).

Similarly, decreased food intake is not due to fever because endotoxin-induced anorexia and fever can be separated using antipyretics (152). Under certain circumstances, IL-1 induces fever but not anorexia (85). Furthermore the time course of fever and anorexia is dissociated (66,77). Increased sleep may contribute to decreased feeding, but it may not be a decisive factor, because potent somnogenic peptides lack anorectic activities (43), and anorexia is not always accompanied with decreased water intake, as would be expected if the decreased consummatory behavior was due to a general suppression of motor activity.

In conclusion, much evidence substantiates the role of cytokines in regulating behavioral and autonomic function during pathologies. Despite major efforts and a growing body of data, two intriguing questions for neuroscientists still remain unanswered: What is the exact role of central cytokines in the regulation of physiological processes under normal conditions? Through which interface mechanisms can peripheral, blood-borne cytokines affect functions that are ultimately under the regulation of the CNS?

ACKNOWLEDGMENTS: This work was supported in part by National Institutes of Health grants NS-25378, NS-27250, NS-30514, and NS-31453, and the Office of Naval Research grant N00014–90-J-1069.

REFERENCES

1. Krueger JM, Majde JA. Sleep as a host defense: its regulation by microbial products and cytokines. Clin Immunol Immunopathol 1990;57:188–199.

2. Krueger JM, Obál F Jr, Opp M, Toth L, Johannsen L, Cady AB. Somnogenic cytokines and models concerning their effects on sleep. Yale J Biol Med 1990;63:157–172.

3. Kluger MJ. Fever: role of pyrogens and cryogens. Physiol Rev 1991;71:93–127.

4. Toth LA, Krueger JM. Effects of microbial challenge on sleep in rabbits. FASEB J 1989;3:2062–2066.

5. Toth LA, Krueger JM. Somnogenic, pyrogenic, and hematologic effects of experimental pasturellosis in rabbits. Am J Physiol 1990;258:R536–R542.

6. Johannsen L, Toth LA, Rosenthal RS, et al. Somnogenic, pyrogenic, and hematologic effects of bacterial peptidoglycan. Am J Physiol 1990;259:R182–R186.

7. Johannsen L, Wecke J, Obál F Jr, Krueger JM. Macrophages

produce somnogenic and pyrogenic muramyl peptides during digestion of staphylococci. Am J Physiol 1991;260: R126–R133.

8. Buchwald D, Sullivan JL, Komaroff AL. Frequency of chronic active Epstein-Barr infection in a general medical practice. JAMA 1987;257:2303–2307.

9. Norman S, Shaukat M, Way K, Cohn M, Resnick C. Alterations in sleep architecture in asymptomatic HIV sero-positive patients. Sleep Res 1987;16:494.

10. Norman SE, Chediak AD, Kiel M, Cohn MA. Sleep disturbances in HIV-infected homosexual men. AIDS 1990;4: 775–781.

11. Kimura-Takeuchi M, Majde JA, Toth LA, Krueger JM. Influenza virus-induced changes in rabbit sleep and acute phase responses. Am J Physiol 1992;263:R1115–R1121.

12. Toth LA, Tolley EA, Krueger JM. Sleep as a prognostic indicator during infectious disease in rabbits. Proc Soc Exp Biol Med 1993; 201:179–192.

13. Brown R, Pang G, Husband AJ, King MG. Suppression of immunity to influenza virus infection in the respiratory tract following sleep disturbance. Reg Immunol 1989;2: 321–325.

14. Everson CA. Sustained sleep deprivation impairs host defense. Am J Physiol 1993;265:R1148–R1154.

15. Krueger JM, Walter J, Dinarello CA, Wolff SM, Chedid L. Sleep-promoting effects of endogenous pyrogen (interleukin-1). Am J Physiol 1984;246:R994–R999.

16. Shoham S, Davenne D, Cady AB, Dinarello CA, Krueger JM. Recombinant tumor necrosis factor and interleukin 1 enhance slow-wave sleep. Am J Physiol 1987;253:R142–R149.

17. Obál F Jr, Opp M, Cady AB, et al. Interleukin 1α and an interleukin 1β fragment are somnogenic. Am J Physiol 1990;259:R439–R446.

18. Grenfell S, Smithers N, Witham S, Shaw A, Graber P. Analysis of mutations in the putative nuclear localization sequence of interleukin-1β. Biochem J 1991;280:111–116.

19. Opp M, Postlethwaite AE, Seyer A, Krueger JM. Interleukin 1 receptor antagonist blocks somnogenic and pyrogenic responses to an interleukin 1 fragment. Proc Natl Acad Sci USA 1992;89:3726–3738.

20. Tobler I, Borbely AA, Schwyzer M, Fontana A. Interleukin-1 derived from astrocytes enhances slow wave activity in sleep EEG of the rat. Eur J Pharmacol 1984;104:191–192.

21. Opp MR, Obál F Jr, Krueger JM. Interleukin-1 alters rat sleep: temporal and dose-related effects. Am J Physiol 1991;260:R52–R58.

22. Susic V, Totic S. "Recovery" function of sleep: effects of purified human interleukin-1 on the sleep and febrile response of cats. Met Brain Dis 1989;4:73–80.

23. Friedman EM, Boinski S, Coe CL. Interleukin-1 induces sleep-like behavior and alters cell structure in juvenile rhesus macaques. Am J Primatol 1994 (in press).

24. Kapás L, Payne L, Obál F Jr, Opp M, Johannsen L, Krueger JM. Sleep in diabetic rats: effects of interleukin 1. Am J Physiol 1991;260:R995–R999.

25. Opp MR, Krueger JM. Interleukin 1-receptor antagonist blocks interleukin 1-induced sleep and fever. Am J Physiol 1991;269:R453–R457.

26. Opp MR, Obál F Jr, Krueger JM. Effects of α-MSH on sleep,

behavior, and brain temperature: interactions with IL-1. Am J Physiol 1988;255:R914–R922.

27. Walter JS, Meyers P, Krueger JM. Microinjection of interleukin-1 into brain: separation of sleep and fever responses. Physiol Behav 1989;45:169–176.

28. Krueger JM, Obál F Jr. Neuronal group theory of sleep function. J Sleep Res 1993;2:63–69.

29. Hayaishi O. Molecular mechanisms of sleep-wake regulation: roles of prostaglandins D_2 and E_2. FASEB J 1991; 5:2575–2581.

30. Kapás L, Opp M, Kimura-Takeuchi M, Krueger JM. Peripheral prostaglandins do not mediate the hypnogenic effects of interleukin 1. Sleep Res 1991;20A:35.

31. Kapás L, Krueger JM. Effects of naloxone pretreatment on interleukin 1-induced sleep and fever. Sleep Res 1993;22: 435.

32. Kapás L, Shibata M, Kimura, Krueger JM. Inhibition of nitric oxide synthesis suppresses sleep in rabbits. Am J Physiol 1994;266:R151–157.

33. Kapás L, Kimura M, Fang J, Krueger JM. Microinjection of nitric oxide synthesis inhibitor into the brain stem suppresses sleep in rats. Soc Neurosci Abstr 1993;19:1814.

34. Payne LC, Obál F Jr, Opp MR, Krueger JM. Stimulation and inhibition of growth hormone secretion by interleukin-1β: the involvement of growth hormone-releasing hormone. Neuroendocrinology 1992;56:118–123.

35. Fang J, Obál F Jr, Payne L, Krueger JM. Growth hormone-releasing hormone is involved in interleukin-1 induced sleep in rats. Soc Neurosci Abstr 1993;16:573.

36. Opp MR, Krueger JM. Somnogenic actions of interleukin-2: real or artifact. Sleep Res 1994;23:26.

37. Opp M, Obál F Jr, Cady AB, Johannsen L, Krueger JM. Interleukin-6 is pyrogenic but not somnogenic. Physiol Behav 1989;45:1069–1072.

38. Opp M, Obál F Jr, Krueger JM. Corticotropin-releasing factor attenuates interleukin 1-induced sleep and fever in rabbits. Am J Physiol 1989;257:R528–R535.

39. Moldofsky H, Lue FA, Eisen J, Keystone E, Gorczynski RM. The relationship of interleukin-1 and immune functions to sleep in humans. Psychosom Med 1986;48:309–318.

40. Lue FA, Bail M, Gorczynski R, Moldofsky H. Sleep and interleukin-1-like activity in cat cerebrospinal fluid. Sleep Res 1987;16:51.

41. Opp MR, Krueger JM. An interleukin-1 receptor antagonist blocks interleukin-1 induced sleep and fever. Am J Physiol 1991;260:R453–R457.

42. Opp MR, Krueger JM. Interleukin-1 antibodies reduce NREMS and attenuate NREMS rebound after sleep deprivation in the rabbit. Sleep Res 1992;21:323.

43. Kapás L, Hong L, Cady AB, et al. Somnogenic, pyrogenic, and anorectic activities of tumor necrosis factor α (TNFα), and TNFα fragments. Am J Physiol 1992;263:R708–R715.

44. Kapás L, Krueger JM. Tumor necrosis factor-β induces sleep, fever, and anorexia. Am J Physiol 1992;263:R703–R707.

45. Eck MJ, Sprang SR. The structure of tumor necrosis factor-α at 2 6 A resolution. J Biol Chem 1989;264:17595–17605.

46. Breder CD, Saper CB. Tumor necrosis factor immunoreac-

tive innervation in the mouse brain. Soc Neurosci Abstr 1988;14:1280.

47. Krueger JM, Walter J, Davenne D, Shoham S, Dinarello C. Interferon α_2 enhances slow-wave sleep in rabbits. Soc Neurosci Abstr 1985;11:1283.

48. Krueger JM, Dinarello CA, Shoham S, Davenne D, Walter J, Kubillus S. Interferon alpha-2 enhances slow-wave sleep in rabbits. Int J Immunopharmacol 1987;9:23–30.

49. Kimura-Takeuchi M, Majde JA, Toth LA, Krueger JM. Effects of recombinant human interferons on sleep in rabbits. Sleep Res 1993;22:36.

50. Birmanns B, Saphier D, Abramsky O. α-Interferon modifies cortical EEG activity: dose-dependence and antagonism by naloxone. J Neurol Sci 1990;100:22–26.

51. De Sarro GB, Masuda Y, Ascioti C, Audino MG, Nistico G. Behavioural and ECoG spectrum changes induced by intracerebral infusion of interferons and interleukin-2 in rats are antagonized by naloxone. Neuropharmacology 1990; 29:167–179.

52. Reite M, Laudenslager M, Jones J, Crnic L, Kaemingk K. Interferon decreases REM latency. Biol Psychiatry 1987;22: 104–107.

53. Cerami A, Ikeda Y, Le Trang N, Hotez PJ, Beutler B. Weight loss associated with an endotoxin-induced mediator from peritoneal macrophages: the role of cachectin (tumor necrosis factor). Immunol Lett 1985;11:173–177.

54. Patton JS, Peters PM, McCabe J, et al. Development of partial tolerance to the gastrointestinal effects of high doses of recombinant tumor necrosis factor-α in rodents. J Clin Invest 1987;80:1587–1596.

55. Hoshino E, Pichard C, Greenwood CE, et al. Body composition and metabolic rate in rat during a continuous infusion of cachectin. Am J Physiol 1991;260:E27–E36.

56. Socher SH, Friedman A, Martinez D. Recombinant human tumor necrosis factor induces acute reductions in food intake and body weight in mice. J Exp Med 1988;167:1957–1962.

57. Mahony SM, Tisdale MJ. Induction of weight loss and metabolic alterations by human recombinant tumour necrosis factor. Br J Cancer 1988;58:345–349.

58. van Miert ASJPAM, van Duin CTM, Wensing TH. Fever and acute phase response induced in dwarf goats by endotoxin and bovine and human recombinant tumour necrosis factor alpha. J Vet Pharmacol Ther 1992;15:332–342.

59. Michie HR, Sherman ML, Spriggs DR, Rounds J, Christie M, Wilmore DW. Chronic TNF infusion causes anorexia but not accelerated nitrogen loss. Ann Surg 1989;209:19–24.

60. Oliff A, Defeo-Jones D, Boyer M, et al. Tumors secreting human TNF/cachectin induce cachexia in mice. Cell 1987; 50:555–563.

61. Mullen BJ, Harris RB, Patton JS, Martin RJ. Recombinant tumor necrosis factor-alpha chronically administered in rats: lack of cachectic effect. Proc Soc Exp Biol Med 1990; 193:318–325.

62. Darling G, Fraker DL, Jensen JC, Gorschboth CM, Norton JA. Cachectic effects of recombinant human tumor necrosis factor in rats. Cancer Res 1990;50:4008–4013.

63. Tracey KJ, Wei H, Manogue KR, et al. Cachectin/tumor ne-

crosis factor induces cachexia, anemia, and inflammation. J Exp Med 1988;167:1211–1227.

64. Fong Y, Moldawer LL, Marano M, et al. Cachectin/TNF or IL-1α induces cachexia with redistribution of body proteins. Am J Physiol 1989;256:R659–R665.

65. Stovroff MC, Fraker DL, Swedenborg JA, Norton JA. Cachectin/tumor necrosis factor: a possible mediator of cancer anorexia in the rat. Cancer Res 1988;48:4567–4572.

66. Plata-Salaman CR, Oomura Y, Kai Y. Tumor necrosis factor and interleukin-1β: suppression of food intake by direct action in the central nervous system. Brain Res 1988;448: 106–114.

67. Fantino M, Wieteska L. Evidence for a direct central anorectic effect of tumor-necrosis-factor-alpha in the rat. Physiol Behav 1993;53:477–483.

68. Bodnar RJ, Pasternak GW, Mann PE, Paul D, Warren R, Donner DB. Mediation of anorexia by human recombinant tumor necrosis factor through a peripheral action in the rat. Cancer Res 1989;49:6280–6284.

69. Tracey KJ, Morgello S, Koplin B, Fahey TJ III, Fox J, Aledo A. Metabolic effects of cachectin/tumor necrosis factor are modified by site of production. J Clin Invest 1990;86: 2014–2024.

70. Mahony SM, Tisdale MJ. Role of prostaglandins in tumour necrosis factor induced weight loss. Br J Cancer 1989;60: 51–55.

71. McCarthy DO, Daun JM. The effects of cyclo-oxygenase inhibitors on tumor-induced anorexia in rats. Cancer 1993; 71:486–492.

72. McCarthy DO, Kluger MJ, Vander AJ. Suppression of food intake during infection: is interleukin involved? Am J Clin Nutr 1985;42:1179–1182.

73. Shimomura Y, Shimizu H, Takahashi M, et al. Effects of peripheral administration of recombinant human interleukin-1 beta on feeding behavior of the rat. Life Sci 1990;47: 2185–2192.

74. Shimomura Y, Inukai T, Kuwabara A, et al. Enhanced sensitivity to anorexia and consumption of drinking water induced by interleukin-1β in obese yellow mice. Eur J Pharmacol 1991;209:15–18.

75. Moldawer LL, Andersson C, Gelin J, Lunkholm KG. Regulation of food intake and hepatic protein synthesis by recombinant-derived cytokines. Am J Physiol 1988;254: G450–G456.

76. Masotto C, Caspani G, De Simoni MG, et al. Evidence for a different sensitivity to various central effects of interleukin-1β in mice. Brain Res Bull 1992;28:161–165.

77. van Miert AS, Kaya F, van Duin CT. Changes in food intake and forestomach motility of dwarf goats by recombinant bovine cytokines (IL-1 beta, IL-2) and IFN-gamma. Physiol Behav 1992;52:859–864.

78. Mrosovsky N, Molony LA, Conn CA, Kluger MJ. Anorexic effects of interleukin 1 in the rat. Am J Physiol 1989;257: R1315–R1321.

79. Otterness IG, Seymour PA, Golden HW, Reynolds JA, Daumy GO. The effects of continuous administration of murine interleukin-1 in the rat. Physiol Behav 1988;43: 797–804.

80. Hermus RM, Sweep CG, van der Meer MJ, et al. Continuous infusion of interleukin-1 beta induces a nonthyroidal

illness syndrome in the rat. Endocrinology 1992;131: 2139–2146.

81. Otterness IG, Golden HW, Seymour PA, Eskra JD, Daumy GO. Role of prostaglandins in the behavioral changes induced by murine interleukin 1 alpha in the rat. Cytokine 1991;3:333–338.

82. Weingarten S, Savoldelli D, Langhans W. Enhancement or loss of the hypophagic effect of interleukin-1 upon chronic administration. Physiol Behav 1992;52:831–837.

83. Busbridge NJ, Dascombe MJ, Rothwell NJ. Chronic effects of interleukin-1 beta on fever, oxygen consumption and food intake in the rat. Horm Metab Res 1993;25:222–227.

84. Hellerstein MK, Meydani SN, Meydani M, Wu K, Dinarello CA. Interleukin-1-induced anorexia in the rat. Influence of prostaglandins. J Clin Invest 1989;84:228–235.

85. McCarthy DO, Kluger MJ, Vander AJ. Effect of centrally administered interleukin-1 and endotoxin on food intake of fasted rats. Physiol Behav 1986;36:745–749.

86. Uehara Y, Shimizu H, Shimomura Y, Negishi M, Kobayashi I, Kobayashi S. Effects of recombinant human interleukins on food intake of previously food-deprived rats. Proc Soc Exp Biol Med 1990;195:197–201.

87. Shimizu H, Uehara Y, Shimomura Y, Kobayashi I. Central administration of ibuprofen failed to block the anorexia induced by interleukin-1. Eur J Pharmacol 1991;195:281–284.

88. Plata-Salaman CR, French-Mullen JMH. Intracerebroventricular administration of a specific IL-1 receptor antagonist blocks food and water intake suppression induced by interleukin-1β. Physiol Behav 1992;51:1277–1279.

89. Uehara Y, Shimizu H, Sato N, Mura YS, Mori M. The dipeptide Lys-Pro attenuates interleukin-1β-induced anorexia. Peptides 1993;14:175–178.

90. Uehara Y, Shimizu H, Sato N, Tanaka Y, Shimomura Y, Mori M. Carboxyl-terminal tripeptide of α-melanocyte-stimulating hormone antagonizes interleukin-1-induced anorexia. Eur J Pharmacol 1992;220:119–122.

91. Plata-Salaman CR. Dexamethasone inhibits food intake suppression induced by low doses of interleukin-1 beta administered intracerebroventricularly. Brain Res Bull 1991;27:737–738.

92. Chance WT, Fischer JE. Aphagic and adipsic effects of interleukin-1. Brain Res 1991;568:261–264.

93. Kuriyama K, Hori T, Mori T, Nakashima T. Actions of interferon α and interleukin-1β on the glucose-responsive neurons in the ventromedial hypothalamus. Brain Res Bull 1990;24:803–810.

94. Shimomura Y, Inukai T, Kuwabara S, et al. Both cyclooxygenase and lipoxygenase inhibitor partially restore the anorexia by interleukin-1 beta. Life Sci 1992;51:1419–1426.

95. Oldenburg HS, Rogy MA, Lazarus DD, et al. Cachexia and the acute-phase protein response in inflammation are regulated by interleukin-6. Eur J Immunol 1993;23:1889–1894.

96. Uehara A, Sekiya C, Takasugi Y, Namiki M, Arimura A. Anorexia induced by interleukin 1: involvement of corticotropin-releasing factor. Am J Physiol 1989;257:R613–R617.

97. Plata-Salaman C, Borkoski JP. Interleukin-8 modulates

98. Segall MA, Crnic LS. An animal model for the behavioral effects of interferon. Behav Neurosci 1990;104:612–618.

99. Crnic LS, Segall MA. Behavioral effects of mouse interferons-alpha and -gamma and human interferon-alpha in mice. Brain Res 1992;590:277–284.

100. Langstein HN, Doherty GM, Fraker DL, Buresh CM, Norton JA. The roles of γ-interferon and tumor necrosis factor α in an experimental rat model of cancer cachexia. Cancer Res 1991;51:2302–2306.

101. Crnic LS, Segall MA. Prostaglandins do not mediate interferon-alpha effects on mouse behavior. Physiol Behav 1992;51:349–352.

102. Plata-Salaman CR. Interferons and central regulation of feeding. Am J Physiol 1992;263:R1222–R1227.

103. Matthys P, Dijkmans R, Proost P, et al. Severe cachexia in mice inoculated with interferon-gamma-producing tumor cells. Int J Cancer 1991;49:77–82.

104. Shibata M. Hypothalamic neuronal responses to cytokines. Yale J Biol Med 1990;63:147–156.

105. Bligh J. Temperature regulation in mammals and other vertebrates. New York: North-Holland Publishing, 1973.

106. Magoun HW, Harrison F, Brobeck JR, Ranson SW. Activation of heat loss mechanisms by local heating of the brain. J Physiol 1938;1:101–114.

107. Strom G. Effect of hypothalamic cooling on cutaneous blood flow in the unanesthetized dog. Acta Physiol Scand 1950;21:271–277.

108. Freeman WJ, Davis DD. Effects on cats of conductive hypothalamic cooling. Am J Physiol 1959;197:145–148.

109. Hammel HT, Hardy JD, Fusco MM. Thermoregulatory responses to hypothalamic cooling in unanesthetized dogs. Am J Physiol 1960;198:481–486.

110. Nakayama T, Hammel HT, Hardy JD. Single unit activity of anterior hypothalamus during local heating. Science 1961;134:560–561.

111. Nakayama T, Hammel HT, Hardy JD, Eisenman JS. Thermal stimulation of electrical activity of single units in the preoptic region. Am J Physiol 1963;204:1122–1126.

112. Hardy JD, Hellon RF, Sutherland K. Temperature-sensitive neurons in the dog's hypothalamus. J Physiol 1964;175:242–253.

113. Cunningham DJ, Stolwijk JAJ, Murakami N, Hardy JD. Responses of neurons in the preoptic area to temperature, serotonin, and epinephrine. Am J Physiol 1967;213:1570–1581.

114. Wit A, Wang SC. Temperature-sensitive neurons in preoptic/anterior hypothalamic region: actions of pyrogens and acetylsalicylate. Am J Physiol 1968;215:1160–1169.

115. Eisenman JS. Pyrogen-induced changes in the thermosensitivity of septal and preoptic neurons. Am J Physiol 1969;216:330–334.

116. Schoener EP, Wang SC. Leukocyte pyrogen and sodium acetylsalicylate on hypothalamic neurons in the cats. Am J Physiol 1975;229:185–190.

117. Hori T, Shibata M, Nakashima T, et al. Effects of interleukin-1 and arachidonate on the preoptic and anterior hypothalamic neurons. Brain Res Bull 1988;20:75–82.

118. Shibata M, Blatteis CM. Differential actions of interleukin-1, tumor necrosis factor, and interferon on hypothalamic neurons in vitro. Am J Physiol 1991;261:R1096–R1103.

119. Coceani F, Lee J, Dinarello CA. Occurrence of interleukin-1 in cerebrospinal fluid of the conscious cat. Brain Res 1988;446:245–250.

120. Dinarello CA, Weiner P, Wolf SM. Radiolabeling and disposition in rabbits of purified human leukocytic pyrogen. Clin Res 1978;26:522.

121. Dinarello CA, Cannon JG, Wolf SM. New concepts on the pathogenesis of fever. Rev Infect Dis 1988;10:168–189.

122. Banks WA, Oritz L, Plotkin SR, Kastin AJ. Human interleukin (IL) 1α, murine IL-1α and murine IL-1β are transported from blood to brain in the mouse by a shared saturable mechanism. J Pharmacol Exp Ther 1991;259:988–996.

123. Blatteis CM, Bealer SL, Hunter WS, Llanos-QJ, Ahokas RA. Suppression of fever after lesions of the anteroventral third ventricle in guinea pigs. Brain Res Bull 1983;11:519–526.

124. Stitt JT, Shimada SG. Enhancement of the febrile responses of rats to endogenous pyrogen occurs within the OVLT region. J Appl Physiol 1989;67:1740–1746.

125. McKinley MJ, Clevers J, Denton DA, Oldfield BJ, Penschow J, Rundgren M. Fine structure of the organum vasculosum of the lamina terminalis. In: Gross PM, ed. Circumventricular organs and body fluid, vol 1. Boca Raton, FL: CRC Press, 1987:111–130.

126. Shibata M, Blatteis CM. Human recombinant tumor necrosis factor and interferon affect the neuronal activity of the organum vasculosum laminae terminalis. Brain Res 1991;562:323–326.

127. Shibata M, Blatteis CM. Neurons in the organum vasculosum laminae terminalis respond to tumor necrosis factor and serotonin in slice preparations. In: Mercer JB, ed. Thermal physiology. Amsterdam: Elsevier/Excerpta Medica, 1989:413–414.

128. Matsuda T, Hori T, Nakashima T. Thermal and PGE$_2$ sensitivity of the organum vasculosum lamina terminalis region and preoptic area in rat brain slices. J Physiol 1992;454:197–212.

129. Milton AS, Wendlandt S. Effect on body temperature of prostaglandins of the A, E and F series of injection into the third ventricle of unanesthetized cat and rabbits. J Physiol 1971;218:325–336.

130. Feldberg W, Saxena PN. Fever produced by prostaglandin E$_1$. J Physiol 1971;217:547–556.

131. Flower RJ, Vane JR. Inhibition of prostaglandin synthetase in brain explains the antipyretic activity of paracetamol (4-acetamidophenol). Nature 1972;240:410–411.

132. Feldberg W, Gupta KP. Pyrogen fever and prostaglandin-like activity in cerebrospinal fluid. J Physiol 1973;228:41–53.

133. Schoener EP, Wang SC. Effects of locally administered prostaglandin E$_1$ on anterior hypothalamic neurons. Brain Res 1976;117:157–162.

134. Gordon CJ, Heath JE. The effect of prostaglandin E$_2$ on the firing rate of thermally sensitive and insensitive neurons in the preoptic/anterior hypothalamus of unanesthetized rabbits. Fed Proc 1979;38:1295.

135. Clark MA, Chen M-J, Crooke ST, Bomalask JS. Tumor necrosis factor (cachectin) induces phospholipase A2 activity and synthesis of a phospholipase A2-activating protein in endothelial cells. Biochem J 1988;250:125–132.

136. Rossi V, Breviario F, Ghezzi P, Dejana E, Mantovani A. Prostacyclin synthesis induced in vascular cells by interleukin-1. Science 1985;229:174–176.

137. Milton AS. Endogenous pyrogen initiates fever by a peripheral and not a central action. In: Mercer JB, ed. Thermal physiology. Amsterdam: Elsevier/Excerpta Medica, 1989:377–383.

138. Morimoto A, Long NC, Nakamori T, Murakami N. The effect of prostaglandin E$_2$ on the body temperature of restrained rat. Physiol Behav 1991;50:249–253.

139. Stitt JT. Passage of immunomodulators across the blood-brain barrier. Yale J Biol Med 1990;63:121–131.

140. Moritoki H, Takeuchi S, Hisayama T, Kondoh W. Nitric oxide synthase responsible for L-arginine-induced relaxation of rat aortic ring in vitro may be an inducible type. Br J Pharmacol 1992;107:361–366.

141. Zembowicz A, Hecker M, Macarthur H, Sessa WC, Vane JR. Nitric oxide and another potent vasodilator are formed from N^G-hydroxy-L- arginine by cultured endothelial cells. Proc Natl Acad Sci USA 1991;88:11172–11176.

142. Knowles RG, Moncada S. Nitric oxide as a signal in blood vessels. Trends Biochem Sci 1992;17:399–402.

143. Henry Y, Lepoiver M, Drapier J-C, Ducrocq C, Boucher J-L, Guissani A. EPR characterization of molecular targets for NO in mammalian cells and organelles. FASEB J 1993;7:1124–1134.

144. Wagner DA, Young VR, Tannenbaum SR. Mammalian nitrate biosynthesis: incorporation of ^{15}NH$_3$ into nitrate is enhanced by endotoxin treatment. Proc Natl Acad Sci USA 1983;80:4518–4521.

145. Stuehr DJ, Marletta MA. Mammalian nitrate biosynthesis: mouse marcrophages produce nitrite and nitrate in response to Escherichia coli lipopolysaccharide. Proc Natl Acad Sci USA 1985;82:7738–7742.

146. Amir S, De Blasio E, English AM. N^G-monomethyl-L-arginine co-injection attenuates the thermogenic and hyperthermic effects of E$_2$ prostaglandin microinjection into the anterior hypothalamic preoptic area in rats. Brain Res 1991;556:157–160.

147. Vigne P, Damais C, Frelin C. IL-1 and TNFα induce cGMP formation in C6 astrocytoma cells via the nitridergic pathway. Brain Res 1993;606:332–334.

148. Mollace VM, Colasanti M, Rodino P, Massoud R, Lauro GM, Nistico G. Cytokine-induced nitric oxide generation by cultured astrocytoma cells involves a Ca^{++}/calmodulin-independent NO-synthase. Biochem Biophys Res Commun 1993;191:327–334.

149. Boje KM, Aroa PK. Microglia-produced nitric oxide and reactive nitrogen oxides mediate neuronal cell death. Brain Res 1992;587:250–256.

150. Kandasamy SB, Williams BA. Central effects of dibutyryl cyclic AMP and GMP on the temperature in conscious rabbits. Brain Res 1983;277:311–320.

151. Murray MJ, Murray AB. Anorexia of infection as a mechanism of host defense. Am J Clin Nutr 1979;32:593–596.

152. McCarthy DO, Kluger MJ, Vander AJ. The role of fever in appetite suppression after endotoxin administration. Am J Clin Nutr 1984;40:310–316.

CHAPTER 20

ROLE OF CYTOKINES ON THYROID FUNCTIONS

J. A. Romijn and H. P. Sauerwein

The principal secretory product of the thyroid, thyroxine (T_4), is considered to be biologically inactive, but it is converted in peripheral tissues into the biologically active hormone tri-iodothyronine (T_3). Consequently, plasma T_3 is derived predominantly from peripheral deiodination of the outer ring of T_4, and only to a small extent from direct secretion by the thyroid.

Thyroid hormone metabolism is regulated in a very complex system inside and outside the thyroid gland. In the central nervous system (CNS), the hypothalamus and the pituitary gland produce thyroid-releasing hormone (TRH) and thyroid-stimulating hormone (TSH), respectively. Feedback interactions between the hypothalamus, the pituitary gland, and plasma thyroid hormones, especially T_4, are major mechanisms that regulate secretion of T_4 and T_3 by the thyroid. In addition to this hypothalamic-pituitary-thyroid interaction, intrathyroidal mechanisms regulate thyroid hormone synthesis and secretion. The peripheral conversion of T_4 into T_3 is regulated independently from TSH, and it is an important process that determines the availability of the biologically active hormone T_3.

Thyroid function is affected by many unrelated pathophysiological conditions. In different thyroid diseases, the thyroid may produce excessive or insufficient amounts of thyroid hormone. In thyroid disease, there may also be changes in thyroid morphology, with or without changes in thyroid function. In nonthyroidal illness (NTI), there are profound alterations in thyroid hormone concentra-

tion and metabolism in patients, who are considered to be euthyroid despite changes in the plasma concentrations of the different thyroid hormones outside the normal range. These alterations in thyroid hormone metabolism in otherwise euthyroid patients are referred to as the euthyroid sick syndrome (1).

Cytokines affect the thyroid, and they modulate many regulatory steps in thyroid hormone metabolism. Although cytokines may be involved both in (non)autoimmune thyroid disease and in the euthyroid sick syndrome, there is currently no clear perspective of cytokine-thyroid interaction in relation to separate thyroid disorders, because thyroid hormone metabolism is complex, and it involves multiple levels of regulation. In vitro, the effects of different cytokines on thyroid cells can be studied separately, but interpretation of these data may be difficult in relation to in vivo data. In vivo, the effects of cytokines on thyroid hormone metabolism cannot be evaluated separately, because each cytokine affects the entire cytokine network. Consequently, the pathogenetic role of cytokines in different, nonrelated diseases affecting thyroid function and morphology is far from being completely elucidated.

In this chapter, we summarize the effects of cytokines on the thyroid, not in relation to different thyroid diseases, but in relation to the different levels of regulation of thyroid hormone metabolism. Because most studies of the effects of cytokines on thyroid hormone metabolism have been performed with tumor necrosis factor (TNF), interleukin-1 (IL-1), IL-6, and interferon-γ (IFN-γ), we concentrate on these cytokines.

CYTOKINE RECEPTORS AND CYTOKINE PRODUCTION WITHIN THE THYROID GLAND

The presence of cytokine receptors and local cytokine production within the thyroid is of interest, because cytokines have mainly paracrine effects. Moreover, cytokines profoundly influence thyroid hormone synthesis in vitro, and they induce morphological changes in thyrocytes. These biological activities of cytokines are mediated by binding of cytokines to specific binding sites in thyroid cells. Cytokine binding has been studied in isolated thyrocytes obtained from thyroid glands and in thyroid cell lines, such as FRTL-5 cells. This is a well characterized, differentiated rat thyroid epithelial cell line that depends on TSH for growth, and it responds to stimuli known to affect thyroid cell metabolism. Specific binding sites for TNF have been demonstrated in FRTL-5 cells, as well as in different human thyroid cell lines (2–4). In human thyroid cells, receptors for IL-1, IL-6, and IFN-γ have also been demonstrated (4–6). Expression of cytokine binding sites in thyrocytes is influenced by TSH and cytokines. For instance, TSH appears to up-regulate TNF receptors in FRTL-5 cells (2). TNF-α probably augments IFN-γ binding to normal thyrocytes (4). TNF-α also induces a dose-dependent decrease in the specific binding of TNF-α to thyrocytes, a phenomenon that might be explained by down-regulation of TNF-α cell surface receptors by the cytokine (3).

In addition to expression of specific binding sites for cytokines, thyrocytes are also capable of producing cytokines. Purified thyroid follicular cells from patients with Graves' disease and patients with nontoxic goiter are reported to express high levels of messenger RNA (mRNA) for IL-1 α and IL-6, and they secreted IL-1α and IL-6 spontaneously in one study (7), although the data for IL-1 could not be reproduced in another report (8). Other studies indicate that thyrocytes from patients with Graves' disease, from para-adenomatous thyroid tissue, and from FRTL-5 cells, not only secrete IL-6 spontaneously but also that release of this cytokine is stimulated by TSH and other cytokines (e.g., TNF, IFN-γ, and IL-1)(9–12). Although IL-6 production by thyrocytes is enhanced by IL-1, IL-6 is not merely a second mediator of IL-1 on thyroid cells, because the effects of IL-6 on thyroid cells differ from those of IL-1 (10).

It was recently demonstrated that human thyroid cells from patients with different (non)autoimmune thyroid disorders also produce IL-8 spontaneously. IL-8 production was increased by IL-1. Whereas TSH and TNF had an inconsistent effect, IFN-γ reduced basal levels and IL-1 stimulated IL-8 production (13). The pathophysiological relevance of this observation is unclear, because the effects of IL-8 on thyroid function have not been described.

These data on cytokine production by thyrocytes were obtained ex vivo in isolated thyroid cells. There is also evidence for production of cytokines within the thyroid gland in vivo. In situ hybridization and immunohistochemistry techniques have provided evidence for in vivo production of IFN-γ, TNF-α, IL-1α, IL-1β, and IL-6 in freshly isolated tissue samples of thyroid glands from patients with various thyroid diseases (7,14,15). In these studies, it was shown that cytokine production in vivo is not restricted to infiltrating mononuclear cells in the thyroid, but it also involves thyroid follicular cells (7,14). Moreover, endothelial cells participate in cytokine-thyroid cell interactions. In thyroid glands obtained from patients with Graves' disease, IL-1β has been demonstrated on perifollicular endothelial cells (16), and endothelial cells are able to produce cytokines in response to stimuli (e.g., IL-1). The possibility also exists that cytokines are not only part of the pathophysiological regulation of thyroid functions, but also have a role in thyroid physiology, because IL-6 mRNA and IL-6 protein have been observed in samples of normal thyroid tissue (14).

Thus, thyroid epithelial cells have specific binding sites for multiple cytokines, and they are able to produce several cytokines in vivo and in vitro. These data provide evidence for the possibility of a complicated interaction of cytokines and TSH between plasma, endothelial cells, infiltrating mononuclear cells, and thyroid cells in nonautoimmune thyroid disease and nonthyroidal illness.

METABOLIC EFFECTS OF CYTOKINES IN THYROID CELLS

Synthesis and secretion of thyroid hormone in the thyroid follicles involves multiple sequential steps (Fig. 20–1) (17): (a) active uptake of iodide from plasma; (b) thyroglobulin production; (c) iodination of tyrosyl residues of thyroglobulin catalyzed by thyroid peroxidase (TPO); (d) coupling of iodotyrosin molecules, also catalyzed by TPO, within thyroglobulin, to form T_4 and T_3; (e) proteolysis of thyroglobulin, with release of free iodothyronines and reutilization of iodide; and (f) secretion of T_4 and T_3 into blood. In vitro effects of cytokines on iodide uptake (step a), thyroglobulin and TPO production (involved in steps b–d), protein iodination (step c), and T_3 secretion (step f), have been documented.

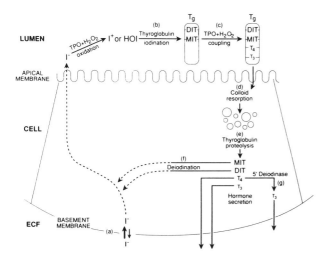

Figure 20–1 Thyroid hormone synthesis and release. Cytokines, such as IL-1, TNF-α, IL-6, and IFN-γ affect the regulation of thyroid hormone metabolism in thyroid cells at multiple levels. Effects of cytokines on iodide transport, TPO, thyroglobulin metabolism, and thyroid hormone secretion have been documented (see pages 318–320). (Adapted from Taurog A. Hormone synthesis: thyroid iodine metabolism. In: Braverman LE, Utiger RD, eds. The thyroid, ed 6. Philadelphia: J. B. Lippincott, 1991:51–97.)

Iodide uptake

Iodide uptake from plasma by thyroid follicle cells is an active TSH-dependent process. In TSH-stimulated thyrocytes, iodide concentrations may be 500-fold higher than plasma iodide concentrations. TSH-stimulated [125J] uptake is inhibited by TNF in a dose-dependent manner in FRTL-5 cells (2,18–20). This inhibition of TSH-stimulated iodide uptake by TNF is found not only in experimental cell lines but also in human thyrocytes (21). These in vitro data are confirmed in vivo, because TNF administration to rats results in decreased thyroid [125J] uptake compared with control animals (22). Comparable in vitro results have been obtained with IL-1: This cytokine inhibits both basal and TSH-stimulated iodine uptake in FRTL-5 cells (18).

The effects of IFN-γ are less clear, and they depend on the system in which it is tested. In FRTL-5 cells, IFN-γ stimulates basal iodide uptake, and it enhances the effects of TSH on iodine uptake (20,23,24). However, in cultured human thyrocytes, TSH-induced [125J] uptake is inhibited in a dose-dependent manner (21). TNF, which inhibits TSH-stimulated iodine uptake, augments the enhancing effect of IFN-γ on TSH-stimulated [125J] uptake in FRTL-5 cells (20), whereas it potentiates the inhibitory effect of IFN-γ in human thyrocytes (21).

The mechanisms underlying the modulations in iodide uptake in thyroid cells by cytokines are not entirely clear.

Because TSH stimulates iodide uptake through binding to receptors, one possibility is that cytokines may affect TSH binding. This potential mechanism has been excluded for the effects of TNF. TNF treatment does not affect TSH binding in human and rat thyroid cells, nor does it compete with TSH for the binding of TSH to its receptor (2). This finding suggests that the effects of at least TNF are on the postreceptor action of TSH: on cyclic adenosine monophosphate (cAMP) levels or on a cAMP-mediated process. Basal and TSH-stimulated generation of cAMP in FRTL-5 cells is not influenced by TNF, but the effects of cAMP in these cells is inhibited by TNF and IL-1, suggesting that the effect of these cytokines is probably distal to cAMP generation. However, in a subsequent study, Pang and colleagues (18) showed that TNF did not inhibit basal and TSH-stimulated generation of cAMP. Although activation of phospholipase A_2 is the mechanism of action of TNF in nonthyroid cell lines, and although the phospholipase A_2 system is present in thyroid cell lines, the influence of TNF on FRTL-5 cells appears to not be mediated by this pathway (18).

From these findings it is evident that the mechanisms of action of cytokines on thyrocytes are still unclear. The nature and mechanisms of interaction between cytokines such as TNF and IFN-γ with respect to the effects on iodide uptake is even more subject to speculation, and they seem to depend at least in part on experimental conditions and the system in which a cytokine is tested.

Thyroglobulin synthesis

Thyroglobulin is a large protein with a molecular weight of 660,000 daltons. Cloning of human thyroglobulin complementary DNA (cDNA) fragments has provided probes that allow analysis of thyroglobulin gene expression in thyrocytes. Thyroglobulin gene expression and secretion by thyrocytes is stimulated by TSH. In isolated thyrocytes obtained from thyroid glands of patients with Graves' disease, expression of TSH-induced thyroglobulin mRNA is inhibited in a dose-related manner by IL-1α and IL-1β, as well as by IFN-γ (24,25). In accordance, IFN-γ decreases basal and TSH-stimulated incorporation of [35S] methionine in thyroglobulin in FRTL-5 cells (26), indicating decreased synthesis of thyroglobulin. Likewise, the TSH-induced release of thyroglobulin is inhibited by IL-1α in a dose-dependent manner in FRTL-5 cells (26). In accordance, in thyrocytes obtained from patients with Graves' disease, IFN-γ inhibits TSH-stimulated thyroglobulin secretion in a dose-dependent manner (27). In thyrocytes obtained from para-adenomatous tissue obtained during thyroidectomies, IL-1 caused dose-dependent suppression of the secretion of thyroglobulin, whereas IL-6 had no effect (10,28).

Thus, thyroglobulin metabolism seems to be inhibited by IL-1 and IFN-γ regardless of the system in which it is tested. IL-6 seems to have no effect.

Iodination

Iodination of tyrosine residues in the thyroglobulin molecule involves multiple steps. Thyroglobulin is transported through the endoplasmic reticular system to the apical part of the thyroid cell, where it interacts with TPO, which is abundantly present in the apical plasma membrane. TPO oxidizes iodide by use of H_2O_2, and it subsequently incorporates oxidized iodide in tyrosines in the thyroglobulin molecule, resulting in the formation of monoiodothyronine (MIT) and, by addition of a second iodide atom, in di-iodothyronine (DIT). TSH stimulates TPO gene expression and content in thyrocytes (17).

Cytokines affect TPO metabolism. TSH-stimulated TPO gene expression is inhibited by IL-α, IFN-γ, and IL-6 in cultured thyrocytes obtained from thyroid glands of patients with Graves' disease (6,29,30). In accordance, IFN-γ reduces basal content and TSH-induced increase of TPO in similarly obtained thyrocytes, indicating that the decrease in TPO gene expression induced by IFN-γ is indeed associated with decreased TPO synthesis (31). Because patients with a TPO defect have hypothyroidism (32), a decrease in TPO content induced by cytokines might affect thyroid function.

The effect of cytokines on iodination has been studied in a model of porcine thyroid follicles (33) and in human thyrocytes (21). In the porcine model, the effect of IL-1 was studied. The results were not very clear because the effects of IL-1 were difficult to interpret due to combined effects of IL-1 concentrations, TSH concentration, and time. Data obtained in the human thyrocytes were straightforward. TNF-α, IL-1, and IFN-γ inhibit de novo synthesis of MIT, DIT, T_3, and T_4, and the combination of cytokines more than additively inhibits TSH-induced [^{125}J] incorporation (21).

Therefore, the different cytokines tested seem to generally have an inhibiting effect on TPO metabolism and iodination.

Thyroid hormone secretion

In addition to the mentioned effects of cytokines on thyroid hormone synthesis, cytokines affect thyroid hormone secretion by thyrocytes, mainly in an inhibitory way. The effects have only been tested in human thyrocytes. IFN-γ inhibits TSH-stimulated secretion, but not basal T_3 secretion, by cultured human thyrocytes (27,34). Likewise, IL-6 inhibited TSH-induced T_3 secretion in a dose-dependent manner (6). Sato and colleagues (21) observed that IFN-γ, TNF-α, and IL-1 inhibit secretion of [^{125}J] T_4 and [^{125}J]T_3 into the medium. These inhibitory effects of cytokines on thyroid hormone secretion are probably at least partially related to the mentioned inhibitory effects on thyroid hormone synthesis.

MITOGENIC EFFECTS OF CYTOKINES ON THYROID CELLS

Mitogenic and morphological effects of cytokines on thyroid cells have been studied in different systems. The results are contradictory, and they seem to be dependent on the system used.

IFN-γ induces a dose-dependent inhibition of tritium thymidine incorporation (a reflection of cell proliferation), DNA content, and cell count in human thyroid cells (34,35). In FRTL-5 cells, the results are contradictory. In some studies, inhibitory effects of IFN-γ on tritium thymidine incorporation were found (20,26), whereas in another study, a stimulatory effect was observed (36).

TNF-α stimulated cell proliferation, measured by tritium thymidine incorporation and paralleled by changes in DNA and protein content in human thyrocytes. As with IFN-γ, the effects of TNF in FRTL-5 cells are not equivocal. The effect of cell age on TNF sensitivity was studied in young and old FRTL-5 cells (36). Although stimulation by TNF of tritium thymidine incorporation paralleled by changes in DNA and protein content were found in young cells, an increase in tritium thymidine incorporation was also found in old cells, but DNA content and cell number decreased dramatically in these cells. Apparently, increasing cell age induces an increase in sensitivity to the cytotoxic effects of TNF (36).

IL-1α and IL-1β stimulate tritium thymidine incorporation into thyrocytes from normal subjects and from patients with Graves' disease (8,24), as well as into FRTL-5 cells (18,37,38). In the presence of TSH, however, IL-1 caused a significant reduction in both tritium thymidine incorporation into FRTL-5 cells (37) and DNA synthesis in papillary, but not follicular, thyroid carcinoma cells (38).

It is evident that some of the data on the effects of cytokines on cell proliferation are conflicting, which may at least partly be explained by differences in experimental conditions or dual control of thyroid cell proliferation by individual cytokines. In this respect, prostaglandins are of interest, because human thyrocytes are able to produce PGE_2 in response to IL-1, and prostaglandins may inhibit cell proliferation. In accordance, indomethacin inhibited thyrocyte PGE_2 release, and it augmented the proliferative response of thyrocytes to IL-1 (8). IL-1 may therefore have both positive and negative effects on growth control. In normal thyrocytes, this dual control would limit uncontrolled cell proliferation.

IMMUNOLOGICAL EFFECTS OF CYTOKINES ON THYROID CELLS

Interest in the effects of IFN-γ was greatly stimulated by the observation of Todd and associates (39), that IFN-γ could induce human leukocyte antigen-DR (HLA-DR) expression on follicular thyroid cells, which are normally negative for HLA-DR molecules (39). These authors previously found that thyroid epithelial cells from patients with autoimmune thyroid diseases strongly express major histocompatibility complex (MHC) class II molecules (or HLA-DR), in contrast to normal thyroid cells (40). Bottazzo and colleagues (41) therefore hypothesized that aberrant HLA-DR expression may cause immunogenic presentation of autoantigens in association with HLA-DR and initiate T-cell activation, which results in autoimmune disease. Thyrocyte HLA-DR expression is not generally (or effectively) induced by nonspecific environmental factors, but it is secondary only to a specific immune assault in autoimmune disease (42).

The effects of IFN-γ on HLA-DR expression of thyroid cells are modulated by TSH, IL-1, and TNF-α, although these factors alone do not affect HLA-DR expression (4,43–45). IL-6 does not affect HLA class I or II expression, neither alone nor in combination with IFN-γ (45).

Intrathyroidal T-cell populations could serve as a source of lymphokines that modulate HLA-DR expression (46). Because the effects of IFN-γ on HLA-DR expression occur at the same concentration and in experimental conditions as those found to be effective on the modulation of metabolic and mitogenic functions of cultured thyrocytes (34), cytokine-thyroid cell interactions may be implicated in initiation or perpetuation of morphological, functional, and immunological changes observed in autoimmune thyroid disease.

EFFECTS OF CYTOKINE ADMINISTRATION ON THYROID HORMONE METABOLISM IN VIVO

In addition to documented in vitro effects on intrathyroidal thyroid hormone synthesis and secretion, administration of cytokines affects in vivo thyroid hormone metabolism. The effects of cytokines on extrathyroidal thyroid hormone metabolism are of special interest with regard to the euthyroid sick syndrome. This syndrome occurs in association with many conditions, such as acute and chronic infectious diseases, surgery, and malignant disorders. These changes in thyroid hormone metabolism are more or less similar and unrelated to the underlying diseases, although a few exceptions exist (e.g., renal fail-

ure, human immunodeficiency virus infection) (1,47). Rather, manifestations of the euthyroid sick syndrome are related to severity of illness (48). Figure 20–2 represents the relative changes in circulating thyroid hormones related to severity of illness. During the initial phases of mild nonthyroidal illness, a decreased plasma T_3 concentration, with a concomitant increase of reverse T_3 concentration, is readily observed. Mild systemic illness may also result in elevated concentrations of total T_4 and free FT_4, especially during recovery of nonthyroidal illness (49). In contrast, in critical illness, T_4 concentrations may become very low, and they are associated with a high mortality (50). Despite profound changes in circulating thyroid hormone concentrations in nonthyroidal illness, plasma TSH concentrations are usually within normal limits, although decreased or slightly increased TSH values are occasionally observed in patients with nonthyroidal illness (49,51). It has been suggested that critical illness may induce secondary hypothyroidism, as evidenced by normal or decreased TSH values in the presence of low T_3/T_4 syndrome. The occurrence of secondary hypothyroidism is disputed, however, because free T_4 and T_3 concentrations are usually within normal range. Nonetheless, there are indications for altered hypothalamic-pituitary-thyroid relationships (51).

It is evident that nonthyroidal illness induces changes in virtually all levels of extrathyroidal regulation of thyroid hormone metabolism (1,48,52). The euthyroid sick syndrome involves changes in central regulation of TSH secretion, thyroid hormone secretion, binding of thyroid hormones to plasma proteins, peripheral uptake of thyroxine, peripheral nondeiodinative pathways, T_3 binding to nuclear receptors, and postreceptor effects of T_3.

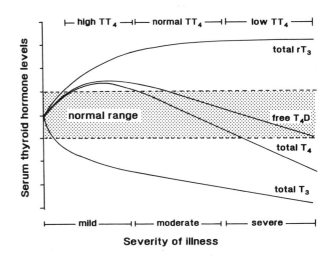

Figure 20–2 Changes in plasma thyroid hormone levels in patients with nonthyroidal illness relative to the severity of illness. (Reproduced by permission from Kaptein EM. Thyroid hormone metabolism in illness. In: Henneman G, ed. Thyroid hormone metabolism. New York: Marcel Dekker, 1986:297–333.)

Recently, it has become apparent that mediators such as cytokines are essential factors in the pathogenesis of both acute and chronic diseases. Although the mechanisms underlying nonthyroidal illness are probably multifactorial, it is possible that these mediators may be involved in the alterations in thyroid hormone metabolism observed in nonthyroidal illness. The effects of cytokines on thyroid hormone metabolism in vivo have been studied both in humans and in animal experiments.

Cytokines are able to modulate major determinants of thyroid hormone metabolism in vivo (Fig. 20–3). In general, these effects of cytokines are dose-dependent and time-dependent. Administration of higher doses of IL-1 and TNF-α to rats and mice has more pronounced effects on thyroid hormone indices than administration of lower doses (53–56). Prolonged administration of IL-1 and TNF-α to rats, however, is associated with down-regulation of the effects on thyroid hormone metabolism, similar to that reported for other biological effects of cytokines (53,56,57). In addition to dose-dependent and time-dependent effects, the effects of cytokines on thyroid hormones depend on species characteristics of thyroid hormone metabolism. For instance, the half-life of thyroxine in rats is much shorter than in humans (14–16 hours vs 8 days). Therefore, changes in thyroxine secretion induced by cytokines are likely to be more rapidly detectable in rodents than in humans.

Administration of TNF and IL-1 to rodents and TNF to humans results in changes of plasma T_3, T_4, and TSH concentrations (53,55–60) (Figs. 20–4 to 20–6). These effects

of cytokines are associated with modulation of the hypothalamic-pituitary-thyroid axis at multiple levels (see Fig. 20–3). Hypothalamic TRH content in rats is decreased by a single dose of TNF and by increasing doses of TNF, but not by multiple injections of low-dose TNF (22). These changes are associated with similar changes in pituitary TSH β-subunit mRNA, but not α-subunit mRNA, as well as with parallel changes in plasma TSH concentrations (22). Thus, the decrease in pituitary TSH secretion induced by TNF is probably related to decreased TRH stimulation, reflected in hypothalamic TRH content. Stimulation of type II 5′-deiodinase activity within the pituitary gland is another explanation for decreased TSH concentrations observed after cytokine administration in vivo. Increased type II 5′-deiodinase activity causes increased conversion of T_4 into T_3 in the pituitary gland, resulting in decreased TSH secretion. IL-1 has been reported to stimulate 5′-deiodinase activity in the brain cortex of rats

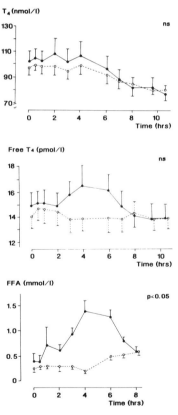

Figure 20–4   Plasma T_4, free T_4, and free fatty acid concentrations (mean ± SE) after intravenous bolus injection of recombinant human TNF (50 µg/m²; *closed circles*) or an equivalent volume of isotonic saline (*open circles*) to 6 healthy subjects. Free T_4 concentrations increased transiently in 5 of 6 subjects after TNF administration. Concomitantly, a transient increase in plasma FFA concentrations was found in all subjects. (Adapted from Van der Poll T, Romijn JA, Wiersinga WM, Sauerwein HP. Tumor necrosis factor: a putative mediator of the euthyroid sick syndrome in man. J Clin Endocrinol Metab 1991;71:1567–1572.)

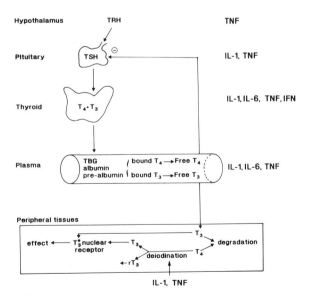

Figure 20–3   Whole body thyroid hormone metabolism. Administration of cytokines modulates the regulation of thyroid hormone metabolism at multiple levels. (Adapted from Wiersinga WM, Krenning EP. Laboratorium diagnostick van hyper-en hypothyreodic. In: Wiersinga WM, Krenning EP: Schildklierziekten. Alphen, The Netherlands: Samson Stafleu, 1988:73–97.)

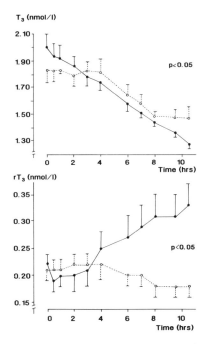

Figure 20–5 Plasma T_3 and rT_3 concentrations (mean ± SE) after intravenous bolus injection of recombinant human TNF (50 µg/m²; *closed circles*) or an equivalent volume of isotonic saline (*open circles*) to 6 healthy subjects. TNF induced a significant decrease in T_3 concentrations and a significant increase in rT_3 concentrations. (Adapted from Van der Poll T, Romijn JA, Wiersinga WM, Sauerwein HP. Tumor necrosis factor: a putative mediator of the euthyroid sick syndrome in man. J Clin Endocrinol Metab 1991;71:1567–1572.)

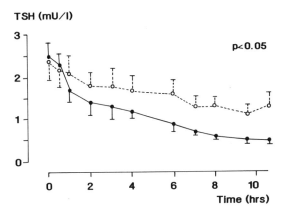

Figure 20–6 Plasma TSH concentrations (mean ± SE) after intravenous bolus injection of recombinant human TNF (50 µg/m²; *closed circles*) or an equivalent volume of isotonic saline (*open circles*) to 6 healthy subjects. TNF induced a significant decrease in TSH concentrations. (Reproduced by permission from Van der Poll T, Romijn JA, Wiersinga WM, Sauerwein HP. Tumor necrosis factor: a putative mediator of the euthyroid sick syndrome in man. J Clin Endocrinol Metab 1991;71:1567–1572.)

(57). The data on the effects of IL-1 on pituitary TSH metabolism are conflicting, because IL-1 administration to mice resulted in an increased pituitary TSH content (58).

In line with the study by Pang and colleagues (22), Sweep and associates (56) showed that continuous, subpyrogenic dose administration of TNF to rats did not affect plasma TSH concentrations or TSH responsiveness to TRH. In humans, a single pyrogenic dose of TNF induced a decline in TSH concentrations (59). These data indicate that high doses of TNF-α decrease TSH secretion in animals and humans, whereas (multiple) low-dose administration of TNF has no effect, at least in animals.

TNF not only affects TSH secretion, but also TSH bioactivity. TNF treatment reduced the binding of pituitary TSH to concanavalin A, indicating that TNF alters the glycosylation of TSH. The altered bioactivity of TSH was confirmed in vitro. TSH with reduced affinity for concanavalin A had reduced metabolic effects on FRTL-5 cells (22).

The effects of IL-1 on regulation of TSH secretion have been studied less extensively than those of TNF, and the results are not equivocal. In vitro, IL-1β stimulates TSH secretion by dispersed pituitary cells (60). However, in rats, a single injection and administration of continuous, high doses of IL-1 are associated with decreased plasma

TSH concentrations (55,57), in contrast to the stimulatory effects of IL-1 in vitro (60). Similar to TNF, continuous administration of low doses of IL-1 did not significantly alter TSH concentrations in rats (55). Despite decreased free T_4 levels, the decrease in plasma TSH concentrations induced by IL-1 was associated with impaired TSH responsiveness to TRH, indicating that the alterations in TSH secretion induced by IL-1 were not merely explained by decreased TRH stimulation, but that other factors must also be involved (55).

The hypothalamic-pituitary-thyroid axis is not only modulated by cytokines at hypothalamic and pituitary gland levels, but also at the thyroid level. In vitro, cytokines have profound effects on thyroid hormone synthesis and secretion, as described previously. These in vitro data are supported by evidence obtained in vivo. Administration of TNF in rats reduced thyroid [^{125}J] uptake, similar to FRTL-5 cells in vitro (22). Furthermore, in TNF- and IL-1–treated rats and mice, the T_3 and T_4 response to TSH was greatly diminished in comparison to pair-fed control animals (53–56). These studies suggest that the function of the thyroid gland is altered by cytokines in vivo.

There are also indications for altered feedback regulation between the thyroid hormones and pituitary TSH secretion. Administration of high doses of TNF in healthy subjects decreased TSH concentrations in the presence of low T_3 concentrations, whereas T_4 and free T_4 concentrations were not significantly changed (59). Similar changes were observed in animals after IL-1 and TNF administration (53,56,57). Therefore, the decrease of plasma TSH concentrations induced by cytokines would not have been expected in the presence of normal pituitary-thyroid feedback regulation.

In the euthyroid sick syndrome, decreased concentrations and decreased binding affinity of plasma proteins binding thyroid hormones are commonly found (50). Cytokines may also affect the concentration of plasma thyroid hormone binding proteins. In vitro, IL-6 caused a dose-dependent and time-dependent decrease in gene expression and secretion of T_4-binding globulin (TBG) by human hepatoblastoma-derived cells (61). In addition, IL-6 induced a decrease in the transcription of other major thyroid hormone-binding proteins, transthyretin and albumin (61). Likewise, TNF-α affects albumin gene expression and albumin synthesis by the liver (62,63). In contrast to humans, in rats, plasma T_4 is predominantly bound to T_4-binding prealbumin (TBPA) and, to a lesser extent, to albumin. Administration of TNF-α and IL-1 to rats results in a transient reduction of TBPA (56,57).

Although cytokines may affect the synthesis of plasma thyroid hormone binding proteins directly, binding affinity of those proteins may be altered in nonthyroidal illness by the induction of circulating factors, such as free fatty acids (FFA) (64). A bolus injection of TNF-α increases plasma FFA levels in association with an increase in free T_4 levels in healthy subjects (59) (see Fig. 20–4). However, an increase of FFA concentrations was not induced by low-dose infusion of TNF in rats, although an increased percentage of free T_4 was observed (56). Cytokines are able to change binding of thyroid hormones to plasma proteins directly or indirectly. This change may be induced by very low doses of cytokines, such as TNF, that do not affect the pituitary-thyroid axis or peripheral thyroid hormone metabolism (56).

In addition to effects on the pituitary-thyroid axis, the thyroid, and plasma proteins, cytokines also modulate peripheral thyroid hormone metabolism. In humans with NTI, serum T_3 levels are decreased, but reverse T_3 levels are, in general, reciprocally increased (1,50). The two key enzymes that regulate peripheral conversion are type I 5'-deiodinase (5'D-I), predominantly found in liver and kidney, and type II 5'-deiodinase (5'D-II), which predominantly resides in brain and pituitary gland. In NTI, 5'D-I activity is impaired, resulting in decreased peripheral conversion of T_4 to T_3 and diminished clearance of rT_3, which causes low serum T_3 and high reverse T_3 levels. In human subjects, TNF administration results in decreased T_3 levels, decreased T_3/T_4 ratios, and increased rT_3 concentrations, which is in line with decreased 5'D-I activity (59) (see Fig. 20–5). In rats, the effects of TNF on deiodinase activity are not completely clear because TNF administration decreases 5'D-I activity after a single bolus, it increases 5'D-I activity after multiple injections, and it does not influence the plasma T_3/T_4 ratio or hepatic 5'D-I activity after low dose continuous administration (22–56). In mice, however, the plasma T_3/T_4 ratio and 5'D-I levels are higher in TNF-treated mice than in pair-fed control animals, an effect opposite to that in

rats (54). IL-1 administration to rats does not affect the T_3/T_4 ratio of 5'D-I activity (55), whereas in IL-1–treated mice, the plasma T_3/T_4 ratio, plasma rT_3 concentrations, and hepatic 5'D-I activity are increased (53). Therefore, the results of both TNF and IL-1 administration on peripheral thyroid hormone metabolism are contradictory, which may to some extent be the result of species differences in peripheral thyroid hormone metabolism in general. Alternatively, there are also dose-dependent or dual effects of TNF and IL-1 on peripheral thyroid hormone metabolism.

In vitro and in vivo, the effects of cytokines on thyroid functions resemble to a great extent the changes observed in nonthyroidal illness. It is therefore tempting to speculate that cytokines are at least partly involved in the pathogenesis of the euthyroid sick syndrome in many unrelated diseases. Nonetheless, this issue is not completely resolved. In general, in the experiments on thyroid hormone metabolism, pharmacological amounts of cytokines were administered, whereas in most nonthyroidal illness, cytokines are hardly detectable in plasma. Although many of the in vivo effects of cytokines can be reproduced in vitro, it is uncertain that the changes induced by cytokines in vivo in thyroid hormone metabolism are direct effects of cytokines or indirect effects induced by systemic illness caused by cytokines. For instance, Chopra and associates (65) observed no appreciable relationship between TNF-α and iodothyronine levels in patients with NTI. However, it is possible that plasma cytokine concentrations are not a good indicator for paracrine cytokine production, and that, as a result, it is unlikely to find such a relationship between cytokines and plasma thyroid hormone concentrations.

There are also discrepancies between the effects of cytokines and nonthyroidal illness. For instance, in IL-1–treated rodents, there is no indication of decreased 5'D-I activity (53,55), although this is a common feature of the euthyroid sick syndrome. An alternative approach to address the relation between NTI and cytokines is to study thyroid hormone metabolism after immunoneutralization of cytokines in an animal model of nonthyroidal illness to examine the role of different cytokines on thyroid hormone metabolism, but studies employing this approach have not been published.

THYROID DYSFUNCTION ASSOCIATED WITH CYTOKINE THERAPY

In general, malignancies are not associated with other changes in thyroid hormone metabolism than those found in the euthyroid sick syndrome. In contrast, thyroid dysfunction has been described, in addition to features of the euthyroid sick syndrome, in a number of clinical trials using cytokine therapy for patients with malignancies or chronic hepatitis. Treatment with IFN-α and high-dose IL-2, alone or in combination with IFN-α or lymphokine-activated killer (LAK) cells, was associated with a remarkably high incidence of de novo thyroid dysfunction (66–71), especially when administered repetitively over a prolonged period (68). Both hyperthyroidism (especially after the start of therapy) and hypothyroidism (after prolonged therapy) have been reported during treatment with IFN-α alone, or during combination therapy with IL-2 and TNF-α or IL-2 and TNF (68,70,72). It has been suggested that this sequential pattern of thyroid hormone abnormalities resembles the pattern found in the clinical course of thyroiditis (67,70). Immunocytochemistry of fine-needle aspiration of the thyroid in these patients revealed changes consistent with autoimmune thyroiditis with a mixed lymphocytic/histiocytic infiltrate and strong staining of thyrocytes for HLA class II antigens (67). However, in contrast to autoimmune thyroiditis, such as Hashimoto's disease, thyroiditis associated with cytokine therapy is self-limited (67). Despite the appealing hypothesis that autoimmunity is responsible for the thyroid dysfunction observed with immunotherapy, the evidence is only circumstantial. In a prospective study, de novo antithyroid antibodies developed in no patients, although thyroid dysfunction developed in virtually all patients (68). Therefore, thyroid dysfunction during immunotherapy may also be secondary to nonspecific, nonautoimmune, toxic mechanisms (68,69). As described in the section on cytokine effects on the thyroid gland, IL-1, TNF, IFN-γ, and IL-6 affect thyroid hormone synthesis and secretion in vitro. IL-2 and IFN-α therapy may induce these cytokines (73), and they are therefore able to interfere indirectly with thyroid hormone metabolism.

CONCLUSIONS

The effects of cytokines on thyroid function and extrathyroidal thyroid hormone metabolism present challenging concepts regarding the pathogenesis of thyroid disorders and the euthyroid sick syndrome. Moreover, cytokines may have a role in the physiological (perhaps paracrine) regulation of thyroid function.

REFERENCES

1. Wartofsky L, Burman KD. Alterations in thyroid function in patients with systemic illness: the "euthyroid sick syndrome." Endocr Rev 1982;3:164–217.

2. Pang XP, Hershman JM, Chung M, Pekary AE. Characterization of tumor necrosis factor-alpha receptors in human and rat thyroid cells and regulation of the receptors by thyrotropin. Endocrinology 1989;125:1783–1788.

3. Deus U, Buscema M, Schumacher H, Winkelmann W. In vitro effects of tumor necrosis factor-α in human thyroid follicular cells. Acta Endocrinol (Copenh) 1992;127:220–225.

4. Buscema M, Todd I, Deuss U, et al. Influence of tumor necrosis factor-α on the modulation by interferon-gamma on HLA class II molecules in human thyroid cells and its effect on interferon-gamma binding. J Clin Endocrinol Metab 1989;69:433–439.

5. Svenson M, Kayser L, Hansen MB, Krogh Rasmussen Å, Bendtzen K. Interleukin-1 receptors on human thyroid cells and on the rat thyroid cell line FRTL-5. Cytokine 1991;3:125–130.

6. Tominaga T, Yamashita S, Nagayama Y, et al. Interleukin-6 inhibits human thyroid peroxidase gene expression. Acta Endocrinol (Copenh) 1991;124:290–294.

7. Grubeck-Loebenstein B, Buchan G, Chantry D, et al. Analysis of intrathyroidal cytokine production in thyroid autoimmune disease: thyroid follicular cells produce interleukin-1 alpha and interleukin-6. Clin Exp Immunol 1989;77:324–330.

8. Kawabe Y, Eguchi K, Shinokara C, et al. Interleukin-1 production and action in thyroid tissue. J Clin Endocrinol Metab 1989;68:1174–1183.

9. Weetman AP, Bright-Thomas R, Freeman M. Regulation of interleukin-6 release by human thyrocytes. J Endocrinol 1990;127:357–361.

10. Rasmussen ÅK, Kayser L, Feldt-Rasmussen U, et al. Interleukin-6 is not a second mediator of interleukin-1 induced suppression of thyroid function in cultured human thyrocytes. Exp Clin Endocrinol 1991;97:179–181.

11. Iwamoto M, Sakihama T, Kimnoea N, Tasaha K, Onaya T. Augmented interleukin-6 production by rat thyrocytes (FRTL-5): effect of interleukin 1β and thyroid stimulating hormone. Cytokine 1991;3:345–349.

12. Kennedy RL, Jones TH, Davies R, Justice SK, Lemoine NR. Release of interleukin-6 by human thyroid epithelial cells immortalized by simian virus 40 DNA transfection. J Endocrinol 1992;133:477–482.

13. Weetman AP, Bennett GL, Wong WLT. Thyroid follicular cells produce interleukin-8. J Clin Endocrinol Metab 1992;75:328–330.

14. Zheng RQH, Abney E, Chu CQ, et al. Detection of interleukin-6 and interleukin-1 production in human thyroid epithelial cells by non-radioactive in situ hybridization and immunohistochemical methods. Clin Exp Immunol 1991;83:314–319.

15. Rutenfranz I, Kruse A, Rink L, Wenzel B, Arnholdt H, Kirchner H. In situ hybridization of the mRNA for interferon-gamma, interferon-α, interferon-β, interleukin-1β and interleukin-6 and characterization of infiltrating cells in thyroid tissues. J Immunol Meth 1992;148:233–242.

16. Miyazaki A, Hanafusa T, Itoh N, et al. Demonstration of interleukin-1β on perifollicular endothelial cells in the thyroid glands of patients with Graves' disease. J Clin Endocrinol Metab 1989;69:738–744.

17. Taurog A. Hormone synthesis: thyroid iodine metabolism. In: Braverman LE, Utiger RD, eds. The thyroid, ed 6. Philadelphia: J. B. Lippincott, 1991:51–97.

18. Pang XP, Hershman JM, Smith V, Pekary AE, Sugawara M. The mechanism of action of tumour necrosis factor-α and interleukin-1 on FRTL-5 rat thyroid cells. Acta Endocrinol (Copenh) 1990;123:203–210.

19. Padwardhan NA, Lombardi A. Effects of tumor necrosis factor on growth and function in FRTL5 cells. Surgery 1991;110:972–977.

20. Zakarija M, Mckenzie JM. Influence of cytokines on growth and differentiated function of FRTL5 cells. Endocrinology 1989;125:1260–1265.

21. Sato K, Satoh T, Shizume K, et al. Inhibition of ^{125}J organification and thyroid hormone release by interleukin-1, tumor necrosis factor-α, and interferon gamma in human thyrocytes in suspension culture. J Clin Endocrinol Metab 1990;70:1735–1743.

22. Pang XP, Hershman JM, Mirell CJ, Pekary AE. Impairment of hypothalamic-pituitary-thyroid function in rats treated with human recombinant tumor necrosis factor-α (cachectin). Endocrinology 1989;125:76–84.

23. Weetman AP. Recombinant gamma-interferon stimulates iodide uptake and cyclic AMP production by FRTL5 thyroid cell line. FEBS Lett 1987;221:91–94.

24. Yamashita S, Kimura H, Ashizawa K, et al. Interleukin-1 inhibits thyrotropin-induced human thyroglobulin gene expression. J Endocrinol 1989;122:177–183.

25. Kury AWC, Lau KS. Interferon-gamma inhibit thyrotropin-induced thyroglobulin gene transcription in cultured human thyrocytes. J Clin Endocrinol Metab 1990;70:1512–1517.

26. Misaki T, Tramontano D, Ingbar SH. Effects of rat gamma- and non-gamma-interferons on the expression of Ia antigen, growth, and differentiated functions of FRTL5 cells. Endocrinology 1988;123:2849–2857.

27. Nagayama Y, Izumi M, Ashizawa K, et al. Inhibitory effect of interferon-gamma on the response of human thyrocytes to thyrotropin (TSH) stimulation: relationship between the response to TSH and the expression of DR antigen. J Clin Endocrinol Metab 1987;64:949–953.

28. Rasmussen ÅK, Bech K, Feldt-Rasmussen U, et al. The influence of Interleukin-1 on the function of in vitro cultured human thyroid cells in monolayers. Acta Endocrinol (Copenh) 1987;281(suppl):93–95.

29. Ashizawa K, Yamashita S, Nagayama Y, et al. Interferon-gamma inhibits thyroidal peroxidase gene expression in cultured human thyrocytes. J Clin Endocrinol Metab 1989;69:475–477.

30. Ashizawa K, Yamashita S, Tobinga T, et al. Inhibition of human thyroid peroxidase gene expression by interleukin 1. Acta Endocrinol (Copenh) 1989;121:465–469.

31. Asakawa H, Hanafusa T, Kobayashi T, Takai S, Kono N, Tarui S. Interferon-gamma reduces the thyroid peroxidase content of cultured human thyrocytes and inhibits its increase by thyrotropin. J Clin Endocrinol Metab 1992;74:1331–1335.

32. Medeiros-Neto GA, Okamura K, Cavaliere H, et al. Familial thyroid peroxidase defect. Clin Endocrinol (Oxf) 1982;17:1–14.

33. Westermark K, Nilsson M, Karlsson FA. Effects of interleukin alpha on porcine thyroid follicles in suspension culture. Acta Endocrinol (Copenh) 1990;122:505–512.

34. Kraiem Z, Sobel E, Sadeh O, Kinarty A, Lahat N. Effects of

35. Zakarija M, Hornicek FJ, Levis S, Mckenzie JM. Effects of gamma-interferon and tumor necrosis factor α on thyroid cells: induction of class II antigen and inhibition of growth stimulation. Mol Cell Endocrinol 1988;58:129–136.

36. Chen G, Pekary AE, Hershman JM. Aging of FRTL-5 rat thyroid cells causes sensitivity to cytotoxicity induced by tumor necrosis factor-α. Endocrinology 1992;131:863–870.

37. Zeki K, Azuma H, Suzuki H, Morimoto I, Eto S. Effects of interleukin-1 on growth and adenosine 3',5'-monophosphate generation of the rat thyroid cell line, FRTL-5 cells. Acta Endocrinol (Copenh) 1991;124:60–66.

38. Mine M, Tramontano D, Chin WW, Ingbar SH. Interleukin-1 stimulates thyroid cell growth and increases the concentration of the c-myc proto-oncogene mRNA in thyroid follicular cells in culture. Endocrinology 1987;120:1212–1214.

39. Todd I, Pujol-Borrell R, Hammond LJ, Bottazzo GF, Feldmann M. Interferon gamma induces HLA-DR expression by thyroid epithelium. Clin Exp Immunol 1985;61:265–273.

40. Hanafusa T, Chiovato L, Domach D, Pujol-Borrell R, Russell RCG, Bottazzo GF. Aberrant expression of HLA-DR antigen on thyrocytes in Graves' disease: relevance for autoimmunity. Lancet 1983;2:1111–1115.

41. Bottazzo GF, Pujol-Borrell R, Hanafusa T, Feldmann M. Role of aberrant HLA-DR expression and antigen presentation induction of endocrine autoimmunity. Lancet 1983;2:1115–1118.

42. Iwatani Y, Gerstein HC, Iitaka M, Row VV, Volpé R. Thyrocyte HLA-DR expression and interferon-gamma production in autoimmune thyroid disease. J Clin Endocrinol Metab 1986;63:695–708.

43. Platzer M, Neufeld DS, Piccinini LA, Davies TF. Induction of rat thyroid cell MHC class II antigen by thyrotropin and gamma-interferon. Endocrinology 1987;121:2087–2092.

44. Piccinini LA, Mackenzie WA, Platzer M, Davies TF. Lymphokine regulation of HLA-DR gene expression in human thyroid cell monolayers. J Clin Endocrinol Metab 1987;64:543–548.

45. Migita K, Eguchi K, Otsubo T, et al. Cytokine regulation of HLA on thyroid cells. Clin Exp Immunol 1990;82:548–552.

46. Del Prete GF, Tiri A, Mariotti S, Pinchera A, Ricci M, Romagnani S. Enhanced production of gamma-interferon by thyroid-derived T cell clones from patients with Hashimoto's thyroiditis. Clin Exp Immunol 1987;69:323–331.

47. Hommes MJT, Romijn JA, Endert E, et al. Hypothyroid-like regulation of the pituitary-thyroid axis in stable human immunodeficiency virus infection. Metabolism 1993;42:556–561.

48. Kaptein EM. Thyroid hormone metabolism in illness. In: Henneman G, ed. Thyroid hormone metabolism. New York: Marcel Dekker, 1986:297–333.

49. Hamblin PS, Dijer SA, Mohr VS, et al. Relationship be-

tween thyrotropin and thyroxine changes during recovery from severe hypothyroxinemia of critical illness. J Clin Endocrinol Metab 1986;62:717–721.

50. Kaptein EM, Weiner JM, Robinson WJ, Wheeler WS, Nicoloff JT. Relationship of altered thyroid hormone indices to survival in nonthyroidal illness. Clin Endocrinol (Oxf) 1982;16:565–574.

51. Romijn JA, Wiersinga WM. Decreased nocturnal surge of thyrotropin (TSH) in nonthyroidal illness. J Clin Endocrinol Metab 1990;70:35–42.

52. Tibaldi JM, Surks MI. Animal models of nonthyroidal disease. Endocr Rev 1985;6:87–102.

53. Fujii T, Sato K, Ozawa M, et al. Effect of interleukin-I (IL-1) on thyroid hormone metabolism in mice stimulation of IL-1 of iodothyronine 5'-deiodinating activity (type I) in the liver. Endocrinology 1989;124:167–174.

54. Ozawa M, Sato K, Han DC, Kawakami M, Tsushima T, Shizume K. Effects of tumor necrosis factor-α/cachectin on thyroid hormone metabolism in mice. Endocrinology 1988;123:1461–1467.

55. Hermus ARMM, Sweep CGJ, van der Meer MJM, et al. Continuous infusion of interleukin-1β induces a nonthyroidal illness syndrome in the rat. Endocrinology 1992; 131:2139–2146.

56. Sweep CGJ, van der Meer MJM, Ross HA, Vranckx R, Visser TJ, Hermus ARMM. Chronic infusion of TNF-α reduces plasma T_4 binding without affecting pituitary-thyroid activity in rats. Am J Physiol 1992;263:E1099–E1105.

57. Dubuis JM, Dayer JM, Siegrist-Kaiser CA, Burger AG. Human recombinant interleukin-1β decreases plasma thyroid hormone and thyroid stimulating hormone levels in rats. Endocrinology 1988;123:2175–2181.

58. Enomoto T, Sugawa H, Kosuji S, Ioue D, Mori T, Imura H. Prolonged effects of recombinant human interleukin-1α on mouse thyroid function. Endocrinology 1990;127: 2322–2327.

59. Van der Poll T, Romijn JA, Wiersinga WM, Sauerwein HP. Tumor necrosis factor: a putative mediator of the euthyroid sick syndrome in man. J Clin Endocrinol Metab 1991;71:1567–1572.

60. Bernton EW, Beach JE, Holaday JW, Smallbridge RC, Fein HG. Release of multiple hormones by direct action of interleukin-1 on pituitary cells. Science 1987;238:519–521.

61. Bartalena L, Farsetti A, Flink IL, Robbins J. Effects of interleukin-6 on the expression of thyroid hormone-binding protein genes in cultured human hepatoblastoma-derived (hep G2) cells. Mol Endocrinol 1988;2:313–323.

62. Perlmutter DH, Dinarello CA, Punsal PI, Colten HR.

Cachectin/tumor necrosis factor regulates hepatic acute-phase gene expression. J Clin Invest 1986;78:1349–1354.

63. Ramadori G, van Damm J, Rider H, Meyer K. Interleukin-6, the third mediator of acute phase reaction, modulates hepatic protein synthesis in human and mouse. Comparison with interleukin 1β and tumor necrosis factor α. Eur J Immunol 1988;12:1259–1264.

64. Chopra IJ, Chua Teco GN, Mead JF, Huang TS, Beredo A, Solomon DH. Relationship between serum free fatty acids and thyroid hormone binding inhibitor in nonthyroidal illness. J Clin Endocrinol Metab 1985;60:980–984.

65. Chopra IJ, Sukane S, Chira Teco GN. A study of the serum concentration of tumor necrosis factor-α in thyroidal and nonthyroidal illness. J Clin Endocrinol Metab 1991;72: 1113–1116.

66. Atkins MB, Mier JW, Parkinson DR, Gould JA, Berkman EM, Kaplan MM. Hypothyroidism after treatment with interleukin-2 and lymphokine-activated killer cells. N Engl J Med 1988;318:1557–1563.

67. Pichert G, Jost LM, Zöbelil, Oderma HB, Pedio G, Stakel RA. Thyroiditis after treatment with interleukin-2 and interferon α-2a. Br J Cancer 1990;62:100–104.

68. Jacobs EL, Clare-Salzer MJ, Chopra IJ, Fylin RA. Thyroid functions abnormalities associated with the chronic outpatient administration of recombinant interleukin-2 and recombinant interferon-alpha. J Immunother 1991;10:448–455.

69. Kung AWC, Lai CC, Wong KL, Tam CF. Thyroid functions in patients treated with interleukin-2 and lymphokine-activated killer cells. Q J Med 1992;82:33–42.

70. Vassilopoulou-Sellin R, Sella A, Dexeus FH, Theriault RL, Pololoff DA. Acute thyroid dysfunctions (thyroiditis) after therapy with interleukin-2. Horm Metab Res 1992;24:434–438.

71. Berris B, Feinman SV. Thyroid dysfunction and liver injury following alpha-interferon treatment of chronic viral hepatitis. Dig Dis Sci 1991;36:1657–1660.

72. Burman P, Tötterman TH, Oberg K, Karlsson FA. Thyroid autoimmunity in patients on long term therapy with leucocyte-derived interferon. J Clin Endocrinol Metab 1986;63: 1086–1090.

73. Reem GF, Yeh NH. Interleukin-2 regulates expression of its receptor and synthesis of gamma interferon by human T lymphocytes. Science 1984;225:429–430.

74. Wiersinga WM, Krenning EP. Laboratorium diagnostiek van hyperen hypothyreoidie. In: Wiersinga WM, Krenning EP: Schildklierziekten. Alphen, The Netherlands: Samson Stafleu, 1988:73–97.

CHAPTER 21

ROLE OF CYTOKINES IN OVARIAN PHYSIOLOGY: INTERLEUKIN-1 AS A POSSIBLE CENTERPIECE IN THE OVULATORY SEQUENCE

Izhar Ben-Shlomo, Arye Hurwitz, Ehud Kokia, Wendy J. Scherzer, Richard M. Rohan, Donna W. Payne, and Eli Y. Adashi

---

Ovarian physiology attracts an ongoing research effort that has revealed a complex network of regulatory mechanisms involving steroid hormones, gonadotropins, growth factors and their cognate binding proteins, and, lastly, cytokines. This chapter reviews the findings concerning the possible role for cytokines in ovarian physiology. Because they are primarily active in inflammatory and inflammatory-like phenomena, cytokines were hypothesized to be involved in the ovulatory process, because the latter bears resemblance to inflammatory processes in several respects (1). The specific focus of this review is interleukin-1 (IL-1), a prominent representative of this group of peptides, and one that has been extensively evaluated in the context of the ovary.

THE INTERLEUKIN-1 SYSTEM

The IL-1 system is composed of ligands (IL-1α, IL-1β) (2–5), receptors (types I and II), receptor antagonist, and soluble receptors (extracellular binding proteins) (6–8). IL-1α and IL-1β are distinct gene products with limited sequence homology (26% in humans), but they interact with the same cell surface receptors with different affinities (9–13). Both must undergo proteolytic cleavage to become active.

For IL-1β, the specific protease involved was identified, cloned, and named convertase. It cleaves the 153-residue, biologically active C-terminal of the nascent 269-residue peptide (14). There are two types of cell surface high affinity, low capacity receptors that are comparable in their recognition (extracellular) and transmembranous sites, but they differ in the cytoplasmic domain (15–17). In humans, the type I receptor possesses a 213-amino acid long intracytoplasmic domain, whereas the type II receptor has a short 29-residue domain. It has been shown that these two receptors act independently, and they do not participate in the formation of a complex composed of a ligand and both receptors (18). This observation lends credibility to the assumption that these two receptors serve two distinct transduction pathways, which is in keeping with the observation that representation of the two receptor types varies from tissue to tissue. Although not currently fully elucidated, signal transduction by both or either of these receptors may involve sphingomyelin hydrolysis, which has also been implicated in tumor necrosis factor-α (TNF-α) signal transduction (19).

A unique feature of the IL-1 system is the existence of a naturally occurring receptor antagonist (IL-1RA), which is similar to IL-1 with regard to both size (152 amino acid residues) and structure (30% amino acid identity) (20–26). It is thought to constitute a temporally dependent, instantaneous regulator of IL-1 action at its cognate receptor level (27).

THE INTRAOVARIAN IL-1 SYSTEM

Although the relevance of IL-1 to ovarian physiology remains uncertain, an increasing body of evidence supports such a possibility. First, measurable amounts of IL-1–like activity have been documented in both porcine (28) and human (29,30) follicular fluid. In vivo studies at the level of the murine, porcine, and human ovary demonstrated IL-1 to exert antigonadotropic (31–37) or steroidogenic (38–42) effects contingent on the experimental circumstances under study. In human follicular fluid, a correlation was found between IL levels and progesterone levels (43). Hence, it is tempting to speculate that locally derived IL-1, possibly of somatic ovarian cell or resident ovarian macrophage origin, may have a role in an intraovarian regulatory loop.

Because IL-1 is an established mediator of inflammation (44) and because ovulation may constitute an inflammatory-like reaction (1), consideration should be given to the possibility that IL-1 might have an intermediary role in the preovulatory developmental cascade and the terminal ovulatory process. Such speculation is supported by the recognition that IL-1 has been shown in multiple (nonovarian) tissues to promote several ovulation-associated phenomena, such as prostaglandin biosynthesis, plasminogen activator production, glycosaminoglycan generation, collagenase activation, and vascular permeability enhancement.

Using an established experimental model capable of stimulating naturally occurring follicular maturation, ovulation, and corpus luteum formation in rats, Hurwitz and colleagues (45) observed low levels of IL-1β RNA in whole ovarian material prior to gonadotropic stimulation. Treatment with pregnant mares' serum gonadotropin (PMSG) for 48 hours resulted in a modest, albeit measurable, increase in the steady-state levels of the ovarian IL-1β message. However, the relative abundance of ovarian IL-1β transcripts following a 6-hour exposure to human chorionic gonadotropin (hCG) produced a 4- to 5-fold increase ($p < 0.05$) over the untreated state at a time point approximately 6 hours prior to projected follicular rupture. Twenty-four and 48 hours following hCG administration, a significant ($p < 0.05$) decrease was noted (relative to the 6-hr peak) to a level comparable to that seen at the conclusion of 48 hours of treatment with PMSG. Cellular localization studies revealed the gonadotropindependent IL-1β mRNA to be theca-interstitial cell–exclusive.

To assess rat ovarian IL-1β gene expression under in vitro circumstances, the same authors (45) set out to determine whether IL-1 may influence the relative level of its own message. Treatment of whole ovarian dispersates with recombinant human IL-1β (10 ng/mL) for 4 and 24 hours resulted in a marked ($p < 0.05$) time-dependent increase (up to 12-fold) in the relative abundance of IL-1β transcripts when compared with untreated control specimens. These observations establish the rat ovarian theca-interstitial cell as a site of IL-1β gene expression, the preovulatory acquisition of which is gonadotropin-dependent. In addition, IL-1β was shown to exert a positive up-regulatory effect on its own expression, an autocrine action potentially concerned with self-amplification. This temporal (potentially self-amplifying) sequence of events provides support for the proposal that intraovarian IL-1β may have an intermediary role in the preovulatory developmental cascade.

Hurwitz and colleagues (46) also studied the human intraovarian IL-1 system using solution hybridization/RNase protection assays. No detectable IL-1 signal was evident in whole ovarian material from days 4 or 12 of an unstimulated menstrual cycle. However, expected protected fragments corresponding to IL-1β (175 bp) transcripts (IL-1β>>IL-1α) were detected in preovulatory follicular aspirates, secured in the course of a gonadotropin-stimulated in vitro fertilization cycle. Preovulatory peripheral monocytes obtained from patients' blood at the time of oocyte retrieval tested negative for both IL-1 transcripts, thereby effectively eliminating the possibility that contaminating peripheral monocytes contribute to IL-1 transcripts detected in preovulatory follicular aspirates. IL-1β transcripts were also detected in cultured forskolin-treated (25 μmol/L) (macrophage-poor) granulosa cells (but not theca-interstitial cells), suggesting (but not conclusively proving) that the granulosa cell may be a site of IL-1β gene expression in humans. The difference noted between this localization and that in the rat is reminiscent of other interspecies differences in cellular expression found previously.

When macrophage-depleted follicular aspirates, prepared by magnetically driven immune sorting and validated by flow cytometry analysis, were tested, a single protected fragment (projected to be 477 bases long) corresponding to type I IL-1 receptor transcripts was detected in whole ovaries from days 4 and 12 of an unstimulated menstrual cycle and in preovulatory follicular aspirates. Type I IL-1 receptor transcripts were also detected in cultured granulosa and theca-interstitial cell preparations, but not in preovulatory peripheral monocytic cells obtained at the time of oocyte retrieval. Treatment of cultured granulosa or theca-interstitial cells with forskolin (25μmol/L) resulted in a 2- to 3-fold increase in the steady-state level of type I IL-1 receptor transcripts. A single protected fragment (147 bases long) corresponding to IL-1RA transcripts was detected in whole ovarian material from day 4 of an unstimulated menstrual cycle, as well as in macrophage-free preovulatory follicular aspirates. No detectable signal was noted in granulosa or theca-interstitial cells cultured in the absence or presence of forskolin.

These results reveal the existence of a complete, highly compartmentalized, hormonally dependent intraovarian IL-1 system replete with ligands, receptor, and receptor antagonists. The apparent midcycle induction of ovarian IL-1 gene expression and the reported ability of IL-1 to promote a host of ovulation-associated phenomena give rise to the speculation that locally derived IL-1 may be an important component of an intraovarian regulatory loop concerned with genesis and maintenance of the preovulatory cascade of follicular events.

Given the well-established preovulatory increase in the intraovarian content of prostaglandin (PG) and its apparent linkage to the ovulatory process (47), demonstration of a stimulatory effect of IL-1 on ovarian PG biosynthesis may provide additional indirect support for the postulate that IL-1 may have a meaningful intermediary role in the preovulatory cascade. Kokia and associates (48) documented the constitutive ability of whole ovarian dispersates to elaborate both prostaglandin E_2 (PGE_2) and prostaglandin $F_{2\alpha}$ ($PGF_{2\alpha}$) in a cell density–dependent fashion, as well as a stimulatory effect of IL-1β on the generation of both PG species (48). The relative abundance of PGE_2 was 2.7- to 3.9-fold higher when compared with $PGF_{2\alpha}$, regardless of the cell density employed.

To define the cellular populations concerned with prostaglandin biosynthesis, increasing cellular densities of whole ovarian dispersates, isolated granulosa cells, or thecainterstitial cells were cultured in the absence or presence of IL-1β (10 ng/mL). All cellular preparations displayed constitutive (albeit relatively limited) cell density–dependent elaboration of PGE_2 in the absence of cytokine stimulation. Whole ovarian dispersates proved substantially ($p < 0.05$) more active in this connection as compared with their isolated granulosa or theca-interstitial cell counterparts, regardless of the size of the cellular inoculum employed (whole ovarian dispersates > granulosa cells > theca-interstitial cells). Treatment with IL-1β resulted in significant ($p < 0.05$) increases in PGE_2 accumulation for all cell densities studied. Ovarian dispersates also displayed substantially ($p < 0.05$) enhanced accumulation of PGE_2 as compared with isolated granulosa or theca-interstitial cells. These measurements were taken to suggest a requirement for cell-cell interaction.

Consequently, reconstitution at a projected physiological ratio of 4:1 (granulosa to theca) was carried out, which revealed synergistic interactions in the elaboration of PGE_2 under both basal and IL-1β–treated circumstances, the magnitude of which proved comparable to that displayed by whole ovarian dispersates. Comparable results were obtained for heterologous coculture experiments using transwell dual-chamber technology, which precludes direct cellular contact while ensuring that media will be shared by the cellular populations under study. These experiments revealed that optimal ovarian prostaglandin biosynthesis requires heterologous, contact-independent (presumably humorally mediated) cell-cell interaction.

A recent study by Brännstrom and coworkers (49) tested the possible participation of macrophages in the function of the IL-1 system during critical stages of follicular development and rupture. Specific immunohistochemical techniques revealed a remarkable increase in the number of resident macrophages in the theca-interstitial compartment of preovulatory follicles. Because they are a well-documented source of IL-1 bioactivity, these macrophages were postulated to have a meaningful role in the preovulatory increase in the component of the intraovarian IL-1 system. In a further attempt to elucidate the dynamic role of IL-1β, these authors made use of the in vitro perfused rat ovary model (41). After gonadotropic stimulation, rat ovaries were perfused with various substances. It was demonstrated that IL-1β synergizes with luteinizing hormone (LH) in the shedding of oocytes, whereas by itself it caused ovulation of a very small number of oocytes. The authors concluded that IL-1β induces ovulation in the rat. However, these results should be viewed with caution, because the number of oocytes shed in these experiments was small (3–4/ovary with LH trigger, and 9–11/ovary with the addition of IL-1β) in comparison to the in vivo numbers of oocytes shed by rats (20–30 oocytes/ovary). In addition, only 5 animals were tested in each group. These observations, however, bring evaluation of IL-1 in ovarian physiology a step closer to the real in vivo situation.

This information, in addition to the demonstration of gonadotropin-dependent midcycle induction of IL-1 transcripts, supports the view that IL-1 may be the centerpiece of an intraovarian regulatory loop concerned with the promotion of key preovulatory events. In this regard, we observed IL-1β–induced nitric oxide production by rat ovarian cell cultures (Ben-Shlomo I, et al., unpublished observations). In view of the multiplicity of nitric oxide effects in other tissues, it could be a possible participant in the IL-1β ovarian regulatory loops.

Despite the apparent preliminary nature of the observations cited herein, there is every reason to believe that continued investigation will provide new and meaningful insight relevant to the understanding of the complex interactions between the various cellular components of the ovary. If recent progress is any indication, the next decade may reveal that intraovarian cytokine messengers, as well as a host of growth factors, have major roles throughout the ovarian life cycle.

ACKNOWLEDGMENT: This work was supported in part by National Institutes of Health Grant HD-30288 (E.Y.A.).

REFERENCES

1. Espey L. Ovulation of an inflammatory reaction—a hypothesis. Biol Reprod 1990;22:73–106.

2. Nathan C, Sporn M. Cytokines in context. J Cell Biol 1991;113:981–986.

3. Trotta PP. Cytokines: an overview. Am J Reprod Immunol 1991;25:137–141.

4. Kennedy RL, Jones TH. Cytokines in endocrinology: their roles in health and in disease. J Endocrinol 1991;129:167–178.

5. Harrison LC, Campbell IL. Cytokines: an expanding network of immuno-inflammatory hormones. Mol Endocrinol 1988;2:1151–1156.

6. Dower SK, Wignall JM, Schooley K, et al. Retention of ligand binding activity by the extracellular domain of the IL-1 receptor. J Immunol 1989;142:4314–4320.

7. Symond JA, Duff FW. A soluble form of the interleukin-1 receptor produced by a human B cell line. FEBS Lett 1990; 272:133–136.

8. Giri JG, Newton RC, Horuk R. Identification of soluble interleukin-1 binding protein in cell-free supernatants. J Biol Chem 1990;265:17416–17419.

9. Lomedico PT, Guber U, Hellmann CP, et al. Cloning and expression of murine interleukin-1 cDNA in escherichia coli. Nature 1984;312:458–462.

10. March CJ, Mosley B, Larsen A, et al. Cloning, sequence and expression of two distinct human interleukin-1 complementary DNAs. Nature 1985;315:641–647.

11. Bird TA, Sakatvala J. Identification of a common class of high affinity receptors for both types of porcine interleukin-1 on connective tissue cells. Nature 1986;324:263–266.

12. Kilian PL, Kaffka KL, Stern AS, et al. Interleukin-1α and interleukin-1β bind to the same receptor on T cells. J Immunol 1986;136:4509–4514.

13. Dower SK, Kronheim SR, Hopp TP, et al. The cell surface receptors for interleukin-1α and interleukin-1β are identical. Nature 1986;324:266–268.

14. Cerretti DP, Kozlosky CJ, Mosley B, et al. Molecular cloning of the IL-1 converting enzyme. Science 1992;256:97–99.

15. McMahan CJ, Slack JL, Mosley B, et al. A novel IL-1 receptor, cloned from B cells by mammalian expression, is expressed in many cell types. EMBO J 1991;10:2821–2832.

16. Sims JE, March CJ, Cosman D, et al. cDNA expression cloning of the IL-1 receptor, a member of the immunoglobulin superfamily. Science 1988;241:585–588.

17. Sims JE, Acres B, Grubin CE, et al. Cloning the interleukin-1 receptor from human T cells. Proc Natl Acad Sci USA 1989;86:8946–8950.

18. Slack J, McMahan CJ, Waugh S, et al. Independent binding of interleukin-1α and interleukin-1β to type I and type II interleukin-1 receptors. J Biol Chem 1993;268:2513–2524.

19. Mathias S, Younes A, Kan C-C, Orlow I, Joseph C, Kolesnick RN. Activation of the sphingomyelin signaling pathway in intact EL4 cells and in a cell-free system of IL-1β. Science 1993;259:519–522.

20. Eisenberg SP, Brewer MT, Verderber E, Heimdal P, Brandhuber BJ, Thompson RC. Interleukin-1 receptor antagonist is a member of the interleukin-1 gene family: evolution of a cytokine control mechanism. Immunology 1991; 88:5232–5236.

21. Shuck ME, Eessalu TE, Tracey DE, Bienkowski MJ. Cloning, heterologous expression and characterization of murine interleukin-1 receptor antagonist protein. Eur J Immunol 1991;21:2775–2780.

22. Haskill S, Martin G, Van Le L, Morris J. cDNA cloning of an intracellular form of the human interleukin-1 receptor antagonist associated with epithelium. Proc Natl Acad Sci USA 1991;88:3681–3685.

23. Eisenberg SP, Evans RJ, Arend WP, et al. Primary structure and functional expression from complementary DNA of a human interleukin-1 receptor antagonist. Nature 1990; 343:341–346.

24. Hannum CH, Wilcox CJ, Arend WP, et al. Interleukin-1 receptor antagonist activity of a human interleukin-1 inhibitor. Nature 1990;343:336–340.

25. Carter DB, Deibel MB Jr, Dunn CJ, et al. Purification, cloning, expression and biological characterization of an interleukin-1 receptor antagonist protein. Nature 1990;344: 633–638.

26. Matsushima H, Roussel MF, Matsushima K, Hishinuma A, Sherr CJ. Cloning and expression of murine interleukin-1 receptor antagonist in macrophages stimulated by colony-stimulating factor 1. Blood 1991;78:616–623.

27. Dripps DJ, Brandhuber BJ, Thompson RC, Eisenberg SP. Interleukin-1 (IL-1) receptor antagonist binds to the 80kDa IL-1 receptor but does not initiate IL-1 signal transduction. J Biol Chem 1991;266:10331–10336.

28. Takakura K, Taii S, Fukuoka M, et al. IL-1 receptor/p55 (Tac)-inducing activity in porcine follicular fluid. Endocrinology 1989;125:618–623.

29. Khan SA, Schmid K, Hallin P, Paul RD, Geyter CD, Nieschlag E. Human testis cytosol and ovarian follicular fluid contains high amounts of interleukin-1-like factor(s). Mol Cell Endocrinol 1988;58:221–230.

30. Wang LJ, Norman RJ. Concentrations of immunoreactive interleukin-1 and interleukin-2 in human preovulatory follicular fluid. Hum Reprod 1992;7:147–150.

31. Gottschall PE, Uehara A, Hoffman ST, Arimura A. Interleukin-1 inhibits FSH-induced differentiation in rat granulosa cells in vitro. Biochem Biophys Res Commun 1987;149: 502–509.

32. Gottschall PE, Katsuura G, Arimura A. Interleukin-1 beta is more potent than interleukin-1 alpha in suppressing follicle-stimulation hormone-induced differentiation of ovarian granulosa cells. Biochem Biophys Res Commun 1989; 163:764–770.

33. Kasson BG, Gorospe WC. Effects of interleukins-1, -2, and -3 on follicle stimulating hormone induced differentiation of rat granulosa cells. Mol Cell Endocrinol 1989;62:103–111.

34. Fukuoka M, Mori T, Taii S, Yasuda K. Interleukin-1 inhibits luteinization of porcine granulosa cells in culture. Endocrinology 1988;122:367–369.

35. Yasuda K, Fukuoka M, Taii S, Takakura K, Mori T. Inhibitory effects of interleukin-1 on follicle stimulating hormone induction of aromatase activity, progesterone secretion, and functional luteinizing hormone receptors in cultures of porcine granulosa cells. Biol Reprod 1990;43: 905–912.

36. Fukuoka M, Taii S, Yasuda K, Takakura K, Mori T. Inhibitory effects of interleukin-1 on luteinizing hormone-stimulated adenosine 3′,5-monophosphate accumulation by cul-

tured porcine granulosa cells. Endocrinology 1989;125:136–143.

37. Gottschall PE, Katsuura G, Arimura A. Interleukin-1 suppresses follicle-stimulating hormone-induced estradiol secretion from cultured ovarian granulosa cells. J Reprod Immunol 1989;15:281–290.

38. Nakamuar Y, Kato H, Terranova PF. Interleukin-1α increases thecal progesterone production of preovulatory follicles in cyclic hamster. Biol Reprod 1990;43:169–173.

39. Barak V, Yanai P, Treves AJ, Roisman I, Simon A, Laufer N. Interleukin-1: local production and modulation of human granulosa luteal cells steroidogenesis. Fertil Steril 1992;58:719–725.

40. Fujiwara H, Iwai M, Takakura K, Kanzaki H, Mori T. Cytokine modulation of progesterone and estradiol secretion in cultures of luteinized human granulosa cells. J Clin Endocrinol Metab 1992;75:254–258.

41. Brannstrom M, Wang L, Norman RJ. Ovulatory effect of interleukin-1β on the perfused rat ovary. Endocrinology 1993;132:399–404.

42. Brannstrom M, Wang L, Norman RJ. Effects of cytokines on prostaglandin production and steroidogenesis of incubated preovulatory follicles of the rat. Biol Reprod 1993;48:165–171.

43. Barak V, Mordel N, Holzer H, Zajicek G, Treves AJ, Laufer N. The correlation of interleukin-1 and tumour necrosis factor to oestradiol, progesterone and testosterone levels in periovulatory follicular fluid of in vitro fertilization patients. Hum Reprod 1992;7:462–464.

44. Dinarello CA. Biology of interleukin-1. FASEB J 1988;2:108–115.

45. Hurwitz A, Ricciarelli E, Botero L, Roham RM, Hernandez ER, Adashi EY. Endocrine- and autocrine-mediated regulation of rat ovarian (theca-interstitial) interleukin-1β gene expression: gonadotropin-dependent preovulatory acquisition. Endocrinology 1992;129:3427–3429.

46. Hurwitz A, Loukides J, Ricciarelli E, et al. The human intraovarian interleukin-1 (IL-1) system: highly-compartmentalized and hormonally-dependent regulation of the genes encoding IL-1, its receptor, and its receptor antagonist. J Clin Invest 1992;89:1746–1754.

47. Poyse NL. Prostaglandin and ovarian function. In: Hiller K, ed. Advances in eicosanoid research. London: MTP Press Ltd., 1987:1–29.

48. Kokia E, Hurwitz A, Ricciarelli E, et al. Interleukin-1 stimulates ovarian prostaglandin biosynthesis: obligatory role for heterologous contact-dependent cell-cell interaction. Endocrinology 1992;130:3095–3097.

49. Brannstrom M, Mayhofer G, Robertson SA. Localization of leukocyte subsets in the rat ovary during the periovulatory period. Biol Reprod 1993;48:277–286.

CHAPTER 22

ROLE OF CYTOKINES IN OXIDATIVE DAMAGE

Eric D. Whitman, Gerard M. Doherty, Gary R. Peplinski, Jeffrey A. Norton

The aerobic environment offers many advantages to mammalian cells. In contrast to the anaerobic environment, cellular energy production, through oxidative phosphorylation, much more efficiently produces adenosine triphosphate (ATP) for use in various intracellular processes. An inherent danger in this environment is the partial reduction of molecular oxygen and the consequent formation of highly reactive oxygen compounds, or free radicals. These substances can be toxic to both normal and abnormal cells, but they are counteracted by intracellular and extracellular defense systems in the body. When these adaptive antioxidant defenses are overwhelmed, cellular damage and, potentially, cellular mutation or destruction occurs.

The role of cytokines in the oxidative damage of cells has been extensively investigated in vitro for various cellular systems. Several cytokines, principally tumor necrosis factor (TNF), interleukin-1 (IL-1), and interferon-γ (IFN-γ), appear to cause, either directly or indirectly, the production of reactive oxygen species (ROS). However, the full in vivo significance of cytokine-induced oxidative damage is largely unknown.

In this chapter we discuss the role of cytokines in cellular oxidative damage. First, the mechanisms of oxidative damage, including the existing cellular defense system of antioxidants, are outlined to provide a structural background for the remainder of the chapter. In the second portion of the chapter, the role of cytokines in the production of ROS is discussed, with emphasis on the re-

search performed in this area on the way cytokines interact with different cell types to lead to ROS release. In the final section of this chapter, we discuss the in vivo implications of cytokine-induced oxidative damage.

THE ORIGIN OF REACTIVE OXYGEN SPECIES

Oxygen-containing molecules or molecular fragments with a single, unpaired electron in the outer atomic orbital are powerful oxidants, known as free radicals (1). These ROS can be formed by the transfer of an electron to or from the molecule in question. The resulting compound is highly reactive; it "quenches" itself almost instantaneously by accepting another electron from a neighboring molecule to regain its neutral status with fully filled, paired, outer electron shells. Thus, another term for ROS is *reactive oxygen intermediates* (ROI), which emphasizes their short half-life. Experimentally, the transient nature of these molecules is emphasized by our ability to only measure the byproducts of their existence.

The primary oxygen free radicals involved in cellular systems are the superoxide anion ($O_2\cdot$) and the hydroxyl radical (HO$\cdot$). Other ROS include singlet oxygen ($^1O_2$; usually formed on stimulation of O_2 by illumination), perhydroxy radical (HO$_2\cdot$), and hypohalides formed by the interaction of chloride with hydrogen peroxide

(H_2O_2) and myeloperoxidase (e.g., HOCl). H_2O_2, although not technically a free radical, is also an ROS, in that it can interact with many of the mentioned ROS either to restore their neutral, paired, electron status, or to form new ROI. All can be significant initiators of oxidative damage to the cell (1,2) because of their reactivity.

The source of most, if not all, cellular ROS generation in a normal oxidation state (nonstressed) is the mitochondrial respiratory chain (3). The reduction of molecular oxygen to water by the respiratory chain results in a very small (3–5%) leak of electrons from the microsomal cytochrome P-450 complex. Molecular oxygen is partially reduced by these electrons to produce ROS as depicted in the following equations.

$$O_2 + e^- \rightarrow O_2\bullet \qquad (1)$$

$$O_2\bullet + e^- \rightarrow O_2^{2-} + 2H^+ \Rightarrow H_2O_2 \qquad (2)$$

$$O_2\bullet + H^+ \rightarrow HO_2\bullet \qquad (3)$$

Superoxide ($O_2\bullet$) is produced in the greatest amount, and it may undergo further reactions, as shown.

Most of the $O_2\bullet$ produced is reduced by a process called dismutation, which forms H_2O_2:

$$2O_2\bullet + 2H^+ \rightarrow H_2O_2 + O_2 \qquad (4)$$

This reaction occurs spontaneously, but the superoxide dismutase (SOD) enzymes, which will be more fully discussed in a later section, change the equilibrium of the chemical reaction, so that more of the free radical is eliminated. Superoxide anion that is not reduced to H_2O_2 can undergo a number of reactions, most importantly the conversion of oxidized iron (Fe^{3+}) to its reduced form.

$$O_2\bullet + Fe^{3+} \rightarrow Fe^{2+} + O_2 \qquad (5)$$

Iron or copper in the reduced state can catalyze the Fenton reaction, first described in 1894 (4).

$$Fe^{2+} (Cu^+) + H_2O_2 \rightarrow Fe^{3+} (Cu^{2+}) + HO\bullet + OH- \qquad (6)$$

Combining these two reactions illustrates the potential interaction between $O_2\bullet$ and H_2O_2 in the presence of an iron catalyst, which is the Haler-Weiss reaction (5).

$$H_2O_2 + O_2\bullet \rightarrow O_2 + HO\bullet + OH- \qquad (7)$$

This in vivo reaction forms the hydroxyl radical, HO•, the most toxic ROS to biological materials. HO• is able to react with various molecules, including amino acids, phospholipids, DNA, and sugars. Therefore, its toxicity can include cell membrane, protein, and nucleic acid damage.

The hypohalides hydrochlorous acid (HOCl) and N-chloroamine (RNHCl) are ROS that can also cause cellular damage. Halide oxidation occurs when H_2O_2 forms a substrate-enzyme complex with the enzyme myeloperoxidase. Chloride ions serve as electron donors, and they are oxidized to their corresponding acids.

$$Cl^- + H_2O_2 + H^+ \rightarrow HOCl + H_2O \qquad (8)$$

The hypohalides are extremely reactive, and they are readily bacteriocidal or cytotoxic (2,6).

Xanthine dehydrogenase is an enzyme present in most cells that transfers electrons to nicotinamide adenine dinucleotide (NAD^+) during oxidation of xanthine or hypoxanthine to uric acid. By sulfhydryl oxidation or calcium-dependent proteolysis, the enzyme can be converted to xanthine oxidase, which uses molecular oxygen as an electron acceptor (7). This may be another mechanism by which ROS are generated in cells.

The respiratory burst

In the preceding paragraphs, we described the production of ROS by cells in the resting state. Although potentially harmful to normal host tissues, these ROS are generally counteracted by native defense mechanisms, including SOD and others, that are discussed later in the chapter. However, when stimulated by various agonists, including bacteria, yeast, some proteins, antibody-antigen complexes, phorbol esters, or cytokines, neutrophils and macrophages (i.e., phagocytes) can become "activated" to produce ROS. This rapid and extensive response to phagocytic stimulation, characterized by an immediate increase in oxygen consumption and production of ROI, is called the *respiratory burst* (5,8).

The initial features of the respiratory burst are an increase in nonmitochondrial (9) oxygen consumption, accompanied by increased utilization and oxidation of glucose via the hexose monophosphate shunt (2). This process is mediated by the enzyme NADPH oxidase, which is activated from its resting state when stimulated by the appropriate extracellular material (10,11). This enzyme oxidizes NADPH to $NADP^+$ to produce superoxide.

$$NADPH + H+ + 2O_2 \rightarrow NADP^+ + 2H^+ + 2O_2\bullet \qquad (9)$$

$O_2\bullet$ may undergo dismutation, forming H_2O_2, or react with previously formed H_2O_2 in the Haler-Weiss reaction to produce the highly toxic hydroxyl radical, HO•. The production of $O_2\bullet$ alone does not appear to cause cellular injury, which supports the finding that HO• is necessary for oxidative damage (12). Some ROS, such as H_2O_2, can permeate membranes to oxidize molecules in the extracellular compartment in the presence of reduced iron molecules (Fe^{2+}), halides, and myeloperoxidase.

The respiratory burst has been implicated in several in vivo situations, particularly the host response to inflammation, infection, and tumor. The clinical ramifications of this relationship are discussed in a later section of this chapter.

The effect of the ROS produced can be classified chemically or biologically. The chemical effects of the ROS produced during the respiratory burst are divided into three major types of interactions: radical addition, electron transfer, and atom abstraction (13) (Table 22–1). In all cases, a new free radical, with an unpaired electron, is formed. Thus, the existence of ROS can persist as a chain reaction, propagated to other molecules until a stable compound results. Eventually, a paired-electron, stable compound is formed, and the chain reaction is halted.

The biological effects of the respiratory burst of ROS have been divided into four categories: defensive, toxic, proinflammatory, and modulatory (5). Defensive effects are targeted toward foreign organisms, such as bacteria, parasites, yeast (14,15), and, potentially, tumor cells. Toxic effects include damage to cell membranes, functional proteins, and nucleic acids. The inflammatory effects of ROS appear to involve many of the changes seen in severe inflammatory clinical disorders, such as septic shock and adult respiratory distress syndrome (ARDS), in which there is increased vascular permeability and release of multiple vasoactive proteins. Finally, the modulatory effects of ROS are due to the direct toxicity of the ROS to various enzymes (5).

Mechanisms of cellular damage

The free radical theory of cellular oxidative injury suggests that production of ROS, if unchecked by antioxidant defense mechanisms, leads to oxidation of cellular constituents and eventual destruction of cellular function.

TABLE 22–1   THREE MAJOR TYPES OF RADICAL INTERACTIONS WITH BIOLOGICAL MOLECULES

Radical addition
  $R\bullet + H_2C=CX \rightarrow H(R)C-C\bullet X$
Electron transfer
  $R\bullet + O_2 \rightarrow R^+ + O_2\bullet$
Atom abstraction
  $R\bullet + H_3C-CH_2-CH_3 \rightarrow RH + H_3C-C\bullet H-CH_3$

Compelling evidence supporting this theory derives from genetic manipulation experiments. SOD, an ROS scavenger enzyme, reacts with $O_2\bullet$ to form H_2O_2 via dismutation (Eq. 4). Strains of *Escherichia coli* bacteria with a mutated, defective SOD gene are unable to produce this enzyme. These bacteria grow well in an anaerobic environment, but slowly, with increased spontaneous mutations in an oxygen-rich medium (16). All deleterious oxygen-associated effects observed are reversed by introduction of a plasmid bearing a functional SOD gene (17).

Targets of oxidative damage include proteins, lipids, and DNA. In general, oxidative damage to specific amino acids within a protein is dictated by the catalytic iron or copper binding sites where HO• is produced. Arginine, histidine, proline, and lysine are most sensitive to oxidative damage (18). Sulfhydryl groups on methionine and cysteine are oxidized to form radicals.

$$\text{Protein-SH} + \text{HO}\bullet \rightarrow \text{protein-S}\bullet + H_2O \qquad (10)$$

These radicals induce conformational changes in proteins, with consequent alteration of protein function. Radicals link together, forming intramolecular disulfide bridges,

$$\text{Protein-S}\bullet + \text{protein-S}\bullet \rightarrow \text{protein-S-S-protein} \qquad (11)$$

as well as intermolecular protein dimerization and, ultimately, protein function loss, fragmentation, or both (19,20). Oxidation at the active site of a protein may defunctionalize the protein entirely. Oxidized proteins can also be degraded to individual amino acids by a unique class of "neutral proteases" (21).

One of the most critical results of cellular oxidation is lipid peroxidation. ROS react with the electron-rich double bonds of unsaturated lipids within plasma and organelle membranes to form lipid radicals.

$$CH_2 = CX + HO\bullet \rightarrow CH_2 = C\bullet X + H_2O \qquad (12)$$

These radicals then react with molecular oxygen.

$$CH_2 = C\bullet X + O_2 \rightarrow CH_2 = C(O_2\bullet)X \qquad (13)$$

Peroxy radicals result, which may diffuse in the plane of the membrane to extract electrons from other molecules in the presence of a metal catalyst (22). Bilayer integrity is lost and lipid fluidity is altered. Cleavage of carbon bonds during lipid peroxidation results in the formation of aldehydes, which are very biologically active molecules that have been shown to inhibit platelet aggregation and adenyl cyclase activity (23).

ROS reaction with DNA results in a variety of potentially unstable intramolecular and intermolecular chemical alterations. Purification of human DNA from irradiated cells has revealed single- and double-stranded DNA disruptions. Sequencing studies of DNA after treatment with bleomycin, a chemical that generates ROS when bound to DNA in the presence of iron, revealed strand breaks as well as base misincorporations and deletions (24). A stable derivative of guanine, 8-hydroxyguanine (OH⁸Gua), has been identified in DNA in vitro after treatment with a variety of agents known to produce hydroxyl radicals (25). OH⁸Gua formation leads to extensive mispairing with itself and, to a lesser extent, with its immediately neighboring normal bases, causing G → T and A → C transversions in vitro and in vivo in *E. coli* (26). HO• also forms radiation-induced DNA histone-protein crosslinks (27). All these alterations in DNA may be of importance in mutagenesis and eventual cell death (28).

DEFENSES AGAINST OXIDATIVE CELLULAR DAMAGE

Cellular survival in an atmosphere containing oxygen requires defense mechanisms to cope with the highly reactive oxygen species that are formed in small but dangerous quantities. Once formed, free radicals follow one of three pathways (Fig. 22–1). They may react with cellular components, including membrane lipids, cellular proteins, or nucleic acids, thus causing damage to the component and, potentially, cellular dysfunction (29,30). ROS can also react with some cellular and extracellular compounds that are chemically stable after the reaction, thus eliminating the risk of damage to cells. These ROS scavengers include Vitamin E (isomers of tocopherol), Vitamin C (ascorbic acid), Vitamin A (β-carotene and retinol), and uric acid (Table 22–2). Finally, some specific enzymatic systems have evolved to detoxify ROS and to prevent cellular damage. These systems include the enzymes catalase, glutathione peroxidase, and the superoxide dismutases (Table 22–2).

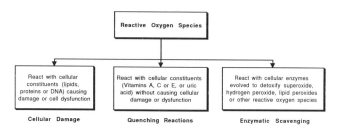

Figure 22–1 Pathways of biological reactive oxygen species. The three potential types of interactions of ROI are shown.

ROS scavenger compounds

Quantitatively, the most important intracellular ROS scavenger agent is Vitamin E. A series of naturally occurring tocopherols have Vitamin E activity; the most preva-

TABLE 22–2   ACTIVE AGENTS IN REACTIVE OXYGEN SPECIES SCAVENGING

Agent	Location	Function
Vitamin E (tocopherol)	Cell membranes	Reduces lipophilic ROS
Vitamin C (ascorbic acid)	Cytoplasm, plasma	Reduces ROS and oxidized tocopherols
Vitamin A (β-carotene, retinol)	Cell membranes, especially liver	Singlet oxygen scavenger; inhibits lipid peroxidation
Uric acid	Plasma	Reduces singlet oxygen and hydroxyl radical
Catalase	Cytoplasm, peroxisomes	Catalyzes reduction of H_2O_2, oxidation of others (ethanol, phenols)
Glutathione	Cytoplasm	Electron donor for enzymatic reduction of H_2O_2, lipid peroxides, disulfides
Glutathione peroxidase	Cytoplasm	Catalyzes glutathione-dependent H_2O_2 reduction
Glutathione reductase	Cytoplasm	Catalyzes NADPH-dependent glutathione disulfide reduction
Copper-zinc superoxide dismutase	Cytoplasm	Catalyzes dismutation of O_2•ion to H_2O_2 and oxygen
Manganous superoxide dismutase	Mitochondria	Catalyzes dismutation of O_2•ion to H_2O_2 and oxygen
Extracellular superoxide dismutase	Plasma	Catalyzes dismutation of O_2•ion to H_2O_2 and oxygen

ROS = reactive oxygen species.

lent is α-tocopherol (5,7,8-trimethyltocol), which accounts for approximately 90% of tocopherols in animal tissues and is the most active in bioassays. Vitamin E acts as an electron donor to reduce the ROS or the peroxidation products of unsaturated fatty acids. Because of its lipid solubility, Vitamin E is located and active in cellular constituent membranes, including mitochondrial, nuclear, and endoplasmic reticulum membranes. In its location, it protects the membrane lipids from oxidation. In animals made Vitamin E–deficient by dietary manipulation, toxic oxidation products, particularly of fatty acids, are detected. Supplementation with unrelated antioxidants, such as synthetic antioxidants, selenium, and the coenzyme Q group, can prevent or reverse the symptoms of Vitamin E deficiency (31). Thus, the crucial function of Vitamin E appears to be its antioxidant effect, and its lipid solubility dictates that this function will be in the cell membranes.

Vitamin C or ascorbic acid is another ubiquitous, nonspecific, intracellular antioxidant that is important in cellular function and in the defense against ROS. Ascorbic acid is readily and reversibly oxidized to dehydroascorbic acid, and it is active in many cellular processes as an electron donor, including collagen, steroid, and carnitine synthesis; folic-to-folinic acid conversion; and tyrosine metabolism. Ascorbic acid is abundant in the cytoplasm and the plasma, and, as a nonspecific reducing agent, it is available to scavenge water-soluble ROS. It may also reduce oxidized tocopherols, thus returning scavenging activity to oxidized Vitamin E (31,32).

Beta-carotene, or provitamin A, is the most active carotenoid found in plants, and it provides approximately one half of the average Vitamin A intake in adults in the United States. Beta-carotene is absorbed in the intestine, and it is oxidized to retinal, which can then be further oxidized to retinoic acid or reduced to retinol. Retinol is the ubiquitous Vitamin A form in humans. Both β-carotene and retinol can function as reducing agents to scavenge ROS or lipid peroxides. Like Vitamin E, Vitamin A is lipid-soluble, and it is membrane-associated intracellularly. It is especially concentrated in the membranes of the Golgi apparatus and in the endoplasmic reticulum of hepatocytes. Vitamin A is therefore able to limit lipid peroxidation in cell membranes, especially in the metabolically active hepatocytes. In plasma, retinol is transported by a retinol-binding protein; its role as an ROS scavenger in plasma is not clear (31,33).

Uric acid is present in plasma at approximately 300 μmol/L. It can react with singlet $^1O_2$ and HO•, acting as an ROS scavenger. This process protects hemoglobin from peroxide oxidation and red blood cells from lipid peroxidation in some experimental systems. Its ubiquity and water-solubility make it an important ROS scavenger in the extracellular space, which has relatively less ROS defensive capacity (31).

Reactive oxygen species enzymatic scavenger systems

Three enzymatic pathways have developed that specifically detoxify ROS to prevent cellular damage: catalase, glutathione peroxidase, and SOD systems. The first two catalyze H_2O_2 breakdown. H_2O_2, as described, is not a free radical, but it can participate in chemical reactions that produce highly damaging products. Therefore, lowering the concentration of H_2O_2 is important in prevention of oxidative injury.

The first of these enzymatic scavenger systems is based on catalase. Catalase is ubiquitous in cellular cytoplasm, and it is especially abundant in peroxisomes. It utilizes the H_2O_2 generated by the reactions described earlier to oxidize other substrates, such as phenols, formic acid, formaldehyde, and ethanol (Fig. 22–2, reaction 1). This process is especially important in hepatocytes and kidney cells, where elimination of both the H_2O_2 and the oxidized substance is important. Catalase can also convert excess H_2O_2 to water and molecular oxygen (see Fig. 22–2, reaction 2). Catalase can therefore detoxify hydrogen peroxide to prevent uncontrolled peroxidation of cellular components or creation of other ROS (31,34).

Glutathione peroxidase catalyzes a similar reaction using the tripeptide glutathione as a reducing agent. High concentrations of glutathione are present in the cytoplasm, where it can participate in the reaction to eliminate excess H_2O_2. Glutathione is kept reduced by cytoplasmic NADPH (10), which donates electrons (catalyzed by glutathione reductase) to oxidized glutathione to

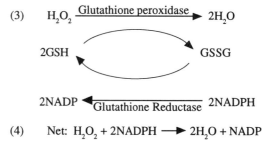

Catalase Pathway

$$(1) \quad H_2O_2 + RH_2 \xrightarrow{\text{catalase}} R + 2H_2O$$

R=ethanol, phenols, formic acid

$$(2) \quad 2H_2O_2 \xrightarrow{\text{catalase}} 2H_2O + O_2$$

Glutathione Pathway

$$(3) \quad H_2O_2 \xrightarrow{\text{Glutathione peroxidase}} 2H_2O$$

2GSH → GSSG

2NADP ← $\overline{\text{Glutathione Reductase}}$ 2NADPH

$$(4) \quad \text{Net: } H_2O_2 + 2NADPH \longrightarrow 2H_2O + NADP$$

Figure 22–2 Chemical enzymatic scavenging of hydrogen peroxide. Equations 1 and 2 show catalase enzyme system; equations 3 and 4 describe the glutathione reductase system.

convert any disulfide bonds back to cysteine residues (see Fig. 22–2, reaction 3). The net effect is donation of electrons from NADPH to H_2O_2, which forms water and NADP (see Fig. 22–2, reaction 4). This activity detoxifies H_2O_2 to prevent cellular damage, similar to the effect of the catalase system (31,34).

At its usual low, cytoplasmic concentration, H_2O_2 is preferentially metabolized by the glutathione peroxidase pathway, because of the more favorable kinetics of this enzyme compared with catalase. However, catalase activity increases with increasing concentration of H_2O_2. Also, because catalase is concentrated in peroxisomes, most H_2O_2 detoxification there is catalase-mediated. Therefore, these two pathways appear to be complementary; the predominant pathway is dependent on the H_2O_2 concentration and the intracellular location of the ROS (31).

The SOD family of enzymes are metalloproteins that catalyze the conversion of $O_2\bullet$ to H_2O_2 and molecular oxygen via the process known as dismutation (Eq. 4). The H_2O_2 generated by this dismutation can be further converted by glutathione peroxidase to water, as described, thus causing overall transformation of $O_2\bullet$, an ROS, to water and oxygen, two nontoxic substances, mediated by NADPH (see Fig. 22–2, reaction 2). There are three mammalian forms of SOD: copper-zinc SOD (CuZnSOD), primarily in the cytoplasm; manganous SOD (MnSOD), primarily in mitochondria, and which appears to be the main inducible form of SOD activity; and a high molecular weight extracellular SOD (EC-SOD), which is found mainly in plasma and lung tissue (31,35,36).

The distribution of SOD enzymes in tissues has been studied for various mammals, revealing general patterns of enzyme activity. Notably, the metabolically active tissues of liver and kidney have the highest levels in all species studied. Skeletal muscle, gut, and pancreas generally have much lower levels of enzyme activity. Additional studies have demonstrated that SOD activity can be induced by oxidant stresses, such as hyperoxia, endotoxinemia, or treatment with some cytokines (35,37–41).

The SOD family is the major enzymatic mechanism for cellular protection from $O_2\bullet$. It is far more efficient than the spontaneous reactions that can also detoxify ROS, and the enzyme does not require reduction by another electron donor to return to an active state (as does tocopherol). The SOD activities are distributed at the sites of superoxide production (i.e., CuZnSOD in cytoplasm; MnSOD in mitochondria); there is relatively little SOD activity in plasma. The low plasma SOD activity may be a compromise to allow the activity of endogenous systems that utilize superoxide for cell killing in the extracellular space, such as neutrophils. There are few mechanisms to limit extracellular ROS activity; there is little or no catalase activity, no measurable glutathione, and significantly less SOD activity (mainly EC-SOD) than in intracellular sites. There is less ROS quenching activity as well, be-cause uric acid and ascorbic acid are both relatively inefficient at physiological concentrations. A major inhibitor of extracellular oxidative damage may be the lack of reduced iron to catalyze the formation of $HO\bullet$ from H_2O_2; plasma free iron levels are essentially zero because the iron is transported in plasma by transferrin, in the Fe^{3+} state. Thus, SOD activity may be the main intracellular ROS defense system; other systems are primarily responsible for extracellular ROS. EC-SOD appears to be highly regulated, and it may have an important role in some situations (31,35).

The cellular defense mechanisms against ROS outlined herein are clearly important in cellular survival in an oxygen-containing environment. The evolutionary pressures that have conserved systems, such as catalase and MnSOD from bacteria to humans, and also selected for the development of apparently newer SOD enzymes (i.e., EC-SOD) testify to the requirement for this layer of cellular defense.

CYTOKINES AND REACTIVE OXYGEN SPECIES

The association of cytokines and ROS production has developed along with our understanding of cytokines. The earliest reports regarding the potential interaction of cellular protein products (i.e., cytokines) with ROS and oxidative damage were only able to use cell culture supernatants as the effector media (15,42,43). The availability of purified and recombinant cytokines has enabled investigators to more completely identify the role of various cytokines in the production of ROS and cellular oxidative damage. In this section of the chapter, we discuss the experimental basis for the role of cytokines in the induction of ROS, the effect of various cytokines on different cell types and species, and the known mechanisms by which the cytokines exert their effect.

Experimental methods to measure ROS production

Before discussing the experimental evidence for ROS production by cells following cytokine exposure, it is important to understand the methods used to identify these effects. In general, following experimental treatment, the production of ROS is measured by one of the methods shown in Table 22–3. Most commonly, the production of $O_2\bullet$ is determined by measuring the SOD-inhibitable reduction of cytochrome C. Using well-established methods, absorbance (at 550 nm) of the reaction solution can be used to calculate the amount of $O_2\bullet$ produced (44,45).

TABLE 22–3 MEASUREMENT OF ROS FORMATION

Intermediate Measured	Technique/Comment
$O_2\bullet$	SOD inhibitable reduction of cytochrome C, or cypridine luciferin analog (CLA)-dependent chemiluminescence
H_2O_2	Horseradish peroxidase oxidation of scopoletin, or phenol red
GSSG	NADPH-dependent GSSG reductase enzyme system
Malondialdehyde (MDA)	End product of lipid peroxidation

ROS = reactive oxygen species; SOD = superoxide dismutase.

This measurement of $O_2\bullet$ release can also be made continuously (46) to plot the kinetics of the reaction.

Another ROS measured is H_2O_2. Hydrogen peroxide release is most commonly determined by horseradish peroxidase oxidation of scopoletin, which changes the absorbance at 436 nm. An alternative method is to use phenol red instead of scopoletin and reading the absorbance at 610 nm (47). The other two measuring systems noted, glutathione reductase (GSH-GSSG) and malondialdehyde (MDA) production, are less commonly used, but they appear to give similar results (48).

Early experimental work

In the mid-1970s, it was noted by several investigators that activated phagocytes secreted H_2O_2 (44), and that this release of peroxide could be correlated with effector function (15). The supernatants of spleen cells or lymphocytes were found to markedly increase the ability of macrophages to both secrete H_2O_2 and eliminate infectious pathogens (15,42,43). In a typical set of experiments, Nathan and colleagues (15) at The Rockefeller University in New York collected peritoneal macrophages from mice immunized against *Trypanosoma cruzi,* and then exposed the cultured macrophages to supernatant from the spleen cells of similarly immunized mice. This "spleen cell factor" caused a time- and dose-dependent increase in H_2O_2 and parasitic killing by the cultured macrophages (15). However, the change in macrophage behavior was only noted when the cells were incubated with phorbol myristate acetate (PMA), a compound that stimulates protein kinase C activity.

The first report of ROS release following cytokine stimulation alone was published by Freund and Pick (43) from Tel Aviv University in Israel. In these experiments, guinea pig peritoneal macrophages cultured ex vivo and treated with "lymphokine," the supernatant from concavalin-A–stimulated lymphocytes, were able to secrete increased amounts of H_2O_2 relative to control cells. The production of $O_2\bullet$ was also measured, but it was found to be unchanged after experimental treatment (43).

Evidence for cytokine induction of ROS release

Since these early experiments, much work has been done with purified and, more recently, recombinant cytokines and their effect on ROS release. Table 22–4 lists the experimental evidence for cytokine-induced release of ROS from various cell lines. The cytokines, TNF-α, IL-1α, IL-1β, IFN-γ, and granulocyte- macrophage colony-stimulating factor (GM-CSF) have been shown in multiple experiments to cause release of ROS from a variety of cells. The most common cell type that can produce ROS is the phagocyte (either monocytes/macrophages or polymorphonuclear leukocytes [PMNs]). Other cell types that can produce $O_2\bullet$ or H_2O_2 after cytokine stimulation include rat islet cells, mouse hepatocytes, and human chondrocytes and fibroblasts. Both IL-1α and IL-1β have shown no increase in ROS production in other experimental models (49–52). Although this statement implies that IL-1α and IL-1β may not consistently effect the ROS release of cells (phagocytes and others), it is more likely that the experimental conditions in which these cytokines had no effect were insufficient to enhance ROS production. For instance, in one set of experiments, IL-1α and IL-1β caused release of ROS from monocytes after secondary stimulation with PMA (50). The same conditions were then applied to PMNs, except for the secondary stimulating compound, which was switched to a chemotactic peptide, formyl-methionyl-leucyl-phenylalanine (fMLP). Although fMLP did not stimulate the PMNs to release ROS, PMA, which works through a different mechanism, was not tested for PMNs in that experimental design. It is possible that a different secondary stimulating compound may have caused enhanced ROS release after treatment. Also, the ability of IL-1β or IL-1α to prime PMNs for $O_2\bullet$ release has been measured as 25 to 500× less powerful than TNF-α when assessed in the same model system (51). Thus, the inconsistent conclusions regarding IL-1 and ROS production may be in part due to poor sensitivity of available experimental methods.

To summarize the known effects of various cytokines on ROS production, Table 22–5 lists the cytokines by category: consistent experimental enhancement of ROS release; equivocal, but probable, enhancement; no effect; or inhibition of ROS release. The second category (probable increase in ROS release) includes cytokines that have

TABLE 22–4   CYTOKINE-ASSOCIATED ROS PRODUCTION (IN VITRO)

Cytokine	Species	Cell	Priming	Direct Effect	References
rTNF-α	Human	Monocyte	PMA, fMLP	None	(53,58)
		PMN (suspension)	PMA, fMLP	None	(60,61)
		PMN (adherent)	—	Yes	(12,65)
		Fibroblasts	—	Yes	(100)
		Eosinophils	PMA	Yes	(101)
	rat (hTNF used)	Macrophages (BM)	PMA	None	(49)
		Macrophages (A)	IgG	None	(102)
		PMN	IgG	None	(102)
	Mouse (hTNF used)	Hepatocytes	None	Yes	(48)
		Macrophages (BM)	PMA, Zy	None	(54)
		Macrophages (P)	PMA, Zy	None	(54)
rTNF-β	Human	PMN (adherent)	None	Yes	(12)
rIFN-γ	Human	Macrophages	PMA, fMLP	Yes	(14,53,56,58)
	Rat (rat IFN used)	Macrophages (P)	Zy	None	(103)
	Mouse (muIFN used)	Macrophages (P)	PMA, Zy	None	(54)
		Macrophages (BM)	PMA, Zy	None	(54)
rGM-CSF	Human	PMN	fMLP	Yes	(12,55,63,104)
		Monocytes	PMA, fMLP	None	(53)
	Mouse (mu-GM-CSF used)	Macrophages (P)	PMA, Zy	None	(54)
		Macrophages (BM)	PMA, Zy	None	(54)
rIL-1α	Human	Monocyte	PMA, fMLP	None	(50,58)
		Fibroblasts	None	Yes	(100)
	Mouse (hIL-1α used)	Macrophages (BM)	PMA, Zy	None	(54)
rIL-1β	Human	Monocyte	PMA, fMLP	None	(50,58)
		PMN	fMLP	None	(51)
		Chondrocytes	None	Yes	(52)
rG-CSF	Human	PMN	fMLP	None	(55)
rIL-3	Human	Monocytes	PMA, fMLP	None	(53)

ROS = reactive oxygen species; TNF = tumor necrosis factor; PMA = phorbol myristate acetate; fMLP = formyl-methionyl-leucyl-phenylalanine; PMN = polymorphonuclear leukocyte; IFN = interferon; GM-CSF = granulocyte-macrophage colony-stimulating factor; IgG = immunoglobulin G; P = peritoneal; BM = bone marrow; A = alveolar (macrophages); Zy = zymosan.

shown inconsistent results, such as IL-1α and IL-1β, or those that have not been as extensively investigated as cytokines in the first category. These cytokines, such as IL-3 (53) and G-CSF (54,55), will likely have their roles in the induction of ROS release better defined in the years to come. Although not as extensively investigated as TNF-α and others, the cytokines listed as having no effect are unlikely to cause ROS release, based on the experimental evidence to date (52,56). IL-4 appears to inhibit ROS production in all experimental studies to date (53,57). Reduced $O_2\bullet$ release was correlated with im-

paired phagocytic capability (anti-Leishmanial activity) in human macrophages treated with IL-4 (53).

Mechanisms of cytokine action

The major distinction between the various experimental conditions and outcomes is whether the treated cells produce ROS directly after stimulation with a cytokine, or if a second stimulus, most commonly PMA, is necessary. This phenomenon has been termed *priming* (11). As

TABLE 22-5 CYTOKINE EFFECT ON ROS PRODUCTION

Unequivocal increase in ROS release
TNF-α, TNF-β
IFN-γ
GM-CSF
Probable increase in ROS release
IL-1α
IL-1β
IL-3
G-CSF
No increase in ROS release
IFN-α A
IFN-α D
IFN-β
IL-6
Inhibition of ROS release
IL-4

ROS = reactive oxygen species; TNF = tumor necrosis factor; IFN = interferon; GM-CSF = granulocyte-macrophage colony-stimulating factor; IL = interleukin.

TABLE 22-6 NONCYTOKINES THAT CAUSE ROS RELEASE

Compound	Description
PMA	Protein kinase C activator
fMLP (formyl-methionyl-leucyl-phenylalanine)	Bacterial chemoattractant
A23187	Calcium ionophore
Zymosan	Yeast particle
LPS	Lipopolysaccharide from bacterial cell wall
ConA	Cocanavalin A (mitogen)
C5a	Complement cascade component
Platelet-activating factor	Acetyl-glyceryl-ether-phosphoryl-choline
Immunoglobulin G immune complexes	Antibody-antigen complex
Amphotericin B	Antifungal agent

shown in Table 22–4, many phagocytic and nonphagocytic cells can induce ROS release by themselves. However, addition of a second agent, such as PMA or fMLP, always increases the ROS response, if tested (51). In theory, treatment of cells with cytokines can alter the cellular biochemical status, thus enabling an enhanced ROS production response to a second stimulus. Table 22–6 lists the noncytokine compounds that effectively induce ROS release from cells. Many are nonphysiological, such as PMA or A23187; they cause ROS release through their effect on intracellular biochemical processes. Concanavalin A (ConA) is a mitogen that nonspecifically activates phagocytic cells. The other compounds listed are effective at physiological doses, and they are therefore more relevant to the potential clinical effects of oxidative damage. Zymosan and lipopolysaccharide (LPS) are released by invading fungus and bacteria, respectively, and they exert their effects on cells through a variety of mechanisms. LPS directly stimulates ROS release, and it also mediates increased ROS production or priming for release by causing cells to secrete various cytokines (58). Interaction of cells with complement components, including C5a, opsonized zymosan, or antibody-antigen complexes, can also cause ROS release. Finally, the antifungal agent, amphotericin B, which has direct fungicidal effects, may also work through stimulation of ROS release in the presence of fungal infection (59). Table 22–7 lists the various inhibitors of components of the oxidation-reduction system of the mammalian cell that are used experimentally to define the mechanisms of ROS release.

The mechanism of "priming" cells for ROS release has been investigated in numerous experiments. Initial work on the priming mechanism was accomplished before recombinant or purified cytokines were available and therefore looked only at the effect of PMA, fMLP, and other ROS agonists on various enzyme systems. McPhail and colleagues (11) showed that sequential stimulation with different agonists caused enhanced activation of the NADPH oxidase enzyme system in human PMNs, relative to a single stimulus. This finding suggests that the cellular biochemical mechanisms of the three agents tested (i.e., PMA, fMLP, A23187) are different yet synergistic in their relationship to ROS production. However, if the same agonist (e.g., PMA) was used for both treatments, the NADPH oxidase activity was decreased, implying that the second stimulus could either activate or deactivate the production of ROS, depending on its nature. This desensitization or tolerance to successive identical stimuli occurred with fMLP, A23187, and PMA; NADPH activity was decreased by 80, 100, and 40%, respectively (11). This phenomenon of tolerance induction may have clinical relevance, and it is discussed in a later section in detail.

The biochemical basis of priming has been further investigated using recombinant cytokines. Berkow and associates (60,61) have shown that TNF priming of human PMNs for $O_2\cdot$ release is independent of extracellular sodium or calcium influx, altered arachidonic acid release, activation or translocation of protein kinase C, and pertussis toxin–sensitive G-protein regulation. The kinetics of the NADPH oxidase enzyme system are similarly unal-

TABLE 22–7   EXPERIMENTAL INHIBITORS OF ROS SYSTEMS

System	Inhibitors
Mitochondrial respiratory chain	Rotenone, sodium azide, cyanide
Iron oxidation-reduction	Desferrioxamine (DFO)
Peroxide scavengers	Mannitol, catalase, benzoate, dimethyl sulfoxide
Protein kinase C	H-7, staurosporine
Superoxide dismutase (SOD)	Diethyldithiocarbamic acid (DDC) (Cu, ZnSOD only) Nitroprusside—all SOD
Lipid peroxidation	U78518E, Vitamin E
Microfilament structure	Cytochalasin B
Xanthine oxidase	Xanthine, allopurinol

ROS = reactive oxygen species.

tered, as has been shown in other studies (62). Berkow and associates did identify a time-dependent and TNF-α dose-dependent increase in the phosphorylation of several proteins, most notably a 64-kd band. In work with rhGM-CSF and rhG-CSF, protein kinase C activation and translocation was similarly absent following incubation with either of the growth factors. However, release of membrane-associated arachidonic acid within 5 minutes of the incubation start time was measured, probably indicating interaction of the two factors with membrane-based phospholipases (55). The investigators theorized that the long incubation time necessary for maximal priming by rhGM-CSF, relative to TNF-α, may be necessary to allow build-up of arachidonic acid metabolites to a certain effective threshold level (55,63). Other studies documented an increase in fMLP-specific receptors following rhGM-CSF incubation, which may represent nonspecific up-regulation of potentially costimulatory receptors (63).

In conclusion, the exact mechanisms by which cells are primed by exposure to cytokines to release ROS are largely unknown. It appears that the different cytokines function through a variety of pathways and receptors, but not directly through protein kinase C, or other common mechanisms of cellular activation. The full explanation will likely be a combination of conformational and biochemical changes in enzyme systems not yet identified.

As shown in Table 22–4, some cytokines can directly cause ROS release from certain cell populations without addition of a "priming" agent. The mechanism of this phenomenon has also been investigated in multiple stud-

ies. Initial work was able to connect production of H_2O_2 with dismutation of $O_2\bullet$ by the SOD group of enzymes. In a 1986 study by Freund and Pick (62), production of measurable H_2O_2 was almost totally eliminated by the universal SOD inhibitor, sodium nitroprusside, with conversion of ROS release to $O_2\bullet$. This reaction proved that enzymatic dismutation (Eq. 4) is integrally involved in ROS production following stimulation with "lymphokine," a supernatant of activated lymphocytes. Furthermore, these investigators could attribute all significant dismutation of ROS to MnSOD, as opposed to the CuZn-SOD also present. This distinction was possible with the CuZnSOD inhibitor, diethyldithiocarbamic acid (DDC), which caused a barely perceptible change in the SOD activity of either whole cells or homogenates of cells treated for 72 hours with the lymphokine solution (62). In a separate study, DDC did not inhibit TNF-α–induced cytolysis of L-M murine fibroblasts in vitro, confirming the insignificant role of CuZnSOD in $O_2\bullet$ dismutation (64).

Subsequent investigation has looked at the exact mechanisms whereby any ROS are generated. The ability of PMNs to adhere to a glass wall is associated with ROS release following cytokine stimulation alone (2,65), but nonadherent cells of the same lineage will only produce ROS after a secondary stimulus, such as PMA. Adherent PMNs may otherwise be activated or "primed" by a noncytokine stimulus, and cytokine administration may in fact be a secondary agent in that situation. Activation of the "respiratory burst" by TNF-α in adherent PMNs appears to involve cyclic adenosine monophosphate (AMP) and the cellular microfilament structure, because it is severely inhibited by dibutyryl cyclic AMP (an analog) and cytochalasin B. However, in that experimental model (65), release of ROS was independent of arachidonic acid release and phosphoinositide hydrolysis, both of which had been suggested by other work (5).

Movement of intracellular calcium may also be important in the generation of ROS directly following cytokine stimulation. Tsujimoto and coworkers (66) showed that 8-(diethylamino)-octyl-3,4,5-trimethoxybenzoate hydrochloride, an inhibitor of intracellular calcium mobilization, prevented human neutrophils from releasing ROS in the presence of TNF. Conversely, inhibiting extracellular calcium availability did not significantly change ROS release (66). This article also confirmed the findings of others that cytochalasin B alters the ROS release profile. As noted by other authors (65), this compound, which alters fluidity and function of the cell membrane, impairs the ability of TNF to cause ROS generation. However, the same compound enhances $O_2\bullet$ production following stimulation by fMLP alone (66). This finding again suggests a multifactorial mechanism for ROS generation following stimulation by various compounds.

The exact mechanisms whereby cytokines such as TNF and IL-1 cause the release of ROS remain unknown, not only in the setting of "priming" for secondary stimulation by agents such as PMA and fMLP, but also when the cytokine alone enhances ROS production. As noted, there is much contradictory and negative data published regarding these phenomena. The significant increase in $O_2\bullet$ production and release seen following selected cytokine treatment suggest that cytokines are important cofactors in the "respiratory burst" of neutrophils and macrophages, and they may also sensitize other cells to the effects of that burst (67). In the final section of this chapter, we discuss the clinical implications of the association between cytokines and ROS release.

CLINICAL APPLICATIONS OF CYTOKINE-INDUCED OXIDATIVE DAMAGE

The mechanisms of cellular damage from oxidative processes have been implicated in several pathophysiological states (Table 22–8). Although the extremely reactive nature of ROS makes it difficult to clearly document a causal role in specific clinical situations, ROS have been recognized in experimental models of acute inflammation, autoimmune diseases, hemochromatosis, vascular atheromatous plaques, tissue ischemia, reperfusion injury, pulmonary hyperoxia, sepsis, aging, and cancer (68). Many of these conditions are characterized by activated phagocyte cytokine production and ROS release. Conversely, neutrophils from patients with chronic granulomatous disease of childhood, which are deficient in NADPH oxidase, are unable to kill catalase-producing organisms, and patients suffer from recurrent granulomatous infections. It is hypothesized that the "respiratory burst" is actively involved in these clinical effects, and that cytokines alter the oxidative capacity of this burst phenomenon, as described. For example, phagocytic response to infectious agents is enhanced in vitro by cytokines (14). Furthermore, a recent prospective randomized study demonstrated that IFN-γ, a cytokine that clearly augments ROS release, decreased the incidence of infection in patients with chronic granulomatous disease (69). Rabinovitch and associates (70) showed that isolated rat islet cells exposed to a combination of cytokines exhibited diminished insulin release, increased ROS production, and islet necrosis. The toxic effect in vitro of cytokines on islet cells, mediated by ROS release, has been confirmed in other studies (71).

Despite the in vitro evidence for cytokine-enhanced oxidative burst capacity, in vivo or clinical involvement of cytokines in production of ROS and induction of oxidative damage is less well documented. Table 22–9 lists experiments in which in vivo treatment with recombinant cytokines was followed by in vitro measurement of ROS production. In the first three cases listed, rodents were given recombinant cytokines; macrophages, either peritoneal or alveolar, were then harvested. In all three cases, the macrophages made ROS following stimulation with another compound, but not spontaneously (i.e., no direct effect of the cytokine exposure on ROS release). Nonetheless, the results of these experiments indicate significant in vivo priming of macrophages following cytokine exposure, leading to an enhanced response to infectious agents or particles, such as Histoplasma or zymosan (59).

The final experiments listed evaluated the oxidative response to in vivo cytokines in humans. Sullivan and colleagues (72) examined the oxidative burst capacity of human granulocytes before and after a 12- to 24-hour infusion of recombinant GM-CSF. Increased $O_2\bullet$ release was seen relative to pretreatment values, even without a secondary stimulus, although this number was not statistically significant. However, stimulation in vitro with either fMLP or PMA caused a significant increase in ROS production over that of granulocytes similarly stimulated before GM-CSF treatment ($p < 0.03$, $p < 0.01$, respectively) (72). As stated by the authors, these results suggest

TABLE 22–8   PROPOSED CLINICAL EFFECTS OF CYTOKINE–INDUCED OXIDATIVE DAMAGE

Infectious
    Antifungal
        Candida
        Histoplasma
    Antiparasitic
        Toxoplasma gondii
        Leishmania sp.
        Trypanosoma cruzi
Sepsis
    Vasodilation
    End-organ injury
    ARDS pathogenesis
Cutaneous
    Pathogenesis
        Bullous dermatoses
        Allergic contact dermatitis
        Porphyria
        Lupus erythematosus
Neoplasm
    Carcinogenesis
    Anti-tumor response
Other
    Chronic granulomatous disease
    Diabetes

ARDS = adult respiratory distress syndrome.

TABLE 22–9   CYTOKINE-ASSOCIATED ROS PRODUCTION
(IN VIVO CYTOKINE ADMINISTRATION)

Cytokine	Species	Cell Tested	Priming	Direct Effect	References
rhTNF-α	Rat	Macrophage (A)	PMA	None	(105)
rmuTNF-α	Mouse	Macrophage (P)	Zy, Histo	None	(59)
rmuIFN-γ	Mouse	Macrophage (P)	Zy, Histo	None	(59)
rhGM-CSF	Human	PMN	PMA, fMLP	Minimal	(72,73)
rhG-CSF	Human	PMN	fMLP, PMA	None	(74)
rhTNF-α	Human	PMN	See text	None	(75)

ROS = reactive oxygen species; TNF = tumor necrosis factor; IFN = interferon; GM-CSF = granulocyte-macrophage colony-stimulating factor; PMN = polymorphonuclear leukocyte; PMA = phorbol myristate acetate; fMLP = formyl-methionyl-leucyl-phenylalanine; P = peritoneal; A = alveolar (macrophages); Zy = zymosan; Histo = *H. capsulatum*.

that rhGM-CSF, in addition to its other potential therapeutic benefits, may augment the oxidative burst capacity of granulocytes, and thereby possibly enhance the host's microbicidal and tumoricidal defenses.

Kaplan and associates (73) performed a similar study in 10 patients with widespread carcinoma. After administration of intravenous rhGM-CSF, the ROS release of PMNs increased in response to both fMLP and PMA. PMNs that were not exposed to a secondary agent in vitro had an inconsistent and nonstatistically significant increase in ROS production. Higher doses of GM-CSF generally caused a less intense $O_2\bullet$ release for both stimulants. The enhanced oxidative response was seen after either a bolus or a continuous dose of GM-CSF, and it was again cited as an additional therapeutic benefit of GM-CSF treatment (73).

The effect of rhG-CSF in vivo was investigated by Ohsaka and colleagues (74). Seven adults with lymphoma were given G-CSF (IV for 14 consecutive days), and neutrophils were harvested before, during, and after treatment. Although the patients received different chemotherapy regimens before their G-CSF treatments, as well as different G-CSF doses (to compare other factors), enhanced $O_2\bullet$ release was seen in all patients following treatment and in vitro stimulation with fMLP. Additional in vitro incubation of the harvested cells with G-CSF did not increase the oxidative response in most patients (74). This finding suggests, along with the data from the previous experiment, that there is "unpriming" or tolerance induction with excessive or repetitive exposure to the priming agent.

A similar phenomenon was seen with in vivo TNF-α exposure. Kapp and associates (75) harvested peripheral blood PMNs from patients receiving continuous IV rhTNF-α for 5 days as part of a treatment protocol for metastatic melanoma. The isolated PMN were stimulated with TNF-α, TNF-β, GM-CSF, PMA, opsonized zymosan, and fMLP. Although TNF-α, TNF-β, and PMA stimulated $O_2\bullet$ release on days 1 through 3, by day 4, the PMN oxidative response had returned to baseline. GM-CSF and opsonized zymosan had no effect. The fMLP continued to enhance $O_2\bullet$ release through day 8, but it was maximally stimulatory at day 4. The data suggest that TNF-α primes human PMNs in vivo for enhanced ROS release to different stimuli, but that prolonged continuous exposure to TNF-α may induce a "tolerance," whereby the oxidative burst response to subsequent stimulation is unchanged or even reduced (75).

As described, multiple studies have shown that cytokine exposure in vivo can prime human granulocytes for an enhanced oxidative burst response to a second stimulus. However, the response varies with the dose and duration of cytokine administration, consistent with other effects of these cytokines (76,77). This finding points out the paradoxical nature of cytokine function, particularly as it relates to ROS production.

Cytokines such as TNF-α and IL-1 are highly conserved biologically, and they are capable of causing extreme toxicity, even death, at certain physiological doses. Blockade of IL-1 by the use of its specific receptor antagonist (IL-1RA) (78) and blockade of TNF by the use of TNF antibodies (79,80) reversed the lethal effects of endotoxin, implying that each of these cytokines are partially responsible for the lethal effects of endotoxin (i.e., LPS). Administration of cytokines prior to LPS have also protected against the lethality of LPS (81–84). Thus, both administration of cytokines and strategies to block their effects can be beneficial to the host organism. Because cytokines are ubiquitous, pluripotent, and potentially toxic, the organism needs mechanisms to control or regulate cytokine responses. It is clear that cellular toxicity of TNF and other cytokines is mediated through generation of ROS (85–88). One mechanism of cytokine protection against cellular toxicity associated with agents that induce cytokine production is generation of enzymes to protect against the harmful effects of ROS. A candidate protective enzyme is MnSOD (38,85,88–90).

The mechanism of TNF-α cytotoxicity is unclear, but it may be at least partially mediated through generation of ROS (85–88). The susceptibility of a cell to killing by TNF-α may be influenced by its content of antioxidant enzymes, such as catalase, SOD, and glutathione peroxidase, as described previously. SOD protects cells from the toxicity of $O_2 \cdot$, whereas catalase and glutathione peroxidase scavenge H_2O_2. Eukaryotic cells contain two types of SOD. CuZnSOD is mainly in the cytosol, is constitutively expressed, and is not induced by TNF or other cytokines. MnSOD is found mainly in the mitochondria, and gene expression is induced by TNF-α, TNF-β, IL-1α, and IL-1β (38). MnSOD reduces superoxide to less toxic H_2O_2 and O_2. It is found in a variety of tissues, and it is thought to be an integral part of the cellular resistance to ROS injury. Pretreatment of cells with low levels of either TNF-α or IL-1α confers resistance to subsequent killing.

It has been shown by Wong and colleagues (38,89) that generation of MnSOD is essential for cellular resistance to TNF-α. A human lung cancer cell line, A549, was treated with TNF-α for 12 hours, and expression of different candidate genes for protection against toxic reactive oxygen species was measured (38). TNF-α did not induce expression of catalase, CuZnSOD, glutathione peroxidase, or cytochrome oxidase over constitutive expression. However, TNF-α dramatically increased expression of both the 4-kb precursor and the 1-kb active form of MnSOD. TNF-β, IL-1α, and IL-1β had similar effects on A549 cells, but IFN-α, IFN-γ, IL-2, and IL-6 did not. In a subsequent study, using 293 human kidney cell lines and ME-180, a human cervical carcinoma cell line, overexpression of the gene for MnSOD resulted in increased resistance to TNF-α, and insertion of antisense to MnSOD resulted in increased cellular sensitivity to TNF-α (89).

Block and associates (91) cultured the TNF-sensitive L929 cell line in various concentrations of TNF-α (0 ng/mL, L929-S; 10 ng/mL, L929-R10; 100 ng/mL, L929-R100) continuously for 4 months. Total cellular RNA was extracted for Northern blot analyses and probed with ^{32}P-labeled cDNA for MnSOD, CuZnSOD, and actin. RNA was extracted from endotoxin-stimulated A549 cells and used as a positive control (Fig. 22–3). The results demonstrate that the cellular complement of MnSOD mRNA is increased 20-fold over baseline levels in L929-R100 cells grown in high concentrations of TNF, and to a lesser degree in cells grown in lesser amounts of TNF-α (L929-R10 cells). This study, in addition to the studies of Wong and colleagues (38,89), suggest that MnSOD is an important enzyme in the mechanism of cellular resistance to TNF-α and imply that TNF-α exposure induces cells to produce this enzyme, which is a natural protective mech-

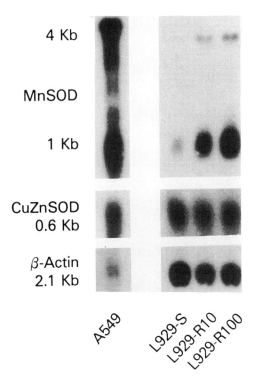

Figure 22–3 Northern blot analysis of RNA from TNF-sensitive and -resistant L929 cells demonstrating increasing quantities of manganous superoxide dismutase (MnSOD) mRNA, with increasing concentrations of TNF-α in culture media (L929-S, no TNF; L929-R10, 10 ng/mL, TNF; L929-R100, 100 ng/mL TNF). Equivalence of mRNA loading is demonstrated by equivalence of signal for CuZnSOD. RNA from endotoxin-stimulated A549 cells is used as a positive control. The figure demonstrates increasing expression of MnSOD mRNA with increasing concentrations of TNF-α. (Reproduced by permission from Block MI, Alexander HR, Buresh C, Norton JA. Acquired resistance to TNF in vitro is associated with increased expression of the gene for MnSOD but not gene amplification. Surg Forum 1991;42:464–467.)

anism to toxic effects of TNF-α. Other studies, however, failed to show an increase in MnSOD production in cells resistant to TNF-α in vitro (92,93).

Whole animal studies also demonstrate that cytokines such as TNF-α and IL-1α induce production of MnSOD, which is able to improve outcome of animals exposed to agents that mediate toxicity through ROS (83,84,94–96). Such agents include endotoxin (84), TNF-α (97), gram-negative sepsis (83,95), and high concentrations of oxygen (96). First, it has been shown that mice treated intravenously with murine TNF-α have increased production of MnSOD in organs (38). Mice were treated with 5 μg muTNF-α; 24 hours later, mRNA was purified from thymus, kidney, bone marrow, and spleen. In each organ, one injection of TNF-α gave increased expression of the gene for MnSOD over nontreated control animals. Subsequently, it has been demonstrated that human IL-1α will also induce the gene for MnSOD in the liver of treated

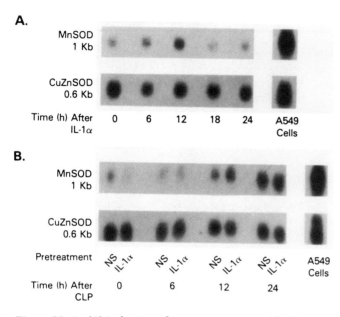

Figure 22–4 (A) Induction of manganous dismutase (MnSOD) in liver of mice at various intervals after IL-1α injection (27 μg/kg IV). (B) Augmented expression of MnSOD in livers of mice after cecal ligation and puncture (CLP) when animals were treated with IL-1 or normal saline 24 hours before CLP. Gene expression of CuZnSOD is constitutive in both A and B, and it is used as a control for equal loading. A549 cells stimulated with endotoxin were used as a positive control for MnSOD expression. (Reproduced by permission from Alexander HR, Jensen JC, Doherty GM, Block MI, Buresh CM, Norton JA. Induction of manganous superoxide dismutase (MnSOD) gene expression by interleukin-1 (IL-1): possible molecular basis for IL-1 protection against lethal sepsis. Surg Forum 1991;42:98.)

animals (Fig. 22–4) (94). Mice were given 27 μg/kg recombinant human IL-1α IV at time 0, and they were killed at various times following treatment. Total cellular RNA was harvested from liver and lung, and it was probed sequentially with ^{32}P-labeled cDNA for MnSOD and CuZnSOD. The blots for the liver are shown in Fig. 22–4. The CuZnSOD gene was constitutively expressed in liver tissue, and it did not change following IL-1α. Expression of MnSOD was maximum 12 hours following administration of IL-1α in both liver (Fig. 22–4) and lung (data not shown). These data indicate that systemic administration of IL-1α (94), like TNF-α (38), can induce tissue expression of the gene for MnSOD.

Because both IL-1α and TNF-α treatment induces expression of MnSOD after in vivo exposure, the next question is whether IL-1 and TNF-α treatment is able to protect against conditions whose toxicity is mediated by ROS. As mentioned, TNF-α mediates part of its toxicity through ROS (85–88). Low-dose IL-1α and TNF-α pretreatment decreased the lethality of TNF-α in experimental studies in mice (Table 22–10) (97). When mice were pretreated with sublethal, nontoxic doses of either IL-1α

TABLE 22–10 CYTOKINE PROTECTION AGAINST TNF LETHALITY IN MICE*

Pretreatment Agent	Pretreatment Dose (μg/kg)	Lethal TNF-α Challenge Dose (μg/kg)	72 hr Survival (%)
Saline	—	130	0
hIL-1α	100	130	92[†]
hTNF-α	30	130	50[†]

*Interval between pretreatment cytokines dose and lethal challenge dose of TNF-α varied from 3 to 8 days, with similar results.
[†]Significantly greater than saline, but not different from each other.
TNF = tumor necrosis factor; IL = interleukin.
Data are from Sheppard BC, Norton JA. Tumor necrosis factor and interleukin-1 protection against the lethal effects of tumor necrosis factor. Surgery 1991;106:698–705.

or TNF-α and subsequently (3–8 days later) challenged with a lethal dose of TNF-α, there was a marked reduction in lethality. Similarly, when mice were pretreated with cytokine and subsequently challenged with endotoxin (LPS), protection was seen (Table 22–11) (81,83,84,95). Furthermore, it was demonstrated that TNF-α pretreatment diminishes the hypotension and tissue injury associated with endotoxin (84). TNF-α pretreatment with multiple injections of cytokine has been shown to decrease lethality, hypotension, and hypothermia of severe gram-negative sepsis in rats (95). Rats pretreated with TNF-α had enhanced levels of MnSOD gene expression in the liver 12 hours following cecal ligation and puncture compared with control animals, implying that cellular expression of this enzyme was responsible for the demonstrated protective effects of TNF-α (Fig. 22–5) (95). The exact same benefit of IL-1α pretreatment in cecal ligation and puncture has been demonstrated (94). Furthermore, the mechanism of the protective effect of IL-1α following cecal ligation and puncture was demonstrated to be enhanced induction of the gene for MnSOD at 12 hours (Fig. 22–4B).

It therefore appears that TNF-α, LPS, and gram-negative sepsis each induce toxicity and death through ROS. IL-1α and TNF pretreatment in sublethal doses rapidly enhances cellular expression of MnSOD, an enzyme that protects cells from ROS (Figs. 22–3, 22–4A). Subsequent exposure of cytokine-pretreated animals to agents that mediate toxicity through ROS, such as cecal ligation and puncture or LPS, results in enhanced expression of cellular MnSOD (Figs. 22–4B, 22–5) and protection against manifestations of toxicity (see Table 22–11).

Expression of TNF-α, IL-6, and IL-1 in the lungs of mice exposed to toxic concentrations of oxygen for several days implicates local production of cytokine as a pos-

TABLE 22–11 CYTOKINE PROTECTION AGAINST ENDOTOXIN LETHALITY IN RODENTS

Species	Pretreatment Agent	Dose of Cytokine (μg/kg)	Time Between Pretreatment Challenge (hr)	LPS Dose (mg/kg)	72-hr Survival (%)
Mice	Saline	—	24	30	17
	hIL-1α	27	24	30	100*
Rat	Saline	—	24	20	25
	hTNF-α	50	24	20	80*

*Significantly greater than saline, but not different from each other.
LPS = lipopolysaccharide; IL = interleukin; TNF = tumor necrosis factor.
Data are from (83,84).

sible cause of oxygen toxicity (Fig. 22–6) (96). The link between inflammatory cytokines and free radicals has also been supported by other investigations. TNF-α and IL-6 can activate macrophages and increase production of $O_2\bullet$ by neutrophils to generate ROS (85–87). Pretreatment of mice with TNF-α afforded protection against subsequent exposure to continuous 100% oxygen and prolongation of survival compared with control mice pretreated with saline (96). Pretreatment with TNF-α was associated with enhanced expression of the gene for MnSOD in lungs of mice exposed to continuous 100% oxygen, implying that this was the mechanism of protection.

It is clear that cytokines, including IL-1 and TNF, are responsible for the lethality of numerous conditions, including endotoxin, gram-negative sepsis, and oxygen toxicity. It is also clear that cytokine induction of ROS and free radicals accounts for much of the cellular death and toxicity. This paradoxical effect of cytokines could be explained by the ability of sublethal doses of cytokines, such as IL-1α and TNF-α, to rapidly induce MnSOD, a protective enzyme that eliminates intracellular $O_2\bullet$ before it can react further and form more toxic compounds, such as HO•. This finding has been used in numerous animal models to demonstrate marked amelioration of lethal injuries (some examples have been provided). Such strategies may be useful in patients who are at high risk for the development of life-threatening infection or other conditions whose toxicity are mediated through ROS.

Another paradoxical effect of cytokines related to ROS release has been shown in the interplay of PMNs, lymphocytes, TNF-α, and tumor cells. TNF-α–treated PMNs can suppress tumor cell proliferation (98), and cause tumor cytolysis in vitro. This activity is blocked by catalase, but not SOD, implying that H_2O_2, but not $O_2\bullet$, is involved in the antitumor effect (99). However, TNF-α–activated PMNs inhibit the tumor cell cytotoxicity of lymphokine-activated killer (LAK) cells and natural killer (NK) cells (98). This inhibition is also reversible by catalase, but not SOD. Thus, the in vivo effect of TNF-α is characterized by

enhanced antitumor efficacy of PMNs, coupled with PMN-mediated reduction in LAK and NK cell function. Both processes involve production of ROS, although there are probably other factors involved. Use of TNF for cancer therapy will need to circumvent this paradoxical effect on the host's antitumor immune defense systems.

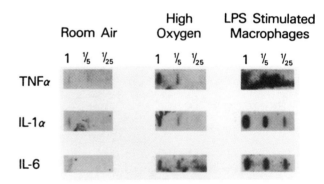

Figure 22–5 Gene expression of MnSOD following cecal ligation and puncture (CLP) in the liver of rTNF-α- or saline-treated rats. Animals were treated with rTNF-α or saline and underwent CLP 24 hours later. RNA was extracted from liver at each time point. At t = 0, before CLP, there is evidence of slightly increased expression of the gene for MnSOD in the liver of rats treated with rTNF compared with control rats. Twelve hours after CLP, clear augmentation of the gene for MnSOD is observed in both control and rTNF-treated rats compared with levels at t = 0. In addition, at 12 hours, MnSOD gene expression is further augmented in the liver of rTNF-treated compared with control rats. After 24 hours, MnSOD gene expression returns to basal levels in both groups. The hepatic gene expression for CuZnSOD and B-actin remain the same before and at each time point after CLP in either rTNF-treated or saline control animals. RNA extracted from A549 cells treated with 0.1 gm LPS served as a positive control for MnSOD gene expression. (Reproduced by permission from Alexander HR, Sheppard BC, Jensen JC, et al. Treatment with recombinant human tumor necrosis factor-alpha protects rats against lethality, hypotension, and hypothermia of gram-negative sepsis. J Clin Invest 1991;88:34–39.)

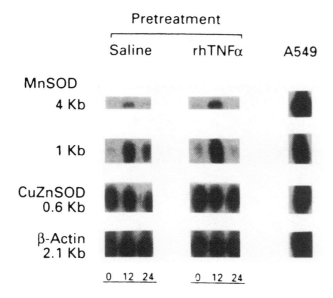

Pretreatment

| | Saline | rhTNFα | A549 |

MnSOD 4 Kb

1 Kb

CuZnSOD 0.6 Kb

β-Actin 2.1 Kb

0 12 24   0 12 24

Hours after CLP

Figure 22–6 Slot blots of mRNA from lungs of mice exposed to room air or high-dose oxygen for 3 days, and slot blots of total RNA from murine macrophages exposed to LPS for 24 hours. Macrophages have marked expression of genes for TNF-α, IL-1α, and IL-6, and they serve as a positive control. mRNA from lungs of mice exposed to high-dose oxygen for 3 days has increased expression of the genes for TNF, IL-1, and IL-6, compared with mRNA from lungs of mice exposed to room air. (Reproduced by permission from Jensen JC, Pogrebniak HW, Pass HI, et al. The role of tumor necrosis factor in oxygen toxicity. J Appl Physiol 1992;72:1902–1907.)

CONCLUSION

ROS, principally $O_2 \bullet$, are produced by granulocytes and other cells in response to various stimuli. $O_2 \bullet$ is rapidly chemically converted to other ROS, such as the very toxic hydroxyl radical and the generally less damaging hydrogen peroxide. Additional reactions that form toxic intermediates or damage cellular components are possible. Several protective enzymatic and cofactor systems exist to protect the cells against low levels of ROS.

The respiratory burst is a massive release of ROS by phagocytes when exposed to chemical or particulate agonists. Several cytokines, principally TNF-α, IL-1, IFN-γ, and GM-CSF, have been shown to enhance the respiratory burst of these cells. This enhancement generally takes the form of "priming" the cells for a greater ROS release after secondary stimulation by cofactors, such as PMA, fMLP, and zymosan. The clinical impact of this priming is not well understood, but preliminary studies with intravenous recombinant TNF-α and GM-CSF indicate that there is an enhanced oxidative burst capacity, and that it varies with dose and duration of cytokine exposure.

ROS have been implicated in the pathogenesis of several clinical disorders. However, the role of cytokines in ROS production and induction of oxidative damage in many of these situations is unclear. It appears that cytokines may have a paradoxical role in many diseases in which low doses of cytokines may be beneficial, but higher doses may lead to injury or death. ROS release is involved in both of these potential outcomes of cytokine therapy. Modulation of cytokine dose and ROS production may have a significant clinical impact in many areas.

REFERENCES

1. Borg DC. Oxygen free radicals and tissue injury. In: Tarr M, Sarrison, F, eds. Oxygen free radicals in tissue damage. Boston: Birkhauser Boston, 1993:12–53.

2. Camussi G, Albano E, Tetta C, Bussolino F. The molecular action of tumor necrosis factor-α. Eur J Biochem 1991;202: 3–14.

3. Turrens JF, Freeman BA, Crapo JD. Hyperoxia increases H_2O_2 release by lung mitochondria and microsomes. Arch Biochem Biophys 1982;217:411–421.

4. Halliwell B, Gutteridge JMC. Oxygen toxicity, oxygen radicals, transition metals and disease. Biochem J 1984;219: 1–14.

5. Rossi F, Bellavite P, Berton G, Grzeskowiak M, Papini E. Mechanism of production of toxic oxygen radicals by granulocytes and macrophages and their function in the inflammatory process. Pathol Res Pract 1985;180:136–142.

6. Albrich JM, McCarthy CA, Hurst JK. Biological reactivity of hypochlorous acid: implications for microbicidal mechanisms of leukocyte myeloperoxidase. Proc Natl Acad Sci USA 1981;78:210–214.

7. Engerson TD, McKelvey TG, Rhyne DB, Boggio EB, Snyder SJ, Jones HP. Conversion of xanthine dehydrogenase to oxidase in ischemic rat tissues. J Clin Invest 1987;79:1564–1570.

8. Henson PM, Johnston RB Jr. Tissue injury in inflammation. Oxidants, proteinases, and cationic proteins. J Clin Invest 1987;79:669–674.

9. Larrick JW, Wright SC. Cytotoxic mechanism of tumor necrosis factor-α. FASEB J 1990;4:3215–3223.

10. Boobis AR, Fawthrop DJ, Davies DS. Mechanisms of cell toxicity. Curr Opin Cell Biol 1990;2:231–237.

11. McPhail LC, Clayton CC, Snyderman R. The NADPH oxidase of human polymorphonuclear leukocytes: evidence for regulation of multiple signals. J Biol Chem 1984;259: 5768–5775.

12. Kapp A, Zeck-Kapp G. Activation of the oxidative metabolism in human polymorphonuclear neutrophilic granulocytes: the role of immuno-modulating cytokines. J Invest Dermatol 1990;95:945–995.

13. Smith CV. Free radical mechanisms of tissue injury. III. Types of radical reactions. In: Moslen MT, Smith CV, eds. Free radical mechanisms of tissue injury. Boca Raton, FL: CRC Press, 1992:6–16.

14. Nathan CF, Murray HW, Wiebe ME, Rubin BY. Identification of interferon-γ as the lymphokine that activates

human macrophage oxidative metabolism and antimicrobial activity. J Exp Med 1983;158:670–689.

15. Nathan C, Nogueira N, Juangbhanich C, Ellis J, Cohn Z. Activation of macrophages in vivo and in vitro. J Exp Med 1979;149:1056–1068.

16. Touati D. Molecular genetics of superoxide dismutases. Free Radic Biol Med 1988;5:393–402.

17. Natvig DO, Imlay K, Touati D, Hallewell RA. Human copper-zinc superoxide dismutase complements superoxide dismutase-deficient Escherichia coli mutants. J Biol Chem 1987;262:14697–14701.

18. Stadtman ER. Metal ion-catalyzed oxidation of proteins: biochemical mechanism and biological consequences. Free Radic Biol Med 1990;9:315–325.

19. Ziegler DM. Role of reversible oxidation-reduction of enzyme thiols-disulfides in metabolic regulation. Annu Rev Biochem 1985;54:305–329.

20. Wolff SP, Dean RT. Fragmentation of proteins by free radicals and its effect on their susceptibility to enzymic hydrolysis. Biochem J 1986;234:399–403.

21. Rivett AJ. Preferential degradation of the oxidatively modified form of glutamine synthetase by intracellular mammalian proteases. J Biol Chem 1985;260:300–305.

22. Girotti A. Mechanisms of lipid peroxidation. J Free Radic Biol Med 1985;1:87–95.

23. Esterbauer H, Cheeseman KH, Dianzani MU, Poli G, Slater F. Separation and characterization of the aldehydic products of lipid peroxidation stimulated by ADP-Fe^{2+} in rat liver microsomes. Biochem J 1982;208:129–140.

24. Teebor GW, Boorstein RJ, Cadet J. The repairability of oxidative free radical mediated damage to DNA: a review. Int J Radiat Biol 1988;54:131–150.

25. Floyd RA, West MS, Eneff KL, Hogsett WE, Tingey DT. Hydroxyl free radical mediated formation of 8-hydroxyguanine in isolated DNA. Arch Biochem Biophys 1988;262:266–272.

26. Cheng KC, Cahill DS, Kasai H, Nishimura S, Loeb LA. 8-hydroxyguanine, an abundant form of oxidative DNA damage, causes G to T and A to C substitutions. J Biol Chem 1992;267:166–172.

27. Mee LK, Adelstein SJ. Predominance of core histones in formation of DNA-protein crosslinks in gamma-irradiated chromatin. Proc Natl Acad Sci USA 1981;78:2194–2198.

28. Loeb LA, James EA, Waltersdorph AM, Klebanoff SJ. Mutagenesis by the autoxidation of iron with isolated DNA. Proc Natl Acad Sci USA 1988;85:3918–3922.

29. Moody CS, Hassan HN. Mutagenicity of oxygen free radicals. Proc Natl Acad Sci USA 1982;79:2855–2859.

30. Svingen BA, O'Neal FO, Aust SD. The role of superoxide and single-oxygen in lipid peroxidation. Photochem Photobiol 1978;28:803–809.

31. Freeman BA, Crapo JD. Free radicals and tissue injury. Lab Invest 1982;47:412–426.

32. Danford DE, Munro HN. Water-soluble vitamins. In: Gilman AG, Goodman AS, Gilman A, eds. The pharmacological basis of therapeutics, ed. 6. New York: Macmillan, 1980:1560–1582.

33. Mandel HG, Cohn VH. Fat-soluble vitamins. In: Gilman AG, Goodman LS, Gilman A, eds. The pharmacological

basis of therapeutics, ed. 6. New York: Macmillan, 1980:1583–1601.

34. Alberts B, Bray D, Lewis J, Raff M, Roberts K, Watson JD. Molecular biology of the cell, ed. 2. New York: Garland Publishing, 1989.

35. Marklund SL. Extracellular superoxide dismutase and other superoxide dismutase isoenzymes in tissues from nine mammalian species. Biochem J 1984;222:649–655.

36. Bannister JV, Bannister WH, Rotilio G. Aspects of the structure, function, and applications of superoxide dismutase. Crit Rev Biochem 1987;22:111–180.

37. White CW, Ghezzi P, McMahon S, Dinarello CA, Repine JE. Cytokines increase rat lung antioxidant enzymes during exposure to hyperoxia. J Appl Physiol 1989;66:1003–1007.

38. Wong GHW, Goeddel DV. Induction of manganous superoxide dismutase by tumor necrosis factor: possible protective mechanism. Science 1988;242:941–944.

39. Dougall WC, Nick HS. Manganese superoxide dismutase: a hepatic acute phase protein regulated by interleukin-6 and glucocorticoids. Endocrinology 1991;129:2376–2384.

40. Warner BB, Burhans MS, Clark JC, Wispe JR. Tumor necrosis factor-α increases Mn-SOD expression: protection against oxidant injury. Am Physiol Soc 1991;260:L296–L301.

41. Marklund SL. Regulation by cytokines of extracellular superoxide dismutase and other superoxide dismutase isoenzymes in fibroblasts. J Biol Chem 1992;267:6696–6701.

42. Nakagawara A, DeSantis NM, Nogueira N, Nathan CF. Lymphokines enhance the capacity of human monocytes to secrete reactive oxygen intermediates. J Clin Invest 1982;70:1042–1048.

43. Freund M, Pick E. The mechanism of action of lymphokines: VIII. Lymphokine-enhanced spontaneous hydrogen peroxide production by macrophages. Immunology 1985;54:35–45.

44. Babior BM, Kipnes RS, Curnutte JT. Biological defense mechanisms: the production by leukocytes of superoxide, a potential bactericidal agent. J Clin Invest 1973;52:741–744.

45. Rosen H, Klebanoff SJ. Chemiluminescence and superoxide production by myeloperoxidase-deficient leukocytes. J Clin Invest 1976;58:50–60.

46. Newburger PE, Chovaniec ME, Cohen HJ. Activity and activation of the granulocyte superoxide-generating system. Blood 1980;55:85–92.

47. Pick E, Keisari Y. A simple colorimetric method for the measurement of hydrogen peroxide produced by cells in culture. J Immunol Methods 1980;38:161–170.

48. Adamson GM, Billings RE. Tumor necrosis factor induced oxidative stress in isolated mouse hepatocytes. Arch Biochem Biophys 1992;294:223–229.

49. Tanner WG, Welborn MB, Shepherd VL. Tumor necrosis factor-α and interleukin-1α synergistically enhance phorbol myristate acetate-induced superoxide production by rat bone marrow-derived macrophages. Am J Respir Cell Mol Biol 1992;7:379–384.

50. Kharazmi A, Neilson H, Bendtzen K. Recombinant interleukin 1α and β prime human monocyte superoxide production but have no effect on chemotaxis and oxidative

burst response of neutrophils. Immunobiology 1988;177: 32–39.

51. Sullivan GW, Carper HT, Sullivan JA, Murata T, Mandell GL. Both recombinant interleukin-1 (beta) and purified human monocyte interleukin-1 prime human neutrophils for increased oxidative activity and promote neutrophil spreading. J Leukocyte Biol 1989;45:389–395.

52. Tawara T, Shingu M, Nobunaga M, Naono T. Effects of recombinant human IL-1β on production of prostaglandin E_2, leukotriene B_4, NAG, and superoxide by human synovial cells and chondrocytes. Inflammation 1991;15:145–157.

53. Ho JH, He SH, Rios MJC, Wick EA. Interleukin-4 inhibits human macrophage activation by tumor necrosis factor, granulocyte-monocyte colony-stimulating factor, and interleukin-3 for antileishmanial activity and oxidative burst capacity. J Infect Dis 1992;165:344–351.

54. Phillips WA, Hamilton JA. Phorbol ester-stimulated superoxide production by murine bone marrow-derived macrophages requires preexposure to cytokines. J Immunol 1989;142:2445–2449.

55. Sullivan R, Griffin JD, Simons ER, et al. Effects of recombinant human granulocyte and macrophage colony-stimulating factors on signal transduction pathways in human granulocytes. J Immunol 1987;139:3422–3430.

56. Nathan CF, Prendergast TJ, Wiebe ME, et al. Activation of human macrophages: comparison of other cytokines with interferon-γ. J Exp Med 1984;160:600–605.

57. Abramson SL, Gallin JI. IL-4 inhibits superoxide production by human mononuclear phagocytes. J Immunol 1990;144:625–630.

58. Szefler SJ, Norton CE, Ball B, Gross JM, Aida Y, Pabst MJ. IFN-γ and LPS overcome glucocorticoid inhibition of priming for superoxide release in human monocytes: evidence that secretion of IL-1 and tumor necrosis factor-α is not essential for monocyte priming. J Immunol 1989;142: 3985–3992.

59. Wolf JE, Massof SE. In vivo activation of macrophage oxidative burst activity by cytokines and amphotericin B. Infect Immun 1990;58:1296–1300.

60. Berkow RL, Dodson MR. Biochemical mechanisms involved in the priming of neutrophils by tumor necrosis factor. J Leukocyte Biol 1988;44:345–352.

61. Berkow RL, Wang D, Larrick JW, Dodson RW, Howard TH. Enhancement of neutrophil superoxide production by preincubation with recombinant human tumor necrosis factor. J Immunol 1987;139:3783–3791.

62. Freund M, Pick E. The mechanism of action of lymphokines: IX. The enzymatic basis of hydrogen peroxide production by lymphokine-activated macrophages. J Immunol 1986;137:1312–1318.

63. Weisbart RH, Golde DW, Clark SC, Wong GG, Gasson JC. Human granulocyte-macrophage colony-stimulating factor is a neutrophil activator. Nature 1985;314:361–363.

64. Watanabe N, Niitsu Y, Neda H, et al. Cytotocidal mechanism of TNF: effects of lysosomal enzyme and hydroxyl radical inhibitors on cytotoxicity. Immunopharmacol Immunotoxicol 1988;10:109–116.

65. Laudanna C, Miron S, Berton G, Rossi F. Tumor necrosis factor-α/cachectin activates the O_2-generating system of human neutrophils independently of the hydrolysis of phosphoinositides and the release of arachidonic acid. Biochem Biophys Res Commun 1990;166:308–315.

66. Tsujimoto M, Yokota S, Vilcek J, Weissman G. Tumor necrosis factor provokes superoxide anion generation from neutrophils. Biochem Biophys Res Commun 1986;137: 1094–1100.

67. Ward PA, Warren JS, Johnson KJ. Oxygen radicals, inflammation, and tissue injury. Free Radic Biol Med 1988;5: 403–408.

68. Moslen MT, Smith CV. Free radical mechanisms of tissue injury. Boca Raton, FL: CRC Press, 1992.

69. Gallin JI, Malech HL, Weening RS, et al. A controlled trial of interferon gamma to prevent infection in chronic granulomatous disease. N Engl J Med 1991;324:509–516.

70. Rabinovitch A, Suarez WL, Thomas PD, Strynadka K, Simpson I. Cytotoxic effects of cytokines on rat islets: evidence for involvement of free radicals and lipid peroxidation. Diabetologia 1992;35:409–413.

71. Mandrup-Poulsen T, Helqvist S, Wogensen LD, et al. Cytokines and free radicals as effector molecules in the destruction of pancreatic beta cells. Curr Top Microbiol Immunol 1990;164:169–193.

72. Sullivan R, Fredette JP, Socinski M, et al. Enhancement of superoxide anion release by granulocytes harvested from patients receiving granulocyte-macrophage colony-stimulating factor. Br J Haematol 1989;71:475–479.

73. Kaplan SS, Basford RE, Wing EJ, Shadduck RK. The effect of recombinant human granulocyte macrophage colony-stimulating factor on neutrophil activation in patients with refractory carcinoma. Blood 1989;73:636–638.

74. Ohsaka A, Kitagawa S, Sakamoto S, et al. In vivo activation of human neutrophil functions by administration of recombinant human granulocyte colony-stimulating factor in patients with malignant lymphoma. Blood 1989;74: 2743–2748.

75. Kapp A, Komann A, Schopf E. Effect of tumour necrosis factor alpha in vivo on human granulocyte oxidative metabolism. Arch Dermatol Res 1991;283:362–365.

76. Beutler B, Cerami A. Tumor necrosis factors: the molecules and their emerging role in medicine. New York: Raven, 1992.

77. Dinarello CA. Biology of interleukin 1. FASEB J 1988;2: 108–115.

78. Alexander HR, Doherty GM, Buresh CM, Venzon DJ, Norton JA. A recombinant human receptor antagonist to interleukin-1 improves survival after lethal endotoxemia in mice. J Exp Med 1991;173:1029–1032.

79. Beutler B, Milsark IW, Cerami A. Passive immunization against cachectin/tumor necrosis factor protects mice from the lethal effect of endotoxin. Science 1985;229:869–871.

80. Tracey KJ, Fong Y, Hesse DG, et al. Anti-cachectin/TNF monoclonal antibodies prevent septic shock during lethal bacteremia. Nature 1987;330:662–664.

81. Sheppard BC, Fraker DL, Norton JA. Prevention and treatment of endotoxin and sepsis lethality with recombinant human tumor necrosis factor. Surgery 1989;106:156–162.

82. Fraker DL, Stovroff MC, Merino MJ, Norton JA. Tolerance to tumor necrosis factor in rats and the relationship to endotoxin tolerance and toxicity. J Exp Med 1988;168:95–105.

83. Alexander HR, Doherty GM, Fraker DL, Block MI, Swedenborg JA, Norton JA. Human recombinant interleukin-1α protection against the lethality of endotoxin and experimental sepsis in mice. J Surg Res 1991;50:421–424.

84. Alexander HR, Doherty GM, Block MI, et al. Single-dose tumor necrosis factor protection against endotoxin induced shock and tissue injury in the rat. Infect Immun 1991;59:3889–3894.

85. Asoh K, Watanabe Y, Mizoguchi H, et al. Induction of manganese superoxide dismutase by tumor necrosis factor in human breast cancer MCF-7 cell line and its TNF-resistant variant. Biochem Biophys Res Commun 1989;162:794–801.

86. Zimmerman RJ, Chan A, Leadon SA. Oxidative damage in murine tumor cells treated in vitro by recombinant human tumor necrosis factor. Cancer Res 1989;49:1644–1648.

87. Zimmerman RJ, Marafino BJ Jr, Chan A, Landre P, Winkelhake JL. The role of oxidant injury in tumor cell sensitivity to recombinant human tumor necrosis factor in vivo. J Immunol 1989;142:1405–1409.

88. Visner GA, Dougall WC, Wilson JM, Burr IA, Nick HS. Regulation of manganese superoxide dismutase by lipopolysaccharide, interleukin-1 and tumor necrosis factor. J Biol Chem 1990;265:2856–2864.

89. Wong GHW, Elwell JH, Oberley LW, Goeddel DV. Manganous superoxide dismutase is essential for cellular resistance to cytotoxicity of tumor necrosis factor. Cell 1989; 58:923–931.

90. Wong GHW, Neta R, Goeddel DV. Protective roles of MnSOD, TNF-α, TNF-β and D-factor (LIF) in radiation injury. In: 2nd International Conference, ed. Eicosanoids and other bioactive lipids in cancer, inflammation and radiation injury. Berlin: Klinikum Steglitz; 1994 (in press).

91. Block MI, Alexander HR, Buresh C, Norton JA. Acquired resistance to TNF in vitro is associated with increased expression of the gene for MnSOD but not gene amplification. Surg Forum 1991;42:464–467.

92. Melendez JA, Baglioni C. Reduced expression of manganese superoxide dismutase in cells resistant to cytolysis by tumor necrosis factor. Free Radic Biol Med 1992;12:151–159.

93. Boss JM, Laster SM, Gooding LR. Sensitivity to tumour necrosis factor-mediated cytolysis is unrelated to manganous superoxide dismutase messenger RNA levels among transformed mouse fibroblasts. Immunology 1991;73:309–315.

94. Alexander HR, Jensen JC, Doherty GM, Block MI, Buresh CM, Norton JA. Induction of manganous superoxide dismutase (MnSOD) gene expression by interleukin-1(IL-1): possible molecular basis for IL-1 protection against lethal sepsis. Surg Forum 1991;42:98.

95. Alexander HR, Sheppard BC, Jensen JC, et al. Treatment with recombinant human tumor necrosis factor-alpha protects rats against the lethality, hypotension, and hypothermia of gram-negative sepsis. J Clin Invest 1991;88:34–39.

96. Jensen JC, Pogrebniak HW, Pass HI, et al. The role of tumor necrosis factor in oxygen toxicity. J Appl Physiol 1992;72:1902–1907.

97. Sheppard BC, Norton JA. Tumor necrosis factor and interleukin-1 protection against the lethal effects of tumor necrosis factor. Surgery 1991;106:698–705.

98. Shau H. Effects of tumor-necrosis-factor-activated neutrophils on tumor cell survival. Immunol Res 1991;10:114–121.

99. Shau H. Characteristics and mechanism of neutrophil-mediated cytostasis induced by tumor necrosis factor. J Immunol 1988;141:234–240.

100. Meier B, Radeke HH, Selle S, et al. Human fibroblasts release reactive oxygen species in response to interleukin-1 or tumor necrosis factor-α. Biochem J 1989;263: 539–545.

101. Slungaard A, Vercellotti GM, Walker G, Nelson RD, Jacob HS. Tumor necrosis factor α/cachectin stimulates eosinophil oxidant production and toxicity towards human endothelium. J Exp Med 1990;171:2025–2041.

102. Warren JS, Kunkel SL, Cunningham TW, Johnson KJ, Ward PA. Macrophage-derived cytokines amplify immune complex-triggered O₂• responses by rat alveolar macrophages. Am J Pathol 1988;130:489–495.

103. Davila DR, Edwards CK, Arkins S, Simon J, Kelley KW. Interferon-γ-induced priming for secretion of superoxide anion and tumor necrosis factor-α declines in macrophages from aged rats. FASEB J 1990;4:2906–2911.

104. Weisbart RH, Kwan L, Golde DW, Gasson JC. Human GM-CSF primes neutrophils for enhanced oxidative metabolism in response to the major physiological chemoattractants. Blood 1987;69:18–21.

105. Mayer AMS, Pittner RA, Lipscomb GE, Spitzer JA. Effect of in vivo TNF administration on superoxide production and PKC activity of rat alveolar macrophages. Am J Physiol 1993;264:L43–L52.

CHAPTER 23

THE ROLE OF CYTOKINES IN AGING

Monte V. Hobbs and David N. Ernst

The evidence assembled challenges the assumption that the processes of senescence require pervasive deteriorative changes that progress inexorably throughout all parts and functions of the organism, from molecules to behavior. On the contrary, most species show relatively few proximal causes of death during senescence, whether senescence occurs rapidly or very slowly. In many life species, senescence involves dysorganizational consequences that emanate from the physiological or organ function level, rather than through diffuse cellular and molecular degenerative changes that spread "upwards."

Caleb E. Finch [1]

After sexual maturity in mammals, the process of aging is accompanied by physiological changes in many organ systems. The rate of change varies widely at the organ, organism, and species levels, and it is likely influenced by genetic as well as environmental factors (1). The immune system of humans exhibits distinct changes (termed *immunosenescence*) in the last quarter of the average lifespan, a period during which the incidence and severity of many infectious diseases and cancers become most prominent (2). That the first set of events is a normal process of aging that causes the second set is a working hypothesis in several laboratories, but it has been difficult to prove due to both intraspecies variation in "physiological age" (versus chronological age) and the

confounding variable of underlying disease among elderly test subjects.

The integrity of the T-cell compartment during aging is a subject that, for several reasons, has received much attention. First, the T-cell group is comprised of various effector and regulatory cells that are involved in essentially all immunologically relevant host responses (3). Second, the T-cell group is itinerant and capable of producing many pleiotropic cytokines (3,4), thus suggesting cryptic relationships with other organ systems. Third, the postpubertal involution of the thymus is a common feature of mammalian aging, and it leads to a dramatic reduction in the export of new mature T cells to the peripheral lymphoid tissues and the recirculating cell pool (5). Fourth, elderly populations exhibit variable (often reduced) cell-mediated and humoral responses to test antigens (Ag) and vaccines (6). Finally, analyses of T cells stimulated in vitro generally reveal age-altered patterns of cell cycle activity and effector function (7,8). Therefore, age-related changes in T-cell function could contribute to a variety of disorders that increase in the elderly, including possible manifestations of immune deficiency (e.g., mortality due to pneumonia or influenza), dysregulation (e.g., autoantibody production and monoclonal gammopathies), or both (e.g., lymphoid and nonlymphoid cancers), and perhaps could contribute to the decline of other organ systems as well.

We review literature on age-related changes that occur in the cytokine circuitry of the T-cell group. In the last few decades, it has become clear that cytokines are key regulators of virtually all physiological processes, and they can influence development, activation, proliferation, or differentiation of most cell types of the body. The emerging information on the properties of individual cytokines and on cell lineage–specific programs of cytokine and cytokine receptor gene expression has helped to clarify how immune responses unfold, and how perturbations in the cytokine circuitry can have pathological consequences. The first part of this chapter is a discussion of contemporary models of T-cell differentiation and effector function, with particular attention to segregation of cytokine programs among the various T-cell subsets. We then attempt to define common patterns of age-related change in the capacity for cytokine production by the T-cell group, and we discuss how these changes relate to progressive alteration in the numerical representation of T-cell subsets. Finally, we discuss how alterations in the homeostasis of the cytokine network could result in inefficient or inappropriate immune responsiveness by the elderly.

CYTOKINE GENE EXPRESSION BY T-CELL SUBSETS

The term *cytokine* refers to a broad group of extracellular signaling proteins that, in general, are produced transiently after cell activation, act locally as autocrine or paracrine regulators of cell function, and exert their effects by binding to specific high-affinity receptors on target cells. During a host's reaction to foreign Ag, the characteristics of the immune response are dictated largely by qualitative, quantitative, and temporal patterns of cytokine gene expression by locally stimulated T cells (3,4). More than 20 cytokine species are known to be produced by activated T cells, including members of the interleukin (IL-1 to IL-6, IL-8 to IL-10, IL-13, IL-14), interferon (IFN-γ, IFN-α), tumor necrosis factor (TNF-α, TNF-β), colony-stimulating factor (GM-CSF, G-CSF, M-CSF), transforming growth factor-β (TGF-β1), chemokine-β (RANTES, MIP-1α, -1β), and other groups. Considering the known properties of each of the cytokines (3,4), the capacity to express this array equips the T-cell group with a vast potential for stimulatory and inhibitory functions.

Virtually all the T-cell–derived cytokines are pleiotropic, and individual cytokines can regulate production and effects of other cytokines. Therefore, to avoid immunological chaos, the immune system has evolved several levels of compartmentalization that allow fine-tuned control over cytokine expression. For example, cytokine production by T cells is Ag-driven, and it is therefore regulated by the number, type, and state of activation of local Ag-presenting cells (APCs), as well as by the clonal frequency

and migratory properties of T cells with receptors (TCRs) specific for the Ag. The cytokine program of a given T cell can then vary based on its degree of activation, on its inclusion in one of the T-cell lineages (e.g., CD4+TCR$_{\alpha\beta}$+, CD8+TCR$_{\alpha\beta}$+, or TCR$_{\gamma\delta}$+ cell) and its state of differentiation within the lineage (e.g., naive versus memory), and on the balance of cytokines and cytokine antagonists in the local milieu.

Naive T-cell subsets

Naive CD4+ and CD8+ cells are generally defined as cells that have survived TCR selection in the thymus but have not yet responded to cognate Ag in the peripheral tissues. Naive cells can be identified in vivo by their unique constellation of membrane molecules, including high levels of the CD62L (L-selectin, MEL-14) adhesion molecule and the high molecular weight (MW) isoforms of CD45 (i.e., CD45RA^{hi}, B^{hi}, or C^{hi}); high (CD4+ cells) or variable (CD8+ cells) levels of the 3G11 ganglioside; intermediate or low levels of the low MW isoform of CD45 (i.e., CD45RO) and the adhesion/signaling receptors CD2, CD44 (Pgp-1), CD54 (ICAM-1), CD58 (LFA-3); and the integrins α3β1 (CD49c/CD29), α4β1 (CD49d/CD29), α5β1 (CD49e/CD29), α6β1 (CD49f/CD29), and αLβ2 (CD11a/CD18, LFA-1) (9–16). This membrane phenotype contributes to the naive T cell's recirculation patterns (e.g., blood → lymphoid tissue → blood) (15), and it may increase the stimulation threshold of the APC T-cell interaction (10).

Naive T cells generally encounter cognate Ag peptides bound to major histocompatibility complex (MHC) class I (CD8+ cells) or class II (CD4+ cells) molecules on APC in organized secondary lymphoid tissues. The ensuing primary response is characterized by clonal expansion, an effector response that clears the Ag from the body, and then disappearance of the effector cells (17). On the basis of data from in vitro models, the initial activation of naive T cells results in a limited program of cytokine gene expression, including IL-2 (10–13,18–20), which could serve primarily as an autocrine factor to facilitate clonal expansion and differentiation. However, the cytokine program of the stimulated T cells eventually diversifies (11,19–21), thus yielding more proficient primary effector cells (11,21).

Memory T-cell subsets

A population of T cells is generated during the primary response and imprints the immune system with a "memory" of the Ag challenge. The more rapid and vigorous response to re-encounter with Ag reflects, in part, an increased frequency of these Ag-reactive T cells. In addition, the memory T cells acquire new phenotypic traits, such as general decreases in membrane expression of MEL-14/L-selectin, high MW isoforms of CD45 and 3G11, and overall increases in expression of CD2, CD44, CD45RO, CD54, CD58, and several of the integrins (9–16). These and other changes are thought to promote access of T cells to a broader range of tissues (both lymphoid and nonlymphoid) (15) and stimulatory APC types (22), and to lower the stimulation threshold of the APC T-cell interaction (10). The clonal lifespan of memory T cells, the existence of short- and long-term memory cells, and the role of persistent or crossreactive Ag in maintaining these populations are issues currently under intensive investigation (17).

Many investigators have attempted to define how the potential for cytokine gene expression changes during T-cell differentiation. One strategy has been to separate "naive" and "memory" T cells based on the expression of one of the surface molecules described, and then to analyze production of cytokines in primary cultures stimulated with strong polyclonal activators. From most studies, it would appear that the naive to memory conversion of CD4+ cells is associated with a generally unchanged potential for IL-2, IL-6, TNF-α, and TNF-β synthesis, as well as an enhanced capacity for IL-1α, IL-3, IL-4, IL-5, IL-10, IFN-γ, and GM-CSF synthesis (10–13,18, 23–27). Similar studies on CD8+ cells have shown that conversion to a memory status is associated with a similar or decreased capacity for IL-2 synthesis, but an increased potential for IL-3 and IFN-γ production (16,18,28,29).

The pattern of expression of each membrane molecule described is cell activation–dependent; thus, the so called in vivo memory pool presumably contains recently activated cells, effector cells, short- and long-term memory cells, and even anergic cells. Moreover, several of the membrane molecules are heterogeneously coexpressed by this cell group, and individual molecules can be either maintained or reacquired at levels similar to those of naive T cells (11,12,14–16,28). For this reason, cells within the phenotypic clusters identified by their coexpression of two or more of the subset-discriminating molecules provide useful candidates for analysis of further cytokine compartmentalization within the non-naive T pool. Unfortunately, few studies of this nature have been performed. For example, Hayakawa and Hardy (12) demonstrated that mouse CD4+ subsets defined by their coexpression of 3G11 and 6C10 differ in their patterns of activation and cytokine gene expression. Bradley and colleagues (21) showed that, following immunization of mice, primary effector CD4+ cells able to help B cells and to produce IL-2, IL-3, IL-4, and IFN-γ reside in the CD45RB^{lo}MEL-14^{lo} fraction. Finally, Mobley and Dailey (28) found that primary effector CD8+ cells, which are cytotoxic and able to produce IFN-γ, are largely restricted to the CD44^{hi}MEL-14^{lo} fraction.

T-cell differentiation in vitro

Studies of primary and secondary stimulation of T cells in vitro have helped to establish the relationship of T-cell differentiation to the changing pattern of cytokine synthesis. Stimulation of naive or naive-predominant CD4+ cells with mitogen or Ag in short-term cultures yields a population that, after secondary stimulation, produces elevated levels of IL-3, IL-4, IL-5, IL-6, IFN-γ, and GM-CSF (11,19,20). These systems can be further compartmentalized by the cytokines present (in addition to IL-2) during primary stimulation. Thus, exogenous IL-4 can drive the differentiation of CD4+ cells able to produce IL-4 (but minimal IFN-γ), whereas TGF-β and IL-12 direct differentiation toward the reciprocal phenotype (IL-4^{lo}IFN-γ^{hi}) (11,20). Moreover, these two pathways appear to be crossinhibitory via the actions of IFN-γ and IL-4, respectively (20). In similar systems, exogenous IL-2 plus IL-4 drives the differentiation of CD8+ cells to produce IL-4 (30) or IL-4, IL-5, and IL-10 (31), whereas IL-2 alone drives the conversion to IFN-γ–producing cells (31).

CD4+ T-cell clones

Many long-term clones of mouse CD4+ cells can be classified as Th1 or Th2 type, based on differences in activation and growth requirements, profiles of cytokine and cytokine receptor gene expression, and patterns of effector function (3,32). Stimulated Th1 clones produce IL-2, IL-3, IFN-γ, TNF-α, TNF-β, and GM-CSF. In keeping with the properties of these cytokines (3,4), Th1 cells function as cytotoxic cells; they induce delayed-type hypersensitivity and macrophage activation, but they provide restricted help for B-cell responses (e.g., immunoglobulin G$_2$a [IgG$_2$a] synthesis). In contrast, stimulated Th2 clones produce IL-1, IL-3, IL-4, IL-5, IL-6, IL-9, IL-10, IL-13, TNF-α, and GM-CSF. Accordingly (3,4), these cells provide help for the production of IgM, IgG$_1$, IgA, and IgE by B cells; induce eosinophilia; and stimulate mast cells. A third clone classification, termed Th0 (33), contains cells with less restricted patterns of cytokine synthesis, but it is not yet clear whether this group represents an intermediate in the Th1 or Th2 pathway or a separate differentiation pathway. Although early work on human CD4+ clones was not supportive of the Th1/Th2 paradigm in that many clones resembled Th0 cells (34), it is clear that Th1- and Th2-like clones can be derived from donors who had undergone repeated exposure to the selecting Ag (35).

There is ample evidence that Th1- and Th2-derived cytokines are involved in a crossregulating network (3,32). For example, IL-4 and IL-10 can inhibit Th1 clone responses, and, along with IL-13, they can inhibit the production of inflammatory cytokines or the killing of intracellular and extracellular pathogens by activated macrophages (a process driven by Th1-derived IFN-γ). In contrast, IFN-γ can inhibit B-cell growth and differentiation (a process driven by several Th2-derived cytokines), and it can suppress Th2 clone responses.

CD8+ T-cell clones

Initially, long-term clones of mouse CD8+ cells were thought to produce a Th1-like pattern of cytokines, including IL-2, IL-3, IFN-γ, TNF-α, TNF-β, and GM-CSF (36), which is consistent with their classic role in viral infections, inflammation, and cytotoxic reactions. However, recent studies on human and mouse CD8+ clones extended this list to include such Th2-related cytokines as IL-4, IL-5, IL-6, and IL-10 (34,37,38). As with the CD4+ clones, CD8+ clones can exhibit cytokine compartmentalization and crossregulatory effects. For example, Inoue and associates (38) described mouse cytotoxic T-lymphocyte (CTL) clones that produce IFN-γ, but not IL-10, as well as other clones (termed Ts) that suppress proliferation of Th1 and Th2 CD4+ cells, in part through the production of IL-10 and IFN-γ, respectively. Salgame and colleagues (37) described two human CD8+ clone types: type 1, which is cytotoxic and produces IFN-γ, but not IL-4; and type 2, which produces IFN-γ and IL-4, the latter of which is thought to suppress activities of Th1 CD4+ cells.

T-cell subsets in vivo

Information generated from the in vitro models described indicates that the T-cell compartment is a dynamic system that features cytokines as the drivers for TCR-triggered cell activation, growth, selective differentiation, effector function, and crossregulation. Moreover, distinct subprograms of cytokine expression and responsiveness segregate among T-cell subsets, thus providing cells individually well-suited for inflammatory or cytotoxic reactions, humoral responses, or suppression.

It has been known for some time that intensities of delayed-type hypersensitivity (DTH) (Th1-like) and humoral (Th2-like) responses can be inversely related (39). Distinctive roles for Th1-like, Th2-like, and CD8+-cell subsets in protective immunity to a variety of bacterial, protozoan, metazoan, and viral infections are increasingly evident, whereas emergence of an inappropriate subset is sometimes associated with disease susceptibility or promotion (3,32,35,37,40–42). In addition, Th1- or Th2-like subsets have been implicated in several immunopathological conditions, including allergic disorders, organ-specific autoimmunity, and allograft rejection (35). Finally (and consistent with the in vitro models), there is evidence that IL-12, IFN-γ, and IL-4 can function in vivo to

preferentially drive Th1 and Th2 cell differentiation, respectively (3,20), although there are still many questions regarding the source and timing of these (and other) cytokines, as well as about the influence of other factors (e.g., differences in MHC genotype, antigen [dose, route, and epitope], and APC type) on the various differentiative pathways.

Other T-cell subsets

The T-cell population utilizing the γ and δ TCR gene segments ($T_{γδ}$ cells) is comprised of a variety of subsets that differ based on their ontogenetic appearance, tissue localization, TCR repertoire, and thymic dependence (43). The function of $T_{γδ}$ cells is not entirely known, but they have been implicated in various normal and pathological immune responses. Analyses of cytokine production by stimulated $T_{γδ}$ cells or clones derived from several sources have shown a very diverse cytokine program overall (including many of the $T_{αβ}$-associated cytokines), as well as heterogeneous expression patterns among $T_{γδ}$ subsets (43).

REPRESENTATION OF T-CELL SUBSETS DURING AGING

On the basis of the models described, the characteristics of a host's T-cell response to Ag is dictated, at one level, by the frequency of Ag-reactive T cells, and, at another level, by the partitioning of the frequency among CD4+ versus CD8+ cells, naive versus memory cells, and the various crossregulating subsets of memory cells. In this regard, nonprotective immune responses could result from an insufficiency of reactive T cells, or, alternatively, from inappropriate downregulation of protective T-cell subsets. In the following sections, we review recent information on age-related changes in the representation of T-cell subsets.

T-cell subpopulations

The postpubertal involution of the thymus progressively diminishes the infusion of new, mature T cells into the peripheral tissues (5). Despite this age-related change, the peripheral T-cell pool exhibits remarkable stability with respect to total T-cell number and representation of CD4+ and CD8+ T-cell subpopulations throughout life, as evidenced by the modest changes reported in studies on humans and animal models (7,8). There is limited information on the distribution of $T_{γδ}$-cell subsets during aging. One report (44) showed an increase with age in the levels of γ-chain mRNA in the thymus, spleen, and lymph nodes of mice.

Subsets of CD4+ and CD8+ Cells

The decreasing replenishment of the periphery with naive T cells, in combination with an extending history of Ag-driven T-cell differentiation, would be expected to result in an altered equilibrium of naive and memory T cells in late life. Several investigators have addressed this possibility by using immunophenotypic criteria to enumerate these subsets in aging humans and mice (Table 23–1). Most studies on the human system analyzed peripheral blood lymphocytes (PBL) and reported age-related decreases in the proportions of CD4+ and CD8+ cells bearing high levels of CD45RA, with concomitant increases in the fractions of CD45RO^{hi}, CD29^{hi}, and LFA-1^{hi} cells. As described in previous sections, this pattern suggests that aging is accompanied by a diminishing reserve of naive cells and an increasing representation of effector, memory, or recently activated cells.

These subset shifts occur in both sexes (46,49,51), and they are evident from birth to very late life, although there is some disagreement as to whether the changes are gradual throughout life (45,47,49) or are more prominent during distinct phases (50). The magnitude of these changes by late life varies somewhat between studies, but it can be quite profound for both CD4+ and CD8+ cells when rigorous criteria are used to define naive and non-naive T cells (e.g., the use of multiple subset markers) (52). In addition, these latter strategies have helped to identify distinct subsets that are rare in early life but increase in number with age, such as the CD45RA^{hi}-

CD45RO^{lo}LFA-1^{hi} and CD45RA^{lo}CD45RO^{hi}LFA-1^{hi} phenotypes among CD8+ cells (52).

Studies on the mouse model system provided a similar picture of the age-related changes in the T-cell subset frequencies. The general trends for splenic CD4+ and CD8+ cells, shown in Table 23–1, are shifts toward lower proportions of CD45RB^{hi}, 3G11^{hi}, and MEL-14^{hi} cells, as well as greater representations of CD44^{hi} cells. As in the human system, these changes are indicative of an increasing memory/effector cell pool at the expense of a diminishing naive cell population. These subset transitions are ongoing throughout life, are evident in blood and a variety of lymphoid tissues, and are apparent in all tested mouse strains.

Simultaneous analysis of multiple subset markers expressed by mouse T cells allowed a clearer view of the emerging and declining populations during aging. For example, Ernst and coworkers (16,53) described phenotypic clusters for naive CD4^{+} (CD45RB^{hi}3G11^{hi}MEL-14^{hi}CD44^{lo}) and CD8+ (CD45RB^{hi}3G11^{var}MEL-14^{hi}-CD44^{lo}) cells in the spleen, and they showed that the proportions of these cells decreased two- to four-fold from young adulthood to old age. These changes were accompanied by marked increases in multiple phenotypes of CD4+ and CD8+ cells, all of which displayed high levels of CD44, but each of which displayed a unique coexpression of CD45RB, 3G11, and MEL-14.

As discussed previously, there is limited information on the segregation of cytokine programs among the complex phenotypes of the memory/effector pools of humans and rodents (12,21,28). Further studies on well-resolved subsets, from both normal and aged donors, should help clarify this issue and should provide models for deciphering the cellular basis for altered immune responsiveness in the elderly.

CYTOKINE PRODUCTION AND RESPONSIVENESS BY T CELLS DURING AGING

Considering that the various T-cell lineages and their component subsets display unique programs of cytokine gene expression, the dramatic age-related changes in the frequencies of T-cell subsets would be expected to alter the overall potential for cytokine production by the T-cell pool. A survey of published reports on this subject is presented.

Interleukin-2

IL-2 is produced mainly by activated T cells (both naive and memory), and it functions as an autocrine and

TABLE 23–1   REPRESENTATION OF T-CELL SUBSETS DURING AGING

Species	Phenotype	Change with Age (Refs)	
		CD4+ Cells	CD8+ Cells
Human	CD45RA^{hi}	↓ (45–50)	↓ (50)
	CD45RO^{hi}	↑ (48,50,51)	↑ (50,51)
	CD29^{hi}	↑ (45–47,49)	↑ (52)
	LFA-1^{hi}	↑ (52)	↑ (52)
Mouse	CD45RB^{hi}	↓ (16,23, 53–56)	↓ (16)
	3G11^{hi}	↓ (12,16,53, 54)	↓ (16)
	MEL-14^{hi}	↓ (16)	↓ (16)
	CD44^{hi}	↑ (16,53–55, 57,58)	↑ (16,57,58)

paracrine factor for T-cell growth and differentiation, as well as a positive regulator of B-cell, macrophage, and natural killer (NK) cell responses (3). Since its discovery almost two decades ago, many investigators have analyzed how aging affects production of this cytokine by T cells in vitro. The studies have focused primarily on three species (human, mouse, and rat), and they have employed a range of tissues (blood, lymph node, spleen), cell preparations (intact lymphoid cells, T cells, CD4+ and CD8+ cells), culture conditions (bulk, limiting dilution analysis), detection methods (bioassay, enzyme-linked immunosorbent assay, mRNA hybridization), and T-cell activators (Ag, alloantigen [allo-Ag], superantigen [sAg], the plant lectins concanavalin A [Con A] and phytohemagglutinin [PHA], anti-CD3 mAb, phorbol esters [e.g., PMA] plus Ca^{2+} ionophores or other coactivators). General findings from the various systems are summarized in Table 23–2.

There is no consensus on the effects of aging on IL-2 production by T cells, although most studies show a similar or decreased capacity in late life. Furthermore, conclusions on this subject have varied within laboratories depending on the strain (71,73,75) and sex (80) of animals, the source of lymphoid tissues (75), the readout for IL-2 production (59), and the choice of cell stimuli (54,56,59,60,69,73,83). Studies showing age-related decreases in IL-2 synthesis often report that the changes are progressive throughout the lifespan (56,62,63,71,78,79,81), and they reflect a diminishing precursor frequency for IL-2–producing cells (55,57,66). These changes are seen at the levels of both transcription and protein secretion, and they affect, at least, the CD4+ subpopulation (54–56). Age-related decreases in IL-2 production by CD4+ cells in these systems may explain their diminished performance in, for example, the provision of help for the development of CD8+ CTL activity (88,89).

Studies of PBL from elderly humans often report a marked heterogeneity in the capacity for inducible IL-2 synthesis among donors, with segregation of hyporesponsive and near-normal (young adult–like) phenotypes (65,84). One report (65) showed that the hyporesponsive PBL, after a short resting period in vitro, could be stimulated to produce normal levels of IL-2. Furthermore, this donor group exhibited elevated levels of constitutive serum IL-2, and it responded poorly to influenza vaccine relative to the near-normal old and normal adult groups. From these data, the authors concluded that the hyporesponsive phenotype results from a hyperactive T-cell compartment in vivo, thus yielding T cells refractory to further stimulation. Consistent with this notion, an earlier report (90) showed that in vitro-rested T cells from elderly humans exhibit enhanced PHA-induced cell cycle activity. If indeed the elderly are prone to T-cell hyperactivity in vivo, perhaps resulting from chronic low-grade infections or inflammation, then the possibility that this phenomenon renders the immune system less responsive to vaccines or pathogens deserves further investigation.

We are still left with the controversy of whether aging results in a decreased capacity for IL-2 synthesis in vitro (see Table 23–2). A recurring pattern in the literature is that the extent of age-related effects, if any, depend on the choice of T-cell stimuli. Most protocols reporting age-related deficits have employed Ag, allo-Ag, sAg, Con A, PHA, or soluble anti-CD3 mAb as the cell activator (54–57,60–64,66–70,72,74,76–81,84). However, when using Ag, it is difficult to discriminate between intrinsic "defects" in a fraction of Ag-specific T cells and changes related to an altered frequency or tissue localization of these cells. Further complications arise in distinguishing Ag that are truly new to the host (thus targeting a naive T-cell group that diminishes with age) from those that elicit contributions from both naive and memory cell pools.

Use of polyclonal stimuli, although intended to circumvent these problems, introduces its own bias. For example, in several in vitro systems, PHA or Con A preferentially stimulates naive T cells (versus memory cells) from normal humans and mice to proliferate and secrete IL-2 (10,12,13,23,55–57). Therefore, age-related deficits in IL-2 synthesis in response to these activators would be expected from the naive-deficient T cells of old donors. In contrast, studies showing little or no effect of aging on IL-2 production employed immobilized forms of anti-CD3 mAb or PMA plus ionophore or other coactivators (24,25,53,54,56,69,71,83). These stimuli appear to be less subset-biased in that they induce high levels of proliferation and IL-2 synthesis by both naive and memory T cells from normal donors (10,12,13,18,23,55–57), and thus would be expected to recruit additional IL-2 production from the memory-predominant T-cell pool of old donors and to lessen the differences between age groups.

One means of resolving these issues is to analyze the IL-2 responses of "subset-matched" T-cell preparations from young and old donors. Two groups have taken this approach. Miller and colleagues (55,57) found that naive

TABLE 23–2   IL-2 PRODUCTION BY T CELLS DURING AGING

| Change with Age | Species (Refs) | | |
	Human	Mouse	Rat
↓	(59–65)	(54–57,66–79)	(80,81)
↔	(59,82–85)	(24,25,53,54, 56,69,71, 73,75)	(80,86,87)
↑	(59)	(75)	

(CD44^{lo}) T cells isolated from young and old mice have equivalent (and high) precursor frequencies for IL-2–producing cells responding to Con A or sAg, whereas the memory (CD44^{hi} or CD45RB^{lo}) T cells from both age groups were relatively inert in this system. Therefore, age-related decreases in the representation of the naive subsets can account for the decreases in IL-2 production by total T cells in response to these stimuli. Nagelkerken and associates (56) similarly found that Con A–induced IL-2 synthesis is more apparent in the naive (CD45RB^{hi}) CD4+ cell fraction, but they reported an age-related deficit in the response of this subset. However, there were no age-related differences in the responses of naive or memory (CD45RB^{lo}) cells when PMA and ionomycin were used for stimulation.

The survey of literature in this section indicates that the effects of aging on IL-2 synthesis are system-dependent, and that interpretation of results is complicated by age-related shifts in the T-cell subset frequencies and by the unique properties of each subset. In view of these findings—and until we know which of the polyclonal stimuli most accurately mimics Ag stimulation of naive and memory cells in vivo—there seems to be little justification in labeling T cells from old donors "intrinsically defective" in their capacity for IL-2 synthesis.

The IL-2 receptor (IL-2R) consists of at least three components, the α-, β-, and γ-chains, whose stoichiometry dictates the binding affinity and signaling capacity of the complex. Genes encoding these components are upregulated following T-cell stimulation, thus increasing the membrane levels of the high-affinity IL-2R complexes (e.g., αβγ) able to transduce signals for T-cell growth and differentiation (91).

Most studies have shown that aging is associated with reduced proliferation by stimulated T cells in vitro (7). However, this age-related deficit persists even when endogenous IL-2 levels are high (24,53,54,56,69,73,75, 80,83,84,87), and it is often not completely restored by exogenous IL-2 (56,61,67,83,84,86,92,93). These findings prompted several laboratories to investigate the integrity of the IL-2R complex on mitogen-stimulated T cells, CD4+ cells, and CD8+ cells from young and old donors. In general, these studies reported age-related decreases in the capacity to bind (61,92–94) and internalize (94) exogenous IL-2, in the expression of the α- (59,60,67,69,94) and β-chains (94), and in the fraction of cells that hyperexpress the high-affinity IL-2R complexes (92,93). As a cautionary note, however, these changes were not observed in one study in the rat system (87). Furthermore, the age-related deficits in IL-2R expression are often not apparent when strong (less subset-biased) polyclonal stimuli are used (69,83), thus following a pattern similar to that of IL-2 production. Again, we are left wondering whether aging compromises the IL-2/IL-2R circuitry or, alternatively, results in increased proportions of T-cell subsets, which, although normal, score poorly relative to naive T cells in certain in vitro assays.

Interferon-γ

IFN-γ is produced mainly by activated T cells and NK cells. As discussed in previous sections, the capacity for IFN-γ gene expression by T cells segregates predominantly with the memory/effector fractions of CD4+ and CD8+ cells, and it may undergo further partitioning within these fractions (e.g., Th1 versus Th2 clones). IFN-γ exhibits many functions in vitro and in vivo (3,104). These functions include antiviral properties; induction of microbicidal activities, FcR$_\gamma$ expression, and inflammatory cytokine release by macrophages and monocytes; upregulation of MHC molecules on several cell types; enhancement of cytotoxic responses by CTL and NK cells; regulation of B-cell growth and differentiation; and preferential induction of Th1-like response patterns and inhibition of Th2-like reactions.

A survey of reports on age-related changes in IFN-γ production by T cells in primary cultures is presented in Table 23–3. Most of the studies in the mouse system have shown that this capacity increases with age. This change is progressive from young adulthood to late life in several mouse strains (16,24,56,103), is evident in spleen and lymph nodes (75), and affects both the CD4+ (24,56) and the CD8+ (16) T-cell groups. In addition, the age-related increase in IFN-γ synthesis is observed with a variety of cell stimuli (e.g., lectins, anti-CD3 mAb, phorbol myristate acetate (PMA) plus ionophore) and assays for cytokine mRNA and protein. The two reports showing decreased IFN-γ synthesis with age used Con A or PHA as the stimulus, again raising the issue of whether the main sources of IFN-γ (memory T cells) were optimally stimulated. In one study using allo-Ag as the stimulus, minimal age-related differences in IFN-γ synthesis were reported,

TABLE 23–3 IFN-γ PRODUCTION BY T CELLS DURING AGING

Change with Age	Species (Refs)	
	Human	Mouse
↓	(59,63,85, 95–97)	(79,98)
↔	(62,82,84,95, 97,99–101)	(102)
↑	(83)	(16,24,25,43, 54,56,70,72, 74,75,103)

and exogenous IL-12 boosted this response similarly in both the young and old groups (102).

Two reports (16,24) showed that the age-related increase in IFN-γ synthesis by T cells is caused by the shift in the T-cell subset frequencies. In an analysis of cytokine production by the naive (CD44^{lo}) and memory (CD44^{hi}) subsets of CD4+ (24) and CD8+ (16) cells during aging, it was found that (a) the capacity to produce IFN-γ always segregates with the memory subsets regardless of donor age, and (b) there is a trend toward age-related increases in the capacity for IFN-γ within the memory T-cell group. These data suggest that age-related increases in the production of this cytokine by the T-cell pool result from conversion to a predominance of memory-like CD4+ and CD8+ cells, and they are perhaps further enhanced by differentiative change within the memory T-cell group.

Even though the capacity for IFN-γ synthesis may be preserved or enhanced with age in mice, other consequences of T-cell subset shifts may preclude its efficient use in vivo. For example, Orme and associates (105) showed that intravenous infection of young mice with a sublethal dose of *Mycobacterium tuberculosis* is followed by increases in splenic, Ag-reactive CD4+ cells able to produce IFN-γ and eventual resolution of the infection. In contrast, old animals unable to contain the infection show a similar capacity for Ag-specific IFN-γ production, but the response is delayed. The authors argue that this lethal delay is due, in part, to altered T-cell trafficking patterns stemming from the changed expression of the MEL-14 and LFA-1 homing/adhesion receptors.

Unfortunately, results from studies on IFN-γ production in the aging human system (see Table 23–3) have not provided a consensus. Conclusions have varied between laboratories using similar culture conditions and assay methods (62,95,96), and within laboratories based on the choice of stimuli (95,97). Notably, one group observed age-related decreases in IFN-γ gene expression even when strong polyclonal activators (e.g., PMA and ionophore) were used (59). The reasons for this variability among human studies and the differences between the human and the mouse systems are unclear, but they could relate to the selection criteria for human donors or to the use of blood (human studies) versus spleen or lymph node (mouse studies). In addition, none of the human studies addressed the potentially confounding effects of other IFN-γ–producing cells (i.e., NK cells) present in the cell cultures or the individual contributions of the CD4+ and CD8+ cell groups. Clearly, more studies using well-defined systems are needed to clarify this important issue.

Considering the possibility that aging results in an increased capacity for IFN-γ synthesis by the T-cell group, it is surprising that few investigators have studied the consequences of this change. One study showed that exogenous IFN-γ (± exogenous IL-2) caused variable enhancement of proliferative responses by PHA-stimulated

T cells from elderly humans (84). Another group (74) found that, in the mouse system, Con A–induced CTL activity in vitro is elevated in the old group, and its development is unaffected by addition of anti-IFN-γ Ab, whereas CTL activity in the young group was significantly enhanced by this treatment. However, it is unclear what cell type (e.g., T, NK, or LAK) was affected by endogenous IFN-γ in this system.

Interleukin-4

As discussed in previous sections, the capacity for IL-4 gene expression by CD4+ cells is elevated as a consequence of the naive to memory/effector conversion, and it may segregate further among these latter subsets (e.g., Th2-like cells). Moreover, IL-4 is thought to contribute to the differentiation and effector functions of Th2-like cells, while antagonizing development and effects of Th1-like cells (3,20).

Most investigators studying the mouse system reported age-related increases in IL-4 production by lymphoid cells, T cells, or CD4+ cells cultured with a variety of stimuli (Table 23–4). As with the other changes in cytokine expression with age, this trait is acquired gradually throughout life (24,56,71,79). Again, this change is consistent with age-related shifts in the T-cell subset composition and the greater potential of memory cells for IL-4 synthesis in primary cultures. However, in a study of pre-activated memory CD4+ cells grown in extended cultures with exogenous IL-2, there appeared to be an age-related decrease in the accumulation of IL-4, due in part to a reduced expansion of cells from old donors (106). These findings raise the interesting possibility that memory T cells from old donors, although exhibiting potent cytokine programs (and effector function) in the short term, may have de-emphasized their programs for clonal expansion (and extended memory).

Two reports on the human system showed severe (63) and modest (97) age-related decreases in IL-4 production by PBL stimulated with mitogenic lectins. However, use

TABLE 23–4   IL-4 PRODUCTION BY T CELLS DURING AGING

Change with Age	Species (Refs)	
	Human	Mouse
↓	(63, 97)	(106)
↔	(97)	
↑		(24,25,53,54, 56,70–73,79)

of PMA plus ionophore in the latter study reversed this trend, thus reinforcing the concept that age-related effects observed in vitro can be stimulus-dependent.

There is limited information on age-related differences in the responsiveness of T cells to IL-4. One study showed that the proliferative response of mouse T cells to a combination of PMA and IL-4 is not impaired with age (107). Another group (56) found that various combinations of exogenous IL-4 and IL-2 enhance the proliferative response of mouse CD4+ cells to Con A or anti-CD3 mAb, but the degree of enhancement was similar between the young and old groups.

Interleukin-3 and GM-CSF

IL-3 and GM-CSF are key regulators of hematopoiesis, and they can enhance the inflammatory activities of mature myeloid cells (3). Almost all the studies on age-related changes in the production of these cytokines have been performed using the mouse model. Both age-related decreases (55,72,76,78) and increases (24,25,71,108) in IL-3 production by mitogen-stimulated lymphoid cells or T cells have been reported. Again, these differences between laboratories appear to relate to the choice of cell stimuli: age-related decreases are usually (55,72,76,78) but not always (71,108) observed when using Con A, sAg, or soluble anti-CD3 mAb, whereas strong polyclonal stimuli, such as immobilized anti-CD3 mAb or PMA plus ionophore, always reveal age-related increases in IL-3 production (24,25,43,71). Analysis of purified T-cell subsets has helped to clarify this issue. For example, Flurkey and associates (55) showed that precursors for IL-3 production in response to Con A or sAg reside almost entirely in the naive T-cell pool, thus explaining why naive-deficient total T cells from old mice produce less IL-3 when cultured with these activators. In contrast, Hobbs and colleagues (24) found that memory (CD44hi) CD4+ cells stimulated with immobilized anti-CD3 mAb produce much greater levels of IL-3 than their naive counterparts, regardless of the age of donor mice. Moreover, these findings are consistent with another study showing that memory CD4+ (and CD8+) cells from normal mice are superior producers of IL-3 when stimulated with PMA plus ionophore (18). Therefore, age-related increases in the representation of memory CD4+ cells can account for the elevated levels of IL-3 production in response to strong polyclonal stimuli. To date, there is no information available on the effects of age on IL-3 production by CD8+ cells.

There are a few reports on age-related changes in GM-CSF production by stimulated T cells. One study in the human system (59) and two in the mouse system (72,78) using intact lymphoid tissues indicate that this capacity may decline with age. However, firm conclusions on this subject must await more detailed analyses of the response patterns of purified T cells and the component subsets.

IL-5, IL-6, and IL-10

IL-5 functions as a growth and differentiation factor for B cells (particularly in the mouse system), and it is a potent inducer of eosinophilia (3). Two laboratories working on the mouse system have shown age-related increases in the production of this cytokine, using either splenocyte cultures stimulated with soluble anti-CD3 mAb (72) or purified splenic CD4+ cells stimulated with immobilized anti-CD3 mAb (24,25,43). Moreover, the latter group found that this change is progressive with age and relates directly to the accumulation of memory (CD44hi) cells with an increased capacity for IL-5 synthesis (24).

IL-6 is produced by many cell types, and it exhibits a very diverse range of activities (3,4), including inductive roles in T-cell growth, B-cell differentiation, and the acute-phase response. Most of the available data on the age-altered production of this cytokine were generated using intact lymphoid cell cultures, thus making it difficult to assess changes specific for T cells. In these studies (in both human and mouse systems), IL-6 production in response to polyclonal T-cell stimuli was shown to increase (100,109,110), decrease (59), or remain unchanged (59,82,110) with age. Age-related differences also appear somewhat stimulus- (59) and tissue-dependent (110). The one study on purified CD4+ cells from mice (24) reported no change with age in the inducible synthesis of this cytokine.

Daynes and coworkers (110) reported that the blood levels of IL-6 and the constitutive production of IL-6 by lymphoid cells in vitro are both increased for old mouse and human donors, although the findings in vitro are not always apparent in other studies (24,59,82,100). If true, however, these data would suggest an increased frequency of immune hyperactivity in the elderly (as discussed for IL-2 [65]), yielding an elevated release of a cytokine with wide-ranging effects on many organ systems.

IL-10 is also produced by many cell types (e.g., activated T cells, B cells, and macrophages), and it has a number of roles in the immune system, many of which involve enhancement of Th2-like responses and down-regulation of inflammatory (Th1-like) responses (3). To our knowledge, only one study addressed the effect of aging on expression of this cytokine (25). The authors reported increases with age in the capacity of CD4+ cells to produce IL-10 in response to anti-CD3 mAb in vitro. Again, this change related directly to the age-related increase in proportions of memory (CD44hi) CD4+ cells (25).

Given the known B-cell–promoting activities of IL-4, IL-5, IL-6, and IL-10 (3,4), the possibility that production of these cytokines by T cells is not impaired, or is even enhanced, in late life would suggest stable or elevated T-helper cell function. Indeed, the level of serum immunoglobulin is generally maintained throughout life, and it is conceivable that T cells contribute to the age-related increase in autoantibody production and the incidence of monoclonal gammopathies. However, in vitro assessments of age-related changes in T-cell help for B-cell responses yielded inconsistent results, showing generally increased (64,111), decreased (112), or unchanged (113,114) T-cell function.

Other cytokines

Zhou and colleagues (109,115) studied the effects of age on the production of TGF-β, a cytokine group with potent suppressive effects on many cells of the immune system (4). They found that constitutive and Con A–induced TGF-β release by mouse splenocytes was increased with age. The authors went on to show that Con A–induced splenocyte proliferation is suppressed by endogenous and exogenous TGF-β, and that cells from old mice may be more sensitive to this effect. Finally, evidence was presented that concomitant age-related increases in IL-6 production could result in enhanced TGF-βR expression by T cells, perhaps explaining their increased sensitivity to TGF-β–mediated effects.

TNF-α and TNF-β exhibit a broad range of properties, most notably as major inflammatory mediators (4). In one study on aging mice (24), the investigators found no change in the capacity for TNF-α and TNF-β synthesis by splenic CD4+ cells activated with anti-CD3 mAb, whereas another group (100) reported age-related increases in TNF-α production by mitogen-stimulated human PBL.

Summary

The survey of literature in this section reveals distinct age-related changes in the cytokine repertoire of the peripheral T-cell pool. In certain studies on rodents, the profiles of cytokine gene expression by T, CD4+, or CD8+ cells in late life are consistent with the prevailing representation of T-cell subsets (i.e., increased memory/naive T-cell ratio) and the known functional attributes of individual subsets. Thus, T cells from old rodents can exhibit unimpaired production of IL-2, IL-6, TNF-α, and TNF-β (cytokines associated with naive and memory T cells) and enhanced production of IL-3, IL-4, IL-5, IL-10, and IFN-γ (cytokines associated predominantly with memory T cells). Realization of these potentials in vitro depends somewhat on the use of strong polyclonal stimuli that recruit cytokine production by memory T cells, although it could be argued that such stimuli mask age-related defects at the level of the accessory cell or the T cell. Similar

trends are evident in some studies in the human system, but, in general, there is less agreement between laboratories. Establishment of rigorous criteria for donor selection and use of highly purified T cells or cell subsets and a range of stimulation protocols should help resolve some of these issues. Finally, with the exception of studies on the IL-2/IL-2R circuitry, there is very limited information on age-related changes in the expression of cytokine receptors and the response to cytokine signals by T cells. Considering the various cytokine-mediated crossregulatory interactions among T-cell subsets, this area of investigation could prove useful.

STRATEGIES FOR IMPROVING IMMUNITY DURING AGING

In view of recent progress on identification and characterization of T-cell subsets, and on how these subsets change in number and function with age, an important question arises: Can we use this information to design prophylactic and therapeutic measures to counter the immune deficiency and dysregulation that accompany aging? Specifically, can we exploit elements of the immune system (e.g., cytokines and cytokine agonists or antagonists) to accomplish this task? Given the humane concern for the quality of life of our increasing elderly population and the tremendous costs for their hospitalization and treatments for established diseases, the interest is great for improving old and designing new clinical approaches to this problem.

In the context of the naive/memory paradigm, the elderly must face their environment with a dearth of naive, relatively undifferentiated T cells, which are needed for responses to new Ag, including neoantigens expressed by infectious agents and tumors. Thus, immunodeficiency could stem from the inability to generate sufficient numbers of new effector cells that mediate primary immune responses and, in the process, to establish adequate numbers of memory cells to deal with subsequent encounters with the eliciting Ag. In addition, it is conceivable that the processes of T-cell selection and maturation are compromised in the involuting thymus, perhaps allowing emigration of naive cells with defective functions or with inappropriate TCR specificities.

The age-associated increase in the representation of memory T cells could benefit the elderly by mediating immune responses against previously encountered Ag. Due to their enhanced access to a variety of tissues, their capacity to amplify TCR signaling via the action of membrane coreceptors, and their diverse programs of cytokine gene expression, memory T cells can effectively guard against reinfection by pathogens. On the down side, the abundance of well-differentiated memory T cells may render the immune system rigid, at the levels of both the TCR repertoire (fixed in the antigenic history of the host) and the reduced plasticity of cell differentiation. Also inherent in this age-related change is the potential for dysregulation, perhaps through discoordinate overproduction of immunoregulatory cytokines that could either suppress the development or expression of appropriate immune responses (e.g., protective Th1-like and CTL responses to viruses or other intracellular parasites) or amplify inappropriate responses (e.g., nonprotective Th2-like responses to *M. leprae*). In this regard, it is important to re-emphasize that IL-4, IL-10, and IFN-γ, known players in the crossregulatory circuits among T-cell subsets, can be produced at high levels by stimulated T cells from old mice.

It is possible that accumulation of T cells with a declining intrinsic responsiveness could contribute to immunosenescence. Nonresponsive cell types could arise from intrinsic defects (e.g., gene mutations) or from peripheral tolerance mechanisms. Whether and how nonresponsive T-cell types could be maintained for long periods and "allowed" to accumulate to a significant degree in the elderly is unclear.

On the basis of the naive/memory paradigm, prophylactic or therapeutic intervention could be focused on either the dwindling numbers of naive T cells or the increasing fraction of memory T cells (or both) during aging. It may be possible to selectively target naive precursor T cells to respond to new pathogens by immunizing with peptides or fusion proteins that bear new protective epitopes (e.g., those that selectively trigger class I [CTL] or II [Th cells] MHC-restricted responses, or even Th1- or Th2-like responses). Moreover, these neoantigens could be carefully designed to exclude epitopes that can (a) generate suppressor cells; (b) crossreact with previously encountered Ag, which could elicit an inappropriately biased regulatory action by memory T cells; or (c) mimic self-Ag to avoid triggering autoimmune responses (to which the elderly seem more prone). The inherent difficulty in these reductionist approaches is that because of genetic differences, not all individuals will respond appropriately to a given vaccine Ag. Thus, there is a need to use peptides that can bind to multiple MHC alleles or even multiple peptides in the hope that some or all will be presented properly. In other cases, it is desirable to boost pre-existent immunity (e.g., to influenza, tetanus, and pneumococcus) carried by the memory T-cell pool, preferably by intermittent vaccination to avoid a chronic hyperactive (and perhaps refractory) state or exhaustive differentiation of the T cells.

Identification of adjuvants that promote processing and retention of Ag after primary vaccination have been sought to help induce and maintain long-term responsiveness. Inclusion of agents that either provide direct growth or differentiative signals (e.g., IL-2, IL-4, IL-12, IL-13) or selectively induce the release of costimulatory factors (e.g., IL-1, IL-6, TNF-α, IL-12) from local APC are currently under scrutiny. Concurrent application of these agents with Ag may selectively guide the development of particular response types (e.g., Th1-, Th2-, or CTL-like responses) deemed to be protective against a given pathogen. Cytokine antagonists (e.g., soluble cytokine receptors or neutralizing anticytokine or anticytokine receptor mAbs) have been successfully used in animal model systems to direct the development of response types, and they may likewise be applied for human use.

As discussed in earlier sections, IL-2 has been most intensively investigated for its capacity to enhance T-cell responses during aging, although in many patients, even high levels of exogenous IL-2 do not restore T-cell–dependent responses. Due to the action of IL-2 on a variety of cell types and organ systems, its capacity to cause shock and pulmonary edema, and the need to provide high local concentrations of IL-2, repetitive application of high IL-2 doses required to boost in vivo responses to Ag is problematic. Thus, newer measures are being developed (e.g., recombinant virus-mediated gene therapy, somatic gene therapy with naked DNA, or transfection of tumor cells with cytokine genes) that can deliver and maintain high local concentrations of IL-2 and other cytokines at appropriate tissue sites.

CONCLUDING REMARKS

Revisiting the quotation at the beginning of this chapter, the age-altered representation of functionally distinct T-cell subsets may indeed be an example of " . . . dysorganizational consequences that emanate from the physiological or organ function level. . . . " Perhaps driven by the biological clock of thymic involution, the dwindling number of naive cells removes from the T-cell group an important component, one that contains the TCR repertoire needed for new Ag and that is flexible in its choice of differentiative pathways. In contrast, prevalence of well-differentiated T cells in late life could lead to polarized, nonprotective response modes to re-encounter with Ag, dictated either by the inappropriate crossregulation among T cells or by the dominant emergence of nonprotective subsets. Although not discussed herein, the T-cell saga during aging is further complicated by potential changes in the distribution and function of APC and by possible changes in the V-region repertoire and subset composition of the B-cell pool. Thus, the aging T-cell compartment must function by a changing set of rules. Understanding these changes should provide insight into the phenomenon of immunosenescence, thereby guiding clinical approaches to this problem.

REFERENCES

1. Finch CE. Longevity, senescence, and the genome. Chicago: University of Chicago Press, 1990.

2. Mittelmark MB. The epidemiology of aging. In: Hazzard WR, Bierman EL, Blass JP, Ettinger WH Jr, Halter JB, eds. Principles of geriatric medicine and gerontology. New York: McGraw-Hill, 1994:135–151.

3. Howard MC, Miyajima A, Coffman R. T-cell-derived cytokines and their receptors. In: Paul WE, ed. Fundamental immunology. New York: Raven, 1993:763–800.

4. Durum SK, Oppenheim JJ. Proinflammatory cytokines and immunity. In: Paul WE, ed. Fundamental immunology. New York: Raven, 1993:801–835.

5. Scollay RG, Butcher EC, Weissman IL. Thymus cell migration: quantitative aspects of cellular traffic from the thymus to the periphery in mice. Eur J Immunol 1980;10:210–218.

6. Schwab R, Walters CA, Weksler ME. Host defense mechanisms and aging. Semin Oncol 1989;16:20–27.

7. Thoman ML, Weigle WO. The cellular and subcellular bases of immunosenescence. Adv Immunol 1989;46:221–260.

8. Miller RA. Aging and the immune system. In: Masoro E, ed. Handbook of the biology of aging. Oxford University Press, 1994.

9. Budd RC, Cerottini J-C, Horvath C, et al. Distinction of virgin and memory T lymphocytes. Stable acquisition of the Pgp-1 glycoprotein concomitant with antigenic stimulation. J Immunol 1987;138:3120–3129.

10. Sanders ME, Makgoba MW, Shaw S. Human naive and memory T cell: reinterpretation of helper-inducer and suppressor-inducer subsets. Immunol Today 1988;9:195–199.

11. Swain SL, Bradley LM, Croft M, et al. Helper T-cell subsets: phenotype, function and the role of lymphokines in regulating their development. Immunol Rev 1991;123:115–144.

12. Hayakawa K, Hardy RR. Murine CD4+ T-cell subsets. Immunol Rev 1991;123:145–168.

13. Akbar AN, Salmon M, Janossy G. The synergy between naive and memory T cells during activation. Immunol Today 1991;12:184–188.

14. Horgan KJ, Ginther Luce GE, Tanaka Y, et al. Differential expression of VLA-α4 and VLA-β1 discriminates multiple subsets of CD4+CD45RO+ "memory" T cells. J Immunol 1992;149:4082–4087.

15. Mackay CR. Migration pathways and immunologic memory among T lymphocytes. Semin Immunol 1992;4:51–58.

16. Ernst DN, Weigle WO, Noonan DJ, McQuitty DN, Hobbs MV. The age-associated increase in IFN-γ synthesis by mouse CD8+ T cells correlates with shifts in the frequencies of cell subsets defined by membrane CD44, CD45RB, 3G11, and MEL-14 expression. J Immunol 1993;151:575–587.

17. Sprent J. T and B memory cells. Cell 1994;76:315–322.

18. Budd RC, Cerottini J-C, MacDonald HR. Selectively increased production of interferon-γ by subsets of Lyt-2+ and L3T4+ T cells identified by expression of Pgp-1. J Immunol 1987;138:3583–3586.

19. Ehlers S, Smith KA. Differentiation of T cell lymphokine gene expression: the in vitro acquisition of T cell memory. J Exp Med 1991;173:25–36.

20. Paul WE, Seder RA. Lymphocyte responses and cytokines. Cell 1994;76:241–251.

21. Bradley LM, Duncan DD, Tonkonogy S, Swain SL. Characterization of antigen-specific CD4+ effector T cells in vivo: immunization results in a transient population of MEL-14⁻, CD45RB- helper cells that secretes interleukin 2 (IL-2), IL-3, IL-4, and interferon γ. J Exp Med 1991;174:547–559.

22. Bradley LM, Croft M, Swain SL. T-cell memory: new perspectives. Immunol Today 1993;14:197–199.

23. Lee WT, Yin X-M, Vitetta ES. Functional and ontogenetic analysis of murine CD45R^hi and CD45R^lo CD4+ T cells. J Immunol 1990;144:3288–3295.

24. Hobbs MV, Weigle WO, Noonan DJ, et al. Patterns of cytokine gene expression by CD4+ T cells from young and old mice. J Immunol 1993;150:3602–3614.

25. Hobbs MV, Weigle WO, Ernst DN. Interleukin-10 production by splenic CD4+ cells and cell subsets from young and old mice. Cell Immunol 1994;154:264–272.

26. van Kooten C, Rensink I, Pascual-Salcedo D, van Oers R, Aarden L. Monokine production by human T cells; IL-1α production restricted to memory T cells. J Immunol 1991;146:2654–2658.

27. McKnight AJ, Barclay AN, Mason DW. Molecular cloning of rat interleukin 4 cDNA and analysis of the cytokine repertoire of subsets of CD4+ T cells. Eur J Immunol 1991;21:1187–1194.

28. Mobley JL, Dailey MO. Regulation of adhesion molecule expression by CD8 T cells in vivo. I. Differential regulation of gp90^MEL-14(LECAM-1), Pgp-1, LFA-1, VLA-4α during the differentiation of cytotoxic T lymphocytes induced by allografts. J Immunol 1992;148:2348–2356.

29. Hirohata S. T8 cell regulation of human B cell responsiveness: regulatory influences of CD45RA+ and CD45RA- T8 cell subsets. Cell Immunol 1991;1333:15–26.

30. Seder RA, Boulay J-L, Finkelman F, et al. CD8+ T cells can be primed in vitro to produce IL-4. J Immunol 1992;148:1652–1656.

31. Erard F, Wild M-T, Garcia-Sanz JA, Le Gros G. Switch of CD8 T cells to noncytolytic CD8-CD4- cells that make TH2 cytokines and help B cells. Science 1993;260:1802–1805.

32. Street NE, Mosmann TR. Functional diversity of T lymphocytes due to secretion of different cytokine patterns. FASEB J 1991;5:171–177.

33. Firestein GS, Roeder WD, Laxer JA, et al. A new murine CD4+ T cell subset with an unrestricted cytokine profile. J Immunol 1989;143:518–525.

34. Paliard X, De Waal Malefijt R, Yssel H, et al. Simultaneous production of IL-2, IL-4, and IFN-γ by activated human CD4+ and CD8+ T cell clones. J Immunol 1988;141:849–855.

35. Romagnani S. Human TH1 and TH2 subsets: regulation of differentiation and role in protection and immunopathology. Int Arch Allergy Immunol 1992;98:279–285.

36. Mosmann TR, Fong TAT. Alloreactive murine CD8+ T cell clones secrete the Th1 pattern of cytokines. J Immunol 1990;144:1744–1752.

37. Salgame P, Abrams JS, Clayberger C, et al. Differing

lymphokine profiles of functional subsets of human CD4 and CD8 T cell clones. Science 1991;254:279–282.

38. Inoue T, Asano Y, Matsuoka S, et al. Distinction of mouse CD8+ suppressor effector T cell clones from cytotoxic T cell clones by cytokine production and CD45 isoforms. J Immunol 1993;150:2121–2128.

39. Parish CR. The relationship between humoral and cell-mediated immunity. Transplant Rev 1972;13:35–66.

40. Yamamura M, Uyemura K, Deans RJ, et al. Defining protective responses to pathogens: cytokine profiles in leprosy lesions. Science 1991;254:277–279.

41. Heinzel FP, Sadick MD, Mutha SS, Locksley RM. Production of interferon γ, interleukin 2, interleukin 4, and interleukin 10 by CD4+ lymphocytes in vivo during healing and progressive murine leishmaniasis. Proc Natl Acad Sci USA 1991;88:7011–7015.

42. Scott P, Kaufmann HE. The role of T-cell subsets and cytokines in the regulation of infection. Immunol Today 1991;12:346–348.

43. Haas W, Pereira P, Tonegawa S. Gamma/delta cells. Ann Rev Immunol 1993;11:637–685.

44. Matsuzaki G, Yoshikai Y, Kishihara K, Nomoto K, Yokokura T, Nomoto K. Age-associated increase in the expression of T cell antigen receptor γ chain genes in mice. Eur J Immunol 1988;18:1779–1784.

45. De Paoli P, Battistin S, Santini GF. Age-related changes in human lymphocyte subsets: progressive reduction of the CD4 CD45R (suppressor inducer) population. Clin Immunol Immunopathol 1988;48:290–296.

46. Pirrucello PJ, Collins M, Wilson JE, McManus BM. Age-related changes in naive and memory CD4+ T cells in healthy human children. Clin Immunol Immunopathol 1989;52:341–345.

47. Warren RP, Yonk LJ, Burger RA, Singh VK. Age-related changes in CD45R+ and CDw29+ helper T cells in human subjects. Aging: Immunol Infect Dis 1990;2:91–94.

48. Beckman I, Dimopoulos K, Xu X, Ahern M, Bradley J. Age-related changes in the activation requirements of human CD4+ T-cell subsets. Cell Immunol 1991;132:17–25.

49. Utsuyama M, Hirokawa K, Kurashima C, et al. Differential age-change in the numbers of CD4+CD45RA+ and CD4+CD29+ T cell subsets in human peripheral blood. Mech Ageing Dev 1992;63:57–68.

50. Cossarizza A, Ortolani C, Paganelli R, et al. Age-related imbalance of virgin (CD45RA+) and memory (CD45RO+) cells between CD4+ and CD8+ T lymphocytes in humans: a study from newborns to centenarians. J Immunol Res 1992;4:118–126.

51. Hayward AR, Lee J, Beverley PCL. Ontogeny of expression of UCHL1 antigen on TCR-1+ (CD4/8) and TCRδ T cells. Eur J Immunol 1989;19:771–773.

52. Okumura M, Fujii Y, Takeuchi Y, Inada K, Nakahara K, Matsuda H. Age-related accumulation of LFA-1high cells in a CD8+CD45RA^hi T cell population. Eur J Immunol 1993;23:1057–1063.

53. Ernst DN, Hobbs MV, Torbett BE, et al. Differences in the expression profiles of CD45RB, Pgp-1, and 3G11 membrane antigens and in the patterns of lymphokine secretion by splenic CD4+ T cells from young and aged mice. J Immunol 1990;145:1295–1302.

54. Hobbs MV, Ernst DN, Torbett BE, et al. Cell proliferation and cytokine production by CD4+ cells from old mice. J Cell Biochem 1991;46:312–320.

55. Flurkey K, Stadecker M, Miller RA. Memory T lymphocyte hyporesponsiveness to non-cognate stimuli: a key factor in age-related immunodeficiency. Eur J Immunol 1992;22:931–935.

56. Nagelkerken L, Hertogh-Huijbregts A, Dobber R, Drager A. Age-related changes in lymphokine production related to a decreased number of CD45RB^hi CD4+ T cells. Eur J Immunol 1991;21:273–281.

57. Lerner A, Yamada T, Miller RA. Pgp-1hi T lymphocytes accumulate with age in mice and respond poorly to concanavalin A. Eur J Immunol 1989;19:977–982.

58. Grossmann A, Maggio-Price L, Jinneman JC, Rabinovitch PS. Influence of aging on intracellular free calcium and proliferation of mouse T-cell subsets from various lymphoid organs. Cell Immunol 1991;135:118–131.

59. Gauchat J-F, de Weck AL, Stadler BM. Decreased cytokine messenger RNA levels in the elderly. Aging: Immunol Infect Dis 1988;1:191–204.

60. Nagel JE, Chopra RK, Chrest FJ, et al. Decreased proliferation, interleukin 2 synthesis, and interleukin 2 receptor expression are accompanied by decreased mRNA expression in phytohemagglutinin-stimulated cells from elderly donors. J Clin Invest 1988;81:1096–1102.

61. Gillis S, Kozak R, Durante M, Weksler ME. Immunological studies of aging: decreased production of and response to T cell growth factor by lymphocytes from aged humans. J Clin Invest 1981;67:937–942.

62. Weifeng C, Shulin L, Xiaomei G, Xuewen P. The capacity of lymphokine production by peripheral blood lymphocytes from aged humans. Immunol Invest 1986;15:575–583.

63. Guidi L, Bartolini C, Frasca D, et al. Impairment of lymphocyte activities in depressed aged subjects. Mech Ageing Dev 1991;60:13–24.

64. Hara H, Negoro S, Miyata S, et al. Age-associated changes in proliferative and differentiative response of human B cells and production of T cell-derived factors regulating B cell functions. Mech Ageing Dev 1987;38:245–258.

65. Huang Y-P, Pechere J-C, Michel M, et al. In vivo T cell activation, in vitro defective IL-2 secretion, and response to influenza vaccination in elderly women. J Immunol 1992;148:715–722.

66. Miller RA. Age-associated decline in precursor frequency for different T cell-mediated reactions, with preservation of helper or cytotoxic effect per precursor cell. J Immunol 1984;132:63–68.

67. Ernst DN, Weigle WO, McQuitty DN, Rothermel AL, Hobbs MV. Stimulation of murine T cell subsets with anti-CD3 antibody: age-related defects in the expression of early activation molecules. J Immunol 1989;142:1413–1421.

68. Thoman ML, Weigle WO. Cell-mediated immunity in aged mice: an underlying lesion in IL-2 synthesis. J Immunol 1982;128:2358–2361.

69. Thoman ML, Weigle WO. Partial restoration of Con A-induced proliferation, IL-2 receptor expression, and IL-2 synthesis in aged murine lymphocytes by phorbol myristate acetate and ionomycin. Cell Immunol 1988;114:1–11.

70. Dobber R, Hertogh-Huijbregts A, Rozing J, Bottomly K, Nagelkerken L. The involvement of the intestinal microflora in the expansion of CD4+ T cells with a naive phenotype in the periphery. Dev Immunol 1992;2:141–150.

71. Kubo M, Cinader B. Polymorphism of age-related changes in interleukin (IL) production: differential changes of T helper subpopulations, synthesizing IL2, IL3 and IL4. Eur J Immunol 1990;20:1289–1296.

72. Daynes RA, Araneo BA. Prevention and reversal of some age-associated changes in immunologic responses by supplemental dehydroepiandrosterone sulfate therapy. Aging: Immunol Infect Dis 1992;3:135–154.

73. Kariv I, Ferguson FG, Confer FL. Age- and strain-related differences in murine spleen cell responses to different activation signals. Cell Immunol 1992;140:67–80.

74. Saxena RK, Saxena QB, Adler WH. Lectin-induced cytotoxic activity in spleen cells from young and old mice. Age-related changes in types of effector cells, lymphokine production and response. Immunology 1988;64:457–461.

75. Kirschmann DA, Murasko DM. Splenic and inguinal lymph node T cells of aged mice respond differently to polyclonal and antigen-specific stimuli. Cell Immunol 1992;139:426–437.

76. Chang M-P, Utsuyama M, Hirokawa K, Makinodan T. Decline in the production of interleukin-3 with age in mice. Cell Immunol 1988;115:1–12.

77. Fong TC, Makinodan T. In situ hybridization analysis of the age-associated decline in IL-2 mRNA expressing murine T cells. Cell Immunol 1989;118:199–207.

78. Cai N-S, Li D-D, Cheung HT, Richardson A. The expression of granulocyte/monocyte colony-stimulating factor in activated mouse lymphocytes declines with age. Cell Immunol 1990;130:311–319.

79. Cillari E, Milano S, Dieli M, et al. Thymopentin reduces the susceptibility of aged mice to cutaneous leishmaniasis by modulating CD4 T-cell subsets. Immunology 1992;76:362–366.

80. Davila DR, Kelley KW. Sex differences in lectin-induced interleukin-2 synthesis in aging rats. Mech Ageing Dev 1988;44:231–240.

81. Wu W, Pahlavani M, Cheung HT, Richardson A. The effect of aging on the expression of interleukin-2 messenger ribonucleic acid. Cell Immunol 1986;100:224–231.

82. Sindermann J, Kruse A, Frercks H-J, Schutz RM, Kirchner H. Investigations of the lymphokine system in elderly individuals. Mech Ageing Dev 1993;70:149–159.

83. Chopra RK, Holbrook NJ, Powers DC, McCoy MT, Adler WH, Nagel JE. Interleukin 2, interleukin 2 receptor, and interferon-γ synthesis and mRNA expression in phorbol myristate acetate and calcium ionophore A23187-stimulated T cells from elderly humans. Clin Immunol Immunopathol 1989;53:297–308.

84. Hessen MT, Kaye D, Murasko DM. Heterogenous effects of exogenous lymphokines on lymphoproliferation of elderly subjects. Mech Ageing Dev 1991;58:61–73.

85. Mariana E, Mariana AR, Mingari MC, Sinoppi M, Facchini A. Lymphokine production in normal old subjects. In: Facchini A, Haaijman JJ, Labo G, eds. Immunoregulation in aging. The Netherlands: J. H. Pasmans Offsetdrukkerij B. V., 1986:101–108.

86. Rosenberg JS, Gilman SC, Feldman JD. Effects of aging on cell cooperation and lymphocyte responsiveness to cytokines. J Immunol 1983;130:1754–1758.

87. Holbrook NJ, Chopra RK, McCoy MT, et al. Expression of interleukin 2 and the interleukin 2 receptor in aging rats. Cell Immunol 1989;120:1–9.

88. Miller RA, Stutman O. Decline, in aging mice, of the anti-2,4,6-trinitrophenyl (TNP) cytotoxic T cell response attributable to loss of Lyt-2-, interleuklin 2-producing helper cell function. Eur J Immunol 1981;11:751–756.

89. Bloom ET. Functional importance of CD4+ and CD8+ cells in cytotoxic lymphocytes activity and associated gene expression. Impact on the age-related decline in lytic activity. Eur J Immunol 1991;21:1013–1017.

90. O'Leary JJ, Jackola DR, Mehta C, Hallgren HM. Enhancement of mitogen response and surface marker analysis of lymphocytes from young and old donors after preliminary incubation in vitro. Mech Ageing Dev 1985;29:239–253.

91. Taniguchi T, Minami Y. The IL-2/IL-2 receptor system: a current overview. Cell 1992;73:5–8.

92. Proust JJ, Kittur DS, Buchholz MA, Nordin AA. Restricted expression of mitogen-induced high affinity IL-2 receptors in aging mice. J Immunol 1988;141:4209–4216.

93. Nagel JE, Chopra RK, Powers DC, Adler WH. Effect of age on the human high affinity interleukin 2 receptor of phytohaemagglutinin stimulated peripheral blood lymphocytes. Clin Exp Immunol 1989;75:286–291.

94. Hara H, Tanaka T, Negoro S, et al. Age-related changes of expression of IL-2 receptor subunits and kinetics of IL-2 internalization in T cells after mitogenic stimulation. Mech Ageing Dev 1988;45:167–175.

95. Rytel MW, Larratt KS, Turner PA, Kalbfleisch JH. Interferon response to mitogens and viral antigens in elderly and young adult subjects. J Infect Dis 1986;153:984–987.

96. Abb J, Abb H, Deinhardt F. Age-related decline of human interferon alpha and interferon gamma production. Blut 1984;48:285–289.

97. Al-Rayes H, Pachas W, Mirza N, Ahern DJ, Geha RS, Vercelli D. IgE regulation and lymphokine patterns in aging humans. J Allergy Clin Immunol 1992;90:630–636.

98. Grasso G, Muscettola M, Stecconi R, Muzzioli M, Fabris N. Restorative effect of thymomodulin and zinc on interferon-gamma production in aged mice. Ann NY Acad Sci 1993; 673:256–259.

99. Cantell K, Strander H, Saxen L, Meyer B. Interferon response of human leukocytes during intrauterine and postnatal life. J Immunol 1968;100:1304–1309.

100. Fagiolo U, Cossarizza A, Scala E, et al. Increased cytokine production in mononuclear cells of healthy elderly people. Eur J Immunol 1993;23:2375–2378.

101. Canonica GW, Ciprandi G, Scordamaglia A, et al. Lymphokine production and T cell proliferation in aged subjects. In: Facchini A, Haaijman JJ, Labo G, eds. Immunoregulation in aging. The Netherlands: J. H. Pasmans Offsetdrukkerij B. V., 1986:95–99.

102. Bloom ET, Horvath JA. Cellular and molecular mechanisms of the IL-12-induced increase in allo-specific murine cytolytic T cell activity. Implications for the age-related decline in CTL. J Immunol 1994;152:4242–4254.

103. Heine JW, Adler WH. The quantitative production of inter-

feron by mitogen-stimulated mouse lymphocytes as a function of age and its effect on the lymphocytes proliferative response. J Immunol 1977;118:1366–1369.

104. Trinchieri G, Perussia B. Immune interferon: a pleiotropic lymphokine with multiple effects. Immunol Today 1985;6:131–136.

105. Orme IM, Griffin JP, Roberts AD, Ernst DN. Evidence for a defective accumulation of protective T cells in old mice infected with Mycobacterium tuberculosis. Cell Immunol 1993;147:222–229.

106. Li SP, Miller RA. Age-associated decline in IL-4 production by murine T lymphocytes in extended culture. Cell Immunol 1993;151:187–195.

107. Thoman ML, Keogh EA, Weigle WO. Response of aged T and B lymphocytes to IL-4. Aging: Immunol Infect Dis 1988;1:245–253.

108. Iwashima M, Nakayama T, Kubo M, Asano Y, Tada T. Alterations in the proliferative responses of T cells from aged and chimeric mice. Int Arch Appl Immunol 1987;83:129–137.

109. Zhou D, Chrest FJ, Adler W, Munster A, Winchurch RA. Increased production of TGF-beta and IL-6 by aged spleen cells. Immunol Lett 1993;36:7–12.

110. Daynes RA, Araneo BA, Ershler WB, Maloney C, Li G-Z, Ryu S-Y. Altered regulation of interleukin-6 production with normal aging: possible linkage to the age-associated decline in dehydroepiandrosterone (DHEA) and its sulfated derivative. J Immunol 1994;150:5219–5230.

111. Ceuppens JL, Goodwin JS. Regulation of immunoglobulin production in pokeweed mitogen-stimulated cultures of lymphocytes from young and old adults. J Immunol 1982;128:2429–2434.

112. Whisler RL, Newhouse YG. Function of T cells from elderly humans: reductions of membrane events and proliferative responses mediated via T3 determinants and diminished elaboration of soluble T-cell factors for B-cell growth. Cell Immunol 1986;99:422–433.

113. Guidizi MG, Biagiotti R, Almerigogna F, et al. Reduced proliferation and immunoglobulin production in vitro by B cells from aged subjects in response to T-cell derived factors. In: Facchini A, Haaijman JJ, Labo G, eds. Immunoregulation in aging. The Netherlands: J. H. Pasmans Offsetdrukkerij B. V., 1986:263–270.

114. Skias D, Reder AT, Bania MB, Antel JP. Age-related changes in mechanisms accounting for low levels of polyclonally induced immunoglobulin secretion in humans. Clin Immunol Immunopathol 1985;35:191–199.

115. Zhou D, Chrest FJ, Adler W, Munster A, Winchurch RA. Age-related changes in the expression of the TGF-β receptor on CD4+ and CD8+ subsets of T cells. Aging: Immunol Infect Dis 1992;3:217–226.

PART 4

ROLE OF CYTOKINES DURING INFECTION

CHAPTER 24

ROLE OF CYTOKINES/LYMPHOKINES IN GRAM-POSITIVE BACTERIAL INFECTIONS

Thomas Miethke, Claudia Wahl, and Hermann Wagner

Gram-positive bacteria, such as staphylococci and streptococci, are well-recognized pathogens for humans. They are responsible for localized suppurative sequelae such as cutaneous abscesses, furuncles, pharyngitis, and impetigo, as well as systemic and live threatening infections, such as osteomyelitis, pneumonia, and septicemia. In three recent studies of sepsis, gram-positive organisms were found to to be causative between 6 and 24% of infections. Both species produce a number of toxins responsible for systemic adverse effects in both humans and experimental animals. Among these toxins are the group of staphylococcal enterotoxins, the toxic shock syndrome toxin, and the streptococcal erythrogenic (pyrogenic) exotoxins. They are proteins with known amino acid sequence, and most are encoded on plasmids, prophages, or transposons. Functionally, some of these toxins act as superantigens, thereby effectively stimulating the immune system in terms of both activation (as well as acute release of cytokines and lymphokines) and immunosuppression. Acute production of large amounts of cytokines represents one mechanism through which these toxins cause severe systemic symptoms, including hypotension, rashes, and shock. This chapter focuses on the properties of these exotoxins (superantigens) and their interactions with the immune system.

DISEASES CAUSED BY GRAM-POSITIVE COCCI

Staphylococci

The pathogenicity of staphylococci is clearly correlated with their ability to produce coagulase. All coagulase-positive strains are grouped as *Staphylococcus aureus*. Coagulase-negative staphylococci are considered facultatively pathogenic, and they cause opportunistic infections. For example, *S. epidermidis* is frequently associated with infections of intravascular catheters. *S. aureus* is responsible for localized suppurative sequelae, such as cutaneous abscesses, as well as severe systemic infections, such as osteomyelitis, pyelonephritis, pneumonia, endocarditis, and septicemia. A number of toxinoses are caused by *S. aureus* due to synthesis of several exotoxins. Exotoxins are responsible for food poisoning; exfoliatin is responsible for a group of diseases collectively termed *scalded skin syndrome,* and toxic shock syndrome toxin-1 (TSST-1) gives rise to toxic shock, a syndrome characterized by high fever, diarrhea, rashes, and multiorgan failure. Menstruating women who use certain types of tampons have an increased risk for development of this disease, and they represent up to 80% of all patients.

Streptococci

Pathogenic strains of streptococci include *S. pneumonia*, which elicits lobar pneumonia; and the b-hemolytic group A and B streptococci, *S. pyogenes* and *S. agalactiae*. Group A streptococci are responsible for localized infections, such as acute pharyngitis, including its suppurative complications, such as paratonsillar abscesses. Other localized infections are erysipelas and impetigo. *S. pyogenes* causes autoimmune diseases such as rheumatic fever and acute glomerulonephritis. The group B streptococci give rise to neonatal infections with meningitis and septicemia. The rash of scarlet fever is caused by lysogenic strains of group A streptococci producing pyrogenic (erythrogenic) exotoxins.

BACTERIAL PRODUCTS INVOLVED IN PATHOGENICITY

Because *S. aureus* and *S. pyogenes* are the most important pathogenes of staphylococci and streptococci, respectively, the discussion of virulence factors focuses on the products of these bacteria. The virulence factors produced are grouped into locally acting enzymes, which for example cleave extracellular matrix proteins of the host or destroy host cells of infected tissues, and exotoxins, which indirectly but systemically affect the infected host by influencing the immune system.

Staphylococcus aureus

ENZYMES: *S. aureus* is well known to synthesize a variety of exoproteins with different enzymatic activities. Coagulase is, as mentioned, characteristic for all strains of *S. aureus,* and it converts fibrinogen to fibrin by forming a complex with coagulase-reacting factor. It is thought that the layer of fibrin protects invasive *S. aureus* in suppurative lesions. In contrast, staphylokinase has the opposite effect: Clots of fibrin are lysed, thereby promoting local spread of bacteria. It is believed that dissemination of *S. aureus* in tissues is amplified by hyaluronidase cleaving the intercellular matrix. Furthermore, a nuclease with endonuclease and exonuclease activity on DNA and RNA, digesting both molecules from cellular debris, and several lipases are also probably responsible for local spread. Four distinct types (α–δ) of hemolysins are produced by strains of *S. aureus,* and they all cause β-hemolysis. The enzymes differ in their red blood cell (RBC) species specificity and mechanism of action. α-Hemolysin also destroys cell types other than RBCs from different mammalian species by a poreforming mechanism similar to the complement system. Thus, phagocytosis of *S. aureus* is impeded by destruction of phagocytes.

EXOTOXINS: Most of the different exotoxins generated by S. aureus are cloned and sequenced. In contrast to the enzymes mentioned, their activities are not confined to the site of a local infection. Instead, they are responsible for systemic responses of the infected host, such as erythroderma, fever, and toxic shock. There are five major serological types of staphylococcal enterotoxins (referred to as SEA–SEE, Table 24–1). Three subtypes of SEC, designated SEC_1, SEC_2, and SEC_3, have been defined due to minor antigenic variation. Although sequence relationships between all enterotoxins are significant, enterotoxins form two subgroups based on sequence homology. Accordingly, SEA is more closely related to SED and SEE, whereas SEB is more similar to SEC_{1-3}. TSST-1 (Table 24–1), is only distantly related to the enterotoxins. Furthermore, enterotoxins are characterized by a disulfide bridge, which creates a short loop that is absent in TSST-1. As is discussed later, this loop is of functional relevance for exotoxins.

All the toxins addressed thus far are generated by cleavage from a larger precursor molecule; the molecular weight (MW) of the mature form of the enterotoxins is approximately 27 kd and 22 kd for TSST-1. Most are encoded by plasmids, prophages, or transposons. The last group of staphylococcal toxins consists of the exfoliatins A and B (Table 24–1), which are produced by different phage groups of S. aureus. ETB is plasmid-encoded, whereas ETA is chromosomal; their MW is approximately 24 kd. Both toxins cleave the stratum granulosum of the epidermis.

Streptococcus pyogenes

ENZYMES: Two β-hemolysins, streptolysin S and O, are generated by S. pyogenes. Streptolysin S is a small peptide with a MW of 2,800 daltons; serum extracts this hemolysin from streptococcal cells, and it destroys not only RBCs, but also phagocytic leukocytes. In contrast to streptolysin S, streptolysin O (MW, 70 kd) is inactivated by oxygen. Similar to the α-hemolytic toxin of S. aureus, streptolysin O creates pores in the membrane of different cell types by a mechanism analogous to the membrane attack complex of complement. Several enzymes thought to be involved in the local spread of group A streptococci, such as streptokinase, deoxyribonuclease, and hyaluronidase, are produced. Streptokinase activates plasminogen to plasmin, which in turn lyses clots of fibrin around streptococci. The four different serological types of deoxyribonuclease are unable to penetrate the membranes of intact cells, but they cleave free DNA from destroyed phagocytes in purulent lesions. Hyaluronidase dissolves the intercellular matrix, as well as the capsule of streptococci.

TABLE 24 –1 SUPERANTIGENS OF GRAM-POSITIVE ORIGIN

Bacterial Strain	Toxin	Molecular Weight (daltons)	Vβ Orientation (Human)	Vβ Orientation (Mouse)
S. aureus	Enterotoxin A	27,100	Vβ1.1; Vβ5.3; Vβ6.3, 6.4, 6.9; Vβ7.3, 7.4; Vβ9.1	Vβ1, Vβ3, Vβ10, Vβ11, Vβ12, Vβ17
	Enterotoxin B	28,300	Vβ3, Vβ12, Vβ14, Vβ15, Vβ17, Vβ20	Vβ3, Vβ7, Vβ8.1, 8.2, 8.3, Vβ17
	Enterotoxin C1	27,500	Vβ12	Vβ3, Vβ8.2, 8.3, Vβ11, Vβ17
	Enterotoxin C2	27,500	Vβ12, Vβ13.1, Vβ13.2, Vβ14, Vβ15, Vβ17, Vβ20	Vβ3, Vβ8.2, Vβ10, Vβ17
	Enterotoxin C3	27,500	Vβ5, Vβ12	Vβ3; Vβ7; Vβ8.1, 8.2, 8.3; Vβ11, Vβ17
	Enterotoxin D	26,300	Vβ5, Vβ12	Vβ3; Vβ7; Vβ8.1, 8.3; Vβ11, Vβ17
	Enterotoxin E	26,400	Vβ5.1; Vβ6.3, 6.4, 6.9; Vβ8.1; Vβ18	Vβ11, Vβ15, Vβ17
	Toxic shock syndrome toxin 1	22,000	Vβ2	Vβ11, Vβ15, Vβ17
	Exfoliatin toxin	24,000	Vβ2	Vβ10, Vβ11, Vβ15
S. pyogenes	Pyrogenic toxin A	25,700	Vβ2, Vβ12, Vβ14, Vβ15	Vβ3, Vβ8.2, Vβ11
	Pyrogenic toxin B	27,000	Vβ8	?
	Pyrogenic toxin C	24,300	Vβ1, Vβ2, Vβ5.1, Vβ10	?
	M-protein	22,000	Vβ2, Vβ4, Vβ8	?

EXOTOXINS: Three serologically distinct types of streptococcal pyrogenic (erythrogenic) exotoxins (SPE A–C; Table 24–1) are recognized. They are responsible for the rash in scarlet fever, as shown by an erythematous reaction after subcutaneous injection of the toxins (Dick test). Similar to the staphylococcal toxins, they induce fever and amplify the systemic effects of lipopolysaccharides derived from gram-negative bacteria. As with the enterotoxins, the mature form of streptococcal toxins is generated by cleavage from a slightly larger precursor form. The MW for the three distinct types ranges from 24 to 27 kd. Comparison of amino acid sequence homology shows that SPE A is more closely related to the staphylococcal enterotoxins than to SPE B or SPE C. The genes for SPE A and probably for SPE C are located on a phage; conflicting results are reported for the location of the gene for SPE B.

INTERACTIONS OF GRAM-POSITIVE BACTERIA WITH THE IMMUNE SYSTEM

Most of the work examining the interaction of gram-positive bacterial products with the immune system of mam-

mals has been done with exotoxins of *S. aureus* and *S. pyogenes*. In particular, the staphylococcal enterotoxins have been extensively used to determine how the immune system deals with these antigens in vivo, as well as in vitro. However, other molecules, such as streptococcal M-protein, lipoteichoic acid, and α-hemolysin of staphylococci, were also shown to interact with cells of the immune system.

Exotoxins (superantigens)

Staphylococcal as well as streptococcal toxins act in minute concentrations ($<10^{-9}$ mol/L) as powerful stimulators (mitogens) for human and murine lymphocytes, in particular T cells. However, the molecular basis of this activation remained obscure for many years and has unfolded only recently.

INTERACTION WITH MAJOR HISTOCOMPATIBILITY COMPLEX CLASS II–POSITIVE CELLS: The specific binding of exotoxins to class II molecules of the major histocompatibility complex (MHC) was a key finding in attempts to elucidate the mechanism of lymphocyte stimulation by these bacterial exoproteins. It was demonstrated that human T-cell clones were activated by bacterial toxins when MHC class II–positive B-cell lines were present in culture. This response could be blocked by monoclonal antibodies directed against class II molecules. The use of MHC class II–negative cell lines, and their transfection with MHC class II genes provided direct proof that MHC class II structures present exotoxins to T cells. Immunoprecipitation experiments revealed that SEA and SEB bind to human leukocyte antigen-DR (HLA-DR) molecules with high affinity. Similar results have been obtained for the other staphylococcal and streptococcal toxins; SEA has the highest affinity to MHC class II structures. However, the different toxins use distinct binding sites on class II molecules. All three classes of human MHC class II molecules, HLA-DR, HLA-DQ, and HLA-DP, bind exotoxins. Their affinity can be ranked; HLA-DR has the highest affinity, followed by HLA-DQ and HLA-DP. The murine class II structures, H2-IE and H2-IA, have a lower affinity than their human counterparts. H2-IE, which represents the murine homologue to HLA-DR, also displays a higher affinity than H2-IA.

In general, the function of MHC class II molecules is presentation of peptides that are derived from processed soluble, foreign proteins (e.g., bacterial proteins). In addition to other cells, macrophages endocytose such proteins and generate peptides, inside lysosomes, which are composed of 15 to 25 amino acids. Thereafter, the peptides interact with the peptide binding groove of MHC class II molecules inside endosomes, and the entire complex is subsequently transported to the cell surface. In contrast, exotoxins follow an exception to this rule. Exotoxins are not processed, but they bind as whole proteins outside the peptide binding pocket of MHC class II structures. This was shown by point mutations of the peptide binding pocket, which interrupted presentation of peptides, but it did not interfere with binding of the exotoxins.

B cells, monocytes, and dendritic cells express MHC class II molecules on their cell surface, and they therefore interact with bacterial exotoxins. Exotoxin class II molecule complexes cause stimulation of monocytes, which in turn leads to production and secretion of interleukin-1 (IL-1) and tumor necrosis factor (TNF). In comparison to lipopolysaccharides, staphylococcal exotoxins are more potent on a molar basis. Costimulation of B cells with enterotoxins and the protein kinase C activator, phorbol myristate acetate (PMA), results in B-cell proliferation. Furthermore, activation of B cells and monocytes with exotoxins increases their adhesiveness, which is an important prerequisite for cell-to-cell contacts during immune responses.

INTERACTION WITH T CELLS: The second key finding to explain the powerful T-cell stimulatory capacity of exotoxins relates to the discovery that the Vβ chain of the T-cell receptor (TCR) is sufficient to recognize the

toxins. The TCR is a heterodimer that consists of an α- and a β-chain. To build up these chains, developing murine T cells can select from 100 different Vα (variable), 50 Jα (joining), 1 Cα (constant), 20 Vβ, 2 Dβ (diversity), 2 Jβ, and 2 Cβ segments in their genome. Including the mechanism of N-region diversity, this rearrangement process yields up to 10^{10} different TCR molecules; therefore, extremely few T cells express the same TCR. Processed antigens bound to the peptide groove of the MHC molecule are recognized by the α- and β-chain of the TCR; hence, very limited numbers of T cells recognize a given peptide antigen. In contrast, the Vβ-chains of the TCR are sufficient to recognize bacterial exotoxins. Because there are only 20 different murine Vβ segments (approximately twice as much in humans), the number of T cells able to respond to a given exotoxin is extremely high. If all Vβ-defined murine T-cell subsets were of the same size, then 5% of all T cells could react. The high frequency of exotoxin-reactive T cells explains why enterotoxins, exfoliating toxins, and TSST-1 generated by S. aureus, as well as the pryogenic exotoxins produced by S. pyogenes, have been termed superantigens.

T cells of mammals are composed of two major subsets: the CD4+ helper and the CD8+ cytotoxic T-cell subset. CD4+ cells recognize processed peptide antigens presented by self-MHC class II molecules (i.e., they are MHC class II–restricted, whereas CD8+ cells are MHC class I–restricted). As mentioned, superantigens interact only with MHC class II structures. Therefore, it could be expected that only CD4+ T cells expressing an appropriate Vβ-chain of the TCR could respond. However, CD8+ T cells become equally well activated. The conclusion is that the rule of MHC restriction is not valid in the case of exotoxins. Furthermore, T cells of a given individual recognize a peptide antigen only in the context of self-MHC molecules, and they do not respond if the same antigen is presented by an allogeneic MHC molecule. In contrast, superantigens can be presented by allogeneic and even xenogeneic MHC class II structures.

Recognition of superantigens bound to MHC class II–positive cells by appropriate T cells causes rapid cell activation. In mice, subcutaneous injection of the superantigen SEB induces IL-2 receptor expression on all Vβ8+ T cells within the local draining lymph node within 4 hours. In addition, the transferrin receptor, another activation marker of T cells, also becomes up-regulated within the same period. Therefore, 25% of all T cells are triggered, because approximately 25% of all murine T cells use the Vβ8-chain to build up the TCR, and are therefore reactive. As a consequence, cell size of responding superantigen reactive T cells increases, and proliferation starts. Two days after administration of SEB, the Vβ8+ T-cell subset nearly doubled. In vitro data show that of the three types of antigen-presenting cells—B cells, monocytes, and dendritic cells—the latter are 10- to 50-

fold more potent in inducing T-cell activation. In vitro, even femtomolar concentrations of superantigens bound to dendritic cells are able to trigger T-cell responses in a Vβ selective fashion.

The currently favored conclusion is that to activate T cells, superantigens have to form a bridge between T cells and antigen-presenting cells (i.e., they are bifunctional; they interact with the Vβ-chain of the TCR and the superantigen bond to an MHC class II molecule) (Fig. 24–1). Soluble superantigens appear to be unable to bind to the appropriate Vβ-TCR. Studies were undertaken to define amino acid residues of superantigens that participate in these interactions. There is evidence that the disulfide loop of SEA and SEB is an important structure for T-cell activation because cleavage of the disulfide bond abrogates the ability of the toxins to stimulate T cells; however, they are still able to bind to MHC class II molecules. In contrast, TSST-1 lacks this loop, but it is still able to bind to antigen-presenting cells and activate T cells. The interaction sites of SEA and SEE with Vβ3 and Vβ11, respectively, have been mapped. Thus, amino acid residues 214, 220, and 221 of SEA, located at the carboxyl terminal end of the molecule, are critical for binding to Vβ3, and the specificity of SEE binding to Vβ11 is determined by residues 220 and 221. The combination of mutational analysis of SEB and the recently resolved crystal structure of the toxin allowed identification of amino acids impor-

tant for TCR or MHC II interactions. Consequently, a TCR, as well as an MHC II binding site could be located on the three-dimensional structure of the superantigen SEB.

In mice, SEB does not cause expansion of all Vβ8+ T cells. Although all Vβ8+ T cells show signs of activation within 4 hours in terms of IL-2 receptor expression, approximately 50% of Vβ8+ T cells become deleted within the first 24 hours after injection. This deletion is caused by a mechanism termed *apoptotic cell death* (apoptosis), which implies that the genome of the cell is cleaved into large 200-bp fragments by activation of endogenous endonucleases. The surviving subset of Vβ8+ T cells commences to proliferate for the following 1 or 2 days. Thereafter, part of the expanded Vβ8+ T cells becomes numerically reduced below pretreatment levels, again as a result of apoptosis. Superantigen reactive T cells behave in a complex manner. After encountering its ligand in vivo, clonal deletion becomes initiated via an apoptotic process. Part of the cells do not enter the apoptotic pathway, but they initiate clonal expansion until a second wave of apoptosis starts.

LYMPHOKINE PRODUCTION: One of the hallmarks of the interaction of superantigens with cells of the immune system is rapid and massive production of an array of cytokines and lymphokines. As outlined, T cells, as well as B cells, monocytes, and dendritic cells, become stimulated; therefore, all are potential sources of cytokines or lymphokines. In general, T-cell–derived lymphokines, such as IL-2, IL-4, IL-5, interferon-γ (IFN-γ), and TNF-β, as well as macrophage-derived cytokines, such as IL-1, IL-6, and TNF-α (which in fact can be produced by several cell types), are produced in vitro and in vivo.

SECRETION OF LYMPHOKINES IN VITRO: Stimulation of human peripheral mononuclear cells with SEA in vitro results in the production of TNF-α (cachectin), TNF-β (lymphotoxin), and IL-6. TNF-α is already generated after 2 to 3 hours after stimulation; peak levels occur after approximately 6 hours. This cytokine is secreted by T cells and monocytes, yet the majority of TNF-α–producing cells are monocytes. A minor fraction of T cells also secretes TNF-α, but at later time points. Compared with TNF-α, TNF-β is generated later in time, and the responsible cell types were almost exclusively CD4+ T cells, and, only to a minor extent, CD8+ T cells. The kinetic of IL-6 secretion was biphasic; monocytes were responsible for an early peak, followed by a T-cell–derived second peak. The capacity of SEA to induce IL-1 in human monocytes was dependent on the presence of T cells, in particular, the CD4+ T-cell subset. In contrast, stimulation of monocytes with lipopolysaccharide is T-cell–independent, and occurs with a faster kinetic. In both instances, IL-1β is produced. Similar results were obtained with TSST-1. In-

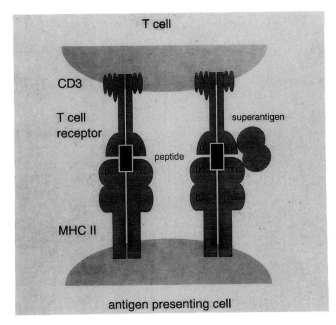

Figure 24–1 Interaction of the T-cell receptor with MHC class II molecules and peptide (left). The peptide is bound to the pocket of the MHC class II molecule formed by the α1 and β1 domains, and both chains of the T-cell receptor recognize the peptide, as well as the MHC class II molecule. Superantigens (right) also bind to MHC class II molecules, but outside the peptide binding groove. Only the β-chain of the T-cell receptor is involved in the recognition of a superantigen.

cubation of highly purified resting human T cells or monocytes with TSST-1 did not result in TNF or IL-1 production. Significant secretion of both cytokines did occur, however, when both cell types were allowed to establish cell-to-cell contacts.

The pattern of lymphokine secretion by T cells after stimulation with superantigens can change. Primary activation of murine CD4+ T lymphocytes with SEB yields high numbers of cells that produce IL-2 and IFN-γ, but it yields low numbers that secrete IL-4, IL-5, and IL-10. Stimulation of the same cells with SEB in the presence of exogenously added IL-4 reduces IFN-γ production, whereas a high fraction of cells produces IL-4 and IL-10. This type of data reflect the presence of two subsets of CD4+ T cells: Th1 (T helper) and Th2 cells, which can be distinguished on the basis of their pattern of lymphokine secretion. Accordingly, Th1 cells preferentially secrete IL-2 and IFN-γ, whereas Th2 cells primarily produce IL-4, IL-5, IL-6, and IL-10.

PRODUCTION OF LYMPHOKINES IN VIVO: Injection of superantigens into mice gives rise to the sequential appearance of several cytokines and lymphokines in the sera of treated animals. In particular, subcutaneous injection of mice with SEB or TSST-1 results in peak levels of TNF as early as 1 hour after treatment. A few hours later, TNF serum levels return to normal values. IL-2 levels peak approximately 2 hours after injection, followed by IL-1 and IL-6 at approximately 4 hours. IFN-γ is the lymphokine with the slowest kinetic; peak values occur at approximately 8 hours (Fig. 24–2). The amounts of cytokines detectable in the sera are amazingly high. Furthermore, the speed of production is surprising because the superantigens are injected subcutaneously into the footpad of mice, but the cytokines and lymphokines measured are serum-borne. This finding means that the whole process of cellular interactions with the superantigen, transcription of cytokine and lymphokine genes, translation of messenger RNA, secretion of the protein, and its systemic spread has to be completed within 1 to 2 hours. The described kinetics of lymphokine induction are very similar to those observed that are provoked by lipopolysaccharides, during which TNF is rapidly produced, followed by IL-1 and IL-6.

TUMOR NECROSIS FACTOR AS A KEY MEDIATOR OF SUPERANTIGEN-INDUCED SHOCK SYMPTOMS: The presence of high amounts of serum-borne cytokines and lymphokines can be fatal. First, rabbits treated with TSST-1 succumb to a shock-like syndrome, and symptoms of significant hemodynamic changes coincide with the presence of TNF-like activity in sera of treated animals. Second, large amounts of recombinant interleukins, such as IL-2, given to cancer patients as an alternative antitumor regimen can elicit se-

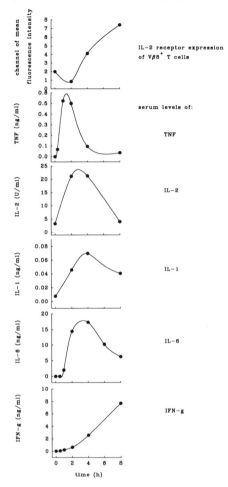

IL-2 receptor expression and kinetics of lymphokine serum levels

Figure 24–2 The kinetic of different cytokine serum levels are depicted after injection of a superantigen (SEB) into mice. The order of appearance is similar to the lipopolysaccharide-provoked cytokine syndrome. The *top panel* illustrates the expression of the IL-2 receptor on Vβ8+ T cells. Cytokines such as TNF and IL-2 are secreted before signs of T-cell activation–like IL-2 receptor expression can be observed.

vere side effects, such as multiorgan dysfunction and cardiovascular failure. In this regard, rodents are more resistant. For example, mice react with weight loss, but they do not present signs of overt disease, even when high doses of superantigens are administered. The intrinsic resistance of mice can be overcome by "sensitizing" the animals. Sensitization can be experimentally achieved by coinjection of D-galactosamine, a substance that interferes with liver cell metabolism. D-galactosamine does not affect the sequelae of the superantigen-provoked cytokine response previously described. Because lethal shock of D-galactosamine–sensitized animals in response to superantigen can be prevented by administration of monoclonal anti-TNF antibodies, TNF may be a key mediator in effecting this syndrome. Furthermore, mutant mice lacking one of the TNF receptors (gp55) exhibit resistance to superantigen-mediated shock. Similar results were obtained when D-galactosamine–sensitized mice were challenged with lipopolysaccharides.

Septic shock induced by gram-negative or gram-positive bacteria therefore differs with regard to the cell type induced to produce lymphokines and cytokines. However, downstream of the producer cells, a similar composition of lymphokines and cytokines may effect similar pathophysiological pathways. Adrenalectomized mice are also sensitive to the lethal effect of superantigens, which points to involvement of glucocorticoids in this shock syndrome. Indeed, high concentrations of glucocorticoids are instantly detectable in the sera of superantigen-treated mice, and blocking glucocorticoid receptors with the drug RU38486, a glucocorticoid and progesterone receptor antagonist, sensitizes mice for the lethal effect of either superantigens or TNF.

The superantigen-induced lethal shock syndrome is triggered via T cells. D-galactosamine–sensitized mice with severe combined immunodeficiency (SCID) who lack T and B cells do not show signs of disease after challenge with superantigens. The absence of symptoms coincides with a lack of TNF in the sera of these animals. However, they are still sensitive to the lethal effects of lipopolysaccharide, and large amounts of serum borne TNF can be measured. Repopulation of SCID mice with T cells restores their sensitivity to superantigens. In addition, the immunosuppressive drug cyclosporin A, which is known to interfere with T-cell activation and therefore lymphokine production, also protects mice from an otherwise lethal challenge with superantigens, and it also prevents the systemic secretion of TNF and IL-2. Compared with lipopolysaccharide-induced shock, the pathophysiology of the superantigen-provoked syndrome is different in that the source of TNF of the former syndrome represents the lipopolysaccharide-activated monocyte, whereas in the latter syndrome, TNF is produced by T cells. Once lymphokine and cytokine production has started, the pathophysiology of both entities appears indistinguishable.

The toxic shock syndrome in humans shares many of the properties just outlined for mice. The disease is mainly caused by the superantigen TSST-1, but it is also caused by some of the staphylococcal exotoxins. In vitro experiments revealed that TSST-1 activates all human T cells expressing the Vβ-2 chain of the TCR, and human leukocytes readily produce an array of cytokines, including TNF, IL-1, and IFN-γ. Furthermore, it has been demonstrated that patients recovering from toxic shock have elevated numbers of Vβ2-expressing T cells, indicating that T cells are involved in the pathogenesis of the disease in humans.

In the pathogenesis of either superantigen- or lipopolysaccharide-induced shock symptoms, TNF displays several functions. First, TNF acts as an endogenous pyrogene, a function shared with IL-1. Second, together with IL-1 and IL-6, the acute-phase response of the liver is triggered, which is thought to enhance nonspecific immunity by increased synthesis of "protective" proteins by hepatocytes, including C-reactive protein, α_2-macroglobulin, fibrinogen, and amyloid A. Third, blood coagulation is activated, resulting in intravascular thrombosis and reduced tissue perfusion. Fourth, TNF reduces the systemic blood pressure. Superantigens are known to activate monocytes and endothelial cells to produce nitric oxide, a potent vasodilator and regulator of systemic blood pressure. Because T-cell–derived TNF, together with IL-1 and IFN-γ, efficiently activate the inducible isoform of the nitric oxide synthetase in macrophages and endothelial cells, the links connecting superantigens with nitric oxide production have been gradually understood.

M-protein

M-proteins are almost unique products of group A streptococci, and they allow further differentiation of this subgroup into more than 80 different serological subtypes. The M-proteins appear to be anchored in the cell membrane, where they traverse the cell wall and give rise to fimbriae protruding from the bacteria. M-proteins are virulence factors that are antiphagocytic. This condition can be shown by treatment of group A streptococci with trypsin, which does not influence the viability of the cells and almost completely removes M-proteins from the cell wall. Trypsin-treated bacteria are easily phagocytosed. Anti-M-protein antibodies are protective, and some seem to be crossreactive to human heart tissues (i.e., myosin). Further research is needed to clearly establish whether this finding relates to the fact that rheumatic fever is provoked by group A streptococci.

M-proteins were recently identified to act as superantigens. Accordingly, a 22-kd fragment of M-type 5 protein preferentially activates human Vβ2+, Vβ4+, and Vβ8+ T cells when presented by MHC class II–positive cells. Thus far, this group of proteins represents a unique superantigen, because they are structural bacterial proteins and not secreted toxins. M-protein–reactive T cells respond with proliferation and IL-2 secretion. Superantigenic properties of M-proteins may lead to activation of potentially autoreactive T cells, which in turn are responsible for autoimmune diseases such as rheumatic fever.

Lipoteichoic acid

The fimbriae of group A streptococci are formed by lipoteichoic acid complexed with M-proteins. Purified lipoteichoic acid isolated from several enterococcal species were able to induce synthesis of IL-1, IL-6, and TNF by human cultured monocytes; lipoteichoic acids from *S. aureus* and *S. pneumoniae* failed to do so.

Infusion of heat-killed *S. epidermidis* into rabbits results in complement activation, elevated serum levels of IL-1β and TNF, hypotension, and multiorgan dysfunction. Culture of blood mononuclear cells with lipoteichoic acid derived from *S. epidermidis* induced production of TNF and IL-1, although the amount induced was 100-fold less than the quantity elicited by lipopolysaccharide. These findings suggest that lipoteichoic acids derived from certain gram-positive bacteria may have a role in vivo similar to that of lipopolysaccharides from gram-negative bacteria.

Staphylococcal α- and β-hemolysin

Staphylococcal α-hemolysin (α-toxin) destroys human platelets and monocytes, in addition to RBCs. Culture of human monocytes with cytotoxic concentrations of these toxins causes the release of large amounts of IL-1. Furthermore, subcytolytic doses result in the release of TNF-α by monocytes. Intravenous injections of α-toxin in monkeys provoke a shock-like syndrome, with cardiovascular collapse and pulmonary edema. These symptoms were paralleled by a decrease in the number of blood platelets. The animals were protected by prior administration of anti-α-toxin hyperimmune globulins, which also abrogated the cytokine release of monocytes cultured in vitro.

Large quantities of β-hemolysin produced by *S. aureus* are also toxic to experimental animals. β-Hemolysin, with a MW of 30 kd, functions as sphingomyelinase C that cleaves sphingomyelin into *N*-acylsphingosine and phosphorylcholine. RBCs of several species, as well as different tissue cells, are lysed dependent on their sphingomyelin content. The mechanism of action of this toxin is interesting because the intracellular signal transduction pathway of TNF-α also involves sphingomyelinase C. Interaction of TNF-α with the smaller TNF receptor, TR55, expressed on the surface of a variety of mammalian cells results in production of *N*-acylsphingosine, which causes activation of the nuclear transcription factor, NF-κB. Because the enzymatic activity of β-hemolysin is similar, the toxin could potentially mimic the intracellular effects of TNF-α.

SUMMARY

Pathogenic gram-positive bacteria, such as *S. aureus* and *S. pyogenes,* contain numerous virulence factors. Among these factors are the more locally acting group of enzymes, such as hyaluronidases and DNAses, which probably act as spreading factors. Virulence factors with systemic importance represent the well-defined group of bacterial superantigens that elicit many responses in vivo caused by infusions of complete bacteria.

This chapter focused on recent findings relating to the influence of virulence factors acting as superantigens, with emphasis on two in vivo phenomenons: lymphokine-cytokine release syndrome and subsequent shock syndrome. Although several conclusions can be drawn from in vitro experiments and experimental animal studies, the transition to human pathophysiology is still speculative, at least in part. However, without doubt, Vβ-selective activation of peripheral T cells by bacterial superantigens occurs in humans, including subsequent acute lymphokine and cytokine release. Definition of the clinical manifestation of a potential lymphokine/cytokine syndrome needs attention. In particular, the potential additive and synergistic effects of lymphokines and cytokines in channeling and targeting peripheral target cells, thereby causing shock symptoms, need to be evaluated.

TCR-Vβ–selective hyperactivation of a large segment of peripheral T cells is believed to have negative consequences on the ability of the immune system to mount antigen (peptide)-specific MHC-restricted T-cell responses. Perhaps the empirical clinical finding of an association of septicemia and shock with immunosuppression will provide an explanation as a result of the systemic effects of immunosuppressive lymphokines released. Candidates could be IL-10 or transforming growth factor-β. Research on the interplay between immune response and bacterial virulence factors, such as superantigens, will help us understand how the immune system performs against "viable bacterial antigens" and faces at the same time the functional consequences triggered by bacterial superantigens.

REFERENCES

1. Beutler B, Milsark IW, Cerami AC. Passive immunization against cachectin/tumor necrosis factor protects mice from lethal effect of endotoxin. Science 1985;22:869–871.

2. Freudenberg MA, Keppler D, Galanos C. Requirement for lipopolysaccharide-responsive macrophages in galactosamine-induced sensitization to endotoxin. Infect Immun 1986;51:891–895.

3. Fleischer B, Schrezenmeier H. T cell stimulation by staphylococcal enterotoxins. Clonally variable response and requirement for major histocompatibility complex class II molecules on accessory or target cells. J Exp Med 1988;167:1697–1707.

4. Jupin C, Anderson S, Damais C, Alouf JE, Parant M. Toxic shock syndrome toxin 1 as an inducer of human tumor necrosis factors and gamma interferon. J Exp Med 1988;167:752–761.

5. Janeway CA Jr, Yagi J, Conrad PJ, et al. T-cell responses to

Mls and to bacterial proteins that mimic its behavior. Immunol Rev 1989;107:61–88.

6. White J, Herman A, Pullen AM, Kubo R, Kappler JW, Marrack P. The V beta-specific superantigen staphylococcal enterotoxin B: stimulation of mature T cells and clonal deletion in neonatal mice. Cell 1989;56:27–35.

7. Fast DJ, Schlievert PM, Nelson RD. Toxic shock syndrome-associated staphylococcal and streptococcal pyrogenic toxins are potent inducers of tumor necrosis factor production. Infect Immun 1989;57:291–294.

8. Marrack P, Kappler J. The staphylococcal enterotoxins and their relatives. *Science* 1990;248:705–711.

9. Marrack P, Blackman M, Kushnir E, Kappler J. The toxicity of staphylococcal enterotoxin B in mice is mediated by T cells. J Exp Med 1990;171:455–464.

10. Galanos C, Freudenberg MA, Reutter W. Galactosmine-induced sensitization of the lethal effects of endotoxin. Proc Natl Acad Sci USA 1979;76:5939–5942.

11. Beutler B, Cerami A. The biology of cachectin/TNF—a primary mediator of the host response. Annu Rev Immunol 1989;7:625–655.

12. Waage A, Espevik T. Interleukin 1 potentiates the lethal effect of tumor necrosis factor alpha/cachectin in mice. J Exp Med 1988;167:1987–1992.

13. Paul NL, Ruddle NH. Lymphotoxin. Annu Rev Immunol 1988;6:407–438.

14. Mollick, JA, Cook RG, Rich RR. Class II MHC molecules are specific receptors for staphylococcus enterotoxin A. Science 1989;244:817–820.

15. Choi Y, Lafferty JA, Clements JR, et al. Selective expansion of T cells expressing V beta 2 in toxic shock syndrome. J Exp Med 1990;172:981–984.

16. Kawabe Y, Ochi A. Programmed cell death and extrathymic reduction of Vbeta8+ CD4+ T cells in mice tolerant to Staphylococcus aureus enterotoxin B. Nature 1991;349:245–248.

17. Miethke T, Wahl C, Echtenacher B, Krammer P, Heeg K, Wagner H. T cell mediated lethal shock triggered in mice by the superantigen staphylococcal enterotoxin B: Critical role of tumor necrosis factor. J Exp Med 1992;175:91–98.

18. Grossman D, Cook RG, Sparrow JT, Mollick JA, Rich RR. Dissociation of the stimulatory activities of staphylococcal enterotoxins for T cells and monocytes. J Exp Med 1990;172:1831–1841.

19. Herman A, Croteau G, Sekaly RP, Kappler J, Marrack P. HLA-DR alleles differ in their ability to present staphylococcal enterotoxins to T cells. J Exp Med 1990;172:709–717.

20. Fraser JD. High-affinity binding of staphylococcal enterotoxins A and B to HLA-DR. Nature 1989;339:221–223.

21. Bhardwaj N, Friedman SM, Cole BC, Nisanian AJ. Dendritic cells are potent antigen-presenting cells for microbial superantigens. J Exp Med 1992;175:267–273.

22. Herman A, Kappler JW, Marrack P, Pullen AM. Superantigens: mechanism of T-cell stimulation and role in immune responses. Annu Rev Immunol 1991;9:745–772.

23. Dellabona P, Peccoud J, Kappler J, Marrack P, Benoist C, Mathis D. Superantigens interact with MHC class II molecules outside of the antigen groove. Cell 1990;62:1115–1121.

CHAPTER 25

ROLE OF CYTOKINES IN SEPTIC SHOCK AND SHOCK-RELATED SYNDROMES

Walton Montegut, Stephen F. Lowry, and Lyle L. Moldawer

Septic shock is the result of severe infection, and it has been estimated to occur in more than 100,000 persons/year nationwide (1). There has been a progressive increase in its incidence, and mortality remains approximately 15 to 40% despite improvements in supportive care (2). Infection is the most frequently recognized cause of morbidity in postoperative patients, and when severe enough, it results in multiple organ system failure (MOSF) (3). The mortality rate of septic shock associated with MOSF is even higher; it exceeds 80% in nearly every reported series (4). Despite significant advances in antimicrobial therapy as well as pulmonary and renal supportive care, a greater understanding of the basic underlying processes that initiate and perpetuate the septic state have only recently begun to be resolved.

Bacterial, viral, and parasitic infections initiate a series of immunological, metabolic, and hemodynamic responses in the host that can only be attributed in part to the classic endocrine hormones such as catecholamines and glucocorticoids. Over the past 10 years, it has been recognized that an additional class of endogenous host mediators, termed *cytokines,* contribute significantly to the pathophysiology of sepsis and to septic shock. Studies have shown that these mediators are responsible for the development of progressive septic complications even after the infected focus has been appropriately treated. Once induced, these proteins are produced by diverse cell types within the local infection, as well as at sites remote from the infection. Cytokines are ca-

pable of mediating a wide range of biological effects, the vast majority of which are beneficial to the host. These effects include stimulation of antimicrobial function, timely healing of wounds, myelostimulation, and mobilization of substrate stores for cell function. This inflammatory cascade is designed to protect the host. However, some of these mediators are capable of inducing adverse effects in the host, and the cascade of humoral and cellular mediators may become temporarily independent of the underlying infection. Current research has demonstrated the role these cytokines have in the inflammatory cascade. We focus on the properties of two pleiotropic cytokines, tumor necrosis factor-α (TNF-α) and interleukin-1 (IL-1), and their roles in sepsis. In addition, the interaction of these proinflammatory cytokines and their naturally produced inhibitors is discussed. Recent studies suggest that the balance between the proinflammatory cytokines and their naturally occurring inhibitors is the prime determinant of cellular responses.

TUMOR NECROSIS FACTOR

TNF-α was first reported in 1975 as a protein that could cause in vivo regression of a murine tumor. Subsequent studies in the 1980s further identified this protein with the development of tissue wasting in cachectic states. It is now known that this 17-kd polypeptide is capable of inducing shock and tissue injury.

TNF-α was first purified and characterized by Aggarwal and colleagues (5). It was initially identified as a polypeptide hormone with a molecular weight of 17 kd, and it is now known to contain 157 amino acids (6). The mature protein contains one intrachair disulfide bond, and it exists predominantly as a trimer in solution (5). It is secreted by a variety of myeloid cells, such as monocytes, lymphocytes, Kupffer cells (7), and peritoneal macrophages (8). Mast cells, endothelial cells, and natural killer cells also synthesize TNF-α. Expression of TNF-α is tightly controlled on a transcriptional as well as a translational level (9). Unstimulated monocytes express low levels of TNF-α messenger RNA (mRNA), and stimulation causes both increased translation and transcription of the mature protein within minutes (9).

Numerous infections and inflammatory stimuli elicit TNF-α synthesis, including bacterial cell wall–derived lipopolysaccharide (LPS), bacterial exotoxins, protozoans, fungi, and viral particles (10). Bacterial infections in rats, rabbits, and baboons cause increased circulating TNF-α levels within minutes, which reach a peak within 90 to 120 minutes (11,12). After a single stimulus, these levels then return to below detectable levels within 4 hours. Further studies demonstrated that bolus infusions of endotoxin in animals and humans induced a similar monophasic peak 1.5 hours after infusion (13).

Despite a frequent ability to detect TNF-α in the circulation of patients or experimental animals following endotoxemia, TNF-α has only been episodically detected in the serum of patients in various disease states (14). It was first identified in patients with parasitic infections, visceral *Leishmaniasis,* and malaria; to this day, the greatest frequency of detecting TNF-α in the circulation has been from patients with parasitic infections (15). Later, TNF-α was identified in meningococcal infection, both in children and adults, and circulating levels greater than 100 pg/mL are associated with increased mortality (16). Furthermore, it has been detected in thermal injury (17), renal allograft rejection (18), and fulminant hepatic failure, although the frequency of detection is often less than 50% (19). Marano and coworkers (20) found that burn patients with sepsis had a higher proportion of detectable circulating TNF than noninfected patients. TNF-α was detectable in only 49% of samples from patients with burn sepsis; 60% of all patients with burn sepsis have TNF-α detectable on one occasion (20). De Groote and associates (21) found that only 29% of patients with documented gram-negative bacteremia had detectable TNF-α. In nearly all studies, there is a positive correlation between circulating TNF-α and mortality. Infection does induce circulating TNF-α, and the frequency of detection is related to severity of the infection (22).

Recently, a greater understanding of the episodic appearance of TNF-α in the circulation has evolved. Not only is TNF-α biosynthesis tightly regulated at the level of gene transcription and translation, but also there is plasma release of natural TNF inhibitors during inflammation. Van Zee and colleagues (23) reported that following endotoxemia, the soluble extracellular chains of the type I (p55) and type II (p75) receptors are shed, and they are capable of inhibiting TNF bioactivity. Critically ill patients also had elevated levels of these proteins. In subsequent in vitro studies, Van Zee and colleagues demonstrated that the levels of p55 and p75 (1–20 ng/mL) were adequate to block the detection of TNF-α in approximately 40% of critically ill patients.

Experimental studies further demonstrated a causal relationship between TNF-α and sepsis. Beutler and associates (24) elicited circulating TNF-α levels in rabbits within 15 minutes of a sublethal intravenous dose of an endotoxin. Levels peaked within 2 hours, and they decreased to baseline within 5 hours. Hesse and coworkers (12) demonstrated the same findings in humans. Administration of endotoxin to humans resulted in detectable TNF-α levels within 30 minutes and peak levels at 1.5 hours after infusion, and these responses occurred temporarily with the appearance of symptoms. These findings have also been confirmed by several groups in humans (13,25), rabbits (26), and rats (27).

More specific effects of TNF were identified following administration of recombinant TNF. High doses of TNF-α in animals can precipitate a syndrome similar to that seen in human septic shock. Acute infusion of high doses of TNF-α in rats results in dose-related hypotension, lactic acidosis, and death (28). Pathological findings were consistent with those found in septic shock (i.e., adrenal necrosis, pulmonary congestion, and intestinal necrosis). Similar findings were produced in canines receiving high-dose infusion of TNF (29). Furthermore, administration of TNF to humans elicits similar metabolic and hemodynamic sequelae, including an increase in glucose and free fatty acid turnover, forearm amino acid efflux, and energy expenditure (30–32). Also, TNF-stimulated expression of a cell surface tissue factor initiates coagulation via generation of thrombin (33). These responses lead to a decrease of activated protein C, thereby increasing the local propensity toward clotting. This finding suggests that TNF may be involved in the disseminated intravascular coagulation seen in sepsis.

Additional evidence for TNF as a mediator of sepsis is obtained from the results of studies in which a blockade of TNF-α was used during bacterial and LPS infusion. Prophylactic administration of a polyclonal rabbit antimouse TNF-α antiserum protected mice from the lethal effects of endotoxins (24). Tracey and associates (34) also demonstrated protection from lethal *Escherichia coli* infusions in nonhuman primates with a monoclonal murine antihuman TNF antibody (34). Treated animals survived for 48 hours, whereas the control animals did not. Also, anti-TNF antibodies attenuated the metabolic consequences of severe bacteremia, such as leukopenia and stress hormone release. Furthermore, the appearance of other cytokines normally seen in sepsis (i.e., IL-1β and IL-6) was blunted (35). These results clearly identified the proximal role of TNF in the inflammatory cascade of sepsis.

Although exaggerated TNF-α production has the capacity to elicit deleterious responses in the host, TNF-α also possesses significant beneficial properties, including the capacity to elicit an endogenous antiviral and antibacterial response. It serves as an endogenous pyrogen with immunostimulatory activity (36). This cytokine promotes the release of neutrophils from the bone marrow, as well as enhanced neutrophil function. It initiates neutrophil margination, transendothelial passage (37), and activation (38), including degranulation, production of superoxide radicals, and release of lysozymes (39), which enhance antibody-dependent cellular cytotoxic and neutrophil-mediated inhibition of functional growth (40). Furthermore, it promotes differentiation of myelogenous cells to monocytes and macrophages, as well as activation of these cells (41). TNF-α also participates in inhibition of intracellular replication of viral and parasitic organisms (42).

INTERLEUKIN-1

IL-1 is another proinflammatory cytokine identified in the inflammatory cascade that contributes to the septic response. This cytokine, which is predominantly synthesized by monocytes and tissue macrophages, is actually a family of at least two distinct proteins, IL-1α and IL-1β. Although the two proteins only share approximately 30% amino acid homology, both species bind to the same surface receptors and produce similar biological responses (43). IL-1 is known under other names, including osteoclast-activating factor, B-cell stimulatory factory, hemopoietin-1, and catabolin (43).

Similar to TNF-α, IL-1 has been shown to be a pluripotent mediator in the pathogenesis of infection, tissue injury, and sepsis. TNF-α induces IL-1 biosynthesis and release from endothelial cells and human monocytes (44). Although IL-1 does not appear capable of inducing irreversible tissue damage on its own, it potentiates many of the biological effects of TNF-α, and administration of IL-1 in vivo induces a reversible shock-like state (45). This state has been demonstrated in both rodent and *Papio*. In the baboon, IL-1 administration induced tachycardia and hypotension (46). Furthermore, IL-6 and IL-8 production was induced during IL-1 administration (47),

and there was also increased production of lactic acid (46). Additional evidence in humans has shown that IL-1 produces neutrophilia, as seen in sepsis (48).

Although these findings do not clearly isolate the role of IL-1 in sepsis, the contribution of exaggerated IL-1 production to the pathway of septic shock was defined in baboons using a receptor antagonist to IL-1 receptors. Fischer and colleagues (49) demonstrated improved survival in nonhuman primates with IL-1 blockade during septic shock due to *E. coli*. By blocking the specific IL-1 cell receptors, there was a clinical improvement in septic parameters. There was less hypotension, less tachycardia, and the animals were more stable clinically. This study further documented the contribution of IL-1 to the clinical symptoms associated with sepsis independent of TNF. Similar results have been obtained by Alexander and coworkers (50) in rats. Despite the independent actions, there is synergistic enhancement of tissue injury between IL-1 and TNF-α. These synergistic mechanisms remain incompletely understood, but they seem to be very important in the induction of septic shock.

CYTOKINE BALANCE AND THE SEPTIC RESPONSE

It has only been recently recognized that the integrated cytokine response to infection and injury is complex, and that, ultimately, tissue responses depend not only on absolute concentrations of TNF-α and IL-1, but also on simultaneous presence of naturally occurring cytokine inhibitors, anti-inflammatory cytokines, and the number of cellular receptors. A pivotal advance in the past 2 years has been discovery and identification of at least two new classes of specific TNF and IL-1 inhibitors that prevent ligand binding to their respective receptors. These include IL-1 receptor antagonist (IL-1Ra), the soluble type II receptor for IL-1 (p68), and the two soluble receptors for TNF (p55 and p75). There has been, however, only a modest exploration into the role that these inhibitors have in modulating the host response to lethal and nonlethal inflammation.

Historically, we used a model of mild endotoxin administration in human volunteers to evaluate the proinflammatory cytokine response. This endotoxin administration results in the release of TNF and IL-1, fever, granulocytosis, tachycardia, and a mild transient hypotension. A schema for this integrated cytokine response encompasses early synthesis and release of TNF and IL-1. This early release of proinflammatory cytokines into the local tissue milieu initiates and orchestrates many of the beneficial responses aimed at improving antimicrobial function and reducing tissue damage. For example, local production of IL-1 and TNF in the liver induces hepatocyte and Kupffer cell IL-6 production, which in combination with IL-1 and TNF-α, reprioritize hepatic metabolism to increase acute-phase protein synthesis and gluconeogenesis (51–53). At the site of tissue injury, local production of these proinflammatory cytokines provokes the release of additional mediators that recruit and activate inflammatory cells via up-regulation of leukocyte and endothelial cell adhesion molecules (54). This process also stimulates fibroblast proliferation (55) and increases local antimicrobial properties (56). In the spleen, locally produced IL-1 can serve as a comitogen (57) and an immune adjuvant, it can increase IL-2 receptor affinity and number, and it can increase macrophage bactericidal function (58,59). In bone marrow, both IL-1 and TNF-α can stimulate the synthesis of other hematopoietic regulators (60,61), promote the release of granulocytes (58), and redirect hematopoietic development along myeloid rather than erythroid pathways (62,63). These early responses mediated by IL-1 and TNF activate host nonspecific immunity and can be considered advantageous to recovering hosts.

However, this initial release of proinflammatory cytokines is ultimately short-lived. For example, following mild endotoxemia in human volunteers, plasma IL-1β and TNF-α levels peak within 4 hours (13,22,64,65). As is discussed, IL-1 activity is mitigated by synthesis and release of IL-1Ra, which interferes with IL-1 binding to its cellular receptors (66). In addition, there is evidence to suggest that shedding of the IL-1 type II receptor (p68) may also occur, and that it prevents IL-1 binding to its cellular receptors.

There is ample evidence that the actions of another proinflammatory cytokine, TNF-α, is also regulated by shedding of the extracellular domains of its cellular receptors. Following a mild endotoxemia, soluble TNF-R I and II concentrations peak 1 to 2 hours after TNF-α administration, and they remain elevated for longer periods (67,68). Recent evocative studies by Porteau and Nathan (69) suggest that release of the TNF-R I (p55) from neutrophils is an active process that does not necessarily involve generation of cellular receptors. The extracellular region of the type I TNF receptor is not only shed from the cell membrane during neutrophil activation (70), but it is also released from neutrophil granules during degranulation. This latter mechanism represents a unique and specific process, independent of ligand binding, by which a specific TNF inhibitor is released during inflammation and neutrophil activation. In the case of TNF, loss of cellular receptors from target tissues serves two purposes: transient desensitization of cells to repeated exposure to TNF-α (71), and formation of receptor-ligand complexes that attenuate peak free TNF-α concentrations and may act as a reservoir to deliver low levels of cytokine over extended periods (72).

A second mechanism by which the host regulates proinflammatory cytokine production and activity is subsequent release of mediators that suppress IL-1 and TNF-α production and increase IL-1Ra release. For example, increased production of prostanoids and the counter-regulatory endocrine response (e.g., cortisol, corticotropin-releasing factor, and α-melanocyte-stimulating hormone) down-regulate IL-1 and TNF-α production and activity (73–75). More recent evidence established that synthesis and release of the anti-inflammatory cytokines (i.e., IL-4, IL-10, and IL-13) also limit the release and effectiveness of earlier proinflammatory cytokine production (76–80). IL-4, IL-10, and IL-13 can down-regulate proinflammatory cytokine release in an autocrine fashion (81–85). In addition, IL-4 and IL-10 can also up-regulate synthesis and release of IL-1Ra, and IL-4 decreases the number of LPS receptors (CD14) on macrophages (81,82).

The net response to an acute nonlethal inflammatory stimulus, when viewed in this integrated manner, is initial release of proinflammatory cytokines, including IL-1 and TNF, that are meant to initiate and integrate the early inflammatory response. This release is followed by release of cytokine inhibitors (IL-1Ra, sIL-1R, and sTNF-R) and anti-inflammatory cytokines (IL-4 and IL-10) that restrict the magnitude and duration of the inflammatory response.

The catastrophic host responses to overwhelming bacterial infections and propagation of the systemic inflammatory response syndrome with multisystem organ dysfunction in ongoing inflammatory processes represent dysregulation of this normal homeostatic process. For example, in acute septic shock due to gram-negative bacteremia or endotoxemia, the magnitude of proinflammatory cytokine response (TNF-α and IL-1) is excessive. The quantities of TNF-α and IL-1 produced are greater than can be mitigated by the release of IL-1Ra- and TNF-soluble receptors. Furthermore, the timing of the release of these cytokine inhibitors is sufficiently delayed in septic shock so that excess proinflammatory cytokines are produced in the reticuloendothelial system. They are also produced in the blood by circulating monocytes and vascular endothelial cells, where their effects on endothelial cells lead to hemodynamic collapse (83).

Similarly, in ongoing inflammatory processes—such as those that occur in hospitalized patients with systemic inflammatory response syndrome (SIRS) or sepsis syndrome or patients with compartmentalized inflammation, such as in rheumatoid arthritis—the mechanisms that ultimately down-regulate proinflammatory cytokine release are ineffective. Under these conditions, chronic production of IL-1β as well as TNF-α, which synergize in their action, may contribute to the progressive synovial damage that occurs. This continued IL-1β production is due in part to the continued external stimuli that the autoimmune process of rheumatoid arthritis invokes. In such cases, repeated or persistent proinflammatory cytokine synthesis (TNF-α, IL-1) contributes to the prostanoid and protease production that occurs. In both septic shock and SIRS, the beneficial aspects of proinflammatory cytokine production (including stimulation of nonspecific host immunity, increased antigen-specific T-cell proliferation, macrophage and natural killer cell bactericidal capacity) are offset by the adverse consequences of continued exposure to elevated TNF-α and IL-1 concentrations.

DETECTION OF IL-1 RECEPTOR ANTAGONIST

The observation that specific inhibitors of IL-1 activity circulate in the blood of infected patients and are excreted in the urine has been known for several years (84,85). Indeed, Spinas and colleagues (86) reported that plasma IL-1 inhibitory activity peaked 4 hours following an endotoxin challenge, and then declined thereafter. Arend and colleagues (66) first identified this inhibitor, and subsequently, Eisenberg and associates (87,88) cloned the gene and revealed that the protein was a member of the IL-1 family but had no agonist properties. IL-1Ra has the distinction of being the only cytokine whose sole known function is to inhibit the actions of another cytokine. Interestingly, the precursor protein of monocyte-derived IL-1Ra contains a signal sequence, and, unlike IL-1α and IL-1β, IL-1Ra is readily secreted (89). An intracellular form of IL-1Ra, the product of alternate mRNA splicing, has also been recently reported in epithelial cells (90). Tissue distribution of IL-1Ra is widespread (19), and IL-1Ra has been recovered in the plasma of critically ill patients and volunteers following endotoxin infusions (92,93). In addition, IL-1Ra mRNA is up-regulated in alveolar macrophages following endotoxin stimulation (94), increased in a variety of tissues following in vivo endotoxin administration (91), and detected in synovial cells of rodents with experimental arthritis (95). Granowitz and colleagues (92) first reported the appearance of IL-1Ra in the blood of human volunteers following experimental endotoxemia, and we have evaluated the appearance of IL-1Ra in the circulation of critically ill patients, volunteers after endotoxemia, and baboons with lethal bacteremia, sublethal endotoxemia, or following IL-1α administration (93).

The data obtained to date confirm that with nonlethal acute inflammatory stimuli, the quantities of IL-1Ra in the systemic circulation are at least 100 times greater than the quantities of IL-1β (or IL-1α); extrapolating from in vitro studies, these quantities appear adequate to block systemic IL-1 actions. However, IL-1 concentrations are significantly higher in the local tissue microenvironment where IL-1 is produced, and they are presumably present in sufficient quantities to initiate local inflammatory responses. Few studies have evaluated tissue concentrations of IL-1Ra. Therefore, the balance between local IL-1 and IL-1Ra concentrations, which ultimately determines net IL-1 activity in tissues, has not been defined.

However, in acute lethal bacterial infections in primates, during which IL-1 production is exaggerated, plasma IL-1Ra concentrations are generally only five- to 10-fold greater than concentrations of IL-1β, and these levels are inadequate to block the systemic (vascular) effects of exaggerated IL-1 production (93). Plasma IL-1Ra concentrations increase significantly with modest sublethal inflammatory stimuli, but levels do not increase further in lethal infections. Similarly, IL-1Ra concentrations are not higher in septic patients that die versus those that survive (93). In contrast, plasma IL-1β concentrations are considerably higher in baboons who die as a result of gram-negative septic shock than in those who survive as a result of nonlethal endotoxemia (94). Waage and associates (95) reported that among patients with meningococcal shock, IL-1 levels were markedly higher in those patients who died. Although the quantities of IL-1Ra are still absolutely greater than the quantities of IL-1β in the circulation, Granowitz and coworkers (96) and McIntyre and associates (97) observed that only 1 to 5% of IL-1 receptor occupancy is required to elicit a maximal IL-1 response, and the affinity of IL-1Ra and IL-1β for their receptors is comparable (88,96). Thus, at least 20- to 100-fold molar excesses of IL-1Ra are required to block the actions of IL-1, and our own in vivo studies suggest that a 1,000-molar excess is required to completely prevent systemic IL-1 responses (97). Circulating IL-1Ra during mild inflammatory stress may thus serve to reduce the systemic responses to localized IL-1 production when plasma appearance of IL-1β is minimal. However, during septic shock, the homeostatic mechanisms in place to offset the pathological sequelae of exaggerated IL-1 production are insufficient to decrease morbidity.

CLINICAL STUDIES WITH ANTI-TNF AND ANTI-IL-1 THERAPIES

Use of monoclonal antibodies and novel soluble TNF receptor–human immunoglobulin G, chimeric fusion proteins to treat patients with sepsis syndrome, are currently under investigation by several pharmaceutical companies. Results to date have shown the monoclonal antibodies to be safe and well tolerated, and they circulate in the plasma with a relatively long half-life (50–54 hr) (98). In a recent report, Fisher and colleagues (99) noted that

TNF antibody was well tolerated in patients despite the development of antimurine antibodies. However, no survival benefit was found for the total study population, but patients with detectable TNF concentrations at study entry appeared to benefit by high dose anti-TNF antibody treatment. These findings suggest that such therapies may have clinical utility in patients in whom evidence of exaggerated TNF production exists.

Recently, results of a Phase II trial of IL-1Ra in patients with sepsis syndrome were reported (100). In an open-label study of 99 patients with sepsis syndrome, IL-1Ra (2.0 mg/kg BW/hr for 72 hr) reduced 28-day, all-cause mortality from 44 to 16%. Preliminary results from a recently completed Phase III, multicenter, randomized, double-blind study, however, could not confirm these initial findings when all patients with sepsis syndrome were included (101). However, in a subgroup of patients with end-organ dysfunction or a predicted risk of mortality greater than 24% (using the APACHE III score), mortality was significantly reduced by IL-1Ra treatment. Clinical trials with IL-1Ra continue in an effort to identify prospectively the optimal patient populations that will benefit from such therapies.

SUMMARY

TNF-α and IL-1 are pleiotropic cytokines involved in both beneficial and adverse responses to acute and chronic inflammation. Not only is the production of TNF-α and IL-1 tightly regulated during inflammation, but also the actions of TNF-α and IL-1 on target tissues are limited by synthesis and release of IL-1Ra, shedding of the IL-1 and TNF receptors, and the numbers of cellular receptors on end tissues. Down-regulation of TNF and IL-1 action is achieved by release of IL-1Ra and the extracellular domain of the IL-1R (p68) or TNF-R (p55 and P75), which compete with cellular receptors for ligand binding. In pathological conditions (e.g., septic shock), excessive production of TNF-α and IL-1 exceeds the capacity of IL-1Ra and shed TNF and IL-1 to block proinflammatory cytokine actions, particularly at the vascular endothelium. Such pathological changes are as much a result of dysregulation between proinflammatory cytokine production and their naturally occurring inhibitors or antagonists as they are a result of excessive production of the mediators themselves. Therapeutic efforts aimed at reducing IL-1–mediated pathology can be aimed both at suppressing the exaggerated production of TNF and IL-1, and at enhancing inhibitor (IL-1Ra, sTNF-R, and sIL-1R) production.

Supported in part by GM-40586, awarded by the National Institute of General Medical Sciences, USPHS.

REFERENCES

1. Bone RC, Fisher CJ, Clemmer TP, et al. A controlled chemical trial of high-dose methylprednisolone in the treatment of severe sepsis and septic shock. N Engl J Med 1987; 317:653–658.

2. Cohn IJ, Burnside GH. In: Schwartz S, Shires G, Spencer F, eds. Infections. (Principles of Surgery, vol 1). New York: McGraw Hill, 1989:1233.

3. Pruitt BAJ. Opportunistic infections in the severely injured patient. In: Gruber D, Walker RI, MacVittie TJ, eds. The pathophysiology of combined injury and trauma. New York: Academic Press, 1987.

4. Gleckman R, Esposito A. Gram-negative bacteremic shock: Pathophysiology, clinical features, and treatment. South Med J 1981;74:335–341.

5. Aggarwal BB, Kohr WJ, Hass PE, et al. Human tumor necrosis factor: production, purification and characterization. J Biol Chem 1985;260:2345–2354.

6. Beutler B, Cerami A. Cachectin: more than a tumor necrosis factor. N Engl J Med 1987;316:379–385.

7. Hese DB, Dauatelis G, Felsen D, et al. Cachectin/tumor necrosis factor gene expression in Kupffer cells. J Leukocyte Biol 1987;42:422.

8. Halme J. Release of tumor necrosis factor-α by human peritoneal macrophages in vivo and in vitro. Am J Obstet Gynecol 1989;161:1718.

9. Beutler B, Krochin N, Milsark IW, et al. Control of cachectin (tumor necrosis factor) synthesis: mechanism of endotoxin resistance. Science 1988;232:977–980.

10. Wong GHW, Gaeddal EV. Tumor necrosis factor alpha and beta inhibit virus replication and synergize with interferons. Nature 1986;23:819–821.

11. Beutler BA, Milsark, IW, Cerami A. Cachectin/tumor necrosis factor: production, distribution and metabolic fate in vivo. J Immunol 1985;166:147–153.

12. Hesse DG, Tracey KG, Fong Y, et al. Cytokine appearance in human endotoxemia and non-human primate bacteremia. Surg Gynecol Obstet 1988;166:147–153.

13. Michie HR, Manogue KR, Spriggs DR, et al. Detection of circulating tumor necrosis factor after endotoxin administration. N Engl J Med 1988;318:1481–1486.

14. Scuderi P, Sterling KE, Lam KS, et al. Raised serum levels of tumour necrosis factor in parasitic infections. Lancet 1986;2:1364–1365.

15. Waage A, Halstensen A, Espevik T. Association between tumor necrosis factor in serum and fatal outcome in patients with meningococcal disease. Lancet 1987;1:355–357.

16. Girardin E, Grau GE, Dayer JM, Roux-Lombard P, Lambert PH. Tumor necrosis factor and interleukin-1 in the serum of children with severe infectious purpurs. N Engl J Med 1988;319:397–400.

17. Drost AC, Burleson DG, Cioffi WG Jr, Jordan BS, Mason AD Jr, Pruitt BA Jr. Plasma cytokines following thermal injury and their relationship with patient mortality, burn size, and time postburn. J Trauma 1993;35:335–339.

18. Maury CPJ, Teppo AM. Raised serum levels of cachectin/tumor necrosis factor alpha in renal allograft rejection. J Exp Med 1987;166:1132–1137.

19. Muto Y, Nouri-Aria KT, Meager A, et al. Enhanced tumor necrosis factor and interleukin-1 fulminant hepatic failure. Lancet 1988;2:72–74.

20. Marano MA, Fong Y, Moldawer LL, et al. Serum cachectin/tumor necrosis factor in critically ill patients with burns correlates with infection and mortality. Surg Gynecol Obstet 1990;170:32–38.

21. de Groote MA, Martin MA, Densen P, Pfaller MA, Wenzel RP. Plasma tumor necrosis factor levels in patients with presumed sepsis: results in those treated with antilipid A antibody vs placebo. JAMA 1989;262:249–251.

22. Cannon JG, Tompkins RG, Gelfand JA, et al. Circulating interleukin-1 and tumor necrosis factor in septic shock and experimental endotoxin fever. J Infect Dis 1990;161:79–84.

23. Van Zee KJ, Kohno T, Fischer E, Rock CS, Moldawer LL, Lowry SF. TNF soluble receptors protect against excessive TNF during infection and injury. Proc Natl Acad Sci USA 1992;89:4845–4849.

24. Beutler A, Milsark IW, Cerami AC. Passive immunization against cachectin/tumor necrosis factor protects mice from lethal effect of endotoxin. Science 1985;229:869–871.

25. Sanchez-Cantu L, Rode HN, Christou NV. Endotoxin tolerance is associated with reduced secretion of tumor necrosis factor. Arch Surg 1989;124:1432–1436.

26. Mathison JC, Wolfson E, Ulevitch RJ. Participation of tumor necrosis factor in the mediation of gram negative bacterial lipopolysaccharide-induced injury in rabbits. J Clin Invest 1988;81:1925–1937.

27. He W, Fong Y, Marano MA, et al. Tolerance to endotoxin prevents mortality in infected thermal injury: association with attenuated cytokine responses. J Infect Dis 1992;165:859–864.

28. Tracey KJ, Beutler B, Lowry SF, et al. Shock and tissue injury induced by recombinant human cachectin. Science 1986;234:470–474.

29. Tracey KJ, Lowry SF, Fahey TJ III, et al. Cachectin/tumor necrosis factor induces lethal shock and stress hormone responses in the dog. Surg Gynecol Obstet 1987;164:415–422.

30. Warren RS, Starnes HF, Gabrilove JL, Oettgen HF, Brennan MF. The acute metabolic effects of tumor necrosis factor administration in humans. Arch Surg 1987;122:1396–1400.

31. Michie HR, Springgs DR, Manogue KR, et al. Tumor necrosis factor and endotoxin induce similar metabolic responses in human beings. Surgery 1988;104:280–286.

32. van der Poll T, Romijn JA, Endert E, Borm JJJ, Büller HR, Sauerwein HP. Tumor necrosis factor mimics the metabolic response to acute infection in healthy humans. Am J Physiol 1991;261:E457–E465.

33. van der Poll T, Büller HR, ten Cate H, et al. Activation of coagulation after administration of tumor necrosis factor to normal subjects. N Engl J Med 1990;322:1622–1627.

34. Tracey KJ, Fong Y, Hesse DG, et al. Anti-cachectin/TNF monoclonal antibodies prevent septic shock during lethal bacteraemia. Nature 1987;330:662–664.

35. Fong Y, Tracey KJ, Moldawer LL, et al. Antibodies to cachectin/tumor necrosis factor reduce interleukin-1 beta

and interleukin-6 appearance during lethal bacteremia. J Exp Med 1989;170:1627–1633.

36. Dinarello CA, Cannon JG, Wolff SM, et al. Tumor necrosis factor (cachectin) is an endogenous pyrogen and induces production of interleukin 1. J Exp Med 1986;163:1433–1450.

37. Moser R, Schleiffenbaum B, Groscurth P, Fehr J. Interleukin 1 and tumor necrosis factor stimulate human vascular endothelial cells to promote transendothelial neutrophil passage. J Clin Invest 1989;83:444–455.

38. Ulich TF, Castillo JD, Keys M, et al. Kinetics and mechanism of recombinant human interleukin 1 alpha and tumor necrosis factor alpha induced changes in circulating numbers of neutrophils and lymphocytes. J Immunol 1987;139:3406–3415.

39. Shalaby MR, Aggarwal BB, Rinderknecht E, et al. Activation of human polymorphonuclear neutrophil functions by interferon gamma and tumor necrosis factors. J Clin Invest 1985;135:2069–2073.

40. Djeu JY, Blanchard DK, Halkias D, et al. Growth inhibition of Candida albicans by human polymorphonuclear neutrophils: activation by interferon-γ and tumor necrosis factor. J Immunol 1986;137:2980–2984.

41. Philip R, Epstein LB. Tumour necrosis factor as immunomodulator and mediator of monocyte cytotoxicity induced by itself, gamma interferon and interleukin 1. Nature 1986;323:86–89.

42. Mestan J, Digel W, Mittnacht S, et al. Antiviral effects of recombinant tumor necrosis factor in vitro. Nature 1986;323:816–819.

43. Dinarello CA. Biology of interleukin 1. FASEB J 1988;2:108–115.

44. Dinarello CA, Cannon JG, Wolff SM, et al. Tumor necrosis factor (cachectin) is an endogenous pyrogen and induces production of interleukin 1. J Exp Med 1986;163:1433–1450.

45. Okusawa S, Gelfand JA, Ikejima T, Connally RJ, Dinarello CA. Interleukin 1 induces a shock-like state in rabbits: synergism with tumor necrosis factor and the effect of cyclooxygenase inhibition. J Clin Invest 1988;81:1162–1172.

46. Fischer E, Marano MA, Barber AE, et al. A comparison between the effects of interleukin-1α administration and sublethal endotoxemia in primates. Am J Physiol 1991;261:R442–R452.

47. Van Zee KJ, DeForde LE, Fischer E, et al. IL-8 in septic shock, endotoxemia, and after IL-1 administration. J Immunol 1991;146:3478–3482.

48. Hawes AS, Fischer E, Marano MA, et al. Comparison of peripheral blood leukocyte kinetics after live Escherichia coli, endotoxin, or interleukin-1α administration. Studies using a novel interleukin-1 receptor antagonist. Ann Surg 1993;218:79–90.

49. Fischer E, Marano MA, Van Zee KJ, et al. Interleukin-1 receptor blockade improves survival and hemodynamic performance in Escherichia coli septic shock, but fails to alter host responses to sublethal endotoxemia. J Clin Invest 1992;89:1551–1557.

50. Alexander HR, Doherty GM, Venzon DJ, Merino MJ, Fraker DL, Norton JA. Recombinant interleukin-1 receptor

antagonist (IL-1ra): effective therapy against gram-negative sepsis in rats. Surgery 1992;112:188–193.

51. Warren RS, Donner DB, Starnes HF Jr, Brennan MF. Modulation of endogenous hormone action by recombinant human tumor necrosis factor. Proc Natl Acad Sci USA 1987;84:8619–8622.

52. Gauldie J, Northemann W, Fey GH. IL-6 functions as an exocrine hormone in inflammation. J Immunol 1990;144:3804–3808.

53. Heinrich PC, Castell JV, Andus T. Interleukin-6 and the acute phase response. Biochem J 1990;265:621–636.

54. Dejana E, Breviario F, Erroi A, et al. Modulation of endothelial cell functions by different molecular species of interleukin-1. Blood 1987;69:695–701.

55. Kohase J, May LT, Tamm I, Vilcek J, Sehgal PB. A cytokine network in human diploid fibroblasts. Mol Cell Biol 1987;7:273–284.

56. Van der Meer JWM, Helle M, Aarden L. Comparison of the effects of recombinant interleukin 6 and recombinant interleukin 1 on nonspecific resistance to infection. Eur J Immunol 1989;19:413–416.

57. Rosenwasser LM, Dinarello CA, Rosenthal AS. Adherent cell function in murine T-lymphocyte antigen recognition. J Exp Med 1979;150:709–715.

58. Merriman CR, Pulliam LA, Kampschmidt RF. Comparison of leukocytic pyrogen and leukocytic endogenous mediator. Proc Soc Exp Biol Med 1977;154:224–233.

59. Czuprynski CJ, Brown JF, Young M, Cooley AJ, Kurtz RS. Effects of murine recombinant interleukin 1 alpha on the host response to bacterial infection. J Immunol 1988;140:962–968.

60. Johnson CS, Keckler DJ, Topper MI, Braunschweiger PG, Furmanski P. In vivo hematopoietic effects of recombinant interleukin-1α in mice. Blood 1989;73:678–683.

61. Bagby GC Jr. Interleukin-1 and hematopoiesis. Blood Rev 1989;3:152.

62. Mochizuki DY, Eisenman JR, Conlon PJ, Larsen AD, Tushinski RJ. Interleukin 1 regulates hematopoietic activity, a role previously ascribed to hematopoietin 1. Proc Natl Acad Sci USA 1987;84:5267–5271.

63. Moldawer LL, Marano M, Wei H, et al. Cachectin/tumor necrosis factor-alpha alters red blood cell kinetics and induces anemia in vivo. FASEB J 1989;3:1637–1643.

64. Fong Y, Marano MA, Moldawer LL, et al. The acute splanchnic and peripheral tissue metabolic response to endotoxin in man. J Clin Invest 1990;85:1896–1904.

65. van Deventer SJH, Büller HR, ten Cate JW, et al. Experimental endotoxemia in humans: analysis of cytokine release and coagulation, fibrinolytic and complement pathways. Blood 1990;76:2520–2526.

66. Arend WP, Joslin FG, Thompson RC, Hannum CH. An IL-1 inhibitor from human monocytes. Production and characterization of biologic properties. J Immunol 1989;143:1851–1858.

67. Van Zee KJ, Kohno T, Fischer E, Rock CS, Moldawer LL, Lowry SF. TNF soluble receptors protect against excessive TNFα during infection and injury. Proc Natl Acad Sci USA 1992;89:4845–4849.

68. Spinas GA, Keller U, Brockhaus M. Release of soluble receptors for tumor necrosis factor in relation to circulating TNF during experimental endotoxemia. J Clin Invest 1992;90:533–536.

69. Porteau F, Nathan CF. Mobilizable intracellular pool of p55 (type 1) tumor necrosis factor receptors in human neutrophils. J Leukocyte Biol 1992;52:122–125.

70. Porteau F, Nathan CF. Shedding of tumor necrosis factor receptors by activated human neutrophils. J Exp Med 1990;172:599–607.

71. Konig M, Wallach D, Resch K, Holtmann H. Induction of hyporesponsiveness to an early post-binding effect of tumor necrosis factor by tumor necrosis factor itself and interleukin-1. Eur J Immunol 1991;21:1741–1745.

72. Aderka D, Engelmann H, Maor Y, et al. Stabilization of the bioactivity of tumor necrosis factor by its soluble receptors. J Exp Med 1992;175:323–329.

73. Hiltz ME, Lipton JM. Anti-inflammatory activity of a COOH-terminal fragment of the neuropeptide alpha-MSH. FASEB J 1989;3:2282–2287.

74. Marcinkiewics J. In vitro cytokine release by activated murine peritoneal macrophages. Cytokine 1991;3:327–332.

75. Luedke CE, Cerami A. Interferon gamma overcomes glucocorticoid suppression of cachectin/tumor necrosis factor biosynthesis by murine macrophages. J Clin Invest 1990;86:1234–1240.

76. Fiorentino DF, Zlotnik A, Mosmann TR, Howard M, O'Garra A. IL-10 inhibits cytokine production by activated macrophages. J Immunol 1991;147:3815–3822.

77. Bogdan C, Vodovotz Y, Nathan C. Macrophage deactivation by interleukin-10. J Exp Med 1991;174:1549–1555.

78. de Waal Malefyt R, Abrams J, Bennett B, et al. Interleukin-10 (IL-10) inhibits cytokine synthesis by human monocytes: an autoregulatory role of IL-10 produced by monocytes. J Exp Med 1991;174:1209–1220.

79. Donnelly RP, Fenton MJ, Kaufman JD, Gerrard TL. IL-1 expression in human monocytes is transcriptionally and posttranscriptionally regulated by IL-4. J Immunol 1991;146:3431–3436.

80. Hart PH, Cooper RL, Finlay-Jones JJ. IL-4 suppresses IL-1 beta, TNF alpha, and PGE2 production by human peritoneal macrophages. Immunology 1991;72:344–349.

81. Vannier E, Miller LC, Dinarello CA. Coordinated anti-inflammatory effects of IL-4: IL-4 suppresses IL-1 production but upregulates synthesis of IL-1 receptor antagonist. Proc Natl Acad Sci USA 1992;89:4076–4080.

82. Ruppert J, Friedrichs D, Xu H, Peters JH. IL-4 decreases the expression of the monocyte differentiation marker CD14, paralleled by an increasing accessory potency. Immunobiology 1991;182:449–464.

83. Vane JR, Anggard EE, Botting RM. Regulatory functions of the vascular endothelium. N Engl J Med 1990;323:27–36.

84. Dinarello CA, Rosenwasser LJ, Wolff SM. Demonstration of a circulating suppressor factor of thymocyte proliferation during endotoxin fever in humans. J Immunol 1981;127:2517–2519.

85. Seckinger P, Lowenthal JW, Williamson K, Dayer J-M, MacDonald HR. A urine inhibitor of interleukin 1 activity that blocks ligand binding. J Immunol 1987;139:1546–1549.

86. Spinas GA, Bloesch D, Kaufmann MT, Keller U, Dayer J-M. Induction of plasma inhibitors of interleukin 1 and TNF-α activity by endotoxin administration to normal humans. Am J Physiol 1990;259:993–997.

87. Eisenberg SP, Evans RJ, Arend WP, et al. Primary structure and functional expression from complementary DNA of a human interleukin-1 receptor antagonist. Nature 1990; 343:341–346.

88. Hannum CH, Wilcox CJ, Arend WP, et al. Interleukin-1 receptor antagonist activity of a human interleukin-1 inhibitor. Nature 1990;343:338–340.

89. Arend WP, Smith MF Jr, Janson RW, Joslin FG. IL-1 receptor antagonist and IL-1β production in human monocytes are regulated differently. J Immunol 1991;147:1530–1536.

90. Haskill S, Martin G, Van Le L, et al. cDNA cloning of an intracellular form of the human interleukin-1 receptor antagonist associated with epithelium. Proc Natl Acad Sci USA 1991;88:3681–3685.

91. Ulich TF, Guo K, Yin S, et al. Endotoxin induced cytokine gene expression in vivo. IV. Expression of Il-1 αβ and IL-1ra mRNA during endotoxemia and endotoxin-initiated local inflammation. Am J Pathol 1992;141:61–68.

92. Granowitz EV, Santos AA, Poutsiaka DD, et al. Production of interleukin-1 receptor antagonist during experimental endotoxemia. Lancet 1991;338:1423–1424.

93. Fischer E, Poutsiaka DD, Van Zee KJ, et al. Interleukin-1 receptor antagonist circulates in experimental inflammation and in human disease. Blood 1992;79:2196–2200.

94. Van Zee K, DeForge L, Fischer E, et al. IL-8 in septic shock, endotoxemia and following IL-1 administration. J Immunol 1991;146:3478–3482.

95. Waage A, Brandtzaeg P, Haltensen A, et al. The complex pattern of cytokines in serum from patients with meningococcal shock: association between IL-6, IL-1 and fatal outcome. J Exp Med 1989;169:333–338.

96. Granowitz EV, Clar BD, Mancilla J, Dinarello CA. Interleukin-1 receptor antagonist competitively inhibits the binding of interleukin-1 to the type II interleukin-1 receptor. J Biol Chem 1991;266:14147–14150.

97. McIntyre KW, Stepan GJ, Kolinsky KD, et al. Inhibition of IL-1 binding and bioactivity in vivo and modulation of acute inflammation of IL-1ra and anti-IL-1 receptor monoclonal antibody. J Exp Med 1991;173:931–939.

98. Wherry J, Pennington JE, Wenzel JP. Tumor necrosis factor and the therapeutic potential of anti-tumor necrosis factor antibodies. Crit Care Med 1993;21(suppl):S436–S440.

99. Fisher CJ Jr, Opal SM, Dhainaut JF, et al. Influence of anti-tumor necrosis factor monoclonal antibody on cytokine levels in patients with sepsis. Crit Care Med 1993;21: 318–327.

100. Fisher CJJ, Slotman GJ, Opal SM, et al. Initial evaluation of human recombinant interleukin-1 receptor antagonist in the treatment of sepsis syndrome: a randomized open label, placebo-controlled multi-center trial. Crit Care Med 1994;22:12–21.

101. Pribble J, Fisher C, Opal S, et al. Human recombinant interleukin-1 receptor antagonist (IL-1ra) increases survival time in patients with sepsis syndrome and end organ dysfunction (abstract). Crit Care Med 1994;22:A192.

CHAPTER 26

ROLE OF CYTOKINES IN MENINGITIS AND OTHER NEUROLOGICAL INFECTIONS

Anders Waage and Trond Sand

The characteristics of immunological and inflammatory reactions in the central nervous system (CNS) are distinctly different from those in other organs. Traditionally, the CNS was seen as an immunologically privileged site because of a relative lack of a lymphatic system and its separation from the blood by the blood-brain barrier (BBB), which, under normal circumstances, is impenetrable to most immunological and inflammatory active substances and restricts the migration of leukocytes. In addition, cells of the CNS express very low levels of the major histocompatibility antigens, which have an important role in induction and regulation of immune responses. The prevailing view has been that immune-competent cells, as well as cells active in the inflammatory reaction, for the most part are recruited from the systemic circulation.

Recently, the profound and ubiquitous influence of cytokines, such as interleukin-1 (IL-1), IL-6, tumor necrosis factor (TNF), and interferon-γ (IFN-γ) on the immune and inflammatory reactions have been established. These cytokines are also produced locally in the CNS and released in the cerebrospinal fluid (CF), and they seem to function as signal molecules in the early development of inflammatory reactions. Although their appearance during inflammatory reactions in the CNS is largely parallel to other locations of the organism, there are distinct characteristics of the cytokine network in the CNS that have been the focus of extensive research.

We review the main areas of this research: What cytokines are actually produced in the CNS and what are their cellular sources? What are the effects of cytokines in the CNS? What is the role of the BBB in relation to cytokines? Furthermore, we analyze the appearance and significance of cytokines in CF in bacterial and viral meningitis and in other CNS infections.

PATHOPHYSIOLOGICAL ASPECTS

The blood-brain barrier

CF is produced by specialized cells of the choroid plexus at a rate of approximately 50 mL/hour, and it is drained into the venous blood by membrane structures, such as arachnoid granulations. The CF freely communicates with the interstitial fluid of the brain tissue via a layer of ependymal cells that lines the ventricles. The interstitial fluid of the brain and the CF therefore constitute a functional compartment separated from the systemic circulation.

The properties of the BBB, the major portion of which is localized to the cerebral capillary endothelium, have attracted much attention. Unlike capillaries in other locations, the capillaries of the brain exhibit rare pinocytosis, and adjacent endothelial cells are fused together by tight junctions or zonulae occludentes (1). This structure provides an effective barrier against macromolecular transport and cell exudation. Only lipid-soluble substances and those transported by carrier-mediated diffusion (e.g., glucose and essential amino acids) traverse the BBB under normal circumstances (2–4). In addition, Na+ and K+ are transported by ion exchange, and the choroid plexus transfers vitamins by active transport.

During immune-mediated and inflammatory events, the normal function of the BBB is lost, leukocytes invade the CNS, the BBB becomes permissive to a number of molecules, and vasogenic edema develops (5–7). It is an old observation that meningitis is accompanied by a marked increase in CF albumin, which leaks across the BBB from plasma.

A number of experimental studies have elucidated the elements of BBB injury during meningitis. An early response (within 4 hr) to meningeal pathogens is an increase in pinocytotic vesicles (8); however, it is questionable whether this increase results in transendothelial transport. Another observation is the opening of the tight intercellular junctions. It can be shown that albumin crosses the barrier by this paracellular pathway (9). Extracted lipopolysaccharide (LPS) from *Haemophilus influenzae* provokes greater BBB permeability than equivalent challenge with the live parent strain (10).

The hallmark of an inflammatory response in the meninges is pleocytosis in the CF. In experimental meningitis, it can be demonstrated that accumulation of leukocytes in CF increases markedly 3 to 4 hours after intracisternal administration of LPS, and a maximum response is reached after 6 to 8 hours (9–11). In contrast, albumin leakage is an early phenomenon that starts at 2 hours, and it attains maximal values after 4 hours.

The diversity of infectious agents capable of inducing meningitis and BBB injury has always suggested the potential for an endogenous host mediator. Both IL-1 and TNF have been identified as such mediators (12,13). In patients with meningitis, intrathecal levels of TNF but not IL-1 correlated with the degree of BBB disruption (14). Furthermore, it has been shown that leakage of albumin across the BBB is inhibited by prior induction of systemic neutropenia, indicating that granulocytes are required to damage the BBB (12).

Do cytokines cross the BBB?

During meningitis, albumin, with a molecular weight of 69 kd, leaks across the BBB. Cytokines, which have a molecular weight between 16 and 30 kd, should consequently be able to cross the permeable BBB, as should most of their polymeric forms.

We examined paired samples of CF and serum from patients with meningococcal disease (15). In patients with meningitis, high levels of TNF and IL-6 in CF were detected. Patients had high levels of albumin in CF, indi-

cating that the BBB was permeable. Despite this finding, no bioactive TNF and low levels of IL-6 were found in serum from the same patients. The findings are mainly consistent with other studies (16,17).

Cytokines produced in the subarachnoid space should cross the BBB to the systemic circulation under these circumstances. However, as a result of leakage to the systemic circulation, there is a dilution factor of 10 to 20. In addition, the cytokines may adhere to tissue and cells in the systemic circulation; furthermore, they may be inactivated by inhibitors and soluble receptors in serum. Although cytokines may leak from CF to blood, these mechanisms apparently are sufficient to neutralize the effect of cytokines in the circulation.

Another important aspect is the existence of trans-BBB induction mechanisms. It has been shown that cisternal administration of IL-1 induced production of IL-6 in blood in rats (18). In fact, this route of administration was more potent than intravenous injection of IL-1, and it was also effective in hypophysectomized or adrenalectomized rats. The hypothalamus-pituitary-adrenal axis is therefore not essential for this effect.

It is reasonable that cytokines cross the BBB when it has become penetrable during inflammation; however, the physiological consequences of this migration are disputable. It is still controversial whether the intact BBB is permissive to cytokines. For instance, fever is induced by cytokines applied centrally as well as peripherally (19). However, in similar experiments, it is difficult to distinguish between leakage or transport of cytokines across the BBB and a trans-BBB induction mechanism. The question of whether cytokines cross the intact BBB is essentially unresolved.

Production of cytokines in the CNS

In experiments in rabbits, we injected meningococcal LPS intracisternally or intravenously, and we measured TNF sequentially in CF and serum (Fig. 26–1) (11). When LPS was given intracisternally, high levels of TNF were detected in CF, and negligible amounts were detected in serum, and vice versa. The important information extracted from this study is (a) TNF is necessarily produced by resident CNS cells, and (b) there is strict compartmentalized production of TNF in the subarachnoid space and the systemic circulation.

What are the cellular sources of cytokines in the CNS? In addition to the neurons, the brain tissue consists of neuroglia cells. There are two broad groups of glia cells: the macroglia, which consist of astrocytes, oligodendrocytes, and ependymal cells; and microglia.

Astrocytes are the most numerous of the glia cells, and they outnumber neurons 10 to 1. They are the most versatile cells within the CNS, and they have a number of

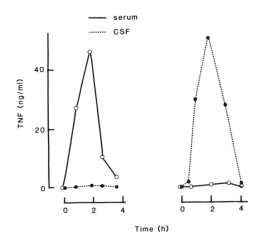

Figure 26-1 Tumor necrosis factor in serum and cerebrospinal fluid after injection of meningococcal lipopolysaccharide (LPS) in the systemic circulation (left) and in the subarachnoid space (right). Five μg LPS was injected intravenously, and 0.5 μg was injected into the subarachnoid space. (Reproduced by permission from Waage A, Halstensen A, Shalaby R, Brantzæg P, Kierulf P, Espevik T. Local production of tumor necrosis factor α, interleukin 1, and interleukin 6 in meningococcal meningitis. J Exp Med 1989;170:1859–1867.)

functions. In this context, two functions are relevant. First, the astrocytes are supposed to contribute to the structural integrity of the BBB as the CNS capillaries are almost completely surrounded by astrocytic end-feet. They may be involved in the formation of tight junctions between adjacent endothelial cells (20). Second, they secrete the cytokines TNF, IL-1, IL-6, and colony-stimulating factors (CSF) (21). Table 26–1 reviews agents able to induce cytokines in astrocytes and microglia.

Microglia comprise approximately 10% of the glia population, and they are considered to be the resident macrophages of the brain. The major subtypes have been denoted ramified, amoeboid, and perivascular microglia. Their main function is phagocytosis, and they are consequently involved in a number of processes. Also, the microglia contribute to the integrity of the BBB (33). Like macrophages in other locations, the microglia produce TNF, IL-1, and IL-6 (see Table 26–1). LPS-induced cytokine production by microglia can be modified by dexamethasone, which inhibits the release of TNF and IL-6, and by pentoxifylline, which inhibits TNF and IL-1, but not IL-6 (34). Furthermore, IFN-γ has the same effect on microglia as on macrophages in other locations because it increases TNF production 20-fold.

From a methodological point of view, it is more convenient to study cell cultures, and most studies are based on this approach. The purity of astrocyte cultures has been a problem in many studies, and the possibility of contaminating microglia has raised a controversy as to whether the astrocytes are the true source of cytokines (28). In vivo, localized production of IL-1 and IL-6 have been

TABLE 26–1   PRODUCTION OF CYTOKINES BY ASTROCYTES AND MICROGLIA*

Inducing Agent	Astrocytes	Microglia	References
LPS	TNF, IL-1, IL-6	TNF, IL-1, IL-6	(22–28)
TNF	IL-6, G-CSF, GM-CSF		(29)
IL-1	TNF, IL-6	IL-6	(24,28,30,31)
IFN-γ	TNF, IL-6	TNF, IL-1	(22,24,26)
Other (virus)	TNF, IL-6		(25,32)

*Results are from primary cultures from human or murine material.
LPS = lipopolysaccharide; TNF = tumor necrosis factor; IL = interleukin; G-CSF = granulocyte colony-stimulating factor.

demonstrated to occur in response to mechanical injury (35). In these experiments, there was evidence that microglia, not astrocytes, were the source of cytokines.

In addition to the resident CNS cells, an inflammatory response implies migration of granulocytes, lymphocytes, and monocytes from the systemic circulation. Among these cells, monocytes and macrophages are major cytokine producers. However, secretion of cytokines from migrating inflammatory cells is necessarily delayed compared with the rapid appearance of TNF, IL-1, and IL-6 in CF after exposure to bacterial products. The initial cytokine response induced by LPS or gram-negative bacteria comes prior to accumulation of leukocytes, and it is consequently caused by resident CNS cells.

Effects of cytokines in the CNS

TNF, IL-1, IL-6, and IFN-γ have numerous effects on CNS cells in addition to induction of the secretion of other cytokines. Some of the effects are summarized in Table 26–2. In addition, TNF, IL-1, and IL-6 have effects on the inflammatory cells (i.e., granulocytes, lymphocytes, and monocytes) that have migrated from the systemic circulation (41).

CLINICAL SYNDROMES

Meningitis

The most common CNS infection is meningitis, which may be caused by a variety of bacteria, parasites, fungus, and viruses. Although many advances in understanding

TABLE 26–2 SOME EFFECTS OF CYTOKINES IN THE CENTRAL NERVOUS SYSTEM*

IL-1

Stimulates astrocyte growth in vitro (36)

Stimulates astrogliosis in vivo (37)

Induces ICAM-1 expression on fetal astrocytes (38)

Induces damage to the blood-brain barrier (BBB) (12)

Induces migration of leukocytes (12,13)

TNF

Increases class 1 MHC on primary astrocytes (39)

Induces ICAM-1 expression on fetal astrocytes (38)

Induces proliferation of astrocytes (40)

Induces damage to BBB (13)

Induces migration of leukocytes (13)

IL-6

Induces proliferation of astrocytes

---

*TNF, IL-1, and IL-6 also induce secretion of other cytokines; see Table 26–1.

MHC = major histocompatibility complex.

and treatment of this disease have been made, morbidity and mortality rates remain high. For instance, in adult patients with pneumococcal meningitis, mortality rates range between 20 and 30%, and they have remained relatively unchanged since the introduction of penicillin. Understanding of the cytokine network in inflammation and immunological reactions has given new insight into the pathophysiology of meningitis, and it has provided the potential for new approaches to treatment.

EXPERIMENTAL MENINGITIS: A number of studies provide information about the production and pathogenetic significance of TNF, IL-1, and IL-6 in bacterial meningitis. These three cytokines are sequentially released in experimental meningitis in rabbits after intracisternal injection of LPS (11). TNF can be detected in CF after 30 minutes, and levels peak after 2 hours (11,42). When whole bacteria preparations were used, the peak level was attained later, and the decline of TNF levels was more gradual (42). IL-1 could be detected after approximately 1 hour, whereas small amounts of IL-6 were found after 3 hours (11). Accumulation of leukocytes in the CF starts later than the initial release of cytokines. When endotoxin was combined with an antiserum to TNF, migration of leukocytes from the systemic circulation was markedly depressed. However, the effect of the antiserum was minimal when it was combined with gram-negative bacteria, indicating that accumulation of leukocytes in this situation is also caused by other mediators (42). In similar experiments with a gram-positive bacteria (Pneumococcus), antibodies to TNF or IL-1 al-

most completely inhibited leukocytosis (43). In a model with meningitis induced by *Candida albicans*, peak levels of TNF in CF were attained 6 hours after intracisternal injection of the fungus (44). After 6 to 10 days of inoculation, a second peak of TNF activity was accompanied by increased CNS inflammation. Fatal outcome was associated with a higher second CF peak of TNF and leukocyte concentrations.

The roles of TNF and IL-1 have been investigated more directly by injection of recombinant cytokines into the CF of experimental animals (12,13,43). This approach confirmed the effect of TNF and IL-1 on accumulation of leukocytes in the CF. Furthermore, both cytokines caused an increase in protein concentration in the CF and a marked increase in brain edema. These cytokines appear to have synergistic effects. In rats, IL-1 had a stronger effect than TNF (12). To test another possible pathogenetic effect of TNF, antiserum to TNF was administered intravenously combined with systemic meningococcal infection (45). Anti-TNF did not influence the invasion of bacteria from the circulation to the CF in these experiments.

In gram-negative meningitis, there seems to be sequential release of TNF, IL-1, and IL-6; TNF and IL-1, possibly via intermediates, may contribute to the meningeal inflammatory response by recruitment of leukocytes and injury to the BBB. However, in vivo, a number of factors are released, and other factors may also be strong inducers of accumulation of leukocytes. TNF is also released in CF during *Candida albicans* meningitis.

DETECTION OF CYTOKINES IN CF IN BACTERIAL MENINGITIS: Detection of cytokines in CF has been extensively reported, and, because the composition of the CF reflects processes in the meninges and the CNS, such observations may have several important implications. During bacterial meningitis, TNF, IL-1, and IL-6, and IL-8 are frequently detected in the CF (Table 26–3). Also, M-CSF and G-CSF, but not GM-CSF, have been detected in CF during bacterial meningitis (57). Most of the studies involve infections with *Neisseria meningitidis*, *Haemophilus influenzae*, and *Streptococcus pneumoniae*. However, the materials also include infections caused by *Escherichia coli*, *Klebsiella* species, *Salmonella*, *Pseudomonas*, *Listeria monocytogenes*, *Staphylococcus aureus*, and *Mycobacterium tuberculosis*.

To evaluate reported concentrations of cytokines, it is important to distinguish between measurements based on immunological reactions and bioactivity, in particular for TNF. Immunoassays may detect complexes of TNF and inhibitors or soluble receptors that are not bioactive. Furthermore, bioactive TNF oligomers may form inactive polymers and monomers that could contribute to the observed discrepancies between immunoreactive and bioactive TNF (58). Results in various studies are therefore not always comparable (59).

TABLE 26–3 CYTOKINES IN CEREBROSPINAL FLUID IN BACTERIAL MENINGITIS

TNF	IL-1	IL-6	IL-8	Reference
3/7*				(46)
		10/18		(47)
4/44	21/42	41/42		(11)
25/27				(48)
79/106	97/102			(49)
1/21	19/21			(50)
15/18				(51)
		4/4		(52)
21/29		24/24		(16)
33/38				(53)
		30/36		(17)
		9/9		(54)
			2/2	(55)
			27/27	(56)

*Number of positive samples/total number of samples.
TNF = tumor necrosis factor; IL = interleukin.

KINETICS OF PRODUCTION/ELIMINATION IN VIVO:

The presence of TNF, IL-1, and IL-6 in the CF in experimental meningitis is transient; clearance occurs within 6 hours in most studies. By sequential sampling of CF from patients with meningitis, information about the kinetics in natural diseases has been obtained. In one study (49), TNF was detected in 53 of 79 samples taken 18 to 30 hours after the positive admission sample. The levels of TNF in the second sample were low. For IL-1, the corresponding number of positive samples taken after 18 to 30 hours was 67 of 97 originally positive samples. In other studies, TNF decreased to levels close to detection limit in samples taken 24 to 48 hours after the initial sample (14,53). TNF has also been detected in CF 4 days after the initial sample (57). Interestingly, antibiotic treatment seemed to increase TNF levels (53). In one patient, IL-6 was barely detectable 16 hours after the initial sample (16), whereas another study found IL-6 in 8 of 11 samples 2 days after start of antibiotics (17).

In conclusion, the total number of patients studied is small, and there is considerable variation in the clearance of TNF, IL-1, and IL-6 that may be detected in CF 18 to 96 hours after the initial positive sample. From a theoretical point of view, the proliferation of gram-negative bacteria in CF, combined with gradual and persisting migration of monocytes from the systemic circulation, should generate a sustained production of monocyte-derived cytokines.

RELATIONSHIP BETWEEN CYTOKINES AND OTHER INFLAMMATORY PARAMETERS:

It is of interest whether CF levels of cytokines correlate with other parameters of inflammation. A number of studies reported positive correlations between the TNF, IL-1, and IL-6 and the parameters leukocyte count, protein, glucose, lactate, C-reactive protein (CRP), neurological complications and sequela, and adverse outcome (11,16,49, 50,53). However, for TNF, lack of correlation with leukocyte count, protein, CRP, and adverse outcome has also been reported (11,48,49,51,53,57). Lack of correlation has also been reported for IL-6 (17). CF levels of IL-8 have been found not to correlate with leukocyte count in CF (56).

Although inconsistencies exist, most data indicate a correlation between early levels of IL-1 and IL-6 in CF and most inflammatory parameters. For TNF, there are discrepancies between studies, and a uniform conclusion cannot be drawn. Generally speaking, interpretation of such correlations should be done with care. A true inflammatory function can only be established by experimental studies and cytokine inhibitory treatment.

Viral meningitis and encephalitis

IL-1, IL-2, IL-6, and IFN-γ have been reported to be produced during viral meningitis, although contradictory results exist. In patients with aseptic meningitis of enteroviral etiology, 89% had detectable CF levels of IL-1 (60). A substantial proportion of patients with either viral meningitis or herpes encephalitis had increased levels of IL-6 in their CF (46,61,62), particularly early in the disease course (46). In contrast, Torre and colleagues (54) did not find elevated CF IL-6 levels in patients with viral meningitis (mainly mumps), whereas high levels were observed in most patients with bacterial meningitis. The lack of IL-6 in this study may be related to mumps virus.

Although IL-6 has been mostly found in infectious CNS disorders, increased levels have also been observed in patients with multiple sclerosis (MS), in inflammatory and noninflammatory neurological disorders (63), and in mice with experimental allergic encephalomyelitis (64).

Chalon and associates (65) found soluble IL-2 receptor (sIL-2R) in the CF of most patients with either aseptic meningitis or herpes virus encephalitis. IL-2 and sIL-2R levels in CF are also detected in other diseases, and they do not discriminate between viral and bacterial meningitis (66). Most studies have reported lack of TNF in CF in viral meningitis (46,60,67), whereas IFN-γ can be detected in CF in viral, but not in bacterial, meningitis (61).

Cytokines are therefore produced in CF in infection of both bacterial and viral etiology; there are, however, differences in the cytokine pattern. First, presence of bioactive TNF is rather specific for a bacterial etiology (16,45,50,60), although immunoreactive TNF may be detected. Second, levels of IL-1 and IL-6 in CF are considerably lower in viral than in bacterial meningitis (16,46,54,60,61).

Few experimental studies have been performed on cytokines in viral meningitis. Frei and colleagues (62) found IL-6 in CF in mice 24 hours after infection with lymphocytic choriomeningitis virus, and they noted a rapid increase after 4 days. IFN-γ was not detected until day 5 or 6 after infection, but levels increased sharply thereafter.

The significance of cytokines in viral meningitis is not clarified. IL-6 may reflect neuroprotective and antigen-eliminating parts of the immune response (32). More experimental studies of the potential role of cytokines in CNS viral infections are needed.

HIV infections in the CNS

CNS macrophages and microglia are the cells that predominantly are infected by human immunodeficiency virus type 1 (HIV-1) during acquired immunodeficiency syndrome (AIDS) dementia and other manifestations of CNS HIV-1 infection. Accordingly, it is not likely that the virus is responsible for clinical symptoms and neuropathological findings during CNS HIV-1 infection (68). The significance of cytokines in this respect has recently been studied by several research groups.

Gallo and colleagues (69) studied 38 patients with HIV-1 infections and found IL-1β in the CF of 58% and IL-6 in the CF of 42% of patients. Neither TNF nor IL-2 were detected, but sIL-2R was most often found in patients with elevated IL-6 and increased intrathecal immunoglobulin G (IgG) synthesis. sIL-2R was also detected in significantly higher serum concentrations in HIV-positive patients as compared with neurological control patients (70), although group differences were not found in CF. The highest levels were observed in patients with HIV-1–related meningitis or opportunistic infections (70).

Mintz and associates (71) investigated sera and CF of children with AIDS. Elevated serum TNF levels (immunoreactive) were found in 15 of the 19 patients with progressive encephalopathy, as compared with only 1 of 12 children without encephalopathy. Elevated levels of TNF in the CF was seldom found in either subgroup, however.

Laurenzi and coworkers (72) found elevated CF levels of IL-6 in 44% of asymptomatic HIV-1 carriers, 48% of patients with multiple sclerosis (MS) and 44% of patients with other neurological disorders. In contrast, more patients with AIDS or AIDS-related complex (80%) and other CNS inflammatory disorders (e.g., aseptic meningi-

tis and neuroborreliosis [75%]) had detectable IL-6 levels in their CF. AIDS patients in the latter study did not have opportunistic infections. Moreover, a relationship between IL-6 and CF IgG could not be confirmed.

In contrast to the negative results reported by Gallo and colleagues (69), Grimaldi and associates (73) were able to detect TNF in 17 of 30 sera and in 22 of 30 CF samples from patients with advanced HIV-1 infections (i.e., group IV B and IV C-1). In patients with primarily CNS involvement, higher TNF levels were seen in CF than in serum. No correlation was found between clinical dementia or demyelination and TNF levels, however.

In cell cultures, it has been shown that HIV-infected macrophages in coculture with astroglia produce TNF and IL-1β, which are neuronotoxic (74,75). IL-6 was not produced (75). Evidence for the presence of TNF in brain parenchyma of HIV-1–positive patients has also been presented (76), whereas IL-1 staining was mainly observed on endothelial cells. Increased CF TNF levels had previously been found in 4 of 6 HIV-1–positive patients, whereas none had detectable IL-6 or IL-1 levels (76). Increased levels of IFN-γ (77) and the macrophage products β2-microglobulin (76) and neopterin (76,77) have also been found in the CF of HIV-1–infected patients. Macrophage activation within the CNS of HIV-1–positive patients is also suggested by the presence of M-CSF in CF (57).

There is accumulating evidence in favor of the concept that neurotoxic effects of cytokines may be directly involved in the pathogenesis of neurological symptoms in HIV-1–infected patients (67,77). TNF may possibly cause diffuse myelin changes of the kind observed in AIDS-related dementia (63,68).

CONCLUSION

Cytokines are signal molecules that initiate, continue, and terminate immunological and inflammatory reactions. These molecules are definitively produced within the CNS, and the expanding knowledge about their production and effects has somewhat modified the concept of the CNS as an immunologically silent site. Production of cytokines within the CNS is most conspicuous, and it has been best studied in bacterial meningitis. An ultimate goal in mediator research is to identify key factors that can be inhibited or enhanced and thereby influence the pathophysiological process. Unfortunately, our current knowledge about cytokine mediators in meningitis or other CNS infections cannot yet be translated into a practical treatment approach. However, combined basic and clinical research in this field has provided a far better understanding of pathophysiological mechanisms.

REFERENCES

1. Brightman MW, Reese TS. Junctions between intimately opposed cell membranes in the verterate brain. J Cell Biol 1969; 40:648–677.

2. Betz AL, Csejtey J, Goldstein GW. Hexose transport and phosphorylation by capillaries isolated from rat brain. Am J Physiol 1979;236:C96–C102.

3. Betz AL, Goldstein GW. Polarity of the blood-brain barrier: neural amino acid transport into isolated brain capillaries. Science 1978;202:225–227.

4. Goldstein GW, Betz AL. Recent advances in understanding brain capillary function. Ann Neurol 1983;14:389–395.

5. Brosnan CF, Claudio J, Martiney JA. The blood-brain barrier during immune responses. Semin Neurosci 1992;4: 193–200.

6. Claudio L, Kress Y, Factor J, Brosnan CF. Mechanisms of edema formation in experimental allergic encephalomyelitis. Am J Pathol 1990;137:1033–1045.

7. Newcombe J, Hawkins CP, Henderson CL, et al. Histopathology of multiple sclerosis lesions detected by magnetic resonance imaging in unfixed postmortem central nervous system tissue. Brain 1991;114:1013–1023.

8. Quagliarello VJ, Long WJ, Scheid WM. Morphologic alterations of the blood-brain barrier with experimental meningitis in the rat. J Clin Invest 1986;77:1084–1095.

9. Quagliarello VJ, Ma A, Strukenbrok H, Palade GE. Ultrastructural localization of albumin transport across the cerebral microvasculature during experimental meningitis in the rat. J Exp Med 1991;174:656–672.

10. Wispelwey B, Lesse AJ, Hansen EJ, Scheld WM. Haemophilus influenzae lipopolysaccharide-induced blood brain barrier permeability during experimental meningitis in the rat. J Clin Invest 1988;82:1339–1346.

11. Waage A, Halstensen A, Shalaby R, Brandtzæg P, Kierulf P, Espevik T. Local production of tumor necrosis factor α, interleukin 1, and interleukin 6 in meningococcal meningitis. J Exp Med 1989;170:1859–1867.

12. Quagliarello VJ, Wispelwey B, Long WJ Jr, Scheld WM. Recombinant human interleukin-1 induces meningitis and blood-brain barrier injury in the rat. J Clin Invest 1991;87: 1360–1366.

13. Ramilo O, Saez-Llorens X, Mertsola J, et al. Tumor necrosis factor α/cachectin and interleukin 1β initiate meningeal inflammation. J Exp Med 1990;172:497–507.

14. Sharief MK, Ciardi M, Thompson EJ. Blood-brain barrier damage in patients with bacterial meningitis: association with tumor necrosis factor-α but not interleukin-1β. J Infect Dis 1992;166:350–358.

15. Waage A, Halstensen A, Espevik T, Brandtzæg P. Compartmentalization of TNF and IL-6 in meningitis and septic shock. Mediators Inflammation 1993;2:23–25.

16. Frei K, Nadal D, Fontana A. Intracerebral synthesis of tumor necrosis factor-α and interleukin-6 in infectious meningitis. Ann NY Acad Sci 1990;594:326–335.

17. Rusconi F, Parizzi F, Garlaschi L, et al. Interleukin 6 activity in infants and children with bacterial meningitis. Pediatr Infect Dis J 1991;10:117–121.

18. de Simoni MG, Sironi M, De Luigi A, Manfridi A, Mantovani A, Ghezzi P. Intracerebroventricular injection of interleukin 1 induces high circulating levels of interleukin 6. J Exp Med 1990;171:1773–1778.

19. Dinarello CA, Cannon JG, Wolff SM. New concepts on the pathogenesis of fever. Rev Infect Dis 1988;10:168–189.

20. Janzer RC, Raff MC. Astrocytes induce blood-brain barrier properties in endothelial cells. Nature 1987;325:253–257.

21. Benveniste EN. Cytokines: influence on glial cell gene expression and function. In: Blalock JE, ed. Neuroimmunoendocrinology, chemical immunology, vol 52. Basel: Karger, 1992:106–153.

22. Fontana A, Kristensen F, Dubbs R, Gemsa D, Weber E. Production of prostaglandin E and an interleukin-1-like factor by cultured astrocytes and C6 glioma cells. J Immunol 1982;129:2413–2419.

23. Roberge FG, Caspi RR, Nusenblatt RB. Glial retinal Müller cells produce IL-1 activity and have a dual effect on autoimmune T helper lymphocytes. J Immunol 1988;140: 2193–2196.

24. Chung IY, Benveniste EN. Tumor necrosis factor-alpha production by astrocytes: induction by lipopolysaccharide, interferon-gamma and interleukin-1. J Immunol 1990;144: 2999–3007.

25. Lieberman AP, Pitha PM, Shin HS, Shin ML. Production of tumor necrosis factor-alpha and other cytokines by astrocytes stimulated with lipopolysaccharide or a neurotropic virus. Proc Natl Acad Sci USA 1989;86:6348–6352.

26. Frei K, Siepl C, Groscurth P, Bodmer S, Schwerdel C, Fontana A. Antigen presentation and tumor cytotoxicity by interferon-gamma treated microglial cells. Eur J Immunol 1987;17:1271–1278.

27. Gulian D. Baker TJ, Shih L, Lachman LB. Interleukin-1 of the central nervous system is produced by ameboid microglia. J Exp Med 1986;164:594–604.

28. Sébire G, Emilie D, Wallon C, et al. In vitro production of IL-6, IL-1β, and tumor necrosis factor-α by human embryonic microglial and neural cells. J Immunol 1993;150: 1517–1523.

29. Malipiero UV, Frei K, Fontana A. Production of hemopoietic colony-stimulating factors by astrocytes. J Immunol 1990;144:3816–3821.

30. Benveniste EN, Sparacio SM, Norris JG, Grenett HE, Fuller GM. Induction and regulation of interleukin-6 gene expression in rat astrocytes. J Neuroimmunol 1990;30:201–212.

31. Bethea JR, Chung IY, Sparacio SM, Gillespie GY, Benveniste EN. Interleukin 1beta induction of tumor necrosis factor gene expression in human astroglioma cells. J Neuroimmunol 1992;36:179–191.

32. Frei K, Malipiero U, Leist T, Zinkernagel R, Schwab M, Fontana A. On the cellular source and function of interleukin 6 produced in the central nervous system in viral diseases. Eur J Immunol 1989;19:689–694.

33. Lassmann H, Vass FK, Hickey WF. Microglial cells are a component of the perivascular glia limitans. J Neurosci Res 1991;28:236–243.

34. Chao CC, Hu S, Close K, et al. Cytokine release from microglia: differential inhibition by pentoxifylline and dexamethasone. J Infect Dis 1992;166:847–853.

35. Woodroofe MN, Sarna GS, Wadhwa M, et al. Detection of

interleukin-1 and interleukin-6 in adult rat brain, following mechanical injury, by in vivo microdialysis: evidence of a role for microglia in cytokine production. J Neuroimmunol 1991;33:227–236.

36. Giulian D, Lachman LB. Interleukin-1 stimulation of astroglial proliferation after brain injury. Science 1985;228: 497–499.

37. Guilian D, Woodward J, Young DG, Krebs JF, Lachmann LB. Interleukin-1 injected into mammalian brain stimulates astrogliosis and neovascularization. J Neurosci 1988;8: 2485–2490.

38. Frohman EM, Frohman TC, Dustin ML, et al. The induction of intracellular adhesion molecule 1 (ICAM-1) expression on human fetal astrocytes by interferon-γ, tumor necrosis factor-α, lymphotoxin, and interleukin-1: relevance to intracerebral antigen presentation. J Neuroimmunol 1989;23:117–124.

39. Lavi E, Suzumura A, Murasko KM, Murray EM, Silberberg DH, Weiss SR. Tumor necrosis factor induces expression of MHC class 1 antigens on mouse astrocytes. J Neuroimmunol 1988;18:245–253.

40. Selmaj KW, Farooq M, Norton WTR, Raine CS, Brosnan CF. Proliferation of astrocytes in vitro in response to cytokines. A primary role for tumor necrosis factor. J Immunol 1990;144:129–135.

41. Steinbeck MJ, Roth JA. Neutrophil activation by recombinant cytokines. Rev Infect Dis 1989;11:549–568.

42. Mustafa MM, Ramilo O, Olsen KD, et al. Tumor necrosis factor in mediating experimental Haemaophilus influenzae type B meningitis. J Clin Invest 1989;84:1253–1259.

43. Saukkonen K, Sande S, Cioffe C, et al. The role of cytokines in the generation of inflammation and tissue damage in experimental gram-positive meningitis. J Exp Med 1990;171: 439–448.

44. Jafari HS, Sàez-Llorens X, Grimprel E, Argylke JC, Olsen KD, McCracken GH Jr. Characteristics of experimental Candida albicans infection of the central nervous system in rabbits. J Infect Dis 1991;164:389–395.

45. Nassif X, Mathison JC, Wolfson E, Koziol JA, Ulevitch RJ, So M. Tumour necrosis factor alpha antibody protects against lethal meningococcaemia. Mol Microbiol 1992;6: 591–597.

46. Leist TP, Frei K, Kam-Hansen S, Zinkernagel RM, Fontana A. Tumor necrosis factor α in cerebrospinal fluid during bacterial, but not viral, meningitis. J Exp Med 1988;167: 1743–1748.

47. Houssiau FA, Bukasa K, Sindic CJM, Van Damme J, Van Snick J. Elevated levels of the 26 K human hybridoma growth factor (interleukin 6) in cerebrospinal fluid of patients with acute infection of the central nervous system. Clin Exp Immunol 1988;71:320–323.

48. McCracken GJ Jr, Mustafa MM, Ramilo O, Olsen KD, Risser RC. Cerebrospinal fluid interleukin 1-beta and tumor necrosis factor concentrations and outcome from neonatal Gram-negative enteric bacillary meningitis. Pediatr Infect Dis J 1989;8:155–159.

49. Mustafa MM, Lebel MH, Ramilo O, et al. Correlation of interleukin-1β and cachectin concentrations in cerebrospinal fluid and outcome from bacterial meningitis. J Pediatr 1989;115:208–213.

50. Mustafa MM, Mertsola J, Ramilo O, Saez-Llorens X, Risser RC, McCracken GH. Increased endotoxin and interleukin 1beta concentrations in cerebrospinal fluid in infants with coliform meningitis and ventriculitis associated with intraventricular gentamycin therapy. J Infect Dis 1989;160: 891–895.

51. Nadal D, Leppert D, Frei K, Gallo P, Lamche H, Fontana A. Tumour necrosis factor-α in infectious meningitis. Arch Dis Child 1989;64:1274–1279.

52. Helfgott DC, Tatter SB, Santhanam U, et al. Multiple forms of IFN-beta/IL-6 in serum and body fluids during acute bacterial infection. J Immunol 1989;142:948–953.

53. Arditi M, Manogue KR, Caplan M, Yogev R. Cerebrospinal fluid cachectin/tumor necrosis factor-α and platelet-activating factor concentrations and severity of bacterial meningitis in children. J Infect Dis 1990;162:139–147.

54. Torre D, Zeroli C, Ferraro G, et al. Cerebrospinal fluid levels of IL-6 in patients with acute infections of the central nervous system. Scand J Infect Dis 1992;24:787–791.

55. Van Meir E, Ceska M, Effenberger F, et al. Interleukin-8 is produced in neoplastic and infectious diseases of the human central nervous system. Cancer Res 1992;52:4297–4305.

56. Halstensen A, Ceska M, Brandtzaeg P, Redl H, Naess A, Waage A. Interleukin-8 in serum and cerebrospinal fluid from patients with meningococcal disease. J Infect Dis 1993;167:471–475.

57. Gallo P, Pagni S, Giometto B, et al. Macrophage-colony stimulating factor (M-CSF) in the cerebrospinal fluid. J Neuroimmunol 1990;29:105–112.

58. Møller B, Mogensen SC, Wendelboe P, Bendtzen K, Munck Petersen C. Bioactive and inactive forms of tumor necrosis factor-α in spinal fluid from patients with meningitis. J Infect Dis 1991;163:886–889.

59. Engelberts I, Stephens S, Francot GJM, van der Linden CJ, Buurman WA. Evidence for different effects of soluble TNF-receptors on various TNF measurements in human biological fluids. Lancet 1991;338:515–516.

60. Ramilo O, Mustafa MM, Porter J, et al. Detection of interleukin 1β but not tumor necrosis factor-α in cerebrospinal fluid of children with aseptic meningitis. Am J Dis Child 1990;144:349–352.

61. Weller M, Stevens A, Sommer N, Melms A, Dichgans J, Wiethölter H. Comparative analysis of cytokine patterns in immunological, infectious, and oncological neurological disorders. J Neurol Sci 1991;104:215–221.

62. Frei K, Leist TP, Meager A, et al. Production of B cell stimulatory factor-2 and interferon γ in the central nervous system during viral meningitis and encephalitis. J Exp Med 1988;168:449–453.

63. Hauser SL, Doolittle TH, Lincoln R, Brown RH, Dinarello CA. Cytokine accumulations in CF of multiple sclerosis patients: frequent detection of interleukin-1 and tumor necrosis factor but not interleukin-6. Neurology 1990;40: 1735–1739.

64. Gijbels K, Van Damme J, Proost P, Put W, Carton H, Billiau A. Interleukin 6 production in the central nervous system during experimental autoimmune encephalomyelitis. Eur J Immunol 1990;20:233–235.

65. Chalon MP, Sindic CJM, Laterre EC. Serum and CSF levels of soluble interleukin-2 receptors in MS and other neuro-

logical diseases: a reappraisal. Acta Neurol Scand 1993;87: 77–82.

66. Schade Larsen C, Bjerager M. Determination of interleukin-2 (IL-2) and soluble IL-2 receptors (S-IL-2R) in serum and cerebrospinal fluid does not discriminate purulent and aseptic meningitis. Scand J Infect Dis 1990;22:327–331.

67. Gallo P, Picinno MG, Krzalic L, Tavolato B. Tumor necrosis factor alpha and neurological diseases. J Neuroimmunol 1989;23:41–44.

68. Merrill JE, Chen ISY. HIV-1, macrophages, glial cells, and cytokines in AIDS nervous system disease. FASEB J 1991; 5:2391–2397.

69. Gallo P, Frei K, Rondorf C, Laxdins J, Tavolato B, Fontana A. Human immunodeficiency virus type 1 (HIV-1) infection of the central nervous system: an evaluation of cytokines in cerebrospinal fluid. J Neuroimmunol 1989; 23:109–116.

70. Griffin DE, McArthur JC, Cornblath DR. Soluble interleukin-2 receptor and soluble CD8 in serum and cerebrospinal fluid during human immunodeficiency virus-associated neurologic disease. J Neuroimmunol 1990;28:97–109.

71. Mintz M, Rapaport R, Oleske JM, et al. Elevated serum levels of tumor necrosis factor are associated with progressive encephalopathy in children with acquired immunodeficiency syndrome. Am J Dis Child 1989;143:771–774.

72. Laurenzi MA, Sidén Å, Persson MAA, Norkrans G, Hagberg L, Chiodi F. Cerebrospinal fluid interleukin-6 activity in HIV infection and inflammatory and noninflammatory diseases of the nervous system. Clin Immunol Immunopathol 1990;57:233–241.

73. Grimaldi LME, Martino GV, Franciotta DM, et al. Elevated alpha-tumor necrosis factor levels in spinal fluid from HIV-1-infected patients with central nervous system involvement. Ann Neurol 1991;29:21–25.

74. Merrill JE, Koyana Y, Zack J, Thomas L, Martin F, Chem ISY. Induction of interleukin-1 and tumor necrosis factor alpha in brain cultures by human immunodeficient virus type 1. J Virol 1992;66:2217–2225.

75. Genis P, Jett M, Bernton EW, et al. Cytokines and arachidonic metabolites produced during human immunodeficiency virus (HIV)-infected macrophage-astroglia interactions: implications for the neuropathogenesis of HIV disease. J Exp Med 1992;176:1703–1718.

76. Tyor WR, Glass JD, Griffin JW, et al. Cytokine expression in the brain during the acquired immunodeficiency syndrome. Ann Neurol 1992;31:349–360.

77. Griffin DE, McArthur JC, Cornblath DR. Neopterin and interferon-gamma in serum and cerebrospinal fluid of patients with HIV-associated neurologic disease. Neurology 1991;41:69–74.

CHAPTER 27

DNA VIRUSES THAT AFFECT CYTOKINE NETWORKS

Grant McFadden

DNA VIRUSES AND CYTOKINES

Viruses that infect vertebrate hosts have been selected through evolutionary pressures to be capable of propagation in the face of an impressive array of immune defense mechanisms (1–7). The ability of a given virus to survive an encounter with an immunocompetent host often depends critically on the extent to which the effector cells and the regulatory molecules that orchestrate the immune response become altered, for example, by virtue of virus replication in immune cells or the activities of viral gene products that modulate the immune network (1,4,5). The consequence of this tug-of-war between virus and host can be recognition and clearance of the virus, unchecked replication leading to disease or death of the host, or establishment of a persistent state, which, at some later date, can result in viral recrudescence and spread if the status of the immune surveillance becomes less effective (2–4,8–10).

In viruses that infect humans, the balance between the host range specificities of the infecting virus and the vigor of the consolidated immune response has a major role in determining whether viruses cause subclinical, latent, or acutely pathogenic infections. In fact, the inability of a host to expeditiously clear a virus infection can be a prelude to secondary disease syndromes, including autoimmune disorders and cancer (10,11). DNA viruses, particularly those that have sufficient genomic size to encode

for more proteins than are minimally required to drive the basic essentials of viral replication, have evolved multiple strategies by which specific virus-encoded gene products interact with elements of the host immune system to retard or inhibit effector molecules that carry out immune clearance (12,13). Some of these viral defense mechanisms, for example, have been targeted at the major histocompatibility complex (MHC)–restricted antigen presentation pathway, which alerts the infected host to the presence of "nonself" viral antigens (5,14–16). This review considers how proteins encoded by DNA viruses can directly affect cytokine elaboration or function and thereby provide some selective advantage for the virus.

It is well known that the cytokine networks that regulate the immune response to pathogens are complex, interactive, and frequently redundant. During the multi-system response to infections by viruses, the roles that individual cytokine activities have can be obscured by the fact that many cytokines operate in ways that can be mutually synergistic or antagonistic, depending on the context of release and site of action (17–19). In theory, any cytokine that stimulates or regulates the various elements of the inflammatory response (e.g., macrophage, natural killer [NK] cells) or the development of acquired immunity (e.g., cytotoxic T cells, helper T cells, B cells) can be classified as "antiviral." Table 27–1 lists the major cytokines that have been frequently implicated as critical in mediating an efficient antiviral response. Of particular importance are the interferons (IFNs), which were first described for their ability to induce the antiviral state in uninfected cells (20–30).

Given the importance of interferons (IFN-α, IFN-β, and IFN-γ) as both antiviral effector molecules and key regulators of the immune response, it is perhaps not surprising that viruses have evolved a variety of strategies to dampen or evade the biological activities of this family of ligands (31–34). In this regard, DNA viruses have been somewhat more successful at such strategies, and they tend to be less sensitive to the effects of IFN than RNA viruses (33,34). A second major cytokine with direct, although poorly understood, antiviral properties is tumor necrosis factor (TNF-α and TNF-β) (35–40), and similar anti-TNF strategies have also been described among DNA viruses (41). All these cytokines are pleiotropic effector molecules with both antiviral and antiproliferative properties, and many are proinflammatory and stimulate monocyte cytotoxicity. Thus, they can be viewed as coparticipants in a more generalized conspiracy of immune molecules that mediates natural and acquired immunity to virus infections.

The ability to analyze the roles of specific antiviral cytokines in the past few years has been aided by the emergence of several technologies that can segregate individual cytokine functions from the overlapping complexities of the immune network. For example, the following experimental strategies have provided important clues as to the relative importance of particular cytokines in the response to individual viruses: (a) utilization of cytokine inhibitors, such as antibodies, soluble receptors, or drug antagonists, to specifically inhibit individual cytokines during virus infection of susceptible hosts (42–46); (b)

infection of transgenic animals bearing knockout lesions in the genes of host cytokines or their receptors (47); (c) virulence studies with viruses, especially vaccinia, that have been engineered to overexpress cellular cytokines at the site of virus infection to assess alterations in pathogenicity (48,49); and (d) analysis of the consequence of inactivating identified viral anticytokine genes by infecting test animals with viruses containing targeted deletions (50).

These studies helped reinforce the importance of anticytokine strategies for viruses to persist in populations of outbred immunocompetent hosts. Unlike RNA viruses, which generally have limited size restrictions on the amount of genetic information that can be contained in any one genome, DNA viruses frequently encode molecular homologues of host cytokines, their receptors, or regulator molecules that modulate cytokine induction or biological activity (12,13). In some instances, it is not entirely clear if these virus genes have arisen from the capture of related cellular genes, possibly via cDNA intermediates, or by convergent evolution into functional mimics of cellular proteins (13,51); in either case, the end result is generation of virus-specific effector/regulator molecules that can alter the host cytokine circuitry sufficiently to favor virus survival. To date, members from five major DNA virus groups have been implicated in such anticytokine strategies (i.e., poxviruses, herpesviruses, adenoviruses, hepadenoviruses, and papovaviruses), and the following sections consider examples utilized by member viruses that infect both humans and related vertebrate host model systems.

TABLE 27–1   PRINCIPAL ANTIVIRAL CYTOKINES

Cytokine	Source	Antiviral Function
IFN-α	Infected leukocytes	Direct antiviral activity; MHC-I up-regulator
IFN-β	Infected nonimmune cells (e.g. fibroblasts)	Similar to IFN-α
IFN-γ	Activated T and NK cells	Direct antiviral activity; MHC-I, II up-regulator; activates macrophages and NK cells
IL-1α and β	Activated APCs	Synergistic with TNF and IFN; stimulates T and B cells
TNF-α	Activated APCs	Direct antiviral activity; synergistic with IL-1, IFN; stimulates T and B cells, neutrophils; MHC-I up-regulator
TNF-β	Activated T cells	Similar to TNF-α
IL-6	Activated T cells and APCs	Stimulates T and B cells; triggers acute-phase responses (with IL-1, TNF)
IL-8 chemokine family (e.g., MCP-1, RANTES, M1P-1α)	Activated T cells and APCs	Attracts and stimulates infiltrating leukocytes

IFN = interferon; MHC = major histocompatibility complex; NK = natural killer cells; IL = interleukin; APC = antigen-presenting cells.

VIRAL PROTEINS WITH HOMOLOGY TO CYTOKINES OR GROWTH FACTORS

In some cases, immune subversion can be carried out with the aid of viral molecules that mimic the actual function of a cellular cytokine by possessing sufficient conformational similarity to the host ligand to be capable of binding to and stimulating the native cellular receptors. To date, this strategy has only been observed for poxviral homologs of two distinct growth factor families and herpesvirus homologs of one particular immunosuppressive cytokine, interleukin-10 (IL-10) (Table 27–2). Although the poxviral growth factors are not, strictly speaking, cytokines, they are closely related regulatory molecules, and they provide a useful paradigm for studying virus/cytokine relationships. As ligand mimics, these molecules illustrate how virus-encoded receptor agonists can function in a positive manner to inappropriately induce a biological response that favors the virus. Although yet to be formally demonstrated, the possibility also exists that certain viral gene products might function as receptor antagonists that bind but inhibit activation of cellular receptors. Given the large number of viral proteins of unknown function that are secreted from the infected cell, particularly in the poxvirus and herpesvirus systems, this remains an attractive, although speculative, hypothesis.

Poxviral growth factors

In 1963 Kato and associates (52), in an attempt to explain how the poxvirus Shope fibroma virus (SFV) caused benign proliferative tumors in rabbits, hypothesized that the virus-infected cells might release a factor that caused uninfected subcutaneous fibroblasts to proliferate by a paracrine-like mechanism. The first suggestion that poxviruses might indeed encode growth factor–like ligands came when computer-assisted database alignment analyses revealed significant homology between a previously sequenced vaccinia early gene, which expressed a 140aa protein designated 19K (53), and the epidermal growth factor (EGF)/transforming growth factor-α (TGF-α) family of growth factors (54–56). The vaccinia protein, now referred to as vaccinia growth factor (VGF), was 45% identical to human EGF (between amino acids 45–89 of VGF), and it maintained all six of the critical cysteine residues required for the characteristic folding domains of the EGF/TGF-α family (57,58). VGF was later shown to be secreted from cells infected with vaccinia as a processed glycoprotein capable of binding to the EGF receptor, inducing tyrosine autophosphorylation and transmitting a proper mitogenic signal, similar to the natural ligands (59–64). Related poxvirus growth factor genes have also been described in *Molluscum contagiosum* (65), variola (66), SFV (67), myxoma virus (68), and malignant rabbit fibroma virus (MRV), a recombinant between Shope fibroma virus and myxoma (69). The growth factor encoded by SFV and MRV (SFGF), and by myxoma (MGF), are also expressed as biologically active ligands for the EGF receptor (70–73), and it is likely that many, if not all, poxviruses encode related growth factors.

Studies using deletion constructs of the growth factor genes in vaccinia, MRV, and myxoma virus indicate that they are dispensable for virus replication in cultured cells, but that they cause attenuated diseases in infected animals (74–77). Importantly, at least in the case of myxoma virus, wild-type levels of virus virulence can be restored by inserting the gene for the cellular TGF-α into the MGF-minus myxoma genome, suggesting that the native targets for the virus ligand in infected tissue are cells bearing the EGF receptor (78). It is likely that the function of the poxviral growth factors is to stimulate, in either an autocrine

TABLE 27–2   VIRAL PROTEINS THAT MIMIC CYTOKINES OR GROWTH FACTORS

Virus	Gene Product	Homologous Cytokine/Growth Factor	Biological Activity
Poxvirus			
Vaccinia	VGF/19K	EGF/TGFa	Yes
SFV/MRV	SFGF	EGF/TGFa	Yes
Myxoma	MGF	EGF/TGFa	Yes
Molluscum contagiosum	McGF	EGF/TGFa	?
Variola	VaGF	EGF/TGFa	?
Poxvirus			
orf	A2R	VEGF	Yes
Herpesvirus			
EBV	BCRF1 (vIL-10)	IL-10	Yes
Equine Herpes (EHV-2)	BCRF1 homolog	IL-10	?

autocrine or paracrine fashion, a mitogenic signal in cells at the infected site to induce host S-phase–dependent functions that would benefit macromolecular synthesis pathways of the virus. These viral growth factors also contribute to the hyperproliferative state in lesions associated with poxviruses that cause benign tumors.

A second poxvirus growth factor, to date only described in the orf poxvirus of sheep, is a homolog of the vascular endothelial growth factor (79). The vascular endothelial growth factor family has a pivotal role in vascularization, tissue remodeling, and angiogenesis (80), but the role that this ligand might have in poxvirus pathogenesis remains to be determined.

EBV vIL-10

In 1990, a new lymphokine, designated cytokine synthesis inhibitory factor, which was defined by its ability to inhibit the release of a variety of cytokines by T cells of the Th1 class, was cloned (81). Interestingly, the deduced sequence of this human ligand was shown to possess a high degree (more than 80% at the amino acid level) of homology with the BCRF1 open-reading frame of Epstein-Barr virus (EBV) (81–83). The cellular ligand, now referred to as IL-10, and the EBV homolog, designated vIL-10, which is expressed late in the EBV lytic pathway, were shown to possess a variety of similar, but not identical, biological properties that suggested they both functioned by repressing certain aspects of the cellular immune system (84–89). For example, vIL-10 inhibits IFN-γ production by T cells and NK cells, and is a macrophage deactivating factor, suggesting that this viral ligand may have an anti-inflammatory role to protect EBV-infected cells from clearance by immune effector cells, particularly of the delayed-type hypersensitivity pathway. In contrast, vIL-10 up-regulates B cells, the natural lymphocyte reservoir of EBV, by stimulating proliferation and differentiation into immunoglobin-secreting plasma cells, suggesting an additional positive role for the ligand in favoring replication of the virus and transformation of B cells into immortalized lines. It has also been suggested that the ability of vIL-10 to enhance secretion of anti-EBV antibodies might actually facilitate uptake of opsonized virions into susceptible cells by Fc receptors (89).

There is no direct evidence for the role of vIL-10 in the propagation of EBV, but it is possible that the viral or host ligand contributes to the generalized immune response perturbations associated with EBV disease, especially infectious mononucleosis and possibly chronic fatigue syndrome. Although the consolidated effects of vIL-10 on the immune recognition of EBV are, under certain conditions, paradoxical (90–92), it is likely that the generalized depression of initiation of the cellular immune response, particularly the activity of antigen-presenting cells (APCs), contributes to either establishment or persistence of EBV latency.

A related vIL-10 gene has also been described in the genome of equine herpesvirus (EHV) type 2 (93), but the role that this gene has in EHV pathogenesis is unknown. However, an animal model for vIL-10 involvement in herpesvirus pathogenesis may prove useful for the study of vIL-10 involvement in EBV-associated diseases in humans.

VIRAL PROTEINS FUNCTIONALLY RELATED TO CYTOKINE RECEPTORS

Cytokines transmit biological information by binding to cellular receptors and initiating signal transduction events that culminate in a biological response (94). One of the ways that some cytokines are believed to be regulated is by elaboration of soluble secreted forms of cellular receptors that can bind and inactivate the extracellular ligands (95,96). In an analogous fashion, one of the emerging strategies for virus intervention of cytokine-mediated immune responses is use of virus-encoded mimics of secreted cytokine receptors that sequester host cytokine ligands before they interact with their cognate cellular receptor. Such viral receptor homologues have been termed *viroceptors* (50) to indicate the generalized strategy of intercepting cytokines important for the antiviral response. Table 27–3 lists the known viroceptors, in addition to other related virus encoded receptor-like molecules, whose function remains to be demonstrated.

Poxviral TNF receptors

Two distinct cellular receptors for TNF-α and TNF-β have been identified, cloned, and sequenced (97–99). These receptors, designated type I and II (or p55 and p75), mediate the antiviral and cytotoxic activities of TNF (100–105), and they are members of a growing superfamily of surface receptors characterized by a four-fold repeat of cysteine-rich extracellular domains (97–100). Database analyses revealed substantial sequence homology between the ligand binding domain of the p75-TNF receptor and the previously sequenced T2 open-reading frame of SFV (100,106). When the T2 gene was independently expressed in transfected cells, the resulting 58-kd protein was found to be secreted into the medium, and it specifically bound TNF-α and TNF-β in a fashion analogous to the secreted forms of the cellular TNF receptors (107). A related poxvirus myxoma, the agent of myxomatosis, was subsequently shown to encode a homologous T2 protein, and targeted deletion analysis of the myxoma-T2 gene indicated that T2 was dispensable for virus growth in tissue cultured cells, but the deletion mutant could only induce

TABLE 27–3   VIRAL HOMOLOGUES OF CYTOKINE RECEPTORS

Virus	Gene Product	Homologous Cytokines/Growth Factor Receptor	Activity of Viral Protein
Poxvirus			
SFV/myxoma	T2	TNF-R (I,II) (p55/p75)	Inhibits TNF-α and TNF-β
Vaccinia	C22L/A53R	TNF-R (I,II) (p55/p75)	(Fragmented genes)
Cowpox	crmB/A53R	TNF-R (I,II) (p55/p75)	Binds TNF-α and TNF-β
Variola	G2R	TNF-R (I,II) (p55/p75)	?
Poxvirus			
SFV/myxoma	T7	IFNγ-R	Inhibits IFN-γ
Vaccinia	B8R	IFNγ-R	Inhibits IFN-γ
Variola	B8R	IFNγ-R	?
Poxvirus			
Vaccinia/cowpox	B15R*	IL-1-R (II) (p60)	Inhibits IL-1β, but not IL-1α
Variola	B14R	IL-1-R (II) (p60)	(Fragmented gene)
Poxvirus			
Vaccinia	B18R**	IL-1-R	No binding of IL-1 or IL-6
		IL-6-R	detected
Herpesvirus			
CMV	US28	Rantes-R/M1P-1α-R and IL-8-R (B)	Binds several chemokines
	US27, UL33	G-protein coupled-R	?
Herpesvirus			
H. saimiri	HVS-15	CD59	?
	ECRF3	IL-8-R (B)	Binds IL-8, GRO/MGSA, and NAP-2
Hepadnavirus			
HBV	env/pre-S1	?	Binds IL-6

*B15R in strain WR (B16R in strain Copenhagen).
**B18R in strain WR (B19R in strain Copenhagen).

an attenuated disease syndrome in infected rabbits (50). Inhibition studies showed that the secreted viral T2 is a potent inhibitor of the cytotoxic functions of rabbit TNF-α suggesting that inactivation of TNF is critical for virus virulence (50,108).

Other poxviral homologues of the TNF receptor super-family have been detected in the genomes of variola (66,109), vaccinia (50,110), and cowpox (111). Vaccinia (strain Copenhagen) contains two TNF receptor–like genes (C22L and A53R), but both exist as only discontinuous open-reading frame fragments (50,110), indicating that at least this strain of vaccinia has lost this particular anti-TNF strategy during its evolution into an attenuated virus vaccine (112). The inhibitory capacity of the myx-

oma T2 protein is highly unique for rabbit TNF (108), suggesting that the ligand specificity of a given poxviral anti-TNF molecule may very well reflect the host in which the virus has evolved. It is not known if T2 functions in infected animals by limiting the direct antiviral or cytotoxic functions of TNF or by dampening its immunoregulatory activities, or both.

Poxviral IFN-γ receptors

While searching for additional poxviral viroceptors that might utilize similar anticytokine strategies against other cellular ligands important for the antiviral response,

Upton and colleagues (113) discovered that the major 37-kd protein secreted from cells infected with myxoma (strain Lausanne) possessed sequence homology with the ligand binding domain of the cellular receptor for IFN-γ. The 37-kd protein, encoded by the T7 gene of both myxoma and SFV, specifically bound and inhibited rabbit IFN-γ, suggesting that IFN-γ was yet another important component of the host antipoxvirus response (113). The poxviral T2- and T7-secreted viroceptors thus represent the first examples of the "star wars" strategy that DNA viruses utilize against extracellular cytokines to combat their own immune destruction (114). Unlike the T2 family of anti-TNF proteins, the homologous T7-like genes in vaccinia (B8R) and variola (B8R) are intact, and they presumably encode functional proteins targeted against the IFN-γ of their respective hosts, which, at least in the case of variola, is humans (66,113).

Poxviral IL-1 receptors

IL-1α and IL-1β are pleiotropic cytokines that regulate the inflammatory process and participate in the early events of the host antiviral response (115,116). Two cellular receptors of IL-1 have been described, each of which recognize both ligands with comparable affinities (117–119). Database analyses revealed that the B15R open-reading frame of vaccinia (strain WR) was structurally similar to the cellular IL-1 receptors, and it had the sequence motifs expected for a secreted glycoprotein (119,120). Unlike the cellular receptors, the expressed B15R protein from vaccinia and cowpox was found to bind only IL-1β, and not IL-1α or IL-1 receptor antagonist (121,122). However, IL-1α is largely cell-associated, and the ability of B15R to bind and inhibit the biological activity of only IL-1β suggests that secreted IL-1 activity is an important contributor to the immune response to poxvirus infection. Vaccinia virus constructs in which the B15R gene has been disrupted have been described by two different groups to have variable effects on pathogenicity (121,122). Inoculation of mice by the intranasal route did not alter mortality levels, but it caused an earlier onset of disease symptoms, possibly due to the increase of available circulating IL-1β ligand brought about by the absence of B15R inhibition (121). In contrast, intracranial inoculation in mice resulted in a two order of magnitude reduction in lethality, thus defining B15R as a virus virulence gene (122). Given, however, that vaccinia virus has no natural vertebrate host—indeed, its origins before being adapted as a live vaccine are relatively obscure (112)—it would be of interest to compare the effect of deletions of B15R homologs from other poxviruses that have a defined pathogenic syndrome in a natural host.

A second poxviral member of this IL receptor superfamily is the vaccinia (strain WR) B18R gene, which encodes a protein found at the surface of infected cells, and secreted as a major soluble antigen (123–126). The B18R sequence has some similarity with the cellular receptors for both IL-1 and IL-6 (120), but binding studies with the B18R protein revealed no interaction with human IL-1α, IL-1β, or IL-6 (121). However, the possibility still remains that B18R could be specific for another, perhaps still unidentified, ligand of this family.

CMV and herpesvirus saimiri receptor homologues

Cytomegalovirus (CMV) is a betaherpesvirus capable of establishing latent infections in myeloid and lymphoid cells that can persist for a lifetime in normal immunocompetent hosts, but can cause serious pathogenicity if an individual acquires deficits in cellular immunity (127,128). There have been numerous suggestions in the literature that CMV might exert immunosuppressive effects by altering the functional cytokine network of the infected host (129–131), but the first clue that virus-encoded gene products might have a direct role in cytokine perturbation came when DNA sequencing studies of the human CMV genome revealed that three gene products, US27, US28, and UL33, were homologous to a large superfamily of G-protein–coupled membrane receptors (132–134). Because the similarity between virus and host genes suggested a common ancestral origin, it was proposed that this represented a case of viral hijacking of receptors (51,133), but whether these open-reading frames exemplify convergent evolution or virus transduction is still debatable. To date, the closest cellular counterpart for these CMV genes is the relationship between US28 and the receptors for macrophage inflammatory protein (MIP)-1α /RANTES (regulated on activation, normal T-expressed and secreted) and for IL-8 (135). All these members carry the signature sequence motifs for seven hydrophobic segments predicted to be membrane-spanning domains, and the N-terminal domains of US28 and the MIP-1α /RANTES receptor are 56% identical, which suggests a common function (135). There are no data on the role of US28 in CMV replication or pathogenesis, but it has been hypothesized that a functional virus receptor capable of binding MIP-1α/RANTES might alter the responsiveness of CMV-infected lymphoid or myeloid cells to stimulation by one or more members of this chemokine family (135).

A second set of herpesvirus/host sequence homologies has been reported for Herpesvirus saimiri, a T-lymphotropic gammaherpesvirus that establishes latent infections in the T cells of the squirrel monkey (136). Sequencing studies of the H. saimiri genome revealed a variety of intriguing similarities with cellular genes, particularly complement control proteins (CCPH), cyclins (ECLF2),

G-protein–coupled receptors (ECRF3), and CD59 (HSV-15) (137–141). The ECRF3 gene bears 30% identity with the IL-8 low-affinity receptor (B), and the expressed viral protein is a functional receptor for IL-8, GRO/MGSA, and NAP-2 (137,139) (Ahuza SK, Murphy P, personal communication).

Hepatitis B IL-6 binding protein

During the analysis of cellular receptors for hepatitis B virus (HBV), Neurath and colleagues (142) observed that the pre-S1 sequence of the viral envelope protein (residues 21–47) specifically bound to the free and membrane-anchored forms of IL-6. HBV can infect peripheral blood lymphocytes, suppress the growth of a variety of hematopoietic progenitor cells, and be reactivated from circulating lymphoid cells by mitogenic activation (143), suggesting that cytokines that regulate these cells could directly affect viral functions. Although not known to possess formal homology with IL-6 receptors, the pre-S1 region of the viral envelope may have a viroceptor-like role in the initial infection of lymphocytes and monocytes or in dampening IL-6 regulatory functions during an early acute-response phase to HBV infection.

VIRAL PROTEINS THAT MODULATE CYTOKINE INDUCTION

Because many antiviral cytokines are rapidly induced by virus infection, one way that viruses can interrupt the cytokine network in a targeted fashion is by down-regulating expression of the cytokine genes or by modifying the synthesis and processing pathways that produce the mature secreted ligand. Table 27–4 lists examples of the different strategies currently known to be employed by specific gene products of DNA viruses. In theory, direct virus intervention could occur by: (a) modulation of key transcriptional factors that are known to regulate cytokine gene transcription (HBV, adenovirus, papillomavirus, several herpesviruses); (b) generalized inhibition of cellular transcription or translation to favor expression of virus genes (many DNA viruses); (c) alteration of post-translational processing or transport pathways through the endoplasmic reticulum (ER) and Golgi; and (d) inhibition of the proteolytic activation of cytokine precursors, intracellularly, at the cell surface, or after secretion into the extracellular spaces (poxviruses). Although mechanism (c) has not yet been formally described for cytokines, several studies detailed the altered processing and transport of cellular MHC proteins in cells infected by CMV (144–147) and of multiple processing defects of cellular proteins induced by papillomaviruses (148);

therefore, this strategy remains at least theoretically possible for the trafficking of specific cytokines. There are also reports of how several DNA viruses (e.g., CMV, HBV) affect key transcriptional regulators, such as NF-κB, by either direct or indirect means (149–152), which could indirectly affect cytokine gene transcription. In other situations, such as following infections of lymphoid cells with a variety of poxviruses, there are perturbations in cytokine secretion profiles that are suspected to be virus-specific, but the underlying mechanisms remain undefined (153,154).

The following section focuses on viral gene products believed to directly inhibit cytokine activation at the level of transcriptional induction and post-translational processing. In some cases, the viral gene products have been identified, but in others, especially the herpesviruses, the regulators remain to be identified.

Poxviral serpins that inhibit proteolytic activation of cytokines

Poxviruses are known to encode multiple members of the serpin (serine protease inhibitor) superfamily, some of which are believed to have direct roles in poxvirus pathogenesis (155,156). Among members of the orthopoxvirus genus, the serpin genes are referred to as *SPI-1* (*B24R* in vaccinia), *SPI-2* (*crmA* or *38K* in cowpox; *B13R* in vaccinia), and *SPI-3* (*K2L* in vaccinia) (157–160). Currently, the SPI-1 gene product has no known function, but SPI-3 has been implicated in cell-to-cell fusion (161–163). Studies of viral growth characteristics on chicken chorioallantoic membranes using a cowpox mutant that lacks the SPI-2 gene demonstrate that virus lesions have a distinctive white pock phenotype because of excessive infiltration with heterophils, suggesting that SPI-2/crmA inhibit some aspect of the chemotactic signal for inflammatory lymphocytes (164–166).

Recently, it has been shown that the crmA/SPI-2 gene product of cowpox is capable of blocking the intracellular proteolytic activation of IL-1β (167), thus providing at least a partial explanation for the increased inflammatory response of cowpox mutants deleted of the SPI-2 serpin gene (166). IL-1β is normally synthesized in an inactive precursor form, which is subsequently cleaved by a cysteine protease during transport to the extracellular environment (168–170). No other intracellular cytokine maturation process has been shown to be affected by SPI-2, but it is reasonable to speculate that other antiviral cytokines that are first synthesized as precursor molecules (e.g., TNF-α) could be targeted by viral serpins as well.

Another related, but distinct, serpin gene, designated *Serp1*, has also been identified in the genome of myxoma virus and malignant rabbit fibroma virus (MRV), and was shown to be required for induction of myxoma/MRV dis-

TABLE 27–4   VIRAL PROTEINS THAT MODULATE CYTOKINE INDUCTION

Virus	Viral Protein	Activity
Poxvirus 　Cowpox 　Vaccinia	SPI-2/crmA/38K SPI-2/B13R	Viral serpin that inhibits intracellular 　proteolytic activation of IL-1β
Poxvirus 　Myxoma/MRV	Serp1	Secreted viral serpin that inhibits extracellular 　(target protease unknown)
Hepadnavirus 　HBV	Nucleocapsid (core/e) Truncated polymerase (terminal protein) X-protein	Represses IFN-β promoter Represses IFN-β induction by dsRNA Transactivates IFN-β promoter
Adenovirus 　Ad5	12S Ela	Inhibits induction of IFN-β and IL-6
Papillomavirus 　BPV-1	E2	Transactivates promoters for GM-CSF, IL-2, 　and IL-3
Herpesvirus 　HSV-1 　EBV 　HHV-6	? ? ?	Inhibits IL-1β and IL-3 induction, but 　up-regulates IL-6 and TNF-α Inhibits TF-α transcription, but up-regulates 　IL-6 Inhibits IL-6 induction, but induces IL-1β and 　TNF-α

ease in infected rabbits (171–172). The Serp1 protein inhibits a variety of serine proteases, including plasmin, urokinase, tissue plasminogen activator, and a member of the complement cascade (173), but its precise molecular target in infected tissues has not been formally identified. The Serp1 protein is secreted from infected cells as a processed glycoprotein, and interferes with some aspect of the inflammatory process (172). One possibility that has been suggested is that Serp1 might interfere with the extracellular proteolytic activation of a cytokine precursor or latent complex; however, the functional significance of such inhibition in terms of regulating inflammation or chemotaxis remains to be investigated. The serpin members are an extremely pleiotropic family of regulators, with a wide range of regulatory activities on the immune response (174,175), and the possibility that they might directly participate in the early inflammatory response to viral infection merits further investigation.

Hepatitis B transactivation/repression of IFN expression

HBV, an extremely important pathogen in humans, is responsible worldwide for hundreds of millions of cases of hepatitis, cirrhosis of the liver, and hepatocarcinoma (176–180). HBV encodes only four major primary translation products, but several of the virus proteins are capable of transactivating or repressing viral and cellular genes (181). Of particular interest for this discussion are the HBV proteins that are capable of regulating the IFN-β promoter, presumably to achieve some measure of protection from the antiviral activity of IFN (33,34). In fact, it has been known for some time that patients chronically infected with HBV are often deficient in IFN induction and responsiveness; in fact, HBV is one of the few viruses (along with certain papillomaviruses) that are amenable to treatment with therapeutic doses of IFN (182–184).

The nucleocapsid gene of HBV is expressed as a nuclear core protein and a secreted form referred to as e-antigen. Transient transfection experiments with individually expressed HBV open-reading frames revealed that both the 21.5-kd core protein and the smaller e-antigen are capable of suppressing induction of the human IFN-β gene by double-stranded RNA (185–187), but the targets for this inhibition remain to be identified. In related experiments, Foster and associates (188) demonstrated that the expressed HBV polymerase could inhibit both the responsiveness of transfected cells to IFN-α and IFN-γ (discussed later) and the induction of IFN-β by double-stranded RNA. The inhibitory activity was most pronounced in transfected cell lines expressing truncated polymerase ("terminal protein"), which lacks reverse transcriptase and RNAse activities, suggesting that the inhibitory domain might be masked in productively infected cells (188). The situation is further complicated by the fact that the HBV-X protein, a potent transactivator of viral and cellular genes (181,189–198), can dramatically up-regulate the IFN-β promoter (199). In cases of coexpression of both X protein and core/e-antigens, the repressive effect of core/e-antigens was dominant (186), suggesting that the effect on the IFN-β promoter by HBV regulatory molecules in infected hepatocytes may very well reflect a summated response to the competing activities of all three viral regulatory proteins.

Adenovirus Ela repression of IFN and cytokine induction

Adenoviruses are ubiquitous in the human population, and they have evolved a variety of strategies to circumvent immune clearance to allow long-term persistence (41,202–204). Adenoviruses are known to have major effects on expression levels of cellular genes in both infected and virus-transformed cells (205,206), and among the major virus transcriptional regulators are the protein products (i.e., 289 and 243 aa) of the Ela gene (207–209). Of relevance to this discussion is the observation that Ela proteins of Ad5 not only interfere with the responsiveness of cells to the effects of IFN-α and IFN-γ (described later), but also they repress the ability of double-stranded RNA to activate the IFN-β promoter (209). Similarly, the Ela proteins were found to down-regulate induction of the IL-6 promoter by a variety of agents, including IL-1, TNF, phorbol ester, and di-butyryl cAMP (210). In both cases, the repression is likely at the level of the transcription factors relevant to each promoter, but the affected molecules have not been defined. The selective advantage for the virus by preventing IFN-β induction is obvious, but inhibition of IL-6 induction may also contribute to viral persistence by dampening the generalized acute-phase response or by preventing IL-6–induced up-regulation of cellular Ela-like proteins (211).

Papillomavirus E2 transactivation of cytokine expression

Papillomaviruses are extensively distributed in the human population; they are the causative agents for a variety of epithelial lesions, and certain subtypes are closely associated with anogenital neoplasia (212–214). Among the important papillomavirus regulatory proteins are the products of the E2 region of the viral genome, which contribute to regulation of both viral and cellular genes (215–217). During studies on transactivation of the GM-CSF promoter by the p40-X gene of human T-lymphotrophic virus type 1 (HTLV-1), it was noticed that the papilloma E2 could functionally substitute for the HTLV-1 transactivator (218,219). This transactivation function of E2 was later shown to be targeted to regulatory sequences that control several other cytokine genes, including IL-2 and IL-3, via consensus motifs that also respond to p40-X of HTLV-1 (220). Although keratinocytes that harbor papillomaviruses secrete a variety of cytokines, including IL-3 and GM-CSF, it is still unclear how E2 up-regulation of these genes might contribute to virus persistence, if indeed this process occurs in infected epithelial tissues.

Herpesviruses perturb cytokine induction

All six classes of herpesviruses that infect humans (HSV-1, HSV-2, EBV, CMV, H. zoster, HHV-6) have evolved sophisticated defense strategies against the immune system (10,221–223). Although it is well established that herpesviruses can cause major dysfunction of cytokine expression (224), almost nothing is known about the relevant viral gene products that mediate these alterations. In the case of HSV-1 infection of activated peritoneal macrophages, reductions in mRNA levels for IL-1β and IL-3, but increases for IL-6 levels, have been described, but it was not established if inhibition was at the level of transcriptional or post-transcriptional processing (224,225). EBV strongly inhibits transcription of the TNF-α gene, but not IL-1, and enhances IL-6 production from infected monocytes and macrophages (224,226), whereas HHV-6 induces both TNF-α and IL-1β, but not IL-6, in peripheral blood mononuclear cells (224,227). Given the importance of cytokines in orchestrating the antiviral response, it is reasonable to conclude that much remains to be uncovered in the area of how herpesvirus regulatory proteins interact with cellular regulatory sequences for these particular cytokines. Exactly how these alterations might achieve selective advantage for the viruses deserves to be more fully investigated.

VIRAL PROTEINS THAT MODULATE CYTOKINE SIGNAL TRANSDUCTION

It has been known for some time that several DNA virus groups, especially hepadnaviruses, certain herpes viruses, SV40, adenoviruses, and poxviruses, can counteract at least some of the direct antiviral effects of IFN and TNF (33,34,41). Although not all the viral proteins that block the responsiveness of cells to these antiviral cytokines have been identified, many virus gene products have been independently expressed in the absence of viral replicative functions and shown to affect specific aspects of cytokine signal transduction pathways. In some cases, the anticytokine activity is a direct property of unique viral RNAs, most notably VAI RNA of adenoviruses and EBER RNA of EBV, which affect the dsRNA-dependent protein kinase pathway of the IFN response (34). This section focuses on the known viral proteins encoded by DNA viruses that can modify cytokine responsiveness (Table 27–5), but it is likely that further examples of this class of

intervention will be discovered when more viral open-reading frames are individually expressed and tested.

Adenovirus proteins that affect cytokine responsiveness

IFN is able to establish the antiviral state only after specific cellular genes are up-regulated by the signal transduction events that follow ligand binding to the type I or type II IFN receptors (228–230). Adenoviruses have evolved a variety of strategies to overcome the effects of IFN downstream of receptor signaling (33,34), one of which is blockade of IFN signal transduction by the Ela gene products (231–232). In cells engineered to over-express the Ela proteins of Ad5, the majority of responses to both type I and type II IFNs were found to be blocked (209,233–235). The Eγ-subunit of transcription factor ISGF-3 (but not Eα) was found to be poorly induced in the presence of Ela, but there are likely more transcription factors that are down-regulated by Ela, given the

TABLE 27–5 VIRAL PROTEINS THAT AFFECT CYTOKINE SIGNAL TRANSDUCTION

Virus	Gene Product	Mechanism
Adenovirus	Ela	Inhibits IFN-α and IFN-γ responsiveness; induces TNF sensitivity
	Elb/19K	Inhibits responsiveness to TNF
	E3/14.7K	Inhibits responsiveness to TNF
	E3/10.4K–14.5K	Inhibits responsiveness to TNF
	E3/10.4K–14.5K	Down-regulates EGF^r INS^r, and IGF^r
Poxvirus		
Vaccinia	E3L	Inhibits IFN response by blocking dsRNA-dep. protein kinase
	K3L	Inhibits IFN response by inhibiting eIF2α phosphorylation
	?A18R?	Affects RNAseL/2′–5′A pathway of IFN response
Herpesvirus		
EBV	EBNA-2	Interrupts IFN-α and IFN-β response downstream of ISGF-3
Hepadnavirus		
HBV	Polymerase (terminal protein)	Inhibits response of IFN-α, IFN-β, and IFN-γ at the level of ISGF-3
Papillomavirus		
HPV16 BPV-1	E5	Stimulates EGF^r, CSF-1^r, and PDGF^r (β)

wide spectrum of IFN-responsive genes that are repressed (209,233,234). Another important consequence of Ela action is to render expressing cells more sensitive to TNF-induced cytolysis (41,203). Although the mechanism by which sensitivity to TNF is exacerbated remains to be deciphered (236), the cytotoxicity of TNF for Ela-bearing cells can be augmented by IL-1, which is frequently coinduced with TNF, and would likely be counterproductive to virus survival in the absence of viral countermeasures (237).

To compensate for this apparently self-destructive trait of Ela, which may be a side product of the extensive range of Ela regulatory activities, adenoviruses utilize at least three sets of viral genes to protect infected cells from TNF killing: Elb/19K, E3/14.7K, and the E3/10.4K–14.5K heterodimer (41,203). Protection from TNF cytolysis by Elb/19K protein is human-specific (238), and it is apparently linked to the ability of Elb to enhance Ela-induced cellular transformation (239). The E3/14.7K protein is a relatively specific inhibitor of TNF cytoxicity, but it does not affect the capacity of TNF to up-regulate MHC class I antigens (240). The protein structural domain that defines E3/14.7K activity has been difficult to map, suggesting the entire protein is required for the TNF protective effects (241).

The heterodimer E3/10.4K–14.5K can prevent TNF cytolysis in the absence of other viral proteins. Both polypeptides are integral membrane proteins that have the additional property of being able to down-regulate a variety of cytokine receptors (242–245). Although the TNF inhibitory effect is probably at the level of signal transduction of the TNF pathway, the E3/10.4–14.5K complex has been shown to down-regulate the receptors for EGF, insulin, and insulin-like growth factor (246–248). It is not known if these down-regulations activate the growth factor transduction pathways to provide a more receptive intracellular environment for viral replication, or whether the function of these proteins is to shield the infected cells from immunoregulatory ligands, such as TGF-α. The E3-encoded proteins that shield adenovirus-infected cells from TNF are up-regulated by TNF (249), suggesting yet another mechanism by which these viruses ensure that TNF effector function is neutralized.

Poxvirus proteins that affect IFN signal transduction

There is abundant evidence to suggest that type I and II IFNs are important for the clearance of poxviruses from infected animals (48,49,250,251), and it is not surprising that these viruses have evolved a variety of strategies to circumvent the effects of IFN (34,156). There is evidence that both the RNAseL/2′-5′A pathway and the double-stranded (ds) RNA-dependent protein kinase (DAI) path-

way that is stimulated in IFN-treated cells can be suppressed by poxviruses, particularly vaccinia (252–256), although all infected cells are not equally susceptible to this repression (156, 257–259). The DAI pathway, which involves phosphorylation and inactivation of eIF-2α by dsRNA-activated protein kinase, has been shown to be inhibited by two vaccinia genes, E3L and K3L, albeit by different mechanisms (260). The E3L proteins, p20 and p25, bind and inhibit dsRNA kinase, thus short-circuiting the phosphorylation activity that leads to translational inhibition (261–263). The K3L protein is a homolog of eIF-2α and interferes with the interaction between eIF-2α and the dsRNA-dependent kinase, thus protecting the cellular translation factor from the inhibitory phosphorylation event (260,264). Consistent with this finding, vaccinia virus in which the K3L gene has been deleted is more sensitive to IFN (265).

Vaccinia is also capable of arresting the RNAseL/2′-5′A pathway of IFN response, but the viral genes responsible remain to be formally identified, although involvement of a viral ATPase or phosphatase has been suggested (252,253,256). Another possible candidate is the A18R gene product, which, when mutated, causes an overwhelming induction of the RNAseL/2′-5′A pathway and results in extensive ribonucleolytic digestion of viral and cellular RNA (266–268). There is some evidence that excessive viral dsRNA is produced by aberrant transcription in the absence of A18R function, which could stimulate the RNAseL/2′-5′A pathway (269), but it is also formally possible that A18R is a helicase that could unwind virus dsRNA to prevent activation of the cellular dsRNA-dependant kinase.

EBV EBNA-2 and HBV polymerase block IFN signal transduction by different mechanisms

Immortalization of B cells by EBV requires the activity of several viral proteins, including EBNA-2, a nuclear phosphoprotein that can transactivate both viral and cellular genes (270). Uninfected B-lymphoid cells that have been transfected with the EBNA-2 gene become resistant to the effects of IFN-α, as measured by the ability to reduce cellular proliferation (271). EBNA-2 functions by blocking IFN-responsive gene induction at the level of transcription, but without affecting ISGF-3, suggesting that inhibition occurs further downstream in the IFN response pathway (272). Unlike the case of Ela of adenoviruses, however, EBNA-2 does not block induction of the antiviral state (271). Thus, EBNA-2 may be more critical for maintenance of virus latency in B cells by shielding transformed cells from IFN-α–mediated growth repression rather than by the protection of the viral replicative machinery from IFN inhibition. It has also been reported that EBNA-2, in conjunction with the EBV latent membrane protein, contributes to up-regulation of the insulin receptor and down-regulation of the insulin-like growth factor receptor in Burkitt's lymphoma cells (273), but it is not known if these effects contribute to virus latency.

In contrast, the hepadnaviruses also confer non-responsiveness to IFN at the level of the induction of the antiviral state (33). Cells transfected with HBV DNA are less sensitive to IFN, as measured by replication of superinfecting Sindbis virus and induction of cellular MHC class I antigens (274). As previously mentioned, the HBV terminal protein mediates the IFN blocking effect, at least in part (188). Both type I and II IFNs are less effective on cells bearing polymerase/terminal protein, and the block is believed to occur at the level of the α-subunit of ISGF-3 (188). Importantly, the terminal protein domain of HBV was recently detected in liver biopsy specimens of patients with chronic HBV who failed to respond to IFN therapy, suggesting that IFN resistance at the clinical level may depend on the nature of polymerase expression in infected hepatocytes (275). This anti-IFN activity by terminal protein would be expected to protect HBV-infected hepatocytes not only from the antiviral state but also from induction of MHC class I antigens by IFN-α, IFN-β, and IFN-γ, and of MHC class II antigens by IFN-γ, thus reducing the recognition of infected cells by CD4$^+$ and CD8$^+$ T lymphocytes (16).

Papillomavirus E5 protein down-regulates receptors for several cytokines and growth factors

Several lines of evidence indicate that papillomaviruses can regulate induction, expression, and activity of a variety of cytokines and their receptors (276–278). Only one papillomavirus protein, encoded by the E5 gene, has been directly associated with regulation of cytokine responsiveness. The E5 proteins of BPV-1 and HPV-16 are small hydrophobic proteins that can potentiate the oncogenic transformation of cells transfected with the genes for certain growth factors and cytokine receptors, especially EGF^r and CSF-1^r (279–281). In the case of BPV E5, the viral oncoprotein binds to a pore-forming component of the vacuolar proton pump (282,283) and activates the receptors for EGF, CSF-1, and platelet-derived growth factor-β (PDGF-β) (279,280,284,285). Ligand-independent stimulation of the PDGF-β receptor by E5 protein has been ascribed to formation of a trimolecular complex between E5, the receptor, and the 16-kd pore component of the proton-ATPase (285). Activation of cellular growth factor receptors in the absence of the cognate ligands may provide a selective advantage for epithelial cells harboring active papillomavirus replication, but the absence of an *in vitro* model system makes this hypothesis difficult to test experimentally.

FUTURE PERSPECTIVES

Cytokine function is only one aspect of the consolidated response to viral infection in a vertebrate host, but extensive use of anticytokine strategies mediated by proteins encoded by DNA viruses affirms the critical role that cytokines have in orchestrating the immune response to pathogenic challenge. Other related aspects of viral defence mechanisms against immune clearance used by the larger DNA viruses include elaboration of virus-specific complement binding proteins, expression of viral Fc receptors, and down-regulation of cellular MHC glycoproteins, all of which aid and augment the strategies described in this review (10–16,156,221–223). More needs to be learned about the genomes of the larger DNA viruses, many of which possess numerous open-reading frames apparently dispensable for virus growth in cultured cells but which likely contribute to virus survival in the immunocompetent host. It seems reasonable to expect that more viral mechanisms specifically designed to counteract host cytokines and other related immunoregulatory molecules will be uncovered.

REFERENCES

1. McChesney MB, Oldstone MBA. Viruses perturb lymphocyte functions: selected principles characterizing virus-induced immunosuppression. Annu Rev Immunol 1987;5: 279–304.

2. Bangham CRM, McMichael AJ. T-cell immunity to viruses. In: Feldman M, Lamb J, Owen MJ, eds. T cells. Baltimore: John Wiley & Sons, 1989:281–310.

3. Virelizier J-L. The immune system: an update for virologists. In: Dimmock NJ, Minor PD, eds. Immune responses, virus infections and diseases. Oxford: IRL Press, 1989:3–14.

4. Whitton JL, Oldstone MBA. Virus-induced immune response interactions. Principles of immunity and immunopathology. In: Fields BN, Knipe DM, Chanock RM, et al, eds. Virology, ed 2. New York: Raven, 1990:369–381.

5. Yewdell JW, Bennink JR. Cell biology of antigen processing and presentation to major histocompatibility complex class I molecule-restricted T lymphocytes. Adv Immunol 1992;52:1–123.

6. Doherty PC. Inflammation in virus infections. Semin Virol 1993;4:117–122.

7. Hartshorn KL, Daignault D, Tauber AI. Phagocyte responses to viral infection. In: Gallin JI, Goldstein IM, Snyderman R, eds. Inflammation: basic principles and clinical correlates. New York: Raven, 1992:1017–1031.

8. Oldstone MBA. Viral persistence. Cell 1989;56:517–520.

9. Oldstone MBA. Molecular anatomy of viral persistence. J Virol 1991;65:6381–6386.

10. Garcia-Blanco MA, Cullen BR. Molecular basis of latency of pathogenic human viruses. Science 1991;254:815–820.

11. zur Hausen H. Viruses in human cancers. Science 1991;254:1167–1173.

12. Gooding LR. Virus proteins that counteract host immune defenses. Cell 1992;61:5–7.

13. Smith GL. Virus strategies for evasion of the host response to infection. Trends in Microbiology 1994;82:80–88.

14. Maudsley DJ, Morris AG, Tomkins PT. Regulation by interferon of the immune response to viruses via the major histocompatibility complex antigens. In: Dimmock NJ, Minor PD, eds. Immune responses, virus infections and diseases. Oxford: IRL Press, 1989:15–33.

15. Maudsley DJ, Pound JD. Modulation of MHC antigen expression by viruses and oncogenes. Immunol Today 1991; 12:429–430.

16. McFadden G, Kane K. How DNA viruses perturb functional MHC expression to alter immune recognition. Adv Cancer Res 1994;63:117–209.

17. Larrick JW, Wright SC. Modulation of viral infections by cytokines. Mol Biother 1992;4:87–94.

18. Bowen JC, Daniel S, Rouse BT. Virus infections and cytokines: can we manage the interactions? Int Rev Immunol 1992;8:33–41.

19. Campbell IL. Cytokines in viral diseases. Curr Opin Immunol 1991;3:486–491.

20. Staeheli P. Interferon-induced proteins and the antiviral state. Adv Virus Res 1990;38:147–200.

21. Jokilik WK. Interferons. In: Fields BN, Knipe DM, Chanock RM, et al, eds. Virology, ed 2. New York: Raven, 1990:383–410.

22. Farrar MA, Schreiber RD. The molecular cell biology of interferon-γ and its receptor. Annu Rev Immunol 1993;11:571–611.

23. Sen GC, Lengyel P. The interferon system. A bird's eye view of its biochemistry. J Biol Chem 1992;267:5017–5020.

24. Landolfo S, Garotta G. IFNγ, a lymphokine that modulates immunological and inflammatory responses. J Immunol Res 1991;3:81–94.

25. Vilcek J. Interferons. In: Sporn MB, Roberts AB, eds. Peptide growth factors and their receptors. New York: Springer-Verlag, 1991:3–38.

26. de Maeyer E, de Maeyer-Guignard J. Interferon-γ. Curr Opin Immunol 1992;4:321–326.

27. Nathan C. Interferon and inflammation. In: Gallin JI, Goldstein IM, Snyderman R, eds. Inflammation: basic principles and clinical correlates. New York: Raven, 1992:265–290.

28. Billiau A, Matthys P. Interferon-γ, more of a cachectin than tumor necrosis factor. Cytokine 1992;4:259–263.

29. Tanaka N, Taniguchi T. Cytokine gene regulation: regulatory cis-elements and DNA binding factors involved in the interferon system. Adv Immunol 1992;52:263–281.

30. de Maeyer E, de Maeyer J. Interferons. In: Thomson A, ed. The cytokine handbook. San Diego: Academic Press, 1991:215–239.

31. Taylor JL, Grossberg SE. Recent progress in interferon research: molecular mechanisms of regulation, action, and virus circumvention. Virus Res 1990;15:1–26.

32. Samuel CE. Antiviral actions of interferon. Interferon-regulated cellular proteins and their surprisingly selective antiviral activities. Virology 1991;183:1–11.

33. Kerr IM, Stark GR. The antiviral effects of the interferons and their inhibition. J Interferon Res 1992;12:237–240.

34. McNair ANB, Kerr IM. Viral inhibition of the interferon system. Pharmacol Ther 1993;56:79–95.

35. Fiers W. Tumor necrosis factor. Characterization at the molecular, cellular and in vivo level. FEBS Lett 1991;285:199–212.

36. Larrick JW, Wright SC. Cytotoxic mechanism of tumor necrosis factor-α. FASEB J 1990;4:3215–3223.

37. Beutler B, Cerami A. The biology of cachectin/TNF—a primary mediator of the host response. Annu Rev Immunol 1989;7:625–655.

38. Vassalli P. The pathophysiology of tumor necrosis factors. Annu Rev Immunol 1992;10:411–452.

39. Ruddle NH. Tumor necrosis factor (TNF-α) and lymphotoxin (TNF-β). Curr Opin Immunol 1992;4:327–332.

40. Vilcek J, Lee TH. Tumor necrosis factor. J Biol Chem 1991;266:7313–7316.

41. Wold WSM, Gooding LR. Region E3 of adenovirus: a cassette of genes involved in host immunosurveillance and virus-cell interactions. Virology 1991;184:1–8.

42. Fernandez-Botran R. Soluble cytokine receptors: their role in immunoregulation. FASEB J 1991;5:2567–2574.

43. Taga T, Kishimoto T. Cytokine receptors and signal transduction. FASEB J 1992;6:3387–3396.

44. Jacobs CA, Beckmann MP, Mohler K, Maliszewski CR, Fanslow WC, Lynch DH. Pharmacokinetic parameters and biodistribution of soluble cytokine receptors. Int Rev Exp Pathol 1993;34B:123–135.

45. Arai K, Lee F, Miyajima A, Miyatake S, Arai N, Yokota T. Cytokines: coordinators of immune and inflammatory responses. Annu Rev Biochem 1990;59:783–836.

46. Pugh-Humphreys RGP, Woo J, Thomson AW. Cytokines and their receptors as potential therapeutic targets. In: Thomson A, ed. The cytokine handbook. San Diego: Academic Press, 1991:357–386.

47. Doherty PC. Virus infections in mice with targeted gene disruptions. Curr Opin Immunol 1993;5:439–483.

48. Ramshaw I, Ruby J, Ramsay A, Ada G, Karupiah G. Expression of cytokine by recombinant vaccinia viruses: a model for studying cytokines in virus infections in vivo. Immunol Rev 1992;127:157–182.

49. Ramsay AJ, Ruby J, Ramshaw IA. A case for cytokines as effector molecules in the resolution of virus infection. Immunol Today 1993;14:155–157.

50. Upton C, Macen JL, Schreiber M, McFadden G. Myxoma virus expresses a secreted protein with homology to the tumor necrosis factor receptor gene family that contributes to viral virulence. Virology 1991;184:370–382.

51. Ross EM. Viral hijack of receptors. Nature 1990;344:707–708.

52. Kato S, Miyamoto H, Takahashi M, et al. Shope fibroma and rabbit myxoma viruses. II. Pathogenesis of fibromas in domestic rabbits. Biken J. 1963;6:135–143.

53. Venkatesan S, Gershowitz A, Moss B. Complete nucleotide sequences of two adjacent early vaccinia virus genes lo-

cated within the inverted terminal repetition. J Virol 1982; 44:637–646.

54. Blomquist MC, Hunt LT, Barker WC. Vaccinia virus 19-kilodalton protein: relationship to several mammalian proteins, including two growth factors. Proc Natl Acad Sci USA 1984;81:7363–7367.

55. Reisner A. Similarity between the vaccinia virus 19K early protein and epidermal growth factor. Nature 1985;313: 801–803.

56. Brown JP, Twardzik DR, Marquardt H, Todaro GJ. Vaccinia virus encodes a polypeptide homologous to epidermal growth factor and transforming growth factor. Nature 1985;313:491–492.

57. Laurence DJR, Gusterson BA. The epidermal growth factor. A review of structural and functional relationships in the normal organism and in cancer cells. Tumor Biol 1990; 11:229–261.

58. Carpenter G, Wahl MI. The epidermal growth factor family. In: Sporn MB, Roberts AB, eds. Peptide growth factors and their receptors. New York: Springer-Verlag, 1991:69–170.

59. Twardzik DR, Brown JP, Ranchalis JE, Todaro GJ, Moss B. Vaccinia virus-infected cells release a novel polypeptide functionally related to transforming and epidermal growth factors. Proc Natl Acad Sci USA 1985;82:5300–5304.

60. Stroobant P, Rice AP, Gullick WJ, Cheng DJ, Kerr IM, Waterfield MD. Purification and characterization of vaccinia virus growth factor. Cell 1985;42:383–393.

61. King CS, Cooper JA, Moss B, Twardzik DR. Vaccinia virus growth factor stimulates tyrosine protein kinase activity of A431 cell epidermal growth factor receptors. Mol Cell Biol 1986;6:332–336.

62. Chang W, Lim JG, Hellström I, Gentry LE. Characterization of vaccinia virus growth factor biosynthetic pathway with an antipeptide antiserum. J Virol 1988;62:1080–1083.

63. Schultz GS, White M, Mitchell R, et al. Epithelial wound healing enhanced by transforming growth factor-α and vaccinia growth factor. Science 1987;235:350–352.

64. Lin Y-Z, Ke X-H, Tam JP. Growth inhibition by vaccinia virus growth factor. J Biol Chem 1990;265:18884–18890.

65. Porter CR, Archard LC. Characterization and physical mapping of Molluscum contagiosum virus DNA and location of a sequence capable of encoding a conserved domain of epidermal growth factor. J Gen Virol 1987;68:673–682.

66. Massung RF, Liu L, Qi J, et al. Analysis of the complete genome of smallpox variola major virus strain Bangladesh-1975. Virology 1994;201:215–240.

67. Chang W, Upton C, Hu S-L, Purchio AF, McFadden G. The genome of Shope fibroma virus, a tumorigenic poxvirus, contains a growth factor gene with sequence similarity to those encoding epidermal growth factor and transforming growth factor alpha. Mol Cell Biol 1987;7:535–540.

68. Upton C, Macen JL, McFadden G. Mapping and sequencing of a gene from myxoma virus that is related to those encoding epidermal growth factor and transforming growth factor alpha. J Virol 1987;61:1271–1275.

69. Upton C, Macen JL, Maranchuk RA, Delange AM, McFadden G. Tumorigenic poxviruses: fine analysis of the recombinant junctions in malignant rabbit fibroma virus, a recombinant between Shope fibroma virus and myxoma virus. Virology 1988;166:229–239.

70. Ye Y, Lin Y-Z, Tam JP. Shope fibroma virus growth factor exhibits epidermal growth factor activities in newborn mice. Biochem Biophys Res Commun 1988;154:497–501.

71. Lin Y-Z, Caporaso G, Chang P-Y, Ke X-H, Tam JP. Synthesis of a biological active tumor growth factor from the predicted DNA sequence of Shope fibroma virus. Biochemistry 1988;27:5640–5645.

72. Lin Y-Z, Le X-H, Tam JP. Synthesis and structure-activity study of myxoma virus growth factor. Biochemistry 1991; 30:3310–3314.

73. Chang W, Macaulay C, Hu S-L, Tam JP, McFadden G. Tumorigenic poxviruses: characterization of the expression of an epidermal growth factor related gene in Shope fibroma virus. Virology 1990;179:926–930.

74. Buller RML, Chakrabarti S, Cooper JA, Twardzik DR, Moss B. Deletion of the vaccinia virus growth factor gene reduces virus virulence. J Virol 1988;62:866–874.

75. Buller RML, Chakrabarti S, Moss B, Frederickson T. Cell proliferative response to vaccinia virus is mediated by VGF. Virology 1988;164:182–192.

76. Opgenorth A, Strayer D, Upton C, McFadden G. Deletion of the growth factor gene related to EGF and TGFα reduces virulence of malignant rabbit fibroma virus. Virology 1992;186:175–191.

77. Opgenorth A, Graham K, Nation N, Strayer D, McFadden G. Deletion analysis of two tandemly arranged virulence genes in myxoma virus, M11L and myxoma growth factor. J Virol 1992;66:4720–4731.

78. Opgenorth A, Nation N, Graham K, McFadden G. Transforming growth factor alpha, Shope fibroma growth factor, and vaccinia growth factor can replace myxoma growth factor in the induction of myxomatosis in rabbits. Virology 1993;192:701–709.

79. Lyttle DJ, Fraser KM, Fleming SB, Mercer AA, Robinson AJ. Homologues of vascular endothelial growth factor are encoded by the poxvirus, orf virus. J Virol 1994;68:84–92.

80. Ferrara N, Houck K, Jakeman L, Leung DW. Molecular and biological properties of the vascular endothelial growth factor family of proteins. Endocr Rev 1992;13:18–32.

81. Moore KW, Vieira P, Fiorentino DF, Trounstine ML, Khan T, Mosmann TR. Homology of cytokine synthesis inhibitory factor (IL-10) to the Epstein-Barr virus gene BCRF1. Science 1990;248:1230–1234.

82. Hsu D-H, de Waal-Malefyt R, Fiorentino DF, et al. Expression of interleukin-10 activity by Epstein-Barr virus protein BCRF1. Science 1990;250:830–832.

83. Vieira P, de Waal-Malefyt R, Dang M-N, et al. Isolation and expression of human cytokine synthesis inhibitory factor cDNA clones: homology to Epstein-Barr virus open reading frame BCRF1. Proc Natl Acad Sci USA 1991;88:1172–1176.

84. Howard M, O'Garra A. Biological properties of interleukin-10. Immunol Today 1992;13:198–200.

85. Zlotnik A, Moore KW. Interleukin 10. Cytokine 1991;3: 366–371.

86. Howard M, O'Garra A, Ishida H, de Waal-Malefyt R, de Vries, J. Biological properties of interleukin 10. J Clin Immunol 1992;12:239–247.

87. de Waal-Malefyt R, Yssel H, Roncarolo, M-G, Spits H, de

Vries JE. Interleukin-10. Curr Opin Immunol 1992;4:314–320.

88. Moore KW, Rousset F, Banchereau J. Evolving principles in immunopathology: interleukin 10 and its relationship to Epstein-Barr virus protein BCRF1. Semin Immunopathol 1991;13:157–166.

89. Moore KW, O'Garra A, de Waal-Malefyt R, Vieira P, Mosmann TR. Interleukin-10. Annu Rev Immunol 1993; 11:165–190.

90. Stewart JP, Rooney CM. The interleukin-10 homology encoded by Epstein-Barr virus enhances the reactivation of virus-specific cytotoxic T cell and HLA-unrestricted killer cell responses. Virology 1992;191:773–782.

91. Niiro H, Otsuka T, Abe M, et al. Epstein-Barr virus BCRF1 gene product (viral interleukin 10) inhibits superoxide anion production by human monocytes. Lymphokine Cytokine Res 1992;11:209–214.

92. de Waal-Malefyt R, Haanen J, Spits H, et al. Interleukin 10 (IL-10) and viral IL-10 strongly reduce antigen-specific human T cell proliferation by diminishing the antigen-presenting capacity of monocytes via downregulation of class II major histocompatibility complex expression. J Exp Med 1991;174:915–924.

93. Rode HJ, Janssen W, Rösen-Wolff P, et al. The genome of equine herpesvirus type 2 harbors an interleukin 10 (Il-10)-like gene. Virus Genes 1993;7:111–116.

94. Miyajima A, Kitamura T, Harada N, Yokota T, Arai K. Cytokine receptors and signal transduction. Annu Rev Immunol 1992;10:295–331.

95. Fernandez-Botran R. Soluble cytokine receptors: their role in immunoregulation. FASEB J 1991;5:2567–2574.

96. Jacobs CA, Beckmann MP, Mohler K, et al. Pharmacokinetic parameters and biodistribution of soluble cytokine receptors. In: Richter GW, Solez K, Ryffel B, eds. Int Rev Exp Pathol vol 34. San Diego: Academic Press, 1993:123–135.

97. Sprang S. The divergent receptors for TNF. TIBS 1990;15:366–368.

98. Loetscher H, Steinmetz M, Lesslauer W. Tumor necrosis factor: receptors and inhibitors. Cancer Cells 1991;3:221–226.

99. Tartaglia LA, Goeddel DV. Two TNF receptors. Immunol Today 1992;13:151–153.

100. Smith CA, Davis T, Anderson D, et al. A receptor for tumor necrosis factor defines an unusual family of cellular and viral proteins. Science 1990;248:1019–1023.

101. Loetscher H, Pan Y-CE, Lahm H-W, et al. Molecular cloning and expression of the human 55 kd tumor necrosis factor receptor. Cell 1990;61:351–359.

102. Schall TJ, Lewis M, Koller KJ, et al. Molecular cloning and expression of a receptor for human necrosis factor. Cell 1990;61:361–370.

103. Heller RA, Song K, Fan N, Chang DJ. The p70 tumor necrosis factor receptor mediates cytotoxicity. Cell 1992;70:47–56.

104. Wong GHW, Tartaglia LA, Lee MS, Goeddel DV. Antiviral activity of tumor necrosis factor (TNF) is signaled through the 55-kDa receptor, type I TNF. J. Immunology 1992; 149:3350–3353.

105. Tartaglia LA, Rothe M, Hu Y-F, Goeddel DV. Tumor necro-

sis factor's cytotoxic activity is signaled by the p55 TNF receptor. Cell 1993;73:213–216.

106. Upton C, DeLange AM, McFadden G. Tumorigenic poxviruses: genomic organization and DNA sequence of the telomeric region of the Shope fibroma virus genome. Virology 1987;160:20–30.

107. Smith CA, Davis T, Wignall JM, et al. T2 open reading frame from the Shope fibroma virus encodes a soluble form of the TNF receptor. Biochem Biophys Res Commun 1991; 176:335–342.

108. Schreiber M, McFadden G. The myxoma virus TNF-receptor homologue (T2) inhibits TNFα in a species specific fashion. Virology, 1994 (in press).

109. Shchelkunov SN, Blinov VM, Sandakhchiev LS. Genes of variola and vaccinia viruses necessary to overcome the host protective mechanisms. FEBS Lett 1993;319:80–83.

110. Howard ST, Chan YS, Smith GL. Vaccinia virus homologues of the Shope fibroma virus inverted terminal repeat proteins and a discontinuous ORF related to the tumor necrosis factor receptor family. Virology 1991;180:633–647.

111. Hu F-Q, Smith C, Pickup DJ. Cowpox virus contains two copies of an early gene encoding a soluble secreted form of the type II TNF-receptor. Virology, 1994 (in press).

112. Baxby D. Jenner's smallpox vaccine: the riddle of vaccinia virus and its origin. London: Heineman Educational Books, 1981.

113. Upton C, Mossman K, McFadden G. Encoding a homology of the IFN-γ receptor by myxoma virus. Science 1992; 258:1369–1372.

114. Barinaga M. Viruses launch their own 'Star Wars.' Science 1992;258:1730–1731.

115. Dinarello CA. Interleukin-1. In: Thomson A, ed. The cytokine handbook. San Diego: Academic Press, 1991:47–82.

116. Dinarello CA. Interleukin-1 and interleukin-1 antagonism. Blood 1991;77:1627–1652.

117. Sims JE, March CJ, Cosman D, et al. cDNA expression cloning of the IL-1 receptor, a member of the immunoglobulin superfamily. Science 1988;241:585–589.

118. Sims JE, Acres RB, Grubin CE, et al. Cloning of the interleukin 1 receptor from human T cells. Proc Natl Acad Sci USA 1989;86:8946–8950.

119. McMahan CJ, Slack JL, Mosley B, et al. A novel Il-1 receptor, cloned from B cells by mammalian expression, is expressed in many cell types. EMBO J 1991;10:2821–2832.

120. Smith GL, Chan YS. Two vaccinia virus proteins structurally related to the interleukin-1 receptor and the immunoglobulin superfamily. J Gen Virol 1991;72:511–518.

121. Alcami A, Smith GL. A soluble receptor for interleukin-1β encoded by vaccinia virus: a novel mechanism of virus modulation of the host response to infection. Cell 1992;71:153–167.

122. Spriggs MK, Hruby DE, Maliszewski CR, et al. Vaccinia and cowpox viruses encode a novel secreted interleukin-1-binding protein. Cell 1992;71:145–152.

123. Ueda Y, Ito M, Tagaya I. A specific surface antigen induced by poxvirus. Virology 1969;138:180–182.

124. Ueda Y, Tagaya I. Induction of skin resistance to vaccinia virus in rabbits by vaccinia-soluble early antigens. J Exp Med 1973;138:1033–1043.

125. Ikuta K, Miyamoto H, Kato S. Biochemical studies on early

cell surface antigen induced by vaccinia and cowpox viruses. J Gen Virol 1980;47:227–232.

126. Ueda Y, Morikawa S, Matsuura Y. Identification and nucleotide sequence of the gene encoding a surface antigen induced by vaccinia virus. Virology 1990;177:588–594.

127. Griffiths PD, Grundy JE. Molecular biology and immunology of cytomegalovirus. Biochem J 1987;241:313–324.

128. Stinksi MF. Cytomegalovirus and its replication. In: Fields BN, Knipe DM, eds. Virology, ed 2. New York: Raven, 1990:1959–1980.

129. Rodgers BC, Scott DM, Mundin J, Sissons JGP. Monocyte-derived inhibitor of interleukin 1 induced by human cytomegalovirus. J Virol 1985;55:527–532.

130. Kapasi K, Rice GPA. Cytomegalovirus infection of peripheral blood mononuclear cells: effects on interleukin-1 and -2 production and responsiveness: J Virol 1988;62:3603–3607.

131. Dudding L, Haskill S, Clark BD, Auron PE, Sporn S, Huang E-S. Cytomegalovirus infection stimulates expression of monocyte-associated mediator genes. J Immunol 1989; 143:3343–3352.

132. Chee MS, Bankier AT, Beck S, et al. Analysis of the protein-coding content of the sequence of human cytomegalovirus strain AD169. Curr Top Micro Immunol 1990;154:125–169.

133. Chee MS, Satchwell SC, Preddie E, Weston KM, Barrell BG. Human cytomegalovirus encodes three G protein-coupled receptor homologues. Nature 1990;344:774–777.

134. Bankier AT, Beck S, Bohni R, et al. The DNA sequence of the human cytomegalovirus genome. J DNA Seq Map 1991;2:1–12.

135. Gao J-L, Kuhns DB, Tiffany HL, et al. Structure and functional expression of the human macrophage inflammatory protein 1α/RANTES receptor. J Exp Med 1993;177:1421–1427.

136. Grassmann R, Fleckenstein B, Desrosiers RC. Viral transformation of human T lymphocytes. Adv Cancer Res 1994;63:211–244.

137. Nicholas J, Cameron KR, Honess RW. Herpesvirus saimiri encodes homologues of G protein-coupled receptors and cyclins. Nature 1992;355:362–365.

138. Albrecht J-C, Fleckenstein B. New member of the multi-gene family of complement control proteins in herpesvirus saimiri. J Virol 1992;66:3937–3940.

139. Albrecht J-C, Nicholas J, Biller D, et al. Primary structure of the herpesvirus saimiri genome. J Virol 1992;66:5047–5058.

140. Nicholas J, Cameron KR, Coleman H, Newman C, Honess RW. Analysis of nucleotide sequence of the rightmost 43 kbp of herpesvirus saimiri (HSV) L-DNA: general conservation of genetic organization between HSV and Esptein-Barr virus. Virology 1992;188:296–310.

141. Albrecht J-C, Nicholas J, Cameron KR, Newman C, Fleckenstein B, Honess RW. Herpesvirus saimiri has a gene specifying a homologue of the cellular membrane glycoprotein CD59. Virology 1992;190:527–530.

142. Neurath AR, Strick N, Sproul P. Search for hepatitis B virus cell receptors reveals binding sites for interleukin 6 on the virus envelope protein. J Exp Med 1992;175:461–469.

143. Barnaba V, Balsano F. Immunologic and molecular basis of

viral persistence. The hepatitis B virus model. J Hepatol 1992;14:391–400.

144. Barnes PD, Grundy JE. Down-regulation of the class I HLA heterodimer and β$_2$-microglobulin on the surface of cells infected with cytomegalovirus. J Gen Virol 1992;73:2395–2403.

145. del Val M, Hengel H, Häcker H, et al. Cytomegalovirus prevents antigen presentation by blocking the transport of peptide-loaded major histocompatibility complex class I molecules into the medial-Golgi compartment. J Exp Med 1992;176:729–738.

146. Yamashita Y, Shimokata K, Mizuno S, Yamaguchi H, Nishiyama Y. Down-regulation of the surface expression of class I MHC antigens by human cytomegalovirus. Virology 1993;193:727–736.

147. Gilbert MJ, Riddell SR, Li C-R, Greenberg PD. Selective interference with class I major histocompatibility complex presentation of the major immediate-early protein following infection with human cytomegalovirus. J Virol 1993; 67:3461–3469.

148. O'Banion MK, Winn VD, Settlemen J, Young DA. Genetic definition of a new bovine papillomavirus type 1 open reading frame, E5B, that encodes a hydrophobic protein involved in altering host-cell protein procesing. J Virol 1993; 67:3427–3434.

149. Kowalik TF, Wing B, Haskill S, Azizkham JC, Baldwin AS Jr, Huang E-S. Multiple mechanisms are implicated in the regulation of NF-κβ activity during human cytomegalovirus infection. Proc Natl Acad Sci USA 1993;90:1107–1111.

150. Kekulé AS, Lauer U, Meyer M, Caselmann WH, Hofschneider PH, Koshy R. The preS2/S region of integrated hepatitis B virus DNA encodes a transcriptional transactivator. Nature 1990;343:457–461.

151. Lauer U, Weiss L, Hofschneider PH, Kekulé AS. The hepatitis B virus pre-S/S^t transactivator is generated by 3′ truncations within a defined region of the S gene. J Virol 1992; 66:5284–5289.

152. Meyer M, Caselmann WH, Schlüter V, Schreck R, Hofschneider PH, Baeuerle PA. Hepatitis B virus transactivator MHBs^t: activation of NF-κB, selective inhibition by antioxidants and integral membrane localization. EMBO J 1992;11:2991–3001.

153. Strayer DS, Horowitz M, Leibowitz JL. Immunosuppression in viral oncogenesis. III. Effects of virus infection on interleukin 1 and interleukin 2 generation and responsiveness. J Immunol 1986;137:3632–3638.

154. Stellbrecht KA, Sperber K, Pogo BG-T. Stimulation of lymphokines in Jurkat cells persistently infected with vaccinia virus. J Virol 1992;66:2046–2050.

155. Turner PC, Moyer RW. The molecular pathogenesis of poxviruses. Curr Topics Microbiol Immunol 1990;163: 125–151.

156. Buller RML, Palumbo GJ. Poxvirus pathogenesis. Microbiol Rev 1991;55:80–122.

157. Boursnell MEG, Foulds IJ, Campbell JI, Binns MM. Nonessential genes in the vaccinia virus HindIII K fragments: a gene related to serine protease inhibitors and a gene related to the 37K vaccinia virus major envelope antigen. J Gen Virol 1988;69:2995–3003.

158. Kotwal GJ, Moss B. Vaccinia virus encodes two proteins that are structurally related to members of the plasma ser-

ine protease inhibitor superfamily. J Virol 1989;63:600–606.

159. Smith GL, Howard ST, Chan YS. Vaccinia virus encodes a family of genes with homology to serine proteinase inhibitors. J Gen Virol 1989;70:2333–2343.

160. Pickup PJ, Ink BS, Hu W, Ray CA, Joklik WK. Hemorrhage in lesions caused by cowpox virus is induced by a viral protein that is related to plasma protein inhibitors of serine proteases. Proc Natl Acad Sci USA 1986;83:7698–7702.

161. Law KM, Smith GL. A vaccinia serine protease inhibitor which prevents virus-induced cell fusion. J Gen Virol 1992;73:549–557.

162. Turner PC, Moyer RW. An orthopoxvirus serpin-like gene controls the ability of infected cells to fuse. J Virol 1992; 66:2076–2085.

163. Zhou J, Sun XY, Fernando GJ, Frayer IH. The vaccinia virus K2L gene encodes a serine protease inhibitor which inhibits cell-cell fusion. Virology 1992;189:678–686.

164. Palumbo GJ, Pickup DJ, Frederickson TN, McIntyre LJ, Buller RML. Inhibition of an inflammatory response is mediated by a 38-kDa protein of cowpox virus. Virology 1989;172:262–273.

165. Chua TP, Smith CE, Reith RW, Williamson JD. Inflammatory responses and the generation of chemoattractant activity in cowpox virus-infected tissues. Immunology 1990; 64:202–208.

166. Frederickson TN, Sechler JMG, Palumbo GJ, Albert J, Khairallah LH, Buller ML. Acute inflammatory response to cowpox virus infection of the chorioallantoic membrane of the chick embryo. Virology 1992;187:693–704.

167. Ray CA, Black RA, Kronheim SR, et al. Viral inhibition of inflammation: cowpox virus encodes an inhibitor of the interleukin-1β converting enzyme. Cell 1992;69:597–604.

168. Cerretti DP, Kozlosky CJ, Mosley B, et al. Molecular cloning of the IL-1b converting enzyme. Science 1992;256:97–100.

169. Thornberry NA, Bull HG, Calaycay JR, et al. A novel heterodimeric cysteine protease is required for interleukin-1b processing in monocytes. Nature 1992;356:768–774.

170. Rubartelli A, Bajetto A, Allavena G, Cozzolino F, Sitia R. Post-translational regulation of interleukin 1β secretion. Cytokine 1993;5:117–124.

171. Upton C, Macen JL, Wishart DS, McFadden G. Myxoma virus and malignant rabbit fibroma virus encode a serpin-like protein important for virus virulence. Virology 1990; 179:618–631.

172. Macen JL, Upton C, Nation N, McFadden G. SERP1, a serine proteinase inhibitor encoded by myxoma virus, is a secreted glycoprotein that interferes with inflammation. Virology 1993;145:348–363.

173. Lomas DA, Evans DL, Upton C, McFadden G, Carrell RW. Inhibition of plasmin, urokinase, tissue plasminogen activator, and C_{1s} by a myxoma virus serine proteinase inhibitor. J Biol Chem 1993;268:516–521.

174. Carrell RW, Evans DL. Serpins: mobile conformations in a family of proteinase inhibitors. Curr Opin Struct Biol 1994;2:438–446.

175. Potema J, Korzus E, Travis T. The serpin superfamily of proteinase inhibitors: structure, function, and regulation. J Biol Chem 1994;269:15957–15960.

176. Schröder CH, Zentgraf H. Hepatitis B virus related hepatocellular carcinoma: chronicity of infection—the opening to different pathways of malignant transformation? Biochim Biophys Acta 1990;1032:137–156.

177. Sherker AH, Marion PL. Hepadnaviruses and hepatocellular carcinoma. Annu Rev Microbiol 1991;45:475–508.

178. Slagle BL, Lee T-H, Butel JS. Hepatitis B virus and hepatocellular carcinoma. Prog Med Virol 1992;39:167–203.

179. Buendia MA. Hepatitis B viruses and hepatocellular carcinoma. Adv Cancer Res 1992;59:167–226.

180. Koshy R. Hepatocellular carcinogenesis by hepatitis B virus: a multiplicity of possible pathways. In: Doerfler W, Böhm P, eds. Malignant transformation by DNA viruses. Weinheim: VCH Press, 1992:171–205.

181. Yen TSB. Regulation of hepatitis B virus gene expression. Semin Virol 1993;4:33–42.

182. Müller R. Interferons in chronic viral hepatitis. Hepatogastroenterology 1991;38:4–9.

183. Finter NB, Chapman S, Dowd P, et al. The use of interferon-α in virus infections. Drugs 1991;42:749–765.

184. Dorr RT. Interferon-α in malignant and viral diseases. Drugs 1993;45:177–211.

185. Twu J-S, Lee C-H, Lin P-M, Schloemer RH. Hepatitis B virus suppresses expression of human β-interferon. Proc Natl Acad Sci USA 1988;85:252–256.

186. Twu J-S, Schloemer RH. Transcription of the human beta interferon gene is inhibited by hepatitis B virus. J Virol 1989;63:3065–3071.

187. Whitten TM, Quets AT, Schloemer RH. Identification of the hepatitis B virus factor that inhibits expression of the beta interferon gene. J Virol 1991;65:4699–4704.

188. Foster GR, Ackrill AM, Goldin RD, Kerr IM, Thomas HC, Stark GR. Expression of the terminal protein region of hepatitis B virus inhibits cellular responses to interferons α and γ and double-stranded RNA. Proc Natl Acad Sci USA 1991;88:2888–2892.

189. Twu J-S, Chu K, Robinson WS. Hepatitis B virus X gene activates κB-like enhancer sequences in the long terminal repeat of human immunodeficiency virus 1. Proc Natl Acad Sci USA 1989;86:5168–5172.

190. Zhou D-X, Taraboulos A, Ou J-H, Yen TSB. Activation of class I major histocompatibility complex gene expression by hepatitis B virus. J Virol 1990;64:4025–4028.

191. Hu K-Q, Vierling JM, Siddiqui A. Trans-activation of HLA-DR gene by hepatitis B virus X gene product. Proc Natl Acad Sci USA 1990;87:7140–7144.

192. Aufiero B, Schneider RJ. The hepatitis B virus X-gene product trans-activates both RNA polymerase II and III promoters. EMBO J 1990;9:497–504.

193. Wu JY, Zhou Z-Y, Judd A, Cartwright CA, Robinson WS. The hepatitis B virus-encoded transcriptional trans-activator hbx appears to be a novel protein serine/threonine kinase. Cell 1990;63:687–695.

194. Seto E, Mitchell PJ, Yen TSB. Transactivation by the hepatitis B virus X protein depends on AP-2 and other transcription factors. Nature 1990;344:72–74.

195. Unger T, Shaul Y. The X protein of the hepatitis B virus acts as a transcription factor when targeted to its responsive element. EMBO J 1990;9:1889–1895.

196. Lucito R, Schneider RJ. Hepatitis B virus X protein activates transcription factor NF-κB without a requirement for protein kinase C. J Virol 1992;66:983–991.

197. Maguire HF, Hoeffler JP, Siddiqui A. HBV X protein alters the DNA binding specificity of CREB and ATF-2 by protein-protein interactions. Science 1991;252:842–844.

198. Kekulé AS, Lauer U, Weiss L, Luber B, Hofschneider PH. Hepatitis B virus transactivator HBx uses a tumour promoter signalling pathway. Nature 1993;361:742–745.

199. Twu J-S, Schloemer RH. Transcriptional trans-activating function of hepatitis B virus. J Virol 1987;61:3448–3453.

200. Horwitz MS. Adenoviruses. In: Fields BN, Knipe DM, eds. Virology, ed 2. New York: Raven, 1990:1723–1740.

201. Müllbacher A. Viral escape from immune recognition: multiple strategies of adenoviruses. Immunol Cell Biol 1992;70:59–63.

202. Blair GE, Zhang X. Human adenoviruses: genetics and immunology. In: Thomas DB, ed. Viruses and the cellular immune response. New York: Marcel Dekker, 1993:389–428.

203. Gooding LR, Wold WSM. Molecular mechanisms by which adenoviruses counteract antiviral immune defenses. CRC Rev Immunol 1990;10:53–71.

204. Andiman WA, Robert MF. Adenoviruses. In: Specter S, Bendinelli M, Friedman H, eds. Virus induced immunosuppression. New York: Plenum Press, 1989:59–72.

205. Rosahl T, Doerfler W. Alterations in the levels of expression of specific cellular genes in adenovirus-infected and -transformed cells. Virus Res 1992;26:71–90.

206. Kalvakolanu DVR, Liu J, Hanson RW, Harter ML, Sen GC. Adenovirus E1A represses the cyclic AMP-induced transcription of the gene for phosphoenolpyruvate carboxykinase (GTP) in hepatoma cells. J Biol Chem 1992;267:2530–2536.

207. Shenk T, Flint J. Transcriptional and transforming activities of the adenovirus E1A proteins. Adv Cancer Res 1991;57:47–85.

208. Nevins JR. Transcriptional activation by the adenovirus E1A proteins. Semin Virol 1993;4:25–31.

209. Ackrill Am, Foster GR, Laxton CD, Flavell DM, Stark GR, Kerr IM. Inhibition of the cellular response to interferons by products of the adenovirus type 5 E1A oncogene. Nucleic Acids Res 1991;19:4387–4393.

210. Janaswami PM, Kalvakolanu DVR, Zhang Y, Sen GC. Transcriptional repression of interleukin-6 gene by adenoviral E1A proteins. J Biol Chem 1992;267:24886–24891.

211. Spergel JM, Chen-Kiang S. Interleukin 6 enhances a cellular activity that functionally substitutes for E1A protein in transactivation. Proc Natl Acad Sci USA 1991;88:6472–6476.

212. Howley PM. Papillomavirinae and their replication. In: Fields BN, Knipe DM, eds. Virology, ed 2. New York: Raven, 1990:1625–1650.

213. Shah KV, Howley PM. Papillomaviruses. In: Fields BN, Knipe DM, eds. Virology, ed 2. New York: Raven, 1990: 1651–1676.

214. Zur Hausen H. Human papillomaviruses in the pathogenesis of anogenital cancer. Virology 1991;184:9–13.

215. Sousa R, Dostatni N, Yaniv M. Control of papillomavirus gene expression. Biochim Biophys Acta 1990;1032:19–37.

216. McBride AA, Romanczuk H, Howley PM. The papilloma-

217. Ham J, Sostatni N, Gauthier J-M, Yaniv M. The papillomavirus E2 protein: a factor with many talents. TIBS 1991;16: 440–444.

218. Miyatake S, Seiki M, DeWaal Malefijt R, et al. Activation of T cell-derived lymphokine genes in T cells and fibroblasts: effects of human T cell leukemia virus type I p40^x protein and bovine papilloma virus encoded E2 protein. Nucleic Acids Res 1988;16:6547–6566.

219. Miyatake S, Seiki M, Yoshida M, Arai K-I. T-cell activation signals and human T-cell leukemia virus type I-encoded p40^x protein activate the mouse granulocyte-macrophage colony-stimulating factor gene through a common DNA element. Mol Cell Biol 1988;8:5581–5587.

220. Heike T, Miyatake S, Yoshida M, Arai K, Arai N. Bovine papilloma virus encoded E2 protein activates lymphokine genes through DNA elements, distinct from the consensus motif, in the long control region of its own genome. EMBO J 1989;8:1411–1417.

221. Rinaldo CR. Immune suppression by herpesviruses. Annu Rev Med 1990;41:331–338.

222. Nash AA, Cambouropoulos P. The immune response to herpes simplex virus. Semin Virol 1993;4:181–186.

223. Banks TA, Rouse BT. Herpesviruses—immune escape artists? Clin Infect Dis 1992;14:933–941.

224. Gosselin J, Flamand L, D'Addario M, et al. Modulatory effects of Epstein-Barr, herpes simplex, and human herpes-6 viral infections and coinfections on cytokine synthesis. J Immunol 1992;149:181–187.

225. Wu L, Eisenstein TK, Morahan PS. Effect of herpes simplex virus type 1 infection on cytokine gene expression in activated murine peritoneal macrophages. Adv Exp Med 1992; 312:67–172.

226. Gosselin J, Menezes J, D'Addario M, et al. Inhibition of tumor necrosis factor-a transcription by Epstein-Barr virus. Eur J Immunol 1991;21:203–208.

227. Flamand L, Gosselin J, D'Addario M, et al. Human herpesvirus 6 induces interleukin-1b and tumor necrosis factor alpha, but not interleukin-6, in peripheral blood mononuclear cell cultures. J Virol 1991;65:5105–5110.

228. Williams RG. Transcriptional regulation of interferon-stimulated genes. Eur J Biochem 1991;200:1–11.

229. Kerr IM, Stark GR. The control of interferon-inducible gene expression. FEBS Lett 1991;285:194–198.

230. Williams RG. Signal transduction and transcriptional regulation of interferon-α-stimulated genes. J Interferon Res 1991;11:207–213.

231. Reich N, Pine R, Levy D, et al. Transcription of interferon-stimulated genes is induced by adenovirus particles but is suppressed by E1A gene products. J Virol 1988;62:114–119.

232. Ackrill AM, Blair GE. Interferon-γ regulation of major histocompatibility class I gene expression in rat cells containing the adenovirus 12 E1A oncogene. Virology 1990;174: 325–328.

233. Kalvakolanu DVR, Bandyopadhyay SK, Harter ML, et al. Inhibition of interferon-inducible gene expression by adenovirus E1A proteins: block in transcriptional complex formation. Proc Natl Acad Sci USA 1991;88:7459–7463.

234. Gutch MJ, Reich NC. Repression of the interferon signal

transduction pathway by the adenovirus E1A oncogene. Proc Natl Acad Sci USA 1991;88:7913–7917.

235. Routes JM. Adenovirus E1A inhibits IFN-induced resistance to cytolysis by natural killer cells. J Immunol 1993; 150:4315–4322.

236. Ames RS, Holskin B, Mitcho M, et al. Induction of sensitivity to the cytotoxic action of tumor necrosis factor alpha by adenovirus E1A is independent of transformation and transcriptional activation. J Virol 1990;64:4115–4122.

237. Tsuji Y, Ninomiya-Tsuji J, Torti SV, et al. Augmentation by IL-1α of tumor necrosis factor-α cytotoxicity in cells transfected with adenovirus E1A. J Immunol 1993;150:1897–1907.

238. Gooding LR, Aquino L, Duerksen-Hughes PJ, et al. The E1B 19,000-molecular-weight protein of group C adenoviruses prevents tumor necrosis factor cytolysis of human cells but not of mouse cells. J Virol 1991;65:3083–3094.

239. White E, Sabbatini P, Debbas M, et al. The 19-kilodalton E1B transforming protein inhibits programmed cell death and prevents cytolysis by tumor necrosis factor α. Mol Cell Biol 1992;12:2570–2580.

240. Horton TM, Ranheim TS, Aquino L, et al. Adenovirus E3 14.7K protein functions in the absence of other adenovirus proteins to protect transfected cells from tumor necrosis factor cytolysis. J Virol 1991;65:2629–2639.

241. Ranheim TS, Shisler J, Horton TM, et al. Characterization of mutants within the gene for the adenovirus E3 14.7-kilodalton protein which prevents cytolysis by tumor necrosis factor. J Virol 1993;67:2159–2167.

242. Krajcsi P, Tollefson AE, Anderson CW. The E3-10.4K protein of adenovirus is an integral membrane protein that is partially cleaved between Ala_{22} and Ala_{23} and has a C_{cyt} orientation. Virology 1992;187:131–144.

243. Krajcsi P, Wold WSM. The adenovirus E3-14.5K protein which is required for prevention of TNF cytolysis and for down-regulation of the EGF receptor contains phosphoserine. Virology 1992;187:492–498.

244. Krajcsi P, Tollefson AE, Wold WSM. The E3-14.5K integral membrane protein of adenovirus that is required for down-regulation of the EGF receptor and for prevention of TNF cytolysis is O-glycosylated but not N-glycosylated. Virology 1992;188:570–579.

245. Krajcsi P, Tollefson AE, Anderson CW, et al. The adenovirus E3 14.5-kilodalton protein, which is required for down-regulation of the epidermal growth factor receptor and prevention of tumor necrosis factor cytolysis, is an integral membrane protein oriented with its C terminus in the cytoplasm. J Virol 1992;66:1665–1673.

246. Hoffman BL, Ullrich A, Wold WSM, et al. Retrovirus-mediated transfer of an adenovirus gene encoding an integral membrane protein is sufficient to down regulate the receptor for epidermal growth factor. Mol Cell Biol 1990;10:5521–5524.

247. Tollefson AE, Stewart AR, Yei S, et al. The 10,400- and 14,500-dalton proteins encoded by region E3 of adenovirus form a complex and function together to down-regulate the epidermal growth factor receptor. J Virol 1991; 65:3095–3105.

248. Kuivinen E, Hoffman BL, Hoffman PA, et al. Structurally related class I and class II receptor protein tyrosine kinases are down-regulated by the same E3 protein coded for by human group C adenoviruses. J Cell Biol 1993;120:1271–1279.

249. Körner H, Fritzsche U, Burgert H-G. Tumor necrosis factor α stimulates expression of adenovirus early region 3 proteins: implications for viral persistence. Proc Natl Acad Sci USA 1992;89:11857–11861.

250. Huang S, Hendriks W, Althage A, et al. Immune response in mice that lack the interferon-γ receptor. Science 1993; 259:1742–1745.

251. Karupiah G, Frederickson TN, Holmes KL, Khairallah LH, Buller RML. Importance of interferons in recovery from mousepox. J Virol 1993;67:4214–4226.

252. Rice AP, Roberts WK, Kerr IM. 2-5A accumulates to high levels in interferon-treated, vaccinia virus-infected cells in the absence of any inhibition of virus replication. J Virol 1984;50:220–228.

253. Paetz E, Esteban M. Nature and mode of action of vaccinia virus products that block activation of the interferon-mediated $ppp(A2'p)_nA$-synthetase. Virology 1984;134:29–30.

254. Whitaker-Dowling P, Youngner JS. Characterization of a specific kinase inhibitory factor produced by vaccinia virus which inhibits the interferon-induced protein kinase. Virology 1984;137:171–181.

255. Rice AP, Kerr IM. Interferon-mediated, double-stranded RNA-dependent protein kinase is inhibited in extracts from vaccinia virus-infected cells. J Virol 1984;50:229–236.

256. Rice AP, Kerr SM, Roberts WK, Brown RE, Kerr IM. Novel 2′,5′-oligoadenylates synthesized in interferon-treated, vaccinia virus-infected cells. J Virol 1985;56:1041–1044.

257. Rodriguez J-R, Rodriguez D, Esteban M. Interferon treatment inhibits early events in vaccinia virus gene expression in infected mice. Virology 1991;185:929–933.

258. Degen HJ, Blum D, Grün J, Jungwirth C. Expression of authentic vaccinia virus-specific and inserted viral and cellular genes under control of an early vaccinia virus promoter is regulated post-transcriptionally in interferon-treated chick embryo fibroblasts. Virology 1992;188:114–121.

259. Lee SB, Esteban M. The interferon-induced double-stranded RNA-activated human p68 protein kinase inhibits the replication of vaccinia virus. Virology 1993;193:1037–1041.

260. Davies MV, Chang H-W, Jacobs BL, Kaufman RJ. The E3L and K3L vaccinia virus gene products stimulate translation through inhibition of the double-stranded RNA dependent protein kinase by different mechanisms. J Virol 1993;67:1688–1692.

261. Watson JC, Chang H-W, Jacobs BL. Characterization of a vaccinia virus-encoded double-stranded RNA-binding protein that may be involved in inhibition of the double-stranded RNA-dependent protein kinase. Virology 1991; 185:206–216.

262. Chang H-W, Watson JC, Jacobs BL. The E3L gene of vaccinia virus encodes an inhibitor of the interferon-induced, double-stranded RNA-dependent protein kinase. Proc Natl Acad Sci USA 1992;89:4825–4829.

263. Chang H-W, Jacobs BL. Identification of a conserved motif that is necessary for binding of the vaccinia virus E3L gene products to double-stranded RNA. Virology 1993;194:537–547.

264. Davies MV, Elroy-Stein O, Jagus R, Moss B, Kaufman RJ.

The vaccinia virus K3L gene product potentiates translation by inhibiting double-stranded-RNA-activated protein kinase and phosphorylation of the alpha subunit of eukaryotic initiation factor 2. J Virol 1992;66:1943–1950.

265. Beattie E, Tartaglia J, Paoletti E. Vaccinia-virus-encoded eIF-2α homolog abrogates the antiviral effect of interferon. Virology 1991;183:419–422.

266. Pacha RF, Condit RC. Characterization of a temperature-sensitive mutant of vaccinia virus reveals a novel function that prevents virus-induced breakdown of RNA. J Virol 1985;56:395–403.

267. Cohrs RJ, Condit RC, Pacha RF, Thompson CL, Sharma OK. Modulation of ppp(A2'p)nA-dependent RNase by a temperature sensitive mutant of vaccinia virus. J Virol 1989;63:948–951.

268. Pacha RF, Meris RJ, Condit RC. Structure and expression of the vaccinia virus gene which prevents virus-induced breakdown of RNA. J Virol 1990;64:3853–3863.

269. Bayliss CD, Condit RC. Temperature-sensitive mutants in the vaccinia virus A18R gene increase double-stranded RNA synthesis as a result of aberrant viral transcription. Virology 1993;194:254–262.

270. Sample C, Kieff E. Molecular basis for Epstein-Barr virus induced pathogenesis and disease. Semin Immunopathol 1991;13:133–146.

271. Aman P, von Gabain A. An Epstein-Barr virus immortalization associated gene segment interferes specifically with the IFN-induced anti-proliferative response in human B-lymphoid cell lines. EMBO J 1990;9:147–152.

272. Kanda K, Decker T, Aman P, Wahlström M, von Gabain A, Kallin B. The EBNA2-related resistance towards alpha interferon (IFN-α) in Burkitt's lymphoma cells effects induction of IFN-induced genes but not the activation of transcription factor ISGF-3. Mol Cell Biol 1992;12:4930–4936.

273. Kriauciunas KM, Goldstein BJ, Lipes MA, Kahn CR. Modulation of expression of insulin and IGF-1 receptor by Epstein-Barr virus and its gene products LMP and EBNA-2 in lymphocyte cell lines. J Cell Physiol 1993;154:486–495.

274. Onji M, Lever AML, Saito I, Thomas HC. Defective response to interferons in cells transfected with the hepatitis B virus genome. Hepatology 1989;9:92–96.

275. Foster GR, Goldin RD, Hay A, et al. Expression of the terminal protein of hepatitis-B virus is associated with failure to respond to interferon therapy. Hepatology 1993;17:757–762.

276. Majewski S, Hunzelmann N, Nischt R, et al. TGFβ-1 and TNFα expression in the epidermis of patients with epidermodysplasia verruciformis. J Invest Dermatol 1991;97:862–867.

277. McGlennen RC, Ostrow RS, Carson LF, Stanley MS, Faras AJ. Expression of cytokine receptors and markers of differentiation in human papillomavirus-infected cervical tissues. Am J Obstet Gynecol 1991;165:696–705.

278. Malejczyk J, Malejczyk M, Köck A, et al. Autocrine growth limitation of human papillomavirus type 16-harboring keratinocytes by constitutively released tumor necrosis factor-α. J Immunol 1992;149:2702–2708.

279. Martin P, Vass WC, Schiller JT, Lowy DR, Velu TJ. The bovine papillomavirus E5 transforming protein can stimulate the transforming activity of EGF and CSF-1 receptors. Cell 1989;59:21–32.

280. Leechanachai P, Banks L, Moreau F, Matlashewski G. The E5 gene from human papillomavirus type 16 is an oncogene which enhances growth factor-mediated signal transduction to the nucleus. Oncogene 1992;7:19–25.

281. Pim D. Collins M, Banks L. Human papillomavirus type 16 E5 gene stimulates the transforming activity of the epidermal growth factor receptor. Oncogene 1992;7:27–32.

282. Goldstein DJ, Finbow ME, Andresson T, et al. Bovine papillomavirus E5 oncoprotein binds to the 16K component of vacuolar H+-ATPases. Nature 1991;352:347–349.

283. Goldstein DJ, Kulke R, Dimaio D, Schlegel R. A glutamine residue in the membrane-associating domain of the bovine papillomovirus type 1 E5 oncoprotein mediates its binding to a transmembrane component of the vacuolar H+-ATPase. J Virol 1992;66:405–413.

284. Petti L, Nilson LA, DiMaio D. Activation of the platelet-derived growth factor receptor by the bovine papillomavirus E5 transforming protein. EMBO J 1991;10:845–855.

285. Goldstein DJ, Anderson T, Sparkowski JJ, Schelegel R. The BPV-1 E5 protein, the 16 kDa membrane pore-forming protein and the PDGF receptor exist in a complex that is dependent on hydrophobic transmembrane interactions. EMBO J 1992;11:4851–4859.

CHAPTER 28

ROLE OF CYTOKINES IN THE PATHOGENESIS OF HUMAN IMMUNODEFICIENCY VIRUS INFECTION

Guido Poli and Anthony S. Fauci

GENERAL CONCEPTS OF THE PATHOGENESIS OF HUMAN IMMUNODEFICIENCY VIRUS DISEASE

The acquired immunodeficiency syndrome (AIDS) was originally described in 1981 as a state of profound immune dysfunction; it was characterized by a loss of CD4+ helper T cells and an unusually high frequency of opportunistic diseases (1,2). The etiologic agent of AIDS has been identified as a pathogenic human retrovirus of the lentivirus subfamily known as human immunodeficiency virus (HIV); it exists in 2 major variants: HIV-1 and HIV-2 (3). HIV has been molecularly cloned, and its genes have been characterized. Although the precise pathogenic mechanisms whereby this virus causes AIDS remain unclear, HIV has been intensively studied, and more has been learned about it over a relatively short period compared with other microbial pathogens that have been associated with human diseases for much longer periods.

In addition to CD4+ T lymphocytes, mononuclear phagocytes (MP) are susceptible to HIV infection both in vitro and in vivo, and they have been found to be dysfunctional in HIV-infected individuals (4). The selective cell tropisms of HIV are explained on the molecular level by the ability of one of its envelope components, gp 120, to bind with high affinity to the human CD4 molecule,

which is expressed on the cell surface of a subset of T lymphocytes and MP (1–4). Recently, other cell types, including cells of the central nervous system (CNS), muscle cells, and others, have been shown to be infectable in vitro by HIV via receptors other than the CD4 molecule (3). Furthermore, different types of dendritic cells likely have a prominent role in the pathogenesis of HIV infection. Follicular dendritic cells present in the germinal centers of lymph nodes can trap free virions on their cell surface via Fc or complement receptors, whereas other types of dendritic cells can initiate T-cell–specific immune responses due to their function as "professional" antigen-presenting cells (1).

An important aspect of HIV disease is that it is comprised of complex pathogenic processes that are multifactorial and multiphasic, including a paradoxical state of immune activation overlapping with immunodeficiency (1,2). There are at least 3 distinct phases in the natural history of HIV infection (Fig. 28–1). The initial phase is primary infection, during which the virus enters the body, replicates at high rates, and widely disseminates, particularly to lymphoid tissues. This phase is frequently associated with clinical symptoms of a mononucleosis-like syndrome, and it lasts for a few weeks. With the emergence of a vigorous humoral and cell-mediated immune response, the infected individual usually enters into an asymptomatic phase referred to as "clinical latency," which persists for several years before clinically apparent disease occurs. During this period, little if any virus replication is detectable in peripheral blood mononuclear cells (PBMC), and it is difficult to culture virus from PB; nonetheless, a slow but progressive decline of PB CD4+ T cells is still observed in the majority of individuals. This finding has led to the extreme interpretation that HIV cannot be the sole cause of AIDS, but that other factors of either microbial, immunological, or behavioral nature must be invoked (5). However, it has been recently demonstrated that active HIV replication occurs during all stages of infection, including the phase of "clinical latency," in lymphoid organs such as lymph nodes, adenoids, and tonsils, despite the fact that little or no viral replication is detectable in PBMC (6). These studies do not imply that other elements, such as immune activation, cytokines, and autoimmunity (1,2), cannot have an important role in the pathogenesis of HIV disease, but they underscore the scientific basis of the central role of HIV as the key determinant of this disease.

Another important aspect of the pathogenesis of HIV disease that has emerged from recent studies is the confirmation that, in addition to a state of active virus replication, HIV infection also exists in vivo in a state of latency, not only in the PB compartment (6), but also in the same lymphoid organs that are active sites of HIV replication and virion accumulation (7). In this regard, a much higher ratio (100-fold or more) of latently infected cells than cells actively expressing HIV has been found in lymphoid organs at any given time (7). These in vivo data suggest that spreading of HIV is a highly regulated process and that the long incubation period occurring between the time of primary infection and AIDS (approxi-

mately 10 years) is correlated with low, although persistent, levels of HIV replication.

A direct correlation between the replicative and the cytopathic capacity of HIV and the clinical state derives both from studies in infected individuals (8,9) and from studies in animal models of AIDS. In these latter studies, animals infected with a highly pathogenic variant of the simian immunodeficiency virus (SIV), known as SIV_{pbj14}, which causes an AIDS-like syndrome in macaques, die within weeks of primary infection (10). Their tissues, particularly the gut-associated lymphoid organs, are heavily infiltrated with massively replicating SIV (10). On the other end of the spectrum, infection of macaques with a molecular clone of SIV deleted of the nef gene causes an asymptomatic infection in association with lower levels of virus replication compared with animals infected with wild type (WT) virus (11). Furthermore, animals infected with the nef-deleted SIV not only remain disease-free, but are also protected from a challenge with WT virus (12). These observations suggest that identification of factors of either viral or host nature that determine the state of latency or active expression and spreading of HIV will likely have a major impact on our understanding of the mechanisms of pathogenesis, as well as provide unique opportunities for therapeutic or preventive intervention.

In this context, the complex network of cytokines involved in inflammatory and immunoregulatory responses has an important role in several components of the pathogenesis of HIV infection and AIDS. First, expression and production of several cytokines are dysregulated in HIV-infected patients, potentially contributing to the global immunodeficiency state typical of this disease (Table 28–1). Second, several cytokines have an important role as growth factors for AIDS-associated malignancies, namely B-cell lymphomas and Kaposi's sarcoma (KS), a topic that

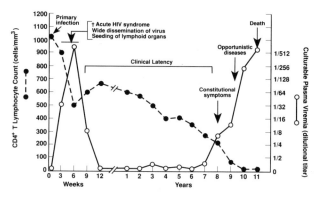

Figure 28–1 Typical course of HIV infection. During the early period after primary infection, there is widespread dissemination of virus and a sharp decrease in the number of CD4 T cells in peripheral blood. An immune response to HIV ensues, with a decrease in detectable viremia followed by a prolonged period of clinical latency. The CD4 T-cell count continues to decrease during the following years, until it reaches a critical level, below which there is a substantial risk for opportunistic diseases.

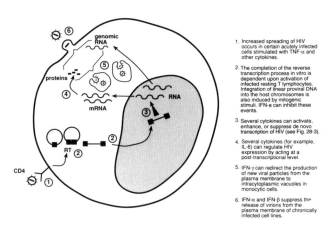

Figure 28–2 Cytokine modulation of HIV life cycle.

TABLE 28–1   HIV INFECTION AND CYTOKINES

Cytokine	In Vivo/Ex Vivo Expression/Production	In Vitro Expression/Production	Effect on HIV Replication
TNF-α/-β	↑	↑	↑
TGF-β	↑	?	↑↓
IL-1	↑	↑	↑
IL-1ra	?	?	↓
IL-2	↓	↓	↑↓
IL-3	↓	?	↑
IL-4	↓↑	?	↑↓
IL-6	↑	↑	↑
IL-7	?	?	↑
IL-8	↑	↑↓	?
IL-10	↑↓	?	↑↓
IL-12	↓	↓	?
IL-13	?	?	↓
GM-CSF	?	↑	↑
M-CSF	?	↓	↑
IFN-α	↓ (↑*)	↓	↓
IFN-β	?	?	↓
IFN-γ	↑↓	↓	↑↓

*Increased levels of "acid-labile IFN-α" are present in HIV-infected individuals.

has been extensively reviewed elsewhere (13,14) and that will not be discussed further. Finally, multiple cytokines can directly regulate the replicative capacity of HIV at multiple levels of its life cycle (Figs. 28–2, 28–3). Certain of these cytokines are produced and secreted by the same cells that are potential targets of HIV infection, providing an example of how infected cells can contribute to the autoregulation of virus expression and spread.

Several recent reviews have provided overviews of the involvement of the cytokine network in HIV infection (15–17). We attempt to summarize the most relevant information regarding each individual cytokine investigated thus far in relationship to HIV disease. Our goal is to provide broad discussions of the importance of each cytokine in the process of HIV infection, as well as to highlight certain general questions to be investigated in the future. Because there have been a large number of reports on the roles of various cytokines in HIV disease, we elected for the sake of space constraints and clarity not to exhaustively report on the total literature in this area. Instead, we chose representative studies on the basis of their originality or relevance to document the important concepts regarding individual cytokines. Because the general characteristics of the cytokines in question, their receptors, and

signal transduction pathways are discussed in other parts of this book, they will not be described unless they are of particular relevance in the specific context of HIV infection.

TUMOR NECROSIS FACTOR-α AND -β

The tumor necrosis factors (TNFs), particularly cachectin/TNF-α, have certainly been the most studied and well characterized cytokines in terms of their potential relevance in HIV infection. TNF-α is used as the reference cytokine in the majority of the studies dealing with the potential role of cytokines as regulators of virus production and spreading, due in large part to its demonstrated molecular mechanism of activation of HIV expression.

TNF-α has been found elevated both in the plasma and the serum (18–21), in cerebrospinal fluid (22–24), and in bronchoalveolar lavage of HIV-infected individuals (25). Certain studies, however, failed to demonstrate increased levels of circulating TNF-α (26). It should be emphasized that accurate detection of immunoreactive or bioactive cytokines, and TNF in particular, in body fluids is biased

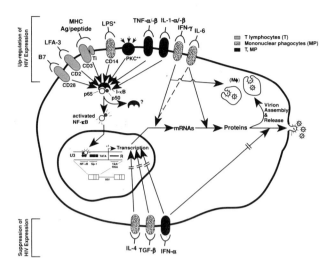

Figure 28–3 Exogenous regulation of HIV-1 expression. Cytokines and other related signaling molecules up-regulate or suppress HIV-1 expression at transcriptional (mostly via NF-κB) and post-transcriptional levels. Only HIV-modulatory cytokines, which have been characterized for their molecular mechanism of action, are represented. The HIV-inductive mechanisms of action of several cytokines, including IL-2 and hemopoietic cytokines such as IL-3, M-CSF, and GM-CSF, remain undefined. For other cytokines known to exert dichotomous effects on virus production depending on the model system used (e.g., IL-4, TGF-β, and IFN-γ), only their most well-defined molecular effects are indicated (see text for details).

by the presence of inhibitors or cytokine-binding molecules, whose levels in the blood are normally higher than those of the related cytokines (27). For example, increased levels of soluble TNF receptors have been observed in HIV-infected individuals (28,29) (Poli G, et al., unpublished observations). In general, PBMC or monocytes isolated from HIV-infected patients have been found to produce higher levels of TNF-α than cells of seronegative control subjects, both in unstimulated conditions and after lipopolysaccharide (LPS) activation (30–36). Some studies also suggested a positive correlation between the levels of TNF production and disease progression (34–36).

Increased expression of TNF-α has also been observed in lung alveolar macrophages (AM) (37–40), macrophages and glial cells infiltrating the retina (41), and macrophages in the spinal cord (42) of HIV-infected individuals. Elevated constitutive production of TNF-α (and interleukin-6 [IL-6]) has also been demonstrated in B lymphocytes obtained from both the PB compartment and, in particular, lymphoid tissues of HIV-infected individuals (43–45). Recombinant (r) gp 120 envelope protein of HIV-1 induced an increased production of both cytokines, as well as Ab, from B lymphocytes of HIV-in-

fected individuals, but not from B cells obtained from HIV-negative individuals, including those affected by autoimmune disorders associated with B-cell activation (44). This effect of gp 120 was not blocked by soluble CD4, indicating that it was not mediated by the CD4 receptor molecule (i.e., not expressed on the surface of B lymphocytes). This observation is consistent with the presence in infected patients of a large pool of B cells expressing gp 120–specific Ab on their surface and primed for the production of anti-HIV gp 120 Ab (46). An independent study reported that gp 120 could induce TNF-α and IL-6 secretion in B lymphocytes from normal individuals in the presence of IL-4 (45). It has also been demonstrated that membrane-bound TNF-α expressed on the surface of CD4+ T-cell clones likely represents an important element in causing or maintaining the state of B-cell activation typical of HIV infection (47). Finally, both CD4+, class II–restricted, and CD8+, class I–restricted cytolytic T lymphocytes (CTL) directed against HIV components have been shown to secrete high levels of TNF-α, TNF-β, and interferon-γ (IFN-γ) during the process of killing target cells (48–50).

Both CD4+ and CD8+ T cells are present in the germinal centers of the lymph nodes of HIV-infected individuals; lymph node germinal centers are among the most important sites of virus replication and accumulation of viral particles (6,7). In this regard, in situ hybridization studies have revealed expression of several cytokines, including TNF-α, in the lymph nodes of HIV-infected individuals (51) (Kotler D, personal communication). Furthermore, higher levels of expression of TNF-α, IL-6, and IFN-γ messenger RNAs (mRNAs) were detected in cells isolated from lymph nodes compared with PBMC throughout the course of HIV infection, including the asymptomatic phase, by semiquantitative reverse transcribed (RT) polymerase chain reaction (PCR) (Graziosi C, et al., personal communication). These findings mirrored the observation that HIV replication is barely detectable in the PB compartment in the early phase of disease, whereas it remains active in lymph nodes and other lymphoid tissues (6).

Because HIV or HIV components, such as gp 120 and the transactivator protein Tat, may induce up-regulation of several genes, including TNF-α (44,45,52–59), it is possible that a continuous cycle of HIV expression and replication is propagated by the chronic expression of proinflammatory cytokines, such as TNF-α. It has been reported that treatment of HIV-infected individuals with the antiviral agent zidovudine (AZT) resulted in decreased levels of TNF-α detectable in the serum (21). In addition, up-regulation of cell surface TNF receptors has been observed in cell lines chronically infected with HIV (60) that appears to be restricted to the p75 receptor molecule in the HL-60–derived OM 10.1 cell line (61). Furthermore, acid labile IFN-α present in the sera of HIV-infected individuals induced cell surface TNF receptors in vitro (30). In contrast, transfection of the HIV-1 tat gene in Raji lymphoblastoid B cells induced both an increased expression of TNF-β (62) and down-regulation of the p75 TNF receptor (63).

Infection with several DNA and RNA viruses leads to an increased susceptibility to the cytotoxic effects of TNF, an effect frequently enhanced by IFN-γ (64). Adenovirus genes have been characterized that confer both susceptibility and resistance to TNF (65,66). An early report indicated that cell lines that were not sensitive to TNF-mediated lysis could be efficiently killed by TNF-α and IFN-γ after infection with HIV, in association with down-regulation of virus expression (67). However, a subsequent study demonstrated that enhancement of TNF-mediated lysis in cells persistently infected with HIV occurred, but in association with increased viral expression (68).

The important question of whether HIV induces a state of increased susceptibility to TNF-mediated lysis still remains open (69). We recently investigated this hypothesis using the U937 (uninfected)/U1 (infected) promonocytic cell systems. We first observed that infected U1 cells were much more sensitive to lysis when treated with TNF-α plus IFN-γ than their uninfected counterpart U937. However, synergistic induction of HIV expression was clearly demonstrable in U1 cells occurring at the same time as the profound cytopathic effects. We could rule out that U1 cells were not killed by the very high levels of virus production because treatments other than TNF-α plus IFN-γ were capable of inducing comparable levels of HIV expression without significant cytopathicity. However, we also observed that several uninfected clones of the parental uninfected cell line U937 showed high susceptibility to lysis by TNF-α plus IFN-γ, similar to infected U1 cells (70).

The possibility of inducing cytotoxic effects in HIV-infected cells without inducing up-regulation of HIV production by selective triggering of the lytic pathway of TNF has been made possible by recent studies on receptor-mediated signal transduction. In fact, it appears that the p75 receptor mediates the TNF-associated cytotoxic effects, whereas the p55 receptor transduces cell activation signals, including up-regulation of HIV transcription (71). Furthermore, mAb directed at other members of the TNF receptor superfamily, such as the Fas antigen, efficiently kills HIV-infected cells without inducing viral expression (72), an observation that we recently confirmed (70). These findings encourage the search for TNF-related molecules with selective cytotoxic activity against HIV-infected cells.

At approximately the same time that the potential antiviral effects of TNF-α and TNF-β were considered, a large body of literature began accumulating that clearly indicated these 2 cytokines were strong inducers of HIV expression. Crude cytokine-enriched supernatants induced

viral expression in latently infected ACH-2 T cells (73). Depletion of TNF-α from the supernatants by specific Ab removed most of the HIV-inductive effect (73), whereas recombinant TNF-α and TNF-β induced HIV expression in ACH-2 cells in a range of concentrations that did not cause substantial cytopathicity (74). A number of other chronically infected cell lines showed similar effects, including U1 (60,75), the Jurkat-derived J1.1 cell line (76), and the HL-60–derived OM10.1 cell line (77). Addition of TNF during the acute phase of viral replication in vitro enhances the formation of syncytia (the result of cell fusion mediated by interaction of the HIV envelope glycoprotein gp 120 and gp41 with the cell membrane of a target CD4+ cell) and increases overall viral production (68,78–82). Induction of viral replication by TNF-α has also been reported in human monocyte-derived macrophages (MDM) acutely infected with HIV (83,84) and macaque macrophages infected with SIV (85). Furthermore, TNF-α has been recently reported to allow in vitro replication of HIV molecular clones defective in an "essential" gene, such as tat (86), or lacking important transcriptional responsive elements in their LTR, such as the Sp-1 binding domains (87) (Poli G, et al., unpublished observations).

Following the demonstration that exogenous TNF could induce HIV expression when added in vitro to cell cultures, it was shown that this cytokine can activate viral production in an autocrine/paracrine fashion in acutely infected cells, such as U937 (81,88), primary PBMC and CD4+ T cells (89,90), and MDM (91). In primary PBMC and purified CD4+ T cells, addition of neutralizing Ab to TNF-α, TNF-β, or IFN-γ was shown to reduce HIV spreading as measured in a syncytium induction scoring assay (89). We recently confirmed and extended these observations in conditions of acute infection where primary PBMC are stimulated with IL-2 in the absence of mitogens. Under these conditions, we clearly observed that blocking of endogenous TNF-α (as well as other cytokines, including IL-1β, IL-6, and IFN-γ), results in substantial suppression, of HIV replication (Kinter AL, et al., unpublished observations). Stimulation of chronically infected U1 and ACH-2 cells with the phorbol ester PMA induced the release of TNF-α in the culture supernatant before the appearance of HIV; more importantly, anti-TNF-α Ab not only suppressed HIV production induced by TNF-α, but also blocked a substantial component of PMA-induced viral expression (60). Furthermore, exogenous TNF-α induces an endogenous TNF-α–mediated loop of HIV expression in chronically infected OM10.1 cells (92).

At the molecular level, TNF-α and TNF-β represent the best characterized examples of cytokine-mediated induction of HIV expression. TNF-α/TNF-β interaction with the p55 receptor on the cell surface leads to activation of the cellular transcription factor NF-κB (71,75,93–96), as described previously for PMA (97). The activated NF-κB complex, usually in the form of the heterodimer p50/p65, can migrate to the cell nucleus and bind to target consensus sequences present in several promoters, including the HIV-1 LTR, which contains 2 repeated NF-κB binding sites in close proximity to the transcription start site (98). Although the functional correlation between TNF stimulation, NF-κB activation, and virus expression is clear, additional steps after activation of NF-κB are likely required for completion of the process of HIV expression. In this regard, TNF-α efficiently activates NF-κB binding activity in primary T-cell clones, but, unlike PMA or antigenic stimulation, this effect does not lead to transactivation of the virus LTR (99). We also observed a discrepancy between the concentrations of TNF required to fully activate HIV expression (usually > 10 U/mL) and the concentrations required to activate NF-κB (as low as 1 U/mL) in U1 cells (Poli G, et al., unpublished observations). Furthermore, short exposure of U1 cells to TNF-α is fully capable of activating NF-κB, but it is insufficient to generate viral production, indicating that both continuous stimulation of the cells and steps other than NF-κB activation are required for production of new virions (Poli G, et al., unpublished observations). Understanding the nature of these additional steps of TNF-mediated induction of virus production may reveal important aspects of the regulation of viral latency and expression in infected cells.

A substantial effort is currently being devoted to discovery and characterization of pharmacological agents capable of interrupting cytokine-dependent HIV replication. Inhibition of the synthesis or effect of TNFs are foremost among these efforts. A recombinant chimeric form of soluble TNF receptor fused to the Fc portion of an immunoglobulin has been recently shown to suppress HIV transcription and expression in chronically infected U1 and ACH-2 cells stimulated with TNF-α (100). A review of this general subject has recently been published (101).

TRANSFORMING GROWTH FACTOR-β

Production of bioactive transforming growth factor-β (TGF-β) from the PBMC of HIV-infected individuals has been reported (102,103). Furthermore, addition of anti-TGF-β1–neutralizing Abs in vitro restored the proliferative responses of both CD4+ T cells and B lymphocytes of HIV-infected individuals (102,103), suggesting the possibility that increased or inappropriate production of TGF-β may have an important role in the immune dysfunction of these cells during the course of HIV infection. These findings are consistent with the profound immunosuppressive effects of TGF-β on virtually every cellular component of the human immune system (104). Expression of TGF-β1 in the brain of HIV-infected patients has been observed in association with infiltrating macrophages or microglial cells infected with HIV (105).

Although the mechanism of up-regulation of TGF-β and other cytokines during HIV infection is unknown, it has been shown that recombinant Tat protein can induce the production of TGF-β1 from bone marrow-derived macrophages, causing inhibition of CFU-GM and BFU-E growth from multipotent CD34+ cells (106). Because infection of CD34+ precursor cells has been described in vivo (107) and several hematological disorders can occur with HIV infection, it is possible that inappropriate expression of TGF-β may be the result of infection of precursor cells in the BM environment. Furthermore, IL-6 (a cytokine that has also been reported to be elevated in HIV-infected individuals) has been shown to decrease proliferative responses of T lymphocytes via induction of TGF-β (108). Similar to TGF-β (106) and TNF-β (62), IL-6 expression is also induced by HIV-1 Tat (109).

Addition of TGF-β to infected cells in vitro resulted in dichotomous effects on HIV replication in both T lymphocytic and MP cells. Enhancement followed by suppression of virus production has been observed in primary T lymphocytes as a consequence of the addition in culture of decreasing amounts of rTGF-β1 (90). In the same study, cocaine was shown to exert an inductive effect in vitro on HIV replication during experiments of viral isolation by means of cocultivation with allogeneic cells. The mechanism of cocaine effect is related to its ability to induce active TGF-β1, as demonstrated by the observation that anti-TGF-β Ab could reverse the stimulatory effect of cocaine (90). Both enhancement and suppression of HIV expression occur in primary MDM infected in vitro with a macrophage tropic strain of HIV as a function of whether the cytokine was added before or several days after infection (110), suggesting that TGF-β may exert opposite effects on MP cells at different stages of infection. However, only up-regulatory effects of the addition of TGF-β to acutely infected U937 cells or primary MDM (111) were reported by an independent laboratory. Under these experimental conditions, TGF-β also caused expansion of the spectrum of viral strains capable of efficient replication in MDM (112).

Only limited information is available on the molecular mechanisms triggered by TGF-β in mediating these different effects in conditions of acute viral replication. A potent suppressive effect of TGF-β has been reported in chronically infected U1 cells stimulated with either PMA or various cytokines (110,113,114). In this cell system, TGF-β was shown to block both HIV transcription and mRNA accumulation induced by PMA. In contrast, TGF-β did not affect TNF-α–induced HIV expression in U1 cells, although it could potently block virus production induced by other cytokines, including IL-1, IL-6, granulo-cyte-macrophage colony-stimulating factor (GM-CSF), and IFN-γ (110,113,114). Because both PMA and TNF-α are known to induce HIV transcription via activation of the cellular transcription factor NF-κB, this finding suggests that TGF-β can selectively block a functional component of PMA capable of inducing NF-κB independently from the release of endogenous TNF-α. In support of this interpretation, we recently observed that TGF-β suppressed the induction of HIV expression in U1 cells sequentially stimulated with certain cytokines and LPS (Goletti D, et al., unpublished observations), a condition that has been previously reported to induce HIV production in U1 cells via activation of NF-κB independently from a TNF-α–mediated autocrine pathway (115,116). In addition, or as an alternative, TGF-β may block an NF-κB–independent pathway of viral transcription triggered by PMA, as described in other cell types (117,118).

INTERLEUKINS

IL-1

Increased levels of IL-1 have been observed in plasma (119,120), cerebrospinal fluid (CSF) (121), skin (122), intestinal mucosa (119,120), and lung epithelial lining fluid (25) of HIV-infected individuals. Furthermore, IL-1β mRNA has been detected in lymph nodes (51,125) (Kotler D, personal communication), as well as in tissue macrophages infiltrating the brain (126,127) or present in the lung alveoli (25,124,128) of seropositive individuals. Increased constitutive and inducible production of IL-1β from PBMC of HIV-infected patients has been reported as a feature of monocyte activation typical of this disease (32,33,124,129). Intraventricular injection of gp 120 into rat brains induced IL-1β production and consequent systemic effects (130), although the nature of the putative gp 120 receptor involved in this interaction has remained undefined.

Local production of IL-1β in the brain, together with that of other proinflammatory cytokines and factors, is hypothesized to contribute to the HIV-induced pathological effects in this organ (4,105,126,127). However, decreased tissue expression of IL-1β mRNA in conjunction with increased levels of TNF-α have been reported in the brains of HIV-infected patients affected by dementia compared with HIV-infected individuals without dementia (131), suggesting a potentially different role of these 2 cytokines in the pathogenesis of HIV-associated CNS disorders. Macrophages and microglia that express IL-1 and TNF-α have been demonstrated in the posterior and lateral funiculi of the thoracic spinal cord; it is believed that

they may be involved in the vacuolar myelopathy associated with HIV infection (42).

Both productive infection of MDM in vitro, as well as incubation of monocytic cells with purified or recombinant (r) gp 120 or gp 120 and gp 41 envelope peptides resulted in the production of IL-1α or IL-1β, or both (52–58,132–137). Similar inductive effects were observed by infecting macaque MDM with SIV (59) and by incubating human monocytes with the OKT4a mAb, but not with OKT4 (54,133). These latter studies suggest that the interaction of gp120 with the CD4 epitope responsible for binding and entry of HIV into target cells was responsible for the production of IL-1β and TNF-α. It has also been reported that only the envelope of certain HIV strains may possess the ability to induce IL-1 and other cytokines (137), suggesting that different viruses may have a different ability to activate the immune system. Furthermore, the HIV-associated protease has been reported to cleave pro-IL-1β into mature IL-1β (138), therefore potentially providing an additional mechanism of activation of IL-1–dependent effects during the course of HIV infection. In addition, other microbial agents concomitantly present in HIV-infected individuals can potentially contribute to an increase in levels of IL-1 and other cytokines, as demonstrated in vitro in normal PBMC acutely infected with the human herpes virus 6 (HHV-6) (139). AZT can block the release of IL-1 from normal monocytes without affecting its synthesis and intracellular accumulation (140), suggesting an additional potential mechanism of action for this antiretroviral compound commonly administered to HIV-infected patients.

Both IL-1α and IL-1β can activate the expression of HIV in vitro. Addition of rIL-1β to primary MDM infected with a macrophage-tropic strain of HIV-1 resulted in increased virus production (56,84,141), an effect that was blocked by IL-4 (84). It has also been suggested that IL-1 and TNF-α may activate HIV replication in MDM in an autocrine manner (56). We recently demonstrated that in a system of acute HIV infection of normal PBMC, in vitro HIV replication was suppressed by blocking the endogenous production of IL-1. This block could be accomplished by anti-IL-1β (but not anti-IL-1α) mAb, by mAb directed at the type I (but not the type II) IL-1 receptor, or by the IL-1 receptor antagonist (IL-1ra) (Kinter AL, et al., unpublished observations).

At the molecular level, IL-1 induction of virus expression, similar to TNF, has been correlated with activation of the cellular transcription factor NF-κB (93,142–145). In addition, IL-1α as well as other cytokines increased the expression of the HIV promoter in MDM derived from transgenic mice carrying an HIV-LTR-CAT transgene (146). We recently observed that IL-1α and IL-1β, similar to TNF-α, directly induced HIV expression in chronically infected U1 cells and synergized in this effect with other cytokines, including IL-4, IL-6, and the glucocorticoid hormone dexamethasone; these effects were blocked by both IL-1Ra and anti-type I (but not anti-type II) IL-1R mAbs (114). However, neither the direct nor the synergistic inductive effects of IL-1 were associated with activation of NF-κB in U1 cells (114), suggesting that steps other than viral transcription were affected by this cytokine, as discussed in detail for IL-6.

IL-1ra

IL-1ra represents the only recognized example to date of a natural selective antagonist of a cytokine; its exclusive function is to block the binding of IL-1a and IL-1β to their cell surface receptors (147). IL-1ra is already being tested in clinical trials as a potential therapeutic modality in conditions characterized by elevated and inappropriate production if IL-1, such as septic shock and rheumatoid arthritis (147,148). IL-1ra expression in vivo has been described by immunohistochemical techniques in tissue macrophages present in the germinal centers of lymph nodes, spleen, and tonsils of uninfected individuals (149), sites that in HIV-infected individuals represent areas of accumulation of both infected cells and extracellular virions (1,6,7). It has also been noted that granulomas of patients with AIDS that are associated with Mycobacterium avium intracellulare contained cells that expressed IL-1Ra, but they were negative for IL-1 immunostaining (149). The previously reported production of a "contra-IL-1" activity by MDM infected in vitro with HIV (150) is likely explained by IL-1ra or a soluble IL-1R–derived molecule.

Given the ability of IL-1 to stimulate HIV replication in vitro, it is not surprising that IL-1ra was found to counteract IL-1 effects, both in chronically infected U1 cells (114) and in PBMC acutely infected with HIV (Kinter AL, et al., unpublished observations). Thus, IL-1ra represents a potential therapeutic agent in HIV infection aimed at inhibiting viral replication, as well as other IL-1–dependent pathological effects associated with increased or inappropriate production of this cytokine.

IL-2

IL-2 is historically the first recognized cytokine of relevance in HIV infection, in that it was an important element in the first successful attempts to isolate the causative agent of AIDS by cocultivation of PBMC from patients with AIDS with allogeneic mitogen-stimulated T-cell blasts (151–153). In addition, early studies conducted in HIV-infected individuals described a defect in IL-2 production after antigen or mitogen stimulation as one of the hallmarks of the immunodeficiency associated with this disease (154–156). A defect of IL-2 production in response to recall antigens has been correlated with an

increase in IL-4 secretion during early-stage HIV infection. This observation was interpreted as an example of pathological Th1/Th2 crossregulation, as supported by the finding that anti-IL-4 Ab could restore IL-2 production (157). Furthermore, in vitro production of IL-2 in response to envelope peptides has been found both in seropositive (158) and seronegative individuals at risk or known to be exposed to HIV (159). In this latter population, this finding has been proposed to be an indicator of a protective Th1-like cellular response; however, no information was provided in that study regarding IFN-γ and IL-4, which are the only cytokines produced exclusively by the CD4+ Th1 and Th2 subsets, respectively (160). Adherent PBMC, predominantly monocytes, from HIV-infected individuals have been shown to produce a 29-kd protein capable of suppressing both IL-2 production and IL-2Rα expression of activated lymphocytes isolated from seronegative donors (161). A previous study correlated such an effect with increased production of the immunosuppressive prostaglandin, PGE_2, by patients' monocytes (162). In contrast to the depressed production of IL-2 observed in the PB compartment, increased levels of IL-2 and soluble IL-2R have been reported in the CSF of HIV-infected individuals in association with increased local Ab production (121,163). IL-2–expressing cells have also been detected in the lymph nodes of HIV-infected individuals, particularly in the germinal centers, although at a frequency comparable to that of hyperplastic nodes obtained from HIV-seronegative patients (51,125). Several studies indicated that increased plasma levels of soluble (s) IL-2R were detectable in HIV-infected individuals, and they represented a potentially useful marker of clinical progression (124,163–166). Increased levels of sIL-2R were positively correlated with progressively increased levels of IL-6 in the plasma of HIV-infected individuals at different stages of disease (164). Furthermore, IL-6 has been shown to increase the levels of sIL-2R shedding from the monocytic cell line THP-1 (167), providing a potential explanation for the presence of this molecule in HIV-infected individuals.

Addition of rIL-2 to cell cultures has been shown to restore the defective natural killer cell activity of HIV-infected individuals (168). Furthermore, addition of rIL-2 to the culture media has been shown to reduce the increased spontaneous mortality of PBMC isolated from HIV-infected individuals (169); in a separate study, IL-2 required the presence of IL-1α to reverse the apoptosis observed in patients' PBMC (170). Neither IL-2 nor IL-4 were able to rescue the defective proliferative capacity of CD8+ anti-HIV cytolytic T-cell clones generated from the PBMC of HIV-infected patients (171).

On the basis of these observations, IL-2 has been administered to HIV-infected patients in an attempt to correct some of the major immune defects associated with HIV infection. In one study, IL-2 appeared to cause a transient state of CD4+ and CD8+ T lymphocytosis, in association with a marked eosinophilia that likely resulted from increased secretion of IL-5 (172). Enhanced cellular responses resembling delayed-type hypersensitivity, with increased local production of IFN-γ, increased natural killer cell (NK) activity, and lymphocyte proliferative responses, have been reported (173). Recently, substantial increases in the numbers of circulating CD4+ T cells have been observed in HIV-infected patients after intermittent administration of rIL-2, without any particular adverse effects (Kovacs J, et al., unpublished observations). No observations of sustained increases in viral replication have been reported in HIV-infected patients treated with IL-2, although clinical progression has been observed in some patients with AIDS-associated KS after treatment with IL-2 and IFN-β (174). However, transient peaks of HIV RNA have been observed recently in the plasma of infected individuals shortly after administration of IL-2, as determined by a branched DNA technique (Lane HC, personal communication). The observation that in vivo administration of IL-2 to cancer patients caused production of both TNF and soluble TNF receptors (175) may be relevant for the clinical use of IL-2 in therapeutic regimens in HIV-infected patients.

It remains to be established whether IL-2 can directly induce HIV replication in T cells, or whether the increased virus production is an indirect consequence of the mitogenic effects of this lymphokine. Infection of resting T cells is demonstrable in vitro, and it leads to a state of nonproductive infection (153,176,177). It has been demonstrated that in vitro infection of resting T cells leads to the accumulation of labile and incomplete products of reverse transcription that can be detected for several hours after infection (178,179). If cell activation occurs within this time frame, the reverse transcription process can be completed, followed by proviral integration and productive viral replication (178,179). This state of "preintegration latency" has not yet been proven to occur in vivo, where full length proviral genomes have been found in latently infected PBMC (180), suggesting that infected cells exist in vivo in a state of partial activation (181,182), as confirmed in macaques infected with SIV (183). In contrast to earlier studies (153,176), direct addition of rIL-2 to PBMC obtained from HIV-seropositive individuals resulted in a substantial increase of HIV replication (182), whereas depletion of IL-2R–positive cells from the total pool of PBMC obtained from healthy volunteers resulted in complete suppression of HIV replication after in vitro infection (177,184,185). We and others (185) observed productive HIV replication in primary PBMC infected in vitro in the presence of IL-2, but in the absence of prestimulation with mitogens (Kinter AL, et al., unpublished observations). In such experimental conditions, HIV replication was largely dependent on the release of several endogenous cytokines, such as IL-1β,

TNF-α, IL-6, IFN-γ (Kinter AL, et al., unpublished observations).

At the molecular level, an inductive effect of IL-2 on the HIV promoter was shown in primary T cells transfected with an HIV-LTR-CAT construct and costimulated with mitogens and antigen-presenting cells (186). However, a separate study utilizing primary T-cell clones transfected with different constructs containing the promoter region of the virus, known as LTR, linked to the reporter gene chloramphenicol acetyl transferase (CAT), showed a profound functional dissociation between T-cell proliferation, activation of NF-κB, and up-regulation of HIV-LTR–dependent transcription under different stimuli. Antigen and PMA stimulation induced the full spectrum of events mentioned, whereas IL-2 stimulation resulted in high levels of cell proliferation, but not induction of NF-κB binding activity or activation of the HIV promoter (99). Similarly, IL-2 was ineffective in activating the virus LTR transfected into cell lines (144). In contrast, IL-2, as well as IL-6, stimulated HIV replication in the monocytic THP-1 cell line, where up-regulation of cell surface IL-2Ra was also observed as a consequence of infection (167). An increase of IL-2Ra has been reported both in monocytes purified from HIV-infected individuals and after in vitro infection or exposure of normal MDM to rgp 120 envelope molecule (187). In contrast, chronically infected cell lines frequently show decreased expression of IL-2 receptors, as well as a decreased capacity to produce IL-2 (76,188). Decreased IL-2 production and proliferative responses of normal T lymphocytes were also found after exposure to HIV that had been inactivated by ultraviolet irradiation, whereas no decrease was observed in the production of IL-1 from autologous monocytes (189). Similar findings were described in both bulk primary T cells and T-cell clones exposed in vitro to rgp 120 (190,191). Finally, a recent study suggested that defective IL-2 production and T-cell proliferation may result as a consequence of increased expression of IFN-γ induced by the HIV-1 nef gene (192). Thus, differential effects of HIV infection on cells of the MP and the T-cell lineage seem to occur in terms of regulation of IL-2/IL-2Rα axis as a function of whether the cells are acutely or chronically infected with HIV.

The possibility of targeting IL-2R expressing cells present in HIV-infected individuals with different types of immunotoxins has been demonstrated in vitro (177,184,185). The specificity of such an approach for eliminating HIV-infected cells without harming uninfected or functionally normal cells remains to be determined.

IL-3

See "Hematopoietic Cytokines."

IL-4

Currently available data conflict with regard to the state of expression of IL-4 during HIV disease. Recent studies described an increased production of this Th2-restricted cytokine during early-stage disease that was correlated with decreased secretion of IL-2 in response to recall antigens (157). Because anti-IL-4 Ab restored IL-2 secretion (157), it was proposed that the observed abnormalities were an indication of a profound unbalance of Th1 and Th2 subsets, with potentially important implications for the pathogenesis of HIV infection (193). In support of this hypothesis, defective secretion of IL-12 has been observed both in PBMC isolated from HIV-infected individuals in response to *Staphylococcus aureus* (SAC) antigen as well as in MDM infected in vitro (194). IL-12 is a cytokine secreted by antigen-presenting cells that is capable of switching the majority of T cells characterized by Th0 or Th2 cytokine profiles toward a Th1/IFN-γ–producing phenotype (195). Increased numbers of cells expressing IL-4 mRNA have been recently described by in situ hybridization technique in lymph nodes of HIV-positive individuals compared with both uninflamed and inflamed nodes of HIV-negative control donors (Kotler D, personal communication). Other studies using in situ hybridization techniques for cytokine mRNAs detected Il-4 in patients' lymph nodes (51), although at levels not higher than those found in reactive lymph nodes obtained from HIV-seronegative individuals. Given the fact that IL-4 has been demonstrated to synergize with gp 120 in the induction of TNF-α and IL-6 from B lymphocytes obtained from normal donors (45), and transfection of the HIV-1 *tat* gene into the Raji lymphoblastoid B-cell line resulted in an increased expression of IL-4 receptors (196), it is likely that HIV or HIV gene products may cooperate with IL-4 in contributing to triggering or maintaining the state of activation of the B-cell compartment during HIV disease (43–47).

In contrast, PCR-based analysis of cytokine mRNA conducted in both PBMC and cells from lymphoid tissues did not detect IL-4 mRNAs, whereas messages for several other cytokines (including TNF-α, IL-6, and IL-10) were readily demonstrated, particularly in lymph node specimens (197). This latter study is consistent with the reported loss of detectable IL-4–producing cells during the course of HIV infection (198–200). Furthermore, it has also been demonstrated that exposure of CD4+ T cells to rgp 120 leads to an impaired ability to provide help to B lymphocytes, in conjunction with a decreased ability to secrete IL-2 and IL-4 (191). Lower levels of IL-4, as well as of IL-1, have also been detected in the brain tissues of demented patients with AIDS compared with patients with AIDS without dementia, whereas TNF-α exhibited the opposite pattern (131),

suggesting a differential role for these cytokines in HIV-associated organ pathology.

With regard to the role of IL-4 in HIV replication, it appears that this cytokine (similar to IL-10, TGF-β, and IFN-γ) may exert different effects as a function of the experimental conditions. IL-4 can induce HIV expression in conjunction with IL-2 in primary human thymocytes, although not in mature PB T cells (201). In one study, IL-4 potentiated the HIV-inductive effect of soluble anti-CD3 mAb, although it was in conjunction with increased levels of cell proliferation (202). In primary MDM, IL-4 induced both cluster formation and HIV replication (203,204). In a separate study, IL-4 enhanced the susceptibility of monocytes freshly isolated from normal donors to be productively infected with HIV (84). However, in the same study, IL-4 also potently suppressed HIV replication in 5-day-old MDM, both in unstimulated conditions and in the presence of HIV-inductive cytokines, such as IL-1, IL-3, GM-CSF, and TNF-α (84). We recently observed suppressive effects of IL-4 on HIV replication when this cytokine was added to IL-2–stimulated PBMC infected in vitro with several strains of HIV-1 (Kinter AL, et al., unpublished observations). IL-4 did not alter the state of relative latency of the chronically infected U1 cell line; however, IL-4 potently synergized with other cytokines, including IL-1, IL-6, and IL-10, in the induction of HIV expression from U1 cells (Weissman D, et al., unpublished observations). In contrast, we also observed that IL-4, similar to TGF-β, could suppress the induction of HIV expression in U1 cells stimulated with LPS (Goletti D, et al., unpublished observations). Thus, IL-4 does not appear to have a unidimensional (suppressive or inductive) effect on HIV expression and replication, but it may manifest dichotomous effects as a function of the experimental conditions and the stimuli used.

IL-6

Similar to TNF-α and IL-1, increased levels of IL-6 have been demonstrated in HIV-infected patients in plasma (205–211), CSF (121,212), and lymph nodes (51,125) (Graziosi C, et al. personal communication; Kotler D, personal communication). A positive correlation was found in some studies between increased levels of IL-6 and elevated production of immunoglobulin (Ig) in plasma (206,208) or CSF (121) that is characteristic of HIV infection. In one study, high levels of IL-6 production were correlated with increased levels of the circulating ICAM-1 adhesion molecule (211). Increased levels of IL-6 have been reported in patients with AIDS with KS compared with other HIV-infected individuals (209); furthermore, both KS and AIDS-associated B-cell lymphomas have been shown to secrete and proliferate in response to IL-6 (13,14). PBMC (124,205), as well as intestinal mononuclear cells obtained from the lamina propria (124), lung AM (128), and B lymphocytes (43–45) isolated from HIV-infected individuals have shown an increased constitutive production of IL-6 compared with uninfected control subjects. In the case of B lymphocytes, IL-6 secretion was further enhanced by rgp120, although not by B-cell mitogens; this effect was not blocked by sCD4 (44), suggesting that cytokine production was triggered via interaction of gp120 with a cell surface Ig receptor (44,45). A separate study did not find increased expression of IL-6 in PBMC or serum of HIV-infected individuals (213), although anti-IL-6 Ab suppressed the high constitutive levels of Ig production typically observed in PBMC obtained from HIV-infected individuals (213).

Increased production of IL-6 has been implicated as a potential cause of the defective proliferative responses of T cells observed during HIV infection, an effect that can be mediated by production of active TGF-β (108). Furthermore, IL-6 has been shown to cause an increased shedding of IL-2R in vitro (167,207); it may therefore be a potential cause of the increased circulating levels of these molecules seen in HIV disease. Finally, elevated levels of IL-6R have been described both in the plasma of HIV-infected patients (214) and after in vitro infection of a promonocytic cell line with HIV (214). Macaques infected with the highly pathogenic variant of SIV known as SIV$_{pbj14}$ (10) produce extremely high levels of this cytokine, whereas primate species that were resistant to the SIV$_{pbj}$ pathogenic effect had much lower levels of circulating IL-6 (10,215). Thus, a close association between replication of pathogenic human and primate lentiviruses and expression of IL-6 emerges from different studies.

In vitro infection of PBMC or exposure of monocytes to certain gp120 envelope proteins resulted in increased secretion of IL-6 (56,137,206,207,216), although some studies did not observe elevation of this or other proinflammatory cytokines during HIV infection (217). Monocytotropic variants of HIV have been found to be more effective in inducing IL-6 secretion from monocytes (206), whereas T cells were not a relevant source of this cytokine in this as well as in an independent study (216). However, rgp 120 and gp 160 have been reported to induce IL-6 production from both normal PBMC and T-cell clones (218). A recent study has shown that the HIV-1 *tat* protein can activate the promoter of IL-6, thereby providing a potential explanation for the observed increased levels of this cytokine (219).

Addition of rIL-6 to primary MDM cultures increases the efficiency of HIV replication (83,141). In macrophages obtained from uninfected macaques, IL-6, unlike TNF-α, did not significantly enhance replication of SIV on a per cell basis, although it increased the cytopathic effect of the virus (85). IL-6, similar to IL-2, augmented the replicative capacity of HIV in the monocytic cell line THP-1 (167), as well as in primary astrocytes (142) and in

one neuroblastoma cell line (220). Furthermore, we recently obtained evidence that IL-6 may drive HIV replication in an autocrine manner, both in PBMC stimulated with IL-2 and in MDM infected with a macrophage tropic strain of HIV (91). IL-6 induces expression of HIV in U1 cells, both alone and in combination with other cytokines, glucocorticoid hormones, and heat (83,114,221) (Poli G, et al., unpublished observations). IL-6 appears to exert both transcriptional and post-transcriptional effects on virus expression in U1 cells; stimulation with this cytokine alone does not usually affect the constitutive levels of HIV transcription, and it does not activate NF-κB, whereas it potently increases the inductive effect of TNF-α on both viral transcription and virion production (83,114,221) (Poli G, et al., unpublished observations). The post-transcriptional effect of IL-6 on HIV expression in U1 cells has been confirmed by recent studies in which a potent synergy on HIV production was induced in U1 cells costimulated with either IL-6 plus IL-1 or IL-6 plus glucocorticoid hormones. Neither induction of NF-κB nor activation of a transfected HIV-LTR-CAT was observed in these conditions (114) (Poli G, et al., unpublished observations).

IL-7

IL-7 is a cytokine with T-cell activating capacity. Its role in HIV infection has not been extensively investigated. In one study, IL-7 was found to strongly synergize with soluble anti-CD3 mAB in the stimulation of virus production from CD8-depleted PBMC isolated from HIV-infected individuals (202). IL-7 up-regulation of virus production, in contrast to IL-4, was not correlated with increased cell proliferation, compared with cells stimulated with anti-CD3 mAb alone (202), suggesting a direct role of IL-7 in the up-regulation of HIV expression.

IL-8

An abnormality of both monocyte and polymorphonuclear leukocyte (PMNL) chemotaxis has been identified early on as an important functional defect in HIV-infected individuals (222–224). However, involvement of chemotactic cytokines in this disease has not yet been extensively investigated. The defective PMNL chemotaxis of HIV-seropositive individuals was up-regulated by supernatant of PBMC obtained from healthy seronegative donors (225); conversely, PMNL of HIV-positive patients increased monokine secretion from normal monocytes in coculture (226). However, neither of these effects was neutralized by anti-IL-8 Ab (225,226). In vitro restoration of the monocyte migratory defect of HIV-infected individuals was accomplished by stimulation with the differentiating agent vitamin D$_3$ (227).

In a single study, in vitro infection of MDM with HIV resulted in the induction of IL-8 mRNA, but protein secretion was decreased (136). Other studies described upregulation of IL-8 secretion as a consequence of HIV infection (56,228). The correlation between the potentially altered production of IL-8 and the defects of phagocyte migratory responses detected in the majority of HIV-infected patients remains to be investigated further.

IL-10

The potential role of IL-10 in HIV disease has recently received considerable attention. Production of IL-10 from stimulated PBMC is elevated in HIV-infected individuals with advanced stages of disease; this finding was interpreted as a functional marker of dysregulation of Th1 and Th2 CD4+ T-cell subsets (157,159,193,229). However, human IL-10 differs substantially from its mouse equivalent in that it is not selectively produced by the Th2 subset of T lymphocytes; it is secreted by a variety of lymphocytic and nonlymphocytic cells, including Th0 and Th1 T cells (160,230). Therefore, in contrast to IL-4, the observation of altered levels of IL-10 in human diseases cannot be interpreted as an absolute indication of dysregulation between Th1 and Th2 CD4+ T-lymphocyte subsets. Furthermore, IL-10 mRNA has been detected by RT-PCR technique in both PBMC and mononuclear cells obtained from lymph nodes of infected individuals, without substantial differences in levels at different stages of disease (197). A recent study described a sharp decrease in the frequency of lymph nodes positive for IL-10 mRNA as detected by in situ hybridization during progression from the asymptomatic phase to AIDS (Kotler D, personal communication).

IL-10 expression and production has been observed in AIDS-associated lymphomas at a frequency much higher than that observed in lymphomas from seronegative individuals (231). Production of IL-10 has been correlated with the presence of Epstein-Barr virus (EBV) (which encodes for a viral homolog of IL-10) in the neoplastic cells (231,232). Cell lines derived from AIDS-associated lymphomas were found to express high levels of IL-10 (232), suggesting that this cytokine, as well as the presence of EBV, can contribute to the state of oligo/polyclonal B-cell activation typical of HIV infection.

Recent studies demonstrated that addition of IL-10 to primary MDM suppresses HIV replication. In one study, this effect was quantitatively correlated with the known ability of IL-10 to inhibit cytokine production from MDM. In particular, IL-10 appeared to exert its suppressive effects on viral spreading by blocking the production of TNF-α and IL-6, which are capable of inducing HIV replication in MDM. In support of this hypothesis, addition of rTNF-α or rIL-6 to MDM cultures infected with

HIV abrogated the IL-10 inhibitory effects (91). A simultaneous and independent study, however, did not show a clear correlation between IL-10 suppressive effects on virus replication and production of endogenous cytokines (219). In contrast to these suppressive effects, IL-10 also enhances HIV replication in MDM cultures when added at concentrations that did not completely block TNF-α and IL-6 production (Weissman D, et al., unpublished observations). When the regulatory effects of IL-10 were tested in chronically infected promonocytic U1 cells, no direct induction of virus expression was observed. However, similar to IL-4 and glucocorticoid hormones (233), IL-10 could potently synergize with other cytokines, including IL-1, IL-4, IL-6, and TNF-α, in the induction of virus expression (Weissman D, et al., unpublished observations). Transcriptional activation of the HIV LTR was also demonstrated in U1 cells costimulated with IL-10 and other cytokines (Weissman D, et al., unpublished observations).

Therefore, although additional studies are required to assign a definitive role to IL-10 in the regulation of HIV production, it is conceivable that this cytokine down-regulates virus production in either experimental or natural conditions in which HIV replication is triggered or sustained by endogenous production of viral-inductive cytokines (i.e., IL-6, and TNF-α) acting in an autocrine/paracrine manner. This model is consistent with the well-described antiinflammatory role of IL-10 (230). However, it is also possible that IL-10 actually enhances the HIV inductive effects of cytokines in experimental or clinical conditions in which these cytokines are either already present or produced by cells not susceptible to the suppressive effect of IL-10. Both a lack of suppressive effects and enhancement of cytokine gene expression by IL-10 has recently been observed in endothelial cells (234).

IL-12

IL-12, a product of B cells and MP, has multiple effects on both T and NK cells (195). Recently, IL-12 has been identified as a major switching factor in the commitment of Th0 CD4+ T cells into Th1-type cells; it was particularly efficient in producing IFN-γ and sustaining a cell-mediated immune response (235). IL-12 has shown in vitro efficacy in correcting the functional defect of NK cells that occurs in HIV-infected patients (168), as previously shown with IL-2 and IFNs. Recently, a defect of IL-12 production has been reported both in monocytes obtained from HIV-infected individuals compared with cells from healthy donors, as well as in MDM from normal donors after in vitro infection with HIV and stimulation with SAC (194). The defect in IL-12 production that occurs during the course of HIV infection may therefore explain the defective production of IFN-γ from

PBMC of infected individuals (168), and it supports the hypothesis that HIV infection is associated with an imbalance of Th1/Th2 regulatory subsets of CD4+ T cells (157,159,193,229).

IL-13

Suppressive effects of IL-13 on HIV replication have recently been reported in human MDM, but not in T-cell blasts (236).

HEMATOPOIETIC CYTOKINES

General dysregulation of hematopoiesis, manifested by varying types and degrees of cytopenias, is not uncommon during HIV disease (237), suggesting that the BM as well as the thymus (1,2,238–240) may represent important targets of infection. BM-derived multipotential CD34+ cells have been successfully infected in vitro (241,242). Over time, these infected cultures become indistinguishable from mature macrophage cultures, harboring very high levels of virions in intracytoplasmic compartments (241). Infection of BM-derived CD34+ cells in vivo has been documented, although it appears to be demonstrable only in patients with very advanced stages of disease or with very low CD4+ cell counts (107). Resident macrophages have been shown to be the main cellular reservoirs of SIV in experimentally infected macaques (243). The possibility that HIV-related gene products, such as the tat protein, may indirectly cause suppressive effects on generation and maturation of myelomonocytic cells has been described (106). Therefore, the effects of hematopoietic cytokines, most frequently studied on mature MDM, also need to be extrapolated to the BM microenvironment, where both direct effects on virus expression in monocytic cells and dysregulatory effects on the maturation of precursor cells may occur. Finally, it is well known that hematopoietic cytokines are not limited in their effects to the immature precursor cells, but that they are potent regulators of mature cell function (244).

Human stem-cell factor

Decreased efficiency of colony formation in soft agar from precursor hematopoietic cells is a common finding in HIV infection. Depletion of CD8+ T cells enhanced the decreased colony-forming capacity of circulating precursor cells (245), whereas in an independent study, neither depletion of this T-cell subset nor addition of IL-3 or GM-CSF could correct this defect (246). Addition of human stem-cell factor (HuSCF) increased the BFU-E, GM-CFU,

and CFU-Mix capacity of circulating precursor cells without altering the levels of HIV replication, the total proliferative capacity of PBMC in response to mitogens and IL-2, or the efficacy of antiviral treatments (247).

IL-3

Limited information is available on the state of IL-3 production during in vivo infection with HIV. Decreased secretion of IL-3 (and IL-4) in response to mitogens or PMA has been reported and correlated with both the stage of disease and the ability of HIV to replicate in culture (198). Addition of IL-3 to MDM cultures exerts inductive effects on virus production (248); this observation was confirmed in subsequent independent studies (84,249), including studies that utilized CD34+ precursor cells as the original source of MDM (242). The inductive effect on HIV production in MDM was correlated with an increased level of cell proliferation (242,249), although independent studies indicated that cell replication is not required for virus production in these cells (250).

It remains to be determined whether a defective production of IL-3 occurs in the BM microenvironment and whether replenishment therapy may lead to reconstitution of certain BM functions in the absence of viral spreading. The observation that AZT blocks HIV replication in both control and IL-3–treated MDM (249) indicates that IL-3 may not induce undesired viral spreading when administered with an antiretroviral agent.

Granulocyte-macrophage colony-stimulating factor

Progressive loss of the capacity of CD4+ T cells to secrete GM-CSF has been reported in HIV-infected individuals (198,251). However, increased levels of GM-CSF have been reported in intravenous drug abusers, regardless of their HIV status (252). Increased levels of GM-CSF have been found in bronchoalveolar lavages of HIV-infected individuals; in addition, increased levels are produced de novo by in vitro stimulation of lung AM with LPS (253). Several clinical protocols utilized GM-CSF to restore certain of the hematological abnormalities associated with this disease; there has been evidence of in vivo efficacy on certain parameters, such as elevation of white blood cell counts (254–256) and increased bactericidal capacity of PMNLs (257). Increased production of superoxide anions and expression of cell surface human leukocyte antigen-DR (HLA-DR) antigens have been reported after GM-CSF administration in conjunction with increased levels of p24 viral Ag in the plasma (254). Other studies using antiretroviral agents in association with GM-CSF have not confirmed that this cytokine caused an increase in the levels of HIV replication in vivo (258,259). In one study, both a decrease of p24 Ag and a prolongation of the time required to isolate HIV from PBMC were observed after administration of GM-CSF to infected patients receiving either AZT or IFN-α (259).

Increased production of GM-CSF, as well as of several proinflammatory cytokines, was observed after incubation of uninfected monocytes with gp 120 envelope protein of some, but not all, HIV-1 strains, an effect that was inhibited by soluble CD4 (137). Furthermore, with the exception of one early report in U937 cells (260) and a study in which treatment with this cytokine decreased the susceptibility of placental macrophages to HIV infection (261), GM-CSF has been demonstrated to enhance HIV replication in both MDM and promonocytic cell lines, such as U937 and U1 (115,116,132,203,248,262–264). In addition, GM-CSF, similar to IL-3, has been shown to increase the levels of HIV replication in BMderived CD34+ cells (242). Up-regulation of virus production by GM-CSF was also documented in lung AM obtained from healthy macaques and infected in vitro with SIV; however, this effect was correlated with increased levels of cell proliferation (85). Pretreatment with GM-CSF has been shown to be necessary for the HIV-inductive effect of LPS in chronically infected U1 cells, an effect mediated by the induction of expression of the cell surface LPS receptor CD14 antigen (115,116). This study has recently been confirmed and extended (Goletti D, et al., unpublished observations). Furthermore, GM-CSF has the ability to synergize with other cytokines, including TNF-α and IL-6, in the induction of virus production in U1 cells (83) (Poli G, et al., unpublished observations). Finally, it has been clearly shown that the viral-inductive effect of GM-CSF may not represent an absolute contraindication for its clinical use, in that an increased efficiency of phosphorylation of AZT as well as of its anti-HIV efficacy has been demonstrated in vitro after treatment of MDM or U937 cells with GM-CSF (262–265).

Macrophage colony-stimulating factor

Little information is available on the production of M-CSF during HIV infection. In one study, detectable levels of this cytokine in the CSF were reported in a variety of neurological conditions, including a minority of patients with the AIDS dementia complex (266). A decrease of M-CSF production as a consequence of in vitro infection with HIV was noted in MDM cultures, in contrast to the increased production of several proinflammatory cytokines (56). M-CSF was found to enhance greatly the susceptibility of MDM to HIV infection and their consequent ability to support high levels of viral replication (264, 267–269). In one study, such inductive effects were cor-

related with an increased expression of the CD4 molecule on the cell surface of treated MDM (269). Most of these studies were conducted with a truncated form of M-CSF, whereas the full-length protein appears to be less or not effective in sustaining HIV replication in MDM. The nature of this functional difference, as well as the molecular mechanisms of M-CSF-inductive effects, have not been fully clarified.

Granulocyte colony-stimulating factor and erythropoietin

Increased plasma levels of erythropoietin (EPO) have been reported in both HIV-negative and HIV-positive homosexual men without any significant correlation with their state of HIV infection or stage of disease (252). Both G-CSF and EPO have been investigated for their ability to correct the abnormal hematological parameters in HIV-infected individuals; these studies demonstrated some clinical efficacy (255,270,271). No evidence of effect on HIV replication has been obtained (255,264,270,271), which is compatible with the lack of evidence that the 2 lineages susceptible to the action of these cytokines are targets for HIV infection. Combination therapy of either G-CSF and EPO with antiretroviral agents is often administered to HIV-infected patients.

INTERFERONS

IFN-α

IFN-α exists as several subspecies (15 or more) (272). In addition, a so called acid-labile IFN-α, previously described in autoimmune diseases such as systemic lupus erythematosus and rheumatoid arthritis, has also been recognized as a marker of HIV infection (273–275). It has also been suggested that acid-labile IFN-α is a dysfunctional IFN that may lead to immune suppression by inhibiting the production or effect of normal IFN (276). Although it is still unclear whether a molecular form corresponding to acid-labile IFN-α truly exists, it has been shown in HIV-infected patients that it is actually a mixture of both IFN-α and IFN-γ (274). Defective synthesis or production of IFN-α has been described in HIV-infected individuals from the mRNA to the protein level in correlation with the stage of disease (34). Furthermore, in vitro infection of MDM has been linked to a defect in IFN-α synthesis (277). In contrast, high levels of IFN-α (which could be accounted for, at least in part, by acid-labile IFN-α) have been frequently reported during HIV infection (278–283). Because gp 120 has been shown to induce IFN from PBMC obtained from normal donors on interaction with the CD4 molecule, it has been proposed that either HIV-associated or shed envelope may represent an important inducer of IFN in vivo (284).

Addition of IFN-α to T-cell blasts infected in vitro with HIV-1 resulted in a profound suppression of virus production, in association with decreased synthesis of viral proteins (285). These studies have been confirmed in acutely infected cell lines (286–292). At the molecular level, it has been demonstrated that IFN-α causes a block in the life cycle of HIV after entry and before or at the beginning of the RT process (290). Furthermore, in studies where cells lines were either permanently or transiently transfected with an IFN-α gene driven by the HIV LTR, a suppressive effect linked to IFN-α expression was observed on a target HIV-1-LTR-CAT reporter system that was correlated with the inhibition of binding of a 45-kd NF-κB complex (291,292). Suppression of the HIV LTR was also observed in neuroblastoma and glioma cell lines treated with IFNs (142). IFN-α is a potent inhibitor of HIV replication in MDM, likely acting at multiple steps of the virus life cycle, including reverse transcription, de novo transcription, and post-transcriptional events (293–297). Furthermore, IFN-α–treated cells appear to produce a significantly less infectious progeny of virions than untreated control cells (293,295), as previously observed in cells infected with other animal viruses, including retroviruses (298). In cell lines chronically infected with HIV, IFN-α appears to suppress production of new virions by affecting the very late phase of particle release from the plasma membrane (299–303), as previously observed with other animal retroviruses (298). This effect of IFN-α does not result in the inhibition of viral antigen shedding from the plasma membrane (302). In vitro synergy between IFN-α and antireverse transcriptase nucleosidic analogs, such as AZT, has been observed (304), providing the basis for the combined use of these 2 agents in clinical trials.

IFN-α is the first cytokine for which a role as an endogenous suppressor factor of HIV replication has been reported. Addition of Ab-neutralizing IFN-α has been shown to increase both the levels of HIV replication and the frequency of positive viral isolation from PBMC of HIV-infected individuals (152,305). Similar effects have been described during acute in vitro infection of the U937 cell line, where treatment with anti-IFN-α or anti-IFN-β Ab caused acceleration of the kinetics of viral replication compared with control cells (81,306).

On the basis of its ability to block different steps in HIV replication in vitro, as well as its relative deficiency in HIV-infected individuals, IFN-α has been administered both alone and in combination with other agents for therapeutic purposes. The original clinical use of IFN-α was actually correlated with its antineoplastic effect against HIV-associated KS; partial and even complete remissions were achieved (307–310). In one of these studies, a decrease in HIV-p24 antigenemia was observed, indicating an in vivo antiviral effect of IFN-α (309). The effect was found to occur in patients with CD4 cell counts above 500/μL, indicating that the antiviral effect of IFN-α could have been caused by its immunostimulatory properties on a relatively healthy immune system, as opposed to a direct antiviral effect. In vitro studies have suggested that the ability of IFN-α to block the spreading of infection in primary PBMC was correlated with the induction of cell-mediated cytotoxicity (311). Several clinical trials have been conducted, including combinations of AZT and CSF (to limit the toxicity observed at the BM level in individuals treated with IFN-α or AZT) (251,252,306–310,312).

IFN-β

Limited studies have been conducted with IFN-β compared with IFN-α, although these 2 molecules have been found to exert similar effects. In vitro restoration of the defective NK cell activity of HIV-infected patients (313) and suppression of HIV replication in primary MDM (293,296) and cell lines (314) have both been reported for IFN-β. Furthermore, as reported for IFN-α, addition of anti-IFN-β Ab to infected cultures resulted in increased levels of virus replication (81), indicating that IFN-β may act as a suppressive endogenous cytokine. A derivative of the U937 cell line that contained a stable IFN-β transgene under the control of a murine MHC gene has shown resistance to HIV infection, an effect that could be reversed by addition of anti-IFN-β–neutralizing Ab to the cultures (315).

A limited number of clinical trials have used IFN-β in HIV-infected patients. No significant changes in the number of HIV proviral copies present in PBMC have been reported after treatment of patients with this agent (316,317). However, an increased plasma half-life of AZT has been observed in regimens of combination therapy with IFN-β (318). Rapid disease progression was observed in 3 of 4 patients with AIDS-associated KS treated with IL-2 and IFN-β (174), although it is more likely that these adverse effects were attributable to IL-2 or IL-2–induced IFN-γ than to IFN-β (173,318).

IFN-γ

It remains a highly controversial issue whether IFN-γ levels are elevated, normal, or depressed during the course of HIV infection. Several studies have described an elevation of either IFN-γ levels or its functionally related molecule, neopterin (a product of IFN-γ–activated macrophages) in the plasma and serum of HIV-infected individuals (319–

323); however, there are conflicting reports on the status of IFN-γ production by cells isolated from HIV-infected patients. Increased constitutive secretion of IFN-γ (and TNF-α) has been observed from PBMC of HIV-infected patients as a function of the stage of disease (35). Furthermore, freshly isolated PBMC from patients, similar to CD8+ CTL clones, produced IFN-γ when challenged in vitro with a proper antigenic peptide (49). However, earlier studies have shown that PBMC obtained from HIV-infected individuals produce less IFN-γ in response to different stimuli (324–329). Similarly, mononuclear cells isolated from the lamina propria of the large bowel showed a decreased constitutive and inducible capacity to secrete IFN-γ; however, they produced levels of IL-1 and IL-6 higher than those observed with cells isolated from uninfected individuals (123). It is likely that some of these discrepancies were due to a variable state of in vivo priming/activation of patients' cells (330) or to the fact that IFN-γ can be secreted by several cell types, such as CD8+ T cells, Th0 and Th1 CD4+ T cells, and NK cells, among others.

Evidence for in vivo production and effects of IFN-γ have been obtained by studies of lung AM obtained from HIV-infected individuals. These cells showed an activated phenotype, as indicated by increased levels of class II antigens expressed on their cell surface, and by their constitutive ability to secrete TNF-α and superoxide anion (331). Of interest, 24 hours of in vitro culture resulted in normalization of some of these parameters, suggesting that AM were indeed preactivated in vivo (331), as further demonstrated by the fact that freshly isolated AM from HIV-infected individuals, but not AM obtained from healthy control donors, expressed mRNA for the IFN-γ–inducible gene IP-10 (331). Increased expression of IFN-γ and neopterin has been reported as a stable marker in the CSF of HIV-infected individuals; these parameters were particularly elevated in the setting of AIDS-associated CNS disorders (332). Lymph nodes of HIV-infected individuals manifested high levels of IFN-γ mRNA (much more abundant than those found in reactive lymph nodes obtained in the germinal centers corresponding to areas infiltrated by CD8+ T lymphocytes) (51,125). Recent RT-PCR studies on cytokine mRNA expression confirmed the presence of increased levels of IFN-γ in lymph node–derived cells compared with PBMC obtained from the same HIV-infected donor (197). The possibility of a direct physical association between HIV and IFN-γ has been suggested by in vitro studies showing that the p17 gag protein could specifically bind IFN-γ (333). A recent intriguing finding is that the HIV-1 nef gene appears to cause several functional abnormalities in T lymphocytes, including down-modulation of the CD4 molecule and suppression of their IL-2–dependent proliferative capacity as a consequence of enhanced production of several cytokines, particularly IFN-γ (192).

IFN-γ has been broadly investigated as an immunostimulating agent capable of restoring some of the defective immune functions associated with HIV infection, including monocyte (334), NK (313,326), and T-cell function (313). IFN-γ, either alone or in combination with TNF-α or other agents, has been administered to HIV-infected patients, with unclear clinical results (334–337).

Addition of IFN-γ to cell cultures undergoing acute in vitro infection has resulted in dichotomous results. Usually, IFN-γ has shown a less pronounced anti-HIV activity than that exerted by IFN-α or IFN-β (286–288). In contrast to the evidence that IFN-α and IFN-β can serve as endogenous negative regulators of HIV replication (81,305,307), it is likely that IFN-γ represents an important endogenous factor that sustains HIV replication in PBMC (89), an observation that we recently confirmed and extended (Kinter AL, et al., unpublished observations). In contrast, anti-IFN-γ Ab increased the expression of HIV in some infected Th1 CD4+ T cell clones (200).

IFN-γ suppressed HIV replication in primary MDM (293,297) and in the monocytic THP-1 and U937 cell lines (167,260), and similar results were obtained with lung AM obtained from healthy macaques and infected in vitro with SIV (85). In one study, both suppressive and inductive effects of IFN-γ were observed on HIV replication in MDM, depending on whether serum was present in the culture medium, an effect that was explained by enhancement of Fc-dependent infection mediated via up-regulation of cell surface Fc receptors by IFN-γ (338). Enhancement, no effect, or suppression of HIV replication has been reported as a function of whether the cells were treated with IFN-γ before, at the same time, or after infection (248); however, no explanation was provided for these opposite effects.

A dichotomous effect of IFN-γ on HIV expression has also been demonstrated in chronically infected U1 cells. IFN-γ directly induced virus production, although this cytokine, at the same time, appeared to inhibit PMA-mediated HIV production (303). This apparent functional dichotomy could be explained by the observation that IFN-γ treatment caused a major redirection of the primary cellular site of virion production from the plasma membrane to intracytoplasmic Golgi-derived compartments (303). Furthermore, similar features of intracytoplasmic vacuole–associated virions were observed in U1 cells co-stimulated with IFN-γ and TNF-α, concomitant with synergistic induction of viral expression and profound cytopathic effects (70). It remains to be established whether similar effects can explain the early dichotomous effects observed with IFN-γ treatment of HIV-infected MDM (248).

Finally, it has also been shown that IFN-γ can inactivate free infectious virus by production of reactive oxygen intermediates (ROI) (339). However, in light of the fact that ROI can lead to increased HIV expression via activation of NF-κB (101,340), it is likely that a multifactorial balance of proviral and antiviral effects is the basis of the conflicting reports on the role of IFN-γ as a regulator of HIV replication.

CONCLUSIONS AND PERSPECTIVES

The cytokine network is intimately involved in the pathogenesis of HIV disease. HIV infection appears to dysregulate the expression of several cytokines in vivo (see Table 28–1); in addition, when virus or viral components, such as gp 120 envelope and *tat*, are added to or transfected into target monocytic or lymphocytic cells, cytokine expression is modulated (Table 28–2). Conversely, several cytokines have demonstrated the capacity to profoundly affect the state of expression and overall spreading of HIV in vitro. Proinflammatory cytokines, such as TNF-α, IL-1, and IL-6, appear to represent potent enhancing factors in the propagation of HIV infection and spreading to new target cells. Other cytokines, such as IFN-α and IFN-β, are potent suppressors of the same process (see Figs. 28–2, 28–3). However, several questions and intriguing findings remain open for further study. It is currently unclear how to interpret the functional dichotomy exerted by certain cytokines, such as TGF-β, IL-4, IL-10, and IFN-γ, on in vitro replication of HIV, and what their ultimate effect

in vivo might be. Furthermore, the recent observation that cytotoxic T lymphocytes can simultaneously kill HIV-infected cells and release cytokines that up-regulate and promote spreading of the virus (30–32,48–50) raises the question whether these cell-mediated immune mechanisms have an exclusively protective role in HIV disease.

It is likely that there are cytokines not yet been investigated, or only begun to be studied in the context of HIV infection, that may have a major role in the pathogenesis of this disease. Among these cytokines are IL-7, IL-9, IL-10, IL-11, oncostatin M, liver (migration) inhibitory factor, and IL-12. In addition, it is possible that other cytokines may become recognized as relevant to HIV infection and offer new insights into the pathogenesis of this disease. Among these latter cytokines are soluble factors elaborated by CD8+ T cells with suppressive activities on either HIV expression (341) or immune function (342), and the recently identified family of vasoactive peptides known as endothelins (343). Furthermore, a number of other physiological or pharmacological agents have already been shown to interact with the cytokine network and to ultimately result in regulatory effects on virus production. A short list of these agents includes vitamins, hormones, other microbes and microbial components, oxidants, and antioxidants (15,101,341,344). Furthermore, cell activation processes mediated by cell-to-cell signaling molecules (including membrane-associated cytokines) and adhesion molecules represent potentially important pathways of regulation of virus expression or

TABLE 28–2   EFFECT OF HIV COMPONENTS ON THE EXPRESSION OF CYTOKINES OR CYTOKINE RECEPTORS

HIV Protein	Function in HIV	Cytokine		Cell Type
gp 120 env	CD4 binding; viral entry	TNF-α	(↑)	MP, B cells
		IL-1β	(↑)	B cells
		IL-2	(↓)	T cells
		IL-6	(↑)	B cells
		GM-CSF	(↑)	MP
		IFN-α	(↑)	PBMC
Tat	Transactivator of viral transcription	TNF-β	(↑)	B cells*
		TNF-R	(↓)	B cells*
		TGF-β	(↑)	MP
		IL-4R	(↑)	B cells*
Nef	CD4 down-modulation; in vivo virulence (SIV)	IL-2	(↓)	T cells
		IL-2R	(↑)	MP
		IFN-γ	(↑)	T cells

*Results obtained in the Raji B cell line.
MP = mononuclear phagocytes.

virus-associated cytopathic effects that may act in synergy with cytokines (1,2,82,344–348). In this context, soluble cytokine receptors have been investigated mostly as markers of disease activity; however, their potentially pathogenic role has not been thoroughly investigated. The fact that cytokine antagonists, such as IL-1Ra or recombinant soluble cytokine receptors, have already provided evidence of in vitro efficacy (100,114) suggests that they may serve as useful agents in regimens of combined treatment.

The molecular mechanisms of cytokine-mediated regulation of virus production are not well understood except for TNF-α and TNF-β, for which there is convincing evidence that their HIV-inductive effects are mediated by activation of the cellular transcription factor NF-κB (See Fig. 28–2). Furthermore, although HIV-1 is the major subtype that causes AIDS throughout the world, HIV-2 is the predominant etiologic agent in certain geographic areas (349). It is generally assumed that HIV-1 and HIV-2 are very similar in their spectrum of target cells and effect; however, recent molecular studies have highlighted substantial differences in their transcriptional regulation directed by the virus LTR (350–352). It remains to be determined whether a different involvement of the cytokine network occurs in individuals infected with HIV-1 versus HIV-2. Similarly, it is important to determine the ability of HIV or SIV to induce or not induce disease in different animal models, such as macaques and chimpanzees, as well as to determine whether these viruses have different capabilities of activating the immune system or the cytokine network. The possibility that functional dysregulation of Th1 and Th2 subsets of CD4+ T lymphocytes may have an important role in the pathogenesis of HIV infection, similar to what has been observed with parasitic diseases, has recently been suggested (193,194,197,200, 229,353), and this idea deserves further investigation. It has been demonstrated that cytokines such as IL-12 may act as important "adjuvants" in determining the type of immune response to microbial agents (195). It is conceivable that similar strategies may be adopted in HIV infection, after understanding whether a "protective" versus a "nonprotective" immune status exists in this disease (354,355).

In conclusion, the ability of HIV to integrate into the host chromosomes represents the essential element that explains the complex and multiple crossregulatory pathways that have been observed between the cells that are targets of HIV infection and the virus. Involvement of the cytokine network in HIV infection and AIDS is an excellent reflection of the intimate relationship between this pathogenic virus and the host. Whether manipulation of the cytokine network will lead to better control of the process of HIV infection remains a fundamental, unanswered question.

ACKNOWLEDGMENTS: We thank Audrey L. Kinter, Jesse S. Justement, Sharilyn K. Stanley, Priscilla Biswas, Drew Weissman, Peter Bressler, Lawrence Fox, and Delia Goletti for helpful discussions, and Ms. Janet S. Bey for typing the manuscript.

REFERENCES

1. Pantaleo G, Graziosi C, Fauci AS. New concepts in the immunopathogenesis of human immunodeficiency virus infection. N Engl J Med 1993;328:327–335.
2. Fauci AS. The multifactorial and multiphasic components of human immunodeficiency virus disease: implications for the design of therapeutic strategies. Science 1993;262:1011–1018.
3. Weiss RA. How does HIV cause AIDS? Science 1993;260:1273–1279.
4. Poli G, Fauci AS. The role of monocyte/macrophages and cytokines in the pathogenesis of HIV infection. Pathobiology 1992;60:246–251.
5. Duesberg PH. AIDS: non-infectious deficiencies acquired by drug consumption and other risk factors. Res Immunol 1990;14:5–11.
6. Pantaleo G, Graziosi C, Demarest JF, et al. HIV infection is active and progressive in lymphoid tissue during the clinically latent stage of disease. Nature (London) 1993;362:355–358.
7. Embretson J, Zupancic M, Ribas JL, et al. Massive covert infection of helper lymphocytes and macrophages by HIV during the incubation period of AIDS. Nature (London) 1993;362:359–362.
8. Shuitemaker H, Koot M, Kootstra NA, et al. Biological phenotype of human immunodeficiency virus type 1 clones at different stages of infection: progression of disease is associated with a shift from monocytotropic to T-cell-tropic virus population. J Virol 1992;66:1354–1360.
9. Groenink M, Fouchier RA, Broersen S, et al. Relation of phenotype evolution of HIV-1 envelope V2 configuration. Science 1993;260:1513–1516.
10. Fultz PN. The pathobiology of SIV infection of macaques. In: Montagnier L, Gougeonn ML, eds. New concepts in AIDS pathogenesis. Marcel Dekker, 1993;59–74.
11. Kestler HW, Ringler DJ, Mori K, et al. Importance of the nef gene for maintenance of high virus loads and for development of AIDS. Cell 1991;65:651–662.
12. Daniel MD, Kirchhoff F, Czajak SC, Sehgal PK, Desrosiers RC. Protective effects of a live attenuated SIV vaccine with a deletion in the nef gene. Science 1992;258:1938–1941.
13. Ensoli B, Barillari G, Gallo RC. Cytokines and growth factors in the pathogenesis of AIDS-associated Kaposi's sarcoma. Immunol Rev 1992;127:147–155.
14. Gill PS. Pathogenesis of HIV-related malignancies. Curr Opin Oncol 1991;3:867–871.
15. Poli G, Fauci AS. Cytokine modulation of HIV expression. Semin Immunol 1993;5:165–173.
16. Farrar WL, Korner M, Clouse KA. Cytokine regulation of human immunodeficiency virus expression. Cytokine 1991;3:531–542.

17. Butera ST, Folks TM. Application of latent HIV-1 infected cellular models to therapeutic intervention. AIDS Res Hum Retrovir 1992;8:991–995.

18. Reddy MM, Sorrell SJ, Lange M, Grieco MH. Tumor necrosis factor and HIV P24 antigen levels in serum of HIV-infected populations. J AIDS 1988;1:436–440.

19. Lahdevirta J, Maury CP, Teppo AM, Repo H. Elevated levels of circulating cachectin/tumor necrosis factor in patients with acquired immunodeficiency syndrome. Am J Med 1988;85:289–291.

20. Mintz M, Rapaport R, Oleske JM, Connor EM, Koenigsberger MR, Denny T, Epstein LG. Elevated serum levels of tumor necrosis factor are associated with progressive encephalopathy in children with acquired immunodeficiency syndrome. Am J Dis Child 1989;143:771–774.

21. De Simone C, Tzantzoglou S, Santini G, et al. Clinical and immunologic effects of combination therapy with intravenous immunoglobulins and AZT in HIV-infected patients. Immunopharmacol Immunotoxicol 1991;13:447–458.

22. Grimaldi LME, Martino GV, Franciotta DM, et al. Elevated alpha-tumor necrosis factor levels in spinal fluid from HIV-1 infected patients with central nervous system involvement. Ann Neurol 1991;29:21–25.

23. Mastroianni CM, Paoletti F, Valenti C, Vullo V, Jirillo E, Delia S. Tumor necrosis factor (TNF-alpha) and neurological disorders in HIV infection. J Neurol Neurosurg Psychiatry 1992;55:219–221.

24. Sharief MK, Ciardi M, Noori MA, et al. Free circulating ICAM-1 in serum and cerebrospinal fluid of HIV-1 infected patients correlate with TNF-α and blood-brain barrier damage. Mediat Inflammation 1992;1:323–328.

25. Biglino A, Forno B, Pollono AM, Ghio P, Albera C. Alveolar immune mediators in HIV-related pneumonia. Different role of IL-2 and IL-1 in inducing lung damage. Chest 1993;103:439–443.

26. Fuchs D, Jager H, Popescu M, et al. Immune activation markers to predict AIDS and survival in HIV-1 seropositives. Immunol Lett 1990;26:75–80.

27. Dinarello CA. Interleukin-1 and tumor necrosis factor and their naturally occurring antagonists during hemodialysis. Kidney Int Suppl 1992;38:68–77.

28. Kalinkovich A, Engelmann H, Harpaz N, et al. Elevated serum levels of soluble tumour necrosis factor receptors (sTNF-R) in patients with HIV infection. Clin Exp Immunol 1992;89:351–355.

29. Godfried MH, van der Poll T, Jansen J, et al. Soluble receptors for tumour necrosis factor: a putative marker of disease progression in HIV infection. AIDS 1993;7:33–36.

30. Lau AS, Der SD, Read SE, Williams BRG. Regulation of tumor necrosis factor receptor expression by acid-labil interferon-α from AIDS sera. AIDS Res Hum Retrovir 1991;7:545–552.

31. Lau LS, Livesey JF. Endotoxin induction of tumor necrosis factor is enhanced by acid-labile interferon-α in acquired immunodeficiency syndrome. Clin Invest 1989;84:738–743.

32. Roux-Lombard P, Modoux C, Cruchaud A, Dayer JM. Purified blood monocytes from HIV-1 infected patients produce high levels of TNF-α and IL-1. Clin Immunol Immunopathol 1989;50:374–384.

33. Hober D, Haque A, Wattre P, Beaucaire G, Mouton Y, Capron A. Production of tumor necrosis factor-alpha (TNF-alpha) and interleukin-1 (IL-1) in patients with AIDS. Enhanced level of TNF-alpha is related to a higher cytotoxic activity. Clin Exp Immunol 1989;78:329–333.

34. Voth R, Rossol S, Klein K, et al. Differential gene expression of IFN-α and tumor necrosis factor-α in peripheral blood mononuclear cells from patients with AIDS related complex and AIDS. J Immunol 1990;144:970–975.

35. Vyakarnam A, Matear P, Meager A, et al. Altered production of tumor necrosis factors alpha and beta and interferon gamma by HIV-infected individuals. Clin Exp Immunol 1991;84:109–115.

36. Hess G, Rossol S, Rossol R, Meyer zum B, Uschenfelde KH. Tumor necrosis factor and interferon as prognostic markers in human immunodeficiency virus (HIV) infection. Infection 1991;2:93–97.

37. Millar AB, Miller RF, Foley NM, Meager A, Semple SJ, Rook GA. Production of tumor necrosis factor-alpha by blood and lung mononuclear phagocytes from patients with human immunodeficiency virus-related lung disease. Am J Respir Cell Mol Biol 1991;5:144–148.

38. Krishnan VL, Meager A, Mitchell DM, Pinching AJ. Alveolar macrophages in AIDS patients: increased spontaneous tumour necrosis factor alpha production in Pneumocystis carinii pneumonia. Clin Exp Immunol 1990;80:156–160.

39. Antinori A, Tamburrini E, Pagliari G, et al. Alveolar macrophages from AIDS patients spontaneously produce elevated levels of TNF-alpha in vitro. Allerg Immunopathol 1992;20:249–254.

40. Israel-Biet D, Cadranel J, Beldjord K, Andrieu JM, Jeffrey A, Even P. Tumor necrosis factor production in HIV-seropositive subjects relationship with lung opportunistic infections and HIV expression in alveolar macrophages. J Immunol 1991;147:490–494.

41. Hofman FM, Hinton DR. Tumor necrosis factor-alpha in the retina in acquired immune deficiency syndrome. Invest Ophthalmol Vis Sci 1992;33:1829–1835.

42. Tyor WR, Glass JD, Baumrind N, et al. Cytokine expression of macrophages in HIV-1 associated vacuolar myelopathy. Neurology 1993;43:1002–1009.

43. Rieckmann P, Poli G, Kehrl JH, Fauci AS. Activated B lymphocytes from human immunodeficiency virus-infected individuals induce virus expression in infected T cells and a promonocytic cell line, U1. J Exp Med 1991;173:1–5.

44. Rieckmann P, Poli G, Fox CH, Kehrl JH, Fauci AS. Recombinant gp 120 specifically enhances tumor necrosis factor-alpha production and lg secretion in B lymphocytes from HIV-infected individuals but not from seronegative donors. J Immunol 1991;147:2922–2997.

45. Boue F, Wallon C, Goujard C, Barre'-Sinoussi F, Galanaud P, Delfraissy JF. HIV induces IL-6 production by human B lymphocytes. Role of IL-4. J Immunol 1992;148:3761–3767.

46. Amadori A, Zamarchi R, Ciminale V, et al. HIV-1-specific T cell activation. A major constituent of spontaneous B cell activation during HIV-1 infection. J Immunol 1989;143:2146–2152.

47. Macchia D, Almerigogna F, Parronchi P, Ravina A, Maggi E, Romagnani S. Membrane tumor necrosis factor-alpha is

involved in the polyclonal B-cell activation induced by HIV-infected human T cells. Nature 1993;363:464–466.

48. Liu AY, Miskovsky EP, Stanhope PE, Siliciano RF. Production of transmembrane and secreted forms of tumor necrosis factor (TNF)-alpha by HIV-1-specific CD4+ cytolytic T lymphocyte clones. Evidence for a TNF-α-independent cytolytic mechanism. J Immunol 1992;148:3789–3798.

49. Jassoy C, Harrer T, Rosenthal T, et al. Human immunodeficiency virus type 1-specific cytotoxic T lymphocytes release gamma interferon, tumor necrosis factor alpha (TNF-alpha) and TNF-beta when they encounter their target antigens. J Virol 1993;67:2844–2852.

50. Harrer T, Jassoy C, Harrer E, Johnson RP, Walker BD. Induction of HIV-1 replication in a chronically infected T-cell line by cytotoxic T lymphocytes. J AIDS 1993;6:865–871.

51. Boyle MJ, Berger MF, Tschuchnigg M, et al. Increased expression of interferon-gamma in hyperplastic lymph nodes from HIV-infected patients. Clin Exp Immunol 1993;92:100–105.

52. Clouse KA, Robbins PB, Fernie B, Ostrove JM, Fauci AS. Viral antigen stimulation of the production of human monokines capable of regulating HIV-1 expression. J Immunol 1989;143:470–475.

53. Molina J-M, Scadden DT, Byrn R, Dinarello CA, Groopman JE. Production of tumor necrosis factor α and interleukin 1β by monocytic cells infected with human immunodeficiency virus. J Clin Invest 1989;84:733–737.

54. Merrill JE, Koyanagi Y, Chen ISY. Interleukin-1 and tumor necrosis factor α can be induced from mononuclear phagocytes by human immunodeficiency virus type 1 binding to the CD4 receptor. J Virol 1989;63:4404–4408.

55. D'Addario M, Roulston A, Wainberg MA, Hiscott J. Coordinate enhancement of cytokine gene expression in human immunodeficiency virus type-1-infected promonocytic cells. J Virol 1990;64:6080–6089.

56. Esser R, von Briesen H, Brugger M, et al. Secretory repertoire of HIV-infected human monocytes/macrophages. Pathobiology 1991;59:219–222.

57. Tyring SK, Cauda R, Tumbarello M, et al. Synthetic peptides corresponding to sequences in HIV envelope gp41 and gp120 enhance in vitro production of interleukin-1 and tumor necrosis factor but depress production of interferon-alpha, interferon-gamma and interleukin-2. Viral Immunol 1991;4:33–42.

58. D'Addario M, Wainberg M, Hiscott J. Activation of cytokine genes in HIV-1 infected myelomonoblastic cells by phorbol ester and tumor necrosis factor. J Immunol 1992; 148:1222–1229.

59. McEntee MF, Gorrell MD, Adams RJ, Narayan O, Pitha P. Tumour necrosis factor and interleukin 6 production during interaction between activated CD4+ lymphocytes and simian immunodeficiency virus-infected macrophages. J Gen Virol 1992;73:1107–1113.

60. Poli G, Kinter A, Justement JS, et al. Tumor necrosis factor α functions in an autocrine manner in the induction of human immunodeficiency virus expression. Proc Natl Acad Sci USA 1990;87:782–785.

61. Butera S, Roberts BD, Leung K, Nabel GJ, Folks TM. Tumor necrosis factor receptor expression and signal

transduction in HIV-1 infected cells. AIDS 1993;7:911–918.

62. Sastri KJ, Reddy HR, Pandita R, Totpal K, Aggarwal BB. HIV-1 tat gene induces tumor necrosis factor-beta (lymphotoxin) in a human B-lymphoblastoid cell line. J Biol Chem 1990;265:20091–20093.

63. Pocsik E, Higuchi M, Aggarwal BB. Down-modulation of cell-surface expression of P80 form of the tumor-necrosis-factor receptor by human immunodeficiency virus-1 tat gene. Lymphokine Cytokine Res 1992;11:317–325.

64. Wong GH, Goeddel DV. Tumour necrosis factors α and β inhibit virus replication and synergize with interferons. Nature 1986;323:819–822.

65. Chen MJ, Holskin B, Strickler J, et al. Induction by E1A oncogene expression of cellular susceptibility to lysis by TNF. Nature 1987;330:581–583.

66. Gooding LR, Elmore LW, Tollefson AE, Brady HA, Wold WS. A 14,700 MW protein from the E3 region of adenovirus inhibits cytolysis by tumor necrosis factor. Cell 1988; 53:341–346.

67. Wong GH, Krowka JF, Stites DP, Goeddel DV. In vitro anti-human immunodeficiency virus activities of tumor necrosis factor-alpha and interferon-gamma. J Immunol 1988;140:120–124.

68. Matsuyama T, Hamamoto Y, Soma G-I, Mizuno D, Yamamoto N, Kobayashi N. Cytocidal effect of tumor necrosis factor on cells chronically infected with human immunodeficiency virus (HIV): enhancement of HIV replication. J Virol 1989;63:2504–2509.

69. Hober D, Lucas B,Wattre P, Capron A, Haque A. TNF-α production by U937 promonocytes is enhanced by factors released from HIV-infected T4 lymphocytes: TNF-α is one of the mediators causing lysis of HIV-infected T4 cells. Clin Immunol Immunopathol 1992;62:168–175.

70. Biswas P, Poli G, Orenstein JM, Fauci AS. Cytokine-mediated induction of human immunodeficiency virus (HIV) expression and cell death in chronically infected U1 cells: do Tumor Necrosis Factor alpha and gamma interferon selectively kill HIV-infected cells? J Virol 1994;68:2598–2604.

71. Kruppa G, Thooma B, Machleidt T, Wiegmann K, Kronke M. Inhibition of tumor necrosis factor (TNF)-mediated NF-kappa B activation by selective blockade of the human 55-kDa TNF receptor. J Immunol 1992;148:3152–3157.

72. Kobayashi N, Hamamoto Y, Yamamoto N, Ishii A, Yonehara M, Yonehara S. Anti-Fas monoclonal antibody is cytocidal to human immunodeficiency virus-infected cells without augmenting viral replication. Proc Natl Acad Sci USA 1990;87:9620–9624.

73. Clouse KA, Powell D, Washington I, et al. Monokine regulation of human immunodeficiency virus-1 expression in a chronically infected human T cell clone. J Immunol 1989; 142:431–438.

74. Folks TM, Clouse KA, Justement J, et al. Tumor necrosis factor alpha induces expression of human immunodeficiency virus in a chronically infected T-cell clone. Proc Natl Acad Sci USA. 1989;86:2365–2368.

75. Griffin GE, Leung K, Folks TM, Kunkel S, Nabel GJ. Activation of HIV gene expression during monocyte differentiation by induction of NF-kappa B. Nature 1989;339:70–73.

76. Perez VL, Rowe T, Justement JS, Butera ST, June CH, Folks

TM. An HIV-1-infected T cell clone defective in IL-2 production and Ca^{2+} mobilization after CD3 stimulation. J Immunol 1991;147:3145–3148.

77. Butera ST, Perez VL, Wu BY, Nabel GJ, Folks TM. Oscillation of the human immunodeficiency virus surface receptor is regulated by the state of viral activation in a CD4+ cell model of chronic infection. J Virol 1991;65:4645–4653.

78. Matsuyama T, Yoshiyama H, Hamamoto Y, et al. Enhancement of HIV replication and giant cell formation by tumor necrosis factor. AIDS Res Hum Retrovir 1989;5:139–146.

79. Michihiko, S, Yamamoto N, Shinozaki F, Shimada K, Soma G, Kobayashi N. Augmentation of in-vitro HIV replication in peripheral blood mononuclear cells of AIDS and ARC patients by tumor necrosis factor. Lancet 1989;1:1206–1207.

80. Lacoste J, D'Addario M, Roulston A, Wainberg MA, Hiscott J. Cell-specific differences in activation of NF-kappa B regulatory elements of human immunodeficiency virus and beta interferon promoters by tumor necrosis factor. J Virol 1990;64:4726–4734.

81. Locardi C, Petrini C, Boccoli G, et al. Increased human immunodeficiency virus (HIV) expression in chronically infected U937 cells upon in vitro differentiation by hydroxyvitamin D3: roles of interferon and tumor necrosis factor in regulation of HIV production. J Virol 1990;64:5874–5882.

82. Gruber MA, Webb DSA, Gerrard TL, Mostowski HS, Vujcic L, Golding H. Re-evaluation of the involvement of the adhesion molecules ICAM-1/LFA-1 in syncytia formation of HIV-1 infected subclones of a CEM T-cell leukemic line. Aids Res Hum Retrovir 1991;7:45–53.

83. Poli G, Bressler P, Kinter A, et al. Interleukin 6 induces human immunodeficiency virus expression in infected monocytic cells alone and in synergy with tumor necrosis factor alpha by transcriptional and post-transcriptional mechanisms. J Exp Med 1990;172:151–158.

84. Schuitemaker H, Kootstra NA, Koppelman MHGM, et al. Proliferation dependent HIV-1 infection of monocytes occurs during differentiation into macrophages. J Clin Invest 1992;89:1154–1160.

85. Walsh DG, Horvath CJ, Hansen-Moosa A, et al. Cytokine influence on simian immunodeficiency virus replication within primary macrophages. Am J Pathol 1991;139:877–887.

86. Popik W, Pitha PM. Role of tumor necrosis factor alpha in activation and replication of the tat-defective human immunodeficiency virus-type 1. J Virol 1993;67:1094–1099.

87. Parrott C, Seidner T, Duh E, et al. Variable role of the long terminal repeat Sp1-binding sites in human immunodeficiency virus replication in T lymphocytes. J Virol 1991;1414–1419.

88. Tadmori W, Mondal D, Tadmori I, Prakash O. Transactivation of human immunodeficiency virus type 1 long terminal repeats by cell surface tumor necrosis factor alpha. J Virol 1991;65:6425–6429.

89. Vyakarnam A, McKeating J, Meager A, Beverley PC. Tumour necrosis factors (α,β) induced by HIV-1 in peripheral blood mononuclear cells potentiate virus replication. AIDS 1990;4;21–27.

90. Peterson PK, Gekker G, Chao CC, Schut R, Molitor TW, Balfour HH. Cocaine potentiates HIV-1 replication in human peripheral blood mononuclear cell cocultures. J Immunol 1991;146:81–84.

91. Weissman D, Poli G, Fauci AS. Interleukin 10 blocks HIV replication in macrophages by inhibiting the autocrine loop of TNF-α and IL-6 induction of virus. AIDS Res Human Retrovir 1994 (in press).

92. Butera ST, Roberts BD, Folks TM. Regulation of HIV-1 expression by cytokine networks in a CD4+ model of chronic infection. J Immunol 1993;150:625–634.

93. Osborn L, Kunkel S, Nabel GJ. Tumor necrosis factor α and interleukin 1 stimulate the human immunodeficiency virus enhancer by activation of the nuclear factor kB. Proc Natl Acad Sci USA 1989;86:2336–2340.

94. Duh EJ, Maury WJ, Folks TM, Fauci AS, Rabson AB. Tumor necrosis factor α activates human immunodeficiency virus type 1 through induction of nuclear factor binding to the NF-κB sites in the long terminal repeat. Proc Natl Acad Sci USA 1989;86:5974–5978.

95. Okamoto T, Matsuyama T, Mori S, et al. Augmentation of human immunodeficiency virus type 1 gene expression by tumor necrosis factor α. AIDS Res Hum Retrovir 1989;5:131–138.

96. Israel N, Hazan U, Alcami J, et al. Tumor necrosis factor stimulates transcription of HIV-1 in human T lymphocytes, independently and synergistically with mitogens. J Immunol 1989;143:3956–3960.

97. Nabel G, Baltimore D. An inducible transcription factor activates expression of human immunodeficiency virus in T cells. Nature 326:711–713.

98. Grilli M, Chiu JS, Lenardo MJ. NF-kB and rel-participants in a multiform transcriptional regulatory system. Int Rev Cytol 1993;143:1–62.

99. Hazan U, Thomas D, Alcami J, et al. Stimulation of a human T-cell clone with anti-CD3 or tumor necrosis factor induces NF-kB translocation but not human immunodeficiency virus 1 enhancer-dependent transcription. Proc Natl Acad Sci USA 1990;87:7861–7865.

100. Howard OMZ, Clouse KA, Smith C, Goodwin RG, Farrar WL. Soluble tumor necrosis factor receptor: inhibition of human immunodeficiency virus activation. Proc Natl Acad Sci USA 1993;90:2335–2339.

101. Poli G, Fauci AS. The effect of cytokines and pharmacologic agents on chronic HIV infection. AIDS Res Human Retrovir 1992;8:191–197.

102. Kekow J, Wachsman W, McCutchan JA, Cronin M, Carson DA, Lotz M. Transforming growth factor β and noncytopathic mechanisms of immunodeficiency in human immunodeficiency virus infection. Proc Natl Acad Sci USA 1990;87:8321–8325.

103. Kekow J, Wachsman W, McCutchan JA, et al. Transforming growth factor-beta and suppression of humoral immune responses in HIV infection. J Clin Invest 1991;87:1010–1016.

104. Kehrl JH. Transforming growth factor β: an important mediator of immunoregulation. Int J Cell Clon 1991;9:438–450.

105. Wahl SM, Allen JB, McCartney-Francis N, et al. Macrophage- and astrocyte-derived transforming growth factor β as a mediator of central nervous system dysfunction in ac-

quired immune deficiency syndrome. J Exp Med 1991;173: 981–991.

106. Zauli G, Davis BR, Re MC, Visani G, Furlini G, La Placa M. Tat protein stimulates production of transforming growth factor-beta 1 by marrow macrophages: a potential mechanism for human immunodeficiency virus-1 induced hematopoietic suppression. Blood 1992;80:3036–3043.

107. Stanley SK, Kessler SW, Justement JS, et al. CD34+ bone marrow cells are infected with HIV in a subset of seropositive individuals. J Immunol 1992;149:689–697.

108. Zhou DH, Munster A, Winchurch RA. Pathologic concentrations of interleukin 6 inhibit T cell responses via induction of activation of TGF-beta. FASEB J 1991;5:2582–2585.

109. Scala G, Ruocco MR, Ambrosino C, et al. The expression of the interleukin 6 gene is induced by the human immunodeficiency virus 1 TAT protein. J Exp Med 1994;179:961–972.

110. Poli G, Kinter AL, Justement JS, et al. Retinoic acid mimics transforming growth factor beta in the regulation of human immunodeficiency virus expression in monocytic cells. Proc Natl Acad Sci USA 1992;89:2689–2693.

111. Lazdins JK, Klimkait T, Woods-Cook K, et al. In vitro effect of transforming growth factor β on progression of HIV-1 infection in primary mononuclear phagocytes. J Immunol 1991;147:1201–1207.

112. Lazdins JK, Klimkait T, Woods-Cook K, et al. The replicative restriction of lymphocytotropic isolates of HIV-1 in macrophages is overcome by TGF-beta. AIDS Res Hum Retrovir 1992;8:505–511.

113. Poli G, Kinter AL, Justement JS, Bressler P, Kehrl JH, Fauci AS. Transforming growth factor β suppresses human immunodeficiency virus expression and replication in infected cells of the monocyte/macrophage lineage. J Exp Med 1991;173:589–597.

114. Poli G, Kinter AL, Fauci AS. Interleukin-1 induces expression of the human immunodeficiency virus alone and in synergy with interleukin-6 in chronically infected U1 cells: inhibition of inductive effects by the interleukin-1 receptor antagonist. Proc Natl Acad Sci USA 1994;91:108–112.

115. Pomerantz RJ, Feinberg MB, Trono D, Baltimore D. Lipopolysaccharide is a potent monocyte/macrophage-specific stimulator of human immunodeficiency virus type 1 expression. J Exp Med 1990;172:253–261.

116. Bagasra O, Wright SD, Seshamma T, Oakes JW, Pomerantz RJ. CD14 is involved in control of human immunodeficiency virus type 1 expression in latently infected cells by lipopolysaccharide. Proc Natl Acad Sci USA 1992;89:6285–6289.

117. Sakaguchi M, Zenzie-Gregory B, Groopman JE, Smale ST, Kim SY. Alternative pathway for induction of human immunodeficiency virus gene expression: involvement of the general transcription machinery. J Virol 1991;65:5448–5456.

118. Antoni BA, Rabson AB, Kinter A, Bodkin M, Poli G. NF-kappa B dependent and independent pathways of HIV activation in a chronically-infected T cell line. Virology 1994;202:684–694.

119. Arditi M, Kabat W, Yogev R. Serum tumor necrosis factor alpha, interleukin 1-beta, p24 antigen concentrations and CD4+ cells at various stages of human immunodeficiency

virus 1 infection in children. Pediatr Infect Dis J 1991;10:450–455.

120. Scott-Algara D, Vuillier F, Marasescu M, DE Saint Martin J, Dighiero G. Serum levels of IL-2, IL-1, TNF-α, and soluble receptor of IL-2 in HIV-1-infected patients. AIDS Res Hum Retrovir 1991;7:381–386.

121. Gallo P, Frei K, Rordorf C, Lazdins J, Tavolato B, Fontana A. Human immunodeficiency virus type 1 (HIV-1) infection of the central nervous system: an evaluation of cytokines in cerebrospinal fluid. J Neuroimmunol 1989;23:109–116.

122. Dreno B, Milpied B, Dutartre H, Litoux P. Epidermal interleukin 1 in normal skin of patients with HIV infection. Br J Dermatol 1990;123:487–492.

123. Kotler DP, Reka S, Clayton F. Intestinal mucosal inflammation associated with human immunodeficiency virus infection. Dig Dis Sci 1993;38:1119–1127.

124. Steffen M, Reinecker HC, Petersen J, et al. Differences in cytokine secretion by intestinal mononuclear cells, peripheral blood monocytes and alveolar macrophages from HIV-infected patients. Clin Exp Immunol 1993;91:30–36.

125. Emilie D, Peuchmaur M, Maillot MC, et al. Production of interleukins in human immunodeficiency virus-1-replicating lymph nodes. J Clin Invest 1990;86:148–159.

126. Genis P, Jett M, Bernton EW, et al. Cytokines and arachidonic metabolites produced during human immunodeficiency virus (HIV)-infected macrophage-astroglia interactions: implications for the neuropathogenesis of HIV disease. J Exp Med 1992;176:1703–1718.

127. Epstein LG, Gendelman HE. Human immunodeficiency virus type 1 infection of the nervous system: pathogenetic mechanisms. Ann Neurol 1993;33:429–436.

128. Twigg HL, Iwamoto GK, Soliman DM. Role of cytokines in alveolar macrophage accessory cell function in HIV-infected individuals. J Immunol 1992;149:1462–1469.

129. Weiss L, Haeffner-Cavaillon N, Laude M, Gilquin J, Kazatchkine MD. HIV infection is associated with the spontaneous production of interleukin-1 (IL-1) in vivo and with an abnormal release of IL-1 alpha in vitro. AIDS 1989;3:695–699.

130. Sundar SK, Cierpial MA, Kamaraju LS, et al. Human immunodeficiency virus glyco-protein (gp 120) infused into rat brain induces interleukin 1 to elevate pituitary-adrenal activity and decrease peripheral cellular immune responses. Proc Natl Acad Sci USA 1991;88:11246–11250.

131. Wesselingh SL, Power C, Glass JD, et al. Intracerebral cytokine messenger RNA expression in acquired immunodeficiency syndrome dementia. Ann Neurol 1993;33:576–582.

132. Folks TM, Justement J, Kinter A, Dinarello CA, Fauci AS. Cytokine-induced expression of HIV-1 in a chronically infected promonocyte cell line. Science 1987;238:800–802.

133. Wahl LM, Corcoran ML, Pyle SW, Arthur LO, Harel-Bellan A, Farrar WL. Human immunodeficiency virus glycoprotein (gp 120) induction of monocyte arachidonic acid metabolites and interleukin 1. Proc Natl Acad Sci USA 1989;86:621–625.

134. Valentin A, Albert J, Svenson SB, Asjo B. Blood derived macrophages produce IL-1, but not TNF-alpha, after infection with HIV-1 isolates from patients at different stages of disease. Cytokine 1992;4:185–191.

135. Yamato K, el-Hajjaoui Z, Simon K, Koeffler HP. Modulation of interleukin-1 beta RNA in monocytic cells infected with human immunodeficiency virus-1. J Clin Invest 1990; 86:1109–1114.

136. Tsai WP, Hirose K, Nara PL, et al. Decrease in cytokine production by HIV-infected macrophages in response to LPS-mediated activation. Lymphokine Cytokine Res 1991; 10:421–429.

137. Clouse KA, Cosentino LM, Weih KA, et al. The HIV-1 gp 120 envelope protein has the intrinsic capacity to stimulate monokine secretion. J Immunol 1991;147:2892–2901.

138. Tomasselli AG, Hui JO, Adams L, et al. Actin, troponin C, Alzheimer amyloid precursor protein and pro-interleukin 1 beta as substrates of the protease from human immunodeficiency virus. J Biol Chem 1991;266:14548–14553.

139. Flamand L, Gosselin J, D'Addario M, et al. Human herpesvirus 6 induces interleukin-1 beta and tumor necrosis factor alpha, but not interleukin-6, in peripheral blood mononuclear cell cultures. J Virol 1991;65:5105–5110.

140. Weiss L, Haeffner-Cavaillon N, Gilquin J, Kazatchkine MD. Zidovudine inhibits functional extracellular monocytic interleukin-1. AIDS 1990;4:255–257.

141. von Briesen H, von Mallinckrodt C, Esser R, et al. Effect of cytokines and lipopolysaccharides on HIV infection of human macrophages. Res Virol 1991;142:197–204.

142. Swingler S, Easton A, Morris A. Cytokine augmentation of HIV-1 LTR-driven gene expression in neural cells. AIDS Res Hum Retrovir 1992;8:487–493.

143. Krasnow SW, Zhang LQ, Leung KY, Osborn L, Kunkel S, Nabel GJ. Tumor necrosis factor-alpha, interleukin 1, and phorbol myristate acetate are independent activators of NF-kappa B which differentially activate T cells. Cytokine 1991;3:372–379.

144. Kobayashi N, Hamamoto Y, Koyanagi Y, Chen IS, Yamamoto N. Effect of interleukin-1 on the augmentation of human immunodeficiency virus gene expression. Biochem Biophys Res Commun 1989;165:715–721.

145. Baldari CT, Macchia G, Massone A, Telford JL. p21ras contributes to HIV-1 activation in T-cells. FEBS Lett 1992; 304:261–264.

146. Leonard J, Khillan JS, Gendelman HE, et al. The human immunodeficiency virus long terminal repeat is preferentially expressed in Langerhans cells in transgenic mice. AIDS Res Hum Retrovir 1989;5:421–430.

147. Dinarello CA, Thompson RC. Blocking IL-1: interleukin 1 receptor antagonist in vivo and in vitro. Immunol Today 1991;12:11.

148. Ohlsson K, Bjork P, Bergenfeldt M, Hageman R, Thompson RC. Interleukin-1 receptor antagonist reduces mortality from endotoxin shock. Nature 1990;348:550–552.

149. Chemsue SW, Warmington KS, Berger AE, Tracey DE. Immunohistochemical demonstration of interleukin-1 receptor antagonist protein and interleukin-1 in human lymphoid tissue and granulomas. Am J Pathol 1992;140: 269–275.

150. Locksley RM, Crowe S, Sadick MD, et al. Release of interleukin 1 inhibitory activity (contral-IL-1) by human monocyte-derived macrophages infected with human immunodeficiency virus in vitro and in vivo. J Clin Invest 1988;82: 2097–2105.

151. Gallo RC, Sarin PS, Gelmann EP, et al. Isolation of human T-cell leukemia virus in acquired immune deficiency syndrome (AIDS). Science 1983;220:865–867.

152. Barre-Sinoussi F, Chermann JC, Rey F, et al. Isolation of T-lymphotropic retrovirus from a patient at risk for acquired immune deficiency syndrome (AIDS). Science 1983;220:868–871.

153. Zagury D, Bernard J, Leonard R, et al. Long-term cultures of HTLV-III–infected T cells: a model of cytopathology of T-cell depletion in AIDS. Science 1986;231:850–853.

154. Lane HC, Siegal J, Rook AH, Masur H, Quinnan GV, Fauci AS. Use of interleukin-2 in patients with the acquired immunodeficiency syndrome (AIDS). J Biol Respir Mod 1984; 3:512–516.

155. Zagury D, Gagne I, Reveil B, et al. Repairing the T-cell defect in AIDS. Lancet 1985;2:449.

156. Schwartz DH, Merigan TC. Interleukin-2 in the treatment of HIV disease. Biotherapy 1990;2:119–136.

157. Clerici M, Hakim FT, Venzon DJ, et al. Changes in interleukin-2 and interleukin-4 production in asymptomatic, human immunodeficiency virus-seropositive individuals. J Clin Invest 1993;91:759–765.

158. Clerici M, Stocks NI, Zajac RA, et al. Interleukin-2 production used to detect antigenic peptide recognition by T-helper lymphocytes from asymptomatic HIV-seropositive individuals. Nature 1989;339:383–385.

159. Clerici M, Giorgi JV, Chou CC, et al. Cell-mediated immune response to human immunodeficiency virus (HIV) type 1 in seronegative homosexual men with recent sexual exposure to HIV-1. J Infect Dis 1992;165:1012–1019.

160. Romagnani S. Human Th1 and Th2 subsets: regulation of differentiation and role in protection and immunopathology. Int Arch Allergy Appl Immunol 1992;98:279–285.

161. Ammar A, Cibert C, Bertoli AM, Tsilivakos V, Jasmin C, Georgoulias V. Biological and biochemical characterization of a factor produced spontaneously by adherent cells of human immunodeficiency virus-infected patients inhibiting interleukin-2 receptor alpha chain (Tac) expression on normal T cells. J Clin Invest 1991;87:2048–2055.

162. Fernandez-Cruz E, Gelpi E, Longo N, et al. Increased synthesis and production of prostaglandin E2 by monocytes from drug addicts with AIDS. AIDS 1989;3:91–96.

163. Ciardi M, Sharief MK, Noori MA, et al. Intrathecal synthesis of interleukin-2 and soluble IL-2 receptor in asymptomatic HIV-1 seropositive individuals. Correlation with local production of specific IgM and IgG antibodies. J Neurol Sci 1993;115:117–122.

164. Honda M, Kitamura K, Matsuda K, et al. Soluble IL-2 receptor in AIDS. Correlation of its serum level with the classification of HIV-induced diseases and its characterization. J Immunol 1989;142:4248–4255.

165. Hofmann B, Nishanian P, Fahey JL, et al. Serum increases and lymphoid cell surface losses of IL-2 receptor CD25 in HIV infection: distinctive parameters of HIV-induced change. Clin Immunol Immunopathol 199;61:212–224.

166. Noronha IL, Daniel V, Schimpf K, Opelz G. Soluble IL-2 receptor and tumour necrosis factor-alpha in plasma of haemophilia patients infected with HIV. Clin Exp Immunol 1992;87:287–292.

167. Tsunetsugu-Yokota Y, Honda M. Effect of cytokines on HIV release and IL-2 receptor expression in monocytic cell lines. J AIDS 1990;3:511–516.

168. Chehimi J, Starr SE, Frank I, et al. Natural killer (NK) cell stimulatory factor increases the cytotoxic activity of NK cells from both healthy donors and human immunodeficiency virus-infected patients. J Exp Med 1992;175:789–796.

169. Pandolfi F, Oliva A, Sacco G, et al. Fibroblast-derived factors preserve viability in vitro of mononuclear cells isolated from subjects with HIV-1 infection. AIDS 1993;7:323–329.

170. Gougeon ML, Laurent-Crawford AG, Hovanessian AG, Montagnier L. Direct and indirect mechanisms mediating apoptosis during HIV infection: contribution to in vivo CD4 T cell depletion. Semin Immunol 1993;5:187–194.

171. Pantaleo G, Koenig S, Baseler M, Lane HC, Fauci AS. Defective clonogenic potential of CD8+ T lymphocytes in patients with AIDS. Expansion in vivo of a nonclonogenic CD3+CD8+DR+CD25– T cell population. J Immunol 1990;144:1696–1704.

172. Teppler H, Kaplan G, Smith K, et al. Efficacy of low doses of the polyethylene glycol derivative of interleukin-2 in modulating the immune response of patients with human immunodeficiency virus type 1 infection. J Infect Dis 1993;167:291–298.

173. McElrath MJ, Kaplan G, Burkhardt RA, Cohn ZA. Cutaneous response to recombinant interleukin 2 in humans immunodeficiency virus 1-seropositive individuals. Proc Natl Acad Sci USA 1990;87:5783–5787.

174. Krigel RL, Padavic-Shaller KA, Rudolph AR, Poiez BJ, Comis RL. Exacerbation of epidemic Kaposi's sarcoma with a combination of interleukin-2 β-interferon: results of a phase 2 study. J Biol Respir Mod 1989;8:359–365.

175. Miles DW, Aderka D, Engelmann H, Wallach D, Balkwill FR. Induction of soluble tumour necrosis factor receptors during treatment with interleukin-2. Br J Cancer 1992;66:1195–1199.

176. Folks TM, Kelly J, Benn S, et al. Susceptibility of normal human lymphocytes to infection with HTLVIII/LAV. J Immunol 1986;136:4049–4053.

177. Bell KD, Ramilo O, Vitetta ES. Combined use of an immunotoxin and cyclosporine to prevent both activated and quiescent peripheral blood T cells from producing type 1 human immunodeficiency virus. Proc Natl Acad Sci USA 1993;90:1411–1415.

178. Zack JA, Arrigo SJ, Weitsman SR, Go AS, Haislip A, Chen IS. HIV-1 entry into quiescent primary lymphocytes: molecular analysis reveals a labile, latent viral structure. Cell 1990;61:213–222.

179. Zack JA, Haislip AM, Krogstad P, Chen IS. Incompletely reverse-transcribed human immunodeficiency virus type 1 genomes in quiescent cells can function as intermediates in the retroviral life cycle. J Virol 1992;66:1717–1725.

180. Bukrinsky MI, Stanwick TL, Dempsey MP, Stevenson M. Quiescent T lymphocytes as an inducible virus reservoir in HIV-1 infection. Science 1991;254:423–427.

181. Schnittman SM, Lane HC, Greenhouse J, Justement JS, Baseler M, Fauci AS. Preferential infection of CD4+ memory T cells by human immunodeficiency virus type 1: evidence for a role in the selective T-cell functional defects observed in infected individuals. Proc Natl Acad Sci USA 1990;87:6058–6062.

182. Todd B, Pope JH, Georghiou P. Interleukin-2 enhances production in 24 hours of infectious human immunodefi-

ciency virus type 1 in vitro by naturally infected mononuclear cells from seropositive donors. Arch Virol 1991;121:227–232.

183. Firpo PP, Axberg I, Scheibel M, Clark EA. Macaque CD4+ T-cell subsets: influence of activation on infection by simian immunodeficiency viruses (SIV). AIDS Res Hum Retrovir 1992;8:357–366.

184. Finberg RW, Wahl SM, Allen JB, et al. Selective elimination of HIV-1 infected cells with an interleukin-2 receptor-specific cytotoxin. Science 1991;252:1703–1705.

185. Ramilo O, Bell KD, Uhr JW, Vitetta ES. Role of CD25+ and CD25– T cells in acute HIV infection in vitro. J Immunol 1993;150:5202–5208.

186. Horvat RT, Wood C. HIV promoter activity in primary antigen-specific human T lymphocytes. J Immunol 1989;143:2745–2751.

187. Allen JB, McCartney-Francis N, Smith PD. Expression of interleukin 2 receptors by monocytes from patients with acquired immunodeficiency syndrome and induction of monocyte interleukin 2 receptors by human immunodeficiency virus in vitro. J Clin Invest 1990;85:192–199.

188. Serpente N, Sitbon M, Vaquero C. Suboptimal and optimal activation signals modulate differently the expression of HIV-1 and cytokine genes. Biochem Biophys Res Commun 1992;182:1172–1179.

189. Amadori A, Faulkner-Valle GP, De Rossi A, Zanovello P, Collavo D, Chieco-Bianchi L. HIV-mediated immunodepression: in vitro inhibition of T-lymphocyte proliferative response by ultraviolet-inactivated virus.

190. Oyaizu N, Chirmule N, Kalyanaraman VS, et al. Human immunodeficiency virus type 1 envelope glycoprotein gp120 produces immune defects in CD4+ T lymphocytes by inhibiting interleukin 2 mRNA. Proc Natl Acad Sci USA 1990;87:2379–2383.

191. Chirmule N, Oyaizu N, Kalyanaraman VS, Pahwa S. Inhibition of normal B-cell function by human immunodeficiency virus envelope glycoprotein, gp120. Blood 1992;79:1245–1254.

192. Fuji Y, Ito M, Ikuta K. Evidence for the role of human-immunodeficiency-virus type-1 NEF protein as a growth inhibitor to CD4+ T-lymphocytes and for the blocking of the NEF function by anti-NEF antibodies. Vaccine 1993;11:837–847.

193. Clerici M, Shearer GM. ATh1 Th2 switch is a critical step in the etiology of HIV infection. Immunol Today 1993;14:107–111.

194. Chehimi J, Starr SE, Frank I, et al. Impaired interleukin 12 production in human immunodeficiency virus-infected patients. J Exp Med 1994;179:1361–1366.

195. Trinchieri G. Interleukin-12 and its role in the generation of Th1 cells. Immunol Today 1993;14:335–338.

196. Puri RK, Aggarwal BB. Human immunodeficiency virus type 1 tat gene up-regulates interleukin 4 receptors on a human B-lymphoblastoid cell line. Cancer Res 1992;52:3787–3790.

197. Graziosi C, Pantaleo G, Gantt KR, et al. Lack of evidence for the dichotomy of T_H1 and T_H2 predominance in HIV-infected individuals. Science 1994;265:248–252.

198. Re MC, Zauli G, Furlini G, Ranieri S, La Placa M. Progressive and selective impairment of IL-3 and IL-4 production

by peripheral blood CD4+ T-lymphocytes during the course of HIV-1 infection. Viral Immunol 1992;5:185–194.

199. Cayota A, Vuillier F, Scott-Algara D, Feuillie V, Dighiero G. Impaired proliferative capacity and abnormal cytokine profile of naive and memory CD4 T cells from HIV-seropositive patients. Clin Exp Immunol 1992;88:478–483.

200. Maggi E, Mazzetti M, Ravina A, et al. Ability of HIV to promote a T_H1 to T_H0 shift and to replicate preferentially in T_H2 and T_H0 cells. Science 1994;265:244–248.

201. Hays EF, Uittenbogaart CH, Brewer JC, Vollger LW, Zack JA. In vitro studies of HIV-1 expression in thymocytes from infants and children. AIDS 1992;6:265–272.

202. Moran PA, Diegel ML, Sias JC, Ledbetter JA, Zarling JM. Regulation of HIV production by blood mononuclear cells from HIV-infected donors: I. Lack of correlation between HIV-1 production and T cell activation. AIDS Res Hum Retrovir 1993;9:455–464.

203. Novak RM, Holzer TJ, Kennedy MM, Heynen CA, Dawson G. The effect of interleukin 4 (BSF-1) on infection of peripheral blood monocyte-derived macrophages with HIV-1. AIDS Res Hum Retrovir 1990;6:973–976.

204. Kazazi F, Mathijs JM, Chang J, et al. Recombinant interleukin 4 stimulates human immunodeficiency virus production by infected monocytes and macrophages. J Gen Virol 1992;73:941–949.

205. Breen EC, Rezai AR, Nakajima K, et al. Infection with HIV is associated with elevated IL-6 levels and production. J Immunol 1990;144:480–484.

206. Birx DL, Redfield RR, Tencer K, Fowler A, Burke DS, Tosato G. Induction of interleukin-6 during human immunodeficiency virus infection. Blood 1990;76:2303–2310.

207. Honda M, Kitamura K, Mizutani Y, et al. Quantitative analysis of serum IL-6 and its correlation with increased levels of serum IL-2R in HIV-induced diseases. J Immunol 1990;145:4059–4064.

208. Rautonen J, Rautonen N, Martin NL, Philip R, Wara DW. Serum interleukin-6 concentrations are elevated and associated with elevated tumor necrosis factor-alpha and immunoglobulin G and A concentrations in children with HIV infection. AIDS 1991;5:1319–1325.

209. de Wit R, Raasveld MH, ten Berge RJ, van der Wouw PA, Bakker PJ, Veenhof CH. Interleukin-6 concentrations in the serum of patients with AIDS-associated Kaposi's sarcoma during treatment with interferon-alpha. J Intern Med 1991;229:539–542.

210. Zauli G, Re MC, Gugliotta L, Furlini G, La Placa M. The elevation of circulating platelets after IFN-alpha therapy in HIV-1 seropositive thrombocytopenic patients correlates with increased plasma levels of IL-6. Microbiologica 1993;16:27–34.

211. Most J, Zangerle R, Herold M. Elevated concentrations of circulating intercellular-adhesion molecule-1 (ICAM-1) in HIV-1 infection. J AIDS 1993;6:221–226.

212. Laurenzi MA, Siden A, Persson MA, Norkrans G, Hagberg L, Chiodi F. Cerebrospinal fluid interleukin-6 activity in HIV infection and inflammatory and noninflammatory diseases of the nervous system. Clin Immunol Immunopathol 1990;57:233–241.

213. Amadori A, Zamarchi R, Veronese ML, et al. B cell activation during HIV-1 infection. II. Cell-to-cell interactions and cytokine requirement. J Immunol 1991;146:57–62.

214. Honda M, Yamamoto S, Cheng M, et al. Human soluble IL-6 receptor: its detection and enhanced release by HIV infection. J Immunol 1992;148:2175–2180.

215. Birx DL, Lewis MG, Vahey M, et al. Association of IL-6 in the pathogenesis of acutely fatal SIV-pbj in pigtailed macaques. AIDS Res Hum Retrovir 1993;9:1123–1129.

216. Nakajima K, Martinez-Maza O, Hirano T, et al. Induction of IL-6 (B cell stimulatory factor-2/IFN-β2) production by HIV. J Immunol 1989;142:531–536.

217. Kornbluth RS, Munis R, Oh PS, Meylan PR, Richman DD. Characterization of a macrophage-tropic HIV strain that does not alter macrophage cytokine production yet protects macrophages from superinfection by vesicular stomatitis virus. AIDS Res Hum Retrovir 1990;6:1023–1026.

218. Oyaizu N, Chirmule N, Ohnishi Y, Kalyanaraman VS, Pahwa S. Human immunodeficiency virus type 1 envelope glycoproteins gp120 and gp160 induce interleukin-6 production in CD4+ T-cell clones. J Virol 1991;65:6277–6282.

219. Saville MW, Taga K, Foli A, Broder S, Tosato, Yarchoan R. Interleukin-10 suppresses human immunodeficiency virus-1 replication in vitro in cells of the monocyte/macrophage lineage. Blood 1994;83:3591–3599.

220. Vesanen M, Wessman M, Salminen M, Vaheri A. Activation of integrated human immunodeficiency virus type 1 in human neuroblastoma cells by the cytokines tumour necrosis factor alpha and interleukin-6. J Gen Virol 1992;73:1753–1760.

221. Stanley SK, Bressler PB, Poli G, Fauci AS. Heat shock induction of HIV production from chronically infected promonocytic and T cell lines. J Immunol 1990;145:1120–1126.

222. Smith PD, Ohura K, Masur H, Lane HC, Fauci AS, Wahl SM. Monocyte function in the acquired immune deficiency syndrome. J Clin Invest 1984;74:2121–2128.

223. Poli G, Bottazzi B, Acero R, et al. Monocyte function in intravenous drug abusers with lymphadenopathy and in patients with acquired immunodeficiency syndrome: selective impairment of chemotaxis. Clin Exp Immunol 1985;62:136.

224. Lazzarin A, Uberti Foppa C, Galli M, et al. Impairment of polymorphonuclear leukocyte function in patients with acquired immunodeficiency syndrome and with lymphadenopathy syndrome. Clin Exp Immunol 1986;65:105.

225. Gabrilovich DI, Shepeleva GK, Serebrovskaya LV, et al. Mononuclear cells from HIV-infected patients produce factors which enhance functional activity of polymorphonuclear neutrophils from healthy subjects. Clin Exp Immunol 1992;89:362–368.

226. Gabrilovich DI, Shepeleva GK, Serebrovskaya LV, Avdeeva LA, Pokrovsky VV. Modification of lymphocyte and monocyte functional activity by polymorphonuclear neutrophils in HIV infection. Scand J Immunol 1993;37:459–467.

227. Girasole G, Wang JM, Pedrazzoni M, et al. Augmentation of monocyte chemotaxis by 1 alpha, 25-dihydroxyvitamin D3. Stimulation of defective migration of AIDS patients. J Immunol 1990;145:2459–2464.

228. Glienke W, von Briesen H, Esser R, Muller S, Andreesen R, Rubsamen-Waigmann H. Expression of macrophage products after in vitro infection of human monocytes/macrophages with HIV. Res Virol 1993;144:35–40.

229. Meyaard L, Schuitemaker H, Miedema F. T-cell dysfunc-

tion in HIV infection: anergy due to defective antigen-presenting cell function? Immunol Today 1993;14:161.

230. Moore KW, Garra AO, Malefyt RW, Vieira P, Mosmann TR. Interleukin-10. Annu Rev Immunol 1993;11:165–190.

231. Emilie D, Touitou R, Raphael M, et al. In vivo production of interleukin-10 by malignant cells in AIDS lymphomas. Eur J Immunol 1992;22:2937–2942.

232. Benjamin D, Knobloch TJ, Dayton MA. Human B-cell interleukin-10: B-cell lines derived from patients with acquired immunodeficiency syndrome and Burkitt's lymphoma constitutively secrete large quantities of interleukin-10. Blood 1992;80:1289–1298.

233. Bressler P, Poli G, Justement JS, Biswas P, Fauci AS. Glucocorticoids synergize with TNF-α in the induction of HIV expression from a chronically infected promonocytic cell line. AIDS Res Hum Retrovir 1993;9:547–551.

234. Sironi M, Munoz C, Pollicino T, et al. Divergent effects of interleukin-10 on cytokine production by mononuclear phagocytes and endothelial cells. Eur J Immunol 1993;23:2692–2695.

235. Hsieh CS, Macatonia SE, Tripp CS, Wolf SF, O'Garra A, Murphy KM. Development of TH1 CD4+ T cells through IL-12 produced by listeria-induced macrophages. Science 1993;260:547–549.

236. Montaner LJ, Doyle AG, Collin M, et al. Interleukin 13 inhibits human immunodeficiency virus type 1 production in primary blood-derived human macrophages in vitro. J Exp Med 1993;178:743–747.

237. Scadden DT, Zon LI, Groopman JE. Pathophysiology and management of HIV-associated hematologic disorders. Blood 1989;74:1455–1463.

238. Bonyhadi ML, Rabin L, Salimi S, et al. HIV induces thymus depletion in vivo. Nature 1993;363:728–732.

239. Aldrovandi GM, Feuer G, Gao L, et al. The SCID-hu mouse as a model for HIV-infection. Nature 1993;363:732–736.

240. Stanley SK, McCune JM, Kaneshima H, et al. Human immunodeficiency virus infection of the human thymus and disruption of the thymic microenvironment in the SCID-hu mouse. J Exp Med 1993;178:1151–1163.

241. Folks TM, Kessler SW, Orenstein JM, Justement JS, Jaffe ES, Fauci AS. Infection and replication of HIV-1 in purified progenitor cells of normal human bone marrow. Science 1988;242:919–922.

242. Kitano K, Abboud CN, Ryan DH, Quan SG, Baldwin GC, Golde DW. Macrophage-active colony-stimulating factors enhance human immunodeficiency virus type 1 infection in bone marrow stem cells. Blood 1991;77:1699–1705.

243. Watanabe M, Ringler DJ, Nakamura M, DeLong PA, Letvin NL. Simian immunodeficiency virus inhibits bone marrow hematopoietic progenitor cell growth. J Virol 1990;64:656–663.

244. Hamilton JA. Colony stimulating factors, cytokines and monocyte-macrophages—some controversies. Immunol Today 1993;14:18–24.

245. Balleari E, Timitilli S, Puppo F, et al. Impaired in vitro growth of peripheral blood hematopoietic progenitor cells in HIV-infected patients: evidence of an inhibitory effect of autologous T lymphocytes. Ann Hematol 1991;63:320–325.

246. Lunardi-Iskandar Y, Georgoulias V, Bertoli AM, et al. Impaired in vitro proliferation of hemopoietic precursors in HIV-1 infected subjects. Blood 1991;78:3200–3208.

247. Miles SA, Lee K, Hutlin L, Zsebo KM, Mitsuyasu RT. Potential use of human stem cell factor as adjunctive therapy for human immunodeficiency virus-related cytopenias. Blood 1991;78:3200–3208.

248. Koyanagi Y, O'Brien WA, Zhao JQ, Golde DW, Gasson JC, Chen ISY. Cytokines alter production of HIV-1 from primary mononuclear phagocytes. Science 1988;241:1673–1675.

249. Schuitemaker H, Kootstra NA, van Oers MH, van Lambalgen R, Tersmette M, Miedema F. Induction of monocyte proliferation and HIV expression by IL-3 does not interfere with anti-viral activity of zidovudine. Blood 1990;76:1490–1493.

250. Weinberg JB, Matthews TJ, Cullen BR, Malim MH. Productive HIV-1$_{BA-L}$ infection of nonproliferating human monocytes. J Exp Med 1991;174:1477–1482.

251. Re MC, Zauli G, Furlini G, et al. GM-CSF production by CD4+ T-lymphocytes is selectively impaired during the course of HIV-1 infection. A possible indication of a preferential lesion of a specific subset of peripheral blood CD4+ T-lymphocytes. Microbiologica 1992;15:265–270.

252. Reddy MM, Grieco MH. Erythropoietin and granulocyte-macrophage colony-stimulating factor (GM-CSF) levels in sera of patients with HIV infection. Int J STD AIDS 1991;2:128–132.

253. Agostini C, Trentin L, Zambello R, et al. Release of granulocyte-macrophage colony-stimulating factor by alveolar macrophages in the lung of HIV-1 infected patients. J Immunol 1992;149:3379–3385.

254. Pluda JM, Yarchoan R, Smith PD, et al. Subcutaneous recombinant granulocyte-macrophage colony-stimulating factor used as a single agent and in an alternating regimen with azidothymidine in leukopenic patients with severe human immuno-deficiency virus infection. Blood 1990;76:463–472.

255. Miles SA. Hematopoietic growth factors as adjuncts to anti-retroviral therapy. AIDS Res Hum Retrovir 1992;8:1073–1080.

256. Levine JD, Allan JD, Tessitore JH, et al. Recombinant human granulocyte-macrophage colony-stimulating factor ameliorates zidovudine-induced neutropenia in patients with acquired immunodeficiency syndrome (AIDS)/AIDS-related complex. Blood 1991;78:3148–3154.

257. Roilides E, Mertins S, Eddy J, Walsh TJ, Pizzo PA, Rubin M. Impairment of neutrophil chemotactic and bactericidal function in children infected with human immunodeficiency virus type 1 and partial reversal after in vitro exposure to granulocyte-macrophage colony-stimulating factor. J Pediatr 1990;117:531–540.

258. Davey RT, Davey VJ, Metcalf JA, et al. A phase I/II trial of zidovudine, interferon-alpha, and granulocyte-macrophage colony-stimulating factor in the treatment of human immunodeficiency virus type 1 infection. J Infect Dis 1991;164:43–52.

259. Krown SE, Paredes J, Bundow D, Polsky B, Gold JW, Flomenberg N. Interferon-alpha, zidovudine, and granulocyte-macrophage colony-stimulating factor: a phase I AIDS clinical trials group study in patients with Kaposi's sarcoma associated with AIDS. J Clin Oncol 1992;10:1344–1351.

260. Hammer SM, Gillis JM, Groopman JE, Rose RM. In vitro modification of human immunodeficiency virus infection by granulocyte-macrophage colony-stimulating factor and gamma interferon. Proc Natl Acad Sci USA 1986;83:8734–8738.

261. Mano H, Chermann JC. Replication of human immunodeficiency virus type 1 in primary cultured placental cells. Res Virol 1991;142:95–104.

262. Perno CF, Yarchoan R, Cooney DA, et al. Replication of human immunodeficiency virus in monocytes. Granulocyte/macrophage colony-stimulating factor (GM-CSF) potentiates viral production yet enhances the antiviral effect mediated by 3′-azido-2′3′-dideoxythymidine (AZT) and other dideoxynucleoside congeners of thymidine. J Exp Med 1989;169:933–951.

263. Perno CF, Cooney DA, Currens MJ, et al. Ability of anti-HIV agents to inhibit HIV replication in monocyte-macrophages or U937 monocytoid cells under conditions of enhancement by GM-CSF or anti-HIV antibody. AIDS Res Hum Retrovir 1990;6:1051–1055.

264. Perno CF, Cooney DA, Gao WY, et al. Effects of bone marrow stimulatory cytokines on human immunodeficiency virus replication and the antiviral activity of dideoxynucleosides in cultures of monocyte/macrophages. Blood 1992;80:995–1003.

265. Hammer SM, Gillis JM, Pinkston P, Rose RM. Effect of zidovudine and granulocyte-macrophage colony-stimulating factor on human immunodeficiency virus replication in alveolar macrophages. Blood 1990;75:1215–1219.

266. Gallo P, Laverda AM, De Rossi A, et al. Immunological markers in the cerebrospinal fluid of HIV-1 infected children. Acta Paediatr Scand 1991;80:659–666.

267. Gendelman HE, Orenstein JM, Martin MA, et al. Efficient isolation and propagation of human immunodeficiency virus on recombinant colony-stimulating factor 1-treated monocytes. J Exp Med 1988;167:1428–1441.

268. Meltzer MS, Nakamura M, Hansen BD, Turpin JA, Kalter DC, Gendelman HE. Macrophages as susceptible targets for HIV infection, persistent viral reservoirs in tissue, and key immunoregulatory cells that control levels of virus replication and extent of disease. AIDS Res Hum Retrovir 1990;6:967–971.

269. Potts BJ, Maury W, Martin MA. Replication of HIV-1 in primary monocyte cultures. Virilogy 1990;175:465–476.

270. Lane HC. The role of immunomodulators in the treatment of patients with AIDS. AIDS 1989;1:181–185.

271. Groopman JE, Feder D. Hematopoietic growth factors in AIDS. Semin Oncol 1992;19:408–414.

272. Jolik WK. Interferons. In: Fields BN, Knipe DM, Chanock RM, eds. Virology. New York: Raven, 1990:383–410.

273. Rinaldo CR, Armstrong JA, Kingsley LA, Zhou S, Ho M. Relation of alpha and gamma interferon levels to development of AIDS in homosexual men. J Exp Pathol 1990;5:127–132.

274. Capobianchi MR, Mattana P, Mercuri F, et al. Acid lability is not an intrinsic property of interferon-alpha induced by HIV-infected cells. J Interferon Res 1992;12:431–438.

275. Rossol S, Voth R, Laubenstein HP, et al. Interferon production in patients infected with HIV-1. J Infect Dis 1989;159:815–821.

276. Hess G, Rossol S, Rossol R, Meyer zum B, Buschenfelde

KH. Tumor necrosis factor and interferon as prognostic markers in human immunodeficiency virus (HIV) infection. Infection 1991;2:93–97.

277. Gendelman HE, Friedman RM, Joe S, et al. A selective defect of interferon α production in human immunodeficiency virus-infected monocytes. J Exp Med 1990;172:1433–1442.

278. Krown SE, Niedzwiecki D, Bhalla RB, Flomenberg N, Bundow D, Chapman D. Relationship and prognostic value of endogenous interferon-α, β2-microglobulin, and neopterin serum levels in patients with Kaposi's sarcoma and AIDS. J AIDS 1991;4:871–880.

279. Grunfeld C, Kotler DP, Shigenaga JK, et al. Circulating interferon-α levels and hypertriglyceridemia in the acquired immunodeficiency syndrome. Am J Med 1991;90:154–162.

280. von Sydow M, Sonnerborg A, Gaines H, Strannegard O. Interferon-alpha and tumor necrosis factor-alpha in serum of patients in various stages of HIV-1 infection. AIDS Res Hum Retrovir 1991;7:375–380.

281. Buimovici-Klein E, McKinley GF, Lange M, et al. Modulation of alpha interferon levels by AZT treatment in HIV-seropositive patients. J Exp Pathol 1992;6:31–39.

282. Grunfeld C, Pang M, Doerrler W, Shigenaga JK, Jensen P, Feingold KR. Lipids, lipoproteins, triglyceride clearance, and cytokines in human immunodeficiency virus infection and the acquired immunodeficiency syndrome. J Clin Endocrinol Metab 1992;74:1045–1052.

283. Hellerstein MK, Grunfeld C, Wu K, et al. Increased de novo hepatic lipogenesis in human immunodeficiency virus infection. J Clin Endocrinol Metab 1993;76:559–565.

284. Capobianchi MR, Ankel H, Ameglio F, Paganelli R, Pizzoli PM, Dianzani F. Recombinant glycoprotein 120 of human immunodeficiency virus is a potent interferon inducer. AIDS Res Hum Retrovir 1992;8:575–579.

285. Ho DD, Hartshorn KL, Rota TR, et al. Recombinant human interferon alpha-A suppresses HTLV-III replication in vitro. Lancet 1985;1:602–604.

286. Yamamoto JK, Barre-Sinoussi F, Bolton V, Pedersen NC, Gardner MB. Human alpha- and beta-interferon but not gamma suppresses the in vitro replication of LAV, HTLV-III, and ARV-2. J Interferon Res 1986;6:143–152.

287. Hartshorn KL, Neumeyer D, Vogt MW, Schooley RT, Hirsch MS. Activity of interferons alpha, beta, and gamma against human immunodeficiency virus replication in vitro. AIDS Res Hum Retrovir 1987;3:125–133.

288. Yamada O, Hattori N, Kurimura T, Kita M, Kishida T. Inhibition of growth of HIV by human natural interferon in vitro. AIDS Res Hum Retrovir 1988;4:287–294.

289. Bednarik DP, Mosca JD, Raj NB, Pitha PM. Inhibition of human immunodeficiency virus (HIV) replication by HIV-trans-activated alpha 2-interferon. Proc Natl Acad Sci USA 1990;86:4958–4962.

290. Shirazi Y, Pitha PM. Alpha interferon inhibits early stages of the human immunodeficiency virus type 1 replication cycle. J Virol 1992;66:1321–1328.

291. Popik W, Pitha PM. Inhibition by interferon of herpes simplex virus type 1-activated transcription of tat-defective provirus. Proc Natl Acad Sci USA 1991;88:9573–9577.

292. Popik W, Pitha PM. Transcriptional activation of the tat-

defective human immunodeficiency virus type-1 provirus: effect of interferon. Virology 1992;189:435–447.

293. Kornbluth RS, Oh PS, Munis JR, Cleveland PH, Richman DD. Interferons and bacterial lipopolysaccharide protect macrophages from productive infection by human immunodeficiency virus in vitro. J Exp Med 1989;169:1137–1151.

294. Gendelman HE, Baca LM, Turpin J, et al. Regulation of HIV replication in infected monocytes by IFN-α. J Immunol 1990;145:2669–2676.

295. Gendelman HE, Baca L, Turpin JA, et al. Restriction of HIV replication in infected T-cells and monocytes by interferon-alpha. AIDS Res Hum Retrovir 1990;6:1045–1049.

296. Hansen BD, Nara PL, Maheshwari RK, et al. Loss of infectivity by progeny virus from alpha interferon-treated human immunodeficiency virus type 1-infected T cells is associated with defective assembly of envelope gp 120. J Virol 1992;66:7543–7548.

297. Meylan PR, Guatelli JC, Munis JR, Richman DD, Kornbluth RS. Mechanisms for the inhibition of HIV replication by interferons-alpha, -beta, and -gamma in primary human macrophages. Virology 1993;193:138–148.

298. Friedman RM, Pitha PM. The effect of interferon on membrane-associated viruses. In: Friedman RM, ed. Interferon: mechanisms of production and action. New York: Elsevier Science, 1984:319–341.

299. Poli G, Orenstein JM, Kinter A, Folks TM, Fauci AS. Interferon-α but not AZT suppresses HIV expression in chronically infected cell lines. Science 1989;244:575–577.

300. Yasuda Y, Miyake S, Kato S, et al. Interferon-α treatment leads to accumulation of virus particles on the surface of cells persistently infected with the human immunodeficiency virus type 1. J AIDS 1990;3:1046–1051.

301. Smith MS, Thresher RJ, Pagano JS. Inhibition of human immunodeficiency virus type 1 morphogenesis in T cells by alpha interferon. Antimicrob Agents Chemother 1991;35:62–67.

302. Fernie BF, Poli G, Fauci AS. Alpha interferon suppresses virion but not soluble human immunodeficiency virus antigen production in chronically infected T-lymphocytic cells. J Virol 1991;65:3968–3971.

303. Biswas P, Poli G, Kinter AL, et al. Interferon-γ modulates the expression of human immunodeficiency virus in persistently infected promonocytic cells by redirecting the production of virions to intracytoplasmic vacuoles. J Exp Med 1992;176:739–750.

304. Dubreuil M, Sportza L, D'Addario M, et al. Inhibition of HIV-1 transmission by interferon and 3′-azido-3′-deoxythymidine during de novo infection of promonocytic cells. Virology 1990;179:388–394.

305. Markham PD, Salahuddin SZ, Veren K, Orndorff SH, Gallo RC. Hydrocortisone and some other hormones ehnance the expression of HTLV-III. Int J Cancer 1986;37:67–72.

306. Mace K, Duc Dodon M, Gazzolo L. Restriction of HIV-1 replication in promonocytic cells: a role for IFN-α. Virology 1989;168:399–405.

307. Gessani S, Puddu P, Varavo B, et al. Role of interferons in the restriction of HIV-1 replication in human monocyte/macrophages. Foum Immunol 1994 (in press).

308. Francis ML, Meltzer MS, Gendelman HE. Interferons in the persistence, pathogenesis, and treatment of HIV infection. AIDS Res Hum Retrovir 1992;8:199–207.

309. Lane HC, Kovacs JA, Feinberg J, et al. Anti-retroviral effects of interferon-α in AIDS-associated Kaposi's sarcoma. Lancet 1988;2:1218–1222.

310. Lane HC, Davey V, Kovacs JA, et al. Interferon-α in patients with asymptomatic human immunodeficiency virus (HIV) infection. Ann Intern Med 1990;112:805–811.

311. Dolei A, Fattorossi A, D'Amelio, Aiuti F, Dianzani F. Direct and cell-mediated effects of interferon-and-on cells chronically infected with HTLV-III. J Interferon Res 1986;6:543–549.

312. Geissler RG, Ottmann OG, Kojouharoff G, et al. Influence of human recombinant interferon-alpha and interferon-gamma on bone marrow progenitor cells of HIV-positive individuals. AIDS Res Hum Retrovir 1992;8:521–525.

313. Poli G, Introna M, Zanaboni F, et al. Natural killer cells in intravenous drug abusers with lymphadenopathy syndrome. Clin Exp Immunol 1985;62:128–135.

314. Williams GJ, Colby CB. Recombinant human interferon-beta suppresses the replication of HIV and acts synergistically with AZT. J Interferon Res 1989;9:709–718.

315. Mace K, Seif I, Anjard C, et al. Enhanced resistance to HIV-1 replication in U937 cells stably transfected with the human IFN-beta gene behind an MHC promoter fragment. J Immunol 1991;147:3553–3559.

316. Oka S, Hirabayashi Y, Mouri H, et al. Beta-interferon and early stage HIV infection. J AIDS 1989;2:125–128.

317. Oka S, Urayama K, Hirabayashi Y, Kimura S, Mitamura K, Shimada K. Human immunodeficiency virus DNA copies as a virologic marker in a clinical trial with beta-interferon. J AIDS 1992;5:707–711.

318. Nokta M, Loh JP, Douidar SM, Ahmed AE, Pollard RB. Metabolic interaction of recombinant interferon-beta and zidovudine in AIDS patients. J Interferon Res 1991;11:159–164.

319. Fuchs D, Hausen A, Reibnegger G, et al. Interferon-γ concentrations are increased in sera from individuals infected with human immunodeficiency virus type 1. J AIDS 1989;2:158–162.

320. Fuchs D, Forsman A, Hagberg L, et al. Immune activation and decreased tryptophan in patients with HIV-1 infection. J Interferon Res 1990;10:599–603.

321. Rinaldo CR, Armstrong JA, Kingsley LA, Zhou S, Ho M. Relation of alpha and gamma interferon levels to development of AIDS in homosexual men. J Exp Pathol 1990;5:127–132.

322. Weissman D, Poli G, Fauci AS. Interleukin-10 blocks HIV replication in macrophages by inhibiting the autocrine loop of TNF-α and IL-6 induction of virus. AIDS Res Human Retrovir 1994 (in press).

323. Reddy MM, McKinley G, Englard A, Grieco MH. Effect of azidothymidine (AZT) on HIV p24 antigen, BETA 2-microglobulin, neopterin, soluble CD8, soluble interleukin-2 receptor and tumor necrosis factor alpha levels in patients with AIDS-related complex or AIDS. Int J Immunopharmacol 1990;12:737–741.

324. Murray HW, Rubin BY, Masur H, Roberts RB. Impaired production of lymphokines and immune (gamma) interferon in the acquired immunodeficiency syndrome. N Engl J Med 1984;310:883–889.

325. Murray HW, Hillman JK, Rubin BY, et al. Patients at risk for AIDS-related opportunistic infections. Clinical manifestations and impaired gamma interferon production. N Engl J Med 1985;313:1504–1510.

326. Rook AH, Hooks JJ, Quinnan GV, et al. Interleukin 2 enhances the natural killer cell activity of acquired immunodeficiency syndrome patients through a gamma-interferon-independent mechanism. J Immunol 1985; 134:1503–1507.

327. Lane HC, Depper JM, Greene WC, Whalen G, Waldmann TA, Fauci AS. Qualitative analysis of immune function in patients with the acquired immunodeficiency syndrome. Evidence for a selective defect in soluble antigen recognition. N Engl J Med 1985;313:79–84.

328. Cauda R, Tyring SK, Tamburrini E, Ventura G, Tambarello M, Ortona L. Diminished interferon gamma production may be the earliest indicator of infection with the human immunodeficiency virus. Virol Immunol 1987;1:247–258.

329. Nokta MA, Pollard RB. Patterns of interferon-gamma production by peripheral blood mononuclear cells from patients with human immunodeficiency virus infection. J Interferon Res 1990;10:173–181.

330. Capsoni F, Minonzio F, Ongari AM, Rizzardi GP, Lazzarin A, Zanussi C. Monocyte-derived macrophage function in HIV-infected subjects: in vitro modulation by rIFN-gamma and rGM-CSF. Clin Immunol Immunopathol 1992;62: 176–182.

331. Buhl R, Jaffe HA, Holroyd KJ, et al. Activation of alveolar macrophages in asymptomatic HIV-infected individuals. J Immunol 1993;150:1019–1028.

332. Griffin DE, McArthur JC, Cornblath DR. Neopterin and interferon-gamma in serum and cerebrospinal fluid of patients with HIV-associated neurologic disease. Neurology 1991;41:69–74.

333. Caruso A, Pollara P, Foresti I, et al. Interferon-gamma is associated with the surface of the human immunodeficiency virus and binds to the gag gene product p17. AIDS Res Hum Retrovir 1989;5:605–612.

334. Murray HW, Scavuzzo D, Jacobs JL, et al. In vitro and in vivo activation of human mononuclear phagocytes by interferon-gamma: studies with normal and AIDS monocytes. J Immunol 1987;138:2457–2462.

335. Murphy PM, Lane HC, Gallin JI, Fauci AS. Marked disparity in incidence of bacterial infections in patients with the acquired immunodeficiency syndrome receiving interleukin-2 or interferon-γ. Ann Intern Med 1988;108:36–41.

336. Ganser A, Brucher W, Brodt HR, et al. Treatment of AIDS-related Kaposi's sarcoma with recombinant gamma-interferon. Onkologie 1986;8:163–166.

337. Agosti JM, Coombs RW, Collier AC. A randomized, double-blind, phase I/II trial of tumor necrosis factor and interferon-gamma for treatment of AIDS-related complex. AIDS Res Hum Retrovir 1992;8:581–587.

338. Degre M, Beck S, Rollag H. Interferon-gamma may enhance infection of blood-derived macrophages with HIV-1 in the presence of HIV-positive serum. APMIS 1992;100:465–469.

339. Ennen J, Kurth R. Interferon-gamma-activated monocytes impair infectivity of HIV particles by an oxygen metabolite-dependent reaction. Immunology 1993;78:171–176.

340. Staal FJT, Ela SW, Roederer M, Anderson MT, Herzenberg LA. Glutathione deficiency and human immunodeficiency virus infection. Lancet 1992;339:909–912.

341. Mackewicz C, Levy JA. CD8+ cell anti-HIV activity: non-lytic suppression of virus replication. AIDS Res Hum Retrovir 1992;8:1039–1050.

342. Sadat-Sowti B, Debre P, Idziorek T, et al. A lectin-binding soluble factor released by CD8+CD57+ lymphocytes from AIDS patients inhibits T cell cytotoxicity. Eur J Immunol 1991;21:737–741.

343. Ehrenreich H, Rieckmann P, Sinowatz F, et al. Potent stimulation of monocytic endothelin-1 production of HIV-1 glycoprotein 120. J Immunol 1993;150:4601–4609.

344. Poli G, Pantaleo G, Fauci AS. Immunopathogenesis of human immunodeficiency virus infection. Clin Infect Dis 1993;17:224–229.

345. Mikovits JA, Raziuddin, Gonda M, et al. Negative regulation of human immune deficiency virus replication in monocytes. Distinctions between restricted and latent expression in THP-1 cells. J Exp Med 1990;171:1705–1720.

346. Asjo B, Cefai D, Debre P, Dudoit Y, Autran B. A novel mode of human immunodeficiency virus type 1 (HIV-1) activation: ligation of CD28 alone induces HIV-1 replication in naturally infected lymphocytes. J Virol 1993;67:4395–4398.

347. Hildreth JEK, Orentas RJ. Involvement of a leukocyte adhesion receptor (LFA-1) in HIV-induced syncytium formation. Science 1989;244:1075–1078.

348. Pantaleo G, Butini L, Graziosi C, et al. Human immunodeficiency virus (HIV) infection in CD4+ T lymphocytes genetically deficient in LFA-1: LFA-1 is required for HIV-mediated cell fusion but not for viral transmission. J Exp Med 1991;173:511–514.

349. Markovitz DM. Infection with the human immunodeficiency virus type 2. Ann Intern Med 1993;118:211–218.

350. Markovitz DM, Hannibal MC, Smith MJ, Cossman R, Nabel GJ. Activation of the human immunodeficiency virus type 1 enhancer is not dependent on NFAT-1. J Virol 1992;66:3961–3965.

351. Hilfinger JM, Clark N, Smith M, Robinson K, Markovitz DM. Differential regulation of the human immunodeficiency virus type 2 enhancer in monocytes at various stages of differentiation. J Virol 1993;67:4448–4453.

352. Arya SK. Human immunodeficiency virus type 2 (HIV-2) gene expression: down-modulation by sequence elements downstream of the transcriptional initiation site. AIDS Res Hum Retrovir 1991;7:1007–1014.

353. Sher A, Gazzinelli RT, Oswald IP, et al. Role of T-cell derived cytokines in the downregulation of immune responses in parasitic and retroviral infection. Immunol Rev 1992;127:183–204.

354. Ada G, HIV. Towards phase III trials for candidate vaccines. Nature 1993;364:489–490.

355. Bolognesi D. The immune response to HIV: implications for vaccine development. Semin Immunol 1993;5:203–214.

CHAPTER 29

ROLE OF CYTOKINES IN FUNGAL INFECTIONS

Elmer Brummer and Faris Nassar

OPPORTUNISTIC
FUNGAL INFECTIONS

Suppression of the immune system during organ and bone marrow transplantation or use of agents with bone marrow cytotoxicity during cancer chemotherapy opens the door to invasion of the host by certain opportunistic fungi. Patients suffering from congenital immunodeficiencies, such as chronic granulomatous disease (CGD) and chronic mucocutaneous candidiasis (CMC), or from the acquired immunodeficiency syndrome (AIDS), are at high risk for infection with particular opportunistic fungi. Opportunistic fungi invade because leukocytes necessary for host defenses have been reduced in number, have subnormal cytokine secretion, or are functionally crippled. Because these immunocompromised conditions are so diverse, the role of cytokines in correcting deficiencies must be tailored to the specific situation.

Transplantation

INTERLEUKIN-2, GRANULOCYTE-, AND GRANULOCYTE-MACROPHAGE COLONY-STIMULATING FACTOR: Steroids, the first-generation immunosuppressants for transplantation, affect both cell-mediated and humoral immunity. Development of newer immunosuppressive agents (e.g., cyclosporine [CsA]) has allowed more selective immune suppression (1). The immunosuppressive mechanism of CsA and FK 506 has been elucidated, and it was reviewed in 1991 by Schreiber (2). CsA binds with high affinity to the protein cyclophilin, and it inhibits signal transduction pathways that lead to T-cell activation. Secretion of interleukin-2 (IL-2) and expression of IL-2 receptors are inhibited by CsA.

Because IL-2 is vital to the development of host defenses against microorganisms, transplantation patients are at risk for various infections. Fortuitously, CsA has microbicidal activity for some fungi (e.g., *Coccidioides immitis* [3] and *Cryptococcus neoformans* [4]). In contrast, immunosuppressed transplantation patients are particularly susceptible to 2 opportunistic fungi: *Aspergillus* species and *Candida albicans*.

ASPERGILLOSIS AND CANDIDIASIS: Aspergillosis was the most common (9 of 10) fungal infection in heart transplantation patients (5); *Candida* infections were the more common fungal infection (22 of 62) in liver transplantation patients (6). Others have reported a high incidence of *Candida* infections (64–83% of fungal infections) in liver transplantation patients (7,8). The mortality rate in liver transplantation patients with candidiasis has been reported to be 50 to 70% (6,8,9).

Candida infections were the most frequent fungal infection (14 of 49) in patients undergoing bone marrow transplantation for aplastic anemia or acute leukemia

(10). Mortality rates of 88% were seen in these situations. In a recent study, 171 of 1,506 bone marrow transplantation patients had invasion candidiasis, with a mortality rate of 39% (11). The frequency of invasion aspergillosis has increased in bone marrow transplantation units in recent years (12–14).

Ordinarily, fungal infections are not a problem in patients immunosuppressed with CsA. Risk factors for acquiring *Aspergillus* infections in transplantation units center around the use of corticosteroids to control rejection episodes, lack of attention to air filtration, and patient isolation (13,15,16). In contrast, acquisition of *Candida* infections in solid organ transplantation was strongly associated with the use of antibiotics to control bacterial infections or steroids to control rejection episodes (8).

During bone marrow transplantation, prolonged neutropenia was found to be the most important risk factor for disseminated candidiasis (11,17). These observations provide a rationale for treatment of marrow transplantation patients with granulocyte colony-stimulating factor (G-CSF) or GM-CSF to enhance recovery of neutrophils after transplantation (18,19).

Cancer: GM-CSF

Opportunistic fungal infections are a serious problem in cancer patients undergoing therapy for leukemias, lymphomas, and solid tumors. *Candida* species and *Aspergillus* species, which are in or on the body or ubiquitous in the environment, respectively, are the main causes of fungal infections in cancer patients.

LEUKEMIAS: The incidence of fungal infection (14%) was similar in acute lymphocytic leukemia (ALL) and acute myelogenous leukemia (AML) patients (20). However, Goodrich and colleagues (11), in 1991, reported that patients with myelogenous leukemia were more likely to acquire fungal infections than patients with aplastic anemia despite their neutropenia predating transplantation. *Candida* species accounted for the majority of fungal infections (70%), and the remaining fungal infections were caused by *Aspergillus* species (30%).

Contributing or predisposing factors for incidence of fungal infections correlated with the use of antileukemic agents, corticosteroids, or antibiotics (20). Granulocytopenia was considered to be the greatest risk factor for acquiring these fungal infections (21). Treatment of such fungal infections in these patients, even with the most potent antifungal agents, has met with only meager success. Reversal of granulocytopenia, careful selection of antibiotics, and discontinuance of steroids coupled with antifungal therapy appears to be the best course of action. G-CSF and GM-CSF have become important cytokines in the reversal of granulocytopenia (18,19).

LYMPHOMAS AND SARCOMAS: In lymphomas and sarcomas, systemic candidiasis was encountered, and it was associated with neutrocytopenia due to cytotoxic chemotherapy (22). Pulmonary aspergillosis can also develop in such patients, but it occurs less frequently than systemic candidiasis (23). The course of action as outlined for ALL and AML is recommended such as reversal of neutrocytopenia with GM-CSF.

Chronic granulomatous disease: IFN-γ

Suppurative bacterial and fungal infections develop in individuals afflicted with CGD. CGD is characterized by polymorphonuclear granulocytes and monocytes that fail to mount an oxidative burst (production of superoxide anion and hydrogen peroxide) during phagocytosis or when stimulated. The molecular basis for CGD has been identified as X-chromosome–linked (65% of patients with CGD) as a defect in membrane cytochrome b_{558}, a component in the NADPH-oxidase system (24). Autosomal recessive inheritance of CGD (34% of patients with CGD) is associated with lack of cytosolic factor required for activation of the oxidative burst (25). Recently, the biochemistry of CGD was reviewed by Smith and Curnette (26).

CANDIDIASIS: The inability of CGD phagocytes to generate an oxidative burst has been reversed (19 of 30 patients) by treatment in vitro with IFN-γ (100 U/mL for 3 days). Moreover, administration of IFN-γ (0.01 mg/m² doses) subcutaneously for 6 days to 3 patients reconstituted defective neutrophil and monocyte bactericidal activity and likely candidacidal activity. This effect was maintained for 20 days after therapy (27). Initial results of a randomized trial of IFN-γ therapy in 128 patients with CGD have recently been reported. A dose of 0.5 mg/m² subcutaneously 3 times per week resulted in a 70% reduction in serious infections (28).

Chronic mucocutaneous candidiasis: transfer factor

CMC is recognized as a complex of defects in which a subset (50%) of patients have endocrine dysfunction in adrenal and parathyroid glands. However, one common denominator is an intriguing immunological condition that results in susceptibility to primarily cutaneous candidiasis.

Cellular immune responses in patients with CMC are depressed, as evidenced by negative delayed-type hypersensitivity (DTH) reactions to recall antigens (mumps, SK-SD, *C. albicans,* and Trichophyton), failure to be sensitized by dinitrochlorobenzene (DNCB), or rejection of heterologous skin grafts (29). Lymphocytes from patients with CMC do not proliferate in one-way mixed lymphocyte cultures or to stimulation with mumps or *Candida* antigens (29).

CUTANEOUS CANDIDIASIS:

Successful immunotherapy with transfer factor (TF) has been documented in several reports (30–33). Successful combination therapy of a patient with CMC with ketoconazole and TF has been reported (34). Despite these encouraging results of immunotherapy of CMC with TF in the 1970s and 1980s, interest in identifying the clinically active component in TF has waned, probably because of the advent of new antifungal agents (e.g., amphotericin B and ketoconazole) and their efficacy in treating CMC (35,36).

AIDS: IFN-γ, IL-2, and M-CSF

Immune deficiency in AIDS is complex, and it varies with stage of disease. In patients with AIDS with low CD4+ T-cell counts (<200/mm^3), peripheral blood mononuclear cells (PBMC) from 13 of 16 patients had impaired proliferative responses and production of lymphokines (IL-2 and IFN-γ) when stimulated with concanavalin A or recall antigens (37,38).

Although T-cell defects in patients with AIDS are severe, monocytes from patients with AIDS responded to activation by IFN-γ (300 U/mL for 3 days), as measured by antimicrobial activity against *Toxoplasma gondii* or *Chlamydia psittaci* (37). Moreover, monocytes from patients with AIDS had normal fungicidal activity against *Cryptococcus neoformans* (75 +/– 3%) and *Aspergillus fumigatus* (68 +/– 2%) (39). However, monocytes from patients with AIDS may have defective accessory cell function for lymphocyte responses (40). Abnormal functional activities (e.g., chemotaxis, bactericidal) of polymorphonuclear neutrophils (PMNs) from patients with AIDS were linked to heat-labile factors in sera from patients with AIDS rather than inherent defects in PMNs (41). However, PMNs from drug addicts with AIDS were defective in phagocytosis and killing of *Candida albicans* (42).

MUCOCUTANEOUS CANDIDIASIS (THRUSH):

C. albicans is part of the normal flora in humans. In patients with AIDS, *Candida albicans* infections present as oral thrush (43); thrush will develop in 80 to 95% of patients with AIDS at some time (44). Thrush is limited to surfaces of mucosal membranes, and its relationship to immune defects has not been established. Although therapies exist for controlling thrush in patients with AIDS (e.g., fluconazole [44]), immune reconstitution with IL-2 alone (45) or IL-2 and IFN-γ (46) have been tried. Cellular immunity was enhanced in these studies; however, there was no evaluation made on the impact of lymphokine immunotherapy on episodes of thrush.

CRYPTOCOCCOSIS:

In an extensive review by Levy and colleagues in 1985 (47), 41 of 315 neurologically symtomatic patients with AIDS with central nervous system (CNS) complications had cryptococcosis. Although cryptococcal meningitis is the most frequent manifestation of infection with *C. neoformans* in AIDS, cryptococcal pneumonia is a significant entity. Twelve of 31 patients with AIDS with cryptococcal infection in one report had cryptococcal pneumonia, and acute-phase mortality was 42% (48).

Therapies exist for treatment of cryptococcosis in AIDS (49); however, the underlying immunological defect that permits infection and dissemination is not known. In the face of relapses after successful primary treatment, oral fluconazole has been used in long-term suppressive therapy of cryptococcosis in AIDS (49). Tissue macrophages may be a privileged site for *C. neoformans*, and relapse may occur from this source. In vitro results indicate that resident murine peritoneal macrophages can be activated by IFN-γ plus lipopolysaccharide (50) or M-CSF (Brummer E, Stevens DA, unpublished data) for enhanced fungistatic activity. Furthermore, activated macrophages can synergize with fluconazole for killing of *C. neoformans*. These data suggest that combination therapy, fluconazole plus an immunomodulator, may be an effective treatment of cryptococcosis in AIDS.

PRIMARY FUNGAL PATHOGENS

Blastomyces dermatitidis

IFN-γ AND IL-4: The possibility that IFN-γ could have a role in host resistance to systemic mycoses was first demonstrated with *B. dermatitidis* (51). Recombinant IFN-γ, at a relatively high concentration (1,000 U/mL), induced a fungicidal state in resident peritoneal macrophages; 34 +/– 1% of *B. dermatitidis* yeast cells were killed in a 4-hour assay. Specific antibody against IFN-γ negated IFN-γ activation of macrophages to kill *B. dermatitidis*. Anti-IFN antibody could also significantly reduce the capacity of supernatants from Con A–stimulated spleen cell cultures to activate macrophages for killing *B. dermatitidis* from 32 to 12% (51).

Pulmonary macrophages could also be activated by INF-γ (1,000 U/mL) to kill yeast-form *B. dermatitidis*. Activated pulmonary macrophages killed 25 +/– 3% of *B. dermatitidis* in a 4-hour assay. Activation of pulmonary macrophages by IFN-γ was abrogated by specific antibody to IFN-γ (52).

In vivo administration of IFN-γ (4 × 10^5 U/mouse intraperitoneally [IP]) 24 hours before lavage of lungs resulted in activation of pulmonary macrophages to kill *B. dermatitidis* (37.5 +/– 0.7% in vitro) (53). The mechanism by which activated macrophages killed *B. dermatitidis* was not dependent on products of the oxidative burst. For example, killing by activated macrophages could not be inhibited by scavengers of superoxide anion, hydrogen peroxide, or hydroxyl radicals (54).

In acute murine pulmonary blastomycosis, spleen cells explanted 3 weeks after infection and stimulated with antigen produced IFN-γ (70 U/mL), but very little IL-4 (5–10 pg/mL). As disease progressed and mortalities mounted, antigen-stimulated spleen cells had an inverse production of IFN-γ (10 U/mL) and IL-4 (142 pg/mL). Peak IL-4 production correlated with peak serum levels of immunoglobulin E (IgE) (6 μg/mL at 3 weeks to 24 μg/mL after 4 weeks of infection) (55) (Fig. 29–1).

Immunization of mice prevented mortalities and arrested progression of the pulmonary infection (55). Nevertheless, a residual low level chronic type of pulmonary infection persisted. Spleen cells from immunized infected mice produced both IFN-γ and IL-4 when stimulated with antigen (55). This effect was observed from 3 to 8 weeks after infection.

These findings indicate that naive mice initially respond to infection with ample production of IFN-γ but, as disease progresses, this response ceases, and IL-4 production increases. In contrast, in a contained smoldering infection, there is dual production of IFN-γ and IL-4, and, in mice cured by treatment with an antifungal agent, low level secretion of these cytokines and antigen-stimulated spleen cells decrease to background levels (55).

Human monocyte-derived macrophages, but not PMN, were fungistatic for *B. dermatitidis* in vitro (56). Supernatants from sensitized peripheral blood mononuclear cell cultures stimulated with antigen increased macrophage fungistatic activity against ingested yeast cells (57). This finding suggested that cytokines present in supernatants enhance the antifungal activity of human monocyte-derived macrophages. The capacity of various purified cytokines to modulate human macrophages for fungicidal activity against *B. dermatitidis* has not been reported. Moreover, the relative production of cytokines (e.g., IFN-γ, IL-4) by antigen-stimulated lymphocytes from patients with active or chronic-type blastomycosis remains to be determined. Results from such studies would be very informative as to the immunoregulatory roles of these cytokines in human blastomycosis.

Histoplasma capsulatum

IFN-γ, GM-CSF, M-CSF, AND IL-3: *H. capsulatum* is capable of replicating intracellularly in resident murine peritoneal macrophages. Activation of macrophages by exposure to IFN-γ (250–500 U/mL) 2 hours before and 16 hours after infection prevented replication of ingested yeast cells by 80% (58). Antibody to IFN-γ not only neutralized IFN-γ activity, but also MAF activity in supernatants from Con A–stimulated T-cell hybridoma cultures. In this system, killing of ingested *H. capsulatum* could not be demonstrated in 22- or 44-hour assays (58).

In an experimental systemic infection model, spleen cells from resistant A/J mice produced 30% more IFN-γ when stimulated with antigen than spleen cells from more susceptible C57B1/6 mice (59). These findings suggest an important role for IFN-γ in resistance to *H. capsulatum*.

H. capsulatum can also replicate intracellularly in human monocyte-derived macrophages (60,61). When peripheral blood monocytes were incubated for 3 days in the presence of IFN-γ (500–1,000 U/mL) and then challenged with yeast cells in tissue culture medium containing 15% fresh human serum, they were fungicidal for *H. capsulatum*. The colony-forming units of ingested or attached yeast cells were significantly reduced (54–58%) by activated macrophage monolayers compared with non-activated macrophage monolayers (61). This reduction was demonstrated in a short-term 2-hour assay. Fungicidal activity was abrogated by superoxide dismutase, but not by azide.

With additional culture time, it was shown that yeast cells that were not killed replicated in macrophages at the same rate as yeast cells in nonactivated macrophage monolayers. This finding suggested that macrophage monolayers were heterogenous and that all macrophages in the monolayer were not activated. Monocytes or monocyte-derived macrophages (cultured for 4–7 days), when exposed to supernatants (40%) from PHA-stimulated peripheral blood mononuclear cells for 24 hours after they

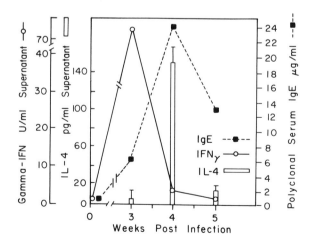

Figure 29–1 IL-4, IgE, and IFN-γ in infected, untreated mice. Serum concentrations of polyclonal IgE (*solid squares*), IFn-γ (*open circles*), and IL-4 (*bars*) in supernatants from antigen-stimulated spleen cell cultures are shown for time points after infection.

had ingested yeast cells, significantly inhibited intracellular replication (62). Possible macrophage-activating cytokines in supernatants were implicated in a subsequent study using recombinant cytokines and an indirect methodology (i.e., ^{3}H-leucine uptake by yeast cells). Monocytes treated with IL-3, GM-CSF, and M-CSF, but not IL-1, IL-2, IFN-γ, tumor necrosis factor-α (TNF-α), or G-CSF, for 3 days inhibited the growth in cocultures in a 24-hour assay (63). It was not clear if inhibited growth was strictly intracellular, because noningested yeast cells were not removed in the assay. IL-3, GM-CSF, or M-CSF did not induce antifungal activity in mature macrophages when tested in the same assay. In another report, when monocyte-derived macrophages or alveolar macrophages were treated with IFN-γ for 3 hours or 3 days, they did not inhibit intracellular replication of ingested yeast cells (61).

Although PMNs inhibit the growth of *H. capsulatum* in cocultures by 77% in 72 hours, killing was not demonstrated (64). Whether cytokines have a role in activating PMNs for enhanced antifungal activity remains to be determined.

Defining the roles for various cytokines in host resistance to histoplasmosis is still in its infancy. Nonetheless, there is clear piece-meal evidence that some cytokines can have protective roles in host resistance to *H. capsulatum*.

Coccidioides immitis

IFN-γ: Pulmonary or peritoneal macrophages that have ingested arthroconidia or endospores of *C. immitis* allow intracellular germination of arthroconidia or growth of endospores into spherules. However, if peritoneal macrophages ingest arthroconidia or endospores in the presence of IFN-γ (1,000 U/mL) followed by culture for 27 hours with IFN-γ present, germination of arthroconidia and growth of endospores are inhibited (65). Inhibition of intracellular growth of *C. immitis* by macrophages in the presence of IFN-γ was shown to be, at least in part, due to killing of endospores or arthroconidia. When pulmonary macrophages ingested arthroconidia or endospores in the presence of IFN-γ, followed by 8 hours of culture in the presence of IFN-γ, CFU were reduced by 50 and 57%, respectively (65). If antibody to IFN-γ was added to macrophages, IFN-γ, and *C. immitis* cultures, reduction of CFU by macrophages was significantly inhibited compared with positive control samples. These data indicate that IFN-γ can have a significant role in host defense against *C. immitis* by activating macrophages to kill this pathogen.

Coculture of human monocytes, sensitized lymphocytes, and arthroconidia of *C. immitis* resulted in killing of arthroconidia (44 +/− 9%) in 6 hours (66). In a different type of assay, the limiting dilution method, monocytes or

macrophages had fungicidal activity against *C. immitis* (67). Additional work is required to determine if IFN-γ given in vivo can activate pulmonary or tissue macrophages to kill *C. immitis* in vitro or affect the outcome of coccidioidomycosis in an animal model.

Paracoccidioides brasiliensis

IFN-γ AND IL-4: IFN-γ at relatively high concentrations (1,000 U/mL) in vitro induced significant fungicidal activity (35%) in peritoneal (68) and pulmonary macrophages (45%) (53) against isolates of *P. brasiliensis* in 4-hour assays. Pulmonary macrophages were also activated in vivo for enhanced killing of *P. brasiliensis* by IP administration of 4×10^5 U IFN-γ 24 hours earlier. Pulmonary macrophages activated in vivo, collected by lavage, and tested in vitro killed *P. brasiliensis* more efficiently than control macrophages (47 vs 25%) (53).

Similar to killing of other thermally dimorphic fungal pathogens by activated macrophages, killing of *P. brasiliensis* did not depend on products of the oxidative burst. This finding was evidenced by the inability of scavengers of superoxide anion, hydrogen peroxide, or hydroxyl radicals to inhibit killing of *P. brasiliensis* by activated peritoneal (69) or pulmonary (53) macrophages.

In long-term 24- to 48-hour cocultures of nonactivated macrophages and *P. brasiliensis,* it was found that ingested yeast cells replicated intracellularly. In contrast, yeast cells ingested by IFN-γ activated macrophages failed to replicate and were killed (100%) in 48 hours (70). These in vitro findings suggest a prominent role for IFN-γ in host resistance to *P. brasiliensis*.

In murine pulmonary disseminated paracoccidioidomycosis, serum IgE levels increased from 0.2 to 10.0 μg/mL by 4 weeks of disease progression. Elevated serum IgE levels were paralleled by increased production of IL-4, but not IFN-γ, by antigen-stimulated lymph node cells. Administration of anti-IL-4 antibody at the time of infection suppressed elevation of serum IgE levels and increased the resistance to pulmonary infection (e.g., 2 $\log_{10}$ fewer CFU/lung at 4 weeks). Treatment of the infection with an antifungal agent eventually cured the infection, and elevated serum IgE levels returned to background. IFN-γ treatment synergized with the antifungal agent in clearing the infection during only the latter stages of treatment (Hostetler JS, et al., unpublished data).

Production of IL-4 appears to have a significant role in the progression of pulmonary disseminated paracoccidioidomycosis. Reversal of IL-4 production with anti-IL-4 antibody, as well as administration of IFN-γ, can have beneficial effects in host resistance to this pathogen.

P. brasiliensis is ingested and grows intracellularly in human monocytes and monocyte-derived macrophages (Moscardi-Bacchi M, et al., unpublished data). Because the pathogenic yeast form remains viable but does not replicate in tissue culture medium, macrophages appear to present a privileged site for the growth of *P. brasiliensis*. Treatment of monocytes or monocyte-derived macrophages with supernatants from mitogen-stimulated peripheral blood mononuclear cells or recombinant IFN-γ for 3 days, followed by infection with yeast cells, resulted in significant inhibition (65–95%) of intracellular replication of *P. brasiliensis*.

REFERENCES

1. Maugh TH. New techniques for selective immune suppression increase transplant odds: cyclosporin A, antilymphocyte serum, and lymphoid irradiation help transplants survive without exposing recipient to hazards of infection. Science 1989;210:44–46.

2. Schreiber SL. Chemistry and biology of immunophilins and their immunosuppressive ligands. Science 1991;251:283–287.

3. Kirkland TN, Fierer J. Cyclosporin A inhibits Coccidioides immitis in vitro and in vivo. Antimicrob Agents Chemother 1983;24:921–924.

4. Mody CA, Toews GB, Lipscomb MF. Treatment of murine cryptococcosis with cyclosporin A in normal and athymic mice. Am Rev Respir Dis 1989;139:8–13.

5. Hoffin JM, Potasman I, Baldwin JC, Oyer PE, Stinson EB, Remington JS. Infectious complications in heart transplant recipients receiving cyclosporine and corticosteroids. Ann Intern Med 1987;106:209–216.

6. Wajszczuk CP, Dummer JS, Ho M, et al. Fungal infection in liver transplant recipients. Transplantation 1985;40:347–353.

7. Schroter GPJ, Hoelscher M, Putnam CW, et al. Fungus infections after liver transplantation. Ann Surg 1977;186:115–122.

8. Castaldo P, Stratta RJ, Wood RP, et al. Clinical spectrum of fungal infections after orthotopic liver transplantation. Arch Surg 1991;126:149–156.

9. Kusne S, Drummer JS, Singh N, et al. Fungal infection after liver transplantation. Transplant Proc 1988;20:650–651.

10. Winston DJ, Gale RP, Meyer DV, Young LS. Infectious complications of human marrow transplantation. Medicine 1979;58:1–31.

11. Goodrich JM, Reed ED, Mori M, et al. Clinical features and analysis of risk factors for invasion candida infection after marrow transplantation. J Infect Dis 1991;164:731–740.

12. Peterson PK, McGlave P, Ramsey N, et al. A prospective study of infectious diseases following bone marrow transplantation: emergence of aspergillus and cytomegalo virus as the major causes of mortality. Infect Control 1983;4:81–89.

13. Scheretz RJ, Belani A, Kramer BS, et al. Impact of air filtration on nosocomial aspergillus infections: unique risk of bone marrow transplant recipients. Am J Med 1987;83:709–718.

14. Barnes RA, Rogers TR. Response rates to a staged antibiotic regimen in febrile neutropenic patients. J Antimicrob Chemother 1988;22:759–763.

15. Opal SM, Asp AA, Canady PB, et al. Efficacy of infection control measures during nosocomial outbreak of disseminated aspergillosis with hospital construction. J Infect Dis 1986;153:634–637.

16. Kusne S, Torre-Cisneros J, Maney R, et al. Factors associated with invasion lung aspergillosis and the significance of positive Aspergillus cultures after liver transplantation. J Infect Dis 1992;166:1379–1383.

17. Body GP. Candidiasis in cancer patients. Am J Med 1984;77:13–19.

18. Teshima H, Ishikawa J, Kitayawa H, et al. Clinical effects of recombinant human granulocyte colony-stimulating factor in leukemic patients: a phase I/II study. Exp Hematol 1989;17:853–858.

19. Aurer I, Ribas A, Gale RP. What is the role of recombinant factors in bone marrow transplantation? Bone Marrow Transplant 1990;6:79–87.

20. Bodey GP. Fungal infections complicating acute leukemia. J Chronic Dis 1966;19:667–687.

21. Gerson SL, Talbot GH, Hurwitz, S, Strom B, Lusk E, Cassileth P. Prolonged granulocytopenia: the major risk factor for invasion pulmonary aspergillosis in patients with acute leukemia. Ann Intern Med 1984;100:345–351.

22. Thaler M, Pastakia B, Shawker TH, O'Leary T, Pizzo PA. Hepatic candidiasis in cancer patients: the evolving picture of the syndrome. Ann Intern Med 1988;108:88–100.

23. Young RL, Bennett JE, Vogel CL, Carbone PP, DeVita VT. Aspergillosis: the spectrum of the disease in 98 patients. Medicine 1970;49:147–173.

24. Ohno Y, Buescher ES, Roberts R, Metcalf JA, Gallin JI. Re-evaluation of cytochrome b and flavinadenine dinucleotide in neutrophils from patients with chronic granulomatous disease and description of a family with probable autosomal recessive inheritance of cytochrome b deficiency. Blood 1986;67:1132–1138.

25. Curnutte JT, Berkow RL, Roberts RL, Shurin SB, Scott JJ. Chronic granulomatous disease due to a defect in the cytosolic factor required for nicotinamide adenine dinucleotide phosphate. J Clin Invest 1988;81:606–610.

26. Smith RM, Curnutte JT. Molecular basis of chronic granulomatous disease. J Am Soc Hematol 1991;77:673–686.

27. Sechler JM, Malech HL, White CJ, Gallin JI. Recombinant human interferon-gamma reconstitutes defective phagocyte function in patients with chronic granulomatous disease of childhood. Proc Natl Acad Sci USA 1988;85:4874–4878.

28. International Collaborative Study Group. Clinical efficacy of recombinant human interferon-gamma in chronic granulomatous disease (abstract). Clin Res 1990;38:46A.

29. Canales L. Middlemas RO, Louro JM, South MA. Immunological observations in chronic mucocutaneous candidiasis. Lancet 1969;1:567–571.

30. Sehulkind ML, Adler WH, Altemeir WA, Ayoub EM. Transfer factor in the treatment of a case of chronic mucocutaneous candidiasis. Cell Immunol 1972;3:606–615.

31. Hitzig WH, Fotonellez HP, Muntener U, Paul S, Spitler LE, Fudenberg HH. Transfer factor: immunologieche

grundlagen und therapeutische erfahrungen. Schweiz Med Wocheusch 1972;102:1237–1244.

32. Valdimarsson H, Holt L, Riches HR, Hobbs JR. Lymphocyte abnormality in chronic mucocutaneous candidiasis. Lancet 1970;1:1259–1261.

33. Littman BH, Rocklin RE, Parkman R, David JR. Transfer factor treatment of chronic mucocutaneous candidiasis: requirement for donor reactivity to Candida albicans. Clin Immunol Immunopathol 1978;9:97–110.

34. Corbeel L, Ceuppens JL, Van den Berghe G, Claeys H, Casteels-Van Daele M. Immunological observations before and after successful treatment of chronic mucocutaneous candidiasis with ketoconazole and transfer factor. Eur J Pediatr 1984;143:45–48.

35. Kirkpatrick CH, Petersen EA, Alling DW. Treatment of chronic mucocutaneous candidiasis with ketoconazole: preliminary results of a double blind clinical trial. Rev Infect Dis 1980;2:599–605.

36. Rosenblatt HM, Byrne W, Ament ME, Graybill JR, Stiehm ER. Successful treatment of mucocutaneous candidiasis with ketoconazole. J Pediatr 1980;97:657–660.

37. Murray HW, Ruben BY, Masur H, Roberts RB. Impaired production of lymphokines and immune (gamma) interferon in the acquired immunodeficiency syndrome. N Engl J Med 1984;310:883–889.

38. Murray HW, Welte K, Jacobs JL, Rubin BY, Mertelsmann R, Roberts RB. Production of an in vitro response to interleukin-2 in acquired immunodeficiency syndrome. J Clin Invest 1985;76:1955–1964.

39. Washburn RG, Tuazon CU, Bennett JE. Phagocytic and fungicidal activity of monocytes from patients with acquired immunodeficiency syndrome. J Infect Dis 1985; 151:565–566.

40. Rich EA, Toossi Z, Fujiwara H, Hanigosky R, Lederman MM, Ellner JJ. Defective accessory function of monocytes in human immunodeficiency virus-related syndromes. J Clin Lab Med 1988;112:174–181.

41. Ellis M, Gupta S, Galant S, et al. Impaired neutrophil function in patients with AIDS or AIDS-related complex: a comprehensive evaluation. J Infect Dis 1988;158:1268–1276.

42. Lazzarin A, Uberti-Foppa C, Galli M, et al. Impairment of polymorphonuclear leukocyte function in patients with acquired immunodeficiency syndrome and with lymphadenopathy syndrome. Clin Exp Immunol 1986;65:105–111.

43. Klein RS, Harris CA, Small CB, Moll B, Lesser M, Freidland CH. Oral candidiasis in high risk patients as the initial manifestation of the acquired immunodeficiency syndrome. N Engl J Med 1984;311:354–358.

44. Stevens DA, Greene I, Lang O. Thrush can be prevented in patients with acquired immunodeficiency syndrome-related complex. Randomized, double-blind, placebo-controlled study of 100 mg oral fluconazole daily. Arch Intern Med 1991;151:2458–2464.

45. Teppler H, Kaplan G, Smith K, et al. Efficacy of low doses of the polyethylene glycol derivative of interleukin-2 in modulating the immune response of patients with human immunodeficiency virus type-1 infection. J Infect Dis 1993;167:291–298.

46. Lane HC, Masur H, Gelmann EP, Fauci AS. Therapeutic approaches to patients with AIDS. Cancer Res 1985;45 (suppl 9):4674S–4676S.

47. Levy RM, Bredesen DE, Rosenblum ML. Neurological manifestations of the acquired immunodeficiency syndrome (AIDS): experience at UCSF and review of the literature. J Neurosurg 1985;64:475–495.

48. Cameron ML, Bartlett JA, Gallis HA, Waskin HA. Manifestations of pulmonary cryptococcosis in patients with acquired immunodeficiency syndrome. Rev Infect Dis 1991; 13:64–67.

49. Sugar AM, Saunders C. Oral fluconazole as suppressive therapy of disseminated cryptococcosis in patients with acquired immunodeficiency syndrome. Am J Med 1988;85: 481–489.

50. Perfect JR, Granger DL, Durack DT. Effect of antifungal agents and gamma-interferon macrophage cytotoxicity for fungi and tumor cells. J Infect Dis 1987;156:316–323.

51. Brummer E, Morrison CJ, Stevens DA. Recombinant and natural gamma-interferon activation of macrophages in vitro: different dose requirements for induction of killing activity against phagocytizable and nonphagocytizable fungi. Infect Immun 1985;49:724–730.

52. Brummer E, Stevens DA. Activation of pulmonary macrophages for fungicidal activity by gamma-interferon or lymphokines. Clin Exp Immunol 1987;70:520–528.

53. Brummer E, Hanson L, Restrepo A, Stevens DA. In vivo and in vitro activation of pulmonary macrophages by IFN-gamma for enhanced killing of Paracoccidioides brasiliensis or Blastomyces dermatitidis. J Immunol 1988; 140:2786–2789.

54. Brummer E, Stevens DA. Fungicidal mechanisms of activated macrophages: evidence for nonoxidative mechanism for killing Blastomyces dermatitidis. Infect Immun 1987; 55:3221–3224.

55. Brummer E, Hanson LH, Stevens DA. IL-4, IgE, and Interferon-gamma production in pulmonary blastomycosis: comparison in mice untreated, immunized, or treated with an antifungal (SCH 39304). Cell Immunol 1994;149: 258–267.

56. Brummer E, Stevens DA. Opposite effect of human monocytes, macrophages, and polymorphonuclear neutrophils on replication of Blastomyces dermatitidis in vitro. Infect Immun 1982;36:297–303.

57. Bradsher RW, Balk RA, Jacobs RF. Growth inhibition of Blastomyces dermatitidis in alveolar and peripheral macrophages from patients with blastomycosis. Am Rev Respir Dis 1987;135:412–417.

58. Wu-Hsieh B, Howard DH. Inhibition of the growth of Histoplasma capsulatum by recombinant murine gamma-interferon. Infect Immun 1987;55:1014–1016.

59. Wu-Hsieh B. Relative susceptibility of inbred mouse strains C57bl/6 and AJ to infection with Histoplasma capsulatum. Infect Immun 1989;57:3788–3792.

60. Fleischmann J, Wu-Hsieh B, Howard DH. The intracellular fate of Histoplasma capsulatum in human macrophages is unaffected by recombinant human interferon-gamma. J Infect Dis 1990;161:143–145.

61. Brummer E, Kurita N, Yoshida S, Hishimura K, Miyaji M. Killing of Histoplasma capsulatum by gamma-interferon

activated human monocyte-derived macrophages: evidence for a superoxide anion dependent mechanism. J Med Microbiol 1991;35:29–34.

62. Newman SL, Gootee L, Bucher C, Bullock WE. Inhibition of intracellular growth of Histoplasma capsulatum yeast cells by cytokine-activated human monocytes and macrophages. Infect Immun 1991;59:737–741.

63. Newman SL, Gootee L. Colony-stimulating factors activate human macrophages to inhibit intracellular growth of Histoplasma capsulatum yeasts. Infect Immun 1992;60:4593–4597.

64. Brummer E, Kurita N, Yoshida S, Nishimura K, Miyaji M. Fungistatic activity of human neutrophils against Histoplasma capsulatum: correlation with phagocytosis. J Infect Dis 1991;164:158–162.

65. Beaman L. Fungicidal activation of murine alveolar macrophages by recombinant gamma-interferon. Infect Immun 1987;55:2951–2955.

66. Beaman L, Pappagianis D. Fate of Coccidioides immitis arthroconidia in human peripheral blood monocyte cultures in vitro. In: Einsten HE, Catanzaro A, eds. Coccidioidomycosis. Washington, DC; National Foundation Infectious Diseases, 1985:170–180.

67. Ample NM, Bejarano GC, Galgiani JN. Killing of Coccidioides immitis by human peripheral blood mononuclear cells. Infect Immun 1992;60:4200–4204.

68. Brummer E, Hanson LH, Restrepo A, Stevens DA. Intracellular multiplication of Paracoccidioides brasiliensis in macrophages: killing and restriction of multiplication by activated macrophages. Infect Immun 1989;57:2289–2294.

69. Brummer E, Hanson LH, Stevens DA. Gamma-interferon activation of macrophages for killing of Paracoccidioides brasiliensis and evidence for nonoxidative mechanisms. Int J Immunopharmacol 1988;10:945–952.

70. Brummer E, Sun SH, Harrison JL, Perlman AM, Stevens DA. Ultrastructure of phagocytosed Paracoccidioides brasiliensis in nonactivated or activated macrophages. Infect Immun 1990;58:2628–2636.

CHAPTER **30**

CYTOKINES AND MALARIA: FOR BETTER OR FOR WORSE

Georges E. Grau and Charlotte Behr

ROLE OF THE IMMUNE STATUS IN EXPRESSION OF MALARIAL PATHOLOGY

Infection with malaria parasites in humans can lead to a wide variety of symptoms, ranging from headaches and mild fever reminiscent of an influenza infection to an extremely severe life-threatening illness. These complications most often include multiorgan failure, even if they seem to be more or less specific for one organ (i.e., renal insufficiency, pulmonary edema, or cerebral malaria [CM]).

Expression of malarial pathology is highly dependent of the host's immune status. Major complications, including CM and severe anemia, appear to be associated with a "*Plasmodium*-naïve immune system," because people at risk for development of severe malaria complications are individuals who contract the disease for the first time, or who have been only slightly exposed to the parasite. This phenomenon is illustrated by the following observations.

The higher frequency of CM in children (most frequently, 1–5 y old) versus adults in endemic areas and the decrease in CM prevalence with age is paralleled by the development of immunity. Epidemiological analyses of humoral immune responses to malaria in Thailand indicate that patients in whom CM develops are less immune than those with acute uncomplicated malaria (1). Thai patients in whom CM develops were mainly adults, rather than children as in Africa, and 65% of patients with CM were not native of endemic provinces, but were immigrants from other parts of Thailand where malaria is not endemic.

CM frequency is also higher in travelers than in people living in endemic areas. Population movements (e.g., Ghana, Papua New Guinea, highlanders moving to the coast, Javan immigrants to West Iran, resettlement of Ethiopian highlanders [2]) are associated with more severe infections.

Decreased cell-mediated immune responses appear to be associated with a reduced prevalence of CM and other complications. For instance, children with severe malnutrition have a lower incidence of CM (3,4). Indeed, various aspects of cell-mediated immunity dysfunctions have been reported in relation with malnutrition (5).

These indirect arguments suggest a role for hyperreactivity of the immune system in the development of malarial complications. Also, in holoendemic areas, a decrease in the intensity and the duration of symptoms with age can be observed, and asymptomatic infections are frequently noted. This absence of symptoms in the presence of a low parasitemia corresponds to the acquisition of a peculiar immunological status called premunition (6). This premunition status is acquired step by step. Initially, protection against clinical manifestations and severe disease is acquired. This first step, corresponding to acquisition of so called clinical immunity, has little effect on the level of parasitemia. Subsequently, resistance to asymptomatic parasitemia develops, but intermittent low-grade parasitemia persists throughout adult life. This second step reflects the "antiparasite immunity" responsible for control of the parasitemia at a low level (7–9). Cytokines, and particularly tumor necrosis factor (TNF), appear to have a critical role in the fine balance between host tissue damage (pathology) and destruction of the parasite (protection). Indeed, they are at the interface between the parasite and the immunocompetent cells (i.e., lymphocytes, natural killer cells, mononuclear phagocytes, endothelial cells), and they modulate the complex interactions between specific and nonspecific immune responses, for better but also for worst.

DUAL EFFECTS OF CYTOKINES IN MALARIA: PATHOLOGY VERSUS PROTECTION

Pathology

IDENTIFICATION OF AN ENDOGENOUS MEDIATOR, TUMOR NECROSIS FACTOR, AS A KEY ELEMENT IN THE PATHOGENESIS OF EXPERIMENTAL CEREBRAL MALARIA: The pathogenesis of CM has been the object of considerable interest, and it remains incompletely understood, although several hypotheses have been proposed (10). The essential pathological feature of severe *Plasmodium falciparum* malaria is sequestration of erythrocytes containing mature forms of the parasite in deep vascular beds. Sequestration is greatest in the brain (11), which may explain why coma is such a prominent feature. This condition is invariably fatal if untreated, and it remains associated with a considerable mortality, even in treated patients. The current opinion is that a combination of host- and parasite dependent–factors contribute not only to the particular pathology of all acute *P. falciparum* attacks, but also to the degree of cerebral involvement.

It is obvious that animal models of malaria do not exactly reproduce the human diseases. However, the parallels that exist between defined antigens of human and rodent parasites, as well as between immunopathogenic pathways in humans and in mouse, may justify the use of such models to orientate further investigations in humans. Although none of the rodent malaria species can be labeled as *P. falciparum*–like by parasitological, morphological, or molecular criteria, infection of mice by *P. berghei* ANKA (PbA) (originally characterized by Josef M. Bafort in Katanga) exhibits important properties of human CM, such as signs of nervous system dysfunction and neurovascular changes. The experimental model for

CM is induced by infection with PbA asexual blood stages in genetically susceptible CBA/Ca mice (12). It consists of a neurologic syndrome occurring 6 to 14 days after infection, and leading to a cumulative mortality of about 90%. Parasitemia at the time of death is consistently low. The neurological manifestations include paralysis (mono-, hemi-, para- or tetraplegia), deviation of the head, tendency to "roll over" after skin stimulation, ataxia and convulsions. The remaining 10% of infected CM-susceptible mice eventually die during the third or fourth week of infection with severe anemia and hyperparasitemia, but without neurologic signs.

This model, akin to human CM, is characterized by petechial hemorrhages that can be evident on macroscopical examination; they are seen in the meninges, the white matter of the cerebrum, the brain stem, and the cerebellum. On histological sections in human CM, "ring hemorrhages" are a key feature. They surround medium size vessels, venules, and even arterioles. The vessel wall is necrotic and the content of the lumen is packed mostly with parasitized red blood cells; leukocytes and fibrin are also occasionally observed. In the mouse model, sequestration of parasitized red blood cells is consistently absent, and the hemorrhages, apparently due to rupture of venules, are constantly associated with a sequestration of leukocytes. The only major differences between human and experimental CM are (1) the absence of knobs on mouse parasitized red blood cells and (2) the nature of cells that are sequestered in brain vessels. Indeed, in malaria-infected mice, the focal arrest of leukocytes, monocytes/macrophages and lymphocytes, in brain vessels is the dominant picture. However, such vascular plugging by mononuclear cells is also seen in lungs from patients with severe falciparum malaria (13) and leukocyte sequestration can also occur in brain vessels during human CM (14–16) (Das et al., personal communication).

The observation that numerous macrophages are present in lymphoid organs and at the site of neurovascular lesions in malaria-infected mice, the fact that TNF is a mediator of acute inflammation, as well as the powerful effects of TNF on endothelial cells led us to explore the role of this molecule in CM. TNF is a hormone with a wide range of biological activities produced principally by activated macrophages (17). Experimental work on rodent malaria over the last few years points to a major role of TNF in CM (Table 30-1).

CYTOKINES AND SEVERE MALARIA: CORRELATION BETWEEN DISEASE SEVERITY AND SERUM TNF IN HUMAN CEREBRAL MALARIA: To evaluate the possible relevance of our findings in the experimental model for CM, we analyzed blood TNF levels in well-characterized Malawian patients. TNF concentrations were measured in serum and in the cerebrospinal fluid (CSF) of children presenting with asexual *P.*

TABLE 30-1   ARGUMENTS FOR A ROLE OF TNF IN EXPERIMENTAL AND HUMAN CEREBRAL MALARIA

Murine CM	Human CM
Serum TNF level and brain TNF mRNA is higher in mice with CM than in malaria-infected mice without neurological complications.	Direct correlation between serum TNF levels and various criteria of disease severity (i.e., hypoglycemia, coma score, sequelae, >4 risk factors) in patients with CM.
TNF administration to PbA-infected, CM-resistant mice triggers the development of CM and acute mortality.	Prognosis related to serum TNF levels on admission.
Immunohistochemical evidence for TNF production in monocytes sequestering in brain vessels of mice succumbing to CM.	Immunohistochemical evidence for TNF production in monocytes sequestering in brain vessels of patients succumbing to CM.
In vivo treatment of malaria-infected mice with polyclonal or monoclonal anti-TNF antibodies prevents CM.	Clinical trial: does murine anti-human TNF monoclonal antibody reduce CM-induced mortality and morbidity?

CM = cerebral malaria; TNF = tumor necrosis factor; PbA = *Plasmodium berghei* ANKA.

falciparum parasitemia during the acute stage of the illness and 1 month later in survivors. The results were then analyzed in relation to the clinical course and the outcome of the illness, as well as to known indicators of severity of *P. falciparum* malaria in children, with particular attention to hypoglycemia (18). Serum concentrations of TNF were elevated in many children with severe *P. falciparum* infection, but they were within normal range 1 month after discharge from hospital in the same patients. A significant correlation existed between the serum TNF level on admission and the severity of the illness: The mean concentrations of TNF were higher on admission in patients who died than in the survivors, as well as in those with four or more *P. falciparum* malaria risk factors than in those patients possessing fewer than four risk factors

(18). The risk factors known to be associated with an adverse outcome include hypoglycemia, a coma score of 0, signs of decerebration or decortication, age less than 3 years, witnessed convulsions, hyperparasitemia, leukocytosis, and an absence of corneal reflexes. Furthermore, the development of sequelae was associated with high TNF levels. Of the eight risk factors identified, three correlated with serum TNF concentrations: hypoglycemia, hyperparasitemia, and age less than 3 years. The highest TNF concentrations were seen in hypoglycemic patients who died shortly after the blood samples had been obtained.

The relation between serum TNF level on admission and outcome was analyzed. Whereas patients with admitting levels under 100 pg/mL had a mortality of less than 5%, mortality increased with serum TNF level, and the 2 patients with serum levels above 1,500 pg/mL died. TNF concentrations in the CSF during the acute neurological phase were found to be slightly but not significantly elevated. However, the highest CSF TNF level was seen in the only lethal case among those studied for CSF.

Thus, TNF may be an important component in the pathogenesis of severe *P. falciparum* malaria, and in particular in the cerebral syndrome and the hypoglycemia that can complicate this disease (18). This association between high serum levels and the severity of *P. falciparum* infection was confirmed in several other studies: It was found that plasma TNF concentrations were higher in Zairian children with *P. falciparum* infection than in 26 severely ill, aparasitemic children (19). Among all parasitemic children, TNF levels increased with increasing levels of parasitemia. On univariate analysis, elevated TNF levels were associated with hyperparasitemia, severe anemia, hypoglycemia, and young age, but not with CM, human immunodeficiency virus type I (HIV-1) seropositivity, or fatal outcome. In this series, however, the mortality rate was low (7%). TNF levels were elevated equally in children with CM and in those with other signs of severe malaria. With multiple linear regression, TNF levels were found to be elevated independently in children with hyperparasitemia and severe anemia. From this study, we concluded that high TNF levels are associated with several manifestations of severe *P. falciparum* malaria, perhaps not specific to CM (19). The close relationship between high blood TNF levels and severity of CM was also reported in European adults (20), in patients from The Gambia (21), and in patients from the Solomon Islands (22).

In a study involving 133 Malawian children with CM, the time-course of plasma TNF concentration and other proinflammatory cytokines closely related to TNF, such as interferon-γ (IFN-γ), interleukin-1 (IL-1), and (IL-6) were examined. IL-1 and IFN-γ were found elevated, but they were not correlated with fever, degree of parasitemia, severity of the disease, and other cytokines. In contrast, plasma IL-6 levels strongly correlate with TNF levels at admission, but they also show comparable kinetics during follow-up, suggesting coordinate production of the two cytokines (23). The same types of results were also found by other investigators (20,21). However, several pieces of evidence indicate that IL-6 might not be directly involved in the pathogenesis of CM. In particular, high IL-6 levels have been also found in uncomplicated malaria (20,23).

In the serum of people suffering an acute malaria attack, without necessarily an association with pathology, several other cytokines can be detected. A recent study has systematically investigated cytokines (amount and kinetics) in human experimental malaria as part of a vaccination experiment (24). These authors detected high levels of IFN-γ in all patients and TNF-α only in those who presented the highest levels of parasitemia. These cytokines were not detectable in the sera of individuals who received the vaccine only. In this particular study, no significant levels of granulocyte-macrophage colony-stimulating factor (GM-CSF), IL-1, or IL-2 were detected. Maybe their results differ slightly from other studies because the patients were treated very early; in these other studies, in addition to IFN-γ (25,26), TNF-α (27), and IL-6, GM-CSF were detectable (28,29). TNF-β was described in the serum of uncomplicated malaria from patients living in an holoendemic area (27), although this cytokine was not detectable in serum of patients with CM (Grau et al., unpublished observations). To our knowledge, this is the first report of raised TNF-β serum levels in a systemic disease. Animal studies by the same authors imply that TNF-β may contribute to the hypoglycemia and to increased serum IL-6 levels observed in malaria. These findings confirm that major T-cell activation takes place during acute malaria.

In addition to P. falciparum infection, P. vivax malaria also gives rise to marked increase in serum TNF levels closely paralleled to the temperature curve, without any cerebral involvement or correlation with lethal outcome (30). The reasons for this phenomenon have been discussed elsewhere (31).

INTERVENTION STUDY: RESPONSE TO MONOCLONAL ANTIHUMAN TNF ANTIBODY IN CHILDREN WITH CM: Because several studies confirmed the observations that circulating TNF levels are significantly higher in CM than in uncomplicated P. falciparum infection, the possibility was raised that therapeutic inhibition of TNF might attenuate some of these pathological processes. A preliminary investigation of murine monoclonal anti-TNF antibody in the treatment of Gambian children with a severe form of CM was undertaken. With conventional therapy, CM is still associated with a fatality rate of approximately 35%. Available data indicate that the anti-TNF monoclonal antibody (mAb) (BC-7), when given in addition to conventional antima-

larial therapy, caused a dose-dependent reduction in fever compared with control subjects (32). Administration of anti-TNF in the context of acute malaria appears to be safe, as indicated by the absence of toxicity and the absence of interference with parasite clearance. Using BC-7, there was a promising trend concerning mortality (which was reduced by almost 50%) and neurological sequelae (which did not appear in treated children). The actual efficacy will be investigated in a large scale study. This observation consolidates the evidence that TNF is involved in the pathogenesis of malaria fever, and it provides the first clear demonstration that specific inhibition of TNF can attenuate the clinical features of infectious disease in humans.

Protective role of cytokines in malaria

If overproduction of cytokines, more precisely of TNF, is a key point in the immunopathology of severe malaria, there are also many experimental data coming from animal models or in vitro culture experiments that demonstrate a potentially protective role for cytokines. This protective effect has been shown to be exerted on pre-erythrocytic, erythrocytic, and sexual stages of malaria parasites.

PARASITICIDAL AND PARASITOSTATIC EFFECTS OF CYTOKINES ON PLASMODIUM PRE-ERYTHROCYTIC AND ERYTHROCYTIC ASEXUAL STAGES: IFN-γ: A protective role of IFN was first suggested against pre-erythrocytic stages. Several IFN inducers protect mice against P. berghei infection. This protection is far greater against sporozoite-induced infections than against blood form-induced infection (33). Administration of mouse or rat IFN-γ, a few hours before sporozoite challenge inhibits, in a dose-dependent manner, the development of exoerythrocytic forms in the liver of mice and rats infected with P. berghei sporozoites (33a), and administration of a neutralizing monoclonal anti-IFN-γ antibody to an immune host can abrogate protective immunity (34). These observations suggest that immunologically induced IFN-γ may be involved in controlling malaria infection under natural conditions.

The mechanisms of action of IFN-γ have been analyzed in vitro: IFN-γ impairs the intrahepatocytic development of P. berghei sporozoites in the human hepatoma cell line HepG2 (35). In the same way, prophylactic treatment with recombinant IFN-γ totally suppresses experimental infection by P. cynomolgi in rhesus monkeys (34). Concerning P. falciparum infection, recombinant IFN-γ inhibits the development of intrahepatic stages in fresh human hepatocytes (36). Moreover, in a prospective longitudinal study conducted in Madagascar, the presence of IFN-γ in the sera of enrolled individuals was correlated to resistance against infection (37). Thus, IFN-γ may inhibit the malaria exoerythrocytic stage in vivo as it does in vitro.

IFN-γ could also act on the erythrocytic stages. Injection of IFN-γ at low doses in P. *chabaudi-adami*–infected mice induced a decrease in the parasitemia (38), and it is toxic when added in vitro to infected erythrocytes (39). Moreover, injection of neutralizing anti-IFN-γ antibodies to P. *chabaudi*–infected mice at the time of parasitemia peak limited the decrease of the parasitemia, but it did not abrogate the ability to clear the parasites (i.e., acquisition of protective immunity) (40). In Aotus monkeys, recent vaccination experiments have shown a correlation between protection and serum IFN-γ levels (41). Directly, IFN-γ induced pyknotic nuclei in cultures of P. *falciparum,* thereby interfering with maturation of schizonts (42).

IL-2:   A direct antiparasite effect of recombinant IL-2, acting not only on the schizont maturation, but also on the segmented mature forms affecting the merozoite liberation, has been described (42).

IL-1-β AND IL-6:   Recombinant human or mouse IL-1-α also protects against the pre-erythrocytic stages of P. *falciparum* malaria (36). It has been postulated that the effect of IL-1 may be mediated in part by C-reactive protein (CRP), an acute-phase protein synthesized by IL-1–stimulated hepatocytes. Evidence for this effect has been obtained with both in vitro and in vivo models of P. *yoelii* infection (43). It has been demonstrated that hepatic IL-1 activity is mediated by secretion of IL-6 (44). Evidence has been obtained that the effect of IL-1 on the hepatic development of P. *falciparum* or P. *yoelii* sporozoites is in part mediated by IL-6, because anti-IL-6 monoclonal antibodies partially neutralize the effect of IL-1 (45).

Various types of experiments have been performed to analyze the mode of action of IL-6 (36). Low doses of IL-1-β injected in C57BL/6 mice infected by P. *berghei* are able to decrease the parasitemia and to also protect the mice against CM, even if these two effects seem not to be linked (46). IL-6 can exert its antimalarial activity by multiple mechanisms. Two mechanisms have been particularly investigated: induction of an oxidative burst and induction of the L-arginine–dependent cytotoxic effector mechanisms (LADEM) (36,47,48).

TNF-α AND TNF-β: If elevated concentrations of TNF can present deleterious effects on patients with acute malaria, as discussed, lower levels of TNF can have beneficial effects. Early experiments suggesting an antiparasite effect mediated by TNF came from the groups of Clark (49) and Taverne (50). They showed that sera from bacillus Calmette-Guerin (BCG)–infected mice 2 hours after injection of lipopolysaccharide (LPS) had a parasiticidal effect on the blood stages of the parasites (i.e., the erythro-

cytic phase of the disease) in vitro and in vivo. Haidaris and colleagues (51) confirmed this effect on P. *falciparum* in vitro cultures. Low doses of TNF-α injected to P. *chabaudi*– as well as P. *yoelii*-infected mice induced a decrease in the parasitemia, without any detectable symptoms and crisis forms (38,40,52). Similarly, TNF infusion before it induces cerebral signs and acute death in CM-resistant mice suppresses the increase in parasitemia in PbA-infected mice (53). More recently, TNF-β was shown able to induce impressive inhibition of H³-glutamine uptake as well as hypoxanthine uptake in a dose-dependent manner (42).

However, beneficial effect of TNF during malaria is not restricted to the erythrocytic stages, because major effects of cytokines are manifested in hepatic and sexual stages of the disease. In experiments using fresh hepatocytes, TNF was not found to have an antiparasite effect at the hepatocyte level, regardless of dose, schedule of administration, and mouse strain used (54). However, it was found that the presence of nonparenchymal cells (NPCs) is a crucial element in the effect of TNF. Addition of NPC to hepatocytes indeed restored the capacity of TNF to modulate parasite hepatic stage development in vitro. In these coculture assays, NPCs essentially consist of pit cells (large granular lymphocytes or natural killer cells), Kupffer cells, T cells, endothelial cells, epithelial cells, fibroblasts, and Ito cells. Some of these cells are known to produce one or several of the following cytokines: IL-1, IFN-γ, and IL-6 (55,56). Supernatants of these cocultures were found to contain markedly elevated IL-6 concentrations after addition of TNF, whereas IL-1 and IFN-γ levels remained undetectable. To confirm that IL-6 is involved in TNF-induced parasite inhibition, anti-IL-6 mAb was added to monocultures and cocultures of hepatocytes. Anti-IL-6 mAb dramatically decreased the TNF-induced inhibition when added 24 hours before sporozoite inoculation (57). These results strongly suggest that IL-6 is a crucial mediator of the observed TNF effect.

Various cytokines, particularly IFN-γ, TNF, and IL-6, whose production is increased during blood-stage malaria (20,25,58–60), might thus modulate the pre-erythrocytic stage of infection. These data further illustrate the interdependence of different stages of development of malaria parasites (54). This dual role of TNF in malaria has to be kept in mind when intervention studies with TNF antagonists are considered.

EFFECT OF TNF AND IFN-γ ON LOSS OF INFECTIVITY OF GAMETOCYTES TO THE MOSQUITOES:

The relationship between cytokine release and the gametocyte infectivity had not been studied until recently. Particular attention was paid to the period of transient loss of infectivity of the parasite to the mosquitoes. Infectivity of malarial infections to mosquitoes is due to the presence of circulating gametocytes, the sexual stages that fertilize in the midgut of a blood-fed mosquito. In several malaria host–parasite systems, it has been noted that peaks of parasitemia are associated with "crisis," characterized by the appearance of morphologically abnormal intraerythrocytic parasites. This peculiar event is synchronous with reduction or loss of infectivity of the parasite to the mosquito, which persists for 4 to 6 days. Neither of these phenomena has been explained.

In the model of *P. cynomolgi* infection in its natural host, the toque monkey, *Macaca sinica,* it has recently been shown that loss of infectivity at crisis is due to death of circulating intraerythrocytic gametocytes mediated by crisis serum (61). In addition, this killing effect in the crisis serum is due to the presence of both TNF and IFN-γ. Indeed, simultaneous addition of rabbit anti-human TNF and anti-human IFN-γ immunoglobulins completely reversed the killing effect of the crisis serum observed in vitro. In contrast, addition of antibodies to either cytokine alone or normal rabbit immunoglobulins had no effect. Conversely, the effects of recombinant human TNF-α and IFN-γ on the viability of healthy infectious gametocytes of *P. cynomolgi* in vitro were tested: Neither cytokine individually nor a combination of both cytokines affected the infectivity of the gametocytes to mosquitoes. However, when either cytokine was added to crisis serum previously depleted of TNF and IFN-γ, the killing effect of the crisis serum was totally restored. These results indicate that TNF and IFN-γ each mediate gametocyte killing independently of the other, but they demonstrate that each cytokine requires the presence of an unknown factor in the crisis serum to mediate this effect.

More recently, additional evidence for a role of TNF in gametocyte killing has been obtained. When studying *P. vivax*–infected subjects, it was found that soon after a paroxysm (i.e., an episode of fever with chills and rigors that coincides with the rupture of erythrocytic schizonts), the serum of malaria non-immune patients mediated killing of parasites (asexual erythrocytic stages and gametocytes). These sera, taken 1 hour after paroxysm, contained elevated TNF concentrations. This in vitro killing effect of human paroxysm sera was completely abrogated by addition of anti-TNF antibodies, and it was restored by addition of recombinant human TNF. When added to normal serum, however, recombinant TNF had no parasite killing effects, indicating, as we had found for monkey crisis serum, that complementary factors present in paroxysm serum, but not in normal serum, were necessary for TNF to kill blood-stage parasites (61). The elevated serum TNF levels and gametocyte killing effects of human serum taken 1 hour after paroxysm are transient. Four hours following a paroxysm, serum TNF levels were decreased in most patients, and the loss of killing effect was dramatic in all patients. Even when recombinant TNF is added to serum taken 4 hours after a paroxysm, it fails to kill gametocytes, thus demonstrating the very

transient presence of complementary factors needed for cytokine-mediated killing of blood-stage parasites (62).

The direct effect of cytokines such as TNF-β and IFN-γ on infected red blood cells observed by Orago and Facer (63) is controversial, and some authors have failed to show any direct antiparasitic effect (42,64,65). The explanation could be that the former study incubated the parasite with cytokines for 48 hours, whereas the latter authors reported a 20-hour incubation period. The precise mechanism of action of these cytokines under these experimental conditions remains unclear. Thus far, nobody has been able to detect any receptor for these cytokines on the surface of the infected red blood cells. However, it is conceivable that some infected erythrocyte surface molecules act as cytokine receptors, as was recently shown for the receptor for *P. vivax* (the Duffy blood group antigen), which is a chemokine (IL-8) receptor (66). An alternative hypothesis would be that cytokines have access to the parasite through a channel. The possible existence of such a channel, a parasitophorous duct, is controversial (67,68).

Concerning the in vivo effect of cytokines on parasitemia, it can be explained by an indirect action of these cytokines. The cytokines would probably induce production of oxygen radicals or nitric oxide (both toxic for the parasite) by some phagocytic mononuclear cells, or neutrophils and even endothelial cells (39,47,69,70). It has been notably shown that IFN-γ, TNF-α, and, to a lesser extent, TNF-β can stimulate neutrophils to phagocytose intraerythrocytic parasites. Other serum factors might also participate, such as some lipid peroxidation products (71) or other unknown factors (61,62).

AMONG THE EFFECTOR MECHANISMS INVOLVED IN HUMAN NATURAL IMMUNITY, WHICH PART IS DUE TO CYTOKINES?

Most of the evidence for the protective role of cytokines is mainly based on experimental models or in vitro experiments. Thus, we still do not know clearly what part is due to cytokines in protective effector mechanisms in human natural acquired immunity. In human malaria, in vivo passive transfer experiments have clearly shown that antibodies have a major role in natural protective immunity. Information from experimental animal models and from in vitro experiments involving human cells indicates that antibodies either act directly by blocking invasion of host cells (hepatocytes or erythrocytes) by the parasites (72–74) or by cooperating with monocytic/macrophagic cells or neutrophils for destruction of the parasite. Several mechanisms have been proposed, such as antibody-dependent cellular cytotoxicity (ADCC), antibody-dependent cellular inhibition (ADCI), opsonization, and phagocytosis (70,75–77). Via some of these mechanisms, antibodies could contribute to long-term control of the parasitemia in immune individuals. Nevertheless, in nonimmune individuals without such protective antibodies, parasitemia levels usually remain low, and only very infrequently do they reach the high levels that can be obtained with virulent strains in some experimental models. Moreover, parasitic "crisis forms" (consisting of degenerative forms of intraerythrocytic malarial parasites and thought to reflect a parasiticidal or parasitostatic activity) have been observed in the blood of nonimmune individuals during the acute phase of infection (78).

The discrepancy between such an ability to control parasitemia and the absence of significant antibody levels might be explained by production of other mediators of the immune response, namely cytokines. As we pointed out earlier, several of the cytokines demonstrating an antiparasitic effect in different experimental systems are detectable in the sera during the malaria acute phase; they therefore could possibly be involved in short-term regulation of the parasitemia (by a direct or an indirect effect on the parasite). However, these cytokines are not detectable in the sera of immune individuals from holoendemic areas harboring low amounts of parasitemia in the absence of symptoms. Due to evident ethical reasons, no information is available about the presence of these cytokines in a particular microenvironment, such as spleen or deep capillaries, where malaria parasites are sequestered, as well as on their possible involvement in long-term control of parasitemia.

REGULATION OF CYTOKINE PRODUCTION

There is now considerable evidence that cytokines participate in both antiparasite protection and parasite-induced pathology, not only in malaria but also in other infectious diseases (79). Cytokines are pleiotropic mediators that can be produced by hematopoietic immunocompetent cells, notably by monocytes/macrophages or T cells, but also by other non-hematopoietic cells such as endothelial cells. These cytokines can be secreted locally or systemically. The outcome of the host-parasite relationship will depend on the nature, kinetics, amount, and sites of production of the cytokines directly or indirectly induced by the parasite.

In human malaria, very little is known concerning the biological events leading to overproduction of cytokines related to severe disease, or about the regulation of production of cytokines that take place during the acquisition of premunition. Understanding of induction of these cytokine productions, as well as in the regulatory phases of the immune response, is an indispensable task to prevent the development of severe malaria. Animal model experiments are irreplaceable for dissecting the immune responses and to help suggest new issues that can be ad-

dressed through human immunoepidemiological studies. For instance, the role of T cells in the pathological events observed in CM or in protective responses has been suggested by studies of experimental murine malaria.

Requirement for T cells in experimental malaria pathology

ESSENTIAL ROLE OF CD4+ T CELLS: The role of T lymphocytes in antimalarial responses has long been recognized, and their involvement in pathology has been suggested by observations that athymic nude mice do not develop CM after infection with PbA (80). Three lines of evidence indicate that helper T lymphocytes have a significant role in the development of murine cerebral malaria (12).

First, in vivo depletion in CD4+ helper/inducer T cells by treatment of *P. berghei*–infected mice with anti-CD4 mAb completely abrogated the occurrence of cerebral malaria, with no modification of the course of infection. Second, thymectomized CBA mice lethally irradiated and reconstituted with T-cell–depleted bone marrow cells (ATxBM mice) are resistant to the development of neurological lesions. Reconstitution of ATxBM CBA mice with CD4+ T cells from normal mice renders these reconstituted mice fully susceptible to the development of neurological complications after infection with *P. berghei*. In contrast, ATxBM mice reconstituted with the CD8+ (Ly.2+) T-cell subset do not die acutely with neurological signs, but they later develop severe anemia and overwhelming parasitemia. Third, earlier mortality with CM is observed after transfer of CD4+/CD8– T cells obtained from mice with cerebral malaria into infected euthymic mice. Another element suggesting the role of T lymphocytes in CM is prevention of the syndrome by low doses of cyclosporine (i.e., doses that are unable to interfere with parasite growth) (81).

MECHANISMS OF TNF OVERPRODUCTION: ROLE OF T-CELL–DERIVED CYTOKINES: To explore the part of the T-cell response in TNF overproduction, selective in vivo blockade of IL-3, GM-CSF, and IFN-γ was investigated in the experimental CM model. Combined treatment with anti-rIL-3 and anti-rGM-CSF antibodies dramatically prevented the development of the neurological syndrome. TNF was not detectable in the serum of mice treated with both antibodies, and it protected against CM. Microscopic examination of brain tissues on day 7 of infection showed that this combined treatment totally prevented intravascular accumulation of mononuclear cells, which is characteristic of mouse CM. Accumulation of macrophages in lymphoid organs, such as spleen red pulp and lymph nodes, which is consistently observed in mice developing CM, was significantly reduced after treatment with both anti-IL-3 and anti-rGM-CSF antibodies (82). As a consequence of CM prevention, the survival of mice receiving the dual treatment with anti-IL-3 and GM-CSF was significantly prolonged: these mice died around the third week of infection, with severe anemia and overwhelming parasitemia, but without CM.

Involvement of IFN-γ in CM is supported by experiments showing that CM and its TNF overproduction can be prevented by treatment of *P. berghei*–infected mice with either polyclonal or monoclonal anti-IFN-γ antibodies (83). Again, this protective effect was seen in the absence of any effect of the anticytokine antibody on the course of parasitemia. In contrast to what is seen with anti-IL-3 and anti-GM-CSF antibodies, anti-IFN-γ antibody treatment did not affect macrophage accumulation within lymphoid organs.

Thus, to explain production of TNF in vivo in CM, one may hypothesize the following. The requirement of CD4+ T cells for CM to develop involves release of at least IL-3 or GM-CSF and IFN-γ, because neutralization of these cytokines prevents markedly elevated blood TNF levels that lead to cerebral vascular lesions. IL-3 and GM-CSF act together by enlarging the pool of mononuclear phagocytes, which is manifested by accumulation of these cells in lymphoid organs. In contrast, IFN-γ is responsible for their activation, thus further stimulating synthesis and release of excessive amounts of TNF. A synergy between IFN-γ and TNF, particularly with respect to effects on endothelial cells, can also be envisaged. IFN-γ is known to up-regulate TNF receptors (84). In addition, TNF has an up-regulating effect on its own synthesis (85), as well as on the increase in TNF mRNA level triggered by IFN-γ (86). At some critical point, this cytokine cascade leads to rapid autoamplification of TNF overproduction that ends in the cerebral vascular lesions of CM.

ANALYSIS OF CYTOKINE GENE EXPRESSION DURING CM: RELATIONSHIP BETWEEN CYTOKINE PRODUCTION IN VITRO AND GENETIC SUSCEPTIBILITY TO CM: There has been a considerable interest in measuring the profile of cytokine production in various infectious disease models, because these profiles were used to define the relative expansion of functionally distinct T-cell subsets (the so called Th1 and TH2 subsets) and their involvement in protection versus pathology. In the murine model of leishmaniasis, for example, it had been suggested that susceptibility to lesions was associated with a predominant Th2 response, whereas resistant strains of mice displayed a Th1 response (87).

The general experimental approach has been to infect mice of the CM-susceptible (CM-S) strain, CBA, and the CM-resistant (CM-R) strain, BALB/c, to isolate spleen or lymph node cells (LNCs) on day 7 of infection with

PbA and to compare their behavior in in vitro restimulations by various stimulants (53). LNCs taken at day 7 of PbA infection in CBA mice proliferated significantly more in response to crude (frozen and thawed) PbA antigen than those of BALB/c mice. There was no PbA-specific proliferation in LNC from uninfected mice from either strain.

We compared production of IFN-γ by these cells. The role of IFN-γ in T-cell–dependent TNF overproduction during CM was indicated by our previous observation that in vivo treatment with anti-IFN-γ mAb was able to protect PbA-infected mice from CM and to prevent the associated TNF overproduction. We found that after restimulation in vitro, LNC from CM-S mice produced dramatically more IFN-γ than those from CM-R mice, in an antigen-specific and a dose-dependent manner. In contrast, lymphoid cells from CM-R mice appear to produce IL-2 and IL-4 in the presence of PbA antigens, whereas cells from CM-S mice do not. These data suggest that the triggering of CM might be a Th1-dependent pathological reaction.

Also, more recently, using Northern blot analysis, we were able to show that TNF mRNA accumulation was significantly higher in mice with CM than in PbA-infected mice, without the cerebral complication (88).

Sources and regulation of cytokines in human malaria

TNF-α–INDUCING *PLASMODIUM* ANTIGENS: TNF, and to a lesser extent IFN-γ, are key cytokines for both pathology and protection in malaria. Thus, characterization and purification of parasite products implicated in the release of such cytokines represent an active area of investigation. It has been shown that malarial products released after schizont rupture and during the reinvasion process can directly stimulate monocytic cells from non-immune individuals to secrete TNF-α, in a manner similar to bacterial endotoxin (LPS) (69,89–93). Furthermore, soluble molecules released by malaria parasites appear to be major TNF-α inducers (90,91,94,95). These soluble antigens from rodent plasmodia are heat-stable molecules, distinguishable from LPS, that trigger TNF release in vitro and in vivo and that can kill D-galactosamine–sensitized mice. Supernatants from cultures of *P. falciparum* contain similar soluble molecules that induce TNF release from both human and mouse macrophages. Crude preparations of these soluble antigens induce T-cell–independent antibodies that specifically block their ability, but not that of endotoxin, to trigger TNF-α secretion (96). Moreover, antisera raised against these so called exoantigens from rodent parasites *P. yoelii* are able to inhibit the ability of exoantigens from *P. falciparum* and *P. vivax*, suggesting communities between the biochemical components implicated in the release of TNF (97).

To characterize further the nature of such parasitic products, enzymatic treatments were undertaken. This TNF-α–inducing activity appeared resistant to proteases and glycosydases but sensitive to the treatment of phospholipase C. Moreover, the activity is specifically inhibited by inositol-1-monophosphate, or phosphatidyl-inositol (93). These results suggest that product activity will depend on an inositolphospholipid structure (89). Recent results suggested that the glycophosphatidyl inositol anchors plasmodial proteins, such as the two major merozoite surface antigens (MSA-1 and MSA-2) (93). These data have led to the interesting concept of antidisease vaccine based on the vaccination by such TNF-α–inducing toxins (98). How such a vaccine could affect the ability of individuals to control the parasitemia remains unanswered.

Although TNF-α–inducing moieties of plasmodial antigens may induce T-cell–independent antibodies, the possibility that such biochemical structures may also activate T cells has not been investigated. In such a context, the MSA-1, MSA-2 molecules, known to contain T-cell epitopes, deserve to be studied in detail. Indeed, the level of T-cell reactivity can profoundly affect the balance between pathology and parasitemia control. In this perspective, the antibody and T-cell reactivity of certain soluble exoantigens, such as the antigenic complex 7 (Ag 7), have been studied in endemic areas. This antigenic complex is known to induce TNF-α when added to monocytes (99,100), and its activity is inhibited by antisera raised against *P. yoelii* exoantigens. It was shown that rural Gambian children acquire antibodies against Ag 7 by approximately 5 to 11 years of age, the period corresponding to acquisition of premunition (i.e., tolerance to significant parasitemia without fever). Concerning the T-cell response, children whose cells produced significant levels of IFN-γ after in vitro restimulation with Ag 7 were more likely to experience clinical manifestations of malaria infection than children whose cells did not produce IFN-γ. Such an Ag 7–induced IFN-γ may exacerbate the LPS-like activity (101).

POLYCLONAL ACTIVATION OF T CELLS (α/β AND γ/δ) DURING FIRST CONTACT WITH THE ERYTHROCYTIC PARASITE STAGE:

Malaria infection is associated with substantial modifications of immunocompetent blood cell populations. Peripheral T-cell numbers are reduced in acute uncomplicated *P. falciparum* malaria (102–104). This T-cell depletion seems very transient because it lasts less than 48 hours (105), and it essentially reflects reallocation of antigen-activated T cells (i.e., cells that have at least a high surface expression for LFA-1) (106). However, immune responsiveness may be profoundly different between individuals who ex-

perience their first malaria attack and those who live in endemic areas. Indeed, activated T-cell numbers (CD3+ HLA-DR+) were found to be lower in malaria-experienced subjects than in Caucasian individuals suffering from their first malaria attack. Likewise, individuals suffering from primary attack showed increased percentages and absolute numbers of T cells bearing γ/δ T-cell receptor in the circulating blood. These T cells are activated, and they express the IL-2 receptor as well as the HLA-DR molecule (107–109). This increase of the γ/δ T-cell population was not observed in individuals from endemic areas suffering from acute malaria (109). In one case of fatal malaria, 40% of γ/δ T cells among CD3+ T cells were found in the red pulp of spleen (110).

In addition to this transient reallocation from the blood to the tissues, a number of parameters give evidence for massive T-cell stimulation: the relative increased blood number of γ/δ T cells; the presence of markers, such as soluble IL-2R or soluble CD8 (which has been detected in malarial serum) (111–113), as well as elevated serum levels of various T-cell–derived cytokines, such as IFN-γ, TNF-β, or GM-CSF. This massive stimulation, together with retention of some T-lymphocyte subsets occurring in deep organs, is a phenomenon previously observed in *P. chabaudi*–infected mice (64,114,115). Such a phenomenon is likely to be more pronounced in individuals with fewer malaria experiences.

The T-cell activation level, the phenotype of activated T cells, as well as the pattern of secreted cytokines can be assessed by in vitro stimulation of peripheral T cells by the whole parasite. These assays have shown that T cells recovered from individuals without any exposure to malaria, compared with T cells of *P. falciparum*–exposed donors, were paradoxically more responsive to lysate of *P. falciparum* blood stages and were massively activated. This lysate selectively induced the outgrowth of a fraction of the T-cell repertoire (approximately 1%) composed of CD4+ α/β T cells and CD4–CD8–T cells expressing the Vγ9/Vδ2 association (116–118). The same association was observed in circulating T-cell populations during acute malaria infection. These T cells activated by this lysate respond in a major histocompatibility complex (MHC)–restricted manner; secrete numerous cytokines, including IFN-γ (119) and TNF-β (120) and can thereby activate monocytes or neutrophils, resulting in parasite destruction (65,121) and short-term control of parasitemia. Thus, T cells showing a cytokine pattern of type 1 could also participate in pathology (122). These results should be discussed in relation with previous observations of a higher capacity of malaria-specific IFN-γ production in nonimmune individuals than in immune subjects (123). Because it is known that nonimmune individuals, such as children in endemic areas or adult visitors from nonendemic areas, are particularly prone to severe complications, these data suggested that a "malaria virgin" immune system is associated with a higher susceptibility to development of malaria complications. These data are consistent with observations in the experimental model of CM, in which T cells from susceptible mice secrete higher level of IFN-γ when restimulated with *P. berghei* lysate than resistant mice.

INFLUENCE OF ENVIRONMENTAL CROSS-REACTING MALARIA ANTIGENS: POSSIBLE PATHOGENIC IMPORTANCE OF THE HOMING OF T CELLS WITH PARTICULAR SPECIFICITIES:

T cells from unexposed individuals that respond at a very high frequency to the blood-stage parasite antigens express the CD45RO phenotype (124). They could be the result of the stimulation by malarial crossreactive antigens with other organisms, as shown for some T-cell clones (125,126). Such crossreactive antigens have been referred to as environmental antigens (127,128). CD45RO+ T cells have different recirculation/distribution patterns, some of which depend on expression of addressins that enable them to home to different tissues. This homing could notably be affected by the site of the first stimulation (129). Thus, according to the attractive hypothesis proposed by Good and Currier (130), depending on T cells' fine specificity (i.e., malaria environmental crossreacting antigens or specific malaria antigens), on the site of stimulation, and on the type of antigen-presenting cell, these T cells could have dramatically different effects. Thus, despite having identical type 1 cytokine patterns, parasite-reactive T cells with different homing patterns could express either pathological or protective functions.

CYTOKINES AND T-CELL STATUS IN LONG-TERM CONTROL OF PARASITEMIA:

Contrasting with the transient effects of circulating cytokines during the acute phase of malaria, little is known about the role of these molecules in long-term control of the parasitemia. It is worth keeping in mind that "chronic malaria" corresponds to a continuous exposure to parasites, rather than persistence of parasites. Until recently, most field studies have only examined the proliferative activities of T cells in individuals living in endemic areas. Numerous recent studies have shown that T-cell proliferation correlates neither with secretion of IFN-γ nor specific serum antibodies (131–134). However, a correlation was found between the presence of IL-4 mRNA in the T cells and the presence of specific antibodies (131,135). In consideration of field constraints, epidemiological confounding factors, or inappropriate choice of antigen, there was no correlation between specific T-cell responses and malaria resistance (136). Studies examining the cytokine pattern in conditions of natural infection could provide insight into whether both Th1 and Th2 are implicated in long-

term control of parasitemia (137) or whether Th1 cytokine patterns would be found in nonimmune individuals, as suggested by Chizzolini and colleagues (123).

SUSCEPTIBILITY VERSUS RESISTANCE TO HUMAN SEVERE MALARIA: IS IT LINKED TO THE GENETICALLY CONTROLLED PRODUCTION CAPACITY OF TNF-α AND TNF-β?

It has recently been reported that the human leukocyte locus, HLABw53, is associated with resistance to severe anemia and CM (138). This preferential association of some HLA loci with resistance to the severe forms of the disease was interpreted by the authors as the result of a different ability of antigen-presenting cells to present some epitopes from the liver stage of malaria to cytotoxic T lymphocytes, which have an important role in providing immunity. In the view that severe malaria might be due to an inappropriate nature or an excessive host immune response leading to immunopathological damages, rather than to a defect of some protective effector mechanisms, another explanation has been proposed by Carter and colleagues (139). They propose that this special haplotype was selected for its reduced ability to induce immunopathological responses. In the PbA model, the outcome of the infection is directly influenced by the mouse strain (i.e., genetic background). Cerebral syndromes develop in some strains and not in others. Recently, murine resistance to development of toxoplasmic encephalitis was found to be correlated to the genetic polymorphism of the TNF-α locus (140). Thus, it is tantalizing to speculate that the preferential association between resistance to severe malaria and HLABw53 could be also related to a cosegregating locus that governs cytokine expression. This locus could map to microsatellite sequences upstream of the coding region for TNF-α and TNF-β, which are located on the same chromosome very close to the HLA locus.

CONSEQUENCES OF TNF OVERPRODUCTION: EFFECTOR MECHANISMS OF TNF-INDUCED TISSUE DAMAGE

TNF is able to induce the release of a large variety of cytokine and noncytokine mediators. To understand what events downstream of TNF could be important in the pathogenesis of severe malaria, the possible involvement of some of these mediators was evaluated in the *P. berghei* model: release of mediators such as IL-6 or nitric oxide, up-regulation of cell-adhesion molecules, as well as a peculiar interaction between endothelial cells and an unexpected effector cell, the platelet.

IL-6: role in hypergammaglobulinemia rather than in cerebral complications

IL-6 is a cytokine with pleiotropic effects on lymphocytes, hepatocytes, and hematopoietic progenitors (141). A variety of cell types can produce IL-6, including monocytes, T-cells, and endothelial cells, which are central to the lesion of CM (142). It has also been shown that synthesis and release of IL-6 can be induced by TNF. Therefore, the possible contribution of IL-6 to the pathogenesis of CM was analyzed. Serum IL-6 levels increased, regardless of the cerebral complications, following parasitemia. Mice treated with anti-TNF or anti-IFN-γ antibodies had no significant increase in serum IL-6 concentrations, whereas the combined treatment with anti-IL-3 and anti-GM-CSF antibodies, which is able to prevent the increase of TNF (82), did not significantly reduce IL-6 production in infected mice. Treatment of PbA-infected mice with anti-IL-6 mAb failed to prevent CM, but it significantly reduced malarial-induced hypergammaglobulinemia (60).

Regarding the origin of IL-6 during malaria infection, a T-cell–dependent pathway is suggested by the ability of anti-IFN-γ mAb treatment to suppress IL-6 production in *Plasmodium*-infected mice (83). However, this by no means indicates that the T cells are the origin of IL-6. At least one signal for IL-6 production may be provided by TNF, because, for example, TNF stimulates IL-6 production by brain macrophages or astrocytes in vitro (143), and second, anti-TNF antibody treatment prevents the increase of IL-6 in serum of *Plasmodium*-infected mice. In malaria, the increase in serum IL-6 can be prevented, either by anti-IFN-γ or by anti-TNF antibody treatment. These data may be discussed in the context of the induction of IL-6 by TNF-β in mice (27). Indeed, the antimouse TNF antibodies available to date, either monoclonal or polyclonal, recognize both TNF-α and TNF-β. In malaria-infected mice, IL-6 production may therefore depend on both these cytokines.

These data suggest that IL-6 is produced in large amounts during malaria infection, but that it does not have a major role in the pathogenesis of CM. However, due to its effects on B cells, IL-6 may be involved in hypergammaglobulinemia and immune complex diseases (e.g., glomerulonephritis observed during malaria infection).

Possible role of nitric oxide

In the context of the analysis of potential effector mechanisms, the pathogenic role of nitric oxide (NO) was evaluated in the murine CM model. NO production has been shown to be triggered by various cytokines, particularly TNF (144), but it is diminished by LPS (145). Involvement of NO in TNF pathology is therefore complex. NO can undoubtedly explain some of the early changes of CM (146), but probably not the end-stage lesion of the disease, which includes brain hemorrhages due to microvascular endothelial cell lesions, because treatment with L-NMMA had an aggravating rather than a protecting effect in mouse CM (147,148). Because the relevance of this model has been questioned, it seems important to stress the point that the mouse model is indeed a model of lethal CM, with brain hemorrhages, a situation that is identical to human CM (16). In view of the role of platelets in CM, two other arguments can suggest that NO has a protective rather than a pathogenic role in CM: NO can reduce platelet aggregation (149), and L-NMMA treatment increases platelet deposition on damaged endothelium in vivo (150).

Role of adhesion molecules

A possible involvement of endothelial cell (EC) adhesion molecules in the pathogenesis of experimental CM was investigated because (a) this syndrome is characterized by an increased adherence of lymphocyte and monocytes to brain venule EC, with resultant vascular damage and focal hemorrhages; (b) TNF is a key mediator, as shown by the anti-TNF antibody effect; and (c) TNF up-regulates the surface expression in EC cultures of various cell adhesion molecules (CAM), such as ICAM-1 (151), the ligand-partner for the lymphocyte and monocyte integrin, LFA-1 (152).

Intercellular adhesion molecule-1 (ICAM-1), as detected by immunofluorescence, is present in high amounts on the EC of brain venules from mice with CM, whereas it is barely detectable on these structures in control mice, either normal mice or those infected with *P. yoelii*, a nonlethal parasite strain that leads neither to increased TNF levels nor to CM. Treatment with a mAb directed against the α-chain (CD11a) of LFA-1, even if given shortly before death, completely protected mice from CM. In sharp contrast, treatment with anti-ICAM-1 mAb was found to be not only inefficient, but very harmful: Mice treated with this mAb died within a few hours with massive hemoptysis (153,154).

One of the possible pathogenic links between TNF and the lesions of human CM is indeed the potential role of this cytokine in the sequestration of parasitized erythrocytes (155), as previously hypothesized (156). Elegant studies by Berendt and colleagues (157) demonstrated that ICAM-1 is one of the molecules involved in cytoadherence of *P. falciparum*–infected erythrocytes, at least in vitro (157). Because TNF, among other cytokines, is known to up-regulate the surface expression of ICAM-1 on endothelial cells (151), it is likely that the markedly high TNF levels observed in patients with CM (18,20) lead to sequestration of parasitized erythrocytes via this pathway. Such a role for surface adhesion molecules is consistent with the finding that in vivo treatment with monoclonal antibodies directed against LFA-1, the ligand of ICAM-1, prevents development of murine CM (153). Moreover, the dramatically rapid effect of anti-LFA-1 mAb in the interruption of incipient murine CM suggests that, in addition to antimalarial drugs and neutralization of excessive TNF production, therapies aimed at preventing cytoadherence via carefully selected targets should be attempted as emergency measures in the critical care of human CM.

Role of platelets

Recent investigations in the murine model of CM allowed proposal of a new effector mechanism of TNF-induced EC lesion. It consists of adhesion of platelets to the surface of EC and subsequent fusion of these platelets into the cytoplasm of EC. This physiological process in vivo (158,159), has been characterized in vitro. Two lines of evidence for fusion have been described: After fusion has been induced in vitro, β-thromboglobulin (β-TG), a platelet-specific protein, is present in the cytoplasm of EC; gpIIb-IIIa, a platelet glycoprotein, is then transferred to the EC surface (Jinning Lou, PhD thesis, Beijing). Platelets were envisaged in the pathogenesis of CM, because there was no clear explanation for the dramatic protective effect of anti-LFA-1 mAb, which protected malaria-infected mice without significantly reducing the number of mononuclear cells in brain vessels (153,154). Recently, it was found that the critical effector of the neurovascular damage of CM is the blood platelet (160).

First, electron microscopic analysis of brains from mice with CM revealed that during CM, platelets adhere to and probably damage brain endothelial cells. Cerebral capillaries and venules contain platelets in dense contact with the endothelium or fusing to damaged brain endothelial cells. The endothelium appears damaged and interrupted by the presence of granules, suggesting the fusion of platelets with endothelium. Monocytes also adhere to brain endothelial cells, but they do not show any dense fusion of the membranes, and the endothelium seems unaffected. Platelets have also been demonstrated as being present in brain vessels in fatal cases of human CM (161).

Second, radiolabeled platelet distribution studies indicated that platelets significantly sequestered in the brain and the lung vasculature during CM. Noncerebral malaria was not associated with cerebral sequestration of platelets.

Third, treatment in vivo with anti-LFA-1 mAb selectively abrogated the cerebral sequestration of platelets; moreover, this effect correlated with prevention of the neurological syndrome. The α-chain (CD11a) and, to a lesser extent, the β-chain (CD18) of the integrin LFA-1 were found to be expressed on platelet membranes.

Fourth, malaria-infected animals rendered thrombocytopenic were significantly protected against CM, further indicating that platelets are central to the pathogenesis of CM.

Thus, a CD11a-dependent interaction between platelets and EC appears pivotal to microvascular damage. Microvascular lesions of CM would thus depend on an integrin-mediated platelet, TNF-induced EC damage (Fig. 30–1). These data suggest a novel mechanism of action for anti-LFA-1 mAb in the neurovascular complications of murine malaria, and they illustrate an unexpected role of platelets in vascular pathology. More recently, involvement of platelets in sepsis-related pathology was also shown (162). Further analysis of the fine mechanisms of this interaction between platelets and EC has been performed in vitro. Cultures of microvascular EC derived from brain, lungs, and other organs allowed identification of several pathways. Platelets indeed modify a number of functions of TNF-activated microvascular EC (Lou et al., unpublished observations). Regulation of the fusion phenomenon is currently under investigation.

CONCLUSIONS

Abnormally activated T cells result in secretion of various cytokines, some of which, such as TNF, have direct toxic effects on vital host structures. TNF-mediated vascular damage certainly involves intricate pathways, utilizing almost all the properties of this cytokine. In addition, the role of platelets in the vascular pathology of CM is an illustration of unexpected TNF properties. Alternatively, involvement of this cell type also provides an explanation for the efficacy of late administration of anti-LFA-1 antibody in CM, and it represents a new mechanism of action

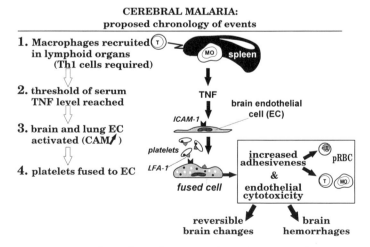

Figure 30–1 Chronology of events in the pathogenesis of experimental cerebral malaria.

of antiintegrin antibodies in vivo. The way in which platelets interact with EC and modify the physiology of these cells represents a possibly important effector pathway of TNF-induced vascular pathology. Likewise, even though in vitro and especially in vivo studies have provided some insights in the extraordinary complexity of cerebral lesions, much remains to be learned about fine malarial pathology. Understanding better the distinct mechanisms of lesions formation remains important to define targets, design relevant parameters to study, and evaluate the side effects of new therapeutic measures. Animal experimentation, particularly in mice, remains an irreplaceable tool to address these major questions and thereby to help improve the status of patients who suffer from severe malaria.

Malarial pathology, at least CM, seems to depend on the very T-cell subset, Th1, that is also capable of mediating protection against infection. The conditions and intensity of stimulation (e.g., type of antigen-presenting cells, nature of the antigen), the duration of activation, and the sites of inappropriate activation of these cells are the crucial parameters that will determine the balance between protection and pathology. Indeed, a critical issue concerning pathology might be preferential homing of some activated Th1 cells in certain microvascular beds. Therefore, the balance between Th1 and Th2 cells, as well as the expression of diverse cell adhesion molecules, are among the deciding parameters that can determine the outcome of the complex host-parasite relationship seen in malaria.

REFERENCES

1. Tharavanij S, Warrell MJ, Tantivanich S, et al. Factors contributing to the development to the cerebral malaria. I. Humoral immune responses. Am J Trop Med Hyg 1984;33:1–11.
2. Warrell DA. Pathophysiology of severe falciparum malaria in man. Parasitology 1987;94:53–76.
3. Edington GM. Cerebral malaria in the gold coast Africa. Four autopsy reports. Ann Trop Med Parasitol 1954;48:300–306.
4. Edington GM. Pathology of malaria in West Africa. Br Med J 1967;1:715–718.
5. Mc Murray DN. Cell-mediated immunity in protein calorie malnutrition. Prog Food Nutr Sci 1984;8:193–228.
7. Christophers SR. The mechanism of immunity against malaria in communities living under hyperendemic conditions. Ind J Med Res 1924;12:273–294.
8. Sinton JA. A summary of our present knowledge of the mechanisms of immunity in malaria. Malaria Inst India 1939;2:71–83.
9. McGregor IA, Smith DA. A health, nutrition and parasitological survey in a rural village Kenaba in west Kiang, The Gambia. Trans R Soc Trop Med Hyg 1952;46:403–427.
10. Phillips RE, Warrell DA. The pathophysiology of severe falciparum malaria. Parasitol Today 1986;2:271–281.
11. McPherson GG, Warrell MJ, White NJ, Looareesuwan S, Warrel DA. Human cerebral malaria. A quantitative ultrastructural analysis of parasitized erythrocyte sequestration. Am J Pathol 1985;119:385–401.
12. Grau GE, Piguet PF, Engers HD, Louis JA, Vassalli P, Lambert PH. L3T4+ T lymphocytes play a major role in the pathogenesis of murine cerebral malaria. J Immunol 1986;137:2348–2354.
13. Duarte MS, Corbett CET, Boulos M, Amato-Neto V. Ultrastructure of the lung in the falciparum malaria. Am J Trop Med Hyg 1985;34:31–35.
14. Polder TW, Jerusalem CR, Eling WMC. Morphological characteristics of intracerebral arterioles in clinical (Plasmodium falciparum) and experimental (Plasmodium berghei) cerebral malaria. J Neurol Sci 1991;101:35–46.
15. Boonpucknavig V, Boonpucknavig S, Udomsangpetch R, Nitiyanant P. An immunofluorescent study of cerebral malaria. Arch Pathol Lab Med 1990;114:1028–1034.
16. Porta J, Carota A, Wildi E, Widmer MC, Margairaz C, Grau GE. Immunopathological changes in human cerebral malaria. Clin Neuropathol 1993;12:142–146.
17. Beutler B, Cerami A. Tumor necrosis, cachexia, shock, and inflammation: a common mediator. Annu Rev Biochem 1988;57:505–518.
18. Grau GE, Taylor TE, Molyneux ME, et al. Tumour necrosis factor and disease severity in children with falciparum malaria. N Engl J Med 1989;320:1586–1591.
19. Shaffer N, Grau GE, Hedberg K, et al. Tumour necrosis factor and severe malaria. J Infect Dis 1991;163:96–101.
20. Kern P, Hemmer CJ, Vandamme J, Gruss HJ, Dietrich M. Elevated tumour necrosis factor alpha and interleukin-6 serum levels as markers for complicated Plasmodium falciparum malaria. Am J Med 1989;87:139–143.
21. Kwiatkowski D, Hill AVS, Sambou I, et al. TNF concentration in fatal cerebral, non-fatal cerebral, and uncomplicated Plasmodium falciparum malaria. Lancet 1990;336:1201–1204.
22. Butcher GA, Garland T, Ajdukiewics AB, Clark IA. Serum tumor necrosis factor associated with malaria in patients in the Solomon Islands. Trans R Soc Trop Med Hyg 1990;84:658–661.
23. Molyneux ME, Taylor TE, Wirima JJ, Grau GE. Tumor necrosis factor, interleukin 6, and malaria. Lancet 1991;337:1098.
24. Harpaz R, Edelman R, Wasserman SS, Levine MM, Davis JR, Sztein MB. Serum cytokine profiles in experimental human malaria. J Clin Invest 1992;90:505–523.
25. Rhodes-Feuillette A, Bellosguardo M, Druilhe P, et al. The interferon compartment of the immune response in human malaria: II. Presence of serum-interferon gamma following the acute attack. J Interferon Res 1985;5:169–178.
26. Brown AE, Webster HK, Teja-isavadharm P, Keeratuthakul D. Macrophage activation in falciparum malaria as measured by neopterin and interferon-gamma. Clin Exp Immunol 1990;82:97–101.
27. Clark IA, Gray KM, Rockett EJ, et al. Increased lymphotoxin in human malarial serum: its ability to increase plasma interleukin-6 and cause hypoglycemia and possible role in malaria pathology. Trans R Soc Trop Med Hyg 1992;86:602–607.

28. Ringwald P, Peyron F, Vuillez JP, Touze JE, Le Bras J, Deloron P. Levels of cytokines in plasma during Plasmodium falciparum attacks. J Clin Microbiol 1991;29:2076–2078.

29. Kremsner PG, Feldmeier H, Zotter GM, et al. Immunological alterations in uncomplicated Plasmodium falciparum malaria. Relationship between parasitemia and indicators of macrophage activation. Acta Trop 1989;46:351–359.

30. Karunaweera ND, Grau GE, Gamage P, Carter R, Mendis K. Dynamics of fever and serum levels of tumor necrosis factor are closely associated during clinical paroxysms in Plasmodium vivax malaria. Proc Natl Acad Sci USA 1992; 89:3200–3203.

31. Grau GE, Piguet PF. TNF in cerebral and non-cerebral malaria. In: Fiers W, Buurman W, eds. TNF: molecular and cellular biology, and clinical relevance. New York: Karger, 1993:162–171.

32. Kwiatkowski D, Molyneux ME, Stephens S, et al. Response to monoclonal anti-TNF antibody in children with cerebral malaria. Q J Med 1993;86:91–98.

33. Jahiel RI, Vilcek J, Nussenzweig RS. Exogenous interferon protects mice against Plasmodium berghei malaria. Nature 1970;227:1350–1351.

33a. Ferreira A, Schofield L, Enea V, et al. Inhibition of development of exoerythrocytic forms of malaria parasites by gamma-interferon. Science 1986;232:881–884.

34. Schofield L, Villaquiran J, Ferreira A, Schellekens H, Nussenzweig RS, Nussenzweig VE. Gamma interferon, CD8+ T cells and antibodies required for immunity to malaria sporozoites. Nature 1987;330:664–666.

35. Schofield L, Ferreira A, Altszuler R, Nussenzweig VE, Nussenzweig RS. Interferon gamma inhibits the intrahepatocytic development of malaria parasites in vitro. J Immunol 1987;139:2020–2025.

36. Mellouk S, Maheshwari RK, Rhodes-Feuillette A, et al. Inhibitory activity of interferons and interleukin 1 on the development of Plasmodium falciparum in human hepatocyte cultures. J Immunol 1987;139:4192–4195.

37. Deloron P, Chougnet C, Lepers JP, Tallet S, Coulanges P. Protective value of elevated serum levels of interferon gamma against exoerythrocytic stages of Plasmodium falciparum. J Clin Microbiol 1991;29:1757–1760.

38. Clark IA, Hunt NH, Butcher GA, Cowden WB. Inhibition of murine malaria Plasmodium chabaudi in vivo by recombinant interferon-γ or tumour necrosis factor, and its enhancement by butylated hydroxyanisole. J Immunol 1987; 139:3493–3496.

39. Shear H, Srinivasan R, Nolan T, Ng C. Role of IFN-γ in lethal and non-lethal malaria in susceptible and resistant murine hosts. J Immunol 1989;143:2038–2044.

40. Stevenson MM, Fong-Tam M, Nowotarski M. Role of interferon-γ and tumour necrosis factor in host resistance to Plasmodium chabaudi AS. Immunol Lett 1990;25:115–122.

41. Herrera MA, Rosero F, Herrera S, et al. Protection against malaria in Aotus monkeys immunized with a recombinant blood-stage antigen fused to a universal T-cell epitope: correlation of serum gamma interferon levels with protection. Infect Immun 1992;60:154–158.

42. Hviid L, Reimert CM, Theander TG, Jepsen S, Bendtzen K. Recombinant human tumour necrosis factor is not inhibitory to Plasmodium falciparum in vitro. Trans R Soc Trop Med Hyg 1988;82:48–49.

43. Pied SD, Nussler A, Pontet M, et al. C-reactive protein protects against pre-erythrocytic stages of malaria. Infect Immun 1989;57:278–282.

44. Helle M, Brakenhoff JP, De Groot ER, Aarden LA. Interleukin-6 is involved in interleukin-1 induced activities. Eur J Immunol 1988;18:957–959.

45. Pied S, Civas A, Berliot-Picard F, et al. Anti-parasitic intercytokine effects of IL-1 and IL-6 on malaria pre-erythrocytic stages: influence of parasite schizogony on IL-6 secretion by liver cells. J Immunol 1994 (in press).

46. Curfs JHAJ, Van der Meer JM, Sauermein SW, Eling WM. Low dosages of interleukin 1 protects mice against lethal cerebral malaria. J Exp Med 1990;172:1287–1291.

47. Ockenhouse CF, Shear HL. Oxidative killing of the intraerythrocytic malaria parasite plasmodium yoelii by activated macrophages. J Immunol 1984;132:424–431.

48. Malhotra K, Salmon D, Lebras J, Vilde JL. Susceptibility of Plasmodium falciparum to a peroxydase-mediated oxygen dependent microbicidal system. Infect Immun 1988;56: 3305–3309.

49. Clark IA, Virolizier JL, Carswell EA, Wood PR. Possible importance of macrophage-derived mediators in acute malaria. Infect Immun 1981;32:1058–1066.

50. Taverne J, Dockrell HM, Playfair JHL. Endotoxin-induced serum factor kills malarial parasites in vitro. Infect Immun 1981;33:83–89.

51. Haidaris CG, Haynes JD, Meltzer MS, Allison AC. Serum containing tumour necrosis factor is cytotoxic for human malaria parasite Plasmodium falciparum. Infect Immun 1983;42:385–393.

52. Taverne J, Tavernier J, Fiers W, Playfair JHL. Recombinant tumour necrosis factor inhibited malaria parasites in vivo but not in vitro. Clin Exp Immunol 1987;67:1–4.

53. Grau GE, Bieler G, Pointaire P, et al. Significance of cytokine production and adhesion molecules in malarial immunopathology. Immunol Lett 1990;25:189–194.

54. Mazier D, Goma J, Pied S, et al. Hepatic phase of malaria—a crucial role as go-between with other stages. Bull WHO 1990;68:126–131.

55. Lotze M, Jirik F, Kabouridis P, et al. B cell stimulating factor 2/interleukin-6 is a costimulant for human thymocytes and T lymphocytes. J Exp Med 1988;167:1253.

56. Katz Y, Strunk RC. Similarities and differences in stimulation of expression of alternative pathway of complement and IFN-beta2/IL-6 genes in human fibroblasts. J Immunol 1989;142:3862–3867.

57. Nussler A, Pied S, Goma J, et al. TNF inhibits hepatic stages in vitro via synthesis of IL-6. Int Immunol 1991;3: 317–321.

58. Sjostrand NO, Eldh J, Samuelson UE, Alaranta S, Klinge E. The effect of L-arginine and ng-monomethyl L-arginine on the inhibitory neurotransmission of the human corpus cavernosum penis. Acta Physiol Scand 1990;140:297–298.

59. Lebbar S, Cavaillon JM, Caroff M, et al. Molecular requirement for interleukin-1 induction by lipopolysaccharide-stimulated monocytes: involvement of the heptosyl-2-keto-3-deoxyoctulosonate region. Eur J Immunol 1986; 16:87–91.

60. Grau GE, Frei K, Piguet PF, et al. Interleukin-6 production in experimental cerebral malaria. Modulation by anti-cytokine antibodies and possible role in hyper gammaglobulinemia. J Exp Med 1990;172:1505–1508.

61. Naotunne TD, Karunaweera ND, Del Giudice G, et al. Cytokines kill malaria parasites during infection crisis: extracellular complementary factors are essential. J Exp Med 1991;173:523–529.

62. Karunaweera ND, Carter R, Grau GE, Kwiatkowski D, Del Giudice G, Mendis KN. Tumour necrosis factor-dependent parasite-killing effects during paroxysms in non-immune Plasmodium vivax malaria patients. Clin Exp Immunol 1992;88:499–505.

63. Orago ASS, Facer CA. Cytokine-induced of Plasmodium falciparum erythrocytic growth in vitro. Clin Exp Immunol 1993;91:287–294.

64. Carlin JM, Jensen JB. Stage- and time-dependent effects of crisis form factor on Plasmodium falciparum in vitro. J Parasitol 1986;72:852–857.

65. Kumaratilake LM, Ferrante A, Rzepczyk C. The role of lymphocytes-T in immunity to Plasmodium falciparum-enhancement of neutrophil-mediated parasite killing by lymphotoxin and IFN-gamma— comparisons with tumor necrosis factor effects. J Immunol 1991;146:762–767.

66. Horuk R, Chitnis C, Darbonne WC, et al. A receptor for the malarial parasite Plasmodium vivax: the erythrocyte chemokine receptor. Science 1993;261:1182–1184.

67. Pouvelle B, Spiegel R, Hsiao L, et al. Direct access to serum macromolecules by intraerythrocytic malaria parasites. Nature 1991;353:73–75.

68. Fugioka H, Aikawa M. Morphological changes of clefts in Plasmodium infected erythrocyte in adverse conditions. Exp Parasitol 1993;76:302–307.

69. Rockett KA, Awburn AW, Cowden WB, Clark IA. Killing of Plasmodium falciparum in vitro by nitric oxide derivatives. Infect Immun 1991;59:3280–3283.

70. Allison AC, Eugui EM. The role of cell-mediated immune response in resistance to malaria, with special references to oxidant stress. Ann Rev Immunol 1983;1:361–392.

71. Rockett KA, Targett GAT, Playfair JHL. Killing of blood stage Plasmodium falciparum by lipid peroxides from tumor necrosis serum. Infect Immun 1988;56:3180–3183.

72. Udomsangpetch R, Lundgren K, Berzins K, et al. Human monoclonal antibodies to Pf155, a major antigen of malaria parasite Plasmodium falciparum. Science 1986;231:57–59.

73. Perrin L, Ramirez E, Lambert PH, Miescher PA. Inhibition of Plasmodium falciparum growth in human erythrocytes by monoclonal antibodies. Nature 1981;289:301–303.

74. Yoshida N, Nussenzweig RS, Potocnjac P, Nussenzweig VE, Aikawa M. Hybridoma produces protective antibodies directed against the sporozoïte stage of malaria parasite. Science 1980;207:71–73.

75. Lunel F, Druilhe P. Effector cells involved in nonspecific and antibody-dependent mechanisms directed against Plasmodium falciparum blood stages in vitro. Infect Immun 1989;1:2043–2049.

76. Bouharoun-Tayoun H, Attanath P, Sabchareon A, Chongsuphajaisiddhi T, Druilhe P. Antibodies that protect humans against Plasmodium-Falciparum blood stages do not on their own inhibit parasite growth and invasion in vitro, but act in cooperation with monocytes. J Exp Med 1990;172:1633–1641.

77. Ferrante A, Kumaratilake L, Rzepczyk C, Dayer JM. Killing of Plasmodium falciparum by cytokine activated effector cells (neutrophils and macrophages). Immunol Lett 1990; 25:179–188.

78. Talafiero WH, Mullingham HW. The histopathology of malaria with special references to the function and the origin of the macrophages in defence. Indian Med Res Mem 1937;29:1.

79. Grau GE, Modlin RL. Immune mechanisms in bacterial and parasitic diseases: protective immunity versus pathology. Curr Opin Immunol 1991;3:480–485.

80. Finley RW, Mackey LJ, Lambert PH. Virulent P. berghei malaria: prolonged survival and decreased cerebral pathology in T-cell deficient nude mice. J Immunol 1982;129: 2213–2218.

81. Grau GE, Gretener D, Lambert PH. Prevention of murine cerebral malaria by low-dose cyclosporin A. Immunology 1987;61:521–525.

82. Grau GE, Kindler V, Piguet PF, Lambert PH, Vassalli P. Prevention of experimental cerebral malaria by anti-cytokine antibodies. Interleukin-3 and granulocyte macrophage colony-stimulating factor are intermediates in increased tumor necrosis factor production and macrophage accumulation. J Exp Med 1988;168:1499–1504.

83. Grau GE, Heremans H, Piguet P, et al. Monoclonal antibody against interferon-gamma can prevent experimental cerebral malaria and its associated overproduction of tumor necrosis factor. Proc Natl Acad Sci USA 1989;86: 5572–5574.

84. Aggarwal BB, Eessalu TE, Hass PE. Characterization of receptors for human tumour necrosis factor and their regulation by gamma-interferon. Nature 1985;318:665–667.

85. Philip R, Epstein LB. Tumour necrosis factor as immunomodulator and mediator of monocyte cytotoxicity induced by itself, gamma interferon and interleukin-1. Nature 1986;323:86–89.

86. Kindler V, Sappino AP, Grau GE, Piguet PF, Vassalli P. The inducing role of tumor necrosis factor in the development of bactericidal granulomas during BCG infection. Cell 1989;56:731–740.

87. Mosmann TR, Coffman RL. TH1 and TH2 cells: different patterns of lymphokine secretion lead to different functional properties. Ann Rev Immunol 1989;7:145–173.

88. Kossodo S, Grau GE. Profile of cytokine production in relation with susceptibility to experimental malaria. J Immunol 1994 (in press).

89. Bate CAW, Taverne J, Roman E, Moreno C, Playfair JHL. Tumour necrosis factor induction by malaria exoantigens depends upon phospholipid. Immunology 1992;75:129–135.

90. Taverne J, Bate CAW, Sarkar DA, Meager A, Rook GAW, Playfair JHL. Human and murine macrophages produce TNF in response to soluble antigens of Plasmodium-falciparum. Parasite Immunol 1990;12:33–43.

91. Bate CAW, Taverne J, Playfair JHL. Soluble malarial antigens are toxic and induce the production of tumour necrosis factor in vivo. Immunology 1989;66:600–605.

92. Bate CAW, Taverne J, Playfair JHL. Detoxified exoantigens and phosphatidylinositol derivatives inhibits tumor necro-

crosis factor induction by malarial exoantigens. Infect Immun 1992;60:1894–1901.

93. Schofield L, Hackett F. Signal transduction in host cells by a glycosylphosphatidylinositol toxin of malaria parasites. J Exp Med 1993;177:145–153.

94. Bate CAW, Taverne J, Playfair JHL. Malarial parasites induce TNF production by macrophages. Immunology 1988; 64:227–231.

95. Taverne J, Bate CA, Playfair JHL. Induction of TNF in vitro as a model for the identification of toxic malaria antigens. Lymphokine Res 1989;8:317–322.

96. Bate CAW, Taverne J, Dave A, Playfair JHL. Malaria exoantigens induce T-independent antibody that blocks their ability to induce TNF. Immunology 1990;70:315–320.

97. Thomas ML. The leukocyte common antigen family. Ann Rev Immunol 1989;7:339.

98. Playfair JHL, Taverne J, Bate CA, Desouza J, Pluta A, Zakian V. The malaria vaccine-anti-parasite or anti-disease. Immunol Today 1990;11:25–27.

99. Jakobsen PH, Baek L, Jepsen S. Demonstration of soluble Plasmodium falciparum antigens reactive with limulus amoebocyte lysate and polymyxin B. Parasite Immunol 1988;10:593–606.

100. Taverne J, Bate CAW, Kwiatkowski D, Jakobsen PH, Playfair JHL. Two soluble antigens of Plasmodium falciparum induce tumour necrosis factor release from macrophages. Infect Immun 1990;58:2923–2928.

101. Riley EM, Jakobsen PH, Allen SJ, et al. Immune response to soluble exoantigens of Plasmodium falciparum may contribute to both pathogenesis and protection in clinical malaria: evidence from a longitudinal, prospective study of semi-immune African children. Eur J Immunol 1991;21: 1019–1025.

102. Ho M, Webster HK, Looareesuwan S, et al. Antigen-specific immunosuppression in human malaria due to Plasmodium falciparum. J Infect Dis 1986;153:763–771.

103. Wells RA, Pavanand K, Zolyomi S, Permpanich B, Macdermott RP. Loss of circulating T lymphocytes with normal levels of B and "null" lymphocytes in Thai adults with malaria. Clin Exp Immunol 1979;35:202–209.

104. Wyler DJ. Peripheral lymphocyte subpopulations in human falciparum malaria. Clin Exp Immunol 1976;23: 471–476.

105. Chougnet C, Tallet S, Ringwald P, Deloron P. Kinetics of lymphocyte subsets from peripheral blood during a Plasmodium falciparum malaria attack. Clin Exp Immunol 1992;90:405–408.

106. Hviid L, Theander GT, Abu-zeid YA, Bayoumi RA, Jensen JB. Transient depletion of T cells with high LFA-1 expression from peripheral blood circulation during acute Plasmodium falciparum malaria. Eur J Immunol 1991;21: 1249–1253.

107. Ho M, Webster HK, Tongtawe P, Pattanapanyasat K, Weidanz WP. Increased gd T cells in acute Plasmodium falciparum malaria. Immunol Lett 1990;25:139.

108. Roussilhon C, Agrapart M, Ballet JJ, Bensussan A. T lymphocytes bearing the gd T cell receptor in patients with acute Plasmodium falciparum malaria. J Infect Dis 1990; 162:283–285.

109. Sarthou JL, Behr C, Roussilhon C, et al. Different patterns

110. Bordessoule D, Gaulard P, Mason DY. Preferential localization of human lymphocytes bearing gd T cell receptors to the red pulp of the spleen. J Clin Pathol 1990;43: 461–464.

111. Ho M, Webster HK, Green B, Looareesuwan S, Kongchareon S, White NJ. Defective production of response to IL2 in acute human falciparum malaria. J Immunol 1988;141:2755–2759.

112. Josimovic-Alasevic O, Feldmeier H, Zwingenberger K, et al. Interleukin 2 receptor in patients with localized and systemic parasitic diseases. Clin Exp Immunol 1988;72: 249–254.

113. Kremsner P, Zotter G, Feldmeier H, et al. Immune response in patients during and after Plasmodium-falciparum infection. J Infect Dis 1990;161:1025–1028.

114. Langhorne J, Simon-Haaraus B. Differential T cell responses to Plasmodium chabaudi in peripheral blood and spleens of C57bl/6 mice during infection. J Immunol 1991;146:2771–2775.

115. Kumararatne DS, Phillips RS, Sinclair D, Parrott DMV, Forrester JB. Lymphocyte migration in murine malaria during the primary patent parasitemia of Plasmodium chabaudi infection. Clin Exp Immunol 1987; 68:65–77.

116. Goerlich R, Häcker G, Pfeffer K, Heeg K, Wagner H. Plasmodium falciparum merozoites primarily stimulate the Vg 9 subset of human gd T cells. Eur J Immunol 1992;21: 2613–2616.

117. Goodier M, Fey P, Eichmann K, Langhorne J. Human peripheral blood gd T cell respond to antigens of Plasmodium falciparum. Int Immunol 1991;4:33–42.

118. Behr C, Dubois P. Preferential expansion of Vg9/Vd2 T cells following stimulations of peripheral blood lymphocytes with extracts of Plasmodium falciparum. Int Immunol 1992;4:361–366.

119. Jaureguiberry G, Ogunkolade W, Bailly E, Rhodes-Feuillette A, Agrapart M, Ballet JJ. Plasmodium falciparum exoprotein stimulation of human T-lymphocytes unsensitized to malaria. J Chromatography 1988;440:385–396.

120. Ferrante A, Staugas REM, Rowan-Kelly B, et al. Production of tumor necrosis factor-alpha and beta by human mononuclear leukocytes stimulated with mitogens, bacteria, and malarial parasites. Infect Immun 1990;58:3996–4003.

121. Kumaratilake LA, Ferrante A, Rzepczyk CM. Tumor necrosis factor enhances neutrophil-mediated killing of Plasmodium falciparum. Infect Immun 1990;58:788–793.

122. Langhorne J, Goodier M, Behr C, Dubois P. Is there a role for gd T cells in malaria? Immunol Today 1992;13:298–299.

123. Chizzolini C, Grau GE, Geinoz A, Schrijvers D. T lymphocyte interferon-gamma production induced by Plasmodium falciparum antigen is high in recently infected non-immune and low in immune subjects. Clin Exp Immunol 1990;79:95–99.

124. Jones R, Hickling JK, Targett GAT, Playfair JHL. Polyclonal in vitro proliferative responses from non-immune donors to Plasmodium falciparum malaria antigens requires

of phenotypic abnormalities in T lymphocyte subpopulations in patterns with acute malaria. International Congress on Malaria and Babesiosis. 1991;111.

UCHL1+ (memory) T cells. Eur J Immunol 1990;20: 307–315.

125. Roussilhon C, Agrapart M, Behr C, Dubois P, Ballet JJ. Interactions of CD4+ and CD8+ human T lymphocytes from malaria-unprimed donors with Plasmodium falciparum schizont stage. Clin Microbiol 1989;27:2544–2551.

126. Currier J, Sattabongkot J, Good M. "Natural" T cells responsive to malaria: evidence implicating immunological cross-reactivity in the maintenance of TCRa/b+ malaria specific responses from non-exposed donors. Int Immunol 1992;4:985–994.

127. Beverley P. Immunological memory in T cells. Curr Opin Immunol 1991;3:355–359.

128. Beverley PCL. Is T-cell memory maintained by crossreactive stimulation? Immunol Today 1990;11:203–205.

129. Mackay RC. Migration pathways and immunologic memory among T lymphocytes. Semin Immunol 1992;4:51–58.

130. Good MF, Currier J. The importance of T cell homing and the spleen in reaching a balance between malaria immunity and immunopathology: the moulding of immunity by early exposure to cross-reactive organisms. Immunol Cell Biol 1992;70:405–410.

131. Troye-Blomberg M, Riley EM, Kabilan L, et al. Production by activated T cells of interleukin-4, but not IFN-gamma is correlated with elevated levels of serum antibodies to activating malaria antigens. Proc Natl Acad Sci USA 1990;87: 5484–5488.

132. Riley EM, Greenwood BM. Measuring cellular immune responses to malaria antigens in endemic populations—epidemiological, parasitological and physiological factors which influence in vitro assays. Immunol Lett 1990;25: 221–229.

133. Riley EM, Ong CSL, Olerup O, et al. Cellular and humoral immune responses to Plasmodium falciparum gametocyte antigens in malaria immune individuals. Limited response to the 48/45 kilodalton surface antigen does not appear to be restricted to MHC restriction. J Immunol 1990;144: 4810–4816.

134. Behr C, Sarthou JL, Rogier C, et al. Antibodies and reactive T cells against the malaria heat-shock protein PF72/HSP70-1 and derived peptides in individuals continuously exposed to Plasmodium falciparum. J Immunol 1992;169: 3321–3330.

135. Riley EM, Allen SJ, Troye-Blomberg M, et al. Association between immune recognition of the malaria vaccine candidate Pf155/RESA and resistance to clinical disease: a prospective longitudinal study in malaria endemic region of West Africa. Trans Soc Trop Med Hyg 1991; 85:436–443.

136. Behr C, Dubois P. Evaluation of human T cell response to malaria antigens in naturally acquired immunity. Res Immunol 1991;142:643–649.

137. Taylor-Robinson AW, Phillips RS, Severn A, Moncada S, Liew FY. The role of TH1 and TH2 cells in a rodent malaria infection. Science 1993;260:1931–1934.

138. Hill AVS, Allsop CEM, Kwiatkowski D, et al. Common West African HLA antigens are associated with protection from severe malaria. Nature 1991;352:595–600.

139. Carter R, Schofield L, Mendis KN. HLA effects in malaria: Increased parasite-killing immunity or reduced immunopathology? Parasitol Today 1992;8:41–42.

140. Freund YR, Sgarlato G, Jacob CH, Suzuki Y, Remington, JS. Polymorphisms in the tumor necrosis factor α (TNF-α) gene correlate with murine resistance to development of toxoplasmic encephalitis and with levels of TNF-α mRNA in infected brain tissue. J Exp Med 1992;175: 683–688.

141. Hirano T, Akira S, Taga T, Kishimoto T. Biological and clinical aspects of interleukin-6. Immunol Today 1990;11: 443–449.

142. Grau GE, Fajardo LF, Piguet PF, Allet D, Lambert PH. Tumour necrosis factor is an essential mediator in murine cerebrale malaria. Science 1987;237:1210–1212.

143. Frei K, Malipiero UV, Leist TP, Zinkernagel RM, Schwab ME, Fontana A. On the cellular source and function of interleukin-6 produced in the central nervous system in viral diseases. Eur J Immunol 1989;19:689–694.

144. Dudek R, Kibbira S, Kahler J, Bing RJ. The effect of immune mediators (cytokines) on the release of endothelium-derived relaxing factor (EDRF) and of prostacyclin by freshly harvested endothelial cells. Life Sci 1992;50: 863–873.

145. Myers PR, Wright TF, Tanner MA, Adams HR. EDRF and nitric oxide production in cultured endothelial cells. Direct inhibition by E. coli-endotoxin. Am J Physiol 1992; 262:H710–H718.

146. Rockett KA, Awburn MM, Aggarwal BB, Cowden WB, Clark IA. In vivo induction of nitrite and nitrate by tumor necrosis factor, lymphotoxin, and interleukin-1: possible role in malaria. Infect Immun 1992;60:3725–3730.

147. Senaldi G, Kremsner PG, Grau GE. Nitric oxide and cerebral malaria. Lancet 1992;340:1554–1555.

148. Kremsner PG, Nussler A, Neifer S, et al. Malaria antigen and cytokine induced production of reactive nitrogen intermediates by murine macrophages: no relevance to the development of experimental cerebral malaria. Immunology 1993;78:286–290.

149. Radomski MW, Palmer RMJ, Moncada S. Modulation of platelet aggregation by L-Arginine nitric oxide pathway. Trends Pharmacol Sci 1991;12:87–88.

150. Herbaczynskacedro K, Lembowicz K, Pytel B. NG-Monomethyl-L-arginine increases platelet deposition on damaged endothelium in vivo—a scanning electron microscopic study. Thromb Res 1991;64:1–9.

151. Rothlein R, Czajkowski M, O'Neil MM, Marlin SD, Mainolfi E, Merluzzi VG. Induction of intercellular molecule 1 on primary and continuous cell lines by pro-inflammatory cytokines. J Immunol 1988;141:1665–1669.

152. Strassman G, Springer T, Adams DO. Studies with antigen associated with the activation of murine mononuclear phagocytes: kinetics of and requirements for induction of lymphocyte function-associated antigen 1 (LFA-1) in vitro. J Immunol 1985;135:147–151.

153. Grau GE, Pointaire P, Piguet PF, et al. Late administration of monoclonal antibody to leukocyte function-antigen 1 abrogates incipient murine cerebral malaria. Eur J Immunol 1991;21:2265–2267.

154. Falanga PB, Butcher EC. Late treatment with anti LFA-1 (CD11a) antibody prevents cerebral malaria in a mouse model. Eur J Immunol 1991;21:2259–2263.

155. Miller LH. Malaria—binding of infected red cells. Nature 1989;341:18.

156. Grau GE, Piguet PF, Vassalli P, Lambert PH. Involvement of tumour necrosis factor and other cytokines in immune-mediated vascular pathology. Int Arch Allergy Appl Immunol 1989;88:34–39.

157. Berendt, AR, Simmons DL, Tansey J, Newbold CI, Marsh K. Intercellular adhesion molecule-1 is an endothelial cell adhesion receptor for Plasmodium falciparum. Nature 1989;341:57–59.

158. Gimbrone MA Jr, Aster RH, Cotran RS, Corkery J, Jandl JH, Folkman J. Preservation of vascular integrity in organs perfused in vitro with a platelet-rich medium. Nature 1969; 222:33–36.

159. Yamazaki H, Fujimoto T, Suzuki H, et al. Interaction of platelets and blood vessels: vascular injuries induced by platelets activation in vivo. Jpn Circ 1992;56: 178–186.

160. Grau GE, Tacchini-Cottier F, Juillard P, Vesin C, Milon G, Piguet PF. An active role for platelets in microvascular pathology of severe malaria 1994;

161. Pongponratn E, Riganti M, Harinasuta T, Bunnag D. Electron microscopic study of phagocytosis in human spleen in falciparum malaria. SE Asian J Trop Med Pub Health 1989;20:31–39.

162. Piguet PF, Vesin C, Ryser JE, Senaldi G, Tacchini-Cottier F, Grau GE. An effector role of platelets in the local or systematic LPS-induced toxicity mediated by CD11/CD18 dependent interaction with the endothelium. Infect Immun 1994 (in press).

CHAPTER 31

ROLE OF CYTOKINES IN PARASITIC INFECTIONS

Venkatachalam Udhayakumar, Patrick J. Lammie, Kathleen A. Dimock, and Altaf A. Lal

It is estimated that more than one third of the human population is victim of parasitic infections, and the annual death toll remains in the millions (1). The life cycle of parasites is complex, and our understanding of their basic biology is primitive. In recent years, however, the study of parasite immunobiology has provided important insights into the different arms of the host immunity directed against the parasite, as well as the parasite's adaptation to host immunity. Discovery of antigenic variation exhibited by Trypanosomes is a classic example (2). Immunological investigations in parasitic disease models have provided important insight into the significance of the dichotomy in cytokine production by Th1 and Th2 cells (3–6). These models have revealed that parasites can exploit shifts in the balance of cytokine production for their own advantage. It has also become clear that the cytokine cascade has a central role in the pathology associated with many parasitic diseases. This discovery will undoubtedly lay foundations for novel immunotherapeutic approaches, as well as for vaccination strategies that are most advantageous to the host.

We focus on recent advances in the field of cytokine biology with reference to parasitic disease models. Because there is limited literature on cytokine regulation in human parasitic infections, we also used selected animal studies to give a broader overview of the field.

ROLE OF CYTOKINES IN PROTECTIVE IMMUNITY AND DISEASE IN INFECTIONS WITH TISSUE-INVADING PARASITES

Parasitic diseases such as leishmaniasis, toxoplasmosis, and Chagas' disease are caused by tissue-invading protozoan parasites (7). Whereas *Leishmania* species have adapted to live within the macrophage, *Toxoplasma gondii* and *Trypanosoma cruzi* can invade any eukaryotic cell regardless of whether it is phagocytic. As a consequence of the adaptation of various parasites to live in different microenvironments, there are obvious differences in the evolution of host protective mechanisms, parasite survival strategies, and the pathology associated with these infections. The ultimate outcome of infection, whether resistance or disease, is influenced by the balance of counter-regulatory cytokines elicited by the parasite. The dual regulatory and effector role of cytokines in determining the outcome of an infection has been best illustrated using experimental *Leishmania major* infection in mice (4,5). Because this model has provided important insights into the crossregulatory mechanisms that may operate within the cytokine network, we focus on it to provide a comprehensive review of how cytokine networks can influence the clinical manifestation of disease in intracellular parasitic infection. Current findings on the role of cytokines in toxoplasmosis and Chagas' disease are also briefly discussed.

Role of cytokines in protective immune mechanisms and disease in leishmaniasis: association of Th1 cells with protection and Th2 cells with disease

Promastigotes of *Leishmania major* invade macrophages and transform into intracellular amastigotes within acidic phagolysosomal compartments. Ultimate destruction of this parasite requires activation of macrophages by cytokines secreted by CD4+ and CD8+ T cells. Detailed immunological studies using *L. major*–infected experimental animals have led to a better understanding of crossregulation in the cytokine network (4,5). Historically, it is well known that genetic background determines the outcome of an experimental infection with *L. major* (8). In genetically resistant mouse strains, such as C3H/HeN, infection with *L. major* causes localized lesions in the skin that heal spontaneously. These mice then develop protective immunity against subsequent infection. However, in susceptible strains, such as BALB/c, *L. major* infection leads to a disseminated visceral disease that eventually kills the infected mice. Furthermore, strong parasite-specific DTH responses develop in resistant strains of mice, with little antibody production, whereas strong antibody responses develop in the susceptible strains, with poor DTH responses (8). Although the genetic basis for this difference has been less clear, an immunological explanation for this phenomenon has emerged from the observation that polarization of Th1 and Th2 CD4+ T cells occurs in mice with different genetic backgrounds following experimental infection with *L. major* (4,5). Three lines of evidence suggest the importance of the Th1/Th2 dichotomy to disease outcome in *L. major* infection in mice: (a) different patterns of cytokine expression in susceptible versus resistant strains of mice, (b) cell transfer experiments involving parasite-specific Th1 or Th2 clones, and (c) in vivo experiments using monoclonal antibodies to neutralize cytokine activities.

DIFFERENT PATTERNS OF CYTOKINE EXPRESSION BY CD4+ T CELLS OF MICE FROM DIFFERENT GENETIC BACKGROUNDS:

In mice that are resistant to *L. major*, the Th1 phenotype has been found to predominate, whereas in susceptible mice, the Th2 phenotype is dominant (5,9–11). This pattern of Th1 and Th2 activation was further confirmed at the molecular level. CD4+ T cells from *L. major*–infected, genetically resistant C57/BL6 strains of mice, and BALB/c mice, which were immunologically manipulated to express the healer phenotype, were shown to express interferon-γ (IFN-γ) but little interleukin-4 (IL-4) messenger RNA (mRNA). In contrast, mice in whom progressive infection developed had CD4+ T cells with IL-4 and IL-10 mRNA, but no IFN-γ transcripts (12,13). Thus, protection was correlated with the development of Th1 cells, whereas susceptibility to the disease was correlated with the production of the Th2 cells.

CELL TRANSFER STUDIES:

The role of Th1 and Th2 cells in conferring protection was further investigated using cell transfer experiments (14). Transfer of *L. major*–specific Th1 clones into naive mice with severe combined immunodeficiency disorders (SCID), which lack mature T and B lymphocytes due to an intrinsic genetic defect, provided protection against *L. major* infection. In the nonreconstituted mice, parasite multiplication was unchecked. Conversely, adoptive transfer of parasite-specific Th2 clones into SCID mice exacerbated lesion development following a challenge infection with *L. major* (14). These T cells were found to persist in the footpad lesions of the recipients 6 weeks after transfer. When these cells were restimulated in vitro, they maintained their characteristic pattern of cytokine secretion.

The complexities of the interaction between the cytokine network, host protective mechanisms, and disease manifestations have become apparent from other studies. In contrast to Holaday and associates (14), Titus and coworkers (15) found evidence for the adoptive transfer of disease using Th1 clones in experimental *L. major* infection. The reason for this apparent contradiction is unclear. However, one critical difference is that Titus and coworkers (15) used syngeneic mice that were depleted of B and T cells, whereas Holaday and associates (14) used SCID mice as recipients.

IN VIVO ADMINISTRATION OF CYTOKINES AND CYTOKINE-SPECIFIC ANTIBODIES:

The role of individual cytokines in the manifestation of disease versus protection has been studied by either direct administration of cytokines or by neutralizing the activity of cytokines with specific antibodies. Injection of anti-IFN-γ antibodies abrogated protective immunity in mice expressing the healer phenotype. However, to be effective, anti-IFN-γ antibodies had to be administered within 1 or 2 weeks after infection (16,17). In these mice, there was a shift in the phenotype of activated CD4+ cells from Th1 to Th2 as early as 3 days following anti-IFN-γ administration (17). Conversely, administration of IFN-γ during *L. major* infection in susceptible mice led to the development of a Th1 rather than a Th2 phenotype. However, there was only a transient difference in the size of the lesions, and the long-term course of the infection was not altered (17). Similarly, *L. major* genetically manipulated to constitutively produce IFN-γ was also found to be ineffective in stimulating susceptible BALB/c mice to resist disease development, despite evidence of significant IFN-γ production (18). These findings indicate that although IFN-γ has a significant role in protection, other factors may also be required to mediate protection.

IL-12, originally named natural killer (NK) cell growth factor, has been shown to favor the commitment of T cells to the Th1 phenotype during the early stages of the immune response (19). The role of IL-12 in regulation of protective immunity and disease has been studied using the experimental model of *L. major* infection (20,21). In vivo administration of IL-12 in susceptible BALB/c mice reduced the parasite burden significantly and induced IFN-γ production. Conversely, administration of anti-IL-12 antibodies was found to induce disease in otherwise resistant C57B1/6 mice. In these mice, disease progression was accompanied by a shift in cytokine secretion to that of Th2 cells, indicating a regulatory role of IL-12 (20,21).

Experiments similar to those described above indicate that IL-4 has a critical role in the disease process in experimental *L. major* infection. Administration of anti-IL-4 antibodies rescued otherwise susceptible mice from cutaneous leishmaniasis (11,22). Similarly, IL-4 injection following *L. major* infection of resistant mice caused a transient but significant shift in the pattern of cytokine secretion from Th1 to Th2. However, this change in the cytokine profile of T cells did not alter the outcome of infection, because these mice were able to self-cure (23). It is apparent that although IL-4 has a significant role in the development of cutaneous murine leishmaniasis, there may be other factors that are also important for the manifestation of disease.

CROSSREGULATION OF EFFECTOR CYTOKINE FUNCTIONS:

Leishmania parasites establish infection within macrophages, and their eventual elimination requires specific activation of macrophages. It has been shown that both IFN-γ and tumor necrosis factor-α (TNF-α) mediate their effects by inducing the production of nitric oxide (NO), which has direct parasiticidal activity (24–26). IL-4, IL-10, and transforming growth factor-β (TGF-β) down-regulate the IFN-γ–induced macrophage functions in vitro and thus may provide a survival advantage for the parasites (27–29). It is not known whether either IL-4 or IL-10 inhibit the antileishmanial activity of macrophages in vivo (30). TGF-β, however, appears to support the survival of the parasite in vivo. TGF-β is produced following *Leishmania* infection, and the virulence of *L. braziliensis* has been correlated with its ability to induce TGF-β (31,32). In the presence of TGF-β, multiplication of *Leishmania* parasites in cultured macrophages increased. Addition of anti-TGF-β antibodies to macrophage cultures decreased leishmanial infection. More importantly, in vivo administration of TGF-β to mice that are resistant to two different species of leishmanial parasites converted the mice to a susceptible phenotype. Conversely, administration of anti-TGF-β antibodies arrested lesion development in susceptible mice. In these mice, anti-TGF-β antibody treatment also shifted the pattern of cytokine production by lymph node cells from a Th2 to a Th1 phenotype (31). These studies suggest that crossregulation of cytokine function may exist in vivo and may have an important role in determining the outcome of *Leishmania* infection.

CD8+ T CELLS AS A SOURCE OF CYTOKINES:

The evidence presented supports the existence of a dichotomy in cytokine production by CD4+ T cells. A similar dichotomy in the pattern of cytokine secretion by human CD8+ T cells has become evident from studies of patients with leprosy (33). CD8+ T cells isolated from skin lesions of lepromatous patients produced IL-4, with little IFN-γ, whereas CD8+ T-cell clones from tuberculoid patients made IFN-γ but not IL-4. Although evidence for the presence of IL-4–secreting CD8+ T cells in murine leishmaniasis is lacking, evidence for a protective role for IFN-γ secreted by CD8+ T cells is building. Initial clues to the role of CD8+ T cells in protection against *L. major* infection came from irradiation experiments conducted in susceptible BALB/c mice. Sublethal irradiation, which depletes CD4+ T cells, converted susceptible BALB/c mice to disease-resistant mice (8). Although there was no ready explanation for these results, it has been recently shown that radioresistant CD8+ T cells were most likely responsible for this protection (34). Furthermore, in immunomodulated BALB/c mice, CD8+ cells were responsible for total IFN-γ and TNF-α production, and these cytokines were important for protection (35,36). The contribution of CD8+ T cells in the production of IFN-γ has also been confirmed in a murine model of *L. amazonensis* infection (37).

CYTOKINE RESPONSES IN HUMAN LEISHMANIASIS:

Studies of leishmaniasis in humans suggest that differential Th1/Th2 activation may have a role in determining the outcome of human infection. In humans with localized cutaneous leishmaniasis (less severe disease), type 1 cytokine transcripts, such as IL-2, IFN-γ, and TNF-β, were predominant in lesions. In contrast, in the chronic and destructive mucocutaneous form of leishmaniasis, both type 1 and type 2 cytokines, with relative abundance of IL-4 mRNA, were found in the lesions (38). Thus, although IL-4 production correlates with susceptibility to severe disease, IFN-γ production correlates with resistance to severe disease.

Leishmania donovani induces a progressive infection that leads to development of severe systemic disease, which may become fatal. Splenomegaly, lymphadenopathy, blockade of the reticuloendothelial system, fever, and weight loss are some notable symptoms. In acute human infections with *L. donovani*, high levels of IL-10 mRNA production have been reported. In these patients, mRNA for IL-2 and IFN-γ increased following treatment. Exogenously added IL-10 was found to inhibit the leishmanial antigen–induced proliferative response of peripheral blood lymphocytes from drug-cured individuals. Addition of anti-IL-10 antibody to peripheral blood lymphocyte (PBL) cultures obtained from patients with acute visceral leishmaniasis increased the proliferative response to leishmanial antigens (39). Thus it appears that progression to chronic disease in human leishmanial infection is associated with expression of Th2 cytokines, as seen in rodents. It remains to be determined whether cytokine-based therapy can be used to treat chronic disease.

Cytokines in the regulation of immunity against Trypanosoma cruzi

Trypanosoma cruzi, a hemoflagellate protozoan, causes Chagas' disease. Infection with this parasite may be acute or chronic. Chronic infection is associated with pathological reactions thought to have an autoimmune basis; the most affected organs are the heart, the esophagus, and the large intestine. Infection with this parasite causes profound immunosuppression in acute infections of mice and humans. The immunosuppression is associated with the lack of IL-2 production and IL-2 receptor expression (40,41). Administration of exogenous cytokines, such as IL-1, IL-2, and granulocyte-macrophage colony-stimulating factor (GM-CSF), can restore immune responsiveness in *T. cruzi*–infected mice (41–43). In vitro replication of this parasite can be effectively controlled by activation of macrophages with IFN-γ, GM-CSF, or TNF-α (44–47). IFN-γ is the most effective among these cytokines in controlling the parasite's replication. IFN-γ mediates its toxic effect by activation of NO in macrophages (4). CD8+ cells may be the source of this cytokine because depletion of this population of lymphocytes increases the susceptibility to disease (48).

IL-4, TGF-β, and IL-10 have been shown to enhance parasite survival by down-regulating the parasite killing mechanisms induced by other cytokines. The ability of IFN-γ to activate macrophages to kill *T. cruzi* was blocked by IL-4, TGF-β, and IL-10 (30,49,50). It appears that these effects are closely related to the ability of these cytokines to inhibit NO production. Thus, these cytokines can work to the advantage of the parasite by inhibiting the production of cytokines such as IFN-γ. The regulatory roles of IL-10 and TGF-β have also been studied by in vivo injection of either TGF-β or anti-IL-10 antibodies (49,50). These studies suggest that TGF-β and IL-10 enhance the susceptibility to *T. cruzi* infection in murine models. Thus, TGF-β given during the course of infection increased the parasitemia, led to early death, and suppressed the protective effects of IFN-γ (49).

The role of cytokines in the development of the tissue pathology associated with chronic infection is unclear. Accumulation of activated CD8+ T cells and TNF-α expressing macrophage-like cells in chagasic hearts from human autopsy material has been demonstrated (51). Because TNF-α has been shown to have a direct role in the process of fibrosis and in activation of cell adhesion molecules that serve as receptors for inflammatory cells, it has been proposed that this finding has some significant implications for the pathology of the disease (51).

Cytokine regulation in Toxoplasma gondii infection

In healthy immunocompetent individuals, *T. gondii* causes very mild acute infection and, very rarely, disease. Latent cyst stages persist in the tissues despite resolution of the acute infection. Immunocompromised individuals are susceptible to acute infection with this parasite, and they can suffer serious central nervous system (CNS) damage or blindness. When the onset of immunodeficiency follows primary infection, reactivation of latent tissue stages similarly leads to severe disease. Thus, *T. gondii* has emerged as a serious opportunistic infection in patients with acquired immunodeficiency syndrome (AIDS) (52). The mechanism underlying this disease process is less clear; however, rodent studies suggest that the immune system has a significant role in pathogenesis.

Cytokines such as IFN-γ and TNF-α have an important role in activation of tissue macrophages and microglial cells to inhibit parasite replication in vitro (53–57). Treatment of *T. gondii*–infected mice with anti-IFN-γ antibodies permits parasite multiplication in the brain, leading to eventual death. These findings suggest that the loss of CD4+ T cells in patients with AIDS, a major, although not exclusive, source for IFN-γ production, may contribute to reactivation of parasites. However, available evidence from rodent studies suggests that depletion of both CD4+ and CD8+ T cells is required (58). Although this finding suggests that CD4+ and CD8+ T cells may act synergistically to produce the IFN-γ needed to control infection, other sources of cytokines needed for protective immunity cannot be completely excluded. Indeed, in vivo administration of IL-12 prolongs the survival of SCID mice infected with *T. gondii* by activating IFN-γ production by NK cells (59).

In *T. gondii*–infected mice, cytokine production in the brain tissue during disease occurrence has been studied by quantitating polymerase chain reaction (PCR)–amplified mRNA transcripts (60,61). Cytokine transcripts for TNF-α, IL-6, and IL-4 were found within 10 days of infection, and by day 15, mRNA for IFN-γ was also found. The continued presence of IFN-γ and TNF-α during later stages of infection did not diminish the severity of disease (60,61). Because IL-4 and IL-10 can inhibit IFN-γ–mediated *T. gondii* killing by macrophages, it can be argued that IL-4 might have inhibited the protective role of IFN-γ in these mice (30,62). If this hypothesis is true, then anti-IL-4 antibodies should provide protection from the disease in these mice. Recent studies show that in advanced stages of AIDS, IL-10 levels increase, whereas the level of type 1 cytokines such as TNF-α decreases (63). It is an intriguing possibility that this shift in the cytokine pattern may favor activation of cysts to release the parasites, thus leading to disease. Despite these studies, it is still unclear why *T. gondii* specifically affects the brain. Additional studies are needed to understand the role of cytokines in the pathology of the disease.

ROLE OF CYTOKINES IN BLOOD-FORM PARASITIC INFECTIONS

Malaria and African sleeping sickness are two major blood-form parasitic infections that can be fatal to humans, and they are of major health concern in the tropical world. Babesiosis is an acute illness caused by *Babesia microti*, which is evolutionarily related to malarial parasites. We restrict our focus to malaria and African sleeping sickness.

African sleeping sickness

African sleeping sickness is caused by *Trypanosoma rhodesiense* and *T. gambiense,* and the tsetse fly is the vector for these parasites. Most of the experimental studies have been done with *T. brucei brucei,* which is the ancestor for these two species of parasites and which does not affect humans. These blood-dwelling parasites can eventually invade the CNS and ultimately lead to progressive loss of brain function, cachexia, and death (8). Because African trypanosomes live extracellularly, they are easy targets for antibody-mediated killing. However, these parasites normally escape from the antibody-mediated immune attack by altering their surface antigens, called variable surface glycoprotein (VSG) (64). Although it is unclear whether cytokines have any direct role in protective immunity, it is apparent that IFN-γ has a significant role in the immunosuppression caused by African trypanosomes. It has been demonstrated that NO and prostaglandins, which are released by IFN-γ–activated macrophages, suppress T-cell responses (65,66). Down-regulation of IL-2 receptors has been frequently found both in humans and mice (67,68). Anti-IFN-γ antibodies

have been shown to abrogate immunosuppression, including restoration of IL-2 receptor expression (66).

More importantly, recent studies have shown that IFN-γ is a growth factor for the trypanosome parasite (69). *T. brucei brucei* releases a lymphocyte triggering factor, which specifically triggers CD8+ T cells to produce IFN-γ. CD8 is the receptor for lymphocyte triggering factor because both anti-CD8 antibodies and soluble CD8 receptors inhibited IFN-γ production. In CD8– mice, *T. brucei brucei* infection caused low parasitemia, and these mice survived longer than CD8+ mice. Neutralization of IFN-γ with specific antibodies suppresses parasite growth in normal mice. These findings suggest that IFN-γ, in contrast to its strong protective role in American trypanosomiasis, serves as a virulence factor in African trypanosomiasis (69). Conversely, in earlier studies, significant levels of circulating IFN-γ were found in resistant but not in susceptible strains of mice (70). The reason for this apparent contradiction is not clear. It is possible that these parasites may use IFN-γ as their growth factor during their extracellular phase, but once phagocytosed by macrophages, they become susceptible to IFN-γ–mediated killing. In *T. rhodesiense*–infected mice, VSG-specific CD4+ T-helper cells that make IFN-γ but not IL-4 have also been identified (71). It remains to be tested whether these effector cells will be advantageous for the parasite or the host.

Cytokine expression in infected mice that manifest chronic meningoencephalitis has also been studied (72). In the brain tissues of affected mice, mRNA for TNF-α, MIP-1, IL-1, and IL-4 were commonly found. Cytokine transcripts for IFN-γ and IL-6 were found only in some of the outbred mice. Despite these findings, the role of these cytokines in the pathology of the disease is not well understood. TNF-α has been found to induce transient brain dysfunction that leads to coma in cancer patients during immunotherapy. Because patients suffering from African trypanosomiasis undergo progressive loss of brain function during terminal stages of infection, it may be worth investigating whether TNF-α has any role in this process.

Role of cytokines in the pathogenesis of cerebral malaria

Because the role of cytokines in malaria has been reviewed in another chapter, we limit our focus to cerebral malaria (CM), which is a major cause for most of the malaria-related deaths. Cerebral malaria is caused by the blood-stage parasites of *Plasmodium falciparum*, and it accounts for 1 to 2 million child deaths annually in Africa alone (73). The role of cytokines in CM has been extensively studied in both humans and mice, and we review how this knowledge will become useful in the development of cytokine-based immunotherapy and antidisease vaccines.

CLINICAL FEATURES OF CM: Cerebral malaria can be defined as a state of altered consciousness in a patient who has *P. falciparum* parasites in the blood and in whom no other cause of altered consciousness can be found (74). The features of CM include impaired consciousness, delirium, abnormal neurological symptoms, and usually convulsions. CM commonly develops over a period of days, but it may also occur rapidly with the onset of coma (74). In malaria-endemic regions, particularly Africa, children in whom antimalarial immunity has not yet developed are the most frequent victims of CM (73). However, nonimmune adults who travel to malaria-endemic regions are at high risk for development of CM. Cytoadherence of parasitized red blood cells (PRBC) in the cerebral microvasculature is a prominent feature in the pathology of human CM (75,76). Pathological studies indicate a higher degree of PRBC trapped in the cerebral microvascular areas of patients with CM (77). The actual cause of death in fatal cases of CM is still unknown.

CYTOKINES IN CM: CLINICAL AND LABORATORY STUDIES: Several clinical studies have attempted to determine the association between serum TNF-α levels and CM (78–80). In a Malawian study, it was shown that the mean serum level of TNF-α was higher in patients with *P. falciparum* infection who died than in those who survived (78). In another study involving children from The Gambia, a similar correlation between serum TNF-α levels and the severity of CM was reported (79). In this study, it was further reported that TNF-α was a better indicator of a fatal outcome in childhood CM than other parameters, such as parasite density and blood glucose levels. Although these studies show an association between serum TNF-α levels and the severity of CM, TNF-α concentrations were also found to be correlated with hyperparasitemia, young age, and anemia (78,80).

The difficulty in drawing general conclusions about the role of a given cytokine in the pathogenesis of CM from this type of clinical study is obvious. In most studies, cytokine levels were measured only when the patients reached the terminal stage of illness, instead of assessing the evolution of cytokine responses from infection to development of disease. To obtain such information, longitudinal epidemiological studies are needed, but there are several difficulties. First, because CM occurs in only approximately 1 to 2% of children living in malaria-endemic areas, thousands of children would have to be enrolled to ensure a sufficient number of patients with CM (73). Second, the onset of CM is unpredictable. Third, in most malaria-endemic areas, it is difficult to rule out the role of other infections or nutritional status on the cytokine cascade (74). Therefore, experimental studies using suitable animal models will be critical to the understanding of the role of the cytokine cascade in CM.

The role of TNF-α in CM has been studied using rodent models. Infection of CBA/Ca mice with *Plasmodium berghei* induces a fatal cerebral disease. In these mice, anti-TNF antibody treatment has been found to abrogate the symptoms of CM (81). However, it is difficult to extrapolate these findings to human CM because this rodent model does not reproduce the pathological features observed in human CM. *Plasmodium coatneyi*, a primate malaria parasite, induces CM in rhesus (*Macaca mulatta*) monkeys (82). The pathological features of CM in this model closely reflect the pathological characteristics of *P. falciparum*–induced CM in humans (82). The cytokine cascade in this nonhuman primate model has not been explored, and this experimental model may be valuable in determining the role of cytokines in CM.

CURRENT THEORIES TO EXPLAIN THE POSSIBLE ROLE OF TNF-α IN THE PATHOGENESIS OF CM: There are at least two theories that explain the role of TNF-α in the pathogenesis of CM. Clark and Cowden (83) proposed that TNF-α may be directly involved in CM by inducing the release of toxic compounds, such as NO, which may cause brain dysfunction. To support this hypothesis, these authors draw parallels between patients with tumors who received TNF-α therapy and patients with CM, both of whom seem to manifest similar neurological symptoms during illness. However, this theory fails to explain why malaria patients with *P. vivax* infections, who likewise produce high serum levels of TNF-α, fail to manifest the symptoms of CM (84).

An alternative hypothesis takes into account the role of TNF-α in inducing the expression of receptors for the cytoadherence of *P. falciparum* on microvascular endothelial cells (81). TNF-α activates expression of cell adhesion molecules such as ICAM-1, VCAM-1, and ELAM-1 on microvascular endothelial cells (85). These molecules on the cerebral microvascular endothelial cells serve as receptors for the binding of parasitized erythrocytes. Despite these findings, it is unclear how cytoadherence of parasites to cerebral microvascular endothelial cells triggers CM.

ROLE OF OTHER PROINFLAMMATORY CYTOKINES IN CM: The role of IL-1 in CM is unclear. Although in one report, plasma levels of IL-1 were found to correlate with severity of disease, others did not find any significant increase of IL-1 in patients with CM (86,87). In rodent studies, one group of investigators claimed that IL-1 treatment prevented CM and reduced parasitemia, whereas others failed to detect IL-1 in mice in which CM developed (86,88).

Serum IL-6 levels have generally been found to increase as the severity of disease increases in human *P. falciparum* infections (87); however, anti-IL-6 therapy does not prevent CM in the *P. berghei*–infected CBA/Ca mice (88). Combined administration of antibodies to GM-CSF and IL-3 or anti IFN-γ antibodies alone has been shown to prevent CM in a rodent model (88). In both instances, it was observed that these antibody treatments reduced TNF-α production, suggesting that GM-CSF, IL-3, and IFN-γ may have roles in CM by modulating the level of TNF-α.

These studies show a significant role for the pro-inflammatory cytokines (TNF-α and others) in the pathology of CM. However, it is not known whether IL-10, IL-4, and TGF-β have some down-regulatory role in the pathogenesis of CM. Understanding their role in pathology and protective immune responses to malaria may be helpful in developing prophylactic and therapeutic approaches to CM.

ROLE OF TNF-α INHIBITORS IN THE TREATMENT OF CM:

Because there is a strong clinical association between TNF-α levels and CM, the role of TNF-α inhibitors in the treatment of CM has been explored in rodent CM. Pentoxifylline and iloprost are potent inhibitors of TNF-α production induced by endotoxins in animals and humans (89–91). Pentoxifylline and iloprost have been shown to prevent *P. berghei*–induced cerebral malaria in CBA/Ca mice (92). Pentoxifylline selectively inhibits the TNF-α production, but not the IL-6 production, induced by malarial antigens in human and murine macrophages (93). In these experiments, it was confirmed that these drugs inhibited TNF-α production in vivo after malaria parasite infection (93). However, use of these drugs in the treatment of human CM has not been explored in detail.

Anti-TNF-α antibodies have been tried as an adjunct for the treatment of human CM in a pilot-scale clinical study (94). Although anti-TNF-α antibodies suppressed the high fever, their beneficial effect could not be established due to a limited sample size. A large scale clinical trial may be needed to determine the therapeutic value of anti-TNF antibodies in CM.

TNF-α–inducing malarial proteins (GPI-toxins) as targets of antidisease vaccine in malaria.

When schizonts rupture out of infected RBCs, a large quantity of soluble antigens is released. Some of these antigens contain phospholipids, which are probably linked to the protein moiety via a glycosyl phosphatidylinositol linkage (95,96). It has been shown that the phospholipid moiety of these proteins can directly activate macrophages to release TNF-α (95). Consistent with this find-

ing, antibodies made against the phospholipids have been shown to block TNF-α production induced by these antigens in vitro (97). Therefore, it has been proposed that an antidisease vaccine targeted to neutralize the TNF-inducing ability of these antigens can be developed. Recent experiments carried out in rodents seem to support this antidisease vaccine concept. In mice, phospholipid coupled to carrier proteins has been shown to induce antibodies that inhibit TNF-α production induced by malarial antigens (98). These mice were also protected from hypoglycemia, which is caused by TNF-α. Therefore, it will be of great interest to test whether the antidisease vaccine can induce protection against CM in humans.

ROLE OF CYTOKINES IN HELMINTH INFECTIONS

Compared with protozoa, helminths present a very different challenge to the immune system in terms of size, antigenic complexity, and lack (in most instances) of replication within the host. Studies of experimental helminth infections have a key role in furthering our understanding of the roles of Th1 and Th2 lymphocyte products in the immune response (5,99). Eosinophilia, mastocytosis, and elevated serum IgE levels, all hallmarks of active helminth infection, are stimulated by cytokine products of Th2 cells (6). These observations have fostered efforts to investigate the relative contribution of Th1 and Th2 lymphocytes to both immunity and disease in helminthic infection.

Experimental infections in intestinal helminths

The immunological basis of worm expulsion in experimentally infected animals has been the subject of both interest and debate for many years; both IgE and mucosal mast cells received a great deal of attention as potential mediators of the effector response (100–103). Although the precise events responsible for the elimination of worms from the gut are still not known, it is clear that these events are T-cell–dependent. In recent studies, two strategies have been employed to study the role of cytokines in protective immunity to intestinal helminths: (a) comparison of cytokine responses in resistant and susceptible strains of mice, and (b) elimination of specific cytokine responses by in vivo administration of anti-cytokine monoclonal antibodies. The results of these studies indicate that expression of a protective or a self-cure response may be host- as well as parasite-specific.

In studies with *Trichuris muris,* cytokine production was examined following infection of resistant and susceptible mouse strains (104,105). Following mitogenic stimulation, mesenteric lymph node cells (MLNC) from resistant BALB/k mice produced high levels of IL-5 and IL-9. In contrast, MLNC from susceptible B10.BR mice produced high levels of IFN-γ and little IL-5 or IL-9 in response to mitogen. These studies led the authors to conclude that the resistant phenotype was associated with the development of a Th2 antiparasite response.

Similar approaches have been applied to the study of *Trichinella spiralis,* with conflicting results. Th1 cells were implicated as the mediators of the protective intestinal immune response in the experiments of Pond and coworkers (106). Susceptible B10.BR mice mounted significantly higher serum IgE and *Trichinella*-specific IgG$_1$ and lower specific IgG$_{2a}$ responses than resistant AKR mice. Resistance was associated with higher levels of parasite antigen-induced IFN-γ and lower production of IL-4 by MLNC. The expression of resistance did not reflect a strict dichotomy between Th1 and Th2 activation in susceptible and resistant strains, however; Th1 and Th2 lymphokine production varied temporally as well as by anatomical compartment (107,108). In contrast, Grencis and colleagues (109) found comparable levels of Th2 cytokines and little IFN-γ production by MLNC from susceptible and resistant mouse strains in response to a *Trichinella* antigen preparation. In light of these conflicting results and the observation that anti-IFN antibody treatment did not affect the rate of worm expulsion (108), the self-cure response in *Trichinella*-infected mice is likely to be a complex process involving the participation of a number of T-cell–dependent mediators (110,111).

The contribution of eosinophils and IgE to antiparasite immunity has been studied in *Heligmosoides*-infected mice by administration of anticytokine or anti-IgE antibodies (112). Anti-IL-5 antibody reduced parasite-induced eosinophilia, but it did not prevent expression of protective immunity. Anti-IL-4 or anti-IL-4 receptor antibody, in contrast, blocked IgE production and inhibited protective immune responses. The relationship between IL-4 and protective immunity was apparently not a function of IgE production, however, because administration of anti-IgE did not prevent worm expulsion. The effect of anti-IL-4 in this model may be related to its effect on mast cells, T lymphocytes, or other cell lineages.

Questions regarding the exact role of mucosal mast cells in the response to intestinal helminths have persisted for nearly 20 years. Use of anti-IL-3 and anti-IL-4 antibodies decreased intestinal mastocytosis by 85 to 90% in *Nippostrongylus*-infected mice, but it did not retard worm elimination (113). In contrast, *Trichinella*-infected mice treated with monoclonal antibody directed against *c-kit*, the receptor for the stem-cell factor, had no mucosal mast-cell response to infection, and they were unable to expel the worms (114). The effect of this monoclonal antibody on other important cell lineages remains undefined, however. It is clear from these studies that a single lymphokine or cell type is unlikely to represent the effector mechanism responsible for parasite expulsion in any of these models. Worm expulsion reflects the congruence of both immunological and physiological events within the gut.

Few studies in humans have been designed to explore the immunological basis of the response directed against intestinal worms. Serological studies indicate the development of antibody responses to *Ascaris* and *Trichuris* (115–117); however, as discussed in greater detail in the section discussing helminth infections in humans, the broad spectrum of the antiparasite isotypic response does not lend itself to any conclusions regarding the predominance of Th1 or Th2 cells in human infection.

Schistosomiasis

Schistosome egg–induced granuloma formation has provided an excellent model to study the induction and modulation of the T-cell–dependent immunopathological processes of granuloma formation and fibrosis (118). T cells from mice with prepatent infections mount Th1 responses to antigens derived from adult worms or schistosomula. The onset of *S. mansoni* egg production is associated with the development of Th2 cells and a prominent IL-10 response, which leads to down-regulation of Th1 activity (119,120). IL-10 production by CD5 B cells can be induced by oligosaccharide residues on egg antigens (121). How this induction of IL-10 may be beneficial to the parasite is unclear.

Depletion studies with monoclonal antibodies have established the key role of IL-4 and IL-5 in granuloma formation and eosinophil recruitment, respectively, in both *S. mansoni* and *S. japonicum* infection (122–125). Anti-IFN-γ, in contrast, had little or no effect on granuloma size in *S. mansoni* infection (122,124), but it did affect granuloma size in *S. japonicum* infection (123). The contribution of IL-2 to granuloma formation is less clear. IL-2 augments granuloma formation in chronically infected mice (126), perhaps, in part, through its effect on IL-5 production (127). In addition, anti-IL-2 reduces granuloma formation and fibrosis in acute infection (128); however, IL-2 mRNA was not found in the granulomatous livers or mesenteric lymph nodes of either acute or chronically infected mice (129). These results imply that the role of IL-2 in cellular activation, expansion, or recruitment may occur at an anatomical site independent of the granuloma and draining lymph nodes.

In models of vaccine-induced immunity, protective responses are generated by Th1 lymphocytes. Following immunization with radiation-attenuated parasites, both spleen cells and lymph node cells produced significant levels of IFN-γ and IL-2 in response to antigens derived from schistosomules (130). Administration of anti-IL-4 or anti-IL-5 to vaccinated animals decreased serum IgE levels and abrogated eosinophilia, respectively, but neither antibody eliminated the protective immunity induced by irradiated cercariae (131). In contrast, anti-IFN-γ antibodies caused a significant reduction in the expression of the protective response in this model (131,132). Repeated immunization with attenuated parasites leads to a partial shift in the pattern of the lymphokine response (130). Production of IL-4 and IL-5 is increased in multiply immunized mice, particularly in draining lymph nodes, whereas splenocytes continue to display Th1 reactivity. Because the magnitude of the protective immune response is not diminished in multiply immunized animals, both Th1 and Th2 responses may contribute to the maximal expression of immunity.

The polar nature of clinical manifestations of many parasitic infections is consistent with the Th1/Th2 paradigm; however, conclusions emanating from experimental models of helminth infections regarding the relationship of lymphokines to protective immunity may not be directly applicable to humans. The nature of exposure and chronicity of human infection differ dramatically from typical experimental models, producing a much more complex immunological picture. Helminth infections in humans persist for years, multiple infections are the rule rather than the exception, and exposure to reinfection is virtually continuous. That this type of antigenic challenge has an effect on the expression of antiparasite immunity is evident from consideration of the clinical manifestations of helminth infection in long-term residents of endemic areas compared with transplants or expatriates. For example, travelers or recent migrants to an endemic area are far more likely to exhibit hyper-reactive syndromes on initial exposure to schistosome or filarial infection than long-term residents (133–135). In filarial infections, these clinical syndromes are characterized by high levels of serum IgE and eosinophilia, and they are consistent with a heightened anti-parasite Th2 response. The absence of comparable clinical syndromes in long-term residents implies that Th2 responses may also be modulated, either by chronic exposure to infective stages or by in utero exposure to parasite antigens or idiotypes directed against these antigens (136,137). Consequently, patterns of antigen-induced lymphokine production may be complex and difficult to reconcile with a strict dichotomy in Th1/Th2 activity.

Nonetheless, human helminth infections have provided insight into the regulation of eosinophilia and IgE responses. Helminth-infected persons had 2.5- and 5-fold more IL-4– and IL-5–producing cells in the PBMC population than uninfected individuals. A direct correlation between these two lymphokines and the frequencies of responding cells suggested that IL-4 and IL-5 regulation were linked (138). IgE production in people with high levels of circulating IgE was correlated with increased frequencies of IL-4–producing cells and parasite antigen–induced production of IL-4. Individuals with lower IgE levels mounted more prominent IFN-γ responses, indicating the importance of the reciprocal relationship of IL-4 and IFN-γ in the regulation of IgE production (139).

Cytokines and protective immunity

Definitive demonstration of protective immunity to schistosomes in humans is problematic. Epidemiological data demonstrate that both parasite prevalence and fecundity decline with age in human populations, suggesting that acquisition of protective immunity is age-dependent. Expression of immunity is thought to be dependent on reciprocal increases and decreases in antilarval IgE and IgG$_4$, respectively (140,141). This finding implies that IgE and IgG$_4$ responses may be differentially regulated.

Arguments regarding the existence of protective immunity in filariasis are also made on epidemiological grounds (142). In Bancroftian filariasis, evidence for protective immunity is found most easily in patients with lymphatic obstruction. In Haiti, persons with elephantiasis have significantly lower microfilaremia and antigenemia than other segments of the population (143) (Addiss DG, et al., unpublished observations). This difference is reflected also in higher proliferative responsiveness to filarial antigens, higher anti-filarial IgG$_2$ levels, and lower antifilarial IgG$_4$ levels among persons with elephantiasis than with microfilaremic individuals, responses that are consistent with preferential stimulation of Th1 cells (143–145). Antifilarial IgG$_4$ and IgE responses were dissociated; IgE levels were higher among patients with disease manifestations, suggesting differential stimulation of these isotypes in vivo (144). In patients with onchocerciasis, parasite antigen stimulated greater production of IL-2 in putatively immune individuals (146). IL-2 production was associated with higher levels of IL-5, suggesting that IL-5 may be involved in the expression of protective immunity.

Do helminth antigens preferentially induce Th2 responses?

The well-established relationship between helminth infection and IgE levels has led to the hypothesis that helminth antigens preferentially stimulate Th2 responses. In experimental models of filariasis, spleen cells from BALB/c mice immunized with radiation attenuated infective larvae (L3) of *Brugia pahangi* produced IL-5 and IL-9 in response to filarial antigen, but little IFN-γ (147). A bias toward Th2 responsiveness was seen also in mice given multiple injections of *B. malayi* microfilarial antigen (148). Similar shifts in responsiveness have also been noted following injection of irradiation attenuated schistosomula, as noted (130). Finkelman and Urban (149,150) proposed that this Th2 bias reflects a general tendency of proteolytic enzymes to induce Th2 responses.

As a practical consequence of the Th2 dominance of antihelminth responses, parasite-induced Th2 cytokines may skew the response to unrelated antigens. When *Schistosoma mansoni*–infected mice are immunized with sperm whale myoglobin, they produce less IL-2 and IFN-γ and more IL-4 following in vitro challenge with myoglobin than uninfected control animals (151). Similarly, the human immunodeficiency virus gp160–specific cytolytic response of spleen cells from mice infected with a vaccinia-gp160 construct was inhibited if the mice were coinfected with *S. mansoni* (152). This type of shift in cellular phenotype reflects the influence of cytokines on lymphocyte maturation during initial activation events. IL-4 and IL-12 are known to stimulate the differentiation of Th0 cells into Th2 and Th1 cells, respectively (19,153–155). Local production of IL-4 by schistosome egg granulomas is therefore likely to skew responses to unrelated antigens. IL-4 also is known to stimulate the differentiation of CD8+ cells into Th2 cytokine producing CD8–CD4– cells, an immunological phenomenon that could amplify further the tendency toward development of Th2 responses (156). The poor DTH responsiveness of individuals with high skin loads of *Onchocerca volvulus* microfilariae to common recall antigens may represent a clinical example of this effect (157,158).

Role of cytokines in establishment of chronic parasitic infections

A characteristic feature of many human helminth infections is their persistence. It is clear from studies of granuloma formation in murine models of schistosomiasis that chronic infections are associated with down-regulation of Th2 responses without a concomitant increase in Th1 responsiveness (129). Similar down-regulatory mechanisms are postulated to occur in chronic helminth infections in humans; in their absence, the re-emergence of responsiveness may lead to the onset of disease. In leprosy, both IL-4 and IL-10 have been proposed as potential mediators of immune regulation in lepromatous patients (33,159). IL-10 is an attractive candidate because of its production by a variety of cell types (160) and its pronounced effect on both Th1 and Th2 lymphocytes (161,162), as well as on macrophage function (160). The inability of all investigators to confirm a central role for IL-10 in the regulation of PBMC responses from all lepromatous leprosy patients may imply the existence of additional mechanisms (tolerance?) to control the expression of immunity in long-term infections (163). The effect of long-term antigen stimulation on the phenotype of lymphokine producing cells is also unclear. Are atypical

cells and patterns of lymphokine production inevitable consequences of chronic stimulation (164)?

UNIFYING PRINCIPLES AND FUTURE DIRECTIONS

Sweeping conclusions regarding the role of cytokines in antiparasite immunity are currently not possible. This uncertainty reflects, at least in part, the growing understanding of the pleiotropic nature of the cytokines, their production by a variety of cell types, and the inherently redundant nature of the immune response. It is clear that we do not know enough about the development of immune responses in vivo in terms of differences in antigen presentation, anatomical compartmentalization of cytokine responses, and the relationship between responses in different compartments.

A great deal of interest has been focused on the relationship between the lymphokine response of the host and the protective or pathological response to parasite infection. To what extent are cytokine responses beneficial to the parasite? Amiri and colleagues (165) demonstrated that schistosomes use TNF-α as a signal for egg production. As discussed, IFN-γ provides a growth signal to African trypanosomes (69). Similar examples of inter-relatedness of host and parasite will no doubt be found in other systems. Understanding the nature of the host-parasite equilibrium is critical to efforts to rationally intervene in the pathway from infection to disease.

REFERENCES

1. Warren KS. The global impact of parasitic disease. In: Englund PT, Sher A, eds. The biology of parasitism: a molecular and immunologic approach. New York: Alan R. Liss, 1988: 3–12.

2. Donelson JE, Rice-Ficht AC. Molecular biology of trypanosome antigenic variation. Microbiol Rev 1985;49:107–125.

3. Mosmann TR, Cherwinski H, Bond MW, Giedlin MA, Coffman RL. Two types of murine helper T cell clone I. Definition according to profiles of lymphokine activities and secreted proteins. J Immunol 1986;136:2348–2357.

4. Sher A, Coffman RL. Regulation of immunity to parasites by T cells and T cell derived cytokines. Annu Rev Immunol 1992;10:385–409.

5. Scott P, Pearce E, Cheever AW, Coffman RL, Sher A. Role of cytokines and CD4+ T cell subsets in the regulation of parasite immunity and disease. Immunol Rev 1989;112: 161–182.

6. Urban JF, Madden KB, Svetic A, et al. The importance of Th2 cytokines in protective immunity to nematodes. Immunol Rev 1992;127:205–220.

7. Cotran RS, Kumar V, Robbins SL, eds. Robbins pathologic basis of disease, ed 4. Philadelphia: W.B. Saunders, 1989.

8. Cox FE, Liew FY. T-cell subsets and cytokines in parasitic infections. Immunol Today 1992;13:445–448.

9. Sadick MD, Locksley RM, Tubbs C, Raff HV. Murine cutaneous leishmaniasis: resistance correlates with the capacity to generate interferon-gamma in response to leishmania antigens in vitro. J Immunol 1986;136:655–661.

10. Boom WH, Liebster L, Abbas AK, Titus RG. Patterns of cytokine secretion in murine leishmaniasis: correlation with disease progression or resolution. Infect Immun 1990;58:3863–3870.

11. Coffman RL, Varkila K, Scott P, Chatelain R. The role of cytokines in the differentiation of CD4$^+$ T cell subsets in vivo. Immunol Rev 1991;123:189–207.

12. Heinzel FP, Sadick MD, Holaday BJ, Coffman RL, Locksley RM. Reciprocal expression of interferon gamma or IL-4 during the resolution or progression of murine leishmaniasis. Evidence for expansion of distinct helper T cell subsets. J Exp Med 1989;169:59–72.

13. Heinzel FP, Sadick MD, Mutha SS, Locksley RM. Production of IFN-γ, IL-2, IL-4 and IL-10 by CD4$^+$ T lymphocytes in vivo during healing and progressive murine leishmaniasis. Proc Natl Acad Sci USA 1991;88:7011–7015.

14. Holaday BJ, Sadick MD, Wang J, et al. Reconstitution of Leishmania immunity in severe combined immunodeficient mice using Th1- and Th2-like cell lines. J Immunol 1991;147:1653–1658.

15. Titus RG, Muller I, Kimsey P, et al. Exacerbation of experimental murine cutaneous leishmaniasis with CD4$^+$ Leishmania major-specific T cell lines or clones which secrete interferon-γ and mediate parasite specific delayed type hypersensitivity. Eur J Immunol 1991;21:559–567.

16. Belosevic M, Finbloom DS, Van Der Meide PH, Slayter M, Nacy CA. Administration of monoclonal anti-IFN-γ antibodies in vivo abrogates natural resistance of C3H/HeN mice to infection with Leishmania major. J Immunol 1989;143:266–274.

17. Scott P. IFN-γ modulates the early development of Th1 and Th2 responses in a murine model of cutaneous leishmaniasis. J Immunol 1991;147:3149–3155.

18. Tobin JF, Reiner SL, Hatam F, et al. Transfected Leishmania expressing biologically active IFN-gamma. J Immunol 1993;150:5059–5069.

19. Hsieh C, Macatonia SE, Tripp CS, Wolf SF, O'Garra A, Murphy KM. Development of T$_H$1 CD4$^+$ T cells through IL-12 produced by listeria-induced macrophages. Science 1993;260:547–549.

20. Sypek JP, Chung CL, Mayor SE, et al. Resolution of cutaneous leishmaniasis: interleukin 12 initiates a protective T helper type 1 immune response. J Exp Med 1993;177:1797–1802.

21. Heinzel FP, Schoenhaut DS, Rerko RM, Rosser LE, Gately MK. Recombinant interleukin-12 cures mice infected with Leishmania major. J Exp Med 1993;177:1505–1509.

22. Sadick MD, Heinzel FP, Holaday BJ, Pu RT, Dawkins RS, Locksley RM. Cure of murine leishmaniasis with anti-interleukin-4 monoclonal antibody. Evidence for a T-cell department, IFN-γ independent mechanism. J Exp Med 1990;171:115–127.

23. Chatelain R, Varkila K, Coffman RL. IL-4 induces a Th-2 response in Leishmania major infected mice. J Immunol 1991;148:1182–1187.

24. Murray HW, Rubin BY, Rothermel CD. Killing of intracellular Leishmania donovani by lymphokine stimulated human mononuclear phagocytes. Evidence that interferon-gamma is the activating lymphokine. J Clin Invest 1983;72:1506–1510.

25. Bogdan C, Moll H, Solbach W, Rollinghoff M. Tumor-necrosis factor-alpha in combination with interferon-gamma, but not with interleukin-4 activates murine macrophages for elimination of Leishmania major amastigotes. Eur J Immunol 1990;20:1131–1135.

26. Liew FY, Li Y, Millot S. Tumor necrosis factor-alpha synergizes with IFN-gamma in mediating killing of Leishmania major through the induction of nitric oxide. J Immunol 1990;145:4306–4310.

27. Liew FY, Millot S, Li Y, Lelchuk R, Chan WL, Ziltener H. Macrophage activation by interferon-gamma from host protective T cells is inhibited by Interleukin(IL)3 and IL4 produced by disease promoting T cells in leishmaniasis. Eur J Immunol 1989;19:1227–1232.

28. Nelson BJ, Ralph P, Green SJ, Nacy CA. Differential susceptibility of activated macrophage cytotoxic effector reactions to the suppressive effects of transforming growth factor-beta 1. J Immunol 1991;146:1849.

29. Spits H, de Wall Malefyt R. Functional characterization of human IL-10. Int Arch Allergy Immunol 1992;99:8–15.

30. Sher A, Gazzinelli RT, Oswald IP, et al. Role of T-cell derived cytokines in the down regulation of immune responses in parasitic and retroviral infection. Immunol Rev 1992;127:183–204.

31. Barral-Netto M, Barral A, Brownell CE, Skeiky YA, Ellingsworth LR, Twardzik DR. Transforming growth factor-beta in leishmanial infection: a parasite escape mechanism. Science 1992;257:545–548.

32. Barral A, Barral-Netto M, Brownell CE, Twardzik DR, Reed SG. Transforming growth factor-beta as a virulence mechanism for Leishmania braziliensis. Proc Natl Acad Sci USA 1993;90:3442–3446.

33. Salgame P, Abrams JS, Clayberger C, Goldstein H, et al. Differing lymphokine profiles of functional subsets of human CD4 and CD8 clones. Science 1991;254:279–282.

34. Hill JO. Reduced numbers of CD4$^+$ suppressor cells with subsequent expansion of CD8$^+$ protective T cells as an explanation for the paradoxical state of enhanced resistance to Leishmania in T cell deficient BALB/c mice. Immunology 1991;72:282–286.

35. Muller I, Pedrazzini TH, Kropf P, Louis JA, Milon G. Establishment of resistance to Leishmania major infection in susceptible BALB/c mice requires parasite specific CD8$^+$ T cells. Int Immunol 1991;3:587–597.

36. Smith LE, Rodrigues M, Russel DG. The interaction betwen CD8$^+$ cytotoxic T cells and Leishmania infected macrophages. J Exp Med 1991;174:499–505.

37. Chan MM. T cell response in murine leishmania mexicana amazonensis infection: production of interferon-gamma by CD8$^+$ T cells. Eur J Immunol 1993;23:1181–1184.

38. Pirmez C, Yamamura M, Uyemura K, Paes-Oliveira M, Conceiçao-Silva F, Modlin RL. Cytokine patterns in the pathogenesis of human leishmaniasis. J Clin Invest 1993;91:139061395.

39. Ghalib HW, Piuvezam MR, Skeiky YA, et al. Interleukin 10 production correlates with pathology in human

Leishmania donovani infections. J Clin Invest 1993;92: 324–329.

40. Rottenberg M, Lindqvist C, Koman A, Segura EL, Orn A. Modulation of both interleukin-2 receptor expression and interleukin 2 production during experimental murine Trypanosoma cruzi infection. Scand J Immunol 1989; 30:65.

41. Reed SG, Inverso JA, Roters SB. Heterologous antibody responses in mice with chronic T. cruzi infection: depressed T helper function restored with supernatants containing IL-2. J Immunol 1984;133:1558.

42. Reed SG, Phil DL, Grabstein KH. Immune deficiency in chronic Trypanosoma cruzi infection: recombinant interleukin-1 restores Th function for antibody production. J Immunol 1989;142:2067.

43. Reed SG, Grabstein KH, Phil DL, Morrissey PJ. Recombinant granulocyte-macrophage colony stimulating factor restores deficient immune responses in mice with chronic Trypanosoma infections. J Immunol 1990;145:1564.

44. Plata F, Wietzerbin F, Pons FG, Falcoff E, Eisen H. Synergistic protection by specific antibodies and interferon against infection by T. cruzi in vitro. Eur J Immunol 1984; 14:930.

45. Reed SG. In vivo administration of recombinant IFN-gamma induces macrophage activation, and prevents acute disease immune suppression and death in experimental Trypanosoma cruzi infections. J Immunol 1988;140:4342.

46. Reed SG, Nathan CF, Phil DL, et al. Recombinant granulocyte-macrophage colony stimulating factor activates macrophages to inhibit Trypanosoma cruzi and release hydrogen peroxide. Comparison to interferon-gamma. J Exp Med 1987;66:1734.

47. De Titto EH, Catterall JR, Remington JS. Activity of recombinant tumor necrosis factor on Toxoplasma gondii and Trypanosoma cruzi. J Immunol 1986;137:1342.

48. Tarleton RL. Depletion of CD8+ T cells increases susceptibility and reverses vaccine-induced immunity in mice infected with Trypanosoma cruzi. J Immunol 1990;144:717–724.

49. Silva JS, Twardzik DR, Reed SG. Regulation of Trypanosoma cruzi infections in vitro and in vivo by transforming growth factor β (TGF-β). J Exp Med 1991;174:539–545.

50. Silva JS, Morrissey PJ, Grabstein KH, Mohler KM, Anderson D, Reed SG. Interleukin 10 and interferon γ regulation of experimental trypanosoma cruzi infection. J Exp Med 1992;175:169–174.

51. Reis DD, Jones EM, Tostes S Jr, et al. Characterization of inflammatory infiltrates in chronic chagasic myocardial lesions: presence of tumor necrosis factor-α+ cells and dominance of granzyme A+, CD8+ lymphocytes. Am J Trop Med Hyg 1993;48:637–644.

52. Frenkel JK. Pathophysiology of toxoplasmosis. Parasitol Today 1988;4:273.

53. Suzuki Y, Orellana MA, Schreiber RD, Remington JS. Interferon-γ: the major mediator of resistance against Toxoplasma gondii. Science 1988;240:516.

54. Chang HR, Grau GE, Pechere JC. Role of TNF and IL-1 in infection with Toxoplasma gondii. Immunology 1990; 69:33.

55. Sibley LD, Adams LB, Fukutomi Y, Krahenbuhl JL. Tumor

necrosis factor-α triggers antitoxoplasmal activity of IFN-γ primed macrophages. J Immunol 1991;147:2340.

56. Chao CC, Hu S, Gekker G, Novick WJ Jr, Remington JS, Peterson PK. Effects of cytokines on multiplication of Toxoplasma gondii in microglial cells. J Immunol 1993;150: 3404–3410.

57. Suzuki Y, Remington JS. The effect of anti-interferon-γ antibody on the protective effect of Lyt-2 immune T cells against toxoplasmosis in mice. J Immunol 1990;144:1954.

58. Gazzinelli R, Xu Y, Cheever A, Sher A. Simultaneous depletion of CD4+ and CD8+ T lymphocytes is required to reactivate chronic infection with Toxoplasma gondii. J Immunol 1992;149:175–180.

59. Gazzinelli RT, Hieny S, Wynn TA, Wolf S, Sher A. Interleukin 12 is required for the T-lymphocyte independent induction of interferon gamma by an intracellular parasite and induces resistance in T cell deficient hosts. Proc Natl Acad Sci USA 1993;90:6115–6119.

60. Hunter CA, Roberts CW, Murray M, Alexander J. Detection of cytokine mRNA in the brains of mice with toxoplasmic encephalitis. Parasite Immunol 1992;14:405–413.

61. Hunter CA, Robert CW, Murray M, Alexander J. Kinetics of cytokine mRNA production in the brains of mice with progressive toxoplasmic encephalitis. Eur J Immunol 1992;22:2312–2317.

62. Gazzinelli RT, Oswald IP, James SL, Sher A. IL-10 inhibits parasite killing and nitrogen oxide production by IFN-γ activated macrophages. J Immunol 1992;148:1792–1796.

63. Clerici M, Shearer GM. A TH1-TH2 switch is a critical step in the etiology of HIV infection. Immunol Today 1993;14: 107–111.

64. Cross GAM. Cellular and genetic aspects of antigenic variation in trypanosomes. Ann Rev Immunol 1990;8:83–110.

65. Sternberg J, McGuigan F. Nitric oxide mediates suppression of T cell responses in murine Trypanosoma brucei infection. Eur J Immunol 1992;22:2741–2744.

66. Darji A, Sileghem M, Heremans H, Brys L, De Baetselier P. Inhibition of T cell responsiveness during experimental infections with Trypanosoma brucei: active involvement of endogenous gamma interferon. Infect Immun 1993; 61:3098–3102.

67. Sileghem M, Darji A, De Baetselier P. In vitro simulation of immunosuppression caused by Trypanosoma brucei. Immunology 1991;73:246–248.

68. Kierszenbaum F, Muthukkumar S, Beltz LA, Sztein MB. Suppression of Trypanosoma brucei rhodesiense of the capacities of human T lymphocytes to express interleukin-2 receptors and proliferate after mitogenic stimulation. Infect Immun 1991;59:3518–3522.

69. Olsson T, Bakhiet M, Hojeberg B, et al. CD8 is critically involved in lymphocyte activation by a T. brucei brucei-released molecule. Cell 1993;72:715–727.

70. De Gee AL, Sonnenfeld G, Mansfield JM. Genetics of resistance to the African trypanosomes. V. Qualitative and quantitative differences in interferon production among susceptible and resistant mouse strains. J Immunol 1985;134:2723.

71. Schleifer KW, Filutowicz H, Schopf LR, Mansfield JM. Characterization of T helper cell responses to the trypanosome variant surface glycoprotein. J Immunol 1993;150: 2910–2919.

72. Hunter CA, Jennings FW, Kennedy PG, Murray M. Astrocyte activation correlates with cytokine production in central nervous system of Trypanosoma brucei brucei-infected mice. J Lab Invest 1992;67:635–642.

73. Greenwood B, Marsh K, Snow, R. Why do some African children develop severe malaria? Parasitol Today 1991;7:277–281.

74. World Health Organization. Severe and complicated malaria. Trans R Soc Trop Med Hyg 1986;80 (suppl):1–50.

75. Trager W, Rudzinska MA, Bradbury PC. The fine structure of Plasmodium falciparum and its host erythrocyte in natural malarial infections in man. Bull WHO 1966;35: 883–885.

76. MacPherson GG, Warrell MJ, White NJ, Looareesuwan S, Warrell DA. Human cerebral malaria. A quantitative ultrastructural analysis of parasitized erythrocytes sequestration. Am J Pathol 1985;119:385–401.

77. Aikawa M, Iseki M, Barnwell JW, Taylor D, Oo MM, Howard RJ. The pathology of human cerebral malaria. Am J Trop Med Hyg 1990;43 (suppl):30–37.

78. Grau GE, Taylor TE, Molyneux ME, et al. Tumor necrosis factor and disease severity in children with falciparum malaria. N Engl J Med 1989;320:1586–1591.

79. Kwiatkowski D, Hill AV, Sambou I, et al. TNF concentration in fatal cerebral, non-fatal cerebral, and uncomplicated Plasmodium falciparum malaria. Lancet 1990;336: 1201–1204.

80. Shaffer N, Grau GE, Hedberg K, et al. Tumor necrosis factor and severe malaria. J Infect Dis 1991;163:96–101.

81. de Kossodo S, Grau GE. Role of cytokines molecules in malaria immunopathology. Stem Cells (Dayt) 1993;11:41–48.

82. Aikawa M, Brown A, Smith CD, et al. A primate model for human cerebral malaria: Plasmodium coatneyi-infected rhesus monkeys. Am J Trop Med Hyg 1992;46:391–397.

83. Clark IA, Cowden WB. Roles of TNF in malaria and other parasitic infections. Immunol Ser 1992;56:365–407.

84. Karunaweera ND, Grau GE, Gamage P, Carter R, Mendis KN. Dynamics of fever and serum levels of tumor necrosis factor are closely associated during clinical paroxysms in Plasmodium vivax malaria. Proc Natl Acad Sci USA 1992; 89:3200–3203.

85. Mantovani A, Bussolono F, Dejana E. Cytokine regulation of endothelial cell function. FASEB J 1992;6:2591–2599.

86. Titus RG, Sherry B, Cerami A. The involvement of TNF, IL-1 and IL-6 in the immune response to protozoan parasites. Immuno Parasitol Today 1991;7:A13–A16.

87. Molyneux ME, Taylor TE, Wirima JJ. TNF and IL-6 in malaria. Lancet 1991;337–1098.

88. Grau GE, Piguet P-F, Pointaire P, Mazier D. Cytokines and malaria: duality of effects in pathology and protection. In: Kunkel SL, Remick DG, eds. Cytokines in health and disease. New York: Marcel Dekker 1992:197–216.

89. Hakin J, Mandell GL, Novick WJ Jr, eds. Pentoxifylline and analogues: effects on leukocyte function. Sommerville: Karger, 1990.

90. Schonharting MM, Scade UF. The effect of pentoxifylline in septic shock—new pharmacological aspects of an established drug. J Med Clin Exp Theoret 1989;20:97–105.

91. Silwa K, Grundmann HJ, Neifer S, et al. Prevention of murine cerebral malaria by a stable prostacyclin analog. Infect Immun 1991;59:3846–3848.

92. Kremser PG, Grundmann H, Neifer S, et al. Pentoxifylline prevents murine cerebral malaria. J Infect Dis 1991; 164:605–608.

93. Prada J, Prager C, Neifer S, Bienzle U, Kremsner P. Production of interleukin-6 by human and murine mononuclear leukocytes stimulated with Plasmodium antigens is enhanced by pentoxifylline, and tumor necrosis factor secretion is reduced. Infect Immun 1993;61:2737–2740.

94. Kwiatkowski D, Molyneux ME, Stephens et al. Anti-TNF therapy inhibits fever in cerebral malaria. Q J Med 1993; 86:91–98.

95. Bate CAW, Taverne J, Roman E, Moreno C, Playfair JHL. Tumour necrosis factor induction by malaria exoantigens depends upon phospholipid. Immunology 1992;75:129–135.

96. Schofield L, Hackett F. Signal transduction in host cells by a glycosylphosphatidylinositol toxin of malaria parasites. J Exp Med 1993;177:145–153.

97. Bate CA, Taverne J, Bootsma HJ, et al. Antibodies against phosphatidylinositol and inositol monophosphate specifically inhibit tumour necrosis factor induction by malaria exoantigens. Immunology 1992;76:35–41.

98. Bate CA, Taverne J, Kwiatkowski D, Playfair JH. Phospholipids coupled to a carrier induce IgG antibody that blocks necrosis factor induction by toxic malaria antigens. Immunology 1993;79:138–145.

99. Finkelman FD, Pearce EJ, Urban JF Jr, Sher A. Regulation and biological function of helminth-induced cytokine responses. Immunoparasitol Today 1991;12:A62–A66.

100. Ogilvie BM, Love RJ. Co-operation between antibodies and cells in immunity to a nematode parasite. Transplant Rev 1974;19:147–168.

101. Woodbury RG, Miller HRP, Huntley JF, Newlands GFJ, Palliser AC, Wakelin D. Mucosal mast cells are functionally active during spontaneous expulsion of intestinal nematode infections in rat. Nature 1984;312:459–461.

102. Hagan P. IgE and protective immunity to helminth infections. Parasite Immunol 1993;15:1–4.

103. Pritchard DI. Immunity to helminths: it too much IgE parasite- rather than host-protective? Parasite Immunol 1993; 15:5–9.

104. Else KJ, Grencis RK. Cellular immune responses to the murine nematode parasite Trichuris muris. I. Differential cytokine production during acute or chronic infection. Immunology 1991;72:508–513.

105. Else KJ, Hultner L, Grencis RK. Cellular immune responses to the murine nematode parasite Trichuris muris. II. Differential induction of TH-cell subsets in resistant versus susceptible mice. Immunology 1992;75:232–237.

106. Pond L, Wassom DL, Hayes CE. Evidence for differential induction of helper T cell subsets during Trichinella spiralis infection. J Immunol 1989;143:4232–4237.

107. Kelly EAB, Cruz ES, Hauda KM, Wassom DL. IFN-γ and IL-5 producing cells compartmentalize to different lymphoid organs in Trichinella spiralis-infected mice. J Immunol 1991;147:306–311.

108. Pond L, Wassom DL, Hayes CE. Influence of resistant and susceptible genotype, IL-1 and lymphoid organ on

Trichinella spiralis-induced cytokine secretion. J Immunol 1992;149:957–965.

109. Grencis RK, Hultner L, Else KJ. Host protective immunity to Trichinella spiralis in mice: activation of Th cell subsets and lymphokine secretion in mice expressing different response phenotypes. Immunology 1991;74:329–332.

110. Wakelin D. Immunogenetic and evolutionary influences on the host-parasite relationship. Dev Comp Immunol 1992;16:345–353.

111. Wakelin D. Allergic inflammation as a hypothesis for the expulsion of worms from tissues. Parasitol Today 1993; 9:115–116.

112. Urban JF Jr, Katona IM, Paul WE, Finkelman FD. Interleukin 4 is important in protective immunity to a gastrointestinal nematode infection in mice. Proc Natl Acad Sci USA 1991;88:5513–5517.

113. Madden KB, Urban JF Jr, Ziltener HJ, Schrader JW, Finkelman FD, Katona IM. Antibodies to IL-3 and IL-4 suppress helminth-induced intestinal mastocytosis. J Immunol 1991; 147:1387–1391.

114. Grencis RK, Else KJ, Huntley JF, Nishikawa SI. The in vivo role of stem cell factor (c-kit ligand) on mastocytosis and host protective immunity to the intestinal nematode Trichinella spiralis in mice. Parasite Immunol 1993;15:55–59.

115. Haswell-Elkins M, Kennedy MW, Maizels RM, Elkins DB, Anderson RM. The antibody recognition profile of naturally infected humans against Ascaris lumbricoides larval ES antigen. Parasite Immunol 1989;11:615–627.

116. Bundy DAP, Lillywhite JE, Didier JM, Simmons I, Bianco AE. Age-dependency of infection status and serum antibody levels in human whipworm (Trichuris trichiura) infection. Parasite Immunol 1991;13:629–638.

117. Needham CS, Bundy DAP, Lillywhite JE, Didier JM, Simmons I, Bianco AE. The relationship between Trichuris trichiura transmission intensity and the age-profiles of parasite-specific antibody isotypes in two endemic communities. Parasitology 1992;105:273–283.

118. Phillips SM, Lammie PJ. Immunopathology of granuloma formation and fibrosis in schistosomiasis. Parasitol Today 1986;2:296–302.

119. Pearce EJ, Caspar P, Grzych J-M, Lewis FA, Sher A. Down regulation of Th1 cytokine production accompanies induction of Th2 responses by a parasitic helminth, Schistosoma mansoni. J Exp Med 1991;173:159–166.

120. Sher A, Fiorentin D, Caspar, P, Pearce EJ, Mossman T. Production of IL-10 by CD4+ T lymphocytes correlates with down-regulation of Th1 cytokine synthesis in helminth infection. J Immunol 1991;147:2713–2716.

121. Palanivel V, Harn DA. LNFPIII stimulated B220+ cells produce IL-10 and may contribute to down regulation of Th1 CD4+ T cells. J Immunol 1993;150:7A.

122. Sher A, Coffman RL, Hieny S, Scott P, Cheever AW. Interleukin-5 (IL-5) is required for the blood and tissue eosinophilia, but not granuloma formation induced by infection with Schistosoma mansoni. Proc Natl Acad Sci USA 1990; 87:61–65.

123. Cheever AW, Xu Y, Sher A, Macedonia JG. Analysis of egg granuloma formation in Schistosoma japonicum-infected mice treated with antibodies to interleukin-5 and gamma interferon. Infect Immun 1991;59:4071–4074.

124. Chensue SW, Terebuh PD, Warmington KS, et al. Role of IL-4 and IFN-γ in Schistosoma mansoni egg-induced hypersensitivity granuloma formation. Orchestration, relative contribution, and relationship to macrophage function. J Immunol 1992;148:900–906.

125. Yamashita T, Boros DL. IL-4 influences IL-2 production and granulomatous inflammation in schistosomiasis mansoni. J Immunol 1992;149:3659–3666.

126. Mathew RC, Ragheb S, Boros DL. Recombinant interleukin-2 therapy reverses diminished granulomatous responsiveness in anti-L3T4 treated S. mansoni infected mice. J Immunol 1990;144:4356–4361.

127. Metwali A, Elliot D, Mathew R, Blum A, Weinstock JV. IL-2 contributes to the IL-5 responses in granulomas from mice infected with Schistosoma mansoni. J Immunol 1993;150: 536–542.

128. Cheever AW, Finkelman FD, Caspar P, Hieny S, Macedonia JG, Sher A. Treatment with anti-IL-2 antibodies reduces hepatic pathology and eosinophilia in Schistosoma mansoni-infected mice while selectively inhibiting T cell IL-5 production. J Immunol 1992;148:3244–3248.

129. Henderson GS, Lu X, McCurley TL, Colley DG. In vivo molecular analysis of lymphokines involved in the murine immune response during Schistosoma mansoni infection. II. Quantification of IL-4 mRNA, IFN- mRNA, and IL-2 mRNA levels in the granulomatous livers, mesenteric lymph nodes, and spleens during the course of modulation. J Immunol 1992;148:2261–2269.

130. Caulada-Benedetti Z, Al-Zamel F, Sher A, James S. Comparison of Th1- and Th2-associated immune reactivities stimulated by single versus multiple vaccination of mice with irradiated Schistosoma mansoni cercariae. J Immunol 1991;146:1655–1660.

131. Sher A, Coffman RL, Hieny S, Cheever AW. Ablation of eosinophil and IgG responses with anti-IL-5 or anti-IL-4 antibodies fails to affect immunity against Schistosoma mansoni in the mouse. J Immunol 1990;145:3911–3916.

132. Smythies LE, Coulson PS, Wilson RA. Monoclonal antibody to IFN-modifies pulmonary inflammatory responses and abrogates immunity to Schistosoma mansoni in mice vaccinated with attenuated cercariae. J Immunol 1992; 149:3654–3658.

133. Beaver PC. Filariasis without microfilaremia. Am J Top Med Hyg 1970;19:181–189.

134. Butterworth AE, Corbett EL, Dunne DW, et al. Immunity and morbidity in human schistosomiasis. In: McAdam KPWJ, ed. New strategies in parasitology. New York: Churchill Livingstone, 1989:193–214.

135. Klion AD, Massougbodji A, Sadeler B-C, Ottesen EA, Nutman TB. Loiasis in endemic and nonendemic populations: immunologically mediated differences in clinical presentation. J Infect Dis 1991;163:1318–1325.

136. Colley DG. Occurrence, roles, and uses of idiotypes and anti-idiotypes in parasitic diseases. In: Cierny J, Hiernaux J, eds. Idiotypic networks and disease. Washington, D.C.: American Society for Microbiology 1990:71–105.

137. Lammie PJ, Hitch WL, Walker EM, Hightower AW, Eberhard ML. Maternal filarial infection as a risk factor for infection in children. Lancet 1991;337:1005–1006.

138. Mahanty S, Abrams JS, King CL, Limaye AP, Nutman TB.

Parallel regulation of IL-4 and IL-5 in human helminth infections. J Immunol 1992;148:3567–3571.

139. King CL, Low CC, Nutman TB. IgE production in human helminth infection. J Immunol 1993;150:1873–1880.

140. Hagan P, Blumenthal UJ, Dunn D, Simpson AJ, Wilkins HA. Human IgE, IgG4, and resistance to reinfection with Schistosoma haematobium. Nature 1991;349:243–245.

141. Capron AR. Immunity to schistosomes. Curr Opin Immunol 1992;4:419–4424.

142. Day, KP, Gregory WF, Maizels RM. Age-specific acquisition of immunity to infective larvae in a bancroftian filariasis endemic area of Papua New Guinea. Parasite Immunol 1991;13:377–390.

143. Lammie PJ, Addiss DG, Leonard G, Hightower AW, Eberhard ML. Heterogeneity in filarial specific immune responsiveness among patients with lymphatic obstruction. J Infect Dis 1993;167:1178–1183.

144. Kurniawan A, Yazdanbakhsh M, van Ree R, et al. Differential expression of IgE and IgG4 specific antibody responses in asymptomatic and chronic human filariasis. J Immunol 1993;150:3941–3950.

145. Yazdanbakhsh M, Paxton WA, Kruize YCM, et al. T cell responsiveness correlates differentially with antibody isotype levels in clinical and asymptomatic filariasis. J Infect Dis 1993;167:925–931.

146. Steel C, Nutman TB. Regulation of IL-5 in onchocerciasis. A critical role for IL-2. J Immunol 1993;150:5511–5518.

147. Bancroft AJ, Grencis RK, Else KJ, Devaney E. Cytokine production in BALB/c mice immunized with radiation attenuated third stage larvae of the filarial nematode, Brugia pahangi. J Immunol 1993;150:1395–1402.

148. Pearlmann E, Hazlett FE, Boom WH, Kazura JW. Induction of murine T-helper-cell responses to the filarial nematode Brugia malayi. Infect Immun 1993;61:1105–1112.

149. Finkelman FD, Urban JF Jr. Cytokines: making the right choice. Parasitol Today 1992;8:311–314.

150. Urban JF Jr, Madden KB, Svetic A, et al. The importance of Th2 cytokines in protective immunity to nematodes. Immunol Rev 1992;127:205–220.

151. Kullberg MC, Pierce EJ, Hieny S, Sher A, Berzofsky JA. Infection with Schistosoma mansoni alters Th1/Th2 cytokine responses to a non-parasite antigen. J Immunol 1992;148:3264–3270.

152. Actor JK, Shirai M, Kullberg MC, et al. Helminth infection results in decreased virus-specific CD8+ cytotoxic T-cell and Th1 cytokine responses as well as delayed virus clearance. Proc Natl Acad Sci USA 1993;90:948–952.

153. Romagnani S. Induction of Th1 and Th2 responses: a key role for the 'natural' immune response? Immunol Today 1992;13:379–381.

154. Seder RA, Paul WE, Davis MM, Fazekas de St. Groth B. The presence of interleukin 4 during in vitro priming determines the lymphokine-producing potential of CD4+ T cells from T cell receptor transgenic mice. J Exp Med 1992; 176:1091–1098.

155. Maggi E, Parronchi P, Manetti R, et al. Reciprocal regulatory effects of IFN-γ and IL-4 on the in vitro development of human Th1 and Th2 clones. J Immunol 1992;148:2142–2147.

156. Erard F, Wild M-T, Garcia-Sanz JA, Le Gros G. Switch of CD8 T cells to noncytolytic CD8-CD4- cells that make Th2 cytokines and help B cells. Science 1993;260:1802–1805.

157. Greene BM, Fanning MM, Ellner JJ. Non-specific suppression of antigen-induced blastogenesis in Onchocerca volvulus infection in man. Clin Exp Immunol 1983;52:259–265.

158. Sobosolay PT, Dreweck CM, Hoffmann WH, et al. Ivermectin-facilitated immunity in onchocerciasis. Reversal of lymphocytopenia, cellular anergy, and deficient cytokine production after single treatment. Clin Exp Immunol 1992;89:407–413.

159. Sieling PA, Abrams JS, Yamamura M, et al. Immunosuppressive roles for IL-10 and IL-4 in human infection. In vitro modulation of T cell responses in leprosy. J Immunol 1993;150:5501–5510.

160. Moore KW, O'Garra A, de Waal Malefyt R, Vieira P, Mosmann TR. Interleukin 10. Ann Rev Immunol 1993; 11:165–190.

161. Del Prete G, De Carli M, Alerigogna F, et al. Human IL-10 is produced by both type 1 helper (Th1) and type 2 helper (Th2) T cell clones and inhibits their antigen-specific proliferation and cytokine production. J Immunol 1993;150:353–360.

162. de Waal Malefyt R, Yssel H, de Vries JE. Direct effects of IL-10 on subsets of human CD4+ T cell clones and resting T cells. J Immunol 1993;150:4754–4765.

163. Mutis T, Kraakman EM, Cornelisse YE, et al. Analysis of cytokine production by Mycobacterium-reactive T cells. Failure to explain Mycobacterium leprae-specific non-responsiveness of peripheral blood T cells from lepromatous leprosy patients. J Immunol 1993;150:4641–4651.

164. Estes DM, Turaga PSD, Sievers KM, Teale JM. Characterization of an unusual cell type (CD4+ CD3–) expanded by helminth infection and related to the parasite stress response. J Immunol 1993;150:1846–1856.

165. Amiri P, Locksley RM, Parslow TG, et al. Tumor necrosis factor restores granulomas and induces parasite egg-laying in schistosome-infected SCID mice. Nature 1992;356:604–607.

CHAPTER 32

DIRECT EFFECT OF CYTOKINES ON MICROORGANISMS

Michel Denis and Reuven Porat

Increasing attention is being given to the importance of cytokines in host resistance to infectious agents, as well as in a variety of physiological and pathophysiological manifestations. It is clear that these molecules will be used as immunoadjuvants in a variety of situations (i.e., immunodeficiency, cancer, and infectious disease). Infectious agents have been exposed to cytokines for thousands of years, and it seems certain that successful pathogens have adapted to their chosen environments. Successful bacterial and parasitic pathogens have adapted remarkably to first-line antibiotics, via, for example, the synthesis and transfer of genes coding for enzymes that confer resistance to these products. Given the fact that bacteria have been exposed to first-line antibiotics in hosts for only the last 50 years, it would make intuitive sense that successful pathogens would have reacted to, and attempted to use, the presence of cytokines in the host's biological fluids to which they have been exposed for so much longer.

We attempt to review some recent evidence that suggests bacteria/parasites and viruses have adapted to cytokine environments. In some cases, microbes use these molecules as growth factors, whereas in other cases (mostly viruses), infectious pathogens capture genetic information for immunosuppressive cytokines or for soluble receptors of cytokines important in host resistance. We begin this chapter with a short review of the indirect antibacterial effect of cytokines, which we believe is important to gain some perspective for subsequent sections.

Most of the information that pertains to the direct effect of cytokines on micro-organisms is relatively recent, and some of it is quite controversial. This is a young, complex, and unclear field of investigation; several more years of study are needed to fully clarify the interaction between microbes and cytokines in the "big picture" of infectious disease.

CYTOKINE IMMUNOTHERAPY

Cytokines regulate a wide variety of cellular functions, and they are active on numerous cell types; they are small molecular weight proteins (1). Many of these metabolites have growth factor activities, such as the lymphocyte growth factors interleukin-2 (IL-2) and IL-4, as well as some others that promote growth and differentiation of uncommitted progenitor cells, such as granulocyte-macrophage colony-stimulating factor (GM-CSF), granulocyte CSF (G-CSF), and IL-3 (2,3). Another group of important cytokines is composed of tumor necrosis factor-α (TNF-α), IL-6, and IL-1 (4); these proinflammatory cytokines mediate responses that occur after an inflammatory or an infectious stimulus.

IL-1, IL-6, and TNF are believed to function as stress hormones of the immune system. They are produced mainly by macrophages and monocytes as a first-line response to infections (5). These three cytokines function individually or in concert as (a) activators of the hepatic acute-phase response involved in production of acute-phase proteins, such as serum amyloid A, C-reactive protein (CRP), fibrinogen, and complement components; (b) endogenous pyrogens responsible for the fever response seen in infections; (c) stimulators of the production of important chemotactic agents, such as IL-8, which is involved in excessive neutrophilia; and (d) leukocyte activators. Indeed, these molecules are involved in increasing the phagocytic and the cytotoxic activity of neutrophils and macrophages, including degranulation of neutrophils and their release of reactive oxygen intermediates (6,7). In addition, they are catabolic agents responsible for redirecting peripheral energy reserves to the acute metabolic demands of the inflammatory response. Obviously, an excess of this response is responsible for the cachexia associated with a number of chronic infectious diseases, such as tuberculosis (8).

One final role for these proinflammatory cytokines is as enhancers of the tissue remodeling that occurs after an infectious episode by virtue of their role in fibroblast proliferation, cartilage and bone resorption, and production of collagenase and protease (8). An obvious side effect of this response is tissue fibrosis, as well as excess tissue destruction, which is observed in chronic infectious diseases (8).

An interesting feature of all cytokines studied thus far are their pleiotropic effects on various cell types. For instance, IL-2, which was originally described as a T-lymphocyte growth factor, how now been shown to possess a wide variety of effects on a large spectrum of cells. IL-2 may contribute to macrophage activation by binding to the P55 receptors present on these cells; it also enhances B-cell growth, causes a polyclonal immunoglobulin M (IgM) response, and it appears to have unexpected effects on vascular cells as well as nerve cells (3,9). These varied effects of any cytokine explain the difficulty of dissecting the impact of cytokine infusion on host resistance to infections or other end-points.

Given their central role in protection against a variety of infectious agents, cytokines have recently been used as adjuvant material in protection against infection. In vivo infusion of high doses of recombinant IL-2 has been shown to protect mice against gram-negative bacterial sepsis (10). Relatively high doses of IL-2 had to be used, and the effect was not clarified, but it appeared to be related to a polyclonal IgM response and enhanced clearance of bacteria from the infected tissues (11). IL-2 has also been used to enhance resistance against a number of more chronic infectious agents, such as mycobacteria (12,13). In a mouse model of the disease, IL-2 has been shown to enhance resistance against *Mycobacterium avium* (14). Similarly to findings in infections with *Escherichia coli*, the exact mechanisms were not clarified. In view of the previously described pleiotropic effects of IL-

2, it may be that this cytokine enhances resistance by stimulating more than one component of the host defense apparatus.

Findings in animal models have culminated in the use of IL-2 as an adjuvant in reconstitution of cutaneous cellular immunity in the setting of lepromatous leprosy (15). In this work, it was shown that IL-2 recapitulated a delayed-type hypersensitivity response, and the authors suggested use of IL-2 as a therapeutic agent in immunosuppressed patients. Indeed, a recent study has shown beneficial effects in the use of IL-2 in severely immunosuppressed patients (16). Low doses of IL-1 are beneficial in host resistance against lethal doses of *Klebsiella;* the mechanism did not appear to involve neutrophils or a corticosteroid response (17). The macrophage growth factor CSF-1 has been shown to enhance the tissue clearance of *Candida albicans* and *Listeria* (18,19), but it paradoxically increased the growth of *Brucella* or *M. avium* in the tissues of mice, presumably by increasing the number of potential intracellular niches for these organisms (20,21).

The T-cell–derived lymphokine interferon-γ (IFN-γ) is an important mediator secreted by the Type 1 subtype of T cells, and, as with other cytokines, it has a variety of effects on numerous cell types. One very well-described effect of IFN-γ is its ability to enhance macrophage microbiostatic or microbicidal effect. This ability appears to be mediated by an increase in the release of microbicidal molecules, such as nitric oxide and reactive oxygen intermediates (22). Stimulation of mouse macrophages with IFN-γ increases the killing of microbes as diverse as *Mycobacteria, Francisella,* and *Leishmania* (22–24). This effect has led to the description of IFN-γ as a molecule that enhances resistance to many infectious agents. Moreover, in vivo experiments with neutralizing monoclonal antibodies have suggested a strong role for IFN-γ in the resistance to *Listeria, Mycobacteria,* and *Salmonella,* as well as others (25–27). In numerous systems, IFN-γ appears to act by increasing macrophage function, which leads to a decrease in bacterial viability in the tissues. However, as mentioned, IFN-γ has a wide variety of effects, including an antiproliferative activity on a number of cells, including T cells.

In a 1989 study of a mouse model of *Candida* infection, a surprising increase in the susceptibility of mice infected with *Candida* was shown when they were treated with IFN-γ (28); it was suggested that this increase was related to a diminished proliferative response of protective T cells. Similarly, another suprising finding in 1990 showed that *Trypanosoma brucei* infections in mice could be therapeutically improved by depleting IFN-γ–producing CD8+ T cells, which suggested a negative role for IFN-γ in the development of resistance to this organism (29).

It has been known for some time that certain forms of immunity are detrimental to the progression of infections caused by certain classes of microbes or parasites. The better known example is infection with the *Leishmania major* parasite. Infection with this protozoan in resistant mice is followed by a strong Th1-like response, with an important IFN-γ secretion, which then enhances macrophage killing of the parasite (30). Conversely, in susceptible hosts, infection appears to induce a Th2-type response, with low levels of IL-2 and IFN-γ and high levels of IL-3, IL-4, and CSF secretion (31). IL-3 and IL-4 have been shown to interfere with the development of macrophage microbicidal activity, presumably via down-regulation of nitric oxide synthase in these cells. This paradigm of resistance mediated by a Th1-like response and susceptibility associated with a Th2-like response has been observed for a number of other infectious agents, such as *Listeria* or *Candida* (32,33). However, a Th2 response, with its associated enhanced IgA response and eosinophil infiltration, is probably an efficient response involved in resistance against a number of gut parasites, such as nematodes (34). Investigations aimed at providing insights into the parameters that govern the Th1/Th2 profile that follows microbial infections could yield important information on the determinants of microbial virulence.

Overall, use of cytokines as immunotherapeutic tools in the setting of infections has given rise to an optimistic view of the use of such reagents. However, it is recognized that there are tremendous problems associated with the eventual use of such material in humans. The recent description of IFN-γ as a positive therapeutic agent in the treatment of chronic granulomatous disease is of considerable interest (35). However, other uses for cytokines are probably limited by the inherent toxicity of such material, their unclear pharmacological behavior, and, probably more importantly, by their pleiotropic effects. Our own studies and the work of other groups have suggested other potential problems, which are outlined in Chapter 33.

INTERACTIONS BETWEEN CYTOKINES AND BACTERIA

In the late 1980s and the early 1990s, it became apparent that there is a striking and unexpected relationship between mammalian cytokines and successful pathogens. This relationship was reviewed by one of us (Michel Denis) in 1991 (36), and we discuss some salient points herein. In a landmark publication, Mazingue and colleagues (37) reported that IL-2, when added to a culture medium of the protozoan *Leishmania*, dramatically increased the growth rate of this parasite. IL-2 could substitute for a growth factor secreted by the protozoan that was eliminated when the parasites were continually washed and reincubated in fresh medium. In this work,

Mazingue and colleagues observed that injection of high doses of IL-2 at the inoculation site in resistant mice infected with *Leishmania* rendered these hosts unexpectedly susceptible. Moreover, the immunosuppressive drug, cyclosporine, rendered susceptible hosts very resistant. Mazingue and colleagues (37) interpreted these data to suggest that *Leishmania* has adapted to the presence of important cytokines, and that it has evolved to use this material as growth factors, which probably constitutes an important virulence factor.

Kongshavn and Ghadirian (38) observed that incubation of *T. musculi* with the cytokine TNF unexpectedly led to a very dramatic increase in the growth rate of this parasite. However, TNF-α–pulsed macrophages were able to kill the parasite. Work by one of us (M.D.) showed that fresh clinical strains of *E. coli* were stimulated to grow in the presence of IL-2 and GM-CSF, whereas TNF-α and IL-4 had no such effect (39). This enhancement of the growth rate was significant only when the bacteria were cultivated in a suboptimal medium, such as fresh serum; bacteria growing in an optimal medium (i.e., bacteriological broth) were not stimulated to grow by cytokines. Enhancement of bacterial growth was seen with yeast-derived or bacteria-derived recombinant cytokines; heat-inactivated or antibody-neutralized cytokines were without effect on bacterial growth rate, suggesting that the enhancement was not simply a nutrient effect. Moreover, addition of excipients to bacteria (i.e., material eluted from a void column that contained small traces of detergents) also had no effect on bacterial growth rate.

A similar phenomenon was described by one of us (Reuven Porat); fresh, clinical important strains of *E. coli* were stimulated in their growth by incubation with the cytokine IL-1 (40). Other findings in the same study showed that a specific IL-1–like receptor structure was present at the bacterial surface. IL-1–mediated enhancement of bacterial growth rate was blocked by including neutralizing doses of an IL-1 receptor antagonist, which occupies the IL-1 receptor without agonist activity. It was estimated that approximately 20,000 to 40,000 IL-1 binding sites were present per *E. coli* bacterium, which suggested the possible involvement of carbohydrate moieties as participants in this binding. Cytokine binding and usage appeared not to be limited to fast-growing bacteria; 1991 reports by Shirasutchi and associates (41) and by one of us (Michel Denis) (42) showed that acquired immunodeficiency syndrome (AIDS)–associated *M. avium* strains were stimulated to grow in the presence of IL-6 (41,42). This enhancement of the growth rate occurred in suboptimal medium; enhancement of growth rate in an optimal medium, such as bacteriological broth, was not significant. Similarly, pulsing of macrophage monolayers infected with *M. avium* with a number of cytokines (e.g., IL-6, CSF-1) led to the super-induced growth of *M. avium* in vitro (43). These findings were interpreted as being relevant to the immunosuppressed state of patients with AIDS, who have very high serum levels of IL-6 and probably of other cytokines. This mechanism may in part be responsible for the unusual susceptibility of patients with AIDS to *M. avium.*

Other important articles in this area include the 1992 work of Barcinski and associates (44). These authors observed that GM-CSF increased the infectivity of the parasite *Leishmania amazonensis* by protecting the promastigote form of this parasite from heat-induced death. Indeed, it appeared that GM-CSF incubation with *Leishmania* enhanced the resistance of this parasite to heat stress, which obviously occurs after infection of mammalian macrophages (44). These authors hypothesized that contact between the cytokines and the bacteria could have triggered a heat-shock response in the parasite.

In 1993, Luo and coworkers (45) reported that TNF-α binds with high affinity receptors to the pathogen *Shigella flexneri.* Binding of the cytokine was inhibited by trypsin treatment, which indicated a protein component. After interaction with TNF-α in solution, *Shigella* became more invasive for epithelial cells in vitro, which suggested that TNF-α/bacteria complexes were interacting with TNF-α receptors present on eukaryotic cells. One of us (Michel Denis) also showed the presence of high affinity receptors at the membrane surface of clinical strains of *M. avium.* Scatchard analysis of receptor interaction showed that AIDS-associated strains had a single receptor species with a kd of 50 nmol/L, and the number of receptors was approximately 10,000/bacterium (46).

In 1993, a complex interplay between leukocytes, cytokines, and parasites was revealed in African trypanosomiasis. It was shown that *Trypanosoma brucei brucei* released a T lymphocyte-triggering factor (TLTF) that induced CD8+ T cells to release IFN-α (47). The released IFN-α was captured by the parasite, and it induced high levels of parasitic growth in vitro. The released TLTF also induced copious production of IL-4 and transforming growth factor-β (TGF-β). Both these cytokines have profound anti-inflammatory activities, including down-regulation of macrophage parasiticidal activity. It can be concluded that *T. brucei brucei* has developed a powerful double-edged virulence mechanism, namely synthesizing a factor that induces the release of a parasitic growth factor (i.e., IFN-γ), as well as inducing a profile of cytokines (i.e., IL-4, TGF-β) that blocks activation of processes associated with clearance of the parasite. The powerful contribution of TLTF to the virulence of *T. brucei brucei* was shown in vivo; monoclonal antibodies against TLTF were injected into infected rats, and it was clear that this approach afforded considerable protection.

These data point to a remarkable adaptation of *T. brucei brucei* to cytokine environments (i.e., evolution of a factor that specifically induces the synthesis of a cyto-

kine that promotes parasitic growth). Identification of molecules such as TLTF is likely to yield interesting therapeutic avenues for a variety of infectious agents. In 1992, it was shown that in a severe combined immunodeficiency (SCID) mouse model of infection with *Schistosoma mansonii*, TNF-α was a crucial cytokine in terms of triggering a granulomatous response (48). Surprisingly, production of eggs in infected hosts was dramatically enhanced by exogenous TNF-α infusion. When schistosome worms were isolated and exposed to TNF-α in vitro, egg production was enhanced, suggesting that the cytokine acted as a signal to the worms to produce eggs. This process indicates adaptation of the parasite to a cytokine environment, signaling a complex physiological process.

Overall, these data suggest that a range of successful pathogens have adapted to the presence of host cytokines by developing binding structures for these molecules, which, in the course of an infection, may act as a sink for protective cytokines and prevent activation of cells with these factors. It is well known that many chronic infectious diseases result in progressive immunosuppression, and it remains to be seen to what extent, if any, bacterial binding of cytokines contributes to this suppression. Moreover, bacteria and parasites have adapted to use these cytokines as growth factors, and they may become important virulence factors in a number of situations. It remains unclear exactly what mechanism was used by bacteria to acquire this phenotype.

In 1989, a study describing a number of important bacterial strains involved in causing pyelonephritis suggested that bacterial strains which infect humans have recruited mammalian DNA coding for proteins that may be important in binding to mucosal surfaces (CD5) (49). This conclusion was based on the strong homology between human and bacterial proteins despite the known high rate of spontaneous mutation of these molecules, which precludes the possibility of a common ancestor. Similarly, receptors for a large number of mammalian molecules at the surface of important pathogens have been described; for example, binding to molecules, such as plasminogen, fibrinogen, and its related fibrin by-products, has been described for *Streptococcus, Haemophilus,* and others (50,51). This type of binding is probably important in preventing an early host response, which limits bacterial dissemination and provides a first-line response to these infectious agents.

It will be of considerable interest to determine the exact mechanism responsible for both binding and growth enhancing effects of cytokines in bacteria and whether bacteria use a signal transduction pathway after binding of these host molecules. As of this writing, there is no information available on the actual mechanism of cytokine enhancement of bacterial or parasitic growth rate. A common finding is that the cytokines do not appear to act as simple nutrients, because heat-inactivation or antibody treatment of cytokines blocked enhancement. Moreover, the growth enhancement occurs in suboptimal media (i.e., tissue culture media), where bacterial growth is not maximal (i.e., not in rich medium). This finding suggests that cytokines may be acting on the bacterial growth rate by triggering mechanisms responsible for acquisition of essential nutrients or microelements, such as iron. Careful study of the effect of cytokines on bacteria in a variety of biochemically defined media could resolve this issue. Also not resolved at this time is the actual percentage of clinically important strains that possess this phenotype. Studies by one of us (Porat R., unpublished observations) have shown that approximately 20% of fresh clinical isolates of E. coli have an enhanced growth rate in the presence of IL-1. Other studies (Denis M, and Ghadirian E, unpublished data) have shown that 7 of 26 AIDS-associated strains of M. avium respond to IL-6.

The exact clinical relevance of these findings is still unclear and probably difficult to ascertain. A number of studies in patients who are receiving infusions of high doses of IL-2 for the treatment of advanced forms of cancer offer some perspective. It has become clear that a large fraction of these patients become very susceptible to infections with a number of opportunistic pathogens, such as Escherichia, Klebsiella, and Staphylococcus (52,53). It is unclear if cytokine use by some of these clinical strains is contributing to this phenomenon. Infusion with large doses of IL-2 is likely to lead to a large number of manifestations. It has been reported that patients receiving high doses of IL-2 had a deficient neutrophil chemotactic response, which may be a crucial parameter in determining the susceptibility to bacterial infections (54). In addition, continuous infusion of IL-2 will likely elicit the production of numerous cytokines that will contribute to breakdown of the integrity of gut mucosal tissues, thereby leading to bacterial translocation. The exact relevance of bacterial binding and usage of cytokines will only become clear after additional studies in experimental animals as well as in freshly derived clinical strains are performed.

IMPLICATIONS FOR CYTOKINE OR ANTICYTOKINE IMMUNOTHERAPY OF BACTERIAL INFECTIONS

In the early 1990s, several studies suggested that a number of cytokines may be involved in down-regulating functions that may be important in determining resistance to infections. For example, the Th2-derived cytokine IL-10 appears to have a pivotal role in down-regulating macrophage microbicidal activity. This effect appears to occur via diminished nitric oxide synthase activity; IL-10 also blocks IFN-γ–mediated enhancement of macrophage microbicidal activity (55). Other cytokines have suppressive activities, such as molecules in the TGF-β family (56). The clear implication of some of these factors in determining susceptibility to infections is shown by in vivo neutralization of these molecules. IL-10 neutralization in a mouse model of M. avium resulted in zero growth of a bacterium that normally grows quite rapidly in the infected tissues (57). In vitro studies showed that as chronic infection developed, there was a progressive decline in splenocyte secretion of IFN-γ and a marked increase in IL-10 release. TGF-β neutralization in a mouse model of Leishmania resulted in dramatically enhanced resistance to this protozoan (58). These data suggest interesting new avenues for immune modulation of bacterial infections. In addition, these data suggest that chronic infectious diseases are associated with down-regulation of the immune response that favors bacterial growth. As mentioned, data on the parasite Trypanosoma has shown that infectious agents have developed efficient ways of skewing the host response toward a profile that evokes the preferential release of cytokines which favor parasite growth, directly or indirectly (47).

Another interesting set of observations is the description, in the early 1990s, of genetic capture and subsequent release by viruses of potentially suppressive cytokines. For example, Epstein-Barr virus, which is responsible for infectious mononucleosis, has the gene for and synthesizes the immunosuppressive cytokine IL-10, which may in part be responsible for the observed immunosuppression seen in mononucleosis and possibly other pathologies (59). Similarly, other viruses synthesize and release soluble receptors for important cytokines, such as TNF-α (60). The human immunodeficiency virus (HIV) has also evolved to use cytokines for its own replication; certain cytokines can induce activation of NF-kβ, a nuclear factor important for transcription of the viral genome. Moreover, the regulatory sequence LTR is a target of NF-kβ, leading to enhanced viral expression. Accordingly, cytokines such as TNF-α, GM-CSF, and IL-6 increase viral expression in leukocytes (61–63). The impact of cytokines on the pathogenesis of AIDs is reviewed elsewhere in this book.

In our view, bacterial, viral, and parasitic adaptations to the presence of cytokines pose new and formidable problems for investigators exploring infectious diseases or the immunotherapeutic potential of cytokines. Approaches based on cytokine intervention must take these factors into account.

ACKNOWLEDGMENTS: Our work was supported by a Medical Research Council-National Health and Welfare Research and Development Joint Program on AIDS, by the Quebec Lung Association, by the Natural Sciences and Engineering Research Council of Canada, and by the "Fonds de la recherche en santé du Québec.

"We thank M Bédard for a careful review of the manuscript, and Dr R. Brzezinski for his helpful insights on bacterial physiology.

REFERENCES

1. Balkwill FR, Burke F. The cytokine network. Immunol Today 1989;10:299–304.

2. Stanley ER. Colony-stimulating factors. In: Stewart WE II, Hadden JW, eds. The lymphokines. Clifton, NJ: Humana, 1981:102–132.

3. Smith KA. Interleukin-2; inception, impact and implication. Science 1989;240:1169–1176.

4. Beutler B, Cerami A. Tumor necrosis, cachexia, shock and inflammation: a common mediator. Annu Rev Biochem 1988;57:505–518.

5. Bone RC. The pathogenesis of sepsis. Ann Intern Med 1991;115:457–469.

6. Dinarello CA. Interleukin-1 and its biologically related cytokines. Adv Immunol 1989;44:153–205.

7. Van Snick J. Interleukin-6; an overview. Annu Rev Immunol 1990;8:253–278.

8. Beutler B, Cerami A. Cachectin and tumor necrosis factor as two sides of the same biological coin. Nature 1986; 320:584–588.

9. Wahl SM, McCartney-Francis N, Hunt DA, Smith PD, Wahl LM, Katona IM. Monocyte interleukin-2 receptor gene expression and interleukin-2 augmentation of microbicidal activity. J. Immunol 1987;139:1342–1347.

10. Chong KT. Prophylactic administration of interleukin-2 protects mice from lethal challenge with Gram-Negative bacteria. Infect Immun 1987;55:668–673.

11. Weyand C, Goronzy J, Fathman CG, Hanley PO. Administration in vivo of recombinant IL-2 protects mice against septic death. J Clin Invest 1987;79:1756–1763.

12. Jeevan A, Asherson GL. Recombinant interleukin-2 limits the replication of Mycobacterium lepraemurium and BCG in mice. Lymphokine Res 1988;7:129–140.

13. Denis M. Cytokine modulation of Mycobacterium lepraemurium infection in mice; important involvement of tumor necrosis factor, interleukin-2 and dissociation from macrophage activation. Int J Immunopharmacol 1991; 13: 889–895.

14. Bermudez LEM, Stevens P, Kolonski P, Wu P, Young LS. Treatment of experimental disseminated Mycobacterium avium infection in mice with recombinant IL-2 and tumor necrosis factor. J Immunol 1988;143:2996–3000.

15. Kaplan G, Kiessling R, Terlemariam S, et al. The reconstitution of cell-mediated immunity in the cutaneous lesions of lepromatous leprosy by recombinant interleukin-2. J Exp Med 1989;169:893–907.

16. Teppler H, Kaplan G, Smith KA, Montana AL, Meyn P, Cohn ZA. Prolonged immunostimulatory effect of low-dose polyethylene glycol interleukin-2 in patients with human immunodeficiency virus type I infection. J Exp Med 1993;177:483–492.

17. Vogels MTE, Sweep CGJ, Hermus ADR, Van der Meer JWM. Interleukin-1 induced nonspecific resistance to bacterial infection in mice is not mediated by glucocorticoids. Antimicrob Agents Chemother 1992;36:2785–2789.

18. Kayashima S, Tsuru S, Shinomiya N, et al. Effects of macrophage colony stimulating factor on reduction of viable bacteria and survival of mice during Listeria monocytogenes infection; characteristics of monocyte subpopulations. Infect Immun 1991; 59:4677–4680.

19. Cenci E, Bartocci A, Puccetti P, Mocci S, Stanley ER, Bistoni F. Macrophage colony-stimulating factor in murine candidiasis; serum and tissue levels during infection and protective effect of exogenous inflammation. Infect Immun 1991;59:868–872.

20. Doyle AG, Halliday WJ, Barnett CJ, Dunn TL, Hume DA. Effect of recombinant human macrophage colony stimulating factor 1 on immunopathology of experimental brucellosis in mice. Infect Immun 1992;60:1465–1472.

21. Denis M. Colony-stimulating factors increase resistance to atypical mycobacteria in resistant mice whereas they decrease resistance in susceptible strains of mice. J Leukocyte Biol 1991;50:296–302.

22. Murray HW. Interferon gamma, the activated macrophage, and host defense against microbial challenge. Ann Intern Med 1988;108:595–608.

23. Titus RG, Kelso A. Louis JA. Intracellular destruction of Leishmania tropica by macrophages activated with macrophage activating factor/interferon. Clin Exp Immunol 1984;55:157–165.

24. Denis M. Interferonγ-treated murine peritoneal macrophages inhibit tubercle bacilli growth via the secretion of reactive nitrogen intermediates. Cell Immunol 1991; 132:150–157.

25. Denis M. Involvement of cytokines in determining resistance and acquired immunity in murine tuberculosis. J Leukocyte Biol 1991;50:495–501.

26. Muotiala A, Makela HP. The role of IFNγ in murine Salmonella Typhimurium infection. Microbiol Pathogenesis 1990; 8:135–141.

27. Buchmeier NA, Schreiber RD. Requirement of endogenous interferon production for resolution of Listeria monocytogenes infection. Proc Natl Acad Sci USA 1985; 82:7404–7408.

28. Garner RE, Kuruganti U, Czarniecki CW, Chiu HH, Domer JE. In vivo immune responses to Candida albicans modified by treatment with recombinant gamma interferon. Infect Immun 1989;57:1800–1808.

29. Bakhiet M, Ollsson T, Van der Meide P, Kristensson K. Depletion of CD8+ T cells suppresses growth of Trypanosoma brucei and interferon γ production in infected rats. Clin Exp Immunol 1990;81:195–199.

30. Heinzel FP, Sadick MD, Holaday BJ, Coffmann RL, Locksley RM. Reciprocal expression of interferon γ or interleukin-4 during the resolution or progression of murine leishmaniasis. Evidence for expansion of distinct helper T cell subsets. J Exp Med 1989;169:59–72.

31. Heinzel FP, Sadick MS, Mutha SS, Locksley RM. Production of interferon γ, IL-2, IL-4 and IL-10 by CD4+ lymphocytes in vivo during healing and progressive murine leishmaniasis. Proc Natl Acad Sci USA 1991;88:7071–7075.

32. Romani L, Mencacci A, Ghohmann U, et al. Neutralizing antibody to interleukin-4 induces systemic protection and T helper type 1-associated immunity to murine candidiasis. J Exp Med 1992;176:19–25.

33. Haak-Frendscho M, Brown JR, Igawa Y, Wagner RD,

Czuprynski CJ. Administration of anti-IL-4 monoclonal antibody 11β11 increases the resistance of mice to Listeria monocytogenes. J Immunol 1992;148:3978–3985.

34. Else KJ, Grencis RK. Cellular immune responses to the murine parasite *Trichuris muris*. Immunology 1991;72:508–513.

35. Curnutte JT. Conventional vs interferon-gamma therapy in chronic granulomatous disease. J Infect Dis 1993;167 (suppl):S8–S12.

36. Denis M, Gregg EO. Cytokines as growth factors for microbes/parasites; a review. Res Microbiol 1991;142:979–983.

37. Mazingue C, Cothez-Detoeuf F, Louis J, Kweider M, Auriault C, Capron A. In vitro and in vivo effects of interleukin 2 on the protozoan parasite *Leishmania*. Eur J Immunol 1989;19:487–491.

38. Kongshavn PAL, Ghadirian E. Enhancing and suppressive effects of tumor necrosis factor/cachectin on Trypanosoma musculi growth. Parasite Immunol 1989;10:581–588.

39. Denis M, Campbell D, Gregg EO. Interleukin-2 and granulocyte-macrophage colony-stimulating factor stimulate growth of a virulent strain of Escherichia coli. Infect Immun 1991;59:1853–1856.

40. Porat R, Clark BD, Wolff SM, Dinarello CA. Enhancement of growth of virulent strains of Escherichia coli by interleukin-1. Science 1991;254:430–432.

41. Shiratsushi H, Johnson JJ, Ellner JJ. Bidirectional effect of cytokines on the growth of Mycobacterium avium within human monocytes. J Immunol 1991;146:3165–3170.

42. Denis M, Gregg EO. Recombinant tumor necrosis factor-alpha decreases whereas recombinant interleukin-6 increases growth of a virulent strain of Mycobacterium avium in human macrophages. Immunology 1991;71:139–141.

43. Denis M. Growth of Mycobacterium avium in human monocytes: identification of cytokines which reduce and enhance intracellular microbial growth. Eur J Immunol 1991;21:391–395.

44. Barcinski M, Schechtman D, Quintao LG, et al. Granulocyte-macrophage colony-stimulating factor increases the infectivity of Leishmania amazonensis by protecting promastigotes from heat-induced death. Infect Immun 1992;60:3523–3527.

45. Luo G, Niesel DW, Shaban RA, Grimm EA, Klimpel GR. Tumor necrosis factor alpha binding to bacteria; evidence for a high affinity receptor and alteration of bacterial virulence properties. Infect Immun 1993;61:830–835.

46. Denis M. Interleukin-6 is used as a growth factor by virulent Mycobacterium avium: presence of specific receptors. Cell Immunol 1992;141:182–188.

47. Olsson T, Bakhiet M, Hojeberg B, et al. CD8 is critically involved in lymphocyte activation by a T. brucei brucei-released molecule. Cell 1993;72:715–727.

48. Amiri R, Locksley RM, Parslow TG, et al. Tumor necrosis factor alpha restores granulomas and induces parasite egg-laying in schistosome-infected SCID mice. Nature 1992;356:604–607.

49. Holmgren A, Branden CL. Crystal structure of chaperone protein Pap D reveals an immunoglobulin fold. Nature 1989;342:248–251.

50. Ullberg M, Kronvall G, Karlsson I, Wiman B. Receptors for human plasminogen on gram-negative bacteria. Infect Immun 1990;58:21–25.

51. Visai L, Speziale P, Bozzini S. Binding of collagens to an enterotoxigenic strain of Escherichia coli. Infect Immun 1990;58:449–455.

52. Murphy PM, Lane C, Gallin JI, Fauci AS. Marked disparity in incidence of bacterial infections in patients with the acquired immunodeficiency syndrome receiving interleukin-2 or interferon γ. Ann Intern Med 1988;108:36–41.

53. Maoleekoonpairoj S, Mittelman A, Sarona S, et al. Lack of protection against bacterial infections in patients with advanced cancer treated by biological response modifiers. J Clin Microbiol 1989;27:2305–2308.

54. Klempner MS, Noring R, Mier JW, Atkins MB. An acquired chemotactic defect in neutrophils from patients receiving interleukin-2 immunotherapy. N Engl J Med 1990;322:959–965.

55. Gazzinelli RT, Oswald IP, James SL, Sher A. IL-10 inhibits parasite killing and nitric oxide production by IFNγ-activated macrophages. J Immunol 1992;148:1792–1796.

56. Gazzinelli RT, Oswald IP, Hieny S, James SL, Sher A. The microbicidal activity of interferon-γ treated macrophages against Trypanosoma cruzi involves an L-arginine-dependent, nitrogen oxide-mediated mechanism inhibitable by interleukin-10 and transforming growth factor-beta. Eur J Immunol 1992;22:2501–2506.

57. Denis M, Ghodirian E. Neutralization of interleukin-10 augments mouse resistance to Mycobacterium avium infections. J Immunol 1993;151:5425–5430.

58. Barral-Netto M, Barral A, Brownell CE, et al. Transforming growth factor-β in leishmanial infection; a parasite escape mechanism. Science 1992;257:545–548.

59. Moore KW, Vieira P, Fiorentino DF, Trounstine ML, Khan TA, Mossmann TR. Homology of the cytokine synthesis inhibitory factor (IL-10) to the Epstein-Barr virus gene BCRF1. Science 1990;248:1230–1234.

60. Upton C, Macen JL, Schreiber M, McFadden G. Myxoma virus expresses a secreted protein with homology to the tumor necrosis factor receptor gene family that contributes to viral virulence. Virology 1991;184:370–382.

61. Folks TM, Justement J, Kinter A, Dinarello CA, Fauci AS. Cytokine-induced expression of HIV-1 in a chronically-infected pro-monocyte cell line. Science 1987;238:800–802.

62. Kotanagi Y, O'Brien WA, Zhao JQ. Cytokines alter production of HIV-1 from primary mononuclear phagocytes. Science 1988;241:1673–1675.

63. Poli G, Bressler P, Kinter A. Interleukin-6 induces human immunodeficiency virus expression in infected monocytic cells alone and in synergy with tumor necrosis factor alpha by transcriptional and post-transcriptional mechanisms. J Exp Med 1990;172:151–158.

PART 5

CYTOKINES AND CANCER

CHAPTER 33

ROLE OF CYTOKINES IN CANCER THERAPY

José Alexandre M. Barbuto and Evan M. Hersh

Cytokines are powerful modulators of diverse cell functions mainly, but not exclusively, within the immune system. As a result of this property, their use represents an attractive approach to the management of cancer. With the advent of recombinant DNA technology, pure cytokines became available in large amounts, which allowed their use in the clinical setting. Some cytokines currently have an established role in cancer therapy (1–3). In this context, cytokines can be grouped into two broad categories: "bone marrow–protective" cytokines and anticancer cytokines. The former group, basically comprised of hematopoietic growth factors, counteracts the toxic myelosuppressive effects of cancer chemotherapy, whereas the latter group includes cytokines that are ultimately (directly or indirectly) cytotoxic to tumor cells. However, cytokines have pleiotropic effects and they frequently show both activities. Hematopoietic growth factors, such as macrophage colony-stimulating factor (M-CSF) and granulocyte-macrophage CSF (GM-CSF), also apparently induce macrophage activation (4–6). Thus, they may have an anticancer effect by inducing cell populations that are cytotoxic to tumor cells. In contrast, many cytokines with anticancer potential such as interleukin-1 (IL-1) (7), IL-3 (8), IL-4 (9), and IL-6 (10), display hematopoietic activity.

This chapter concentrates only on the anticancer role of cytokines, an effect that can be directly mediated by action of the cytokine on cancer cells (11–15), or it can be the consequence of activation of various immune defense mechanisms by the cytokine (16–20).

Because of this latter pathway, therapeutic use of cytokines in cancer treatment poses a different challenge when compared with chemotherapy. For a chemotherapeutic agent, one seeks the maximum tolerated dose (MTD), because it is expected that the drug dose will be directly correlated to tumor cell killing. Cytokines, however, interact in intricate networks: they induce secretion of other cytokines, and very different effects on the immune system can be achieved at different dose levels or when in the presence of other cytokines. Therefore, the optimal biological dose (OBD) (not the MTD) of a cytokine needs to be defined in both preclinical systems and in clinical trials. This OBD will depend on the intended biological effects of the therapy. Different clinical settings with different patient populations may define different OBD of the same cytokine. Hence, clinical trials aimed at definition of OBD of a cytokine should be planned carefully, and they should consider both possible biological effects of the cytokine and their correlation with therapeutic efficacy in disease models and patient immune functions, before and after treatment.

Most of the current experience in cancer treatment with cytokines relies on their systemic use. This route has proven partially successful in some situations, such as use of IL-2 for the treatment of advanced renal-cell carcinoma, malignant melanoma, and lymphomas (21), or use of interferon (IFN) for the treatment of hairy-cell leukemia (22). However, systemic use of cytokines is frequently associated with severe, often limiting toxicities (23,24). An alternative to systemic use of cytokines would be isolated limb perfusion for tumors located in the extremities. This approach has been tested recently, and a 100% response rate was obtained in 23 patients with melanoma or sarcoma, in combination with chemotherapy, tumor necrosis factor-α (TNF-α), IFN-γ, and hyperthermia (25). This study needs confirmation, but even if proven, this approach would still have limited application.

Another locoregional strategy with cytokines is peritumoral or intratumoral injection (26,27). This approach may also be directly cytotoxic or induce an antitumor immune response. Other strategies that attempt to both minimize systemic toxic effects or enhance therapeutic effects are being explored. One of these strategies is molecular bioengineering of cytokines, which attempts construction of hybrid, more effective molecules, with active sites taken from different cytokines. A hybrid molecule, PIXY321, which combines the active sites of GM-CSF and IL-3, is currently being investigated for the treatment of diverse forms of bone marrow suppression (28,29). Also, modification of cytokine molecules so that they maintain their antitumoral effect but show decreased systemic toxicity, a strategy under investigation for TNF-α (30), could prove useful. Another approach, which tries to localize cytokine effects to the tumor site, is genetic alteration of tumor cells to induce cytokine secretion by these modified tumor cells. In many animal models, this **gene therapy** approach has been shown to induce important alterations in the immune recognition of tumors, leading to a markedly heightened antitumor immune response and tumor rejection, without the systemic effects of the produced cytokines (31–33).

Cytokines in cancer treatment have been used alone or in combination with other modalities of biological therapy or in association with chemotherapy. With regard to other aspects of the clinical use of cytokines, studies assessing the effectiveness of their combination with chemotherapeutic agents have not yet fully defined their definitive role.

In general, cytokines induce response in a relatively small percentage (20–30%) of patients, even patients in those malignant disease categories in which they are most effective. Parameters predictive of a response have not been completely defined. In some studies, improvement of patient immune function has been correlated with better responses (34), whereas in others, tumor response and immune activation seem to be independent (35).

INTERFERONS

Interferon was first described as a product of virus-infected cells that induces an antiviral state in other cells

(36). It comprises a series of different proteins that can be grouped into three families: IFN-α, IFN-β, and IFN-γ. Both IFN-α and IFN-β are Type I IFNs, which are acid-stable proteins that act on the same receptor on target cells. IFN-γ, or Type II IFN, is acid-labile, and it acts on a separate receptor on target cells (37). All IFNs can be induced by the action of other cytokines (17,38), but Type I IFNs are usually induced by virus infections; leukocytes produce IFN-α, and fibroblasts and epithelial cells produce IFN-β (37). In contrast, IFN-γ is usually the product of activated T lymphocytes after contact with specific antigens or after polyclonal stimulation with mitogens (39,40).

After interaction with a cell surface receptor, IFN molecules are internalized and degraded, and they initiate a cascade of effects on cell metabolism and gene expression (37,41). The exact mechanisms of IFN action are not perfectly defined, but they involve activation of a series of different pathways, including initial induction of the enzyme 2′-5′-oligoadenylate synthetase and activation of a specific protein kinase (41). Other diverse genes are up-regulated, such as major histocompatibility complex (MHC) antigens (42,43), whereas others are down-regulated, particularly c-myc, c-Ha-ras, and c-src proto-oncogenes (44). The ability of IFNs to induce MHC expression could be used in conjunction with other approaches, such as gene therapy, that attempt to enhance antigen presentation by tumor cells.

As a consequence of IFN interaction with cell receptors, and depending on the cell and IFN types, different effects can be observed. IFNs, mainly IFN-γ, display immune-enhancing properties, which include increased antigen presentation, as well as macrophage, natural killer (NK) cell, and cytotoxic T-lymphocyte activation (37). IFNs are also able to inhibit cell proliferation of both normal and malignant cells (12,45). IFN-α and IFN-β are therefore more potent proliferation inhibitors, and deletion of their genes from chromosome 9 has been observed in human tumors, suggesting a possible role for IFNs as natural tumor inhibitors (46). IFNs also have an antiangiogenic effect, which may have a significant role in IFN activity in some malignancies. This antiangiogenic potential of IFN-α has been directly explored for the management of hemangiomas, and excellent results were achieved (47).

IFNs are the most fully developed of the cytokine classes as cancer therapeutic agents. They have shown activity in several hematological malignancies, as well as in solid tumors. Of the three IFN families, IFN-α is the one with most proven effects, and it is licensed in the United States for treatment of hairy-cell leukemia and Kaposi's sarcoma (KS). IFN-γ has been studied extensively as an anticancer agent, but disappointing results have generally been obtained. Some studies suggest that renal-cell carcinoma may respond to IFN-γ therapy, but this approach still needs to be definitively proven. IFN-β has also been tested, but it did not show striking advantages when compared with IFN-α. It has shown some activity in brain tumors (48); this application is currently under investigation.

IFN-α is usually administered via subcutaneous (SC) or intramuscular (IM) injections, and it has a plasma half-life of 4 to 5 hours (49). However, because its biological effects persist for 2 to 3 days, single daily doses or even a three times a week schedule of administration may be effective, depending on tumor type. Side effects of IFN-α treatment include severe flu-like symptoms (i.e., chills, fever, myalgia, headache, arthralgia), anorexia, fatigue, depression, and mild bone marrow suppression. With higher doses, gastrointestinal effects and neurological and hepatic toxicities are observed (50). The flu-like symptoms are usually responsive to acetaminophen, and the hematological effects are promptly reversed by drug discontinuation, although it is rarely necessary. The white blood cell count commonly decreases into the range of 2,500 cells/mm³ blood, and the platelet count decreases into the range of 100,000/mm³ blood without adverse consequences. Therefore, we usually continue therapy unless counts decrease below these levels.

Most tumor responses are observed at doses of 3 to 5 million units (MU)/day, which are mainly associated with the flu-like symptoms. With continuation of treatment, the severity of the flu-like symptoms subsides, but anorexia, depression, and fatigue may become dose-limiting. In fact, these are the most common, dose-limiting toxicities. To deal with grade III or grade IV toxicities, which require dosage modification, daily therapy should be stopped for 1 week and then restarted at the same dose, but at 3 times/week or every other day. IFN-α toxicity and immune-enhancing effects have been associated with time of day the drug is administered; immune activation is higher and toxicity is lower with evening administration of the drug (51,52). Therefore, a circadian modulated rate of drug delivery has been suggested to enhance immune stimulation and to decrease toxicity (53).

Hematological malignancies that respond to IFN-α treatment include hairy-cell leukemia (54–56), chronic myelogenous leukemia (CML) (57–60), non-Hodgkin's lymphoma (NHL) (61), multiple myeloma (MM) (62,63), and T-cell lymphomas (64). Some solid tumors, such as KS (65,66), renal tumors (67), carcinoid tumors (68), and malignant melanoma (69) also showed objective responses to IFN-α. Myeloproliferative disorders, such as thrombocythemia (70) and polycythemia vera (71), also respond to IFN-α therapy.

Treatment of hairy-cell leukemia with IFN-α was approved by the Food and Drug Administration (FDA) in 1986, and it represented the first approved treatment for human cancer using a recombinant cytokine. Until then, standard treatment for that disease was splenectomy,

which achieved only moderate and temporary improvement of hematological parameters. With this treatment, only 10% of the patients experienced long-lasting benefits (72,73). With the use of IFN-α purified from leukocytes, Quesada and colleagues (22,74) obtained complete or partial remissions in 82% of an initial 22 patients. Virtually all patients showed hematological improvement with normalization of blood counts, even when the bone marrow did not improve. Recombinant IFN-α molecules, which subsequently became available, were evaluated in a series of studies, and they induced responses that ranged between 78 and 100% (54,55,75–78). In these studies, true complete remission developed in only some patients, but even partial responders showed significant improvement of hematological parameters and decreased incidence of infections.

The usual doses for treatment of this neoplasia are low and initially tolerated. In a multicenter study of 212 patients receiving 2 MU/m² 3 times/week, symptoms classified as severe or life-threatening developed in only 16% (56). In fact, some patients can be managed with doses as low as 1 MU daily or 3 times/week. Although the initial treatment schedule is well defined and induces responses in the majority of patients, its ideal duration is not well established. Relapses were observed in 20 to 48% of patients after 12, 18, or 24 months of IFN therapy (79,80). Because prolonged use of IFN-α may be associated with cumulative toxicity, interruption of treatment should be considered after 1 year.

Until recently, IFN-α was the undisputed most effective treatment for hairy-cell leukemia. However, 2′-deoxycoformycin (Pentostatin), an inhibitor of the enzyme, adenosine deaminase, is apparently more effective in the management of this disease. It induced complete responses more frequently, and fewer relapses were observed after its discontinuation (81,82). Results even more encouraging have been obtained with the deoxyadenosine analogue, 2-chlorodeoxyadenosine (83). This drug induced complete remission in 11 of 12 patients initially treated, and it was associated with less toxicity than that induced by Pentostatin. After a single 7-day treatment cycle, long-term remissions were induced (median duration, 15.5 mo). These results indicate that 2-chlorodeoxyadenosine should be the drug of choice for management of hairy-cell leukemia. Randomized trials comparing IFN-α, Pentostatin, and 2- chlorodeoxyadenosine are currently being conducted.

CML is another hematological disease for which IFN-α has shown encouraging results and for which it may become a first line drug. This disease is characterized by an initially indolent chronic course, which lasts 3 to 4 years. Eventually, however, patients enter an accelerated phase; an acute blast crisis then develops, which is refractory to most treatments. During the chronic phase, patients may have elevated white blood cell counts, and immature cells are present in the circulation to various degrees. The cytogenetic hallmark of this disease is the Philadelphia chromosome (Ph[1]), which represents a reciprocal translocation of the long arm of chromosome 22 to chromosome 9 (84). This abnormality is very rarely reversed by chemotherapy, even in responding patients, who experience normalization of blood counts and improvement in bone marrow cellularity. Initial studies of IFN-α purified from leukocytes proved its ability to normalize blood counts in patients with CML (57,85). Its efficacy was confirmed with recombinant forms of the cytokine in a series of studies (58–60,86). Most intriguing, however, was the observation that IFN therapy could induce the suppression of Ph[1] chromosome expression in up to 39% of patients, as described by Kantarjian and associates (86) in a study of 44 patients receiving 5 mU/m²/day. This Ph[1] suppression was confirmed by Southern blot analysis in a limited number of patients (87), suggesting an IFN-induced change in the biological behavior of the disease.

This hypothesis has recently been reinforced by the results of an Italian prospective study of IFN-α2a versus chemotherapy for the treatment of CML (88). In this study, 322 patients were enrolled between 1986 and 1988, and 218 were randomized to receive IFN, whereas 104 received hydroxyurea. Despite an identical response rate in both groups during the first 14 months of treatment, patients in the IFN arm showed a significantly higher level of karyotypic responses (20 vs 0%) and a significantly longer survival (68 vs 53%) after 4 years of treatment. As in other diseases, the mechanism of IFN-α action is unknown in CML, but the lack of response to IFN-α treatment in patients with CML has been correlated with decreased induction of 2′-5′-oligoadenylate synthetase (89). The dose of IFN-α required in patients with CML is substantially higher than in those with hairy-cell leukemia. Thus, during the induction phase of treatment, a dose of 5 mU/m² for several months is necessary. This dose is not tolerated by all patients. Nevertheless, because of its high degree of efficacy, ease of administration, reasonable tolerability, and prolongation of the benign phase, IFN-α should be considered the drug of choice in patients with CML.

IFN-α has been used as a single agent to treat multiple myeloma; responses were achieved in 8 to 18% of patients (90,91). However, IFN-α may have a significant role in MM management after remission has been induced by chemotherapy. Encouraging results have been obtained in different studies, suggesting that IFN-α could prolong relapse-free survival and overall survival in responding patients (62,92). In a recent update on the original study from the Italian Multiple Myeloma Study Group (62), which included 5 more years of follow-up, the impact of IFN-α on overall survival was not confirmed, but the prolongation of relapse-free survival continued to be significant (93). In contrast to these promising results, a large randomized trial, conducted by the Southwest Oncology Group (SWOG) (SWOG myeloma study 8624), did not support the use of IFN in MM (94). In this study involving 508 patients, patients were rerandomized after remission induction to receive IFN maintenance therapy or not. Each group had 96 patients, and after a follow-up of up to 5 years, no differences were noticed in relapse-free survival (median, 11 vs 12 mo) or in overall survival (median, 34 vs 37 mo).

In contrast, a recent randomized trial involving 84 patients with MM claimed an effective role of IFN-α in maintenance therapy (95). All patients were initially treated with high-dose chemotherapy, consolidated with high-dose melphalan, and followed by autologous bone marrow transplantation. They were then randomized to receive maintenance IFN-α or no treatment. Initial chemotherapy induced complete remission in 62 patients. Among these patients, there was significant prolongation of remission in the IFN-treated group, and 53% continued in remission 4 years after treatment. Overall progression-free survival was 39 months in patients receiving IFN-α versus 27 months in the control group. Survival was also significantly better in the IFN arm, with only 1 death vs 6 deaths in the control group. Thus, the degree of initial cytoreduction by chemotherapy may determine the potential utility of IFN-α in this disease. However, with regard to currently available data, IFN-α cannot be recommended for routine remission maintenance in MM, and more studies are still necessary to define its role in this disease.

Lymphomas, including NHLs (61,96) and cutaneous T-cell lymphomas (97,98), have been shown to respond to IFN-α therapy. Response rates varied among different studies, but for both groups of malignancies, they average slightly under 50%. Among NHL, low-grade nodular lymphomas are the most responsive, although mixed and diffuse nodular lymphomas also respond. IFN-β and IFN-γ have also shown some activity against T-cell lymphomas (99,100).

Among solid tumors, the acquired immunodeficiency syndrome (AIDS)–associated KS constitutes the other FDA-approved use of IFN-α for cancer treatment. In this disease, IFN-α achieves responses in 35 to 38% of patients, but much higher doses are required; therefore, it is associated with much more toxicity (66). Improved immune parameters, including enhanced NK cell activity, did not correlate with better responses in patients with KS (35), which probably indicates that IFN-α is active through its antiproliferative properties in KS.

IFN-α is only active in patients with AIDS who have relatively limited KS and in those with CD4+ peripheral blood lymphocyte counts greater than 100/mm³ blood. Because AIDS-related KS is often indolent and rarely life-threatening, these patients may not even require treatment. Furthermore, the very high doses of IFN-α required (36 MU 3 times a week is one recommended common regimen), combined with AIDS-related symptoms of fever, anorexia, fatigue, and weight loss, make IFN-α therapy very toxic and intolerable in this group of patients. Therefore, we do not recommend IFN-α as frontline therapy for KS, and we believe its role may be very limited in the disease.

Malignant melanoma in the metastatic state has been treated with IFN-α; reported responses did not exceed 30%, and treatment duration was (measured in mo) (69,101). In the adjuvant setting, results from a randomized trial using high-dose IFN-α to treat 287 patients with a high risk of relapse have recently been reported (102). This study showed a significant increase in relapse-free survival after surgery, but IFN-α was associated with important toxic effects (including two lethal hepatotoxicities). Furthermore, prolongation of overall survival from 31 to 41 months in the IFN-treated group was not statistically significant. Although the role of IFN-α as a single agent in metastatic disease is limited, its role in the prevention of recurrence after surgical removal of primary tumors or nodal metastasis is considered promising. Several multicenter studies are currently under way to define its role.

IFN-α therapy has a defined role in the management of metastatic renal-cell carcinoma, and it is also being explored as adjuvant therapy for prevention of recurrence or elimination of micrometastases in patients following primary surgery. Numerous studies have been done of IFN-α therapy in metastatic renal-cell carcinoma (103–105), and several reviews have been published (106,107). Generally, daily therapy with high doses of IFN-α (≥ 5 MU/day) resulted in a response rate of approximately 15%, with a duration of approximately 10 months. Occasionally, durable complete remissions are seen (in approximately 5% of treated patients). Best responses are seen in pulmonary and nodal metastases, whereas bone and liver metastases responded less often. Despite these favorable results, a large trial (159 patients) failed to prove a significant impact of IFN-α on overall survival of patients with advanced renal cancer (108), indicating that improved therapeutic approaches are still needed for this malignancy.

Carcinoid tumors have shown objective responses to IFN-α therapy; symptomatic and laboratory improvement occurred in 30 to 60% of patients (68,109). Tumor mass reduction, however, was observed only in a small number of patients. Malignant endocrine pancreatic tumors have also been treated with, and responded to, IFN-α; an objective response rate of 83% was found in one study (110).

Basal-cell carcinomas are very common skin malignancies that can be cured by surgery in approximately 99% of patients. Intralesional administration of IFN-α has been shown to induce complete responses in most patients (111,112). Thus, intralesional use of this cytokine may represent an alternative approach to surgery in patients for whom invasive procedures may be contraindicated.

TABLE 33–1   RECENT CLINICAL TRIALS OF IFN COMBINATIONS FOR CANCER THERAPY

Disease	Drug Combination	No. Patients	Patients RR	Ref.
Metastatic melanoma	IFN-α + 4-drug chemotherapy	45	62%	(115)
	IFN-α + IL-2	14	0	(200)
	IFN-α + 3-drug chemotherapy + IL-2	42	55%	(113)
	IFN-α + cisplatin	42	24%	(114)
Metastatic renal cancer	IFN-α + IL-2	31	42%	(199)
	IFN-α + IL-2 (subcutaneous)	42	12%	(201)
	IFN-α + IL-2	28	11%	(198)
	IFN-α + IL-2	34	12%	(117)
	IFN-α + IL-2	30	30%	(116)
Metastatic colorectal cancer	IFN-α + 5-FU + leucovorin	44	54%	(119)
NHL	IFN-β + IL-2	49	17%	(120)
Advanced esophageal cancer	IFN-α + 5-FU	37	27%	(118)
Cervical cancer	IFN-α + retinoic acid	32	50%	(123)
CML	IFN-α + cytarabine	60	55%	(121)
Advanced cancer	IFN-γ + IL-2	37	5%	(203)
	IFN-γ + IL-2	27	15%	(204)

RR = objective response rate; NHL = non-Hodgkin's lymphoma; CML = chronic myelogenous leukemia; IFN = interferon; IL = interleukin; 5-FU = fluorouracil.

In addition to their use as single agents, IFNs have been used in combination with other cytokines and with chemotherapeutic or differentiation inducing agents in a variety of neoplastic disorders, including malignant melanoma (113–115), renal-cell carcinoma (116,117), esophageal carcinoma (118), colorectal carcinoma (119), lymphoma (120), and CML (121). Some of these studies are summarized in Table 33–1; they illustrate what currently appears to be a very promising area of clinical investigation. The studies that combined IFN-α and IL-2 are discussed later.

Promising results have been observed with the combination of IFN-α and 13-cis-retinoic acid in squamous-cell carcinoma of the skin (122) and the cervix (123,124). Lippman and colleagues (123) recently reported the final results of a Phase II trial of this combination for the management of locally advanced squamous-cell carcinoma of the cervix. A total of 32 patients were enrolled, with disease stages ranging from IB to IVA. The overall major response rate was 50%, with a short time-to-response (≤ 2 mo) and very tolerable toxicities. Although the relapse rate was high (56%) and the time-to-relapse was short (median, 3 mo), this strategy obtained results as good as those obtained by cisplatin-based regimens, without their toxicity levels. This finding indicates the relevance and the need to explore further the combination of IFN-α and 13-cis-retinoic acid, perhaps in combination with active chemotherapy, in the management of this group of malignancies.

Very promising results were also obtained with the combination of IFN-α and chemotherapy for the treatment of metastatic melanoma (113,115). Pyrhönen and coworkers (115) treated 48 patients with metastatic melanoma with a 4-drug chemotherapy regimen followed by IFN-α. They obtained an objective response rate of 62%; six patients (13%) achieved complete remission. Of these six patients, three had continued remission after 7, 18, and 31 months. They also observed that intermittent administration of IFN (2 weeks on and 2 weeks off drug) appeared to be more effective than continuous treatment, and they reported that 4 patients who did not respond to continuous IFN achieved disease regression after IFN administration was switched to this split schedule. In another study, Richard and associates (113) combined IFN-α and IL-2 with a 3-drug chemotherapy regimen plus tamoxifen for the treatment of advanced melanoma, and they obtained response in 55% of the 42 patients included in the trial. Both studies indicate that these cytokines stimulate antitumor immune responses, rather than being directly cytotoxic against the tumor cells. However promising, these studies include limited numbers of patients, and they need to be confirmed in larger randomized trials. It does appear, however, that responses in metastatic melanoma with these combination chemotherapy/IFN-α regimens are consistently close to 60%. In contrast, prior

studies with chemotherapy or with cytokines reported responses in the 20 to 30% range. Therefore, we see this as a major advance in the management of malignant melanoma.

Early studies suggested that the combination of IFN-α and 5-fluorouracil (5-FU) was effective in patients with colorectal cancer (125,126). However, a large multicenter randomized trial that included 245 patients did not support those findings (127). Among the 234 evaluable patients, there was no significant difference between response rates induced by 5-FU alone (21%) and 5-FU plus IFN-α (26%), or in overall survival. These disparities indicate the need for additional studies of this approach in colon cancer.

In CML, where IFN-α has been shown effective as a single agent (88), better results seem to be achievable when IFN-α is combined with chemotherapy, as suggested by Kantarjian and associates (121). The authors studied the combination of IFN-α and low-dose cytarabine in the treatment of advanced stages of CML, and they compared their responses with patients treated previously with IFN-α alone. They treated 40 patients in the late chronic stage and 20 in the accelerated phase of CML. Patients in the late chronic stage responded better to the combination than to IFN alone; 55% achieved complete hematological response (vs 28% with IFN alone), and they had a longer 3-year survival rate (75 vs 48%). These results stress the need for additional evaluation of IFN and chemotherapy combinations.

Thus, IFN-α is well established in our armamentarium of drugs for cancer management, and it has an important role in the therapy of several malignancies. In view of this broad range of activities, IFNs continue to be very interesting cytokines, and future studies should define their role further, mainly in combination with other biological or chemotherapeutic regimens. To elaborate more effective therapeutic approaches, the mechanisms of IFN action in these diverse malignancies should be explored and defined.

INTERLEUKIN-2

Interleukin 2 is the second cytokine studied extensively as a cancer therapeutic agent. It was originally described as the T-cell growth factor (TCGF) (128), and it is able to maintain proliferation of antigen-stimulated T cells (129). As a result of this property, it occupies a central role in the immune system. In addition to effects on T-cell proliferation, IL-2 enhances cytotoxic activity of CD8+ T cells and monocytes (16), and it induces the appearance of broadly cytotoxic cells, known as lymphokine-activated killer (LAK) cells, among peripheral blood mononuclear cell populations (130). It also induces activated B cells to proliferate and secrete immunoglobulin (Ig) (131). Another important effect of IL-2 within the immune system is its ability to stimulate secretion of other cytokines, including IFN-γ, TNF-α, IL-1, and IL-6 (17,18).

The overall stimulatory activity of pharmacological doses of IL-2 on the immune system, mainly its ability to induce LAK cells, motivated investigation of its potential application in cancer therapy (2). LAK cells, which are generated from peripheral blood mononuclear cells cultured in the presence of high concentrations of IL-2, show broad cytotoxic activity against NK cell–resistant tumor targets, they also spare fresh normal cells (130,132). In addition to inducing LAK cells in vitro, administration of high-dose IL-2 to cancer patients in vivo causes the appearance of LAK cell activity in their blood (133). Tumor-infiltrating lymphocytes (TIL), which can be extracted readily from fresh tumor specimens (134) when stimulated by IL-2 in vitro, also show strong cytotoxic activity against tumor target cells (134–136). In contrast to LAK cells, which are derived mainly from cells of the NK cell phenotype and display broad, nonspecific reactivity, TIL are mostly of the T-cell phenotype (137–139), and, in animal models, their cytotoxic activity seems to be tumor-specific and MHC-restricted (140). They may be more effective in the control of tumor growth than LAK cells (141).

The broad cytotoxic activity of IL-2–induced LAK cells against tumor targets provided the rationale for its use in animal models of cancer. Extensive studies were developed that demonstrated the effectiveness of both IL-2 alone and IL-2 plus LAK cells against a variety of tumors, regardless of their immunogenicity (142–146). In these models, the combination of IL-2 and LAK cells was more effective than IL-2 alone, whereas LAK cells alone were ineffective, because they did not survive in vivo without continuous administration of high-dose IL-2 (147,148).

On the basis of these results, Rosenberg and coworkers (149) initiated clinical trials, and, in 1985, they reported the first results of the combination of LAK cells plus high-dose, systemic IL-2. Partial responses were observed in malignant melanoma, renal-cell carcinoma, and colon cancer. This was an important milestone in the development of cancer immunotherapy. The fact that peripheral blood lymphocytes could be removed from a patient with advanced, drug-refractory metastatic cancer, incubated in vitro with IL-2, reinfused into the patient, and induce remission was truly remarkable.

After demonstration of the activity of LAK cells plus IL-2, IL-2 also has been used alone, or in combination with TIL; comparable results were achieved in the same diseases. Most studies were performed with the cytokine being administered to patients via either bolus or continuous intravenous (IV) injection. After a bolus injection, IL-2 has a plasma half-life of 30 to 60 minutes (133). Within minutes of its administration, lymphocytes, including LAK cell precursors, are significantly diminished in the blood, and this lymphopenia persists throughout the treatment cycle (usually 5 days) (133). Simultaneous

to this phenomenon, delayed-type hypersensitivity reactions (150,151) and mitogenic responses to antigens are depressed (133,150). It is believed that the lymphopenia is consequent to migration of the cells into the tissues (152), and increased tumor, skin, myocardial, and portal infiltration by lymphocytes have been observed in treated patients (153,154). After discontinuation of therapy, an intense lymphocytosis is observed (133,155), which has been exploited to provide high numbers of LAK cell precursors in protocols that combine IL-2 and LAK cell therapy.

Although TIL or LAK cell administration are devoid of major untoward effects (156), the overall toxicity of IL-2 administration is extremely high, affecting all organ systems and with important manifestations in virtually all patients treated (21,157–159). This toxicity is important, because LAK or TIL cell therapy is only effective when the cells are given concomitantly with high-dose IL-2. Without the cytokine, their in vivo survival is very limited. Table 33–2 summarizes the major toxicities observed with IL-2 treatment. Chills, nausea, vomiting, and diarrhea develop in most patients. Anemia, thrombocy-

TABLE 33–2   MAJOR TOXIC EFFECTS OF HIGH-DOSE IL-2 THERAPY IN CANCER PATIENTS

Organ System	Toxic Effect
General	Chills and fever; pruritus; edema (symptomatic nerve/vessel compression); weight gain; anaphylaxis; sepsis; death
Hematological	Anemia; thrombocytopenia
Gastrointestinal	Mucositis; nausea and vomiting; diarrhea; colon perforation
Hepatic	Hyperbilirubinemia
Urinary	Oliguria; hematuria; elevated creatinine levels
Respiratory	Respiratory distress; bronchospasm; pleural effusion
Cardiocirculatory	Hypotension; arrythmias; angina; myocardial infarction
CNS	Somnolence; disorientation; coma

IL = interleukin; CNS = central nervous system.
Adapted from (170).

topenia, and eosinophilia are common. Hyperbilirubinemia, hypotension, cardiac arrhythmias, oliguria, and edema are frequently observed, and neuropsychiatric disorders, including confusion, irritability, lethargy, seizures, and coma, have been noted. Several of these disorders, as well as other manifestations of IL-2 toxicity, can be ascribed to an increase in vascular permeability (i.e., the vascular leak syndrome), which could be associated with the IL-2–induced release of other cytokines, including TNF-α, IL-6, and IFN-γ (160–162). Many patients require blood transfusions to correct the anemia, whereas the thrombocytopenia, despite being sometimes intense (<20,000 platelets/mm³), is rarely associated with bleeding. An increased incidence of sepsis (indwelling intravenous access catheter–related) has also been observed, but it can be adequately managed with antibiotics (163–165). Gastrointestinal symptoms are frequent and intense; gastritis, nausea, vomiting, and diarrhea often reach levels that patients do not tolerate. Preventive administration of acetaminophen, ranitidine, cimetidine, and indomethacin to all patients receiving IL-2 is common. Fluid replacement is often necessary, as is use of adrenergic drugs to control hypotension and oliguria. Myocardial infarction has also been associated with high-dose IL-2 treatment. Because of these severe toxicities, patients receiving high-dose IL-2 therapy must be managed in the intensive care unit. Some studies report less severe, but still important, toxicity when IL-2 is administered by continuous infusion (166,167).

An approach that may be effective in controlling IL-2 toxic effects is simultaneous neutralization of other cytokines released by IL-2 infusion into cancer patients. In animal models, administration of neutralizing antibodies against TNF-α was able to diminish toxicity, without negative effects on the antitumoral effects of IL-2 (168). In animal models, pentoxifylline, a drug that inhibits TNF-α release, had similar effects; it decreased IL-2 toxicity, but it maintained its antitumoral efficacy (169).

Several malignancies have been treated with IL-2 alone or with IL-2 plus TIL or LAK cells. An optimal IL-2 administration protocol has not been fully defined with regard to doses, route, or coadministration of agents that can alter toxicity. Similarly, the relative efficiency of IL-2 alone versus IL-2 plus TIL or LAK cells has not been definitively established. Animal studies suggested that the combination of IL-2 and LAK cells was superior to IL-2 administered alone, and initial reports of small numbers of patients seemed to support this observation. However, a prospective randomized trial reported by Rosenberg and colleagues (170) did not confirm this hypothesis. Nevertheless, in another study with a small number of patients with NHL, the IL-2/LAK combination was able to induce responses in 4 of 8 patients, whereas IL-2 alone failed in the 11 patients treated (171). In animal models, TIL were more effective than LAK cells in the control of tumor growth (141). This effect was improved by simultaneous

use of cyclophosphamide (141,172), and it was correlated with TNF-α and IFN-γ release by TIL cocultured with tumor cells (173). Initial clinical trials of TIL cell therapy in limited patient numbers obtained responses in patients that had failed previous therapy with IL-2 (174).

Recently, high-dose IL-2, alone or in combination with LAK cells, was approved by the FDA for therapy of metastatic renal-cell carcinomas. In the largest series of patients treated with this cytokine, Rosenberg and associates (21) obtained a 22% overall response rate in patients with renal-cell cancer treated with IL-2 alone, and a 35% response rate with the IL-2/LAK combination. Of the 12 patients who achieved complete remission, 7 remained free of disease 23 to 34 months following therapy. Other studies obtained similar response rates (175–177). A randomized prospective trial comparing IL-2 versus IL-2/LAK therapy was recently reported by Rosenberg and colleagues (170). No significant difference was observed between response rates in patients treated with IL-2 and LAK cells (33%) versus patients treated with IL-2 alone (24%). Although effective in certain patients, IL-2–based therapy, as outlined, is associated with important toxicity, and patient selection must be stringent.

Some investigators studied subcutaneous administration of IL-2 as a means to reduce toxicity in patients with renal-cell carcinoma to allow inclusion of patients that would not withstand IV therapy (178,179). In a trial including 27 patients, Sleijfer and co-workers (180) included 15 patients with concomitant diseases that would exclude them from IV IL-2 therapy. These conditions included previous myocardial infarction, angina pectoris, cardiac arrhythmias, and cardiac ischemias, among others. One 76-year-old patient with history of vascular disease had a myocardial infarction during therapy and died. Otherwise, overall toxicity in these patients was mild and less intense than that observed with IV therapy. Response rates were 8% for complete remission and 15% for partial remission after 6 weeks of therapy. Duration of remission was also comparable to other studies; the 2 complete remissions lasted 17 and 19 months or more. If this lower toxicity and similar effectiveness are confirmed with higher number of patients compared with high dose IV treatment, subcutaneous administration of IL-2 will prove a relevant improvement in IL- 2 therapy.

Malignant melanoma is another tumor that has been extensively studies, and they have responded to IL-2–based therapy. Rosenberg and associates (21) reported complete and partial remissions in 20 (22%) of 90 patients treated with IL-2 alone or with IL-2 plus LAK cells. No difference in response rates to IL-2 (24%) versus IL-2/LAK (21%) therapy was noted. However, in a prospective randomized trial, a trend to increased survival with the combination IL-2/LAK (18% at 48 mo) versus IL-2 alone (4% at 48 mo) was observed (170). Initial studies suggested that IL-2/TIL therapy might be even more effective against melanoma; a 55% response rate was achieved among the first 20 patients treated with this combination (174). Despite a possible advantage of IL-2/TIL therapy over other IL-2–based therapies (2 responses occurred among 5 patients that previously failed IL-2 therapy), additional studies are needed to explore this hypothesis.

Small numbers of patients with other neoplastic diseases have been treated with IL-2–based protocols. Diseases evaluated include lymphomas, nonsmall-cell lung carcinoma, colorectal carcinoma, and sarcomas. The limited numbers of treated patients preclude any definitive conclusion about the effectiveness of this approach in these malignancies, although some responses have been obtained (21,149,170,171,181).

In summary, IL-2 alone, at either high or moderate doses, is sufficiently active in metastatic renal-cell carcinoma for it to be a prominent part of our armamentarium against this disease. Thus, for renal-cell carcinoma, the biological agents IFN-α and IL-2 are the drugs of choice for metastatic disease. High- dose IL-2 also has enough activity in melanoma to make it a drug that can be used in patients with refractory metastatic disease.

Whether high-dose IL-2 alone or, as implied by some studies, in combination with TIL or LAK cells are more effective is currently unclear. Larger scale, controlled comparative trials are needed to determine this point. The high cost of such trials may preclude their ever being carried out.

Despite the broad cytotoxic activity of LAK cells in vitro, they are ineffective in most clinical situations. The explanation for this phenomenon is not known, but it could be related to a variety of factors. In vitro cytotoxicity of LAK cells against tumor targets is observed at effector-to-target ratios that are not normally achieved by infiltrating lymphocytes within tumors. Furthermore, the tumor microenviroment seems to be adverse for generation of cytotoxic effector cells; tumor infiltrating cells are deficient in their ability to respond to IL-2 (182). TNF-a is a cofactor in LAK cell generation (183–185), and we observed that tumor-infiltrating B lymphocytes frequently produce anti-TNF-α antibodies (186). In addition, the efficacy of adoptive cellular therapy seems to depend more on the ability of effector cells to release cytokines after tumor cell contact than on direct cell cytotoxicity (173). In this situation, cytokine inhibitors within the tumor microenviroment could be of major importance. Either neutralizing antibodies, as suggested by our observations, or other natural inhibitors, including soluble TNF receptors (187,188) or soluble IL-2 receptors (189), which have been shown to be elevated in the serum of some patients with cancer, could protect cancer cells, mainly if produced and released locally. Also, the majority of systemically injected LAK cells do not infiltrate tumor sites; rather, they localize initially to the lungs and later to the spleen and the portal circulation (190–192). This localization could be related to the fact that tumor vessels seem to be deficient

in their ability to initiate leukocyte extravasation (193). Also associated with altered leukocyte-endothelial interactions could be the observation that TIL therapy is more effective when combined with chemotherapy or radiation therapy (172), both of which could cause vascular alterations in the tumor. Finally, the interaction of LAK and tumor cells depends on expression of adhesion molecules on both cell populations, which could be altered during a treatment course, thus allowing the tumor cells to escape LAK cell cytotoxicity.

Therefore, we need better understanding of the tumor microenviroment, including, among other factors, the different populations of infiltrating cells, the local production of cytokines and cytokine inhibitors, as well as the vascular endothelial functions of tumor vessels. This knowledge could improve the low response rates observed with IL-2 therapy, and it could provide another step along the way to the development of more effective cytokine-based immunotherapy.

Another IL-2–based strategy that has been explored is the combination of IL-2 and other cytokines or chemotherapeutic agents for cancer therapy. Available data are not sufficient to establish ideal protocols, but they warrant further investigation.

The combination of IL-2 and IFNs has been the subject of various studies. In vitro observations have demonstrated a supra-additive effect for the sequential use of IFN-α and IL-2–induced LAK cells against melanoma cell lines, even when the cell line used was IFN-α–resistant (194). Accordingly, different investigators confirmed the synergism between these cytokines against tumors in animal models (195–197). These preclinical data led to clinical trials in which the activity of IL-2 in combination with IFN-α was explored (116,117,198–201). In addition, many Phase I and II clinical trials were conducted to investigate IL-2 combinations with diverse other agents, including TNF-α (202), IFN-β (120), IFN-γ (203,204), and chemotherapeutic agents (113,205).

Metastatic renal-cell carcinomas, which are susceptible to either IL-2 or IFN-α alone, have been the subject of many trials using these agents in combination (116,117,198,199). However, the advantages of these combinations have not been definitively proven. In a randomized trial of IL-2 alone versus IL-2 plus IFN-α, 11% of the patients treated with the combination showed an objective response, whereas 17% of those treated with IL-2 alone responded (198). Also, Ilson and colleagues (117) treated 34 patients with the combination, and they obtained a 12% response rate that was associated with high toxicity, including two treatment-related deaths. In contrast to these studies, in which the combination of IL-2 and IFN was not superior to IL-2 alone, Figlin and colleagues (116) and Lipton and associates (199) reported very promising results with the combination. Thirty patients (116) and 39 patients (199) were treated with the combination in an out-patient setting; there were no major toxicities, and response rates of 30 and 33% were achieved, respectively. In another Phase II trial using low-dose, subcutaneous IL-2 and IFN-α, Vogelzang and co-workers (201) obtained a response rate of 12% among their 42 patients, also with modest toxicity. This decreased toxicity constitutes one of the potentially major advantages of this approach. However, conflicting observations among the combination trials stress the need for Phase III randomized studies at the MTD to determine the role of treatment regimens using IL-2 and IFN combinations for the treatment of renal-cell carcinomas.

For the management of malignant melanomas, the combination of IL-2 and IFN at lower doses in an out-patient setting has been inferior to other dose-intensive regimens (200). However, as discussed, Richards and colleagues (113), who combined multidrug chemotherapy, chemomodulation with tamoxifen, IFN and IL-2, obtained a response rate of 55%, as well as a higher frequency of complete remissions and longer duration of responses than with chemotherapy alone. This study emphasizes the potential for this treatment modality.

In summary, combination protocols including IL-2, similar to those including IFN, constitute a significant research area in cytokine-based immunotherapy of cancer. Additional knowledge of cytokine interactions in the cancer patients and inclusion of other cytokines in future studies should increase our ability to utilize immune mechanisms for the control of human malignancies.

TUMOR NECROSIS FACTOR-α

Tumor necrosis factor-α was named for its ability to induce hemorrhagic necrosis of tumors in mice (206); however, it is a pleiotropic cytokine that has been involved in a series of protective and deleterious actions of the immune system (207,208). It has been shown to exert direct cytotoxic effects against tumor cells (11), but as many as two thirds of tumor cell lines tested have been shown to be relatively resistant to TNF-α cytotoxicity (209). TNF-α can produce synergistic effects with different cytokines, such as IFNs (210) and IL-1 (211), and it can induce secretion of a series of different mediators, including IL-1 (212), IL-6 (213), and prostaglandin E_2 (214). Furthermore, TNF-α can induce and regulate the expression of cell adhesion molecules (215) and MHC proteins (216) on endothelial cells and thus alter the composition of cellular tissue infiltrates. It has also been implicated in both the generation and the cytotoxicity of LAK cells and cytotoxic T lymphocytes (183–185,217). In one study of TIL therapy, the ability of these cells to secrete TNF-α and IFN-γ showed a better correlation with efficacy of TIL therapy than Cr^{51}-release cytotoxicity assays (173).

These properties promoted its investigation as a cancer therapeutic agent in a large number of Phase I and II studies. Unfortunately, however, its efficacy has been very limited, and its use is associated with important toxic effects, as exemplified by a recent summary of the SWOG experience (218). Between June 1988 and November 1990, 147 patients were entered in nine Phase II protocols for the treatment of diverse malignancies, including breast, colon, gastric, pancreatic, endometrial, and bladder cancers, as well as multiple myeloma and sarcomas. Only 1 patient among the 127 eligible patients responded (response rate, 0.8%), whereas 13% experienced grade 4 or fatal toxicity. Some of the more common toxicities included chills, fever, malaise, fatigue, nausea, and vomiting. The most serious toxicities were coagulopathies and pulmonary failure. Leukopenia, granulocytopenia, thrombocytopenia, and anemia were also common.

This initial failure of TNF-α in the immunotherapy of cancer reflects the complexity of the cytokine networks in the body, in which TNF has multiple roles. In addition to involved, much more than its name suggests, in a series of immune interactions, it has been implicated as a growth factor for different human tumors (219–222), and TNF inhibitors have been detected in patients with cancer (187,188).

Nevertheless, investigation of TNF-α as an immunotherapeutic agent in cancer should not be abandoned. Recently, Lienard and colleagues (25) investigated intra-arterial administration of high-dose TNF-α in conjunction with melphalan, hyperthermia, and IFN-γ to treat 23 patients with melanoma (19 patients) or sarcoma (five patients). All patients responded, 21 with complete remission and two with partial remission. Eleven of these patients had failed previous local therapy with melphalan alone and one failed therapy with cisplatin. The toxicities observed included neutropenia. thrombocytopenia, hypotension, and kidney failure, but all were reversible. Local TNF toxicity was minimal. Overall survival and disease-free survival at 12 months were 70 and 76%, respectively. These latter results are very encouraging, and they indicate the need for continuous investigation of the role of TNF-α in cancer therapy.

Other approaches also need to be investigated. Attempts to decrease systemic toxicity of TNF-α therapy without diminishing its anticancer effects could lead to substantial advantages. TNF-α mediates its many effects through interaction with two different cellular receptors, p55 and p75 (223). Although interaction with the p75 receptor has been associated with cell cytotoxicity in vitro (224), in vivo experience in murine models suggest that this receptor may be responsible for systemic toxicity rather than tumor cytotoxicity. Human TNF-α binds only to murine p55 TNF receptors (223), and it induces much less systemic toxicity in mice than murine TNF-α, which binds to both receptors. Despite the controversial roles of the different receptors, we can hypothesize that mutant TNF molecules, which are able to interact with one but not the other human receptor, could induce anticancer effects with less systemic toxicity, thus allowing use of higher, more effective TNF-α doses in cancer therapy. Mutant human TNF molecules, which bind selectively to the p55 receptor, have already been described, and they are able to induce cytotoxicity against transformed cells in vitro (30).

Another strategy to decrease toxic effects of TNF-α or to increase its anticancer effects could rely on the use of TNF-α–specific monoclonal antibodies. One study described a monoclonal antibody that potentiated the antitumoral effects of TNF while it decreased endothelial binding of the cytokine (225). Murine monoclonal antibodies that neutralize systemic toxicity without decreasing antitumor activity of TNF-α in animal models have also been described (226). In addition, use of drugs able to decrease TNF-α systemic toxicity could allow use of higher, more efficient TNF-α doses in cancer therapy. Pentoxifylline, a drug that decreases TNF release in the course of IL-2 therapy in mice (169), might also be useful during TNF therapy.

In summary, despite the initial failure of TNF-α as an immunotherapeutic agent for cancer, continuing investigation may generate new or improved approaches for its use. Combination regimens of TNF-α with other cytokines, concomitant use of different TNF toxicity inhibitors, and use of mutant TNF molecules may provide better clinical results than those obtained with TNF-α alone. Certainly, regional therapy with TNF-α is an area that should be explored with high priority, in view of the encouraging clinical results it has already produced.

OTHER CYTOKINES WITH ANTICANCER POTENTIAL

The number of known cytokines is still growing, and many have biological effects that could be advantageous for cancer therapy. Various cytokines have hematopoietic activities that can be very useful in the clinical setting as an adjuvant to dose-intensive chemotherapeutic protocols. These cytokines include IL-1, IL-3, IL-5, IL-6, IL-9, IL-11, erythropoietin, and the various CSFs. Some of these cytokines, such as erythropoietin, G-CSF, and GM-CSF, are already established therapeutic agents licensed for clinical use in the United States, whereas others are still being investigated. In contrast, cytokines can have direct antitumor effects or they can promote immune reactivity against tumors. The cytokines with this potential are the focus of our discussion, and they are listed in Table 33–3.

Many of these anticancer cytokines are already being explored in Phase I or II clinical studies. Obviously, due to the complex nature of their interactions in vivo, we cannot predict from its effects in vitro that a certain cytokine will be useful for cancer therapy in the clinical setting. Similarly, a cytokine may prove valuable in cancer therapy, even if it initially appears devoid of anticancer effects in preclinical systems. Only as a result of con-

TABLE 33–3   OTHER CYTOKINES WITH POTENTIAL DIRECT ANTICANCER ACTIVITY

Cytokine	Effects with Anticancer Potential
Interleukin-1	Macrophage, NK cell, T- and B-cell lymphocyte activation; induction of cytokine production; induction of hemorrhagic necrosis of tumors; direct cytotoxicity against tumor cells; synergism with chemotherapeutic agents (bone marrow stimulation)
Interleukin-4	Antigen-specific cytotoxic T-lymphocytes (CTL) activation; enhancement of MHC antigen expression by tumor cells; tumor cell growth inhibition; potentiation of TNF and IFN-γ antitumor effects
Interleukin-6	Acute-phase reactant production; induction of T-cell proliferation and differentiation; tumor cell growth inhibition (thrombopoietic activity)
Interleukin-7	CTL generation and activation; promotion of LAK cell generation; activation of macrophage tumoricidal activity
Interleukin-12	Potentiation of LAK and NK cell cytolytic activity; facilitation of specific CTL responses; induction of IFN-γ (and TNF) secretion by T and NK cells
M-CSF	Activation of macrophage tumoricidal activity; activation of macrophage free radical production; potentiation of macrophage ADCC; induction of macrophage TNF secretion

NK = natural killer; MHC = major histocompatibility complex; TNF = tumor necrosis factor; IFN = interferon; LAK = lymphokine-activated killer cells; ADCC = antibody dependent cellular cytotoxicity.

tinuous investigation and characterization of the cytokine networks in the human immune system, as well as precise definition of immune system–tumor interactions, will we be able to manipulate effectively the immune system in the cancer patients.

Interleukin-1

Both biochemically distinct types of IL-1 (i.e., IL-1α and IL-1β) have identical biological effects but diverse immunological and inflammatory effects, many of which are similar to those of TNF-α (211). IL-1 has many activating effects on different immune cells, and it induces macrophage cytotoxicity against tumor cell lines (227). IL-1 can also be directly cytotoxic to tumor cells (14,15). In vivo, IL-1 can inhibit the growth of different murine tumors (228,229), and it can cause hemorrhagic necrosis of tumors (228,230). In addition, IL-1 has been shown to synergize with chemotherapeutic agents both in vitro (231) and in vivo (232).

However, IL-1 has been explored in clinical trials mainly as a bone marrow stimulant. Results from animal models indicated radioprotective and chemoprotective actions for IL-1 (7,233,234). In initial clinical trials, cancer patients treated with IL-1 have shown decreased chemotherapy-induced thrombocytopenia and accelerated recovery of platelet counts after high-dose chemotherapy (227,228,235). This effect could make IL-1 an important component of dose-intensive therapeutic regimens.

In one Phase I clinical trial of IL-1, it was shown to induce a 25% response rate in malignant melanoma (236). This observation needs confirmation.

Due to its pleiotropic effects, the role of IL-1 in the immunotherapy of cancer is still difficult to predict. Its hematopoietic effect is promising, but it still needs to be evaluated further with regard to its therapeutic potential and its effects on survival. In contrast, the many immunoenhancing properties of IL-1 could be advantageous in immunotherapeutic settings; however, they need to be balanced with potential deleterious effects, otherwise IL-1 use as an anticancer cytokine could generate disappointing results, similar to the findings of initial TNF-α trials.

Interleukin-4

IL-4 is another cytokine with potential anticancer effects that recently entered clinical studies. Although it inhibits IL-2–induced LAK cell generation (237) and macrophage tumoricidal activity (238), it potentiates differentiation and cytotoxicity of antigen-specific cytotoxic T lymphocytes, including TIL (20). In addition, many tumor cells express IL-4 receptors (239–241); after IL-4 stimulation, they also express higher levels of MHC antigens (242,243), and their growth is inhibited (242–244). An-

other potentially useful effect of IL-4 is its apparent synergism with other anticancer cytokines, such as TNF-α and IFN-γ (245).

Phase I and II clinical trials are currently being conducted to evaluate the clinical potential of this cytokine. To date, solid tumors have been mostly refractory to IL-4 therapy (246–248), whereas some responses have been obtained with hematological malignancies (249). The number of patients treated is still too small to allow any conclusions, but the experimental data support its investigation as an anticancer agent, both as a single agent and in combination with other biological response modifiers.

Interleukin-6

Interleukin-6 displays multilineage hematopoietic activity and T-cell stimulatory effects, and it is involved in the acute-phase reaction (250). Furthermore, it has direct and indirect antitumor effects. Human and murine leukemic cell lines have been shown to have colony growth inhibition and to differentiate in response to IL-6 in vitro (251,252). Breast carcinoma cell lines were also inhibited by the cytokine (253). In animal models, IL-6 promoted the generation of tumor-specific cytotoxic T lymphocytes (254). Metastatic growth of immunogenic murine tumors has been inhibited, and animal survival improved as a result of treatment of tumor-bearing mice with IL-6 (254,255).

These experimental observations support a potential clinical role for IL-6. Its hematopoietic activity, mainly its thrombopoietic potential, could make it a useful agent for bone marrow protection or recovery after myelotoxic regimens. Its antitumoral effects could also lead to significant clinical responses. Initial results from Phase I trials are already being reported in the literature (256).

Macrophage colony-stimulating factor

Macrophage colony-stimulating factor is constitutively produced by bone marrow stromal cells (257), and it supports macrophage growth and differentiation (258). It can also be produced by macrophages and lymphocytes after exposure to inflammatory stimuli (257). In addition to its hematopoietic activity, M-CSF is able to activate different macrophage functions, including cytokine production (5), direct tumor cytostasis and cytolysis (6,259), free radical generation (260), and antibody-dependent cytotoxicity (261). These properties could be advantageous in the treatment of cancer, and M-CSF has shown antitumor activity in animal models (262).

Initial reports from Phase I clinical trials are being published, and they indicate that M-CSF can be administered safely to patients with cancer (263,264). Systemic toxicity has been minimal, with mild decreases in platelet counts. In the study by Sanda and colleagues (263) of 23 patients, 1 patient with renal-cell carcinoma experienced complete regression of pulmonary metastasis and mediastinal adenopathy.

CYTOKINE-RELATED GENE THERAPY OF CANCER

Many cytokines can have direct antitumor effects. Their immunoregulatory potential, however, is what makes cytokines unique as cancer therapeutic agents. Their use may bypass suppressive or defective immunological mechanisms, and it may obtain effective antitumor immune responses.

However, within the microenviroment, where immune cells and antigens interact, cytokines regulate cellular responses and the development of immune response. Frequently, when cytokines reach high systemic levels, they have already lost their homeostatic functions. Septic shock is a good example of such pathological conditions. In this situation, cytokines are no longer effective immunoregulatory molecules, but they have key roles in the pathophysiology of the disorder and they seem to be more deleterious than not (265,266). The systemic toxicity associated with the clinical use of cytokines is therefore not surprising.

Ideally, cytokine therapy should be concentrated in the microenviroment, where the immune response is supposed to develop. When dealing with cancer, regional perfusion of tumors with cytokines is a possibility; however, this approach has limited application. Another novel approach is **gene therapy**, which became possible as a result of the technical developments in molecular biology.

Cytokines can be used in gene therapy protocols in two different ways. One approach introduces antitumor cytokine genes, such as TNF-α, into tumor-infiltrating lymphocytes of the patient. After reintroduction into the patient's circulation, these cells will perhaps infiltrate the tumor again and initiate local secretion of high levels of the cytokine. This approach is currently being explored by Rosenberg and colleagues (2,267).

Another possible strategy, which has also been intensely explored, is genetic modification of tumor cells. Tumor cells are removed from the patient and a cytokine gene is introduced. Cells secreting the cytokine gene are then reintroduced into the patient. The goal is modification of cytokine concentrations at the site of an immune response; however, the modified cells do not have to localize to a specific site, because they should carry the antigens that will induce the immune response.

Many animal models showed that this approach can generate potent immune responses against tumor cells modified with different cytokine genes. These genes include IL-1 (268), IL-2 (269), IL-4 (270,271), IFN-γ (33), IL-6 (272), IL-7 (273,274), and TNF-α (32). Furthermore, vaccination of MBT-2 bladder carcinoma–bearing mice with irradiated, IL-2–producing MBT-2 cells was able to cause regression of orthotopically implanted tumors (275). Similar results showing that established tumors could be affected by cytokine-modified tumor vaccines have been obtained in other animal models, including the Lewis lung carcinoma (276) and a spontaneous murine renal-cell carcinoma (271). In this latter model, Golumbek and colleagues (271) showed that IL-4–transfected tumor cells were rejected in a predominantly T-cell–independent manner; however, at the same time, they were able to induce systemic T-cell immunity. This immunity was tumor-specific, and it could mediate the regression of established parental tumors.

These preclinical studies motivated initiation of a series of Phase I and II clinical trials with different cytokine-modified tumor cells. Whether this approach will be able to effectively modify the established relationship between evolving human tumors and the immune system still needs to be determined.

CONCLUSIONS

Cancer therapy with the use of cytokines constitutes an important field in clinical oncology. In addition to the established use of hematopoietic growth factors as bone marrow protectants; IFN-α for hairy-cell leukemia, KS, and renal-cell carcinoma; and IL-2 for metastatic renal-cell carcinoma, continuous clinical investigation may lead to new indications for cytokine-based cancer therapy.

Results from clinical trials support the use of IFN-α in other malignancies, including CML (both as a single agent and in combination with chemotherapy), squamous-cell carcinomas of the skin and the cervix (in combination with retinoic acid), and malignant melanomas (in combination with chemotherapy and IL-2). TNF-α may prove valuable in regional therapy of melanomas and sarcomas if the promising published results are confirmed. Furthermore, combinations of IL-2 and IFN-α may achieve effective results at less toxic doses in renal-cell carcinomas. Other protocols, using anticancer cytokines alone, in combination, or with chemotherapy, are an active area of investigation, but clinical results do not yet allow definitive conclusions. The role, if any, of gene therapy of cancer with cytokine genes has yet to be defined.

Although established treatments incorporating the use of cytokines are still few, they illustrate the potential of this therapeutic modality. We still need to define more precisely normal cytokine physiology and the role cytokines have in tumor-hose interactions. This knowledge, in addition to clinical experience obtained in Phase I and II trials, should lead to more effective use of cytokines in cancer management.

REFERENCES

1. Hansen RM, Borden EC. Current status of interferons in the treatment of cancer. Oncology 1992;6:19–24.

2. Rosenberg SA. The immunotherapy and gene therapy of cancer. J Clin Oncol 1992;10:180–199.

3. Rubin JT. Interleukin-2: its biological and clinical application in patients with cancer. Cancer Invest 1993;11:460–472.

4. Weisbart RH, Gasson JC, Golde DW. Colony- stimulating factors and host defense. Ann Intern Med 1989;110:297–303.

5. Warren MK, Ralph P. Macrophage growth factor CSF-1 stimulates human monocyte production of interferon, tumor necrosis factor and colony-stimulating activity. J Immunol. 1986;137:2281–2285.

6. Ralph P, Nakoinz I. Stimulation of macrophage tumoricidal activity by the growth and differentiation factor CSF-1. Cell Immunol 1987;105:270–279.

7. Gasparetto C, Laver J, Abbound M, et al. Effects of interleukin 1 on hematopoietic progenitors: evidence of stimulatory and inhibitory activities in a primate model. Blood 1989;74:547–550.

8. Ihle JN. Interleukin-3 and hematopoiesis. Chem Immunol 1992;51:65–106.

9. Broxmeyer HE, Lu L, Cooper S, et al. Synergistic effects of purified recombinant human and murine B cell growth factor-1 / IL-4 on colony formation in vitro by hematopoietic progenitor cells. J Immunol 1988;141:3852–3862.

10. Ikebuchi K, Ihle JN, Hirai Y, et al. Synergistic factors for stem cell proliferation: further studies of the target stem cells and the mechanism of stimulation by interleukin-1, interleukin-6, and granulocyte colony-stimulating factor. Blood 1988;72:2007–2014.

11. Sugarman BJ, Aggarwal BB, Haas BE, et al. Recombinant human tumor necrosis factor-alpha: effects on proliferation of normal and transformed cells in vitro. Science 1985; 230:943–945.

12. Salmon SE, Durie BGM, Young L, et al. Effects of cloned human leukocyte interferons in the human stem cell assay. J Clin Oncol 1983;1:217–225.

13. Taylor CW, Grogan TM, Salmon SE. Effects of interleukin-4 on the in vitro growth of human lymphoid and plasma cell neoplasms. Blood 1990;75:1114–1118.

14. Onozaki K, Matsushima K, Aggarwal BB, et al. Interleukin-1 as a cytocidal factor for several tumor cell lines. J Immunol 1985;135:3962–3968.

15. Lachman LB, Dinarello CA, Llanska ND, et al. Natural and recombinant human interleukin-1β is cytotoxic for human melanoma cells. J Immunol 1986;136:3098–3103.

16. Malkovsky M, Loveland B, North M, et al. Recombinant interleukin-2 directly augments the cytotoxicity of human monocytes. Nature 1987;325:262–265.

17. Heslop HE, Gottlieb DJ, Bianchi ACM, et al. In vivo induction of gamma interferon and tumor necrosis factor by interleukin 2 infusion following intensive chemotherapy or autologous marrow transplantation. Blood 1989;74:1374–1380.

18. Kasid A, Director EP, Rosenberg SA. Induction of endogenous cytokine mRNA in circulating peripheral blood mononuclear cells by IL-2 administration to cancer patients. J Immunol 1989;143:736–739.

19. Rosenberg SA, Spiess PJ, Schwartz S. In vivo administration of IL-2 enhances specific alloimmune responses. Transplantation 1983;35:631–634.

20. Kawakami Y, Rosenberg SA, Lotze MT. Interleukin 4 promotes the growth of tumor infiltrating lymphocytes cytotoxic for human autologous melanoma. J Exp Med 1989;168:2183–2191.

21. Rosenberg SA, Lotze MT, Yang JC, et al. Experience with the use of high-dose interleukin-2 in the treatment of 652 cancer patients. Ann Surg 1989;210:474–485.

22. Quesada JR, Reuben J, Manning JT, et al. Alpha interferon for induction of remission in hairy cell leukemia. N Engl J Med 1984; 310:15–18.

23. Siegel JP, Pari RK. Interleukin-2 toxicity. J Clin Oncol 1991;9:694–704.

24. Quesada JR, Talpaz M, Rios A, et al. Clinical toxicity of interferons in cancer patients: a review. J Clin Oncol 1986; 4:234–243.

25. Lienard D, Ewalenko P, Delmotte JJ, et al. High-dose recombinant tumor necrosis factor alpha in combination with interferon gamma and melphalan in isolation perfusion of the limbs for melanoma and sarcoma. J Clin Oncol 1992;10:52–60.

26. Mavligit GM, Zukiwski AA, Gutterman JU, et al. Splenic versus hepatic artery infusion of interleukin-2 in patients with liver metastasis. J Clin Oncol 1990;8:319–324.

27. Fetell MR, Housepian EM, Oster MW, et al. Intratumor administration of beta-interferon in recurrent malignant gliomas. A phase I clinical and laboratory study. Cancer 1990;65:78–83.

28. Vadhan-Raj S, Papadoupoulos N, Burgess M, et al. Optimization of dose and schedule of PIXY321 (GM-CSF/IL-3 fusion protein) to attenuate chemotherapy (CT)-induced multilineage myelosuppression in patients with sarcoma (abstract). Proc Am Soc Clin Oncol 1993;12:470.

29. Miller L, Smith J II, Urba W, et al. A phase I study of an IL-3/GM-CSF fusion protein (PIXY321) and high dose carboplatin (CBDCA) in patients with advanced cancer (abstract). Proc Am Soc Clin Oncol 1993;12:138.

30. Ostade XV, Vandenabeele P, Everaerdt B, et al. Human TNF mutants with selective activity on the p55 receptor. Nature 1993;361:266–269.

31. Yu JS, Wei MX, Chiocca EA, et al. Treatment of glioma by engineered interleukin-4 secreting cells. Cancer Res 1993; 53:3125–3128.

32. Blankenstein T, Qin Z, Uberla K, et al. Tumor suppression after tumor cell-targeted tumor necrosis factor α gene transfer. J Exp Med 1991;173:1047–1052.

33. Watanabe Y, Kuribayashi K, Miyatake S, et al. Exogenous expression of mouse interferon γ cDNA in mouse neuroblastoma C1300 cells results in reduced tumorigenicity by augmented anti-tumor immunity. Proc Natl Acad Sci USA 1989;89:9456–9460.

34. Kosmidis PA, Baxevanis CN, Tsavaris N, et al. The prog-

nostic significance of immune changes in patients with renal cell carcinoma treated with interferon alfa-2b. J Clin Oncol 1992;10:1153–1157.

35. Krown SE, Real FX, Cunningham-Rundles S, et al. Preliminary observations of the effect of recombinant leukocyte A interferon in homosexual men with Kaposi's sarcoma. N Engl J Med 1983;308:1071–1076.

36. Isaacs A, Lindenmann J. Virus interference: I. The interferon. Proc R Soc Lond (Biol) 1957;147:258–267.

37. Kurzrock R, Talpaz M, Gutterman JU. Interferons - α, β, γ: basic principles and preclinical studies. In: DeVita VT, Hellman S, Rosenberg SA, eds. Biologic therapy of cancer. Philadelphia: J.B. Lippincott, 1991;247–274.

38. Taniguchi T. Regulation of cytokine gene expression. Ann Rev Immunol 1988;6:439–464.

39. Epstein LB, Gupta S. Human T lymphocyte subset production of immune (gamma) interferon. J Clin Immunol 1981;1:186–194.

40. Chang T, Testa D, Kung PC, et al. Cellular origin and interactions involved in gamma-interferon production induced by OKT3 monoclonal antibody. J Immunol 1983;128:585–589.

41. Samuel CE. Mechanism of the antiviral action of interferons. Prog Nucleic Acids Res Mol Biol 1988;35:27–72.

42. Fellous M, Nir U, Wallach D, et al. Interferon-dependent induction of mRNA for the major histocompatibility antigens in human fibroblasts and lymphoblastoid cells. Proc Natl Acad Sci USA 1982;79:3082–3086.

43. Kurzrock R, Quesada JR, Talpaz M, et al. Phase I study of multiple dose intramuscularly administered recombinant gamma interferon. J Clin Oncol 1986;4:1101–1109.

44. Clemens MJ. Molecular mechanisms of interferon action. Br J Clin Prac 1988;62(suppl):5–12.

45. Kimchi A. Autocrine interferon and the suppression of the c-myc nuclear oncogene. Interferon 1987;8:86–110.

46. Diaz MO, Ziemin S, Le Beau MM, et al. Homozygous deletion of the α- and β-interferon genes in human leukemia and derived cell lines. Proc Natl Acad Sci USA 1988;85:5259–5263.

47. Folkman J. Successful treatment of an angiogenic disease. N Engl J Med 1989;320:1211–1212.

48. Nagali M, Arai T. Clinical effects of interferon in malignant brain tumors. Neurosurg Rev 1984;7:55–64.

49. Dorr RT. Interferon-α in malignant and viral diseases. A review. Drug 1993;45:177–211.

50. Jones GJ, Itri LM. Safety and tolerance of recombinant interferon alfa-2a (Roferon-A) in cancer patients. Cancer 1986;57:1709–1715.

51. Abrams PG, McClamrock E, Foon KA. Evening administration of alpha interferon. N Engl J Med 1985;312:443–444.

52. Levi F, Canon C, DiPalma M, et al. When should the immune clock be reset. From circadian pharmacodynamics to temporally optimized drug delivery. Ann NY Acad Sci 1991;618:312–329.

53. Déprés-Brummer P, Levi F, Di Palma M, et al. A phase I trial of 21-day continuous venous infusion of α-interferon at circadian rhythm modulated rate in cancer patients. J Immunother 1991;10:440–447.

54. Foon KA, Maluish AE, Abrams PG, et al. Recombinant leu-

kocyte A interferon therapy for advanced hairy cell leukemia. Am J Med 1986;80:351–356.

55. Quesada JR, Hersh EM, Manning JT, et al. Treatment of hairy cell leukemia with recombinant α-interferon. Blood 1986;68:493–497.

56. Thompson JA, Fefer A. Interferon in the treatment of hairy cell leukemia. Cancer 1987;59:605–609.

57. Talpaz M, McCredie KB, Mavligit GM, et al. Leukocyte interferon-induced myeloid cytoreduction in chronic myelogenous leukemia. Blood 1983;62:689–692.

58. Niederle N, Kloke O, Osieka R, et al. Interferon alpha-2b in the treatment of chronic myelogenous leukemia. Semin Oncol 1987;14:29–35.

59. Alimena G, Morra E, Lazzarino M, et al. Interferon alpha-2b as therapy for Ph' positive chronic myelogenous leukemia: a study of 82 patients treated with intermittent or daily administration. Blood 1988;72:642–647.

60. Werter M, de Witte R, Janssen J, et al. Recombinant human interferon alpha-induced cytoreduction in chronic myelogenous leukemia. Blut 1988;56:209–212.

61. Foon KA, Sherwin SA, Abrams PG, et al. Treatment of advanced non-Hodgkin's lymphoma with recombinant leukocyte A interferon. N Engl J Med 1984;311:1148–1152.

62. Mandelli F, Avvisati G, Amadori S, et al. Maintenance treatment with recombinant interferon alpha-2b in patients with multiple myeloma responding to conventional induction chemotherapy. N Engl J Med 1990;322:1430–1434.

63. Salmon SE, Beckord J, Pugh RP, et al. Alpha-interferon for remission maintenance: preliminary report on the Southwestern Oncology Group Study. Semin Oncol 1991;18 (suppl 7):33–36.

64. Kohn EC, Steis RG, Sausville EA, et al. Phase II trial of intermittent high-dose recombinant interferon alpha-2a in mycosis fungoides and the Sezary syndrome. J Clin Oncol 1990;8:155–160.

65. Volberding PA, Mitsuyasu RT, Golando JP, et al. Treatment of Kaposi's sarcoma with interferon alpha-2b (INTRON A). Cancer 1987;59:620–625.

66. Real FX, Oettgen HF, Krown SE. Kaposi's sarcoma and the acquired immunodeficiency syndrome: treatment with high and low doses of recombinant leukocyte A interferon. J Clin Oncol 1986;4:544–551.

67. Sarna G, Figlin R, de Kernion J. Interferon in renal cell carcinoma: the UCLA experience. Cancer 1987;59:610–612.

68. Moertel CG, Rubin J, Kvols L. Therapy of metastatic carcinoid tumor and the malignant carcinoid syndrome with recombinant leukocyte A interferon. J Clin Oncol 1989;7:865–868.

69. Creagan ET, Ahmann DL, Green SJ, et al. Phase II study of recombinant leukocyte A interferon (rIFN-αA) in disseminated malignant melanoma. Cancer 1984;54:2844–2849.

70. Giles FJ, Singer CRJ, Gray AG, et al. Alpha-interferon therapy for essential thrombocythemia. Lancet 1988;2:70–72.

71. Silver RT. A new treatment for polycythemia vera: recombinant interferon alpha. Blood 1990;76:664–665.

72. Flandrin G, Sigaux F, Sebahoun G, et al. Hairy cell leukemia: clinical presentation and follow-up of 211 patients. Semin Oncol 1984;11:458–471.

73. Golomb HM, Ratain MJ, Vardiman JW. Sequential treat-

ment of hairy cell leukemia: a new role for interferon. In: DeVita VT, Hellman S, Rosenberg SA, eds. Important advances in oncology. Philadelphia: JB Lippincott, 1986:311–321.

74. Quesada JR, Hersh EM, Gutterman JU. Treatment of hairy cell leukemia with alpha interferon (abstract). Proc Am Soc Clin Oncol 1984;3:207.

75. Ratain MJ, Golomb HM, Vardiman JW, et al. Treatment of hairy cell leukemia with recombinant alpha-2 interferon. Blood 1985;65:644–648.

76. Jacobs AD, Champlin RE, Golde DW. Recombinant α-2-interferon for hairy cell leukemia. Blood 1985;65:1017–1020.

77. Thompson JA, Brady J, Kidd P, et al. Recombinant alpha-2-interferon in the treatment of hairy cell leukemia. Cancer Treat Rep 1985;69:791–793.

78. Huber C, Flener R, Gastl G. Interferon-alpha-2c in the treatment of advanced hairy cell leukemia. Oncology 1985;42:7–9.

79. Golomb HM, Ratain MJ, Fefer A, et al. Randomized study of the duration of treatment with interferon alfa-2b in patients with hairy cell leukemia. J Natl Cancer Inst 1988;80:369–373.

80. Berman E, Heller G, Kempin S, et al. Incidence of response and long-term follow-up in patients with hairy cell leukemia treated with recombinant interferon alpha-2a. Blood 1990;4:839–845.

81. Johnston JB, Eisenhauer E, Corbett WEN, et al. Efficacy of 2′-deoxycoformycin in hairy cell leukemia: a study of the national cancer institute of Canada clinical trials group. J Natl Cancer Inst 1988;80:765–769.

82. Kraut EH, Bouroncle BA, Grever MR. Pentostatin in the treatment of advanced hairy cell leukemia. J Clin Oncol 1989;7:168–172.

83. Piro LD, Carrera CJ, Carson DA, et al. Lasting remissions in hairy cell leukemia induced by a single infusion of 2-chlorodeoxyadenosine. N Engl J Med 1990;322:1117–1121.

84. Stam K, Heisterkamp N, Grosveld G, et al. Evidence of a new chimeric bcr/c-abl mRNA in patients with chronic myelocytic leukemia and the Philadelphia chromosome. N Engl J Med 1985;313:1422–1429.

85. Talpaz M, Mavligit GM, Ketting M, et al. Human leukocyte interferon to control thrombocytosis in chronic myelogenous leukemia. Ann Intern Med 1983;99:789–792.

86. Kantarjian HM, Talpaz M, Gutterman JU. Biologic therapy of chronic myelogenous leukemia. Oncology 987;1:35–40.

87. Yoffe G, Blick M, Kantarjian HM, et al. Molecular analysis of interferon-induced suppression of Philadelphia chromosome in patients with chronic myeloid leukemia. Blood 1987;69:961–963.

88. Zuffa E, Italian Cooperative Study Group on Chronic Myeloid Leukemia. A prospective study of interferon alpha-2A vs chemotherapy in chronic myeloid leukemia (CML): karyotypic response and survival (abstract). Proc Am Soc Clin Oncol 1993:12:300.

89. Rosenblum MG, Maxwell BL, Talpaz M, et al. In vivo sensitivity and resistance of chronic myelogenous leukemia cells to α-interferon: correlation with receptor binding and induction of 2′-5′-oligoadenylate synthetase. Cancer Res 1986;46:4848–4852.

90. Wagstaff J, Scarffe JH, Crowther D. Interferon in the treatment of multiple myeloma and the non-Hodgkin's lymphomas. Cancer Treat Rev 1985;12(suppl B):39–44.

91. Costanzi JJ, Cooper MR, Scarffe JH, et al. Phase II study of recombinant alpha-2-interferon in resistant multiple myeloma. J Clin Oncol 1985;3:654–659.

92. Westin J. Interferon therapy during the plateau phase of multiple myeloma: an update of a Swedish multicenter study. Semin Oncol 1991;18(suppl 7):33–36.

93. Avvisati G, Boccadoro M, Petrucci MT, et. al. Interferon alpha as maintenance treatment in multiple myeloma: the Italian experience (abstract). IV International Workshop on Multiple Myeloma, Rochester, MN, October 2–5, 1993.

94. Salmon SE, Crowley J. Evaluation of interferon (IFN) in maintenance therapy for myeloma (abstract). IV International Workshop on Multiple Myeloma, Rochester, MN, October 2–5, 1993.

95. Cunningham D, Powless R, Malpas JS, et al. A randomized trial of maintenance therapy with intron-A following high dose melphalan and ABMT in myeloma (abstract). Proc Am Soc Clin Oncol 1993;12:364.

96. Horning SJ, Merigan TC, Krown SE, et al. Human interferon alpha in malignant lymphoma and Hodgkin's disease: results of the American Cancer Society trial. Cancer 1985;56:1305–1310.

97. Bunn PA Jr, Foon KA, Ihde DC, et al. Recombinant leukocyte A interferon: an active agent in advanced cutaneous T-cell lymphomas. Ann Intern Med 1984;101:484–487.

98. Kemme DJ, Bunn PA Jr. State of the art therapy of mycosis fungoides and Sezary syndrome. Oncology 1992;6:31–42.

99. Kaplan EH, Rosen ST, Norris DB, et al. Phase II study of recombinant human interferon-gamma in cutaneous T-cell lymphoma (CTCL). J Natl Cancer Inst 1990;82:208–212.

100. Tamura K, Makino S, Araki Y, et al. Recombinant interferon beta and gamma in the treatment of adult T-cell leukemia. Cancer 1987;59:1059–1062.

101. Hersey P, MacDonald M, Hall C, et al. Immunological effects of recombinant interferon alpha-2a in patients with disseminated melanoma. Cancer 1986;57:1666–1674.

102. Kirkwood JM, Hunt M, Smith T, et al. A randomized controlled trial of high-dose IFN alpha-2b for high-risk melanoma: the ECOG trial EST-1684 (abstract). Proc Am Soc Clin Oncol 1993;12:390.

103. Quesada JR, Rios A, Swanson DA, et al. Antitumor activity of recombinant-derived interferon alpha in metastatic renal cell carcinoma. J Clin Oncol 1985;3:1522–1528.

104. Umeda T, Niijima T. Phase II study of alpha interferon on renal cell carcinoma. Cancer 1986;58:1231–1235.

105. Muss HB, Costanzi JJ, Leavitt R, et al. Recombinant alpha interferon in renal cell carcinoma: a randomized trial of two routes of administration. J Clin Oncol 1987;5:286–291.

106. Stahl M, Wilke HJ, Seeber S, et al. Cytokines and cytotoxic agents in renal cell carcinoma: a review. Semin Oncol 1992;19(suppl 4):70–79.

107. Muss HB. Interferon—clinical applications: renal cell carcinoma. In: De Vita VT, Hellman S, Rosenberg SA, eds. Biologic therapy of cancer. Philadelphia: JB Lippincott, 1991:298–311.

108. Minasian LM, Motzer RJ, Gluck L, et al. Interferon alfa-2a in advanced renal cell carcinoma: treatment results and survival in 159 patients with long-term follow-up. J Clin Oncol 1993;11:1368–1375.

109. Oberg K, Funa K, Alm G. Effects of leukocyte interferon on clinical symptoms and hormone levels in patients with mid-gut carcinoid tumors and carcinoid syndrome. N Engl J Med 1983;309:129–133.

110. Eriksson B, Oberg K, Alm G, et al. Treatment of malignant endocrine pancreatic tumors with human leukocyte interferon. Cancer Treat Rep 1987;71:31–37.

111. Greenway HT, Cornell RC, Tanner DJ, et al. Treatment of basal cell carcinoma with intralesional interferon. J Am Acad Dermatol 1986;15:437–443.

112. Edwards L, Tucker SB, Perednia D, et al. The effect of an intralesional sustained-release formulation of interferon alpha-2b on basal cell carcinomas. Arch Dermatol 1990; 126:1029–1032.

113. Richards JM, Mehta N, Ramming K, et al. Sequential chemoimmunotherapy in the treatment of metastatic melanoma. J Clin Oncol 1992;10:1338–1343.

114. Margolin KA, Doroshow JH, Akman SA, et al. Phase II trial of cisplatin and α-interferon in advanced malignant melanoma. J Clin Oncol 1992;10:1574–1578.

115. Pyrhönen S, Hahka-Kemppinen M, Muhonen T. A promising interferon plus four-drug chemotherapy regimen for metastatic melanoma. J Clin Oncol 1992;12:1919–1926.

116. Figlin RA, Belldegrun A, Moldawer N, et al. Concomitant administration of recombinant human interleukin-2 and recombinant interferon alfa-2a: an active outpatient regimen in metastatic renal cell carcinoma. J Clin Oncol 1992; 10:414–421.

117. Ilson DH, Motzer RJ, Kradin RL, et al. A phase II trial of interleukin-2 and interferon alfa-2a in patients with advanced renal cell carcinoma. J Clin Oncol 1992;10:1124–1130.

118. Kelsen D, Lovett D, Wong J, et al. Interferon alfa-2a and fluorouracil in the treatment of patients with advanced esophageal cancer. J Clin Oncol 1992;10:269–274.

119. Grem JL, Jordan E, Robson ME, et al. Phase II study of fluorouracil, leucovorin, and interferon alfa-2a in metastatic colorectal carcinoma. J Clin Oncol 1993;11:1737–1745.

120. Duggan DB, Santarelli MT, Zamkoff K, et al. A phase II study of recombinant interleukin-2 with or without recombinant interferon-β in non-hodgkin's lymphoma. A study of the cancer and leukemia group B. J Immunother 1992; 12:115–122.

121. Kantarjian HM, Keating M, Estey EH, et al. Treatment of advanced stages of Philadelphia chromosome-positive chronic myelogenous leukemia with interferon-α and low dose cytarabine. J Clin Oncol 1992;10:772–778.

122. Lippman SM, Parkinson DR. 13-cis-retinoic acid and interferon alpha-2a: effective combination therapy for advanced squamous cell carcinoma of the skin. J Natl Cancer Inst 1992;85:235–241.

123. Lippman SM, Kavanagh JL, Paredes-Espinoza M, et al. 13-cis-retinoic acid plus interferon-α2a in locally advanced squamous cell carcinoma of the cervix. J Natl Cancer Inst 1993;85:499–500.

124. Lippman SM, Kavanagh JL, Paredes-Espinoza M, et al. 13-cis-retinoic acid plus interferon alpha-2a: highly active systemic therapy for squamous cell carcinoma of the cervix. J Natl Cancer Inst 1992;84:241–245.

125. Wadler S, Schwartz EL, Goldman M, et al. Fluorouracil and recombinant alpha-2a interferon: an active regimen against advanced colorectal carcinoma. J Clin Oncol 1989;7: 1769–1775.

126. Pazdur R, Ajani J, Patt YZ, et al. Phase II study of fluorouracil and recombinant interferon alpha 2-a in previously untreated advanced colorectal carcinoma. J Clin Oncol 1990; 8:2027–2031.

127. York M, Greco FA, Figlin RA, et al. A randomized phase III trial comparing 5-FU with or without interferon alpha 2a for advanced colorectal cancer (abstract). Proc Am Soc Clin Oncol 1993;12:200.

128. Morgan DA, Ruscetti FW, Gallo RC. Selective in vitro growth of T lymphocytes from normal human bone marrows. Science 1976;193:1007–1008.

129. Smith KA. Interleukin-2: inception, impact and implications. Science 1988;240:1169–1176.

130. Grimm EA, Mazumder A, Zhang HZ, et al. Lymphokine-activated killer cell phenomenon: lysis of natural killer-resistant fresh solid tumor cells by interleukin-2 activated autologous human peripheral blood lymphocytes. J Exp Med 1982;155:1823–1841.

131. Nakanishi K, Malek TP, Smith KA, et al. Both interleukin 2 and a second T-cell derived factor in EL-4 supernatant have activity as differentiation factors in IgM synthesis. J Exp Med 1984;160:1605–1621.

132. Vujanovic NL, Herberman RB, Hiserodt JC. Lymphokine-activated killer cells in rats: analysis of tissue and strain distribution, ontogeny and target specificity. Cancer Res 1988;48:878–883.

133. Lotze MT, Matory YL, Ettinghausen SE, et al. In vivo administration of purified human interleukin-2. Half life, immunologic effects and expansion of peripheral lymphoid cells in vivo with recombinant IL-2. J Immunol 1985;135: 2865–2875.

134. Topalian SL, Muul LM, Solomon D, et al. Expansion of human tumor infiltrating lymphocytes for use in immunotherapy trials. J Immunol Methods 1987;102:127–141.

135. Muul LM, Spiess PJ, Director EP, et al. Identification of specific cytolytic immune responses against autologous tumors in humans bearing malignant melanoma. J Immunol 1987;138:989–995.

136. Rabinowich H, Cohen R, Bruderman I, et al. Functional analysis of mononuclear cells infiltrating into tumors: lysis of autologous tumor cells by cultured infiltrating lymphocytes. Cancer Res 1987;47:173–177.

137. Vose BM, Moore M. Human tumor-infiltrating lymphocytes: a marker of host response. Semin Hematol 1985;22: 27–40.

138. Itoh K, Tilden AB, Balch CM. Interleukin-2 activation of cytotoxic T lymphocytes infiltrating into human metastatic melanomas. Cancer Res 1986;46:3011–3017.

139. Whiteside TL, Miescher S, Hurlimann J, et al. Clonal analysis and in situ characterization of lymphocytes infiltrating human breast carcinomas. Cancer Immunol Immunother 1986;23:169–178.

140. Barth RJ, Bock SN, Mulé JJ, et al. Unique murine tumor associated antigens identified by tumor infiltrating lymphocytes. J Immunol 1990;144:1531–1537.

141. Rosenberg SA, Spiess PJ, Lafreniere R. A new approach to the adoptive immunotherapy of cancer with tumor-infiltrating lymphocytes. Science 1986;233:1318–1321.

142. Mazumder A, Rosenberg SA. Successful immunotherapy of NK-resistant established pulmonary melanoma metastases by the intravenous adoptive transfer of syngeneic lymphocytes activated in vitro by interleukin-2. J Exp Med 1984; 159:495–507.

143. Mulé JJ, Shu S, Schwarz SL, et al. Adoptive immunotherapy of established pulmonary metastases with LAK cells and recombinant interleukin-2. Science 1984;225:1487–1489.

144. Lafreniere R, Rosenberg SA. Successful immunotherapy of murine experimental hepatic metastases with lymphokine-activated killer cells and recombinant interleukin-2. Cancer Res 1985;45:3735–3741.

145. Rosenberg SA, Mulé JJ, Spiess PJ, et al. Regression of established pulmonary metastases and subcutaneous tumor mediated by the systemic administration of high dose recombinant IL-2. J Exp Med 1985;161:1169–1188.

146. Lafreniere R, Rosenberg SA. Adoptive immunotherapy of murine hepatic metastases with lymphokine activated killer (LAK) cells and recombinant interleukin-2 (RIL-2) can mediate the regression of both immunogenic and non-immunogenic sarcomas and an adenocarcinoma. J Immunol 1985;135:4273–4280.

147. Ettinghausen SE, Lipford EH, Mulé JJ, et al. Systemic administration of recombinant interleukin-2 stimulates in vivo lymphoid cell proliferation in tissues. J Immunol 1985;135:1488–1497.

148. Ettinghausen SE, Lipford EH, Mulé JJ, et al. Recombinant interleukin-2 stimulates in vivo proliferation of adoptively transferred lymphokine activated killer (LAK) cells. J Immunol 1985;135:3623–3635.

149. Rosenberg SA, Lotze MT, Muul LM, et al. Observations on the systemic administration of autologous lymphokine-activated killer cells and recombinant interleukin-2 to patients with metastatic cancer. N Engl J Med 1985;313: 1485–1492.

150. Wiebke EA, Rosenberg SA, Lotze MT. Acute immunologic effects of interleukin-2 therapy in cancer patients: decreased delayed type hypersensitivity response and decreased proliferative response to soluble antigens. J Clin Oncol 1988;6:1440–1449.

151. Kradin RL, Kurnick JT, Preffer FI, et al. Adoptive immunotherapy with IL-2 results in the loss of delayed type hypersensitivity responses and the development of immediate hypersensitivity to recall antigens. Clin Immunol Immunopathol 1989;50:184–195.

152. Lotze MT, Rosenberg SA. Interleukin-2: clinical applications. In: De Vita VT, Hellman S, Rosenberg SA, eds. Biologic therapy of cancer. Philadelphia: JB Lippincott, 1991: 159–177.

153. Kragel AH, Travis WD, Feinberg L, et al. Pathologic findings associated with interleukin-2 based immunotherapy for cancer: a postmortem study of 19 patients. Hum Pathol 1990;21:493–502.

154. Gaspari AA, Lotze MT, Rosenberg SA, et al. Dermatologic changes associated with interleukin-2 administration. JAMA 1987;258:1624–1629.

155. Ellis TM, Creekmore SP, McMannis JD, et al. Appearance and phenotypic characterization of circulating Leu 10+ cells in cancer patients receiving recombinant interleukin-2. Cancer Res 1988;48:6597–6602.

156. Rosenberg SA. Immunotherapy of cancer by systemic administration of lymphoid cells plus interleukin-2. J Biol Response Mod 1984;3:501–511.

157. Lee RE, Lotze MT, Skibber JM, et al. Cardiorespiratory effects of immunotherapy with interleukin-2. J Clin Oncol 1989;7:7–20.

158. Denikoff KD, Rubinow DR, Papa MZ, et al. The neuropsychiatric effects of treatment with interleukin-2 and lymphokine activated killer cells. Ann Intern Med 1987; 107:293–300.

159. Belldegrun A, Webb DE, Austin HA, et al. Effects of interleukin-2 on renal function in patients receiving immunotherapy for advanced cancer. Ann Intern Med 1987;106: 817–822.

160. Edwards MJ, Abney DL, Heniford BT, et al. Passive immunization against tumor necrosis factor inhibits interleukin-2 induced microvascular alterations and reduces toxicity. Surgery 1992;112:480–486.

161. Mier JW, Vachino G, van der Meer JW, et al. Induction of circulating tumor necrosis factor (TNF α) as the mechanism for the febrile response to interleukin-2 (IL-2) in cancer patients. J Clin Immunol 1988;8:426–436.

162. Weidmann E, Bergmann L, Stock J, et al. Rapid cytokine release in cancer patients treated with interleukin-2. J Immunother 1992;12:123–131.

163. Hartmann LC, Urba WJ, Steis RG, et al. Use of prophylactic antibiotics for prevention of intravascular catheter-related infections in interleukin-2 treated patients. J Natl Cancer Inst 1989;81:1190–1193.

164. Bock SL, Lee RE, Fisher B, et al. A prospective randomized trial evaluating prophylactic antibiotics to prevent triple-lumen catheter-related sepsis in patients treated with immunotherapy. J Clin Oncol 1990;8:161–169.

165. Pockaj BA, Topalian SL, Steinberg SM, et al. Infectious complications associated with interleukin-2 administration: a retrospective review of 935 treatment courses. J Clin Oncol 1993;11:136–147.

166. West TH, Tauer KW, Yanelli JR, et al. Constant infusion recombinant interleukin-2 in adoptive immunotherapy of advanced cancer. N Engl J Med 1987;316:898–905.

167. Thompson JA, Lee DS, Lindgren CG, et al. Influence of dose and duration of infusion of interleukin-2 on toxicity and immunomodulation. J Clin Oncol 1988;6:669–678.

168. Fraker DL, Langstein HN, Norton JA. Passive immunization against tumor necrosis factor partially abrogates interleukin-2 toxicity. J Exp Med 1989;170:1015–1020.

169. Edwards MJ, Heniford BT, Klar EA, et al. Pentoxifylline inhibits interleukin-2-induced toxicity in C57BL/6 mice but preserves antitumor efficacy. J Clin Invest 1992;90:637–641.

170. Rosenberg SA, Lotze MT, Yang JC, et al. Prospective randomized trial of high-dose interleukin-2 alone or in conjunction with lymphokine-activated killer cells for the treatment of patients with advanced cancer. J Natl Cancer Inst 1993;85:622–632.

171. Weber JS, Yang JC, Topalian SL, et al. The use of interleukin-2 and lymphokine-activated killer cells for the treatment of patients with non-Hodgkin's lymphoma. J Clin Oncol 1992;10:33–40.

172. Cameron RB, Spiess PJ, Rosenberg SA. Synergistic antitumor activity of tumor infiltrating lymphocytes, interleukin 2 and local tumor irradiation—studies on the mechanism of action. J Exp Med 1990;171:249–263.

173. Barth RJ, Mulé JJ, Spiess PJ, et al. Interferon γ and tumor necrosis factor have a role in tumor regressions mediated by murine CD8+ tumor infiltrating lymphocytes. J Exp Med 1991;173:647–658.

174. Rosenberg SA, Packard BS, Aebersold PM, et al. Use of tumor-infiltrating lymphocytes and interleukin-2 in the immunotherapy of patients with metastatic melanoma. N Engl J Med 1988;319:1676–1680.

175. Weiss GR, Margolin KA, Aronson FR, et al. A randomized phase II trial of continuous infusion interleukin-2 or bolus injection interleukin-2 plus lymphokine-activated killer cells for advanced renal cell carcinoma. J Clin Oncol 1992;10:275–281.

176. Thompson JA, Shulman KL, Benyunes MC, et al. Prolonged continuous intravenous infusion interleukin-2 and lymphokine activated killer-cell therapy for metastatic renal cell carcinoma. J Clin Oncol 1992;10:960–968.

177. Geertsen PF, Hermann GG, von der Maase H, et al. Treatment of metastatic renal cell carcinoma by continuous intravenous infusion of recombinant interleukin-2: a single-center phase II study. J Clin Oncol 1992;10:753–759.

178. Whitehead RP, Ward D, Hemingway L, et al. Subcutaneous recombinant interleukin-2 in a dose escalating regimen in patients with metastatic renal cell adenocarcinoma. Cancer Res 1990;50:6708–6715.

179. Stein RC, Malkovska V, Morgan S, et al. The clinical effects of prolonged treatment of patients with advanced cancer with low-dose subcutaneous interleukin-2. Br J Cancer 1991;63:275–278.

180. Sleijfer DTh, Janssen RAJ, Buter J, et al. Phase II study of subcutaneous interleukin-2 in unselected patients with advanced renal cell cancer on an outpatient basis. J Clin Oncol 1992;10:1119–1123.

181. Bernstein ZP, Goldrosen MH, Vaickus L, et al. Interleukin-2 with ex vivo activated killer cell: therapy of advanced non-small-cell lung cancer. J Immunother 1991;10:383–387.

182. Miescher S, Stoeck M, Qiao L, et al. Preferential clonogenic deficit of CD8 positive T lymphocytes infiltrating human solid tumors. Cancer Res 1988;48:6992–6998.

183. Chouaib S, Bertoglio J, Blay JY, et al. Lymphokine activated killers generation pathways: synergy between tumor necrosis factor and interleukin 2. Proc Natl Acad Sci USA 1988;85:6875–6879.

184. Blay JY, Bertoglio J, Fradelizi D, et al. Functional interactions of IL-2 and TNF in the differentiation of LGL into LAK effectors. Int J Cancer 1989;44:598–604.

185. Shimizu Y, Iwatsuki S, Herberman RB, et al. Effects of cytokines on in vitro growth of tumor infiltrating lymphocytes obtained from primary and metastatic liver tumors. Cancer Immunol Immunother 1991;32:280–288.

186. Barbuto JAM, Punt CJA, Grimes WJ, et al. Production of neutralizing antibodies to tumor necrosis factor by human tumor-infiltrating B lymphocytes (abstract). Proc Am Assoc Cancer Res 1993;34:484.

187. Martinet N, Charles T, Vaillant P, et al. Characterization of a tumor necrosis factor-alpha inhibitor activity in cancer patients. Am J Respir Cell Mol Biol 1992;6:510–515.

188. Digel W, Porzsolt F, Schmid M, et al. High levels of circulating soluble receptors for tumor necrosis factor in hairy cell leukemia and type B chronic lymphocytic leukemia. J Clin Invest 1992;89:1690–1693.

189. Abbate I, Correale M, Gargano G, et al. Tumor necrosis factor and soluble interleukin-2 receptor: two immunological biomarkers in female neoplasms. Eur J Gynaecol Oncol 1992;13:92–96.

190. Hornung RL, Salup RR, Wiltrout RH. Tissue distribution and localization of IL-2 activated killer cells after adoptive transfer in vivo. In: Lotzova E, Herberman RB, eds. Interleukin-2 and killer cells in cancer. Boca Raton, FL: CRC Press, 1990:245–258.

191. Maghazachi AA, Herberman RB, Vujanovic NL, et al. In vivo distribution and tissue localization of high purified rat lymphokine activated killer cells. Cell Immunol 1988;115:179–193.

192. Felgar RE, Hiserodt JC. In vivo migration patterns of highly purified adherent lymphokine activated killer cells in tumor bearing rats. Cell Immunol 1992;141:32–46.

193. Wu NZ, Klitzman B, Dodge R, et al. Diminished leukocyte-endothelium interaction in tumor microvessels. Cancer Res 1992;52:4265–4268.

194. DiRaimondo F, LaPushin R, Hersh EM. Synergism between alpha-interferon and interleukin-2-activated killer cells: in vitro studies. Acta Haemat 1987;78(suppl 1):77–83.

195. Brunda MJ, Bellantoni D, Sulich V. In vivo antitumor activity of combinations of interferon-α and interleukin-2 in a murine model. Correlation of efficacy with the induction of cytotoxic cells resembling natural killer cells. Int J Cancer 1987;40:365–371.

196. Rosenberg SA, Schwartz S, Spiess PJ. Combination immunotherapy for cancer: synergistic antitumor interactions of interleukin-2, alpha-interferon, and tumor-infiltrating lymphocytes. J Natl Cancer Inst 1988;80:1393–1397.

197. Cameron RB, McIntosh JK, Rosenberg SA. Synergistic antitumor effects of combination immunotherapy with recombinant interleukin-2 and a recombinant hybrid α-interferon in the treatment of established murine hepatic metastases. Cancer Res 1988;48:5810–5817.

198. Atkins MB, Sparano J, Fisher RI, et al. Randomized phase II trial of high-dose interleukin-2 either alone or in combination with interferon alfa-2b in advanced renal cell carcinoma. J Clin Oncol 1993;11:661–670.

199. Lipton A, Harvey H, Givant E, et al. Interleukin-2 and interferon-α-2a outpatient therapy for metastatic renal cell carcinoma. J Immunother 1993;13:122–129.

200. Whitehead RP, Figlin R, Citron ML, et al. A phase II trial on concomitant human interleukin-2 and interferon-α-2a in patients with disseminated malignant melanoma. J Immunother 1993;13:117–121.

201. Vogelzang NJ, Lipton A, Figlin RA. Subcutaneous interleukin-2 plus interferon alfa-2a in metastatic renal cancer: an outpatient multicenter trial. J Clin Oncol 1993;11:1809–1816.

202. Negrier MS, Pourreau CN, Palmer PA, et al. Phase I trial of recombinant interleukin-2 followed by recombinant tumor necrosis factor in patients with metastatic cancer. J Immunother 1992;11:93–102.

203. Taylor CW, Chase EM, Whitehead RP, et al. A Southwest Oncology Group phase I study of the sequential combination of recombinant interferon-γ and recombinant interleukin-2 in patients with advanced cancer. J Immunother 1992;11:176–183.

204. Viens P, Blaise D, Stoppa AM, et al. Interleukin-2 in association with increasing doses of interferon-gamma in patients with advanced cancer. J Immunother 1992;11:218–224.

205. Bukowski RM, Sergi JS, Budd GT, et al. Phase I trial of continuous infusion interleukin-2 and doxorubicin in patients with refractory malignancies. J Immunother 1991;10:432–439.

206. Carswell EA, Old LJ, Kassel R, et al. An endotoxin-induced serum factor that causes necrosis of tumors. Proc Natl Acad Sci USA 1975;72:3666–3670.

207. Beutler B, Cerami A. The biology of cachectin/TNF—a primary mediator of the host response. Ann Rev Immunol 1989;7:625–655.

208. Vassalli P. The pathophysiology of tumor necrosis factors. Ann Rev Immunol 1992;10:411–452.

209. Haranaka K, Satomi N. Cytotoxic activity of tumor necrosis factor (TNF) on human cancer cells in vitro. J Exp Med 1981;51:191–194.

210. Williamson BD, Carswell EA, Rubin BY, et al. Human tumor necrosis factor produced by human B cell lines: synergistic cytotoxic interactions with human interferon. Proc Natl Acad Sci USA 1983;80:5397–5401.

211. Le J, Vilcek J. Tumor necrosis factor and interleukin 1: cytokines with multiple overlapping biological activities. Lab Invest 1987;56:234–248.

212. Le J, Weinstein D, Gubler U, et al. Induction of membrane-associated interleukin 1 by tumor necrosis factor in human fibroblasts. J Immunol 1987;138:2137–2142.

213. Van Damme J, Opdenakker G, Simpson RJ, et al. Identification of the human 26-kD protein, interferon-beta 2 (IFN-beta 2), as a B cell hybridoma / plasmacytoma growth factor induced by interleukin 1 and tumor necrosis factor. J Exp Med 1987;165:914–919.

214. Dayer JM, Beutler B, Cerami A. Cachectin/tumor necrosis factor stimulates collagenase and prostaglandin E2 production by human synovial cells and dermal fibroblasts. J Exp Med 1985;162:2163–2168.

215. Pober JS. Cytokine-mediated activation of vascular endothelium. Physiology and pathology. Am J Pathol 1988;133:426–433.

216. Collins T, Lapierre LA, Fiers W, et al. Recombinant tumor necrosis factor increases mRNA levels and surface expression of HLA-A,B antigens in vascular endothelial cells and dermal fibroblasts in vitro. Proc Natl Acad Sci USA 1986;83:446–450.

217. Chong AS-F, Scuderi P, Grimes WJ, et al. Tumor targets stimulate IL-2 activated killer cells to produce interferon-γ and tumor necrosis factor. J Immunol 1989;142:2133–2139.

218. Hersch EM, Metch BS, Muggia FM, et al. Phase II studies of recombinant human tumor necrosis factor alpha in patients with malignant disease: a summary of the Southwest Oncology Group experience. J Immunother 1991;10:426–431.

219. Lachmann LB, Brown DC, Dinarello CA. Growth-promoting effect of recombinant interleukin 1 and tumor necrosis factor for a human astrocytoma cell line. J Immunol 1987;138:2913–2916.

220. Goillot E, Combaret V, Ladenstein R, et al. Tumor necrosis factor as an autocrine growth factor for neuroblastoma. Cancer Res 1992;52:3194–3200.

221. Schiller JH, Bittner G, Spriggs DR. Tumor necrosis factor, but not other hematopoietic growth factors, prolongs the survival of hairy cell leukemia cells. Leuk Res 1992;16:337–346.

222. Cordingley FT, Bianchi A, Hoffbrand AV, et al. Tumor necrosis factor as an autocrine tumor growth factor for chronic B cell malignancies. Lancet 1988;1:969–971.

223. Tartaglia LA, Goeddel DV. Two TNF receptors. Immunol Today 1992;13:151–153.

224. Heller RA, Song K, Fan N, et al. the p70 tumor necrosis factor receptor mediates cytotoxicity. Cell 1992;70:47–56.

225. Rathjen DA, Furphy LJ, Aston R. Selective enhancement of the tumour necrotic activity of TNF alpha with monoclonal antibody. Br J Cancer 1992;65:852–856.

226. McLaughlin PJ, Elwood NJ, Russell SM, et al. Properties of monoclonal antibodies to human tumor necroses factor alpha (TNF alpha). Anticancer Res 1992;12:1243–1246.

227. Onozaki K, Matsushima K, Kleinerman ES, et al. Role of interleukin-1 (IL-1) in promoting human mediated tumor cytotoxicity. J Immunol 1985;135:314–320.

228. Braunschweiger PG, Johnson CS, Kumar N, et al. Antitumor effects of recombinant human interleukin-1α in RIF-1 and PancO2 solid tumors. Cancer Res 1988;48:6011–6016.

229. North RJ, Neubauer RH, Huang JJH, et al. Interleukin 1-induced T cell-mediated regression of immunogenic murine tumors. Requirement for an adequate level of already acquired host concomitant immunity. J Exp Med 1988;168:2031–2043.

230. Johnson CS, Chang MJ, Braunschweiger PG, et al. Acute hemorrhagic necrosis of tumors induced by interleukin-1α: effects independent of tumor necrosis factor. J Natl Cancer Inst 1991;83:842–848.

231. Usui N, Mimnaugh EG, Sinha BK. Synergistic antitumor activity of etoposide and human interleukin-1 α against human melanoma cells. J Natl Cancer Inst 1989;81:1904–1909.

232. Nakamura S, Kashimoto S, Kajikawa F, et al. Combination effect of recombinant human interleukin-1 α with antitumor drugs on syngeneic tumors in mice. Cancer Res 1991;51:215–221.

233. Neta R, Douches S, Oppenheim JJ. Interleukin-1 is a radioprotector. J Immunol 1986;136:2483–2485.

234. Moore MAS, Warren DJ. Synergy of interleukin-1 and granulocyte colony-stimulating factor: in vivo stimulation of stem cell recovery and hematopoietic regeneration following 5-fluorouracil treatment of mice. Proc Natl Acad Sci USA 1987;84:7134–7138.

235. Smith JW, Longo DL, Alvord G, et al. The effects of treatment with interleukin-1α on platelet recovery after high-dose carboplatin. N Engl J Med 1993;328:756–761.

236. Starnes HF Jr, Hartman G, Torti F, et al. Recombinant human interleukin-1b (IL-1b) has antitumor activity and acceptable toxicity in metastatic malignant melanoma (abstract). Proc Am Soc Clin Oncol 1991;10:292.

237. Spits H, Yssel H, Paliard X, et al. IL-4 inhibits IL-2-mediated induction of human lymphokine activated killer cells, but not the generation of antigen-specific cytotoxic T lymphocytes in mixed lymphocyte cultures. J Immunol 1988; 141:29–36.

238. Hudson MM, Markowitz AB, Gutterman JU, et al. Effect of recombinant human IL-4 on human monocyte activity. Cancer Res 1990;50:3154–3158.

239. Wagteveld AJ, Zanten AKV, Esselink MT, et al. Expression and regulation of IL-4 receptors on human monocytes and acute myeloblastic leukemia cells. Leukemia 1991;5:782–788.

240. Puri RK, Ogata M, Leland P, et al. Expression of high affinity IL-4 receptors on murine sarcoma cells and receptor mediated cytotoxicity of tumor cells to chimeric protein between IL-4 and Pseudomonas exotoxin. Cancer Res 1991;51:3011–3017.

241. Obiri NI, Siegel JP, Puri RK. Expression of high affinity interleukin 4 receptors on human renal cell carcinoma cells and inhibition of tumor cell growth in vitro by IL-4. J Clin Invest 1993;91:88–93.

242. Hoon DSB, Banez M, Okun E, et al. Modulation of human melanoma cells by interleukin-4 and in combination with γ-IFN or α-tumor necrosis factor. Cancer Res 1991; 51:2002–2008.

243. Hoon DSB, Okun E, Banez M, et al. Interleukin-4 and with γ-interferon or tumor necrosis factor inhibits cell growth and modulates cell surface antigens on human renal cell carcinomas. Cancer Res 1991;51:5687–5693.

244. Toi M, Bicknel R, Harris AL. Inhibition of colon and breast carcinoma cell growth by interleukin-4. Cancer Res 1992; 52:275–279.

245. Totpal K, Aggarwal BB. Interleukin-4 potentiates the antiproliferative effects of tumor necrosis factor on various tumor cell lines. Cancer Res 1991;51:4266–4270.

246. Lotze MT. In vivo administration of recombinant human interleukin 4 to patients with cancer (abstract). J Cell Biochem 1991;33(suppl F).

247. Markowitz A, Kleinerman E, Hudson M, et al. Phase I study of recombinant IL-4 in patients with advanced cancer (abstract). Blood 1989;74(suppl):146a.

248. Taylor CW, Hultquist KE, Taylo AM, et al. Imunopharmacology of recombinant human interleukin-4 administered by the subcutaneous route in patients with malignancy (abstract). Blood 1992;76(suppl):221a.

249. Maher D, Boyd A, McKendrick J, et al. Rapid response of B cell malignancies induced by interleukin 4 (abstract). Blood 1990;76(suppl):93a.

250. Van Snick J. Interleukin-6: an overview. Ann Rev Immunol 1990;8:253–278.

251. Miyaura C, Onozaki K, Akiyama Y, et al. Recombinant human interleukin-6 (B-cell stimulatory factor 2) is a potent inducer of differentiation of mouse myeloid leukemia cells (M1). FEBS Lett 1988;234:17–21.

252. Onozaki K, Akiyama Y, Okano A, et al. Synergistic regulatory effects of interleukin-6 and interleukin-1 on the growth and differentiation of human and mouse myeloid leukemia cell lines. Cancer Res 1989;49:3602–3607.

253. Chen L, Mory Y, Zilberstein A, et al. Growth inhibition of human breast carcinoma and leukemia / lymphoma cell lines by recombinant interferon-β2. Proc Natl Acad Sci USA 1988;85:8037–8041.

254. Mulé JJ, Custer MC, Travis WD, et al. Cellular mechanisms of the antitumor activity of recombinant IL-6 in mice. J Immunol 1992;148:2622–2629.

255. Mulé JJ, McIntosh JK, Jablons DM, et al. Antitumor activity of recombinant interleukin 6 in mice. J Exp Med 1990; 171:629–636.

256. Weber J, Yang JC, Topalian SL, et al. Phase I trial of subcutaneous interleukin-6 in patients with advance malignancies. J Clin Oncol 1993;11:499–506.

257. Hunt P, Robertson D, Weiss D, et al. A single bone marrow-derived stromal cell type supports the in vitro growth of early lymphoid and myeloid cells. Cell 1987;48:997–1007.

258. Stanley ER, Heard PM. Factors regulating macrophage production and growth. Purification and some properties of the colony stimulating factor from medium conditioned by mouse L cells. J Biol Chem 1977;252:4305–4312.

259. Wing EJ, Waheed A, Shadduck RK, et al. Effect of colony stimulating factor on murine macrophages. Induction of antitumor activity. J Clin Invest 1982;69:270–276.

260. Wing EJ, Ampel NM, Waheed A, et al. Macrophage colony-stimulating factor (M-CSF) enhances the capacity of murine macrophages to secrete oxygen reduction products. J Immunol 1985;135:2052–2056.

261. Nakoniz I, Ralph P. Stimulation of macrophage antibody-dependent killing of tumor targets by recombinant lymphokine factors and M-CSF. Cell Immunol 1988;116:331–340.

262. Bock SN, Cameron RB, Kragel P, et al. Biologic and antitumor effects of recombinant human macrophage stimulating factor in mice. Cancer Res 1991;51:2649–2654.

263. Sanda MG, Yang JC, Topalian SL, et al. Intravenous administration of recombinant human macrophage colony-stimulating factor to patients with metastatic cancer: a phase I study. J Clin Oncol 1992;10:1643–1649.

264. Zamkoff KW, Hudson J, Groves ES, et al. A phase I trial of recombinant human macrophage colony-stimulating factor by rapid intravenous infusion in patients with refractory malignancy. J Immunother 1992;11:103–110.

265. Beutler B, Cerami A. The common mediator of shock, cachexia, and tumor necrosis. Adv Immunol 1988;42:213–229.

266. Tracey KJ, Cerami A. Tumor necrosis factor and regulation of metabolism in infection: role of systemic versus tissue levels. Proc Soc Exp Biol Med 1992;200:233–239.

267. Rosenberg SA, Aebersold P, Cornetta K, et al. Gene transfer into humans—immunotherapy of patients with advanced melanoma, using tumor-infiltrating lymphocytes modified by retroviral gene transduction. N Engl J Med 1990; 323:570–578.

268. Douvdevani A, Huleihel M, Zöller M, et al. Reduced tumorigenicity of fibrosarcomas which constitutively generate IL-1 α either spontaneously or following IL-1α gene transfer. Int J Cancer 1992;51:822–830.

269. Fearon ER, Pardoll DM, Itaya T, et al. Interleukin-2 production by tumor cells bypasses T helper function in the generation of an antitumor response. Cell 1990;60:397–403.

270. Tepper RI. The tumor-cytokine transplantation assay and the antitumor activity of interleukin-4. Bone Marrow Transplant 1992;9(suppl 1):177–181.

271. Golumbek PT, Lazenby AJ, Levitsky HI, et al. Treatment of established renal cancer by tumor cells engineered to secrete interleukin-4. Science 1991;254:713–716.

272. Mullen CA, Coale M, Levy AT, et al. Fibrosarcoma cells transduced with the IL-6 gene exhibit reduced tumorigenicity, increased immunogenicity and decreased metastatic potential. Cancer Res 1992;52:6020–6024.

273. Hock H, Dorsch M, Diamantstein T, et al. Interleukin-7 induces CD4+ T cell-dependent tumor rejection. J Exp Med 1991;174:1291–1298.

274. Hock H, Dorsch M, Kunzendorf U, et al. Mechanisms of rejection induced by tumor cell-targeted gene transfer of interleukin-2, interleukin-4, interleukin-7, tumor necrosis factor, or interferon γ. Proc Natl Acad Sci USA 1993;90: 2774–2778.

275. Connor J, Bannerji R, Saito S, et al. Regression of bladder tumors in mice treated with interleukin-2 gene-modified tumor cells. J Exp Med 1993;177:1127–1134.

276. Porgador A, Tzehoval E, Katz A, et al. Interleukin 6 gene transfection into Lewis lung carcinoma tumor cells suppresses the malignant phenotype and confers immunotherapeutic competence against parental metastatic cells. Cancer Res 1992;52:3679–3686.

CHAPTER 34

AUTOCRINE AND PARACRINE ROLE OF CYTOKINES AS GROWTH FACTORS FOR TUMORIGENESIS

Sachiko Suematsu and Tadamitsu Kishimoto

In vitro cell culture system has revealed that the growth of cells is regulated by a variety of cytokines or growth factors, and it is assumed that these same factors control normal cell growth in vivo as well. Abnormal growth of cells is one of the most fundamental characteristics that define tumor or cancer. To explain autonomous growth property of malignant cells, the notion of "autocrine secretion" of growth factor was proposed (1). Since then, many studies concerning autocrine secretion and cancer have been reported, and the original "autocrine hypothesis" can be revised according to certain important new findings (2). Although uncontrolled autocrine growth factor production alone may cause hyperplasia of phenotypically normal cells, it should be an essential element for multistep processes of tumorigenesis, in concert with other genetic perturbations. In addition to malignant transformation, support of autocrine or paracrine growth signals is supposed to be required for tumor progression, including tumor mass formation, tumor stem-cell expansion, and cancer metastasis.

We summarize autocrine and paracrine actions of cytokines involved in tumorigenic transformation of cells, progression of malignancy of cancer cells, and cancer metastasis. Several growth factors that might not be included among the cytokines, such as platelet-derived growth factor (PDGF) and transforming growth factors (TGFs), are discussed because of their "cytokine-like" activities and important roles in tumorigenesis. We discuss interleukin-6 (IL-6) in detail as a clinical target to prevent autocrine growth of plasma-cell neoplasias during therapy.

MECHANISMS OF AUTOCRINE STIMULATION

It has been well known that transformed or cancer cells have autonomous growth capacity, which contributes to their malignant behavior, such as tumor cell invasion and metastasis. In general, malignant cells require fewer exogenous growth factors for optimal growth than normal cells, and they grow autonomously. In 1980, Sporn and Todaro (1) proposed the "autocrine hypothesis" to explain this phenomenon: cells could become transformed by endogeneous production of growth factors acting on their producer cells via functional external receptors on the same cells (Fig. 34–1A). Other than uncontrolled production of growth factors, there can be several ways in which cell growth becomes autonomous, such as abnormal expression of growth factor receptors, disturbances of postreceptor signal transduction, and reduced inhibitory effects on cell growth. It has been revealed that some oncogenes are involved in these aspects and that they enhance autocrine pathways which contribute to carcinogenesis (3). The *sis* oncogene encodes the B chain of PDGF; the int-2, hst/K-FGF and FGF-5 genes code for the members of the fibroblast growth factor (FGF) family; the fms gene encodes the gene for colony-stimulating factor-1 (CSF-1) receptor; the erb B oncogene codes for a truncated form of the receptor for epidermal growth factor (EGF); and the ras gene product is a critical component of intracellular mitogenic signaling pathways. Activation of these oncogenes is supposed to lead to continuous autocrine stimulation of mitogenic signaling, which results in uncontrolled growth of cells.

It has been suggested that autocrine growth signals are transduced not only through cell surface receptor, but also through intracellular receptor (Fig. 34–1B). In fact, antibodies to growth factors can inhibit autonomous growth of malignant cells to a certain extent. However, in many cases, growth inhibition by antibodies was shown to be partial or incomplete (4–6). Furthermore, addition of exogenous growth factor could not transform normal cells (7). These observations suggest that external growth factor production may not be necessary for cell growth or transformation, as well as existence of intracellular interaction of growth factor and its receptor. There is direct evidence that supports the "intracellular autocrine" mechanism. A four amino acid endoplasmic retention signal, Lys-Asp-Glu-Leu (KDEL) was added to the carboxyl terminus of PDGF (8) and IL-3 (9) to prevent the growth factor from being secreted from cells. Transfection of the modified growth factor could induce transformation of cells without any detectable secretion of the growth factor.

Another version of the autocrine concept is that autocrine stimulation can act in an inhibitory manner, which may be described as "negative autocrine stimulation" (10). In considering growth inhibitory action of TGF-β produced by tumor cells, loss of responsiveness to such growth inhibitory factors could induce uncontrolled autonomous growth of cells (this "negative autocrine hypothesis" is discussed in the section concerning TGF-β in this chapter).

The autocrine hypothesis is often discussed in association with genesis of cancer; however, autocrine secretion is not restricted to malignant cells. In inflammation and tissue repair processes, normal cells, such as macrophages, lymphocytes, fibroblasts, and vascular smooth muscle cells. also respond to autocrine growth stimulation (11). In these physiological states, autocrine production of growth factor is under control, in contrast to cancer, in which continuous autocrine growth factor production is observed.

PARACRINE STIMULATION INVOLVED IN TUMORIGENESIS

Paracrine stimulation (i.e., growth stimulation of cells by growth factors produced by the other cells) is also suggested to be involved in tumorigenesis (Fig. 34–1C). Paracrine secretion of certain growth factors for cancer surrounding cells, such as fibroblasts and vascular smooth muscle cells, has been found to induce tumor stroma formation, which may establish a microenvironment for tumor progression, including tumor cell invasion and metastasis. PDGF is a potent mitogen for fibroblasts and endothelial cells, and it is suggested to have a role in connective tissue stroma formation (12). TGF-β is shown to stimulate extracellular matrix formation, and it is supposed to be important in formation of tumor stroma composed of several elements, such as inflammatory cells, newly formed blood vessels, and connective tissue (13). Paracrine secretion of growth factors is also an important factor in understanding the immmune system composed of a variety of actions of macrophages, lymphocytes, and granulocytes. In tumorigenetic processes, TGF-β suppresses growth and function of lymphocytes (14), which may result in impairment of immune surveillance and indirect support of tumor progression.

Another aspect of paracrine stimulation in tumorigenesis is that it may induce activation of an autocrine loop. For instance, TGF-β is synthesized by most cell types, almost all cells have its receptor, and it is known to be secreted in an inactive latent form (14). Therefore, activation of latent TGF-β may be a critical step in control of autocrine stimulation of TGF-β.

AUTOCRINE AND PARACRINE STIMULATION IN TUMOR METASTASIS

Tumors with a highly malignant phenotype metastasize to near and distant sites by a sequential process of tumor

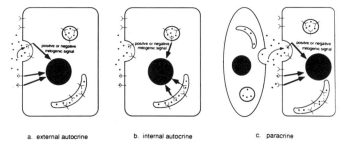

a. external autocrine   b. internal autocrine   c. paracrine

Figure 34–1 Three different patterns of growth factor stimulation. (A) The growth factor (thick dots) is secreted from a cell, and it activates its receptor at the cell surface. (B) The growth factor activates its receptor in the Golgi apparatus or in secretory vesicles. (C) The growth factor secreted from a cell activates its receptor on the other cell surface.

cell migration away from primary tumor site, transportation through blood or lymph vessels, and proliferation at secondary sites (15,16). Because each tumor cell could be growth-stimulated by growth factors produced by neighboring cells if they stay in the primary tumor, migration away from the primary tumor is unnecessary and inconvenient for cancer cells. In fact, low malignancy grade tumors rarely metastasize. For successful formation of metastases, tumor cells must produce and respond to autocrine growth factor. Recent data demonstrated that in many cancers, the metastatic phenotype may be associated with autonomous growth of cells. Human melanoma cell lines were consecutively selected for their invasive capacity through a reconstructed basement membrane, and some were shown to grow more rapidly in serum- and growth factor–free medium than their parental cell lines. One of these variant cell lines with the highest invasive capacity in vitro was metastatic in nude mice. In addition, variant cell lines selected in growth factor–free medium from primary melanoma cell lines showed higher invasive phenotype in vitro and in vivo (17).

Metastatic cells also respond to paracrine growth factors and inhibitors produced by component cells in secondary sites. Cornil and associates (18) demonstrated that growth of human melanoma cells was affected by interaction with normal fibroblasts. Melanoma cells derived from the early stage were growth-inhibited by coculture with normal fibroblasts. In contrast, melanoma cell lines from primary lesions of advanced metastatic melanomas or metastatic sites were found to be growth-stimulated in the presence of fibroblasts. Because the same effects on the growth of melanoma cells were observed by addition of supernatant from fibroblast cultures, it has been suggested that melanoma cell growth was affected by soluble stimulatory and inhibitory growth factors.

With regard to primary tumors, paracrine stimulation produced by metastatic tumor cells for certain kinds of cells that will form tumor stroma at secondary sites must be necessary for the microenvironment for tumor growth.

CYTOKINES INVOLVED IN ONCOGENE-RELATED AUTOCRINE GROWTH MECHANISMS

Platelet-derived growth factor

PROPERTIES OF PDGF AND ITS RECEPTORS: Platelet-derived growth factor is a major mesenchymal cell growth factor originally purified from human platelets, and it has been found to be produced by a wide variety of normal cells and transformed cells (19,20). PDGF is a dimeric, approximately 30-kd protein composed of disulphide-bonded A and B polypeptide chain, and all three dimeric isoforms (PDGF-AA, PDGF-AB, and PDGF-BB) have been identified and purified from platelets and transformed cells. Both PDGF chains are synthesized as precursor molecules, and they undergo dimerization and proteolytic processing after synthesis. The isoforms were found to have different functional activities and secretory behaviors. Whereas PDGF-AA and PDGF-AB are rapidly secreted after synthesis, PDGF-BB remains associated with the producer cell. These isoforms were shown to interact with two different PDGF receptor types (21): the α-receptor binds all three isoforms with high and approximately equal affinities, and the β-receptor binds PDGF-BB with high affinity, and PDGF-AB with low affinity. The two receptor types are structurally and functionally related, and both have an intracellular tyrosine kinase domain.

It is supposed that PDGF is involved in tissue repair processes and regulation of cell growth and differentiation during embryonal development. PDGF may also be involved in several pathological processes, including atherosclerosis, tissue fibrosis, and malignancies (19,20).

PDGF IN MALIGNANT TRANSFORMATION: PDGF was the first peptide growth factor shown to be directly implicated in the autocrine hypothesis of oncogenesis (22). Simian sarcoma virus (SSV)–transformed cells produce a PDGF-like peptide that binds to the PDGF receptor, and it is recognized by anti-PDGF antibodies (23–26). It has been demonstrated that the normal counterpart of the oncogene v-sis of SSV is the cellular gene that encodes the β chain of PDGF. The amino acid sequence of the PDGF β chain was found to be similar to the sequence of the transforming protein p28[sis] coded by v-sis of SSV (27,28). It was revealed that only cells that possess the PDGF receptor can be transformed by SSV (29). Moreover, anti-PDGF antibodies have been found to inhibit transformation by SSV (4,5). The growth rate of SSV-transformed cells in athymic nude mice was correlated with levels of PDGF secreted by the cells (4).

These data suggest autocrine roles for PDGF in malignant transformation. Transfection experiments using retroviral expression vectors revealed that the PDGF B chain has far more transforming potential than the A chain (30). Transfection of a nonreceptor-binding mutant PDGF A chain was shown to inhibit the transformed phenotype of the c-sis/PDGF B chain expressing NIH 3T3 cells (31). The affinity of the mutant/wild-type A chain heterodimer for the PDGF α-receptor was decreased compared with that of the wild-type PDGF A chain homodimer, suggesting the possibility of formation of a low-affinity mutant PDGF-A/PDGF-B heterodimer at the expense of the synthesis of a high-affinity PDGF-BB homodimer, which may cause inhibition of the transformed phenotype.

INTERNAL AUTOCRINE MECHANISM OF PDGF:

Whereas the PDGF receptor is found to be essential for sis-induced transformation (29), the site where autocrine activaton of the receptor takes place has been the subject of controversy (22). In fact, PDGF antibodies cannot reverse completely sis-induced transformation (4,5), and addition of purified PDGF does not transform normal cells (7), suggesting that external growth factor may not be essential for transformation and that ligand-receptor interaction may occur in the intracellular compartment. Autophosphorylated PDGF receptor in v-sis–transformed normal rat kidney (NRK) cells has been shown to be insensitive to trypsin treatment and to be unaffected by suramin, in contrast to activated cell surface receptor (32). Bejcek and colleagues (8) demonstrated that mutant v-sis protein designed to be retained within the endoplasmic reticulum and the Golgi complex could transform NRK cells without extracellular secretion of v-sis. However, Hannink and Donoghue (33) have shown that autocrine stimulation of the PDGF receptor is prevented in v-sis–transfected cells by monensin or suramin treatment, which prevent transport of proteins to the cell surface, suggesting that interaction of v-sis protein and the PDGF receptor occurs at the cell surface.

AUTOCRINE AND PARACRINE ROLES IN SPONTANEOUS HUMAN TUMORS:

A possible autocrine role of PDGF in the genesis of spontaneous human tumors has also been suggested. Northern blot hybridization using probes for both PDGF chains and both PDGF receptors demonstrated coexpression of PDGF and PDGF receptor in human glioma (34,35) and sarcoma (36) cell lines. Analysis of human malignant glioma biopsy specimens by in situ hybridization and immunohistochemistry has demonstrated that presence of both autocrine and paracrine loops in malignant glioma (37). Furthermore, circumstantial evidence for two distinct autocrine loops through PDGF α-receptor and β-receptor was provided (37). Expression of PDGF-A and PDGF-B chains was found to be consistent with malignancy grade. Glioma cells were found to coexpress PDGF-A and the α-receptor, whereas expression of the β-receptor was very low in glioma cells, and concomitant expression of PDGF-B and the β-receptor was found in the endothelial cells of hyperplastic capillaries. These results suggest the existence of autocrine activation of the PDGF α-receptor in glioma cells, as well as paracrine and autocrine activation of the PDGF β-receptor in capillary cells.

There are several examples of PDGF receptor–negative human tumor cells that produce PDGF but have no PDGF receptors (e.g., mammary carcinoma cell lines [38,39], melanoma cell lines [40], and lung carinoma cell lines

[41]). Considering the mitogenic activity of PDGF for fibroblasts and endothelial cells, PDGF may contribute to the formation of a supporting connective tissue stroma via a paracrine mechanism. It was demonstrated that PDGF B chain cDNA-transfected human WM9 melanoma cells induced formation of tumor connective tissue stroma with newly generated blood vessels when they were subcutaneously transplanted into athymic nude mice. Tumors from mice transplanted with the vector-transfected WM9 cells were found to contain large necrotic areas and little blood vessels (42).

Transforming growth factor-α

ISOLATION AND CHARACTERIZATION:

Transforming growth factor-α is a secreted polypeptide that was initially detected in the culture medium of retrovirus-transformed fibroblasts (43). The term *transforming* originated from the observation that TGF-α stimulates anchorage-independent growth in certain cells, but it is now known that TGF-α induces transformation in synergy with TGF-β (44). TGF-α shares structural and functional similarity with EGF, and it binds to the EGF receptor to produce a mitogenic stimulus (45). EGF recpetor was shown to be encoded by the erb B oncogene (46), and it has an intrinsic tyrosine kinase activity, which is common in many growth factor receptors for transducing the mitogenic signal (3).

TGF-α is produced by a number of transformed cell lines, and it is found in tissues and cell lines from human tumors, mostly carcinomas. Recently, it has been demonstrated that TGF-α is detected in nontransformed cells (47). In situ hybridization analysis revealed that TGF-α is also expressed in normal tissue (i.e., developing fetus [48], adult brain [49], and skin keratinocytes [50]). TGF-α is synthesized as a membrane-bound 159 or 160 amino acid precursor; the active 50 amino acid molecule is released from the cell membrane after specific proteolysis (51,52). It has been shown that membrane-bound TGF-α precursor can also activate EGF receptor on adjacent cells, which mediates mitogenic stimulation (53–55). Expression of TGF-α precursor in a bone marrow stromal cell line was found to support attachment and proliferation of a certain hematopoietic progenitor cell line that could not adhere to normal stroma (55). The authors proposed the term *juxtacrine* to designate this mode of intercellular stimulation mediated by binding of a membrane-anchored growth factor to its receptor on an adjacent cell.

TGF-α IN TUMORIGENESIS:

Overexpression of TGF-α has been demonstrated to be associated with neoplastic transformation in a wide array of transformed cells and tumors. In fact, TGF-α was originally detected in culture medium of retrovirally transformed fibroblasts and it was shown to be able to reversibly transform immortalized NRK fibroblasts (43). Since then, it has been demonstrated that TGF-α expression can be induced in cultured cells transformed by several viral and cellular oncogenes (55–60) or by treatment with carcinogens (61). Transformation by the ras oncogene leads to induction of TGF-α expression (56,57). In addition, transformation of fibroblasts by simian virus 40 (SV40) (58) or polyoma virus (59) results in TGF-α secretion, suggesting that several other oncogenes also regulate TGF-α gene expression.

Transfection of TGF-α cDNA into immortalized Rat-1 (62) and NRK (63) fibroblasts induced their transformed phenotype, which was estimated as colony formation in soft agar and tumorigenicity in nude mice. The transformation was reversed by addition of TGF-α antibodies. However, in NIH 3T3 fibroblasts, overexpression of TGF-α did not result in transformation of the cells (64). Di Marco and coworkers (65) demonstrated that overexpression of TGF-α can induce transformation of NIH 3T3 fibroblasts, but only with concomitant high expression of the EGF receptor.

Several experiments using transgenic mice have demonstrated that overexpression of TGF-α can initiate and accelerate tumorigenesis in several organs, including mammary gland, pancreas, liver, and coagulation gland (66–68).

TGF-α expression has been found also in various human tumors (69). Consistent expression of TGF-α was observed in squamous-cell carcinomas and renal-cell carcinomas, and a majority of mammary carcinomas also express the TGF-α gene. In many cases, overproduction of TGF-α is accompanied by overexpression of EGF receptor, suggesting the possibility of an autocrine loop in spontaneous human tumors.

CYTOKINES AS NEGATIVE AUTOCRINE GROWTH FACTORS FOR TUMORIGENESIS

Transforming growth factor-β

CHARACTERIZATION OF TGF-β AND ITS RECEPTORS: Transforming growth factor-β is the prototype of a large family of multifunctional peptides that currently consists of five members, termed TGF-β_1 through TGF-β_5 (14,70). It was initially identified by its ability to induce NRK fibroblasts to proliferate in soft agar in the presence of epidermal growth factor (71). The original isolation of TGF-β from human platelets resulted in the identification of a single form of the peptide, a homodimer with a molecular weight of 25 kd, TGF-β_1 (72). The

five isoforms of TGF-β share similar biological activities, at least in certain cell lines.

TGF-β is secreted from cultured cells in a biologically inactive form that will not bind to cellular receptor (73–75). This latent form of TGF-β can be activated by acidification, alkalinization, and treatment with chaotropic agents (76,77). Because TGF-β is synthesized by most cell types and almost all cells have TGF-β receptors, physiological control of activation of latent TGF-β is important in both paracrine and potential autocrine actions of TGF-β (70).

Membrane receptor labeling assays in a variety of cells have revealed that there are about 10 membrane-associated TGF-β binding proteins (78). Almost all cells have cell surface receptor or binding protein for TGF-β (79, 80). Of these binding proteins, glycoproteins of 53 and 75 kd, termed *type I* and *type II receptors,* respectively, were suggested to mediate functions of TGF-β (81,82). Recently, type I and type II receptors were molecularly cloned, and they were shown to have a cytoplasmic serine/threonine kinase domain (83,84). Another TGF-β binding protein of known structure is a 280-kd betaglycan, termed *type III receptor* (85). It is currently unclear whether type III receptors function as signaling receptors.

TGF-β has been shown to be highly pleiotropic (14, 70). Depending on culture conditions, TGF-β can act to either stimulate or inhibit cellular proliferation, cellular differentiation, or cellular function. Although TGF-β was identified by its ability to induce cell growth of normal fibroblasts in soft agar, only a few types of mesenchymal cells actually proliferate in response to TGF-β. In fact, TGF-β has been revealed to be a potent inhibitor of proliferation in many cell types, including selected cell types of mesenchymal and myeloid origin, as well as nearly all epithelial, lymphoid, and endothelial cells (14).

TGF-β is assumed to be involved in both physiological and pathological states: inflammation and tissue repair, embryogenesis, formation of bone and cartilage, control of immune function, genesis of several diseases accompanying fibrosis, and carcinogenesis (86,87).

POSSIBLE ROLES OF TGF-β IN TUMORIGENESIS: TGF-β has been suggested to be involved in several aspects in tumorigenesis: (a) TGF-β inhibits immune functions and it may decrease immune surveillance for tumor development; (b) TGF-β stimulates tumor growth indirectly via paracrine effects on stromal element of the tumor; and (c) TGF-β acts as a negative autocrine growth factor for tumor cells.

TGF-β is the most potent known endogenous suppressant of lymphocyte proliferation and function (86). It directly or indirectly inhibits proliferation and function of immune competent cells, and it is suggested to control the immune system by suppressing excessive immune reactions. These immune suppressive effects of TGF-β may result in impairment of immune surveillance and indirect support of tumor progression.

TGF-β is important in formation of tumor stroma composed of several elements, such as inflammatory cells, newly formed blood vessels, and connective tissue (87). Many tumor cells secrete higher amounts of TGF-β than normal cells, and such increased TGF-β may contribute to tumor development and progression via its paracrine effects on chemotaxis, neovascularization, and extracellular matric formation.

NEGATIVE AUTOCRINE EFFECT OF TGF-β IN TUMOR DEVELOPMENT: In considering the growth inhibitory effect of TGF-β produced by tumor cells, several investigators proposed the "negative autocrine theory" in tumorigenesis: loss of responsiveness to growth inhibitory factors produced by tumor cells may contribute to the uncontrolled growth characteristics of neoplasms (2,10). As described, most normal cells are growth-inhibited by TGF-β, whereas many transformed and cancer cells, including bronchial carcinoma cells (88), squamous-cell carcinomas (89), leukemia cells (90), pheochromocytoma cells, neuroblastoma cells, retinoblastoma cells (91), and breast carcinoma cells (92,93), lack growth inhibition by TGF-β. Tumor cells might lose their responsiveness to TGF-β in several ways (87): (a) cells could lose their receptors for TGF-β; (b) cells could lose the ability to activate the latent form of TGF-β; and (c) altered signaling mechanisms could result in an inability to properly interpret the signal generated by interaction of TGF-β with its receptor. There are several examples for the first mechanism: certain leukemia cell lines, pheochromocytoma cells, retinoblastoma cells, and breast carcinoma cells were found to lack one or more of these receptors for TGF-β (90–93). For the second mechanism, growth of A-549 human lung carcinoma cells, which have a high amount of latent TGF-β producer cells and proliferate at a high rate, was shown to be inhibited by activated TGF-β after treatment with acid (94). The responsiveness of these cells to TGF-β is supposed to be based on loss of mechanisms of activation of latent TGF-β. Some nonresponsive cell lines that have normal or higher levels of TGF-β receptor are examples of the third mechanism (95,96).

There is evidence to support the notion of a negative autocrine effect of TGF-β in tumorigenesis. Addition of neutralizing TGF-β antibodies can induce proliferation or enhancement of anchorage-independent growth of certain cell lines (97,98). Furthermore, it was demonstrated that reduced levels of TGF-β_1 transcript correlated with disease progression of bladder carcinoma, even if the sample size was small (99). Wu and associates (100) demonstrated a negative autocrine effect of TGF-β more directly. Transfection of human TGF-β_1 antisense

mRNA expression vector into a human colon carcinoma cell line resulted in increased anchorage-independent growth of cells and enhanced tumorgenicity in athymic mice (100).

AUTOCRINE GROWTH FACTORS AS A TARGET FOR TUMOR THERAPY

Interleukin-6

Interleukin-6 is a multifunctional cytokine that is supposed to have a central role in host defense mechanisms, including immune responses, acute-phase reactions, and hematopoiesis (101–103). Abnormal production of IL-6 has been hypothesized to be involved in the generation of several chronic diseases, such as autoimmune diseases and cancers. Diseases related to abnormal IL-6 production are summarized in Table 34–1. Myeloma/plasmacytoma is one of the malignancies for which IL-6 is considered to act as an autocrine growth factor in pathogenesis (104,105). In addition to diagnostic application of

TABLE 34–1   ABNORMAL IL-6 EXPRESSION AND DISEASES

Acute inflammatory disorders
  Meningitis
  Intrauterine infection
  Acute transplant rejection
  Acute hepatitis
  Burns
  Surgical trauma
Chronic diseases
  Rheumatoid arthritis
  Mesangial proliferative glomerulonephritis
  Psoriasis
  Castleman's disease
  Multiple sclerosis
  Systemic lupus erythematosus
  Alzheimer's disease
  Cachexia
  Alcoholic hepatitis
Neoplasms
  Multiple myeloma/plasmacytoma
  Leukemia
  Kaposi's sarcoma
  Renal-cell carcinoma
  Pheochromocytoma
  Cardiac myxoma

IL-6, therapeutic application of IL-6 inhibitor for the disease has been challenging.

IL-6 PROTEIN AND ITS PRODUCTION: Interleukin-6 is a pleiotropic cytokine that was originally identified as a factor in the culture medium of mitogen-stimulated mononuclear cells, which induce antibody production in activated B cells (101–103). For its pleiotropic functions, IL-6 was formerly described as B-cell stimulatory factor 2 (BSF-2), interferon-β_2 (IFFN-β_2), a 26-kd protein, hybridoma/plasmacytoma growth factor (HPGF), and hepatocyte-stimulating factor (HSF). It is a glycoprotein with molecular weight heterogeneity from 21 to 28 kd, depending on the degree of glycosylation. IL-6 is produced by various types of cells, such as macrophages, T cells, B cells, fibroblasts, bone marrow stromal cells, keratinocytes, mesangial cells, endothelial cells, and certain tumor cells. The production of IL-6 is regulated by a variety of stimuli. Lipopolysaccharide (LPS) enhances IL-6 production in monocytes and fibroblasts, whereas glucocorticoids inhibit it. Peptide growth factors such as IL-1, tumor necrosis factor (TNF), IL-2, IFN-β, and PDFG induce IL-6 production. Various virus infections also induce IL-6 production in certain cells.

IL-6 RECEPTOR SYSTEM: The IL-6 receptor system consists of the 80-kd IL-6 receptor (IL-6R) and a 130-kd signal transducer (gp130) (106). Human IL-6R consists of 449 amino acids, and the first domain of 90 amino acids has an immunoglobin (Ig)-like domain (107). The Ig-like domain of IL-6R is not involved in IL-6 binding or IL-6 signal transduction, and the cytoplasmic domain of IL-6R is not required for IL-6 signal transduction (108). Binding of IL-6 to IL-6R triggers the association of IL-6R with a second membrane glycoprotein, gp130, which is a member of the cytokine receptor family (109); gp130 lacks IL-6 binding activity, but it is involved in the formation of high-affinity IL-6 binding sites through its association with IL-6R. Soluble IL-6R and IL-6 complex induce homodimerization of gp130 and tyrosine-specific phosphorylation of gp130 (110). It has been demonstrated that gp130 acts as a common signal transducer among several cytokines, such as ciliary neurotrophic factor (CNTF), leukemia inhibitory factor (LIF), and oncostatin M (OM), illustrating a mechanism for the functional redundancy of cytokines.

IL-6 IS A POTENTIAL AUTOCRINE GROWTH FACTOR IN MURINE PLASMACYTOMAGENESIS: Myeloma/plasmacytoma is a B-cell neoplasia characterized by malignant proliferation of plasma cells that produce a monoclonal Ig that can be detected in serum or urine (111). In murine models, plasmacytoma can be induced in BALB/c mice by intraperitoneal injection of mineral oil or pristane, which induce chronic inflammation in peritoneal cavities (112). Plasmacytomas appear in association with pristane-induced inflammatory granulomatous tissue, which is found to produce IL-6. In fact, IL-6 was formerly known as HPGF, and in vitro growth of murine plasmacytomas was found to depend on IL-6 (113). Overexpression of the IL-6 and the IL-6R gene was reported in several murine plasmacytoma cell lines. MCP11 cells were found to constitutively produce IL-6 due to insertion of an intracisternal A particle (IAP) retrotransposon 18 bp upstream of the 5′-transcriptional start site of the IL-6 gene (114). Enhanced expression of IL-6R was observed in a P3U1 cell line established from a mineral oil–induced BALB/c plasmacytoma, in which the intracytoplasmic region of IL-6R was replaced with part of the long terminal repeat (LTR) of the IAP gene (115). Transfection of IL-6 cDNA was shown to increase the tumorigenicity of an IL-6–dependent B-cell hybridoma and a mouse plasmacytoma (116,117). Furthermore, the increased tumorigency was inhibited by administration of antibodies directed against IL-6 or against its receptor (117). These data suggest possible autocrine roles of IL-6 in the development of murine plasmacytomas.

For another murine model, transgenic mice were generated by introducing the human IL-6 gene fused with the Ig heavy chain enhancer (Eμ-IL-6) into C57BL/6 mouse eggs (118). IL-6 transgenic mice showed massive splenomegaly and lymph node swelling, and they died within several months. Histological analysis revealed that spleen, lymph nodes, and thymus were filled with compactly arranged plasma cells. Although these histological findings were indistinguishable from those of plasmacytoma, the proliferated plasma cells were neither monoclonal nor transplantable to syngeneic mice, suggesting that overexpression of IL-6 induced lethal plasmacytosis but not plasmacytoma in C57BL/6 IL-6 transgenic mice. As described, plasmacytoma can be induced in BALB/c mice by intraperitoneal injection of pristane, but the C57BL/6 strain is resistant to plasmacytoma development (112). Some IL-6 transgenic mice backcrossed to BALB/c mice developed monoclonal malignant plasmacytomas carrying t(12;15) chromosomal translocation (119), which is commonly observed in pristane-induced murine plasmacytomas, and it results in c-myc gene rearrangement (112). These experiments using transgenic mice suggest that autocrine stimulation of IL-6 can induce malignant transformation of plasma cells in concert with certain other factors, such as a BALB/c genetic background and oncogenes (Fig. 34–2).

POSSIBLE AUTOCRINE ROLE OF IL-6 IN THE GENESIS OF HUMAN PLASMA CELL NEOPLASIAS: In human studies, Kawano and associates (120) demonstrated the possible autocrine role of IL-6 in the pathogenesis of human multiple myelomas based on following observations: (a) IL-6 induces in vitro growth of

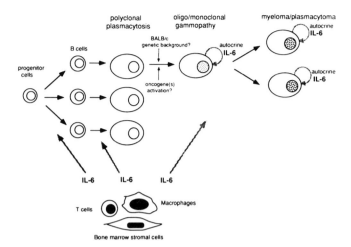

Figure 34–2 Involvement of IL-6 in a multistep tumorigenesis of myloma/plasmacytoma. Paracrine stimulation of IL-6 can initially induce polyclonal plasmacytosis. During the stage of plasmacytosis, a small compartment of plasma cells or precursor cells could induce production of IL-6 and its receptor and grow autonomously. This autocrine production of IL-6 may be induced by activation of certain oncogenes. Autocrine stimulation of IL-6 could stimulate tumorigenic transformation of plasma cells further. Fully transformed myeloma/plasmacytoma cells do not need exogenous IL-6 any longer for their proliferation.

myeloma cells freshly isolated from patients with multiple myeloma; (b) myeloma cells express the IL-6R; (c) myeloma cells produce IL-6; and (d) in vitro growth of myeloma cells is inhibited by anti–IL-6 antibody. Klein and associates (121) also demonstrated that IL-6 is a major growth factor for myeloma cells isolated from patients with myeloma but that it acts in a paracrine fashion. In their report, bone marrow stromal cells are shown to be the major source of IL-6 in patients with myeloma. They could not detect IL-6 expression in human myeloma cell line U266. In support of the existence of an IL-6–mediated autocrine loop, Freeman and colleagues (122) showed IL-6 mRNA expression in all tissue biopsies investigated from myelomas and plasma-cell leukemias. Furthermore, addition of a neutralizing anti-IL-6 monoclonal antibody or IL-6 antisense oligonucleotides inhibits U266 proliferation; these effects are reversed by adding IL-6 (123). They detected IL-6 mRNA in U266 cells only after amplification of the reverse-transcribed mRNA by polymerase chain reaction, indicating that vanishingly low amounts of IL-6 are sufficient for autocrine growth of the cell line.

An autocrine transformation mechanism is suggested in Epstein-Barr virus (EBV)–transformed B lymphoblastoid cell lines. The continuous proliferation of EBV-infected B cells appears to depend on autocrine secretion of cytokines, including IL-1 and IL-6 (124). Transfection of IL-6 gene into EBV-transformed B cells induces an altered pattern of cell growth to a malignant phenotype,

such as cell proliferation in soft agar and tumorigenicity in nude mice (125). Possible autocrine activity of IL-6 was also demonstrated in the pathogenesis of non-Hodgkin's lymphoma, chronic B lymphatic leukemia, and acute myeloid leukemia (126–128).

DIAGNOSTIC AND THERAPEUTIC IMPLICATION OF IL-6 IN PLASMA CELL NEOPLASIAS: An increased serum IL-6 level is a potential dianostic marker in patients with plasma-cell neoplasias. Significant serum IL-6 levels (>5 U/ml estimated by bioassay) were detected in 35% of 85 patients with overt multiple myeloma and 100% of 11 patients with plasma-cell leukemia, whereas elevated levels were detected in only 3% of 35 patients with monoclonal gammopathy of undetermined significance or smoldering myeloma. In addition, serum levels of IL-6 were related to disease activity in patients with overt multiple myeloma (129). Zhang and coworkers (130) reported that the dependence of myeloma cell proliferation on IL-6 in vitro correlates with the in vivo myeloma cell labeling index (i.e., percentage of myeloma cells in the S-phase). Furthermore, it was demonstrated that patients with myeloma whose serum IL-6 levels were below 7 pg/mL survive significantly longer than those with IL-6 concentrations of 7 pg/mL or higher. The 50% survival rate of patients with lower IL-6 levels was 53.7 months, whereas it was only 2.7 months in patients with high IL-6 levels (131). Measurement of serum IL-6 levels and in vitro IL-6 responsiveness may be useful to assess disease severity and response to therapy for plasma-cell neoplasias.

Anti–IL-6 antibody or anti–IL-6R antibody could be used as therapeutic agents for plasma-cell neoplasias. It was demonstrated that anti–IL-6 antibodies inhibited in vitro proliferation of myeloma cells isolated from myeloma bone marrow (120,121). Klein and associates (132) reported a clinical trial of anti–IL-6 monoclonal antibody in a patient with primary plasma-cell leukemia resistant to chemotherapy. The patient was treated with murine anti-IL-6 monoclonal antibodies for 2 months. Serum IL-6 levels were undetectable, and C-reative protein (CRP) levels returned to normal during a 2-month course of treatment. The patient's hypercalcemia and hypergammaglobulinemia were significantly reduced during treatment. No immune response against anti–IL-6 antibody was detected at the end of treatment. Furthermore, no major side effects were noticed during the anti–IL-6 treatment. Although in vitro proliferation of the myeloma cells isolated after treatment was still completely dependent on IL-6 and was inhibited by the anti–IL-6 antibody, a significant myeloma cell proliferation was again detected at the end of treatment. The development of in vivo resistance to IL-6 antibody treatment is being investigated. Mouse anti-human IL-6R antibody was shown to inhibit in vivo growth of human myeloma cells inoculated into mice with severe combined immunodeficiency (133). A humanized anti-human IL-6 antibody was generated to prevent immune response against the antibody administered in patients (134). This reshaped anti–IL-6R antibody was shown to have strong antitumor cell activity against multiple myeloma cells, as well as the original antibody. These antibodies may become effective tools in therapy for multiple myeloma and other IL-6–related diseases.

Chimeric toxin consisting of human IL-6 fused to *Pseudomonas* exotoxin may be useful in the selective elimination of myeloma cells. The chimeric toxin was shown to be specifically cytotoxic to myeloma cell lines with high numbers of IL-6R, but it has no effect on IL-6R–negative cells in vitro (135). Considering the possible clinical utility of the chimeric toxin, its in vitro cytotoxic effect for bone marrow cells from 15 patients with myeloma was tested (136). Cells from five patients were very sensitive to the IL-6-toxin, and cells from three patients showed moderate sensitivity. The remaining seven samples showed little or no sensitivity. Normal bone marrow cells were shown to be resistant to the IL-6 toxin. Although toxicity of the chimeric toxin for normal cells and the effective dose for malignant cells should be investigated further, the IL-6 toxin may be useful, especially in ex vivo marrow purging, for selected patients with multiple myeloma who are candidates for autologous bone marrow transplantation.

REFERENCES

1. Sporn MB, Todaro GJ. Autocrine secretion and malignant transformation of cells. N Engl J Med 1980;303:878–880.

2. Sporn MB, Roberts AB. Autocrine secretion - 10 years later. Ann Intern Med 1992;117:408–414.

3. Aaronson SA. Growth factors and cancer. Science 1991; 254:1146–1153.

4. Huang JS, Huang SS, Deuel TF. Transforming protein of simian sarcoma virus stimulates autocrine growth of SSV-transformed cells through PDGF cell-surface receptors. Cell 1984;39:79–87.

5. Johnsson A. Betsholtz C, Heldin C-H, Westermark B. Antibodies against platelet-derived growth factor inhibit acute transformation by simian sarcoma virus. Nature 1985;317: 438–440.

6. Rosenthal A., Lindquist PB, Bringman TS, Goeddel DV, Derynck R. Expression of rat fibroblasts of a human transforming growth factor-α cDNA results in transformation. Cell 1986;46:301–309.

7. Assoian RK, Grotendorst GR, Miller DM, Sporn MB. Cellular transformation by coordinated action of three peptide growth factors from human platelets. Nature 1984;309: 804–806.

8. Bejcek BE, Li DY, Deuel TF. Transformation by v-sis occurs by an internal autoactivation mechanism. Science 1989;245:1496–1499.

9. Dunbar CE, Browder TM, Abrams JS, Nienhuis AW.

10. COOH-terminal-modified interleukin-3 is retained intracellularly and stimulates autocrine growth. Science 1989; 245:1493–1496.

10. Sporn MB, Roberts AB. Autocrine growth factors and cancer. Nature 1985;313:745–747.

11. Sporn MB, Roberts AB. Peptide growth factors and inflammation, tissue repair, and cancer. J Clin Invest 1986;78: 329–332.

12. Westermark B, Helden C-H. Platelet-derived growth factor in autocrine transformation. Cancer Res 1991;51:5087–5092.

13. Roberts AB, Thompson NL, Heine U, Flanders C, Sporn MB. Transforming growth factor-β: possible roles in carcinogenesis. Br J Cancer 1988;57:594–600.

14. Roberts AB, Sporn MB. The transforming growth factor-βs. In: Sporn MB, Roberts AB, eds. Peptide growth factors and their receptors I. Heidelberg: Springer-Verlag, 1990:419–472.

15. Liotta LA, Stetler-Stevenson WG. Tumor invasion and metastasis: an imbalance of positive and negative regulation. Cancer Res 1991;51(suppl 18):5054s–5059s.

16. Nicolson GL. Cancer progression and growth: relationship of paracrine and autocrine growth mechanisms to organ preference of metastasis. Exp Cell Res 1993;204:171–180.

17. Kath R, Jambrosic JA, Holland L, Rodeck U, Herlyn M. Development of invasive and growth factor-independent cell variants from primary human melanomas. Cancer Res 1991;51:2205–2211.

18. Cornil I, Theodorescu D, Man S, Herlyn M, Jambrosic J, Kerbel RS. Fibroblast cell interactions with human melanoma cells affect tumor cell growth as a function of tumor progression. Proc Natl Acad Sci USA 1991;88:6028–6032.

19. Heldin C-H, Westermark B. Platelet-derived growth factor: three isoforms and two receptor types. Trends Genet 1989; 5:108–111.

20. Heldin C-H, Westermark B. Platelet-derived growth factor: mechanism of action and possible in vivo function. Cell Reg 1990;1:555–566.

21. Heldin C-H, Westermark B. Signal transduction by the receptors for platelet-derived growth factor. J Cell Sci 1990; 96:193–196.

22. Westermark B, Heldin C-H. Platelet-derived growth factor in autocrine transformation. Cancer Res 1991;51:5087–5092.

23. Deuel TF, Huang JS, Huang SS, Stroobant P, Waterfield MD. Expression of a platelet-derived growth factor-like protein in simian sarcoma virus transformed cells. Science 1983;221:1348–1350.

24. Bowen-Pope DF, Vogel A, Ross R. Procution of platelet-derived growth factor-like molecules and reduced expression of platelet-derived growth factor receptors accompany transformation by a wide spectrum of agents. Proc Natl Acad Sci USA 1984;81;2396–2400.

25. Owen AJ, Pantazis P, Antoniades HN. Simian sarcoma virus-transformed cells secrete a mitogen identical to platelet-derived growth factor. Science 1984;225:54–56.

26. Garrett JS, Coughlin SR, Niman HL, Tremble PM, Giels GM, Williams LT. Blockade of autocrine stimulation in simian sarcoma virus-transformed cells reverses down-reg-

ulation of platelet-derived growth factor receptors. Proc Natl Acad Sci USA 1984;81:7466–7470.

27. Waterfield MD, Scrace GT, Whittle N, et al. Platelet-derived growth factor is structurally related to the putative transforming protein p28^{sis} of simian sarcoma virus. Nature 1983;304:35–39.

28. Doolittle RF, Hunkapiller MW, Hood LE, Devare SG, Robbins KC, Aaronson SA, Antoniades HN. Simian sarcoma virus onc gene, v-sis, is derived from the gene (or genes) encoding a platelet-derived growth factor. Science 1983;221:275–277.

29. Leal F, Williams LT, Robbins KC, Aaronson SA. Evidence that the v-sis gene product transforms by interaction with the receptor for platelet-derived growth factor. Science 1985;230:327–330.

30. Bywater M, Rorsman F, Bongcam-Rudloff E, et al. Expression of recombinant platelet-derived growth factor A- and B-chain homodimers in rat-1 cells and human fibroblasts reveals differences in protein processing and autocrine effects. Mol Cell Biol 1988;8:2753–2762.

31. Vassbotn FS, Andersson M, Westermark B, Heldin C-H, Östman A. Reversion of autocrine transformation by a dominant negative platelet-derived growth factor mutant. Mol Cell Biol 1993;13:4066–4076.

32. Keating MT, Williams LT. Autocrine stimulation of intracellular PDGF receptors in v-sis-transformed cells. Science 1988;239:914–916.

33. Hannink M, Donoghue DJ. Autocrine stimulation by the v-sis gene product requires a ligand-receptor interaction at the cell surface. J Cell Biol 1988;107:287–298.

34. Nistér M, Libermann TA, Betsholtz C, et al. Expression of messenger RNAs for platelet-derived growth factor and transforming growth factor-alpha and their receptors in human malignant glioma cell lines. Cancer Res 1988;48:3910–3918.

35. Nistér M, Claesson-Welsh L, Eriksson A, Heldin C-H, Westermark B. Differential expression of PDGF receptors in human malignant glioma cell lines. J Biol Chem 1991;266:16755–16763.

36. Leveen P, Claesson-Welsh, Heldin C-H, Westermark B, Betsholtz C. Expression of messenger RNAs for platelet-derived growth factor and its receptors in human sarcoma cell lines. Int J Cancer 1990;46:1066–1070.

37. Hermanson M, Funa K, Hartman M, et al. Platelet-derived growth factor and its receptors in human glioma tissue: expression of messenger RNA and protein suggests the presence of autocrine and paracrine loops. Cancer Res 1992;52:3213–3219.

38. Rozengurt E, Sinnett-Smith J, Taylor-Papadimitriou J. Production of PDGF-like growth factor by breast cancer cell lines. Int J Cancer 1985;36:247–252.

39. Perez R, Betsholtz C, Westermark B, Heldin C-H. Frequent expression of growth factors for mesenchymal cells in human mammary carcinoma cell lines. Cancer Res 1987;47:3425–3429.

40. Westermark B, Johnsson A, Paulsson Y, et al. Human melanoma cell lines of primary and metastatic origin express the genes encoding the chains of platelet-derived growth factor (PDGF) and produce a PDGF-like growth factor. Proc Natl Acad Sci USA 1986;83:7197–7200.

41. Soderdahl G, Betsholtz C, Johansson A, Nilsson K, Bergh J.

Differential expression of platelet-derived growth factor and transforming growth factor genes in small- and non-small-cell human lung carcinoma lines. Int J Cancer 1988;41:636–641.

42. Forsberg K, Valyi-Nagy I, Heldin C-H, Merlyn M, Westermark B. Platelet-derived growth factor (PDGF) in oncogenesis: development of a vascular connective tissue stroma in xenotransplanted human melanoma producing PDGF-BB. Proc Natl Acad Sci USA 1993;90:393–397.

43. De Larco JE, Todaro GJ. Growth factors from murine sarcoma virus-transformed cells. Proc Natl Acad Sci USA 1978;75:4001–4005.

44. Anzano MA, Roberts AB, Swith JM, Sporn MB, De Larco JE. Sarcoma growth factor from conditioned medium of virally transformed cells is composed of both type α and type β transforming growth factors. Proc Natl Acad Sci USA 1983;80:6264–6268.

45. Derynck R. Transforming growth factor α. Cell 1988;54:593–595.

46. Downward J, Yarden Y, Mayes E, et al. Close similarity of epidermal gorwth factor receptor and v-erb-B oncogene protein sequences. Nature 1984;307:521–527.

47. Derynck R, Lindquist PB, Bringman TS, et al. Expression of the transforming growth factor-α gene in tumor cells and normal cells. Cancer Cells 1989;7:297–301.

48. Wilcox JN, Derynck R. Developmental expression of transforming growth factor-alpha and -beta in mouse fetus. Mol Cell Biol 1988;8:3415–3422.

49. Wilcox JN, Derynck R. Localization of cells synthesizing transforming growth factor-alpha mRNA in the mouse brain. J Neurosci 1988;8:1901–1904.

50. Coffey RJ, Derynck R, Wilcox JN, et al. Production and auto-induction of transforming growth factor-α in human keratinocytes. Nature 1987;328:817–820.

51. Derynck R, Roberts AB, Winkler ME, Chen EY, Goeddel DV. Human transforming growth factor-α: precursor structure and expression in E.coli. Cell 1984;38:287–297.

52. Lee DC, Rose TM, Webb NR, Todaro GJ. Cloning and sequence analysis of a cDNA for rat transforming factor-α. Nature 1985;313:489–491.

53. Wong ST, Winchell LF, McCune BK, et al. The TGF-α precursor expressed on the cell surface binds to the EGF receptor on adjacent cells, leading to signal transduction. Cell 1989;56:495–506.

54. Brachmann R, Lindquist PB, Nagashima M, et al. Transmembrane TGF-α precursors activate EGF/TGF-α receptors. Cell 1989;56:691–700.

55. Anklesaria P, Teixidó J, Laiho M, Pierce JH, Greenberger JS, Massagué J. Cell-cell adhesion mediated by binding of membrane-anchored transforming growth factor α to epidermal growth factor receptors promotes cell proliferation. Proc Natl Acad Sci USA 1990;87:3289–3293.

56. Ozanne B, Fulton RJ, Kaplan PL. Kirsten murine sarcoma virus transformed cell lines and a spontaneously transformed rat cell line produce transforming growth factors. J Cell Physiol 1980;105:163–180.

57. Salmon DS, Perroteau I, Kidwell WR, Tum J, Derynck R. Loss of growth responsiveness to epidermal growth factor and enhanced production of alpha-transforming growth factors in ras-transformed mouse mammary epithelial cells. J Cell Physiol 1987;130:397–409.

58. Kaplan PL, Topp WC, Ozanne B. Simian virus 40 induces the production of a polypeptide transforming growth factor(s). Virology 1981;108:484–490.

59. Kaplan PL, Ozanne B. Polyoma virus-transformed cells produce transforming growth factor(s) and grow in serum-free medium. Virology 1982;123:372–380.

60. Liu C, Tsao M-S, Grisham JW. Transforming growth factors produced by normal and neoplastically transformed rat liver epithelial cells in culture. Cancer Res 1988;48:850–855.

61. Raymond VW, Lee DC, Grisham JW, Earp HS. Regulation of transforming growth factor α messenger RNA expression in a chemically transformed rat hepatic epithelial cell line by phorbol ester and hormones. Cancer Res 1989;49:3608–3612.

62. Rosenthal A, Lindquist PB, Bringman TS, Goeddel DV, Derynck R. Expression of rat fibroblasts of a human transforming growth factor-α cDNA results in transformation. Cell 1986;46:301–309.

63. Watanabe S, Lazar E, Sporn MB. Transformation of normal rat kidney (NRK) cells by an infectious retrovirus carrying a synthetic rat type α transforming growth factor gene. Proc Natl Acad Sci USA 1987;84:1258–1262.

64. Finzi E, Gleming T, Segatto O, et al. The human transforming growth factor type α coding sequence is not a direct-acting oncogene when overexpressed in NIH 3T3 cells. Proc Natl Acad Sci USA 1987;84:3733–3737.

65. Di Marco E, Pierce JH, Fleming TP, et al. Autocrine interaction between TGFα and the EGF-receptor: quantitative requirements for induction of the malignant phenotype. Oncogene 1989;4:831–838.

66. Sandgren EP, Luetteke NC, Palmiter RD, Brinster RL, Lee DC. Overexpression of TGFα in transgenic mice: induction of epithelial hyperplasia, pancreatic metaplasia, and carcinoma of the breast. Cell 1990;61:1121–1135.

67. Jhappan C, Stahle C, Harkins RN, Fausto N, Smith GH, Merlino GT. TGFα overexpression in transgenic mice induces liver neoplasia and abnormal development of the mammary gland and pancreas. Cell 1990;61:1137–1146.

68. Matsui Y, Halter SA, Holt JT, Hogan BLM, Coffey RJ. Development of mammary hyperplasia and neoplasia in MMTV-TGFα transgenic mice. Cell 1990;61:1147–1155.

69. Derynck R, Goeddel DV, Ullrich A, et al. Synthesis of mRNAs for transforming growth factors-α and β and the epidermal growth factor by human tumors. Cancer Res 1987;47:707–712.

70. Barnard JA, Lyons RM, Moses HL. The cell biology of transforming growth factor β. Biochim Biophys Acta 1990;1032:79–87.

71. Roberts AB, Anzano MA, Lamb LC, Smith JM, Sporn MB. New class of transforming growth factors potentiated by epidermal growth factor. Proc Natl Acad Sci USA 1981;78:5339–5343.

72. Assoian RK, Komoriya A, Meyers CA, Miller DM, Sporn MB. Transforming growth factor-beta in human platelets. J Biol Chem 1983;258:7155–7160.

73. Pircher R, Jullien P, Lawrence DA. β-Transforming growth factor is stored in human blood platelets as a latent high molecular weight complex. Biochem Biophys Res Commun 1986;136:30–37.

74. Miyazono K, Hellman U, Wernstedt C, Heldin C-H. Latent high molecular weight complex of transforming growth factor β1. J Biol Chem 1988;263:6407–6415.

75. Wakefield LM, Smith DM, Flanders KC, Sporn MB. Latent transforming growth factor-β from human platelets. J Biol Chem 1988;263:7646–7654.

76. Lawrence DA, Pircher R, Jullien P. Conversion of a high molecular weight latent β-TGF from chicken embryo fibroblasts into a low molecular weight active β-TGF under acidic conditions. Biochem Biophys Res Commun 1985;133:1026–1034.

77. Lyons RM, Keski-Oja J, Moses HL. Proteolytic activation of latent transforming growth factor-β from fibroblast-conditioned medium. J Cell Biol 1988;106:1659–1665.

78. Miyazono K, Dijke PT, Ichijo H, Heldin CH. Receptors for transforming growth factor-β. Abv Immunol 1994;55:181–220.

79. Frolik CA, Wakefield LM, Smith DM, Sporn MB. Characterization of a membrane receptor for transforming growth factor-β in normal rat kidney fibroblasts. J Biol Chem 1984;259:10995–11000.

80. Tucker RF, Branum EL, Shipley GD, Ryan RJ, Moses HL. Specific binding to cultured cells of ^{125}I-labeled type β transforming growth factor from human platelets. Proc Natl Acad Sci USA 1984;81:6757–6761.

81. Laiho M, Weis FMB, Massagué J. Concomitant loss of transforming growth factor (TGF)-β receptor types I and II in TGF-β-resistant cell mutants implicates both receptor types in signal transduction. J Biol Chem 1990;265:18518–18524.

82. Laiho M, Weis FMB, Boyd FT, Ignotz RA, Massagué J. Responsiveness to transforming growth factor-β restored by complementation between cells defective in TGF-β receptors I and II. J Biol Chem 1991;266:9108–9112.

83. Lin HY, Wang X-F, Ng-Eaton E, Weinberg RA, Lodish HF. Expression cloning of the TGF-β type II receptor, a functional transmembrane serine/threonine kinase. Cell 1992;68:775–785.

84. Franzén P, Dijke TP, Ichijo H, Schultz P, Heldin CH, Miyazono K. Cloning of a TGF-β type I receptor that forms a heteromeric complex with the TGF-β type II receptor. Cell 1993;75:681–692.

85. López-Casillas F, Cheifetz S, Doody J, Andres JL, Lane WS, Massagué J. Structure and expression of the membrane proteoglycan betaglycan, a component of the TGF-β receptor system. Cell 1991;67:785–795.

86. Sporn MB, Roberts AB. Transforming growth factor-β. Multiple actions and potential clinical applications. JAMA 1989;262:938–941.

87. Roberts AB, Thompson NL, Heine U, Flanders C, Sporn MB. Transforming growth factor-β: possible roles in carcinogenesis. Br J Cancer 1988;57:594–600.

88. Jetten AM, Shirley JE, Stoner G. Regulation of proliferation and differentiation of respiratory tract epithelial cells by TGF-β. Exp Cell Res 1986;167:539–549.

89. Reiss M, Sartorelli AC. Regulation of growth and differentiation of human keratinocytes by type β transforming growth factor and epidermal growth factor. Cancer Res 1987;47:6705–6709.

90. Keller JR, Sing GK, Ellingsworth LR, Ruscetti FW. Transforming growth factor-β: possible roles in the regulation of

normal and leukemic hematipoietic cell growth. J Cell Biochem 1989;39:79–84.

91. Kimchi A, Wang X-F, Weinberg RA, Cheifetz S, Massagué J. Absence of TGF-β receptors and growth inhibitory responses in retinoblastoma cells. Science 1988;240:196–198.

92. Arteaga CL, Tandon AK, von Hoff DD, Osborne CK. Transforming growth factor β: potential autocrine growth inhibitor of estrogen receptor-negative human breast cancer cells. Cancer Res 1988;48:3898–3904.

93. Zugmaier G, Ennis BW, Deschauer B, et al. Transforming growth factors type β1 and β2 are equipotent growth inhibitors of human breast cancer cell lines. J Cell Physiol 1989;141:353–361.

94. Wakefield LM, Smith DM, Masui T, Harris CC, Sporn MB. Distribution and modulation of the cellular receptor for transforming growth factor-β. J Cell Biol 1987;105:965–975.

95. Chinkers M. Isolation and characterization of mink lung epithelial cell mutants resistant to transforming growth factor-β. J Cell Physiol 1987;130:1–5.

96. Hampson J. Ponting ILO, Roberts AB, Dexter TM. The effects of TGF-β on haemopoietic cells. Growth Factors 1988;1:193–202.

97. Arteaga CL, Coffey RF Jr, Dugger TC, McCutchen CM, Moses HL, Lyons RM. Growth stimulation of human breast cancer cells with anti-transforming growth factor β antibodies: evidence for negative autocrine regulation by tranforming growth factor β. Cell Growth Differ 1990;1:367–374.

98. Hafez MM, Infante D, Winawer S, Friedman E. Transforming growth factor-β₁ acts as an autocrine-negative growth regulator in colon enterocytic differentiation but not in goblet cell maturation. Cell Growth Differ 1990;1:617–626.

99. Coombs LM, Pigott DA, Eydmann ME, Proctor AJ, Knowles MA. Reduced expression of TGFβ is associated with advanced disease in transitional cell carcinoma. Br J Cancer 1993;67:578–584.

100. Wu S, Theodorescu D, Kerbel RS, et al. TGF-β₁ is an autocrine-negative growth regulator of human colon carcinoma FET cells in vivo as revealed by transfection of an antisense expression vector. J Cell Biol 1992;116:187–196.

101. Kishimoto T. The biology of interleukin-6. Blood 1989;74:1–10.

102. Van Snick J. Interleukin 6: an overview. Annu Rev Immunol 1990;8:253–278.

103. Akira S, Taga T, Kishimoto T. Interleukin-6 in biology and medicine. Adv Immunol 1993;54:1–78.

104. Hirano T. Interleukin 6 (IL-6) and its receptor: their role in plasma cell neoplasias. Int J Cell Cloning 1991;9:166–184.

105. Akira S, Kishimoto T. The evidence for interleukin-6 as an autocrine growth factor in malignancy. Semin Cancer Biol 1992;3:17–26.

106. Kishimoto T, Akira S, Taga T. Interleukin-6 and its receptor: a paradigm for cytokines. Science 1992;258:593–597.

107. Yamasaki K, Taga T, Hirata Y, et al. Cloning and expression of the human interleukin-6 (BSF-2/IFNβ2) receptor. Science 1988;241:825–828.

108. Taga T, Hibi M, Hirata Y, et al. Interleukin-6 triggers the association of its receptor with a possible signal transducer, gp130. Cell 1989;58:573–581.

109. Hibi M, Murakami M, Saito M, Hirano T, Taga T, Kishimoto T. Molecular cloning and expression of an IL-6 signal transducer, gp 130. Cell 1990;63:1149–1157.

110. Murakami M, Hibi M, Nakagawa N, et al. IL-6-induce homodimerization of gp130 and associated activation of a tyrosine kinase. Science 1993;260:1808–1810.

111. Barlogie B, Epstein J, Selvanayagam P, Alexanian R. Plasma cell myeloma-new biological insights and advanced in therapy. Blood 1989;73:865–879.

112. Potter M. Genetics of susceptibility to plasmacytoma development in BALB/c mice. Cancer Surv 1984;3:247–264.

113. Nordan RP, Potter M. A macrophage-derived factor required by plasmacytomas for survival and proliferation in vitro. Science 1986;233:566–569.

114. Blankenstein T, Qin Z, Li W, Diamanstein T. DNA rearrangement and constitutive expression of the interleukin 6 gene in a mouse plasmacytoma. J Exp Med 1990;171:965–970.

115. Sugita T, Totsuka T, Saito M, et al. Functional murine interleukin 6 receptor with the intracisternal A particle gene product at its cytoplasmic domain. J Exp Med 1990;171:2001–2009.

116. Tohyama N, Karasuyama H, Tada T. Growth autonomy and tumorigenicity of interleukin-6R-dependent B cells transfected with interleukin-6 cDNA. J Exp Med 1990;171:389–400.

117. Vink A, Coulie P, Warnier G, et al. Mouse plasmacytoma growth in vivo: enhancement by interleukin 6 (IL-6) and inhibition by antibodies directed against IL-6 or its receptor. J Exp Med 1990:172:997–1000.

118. Suematsu S, Matsuda T, Aozasa K, et al. IgG1 plasmacytosis in interleukin 6 transgenic mice. Proc Natl Acad Sci USA 1989;86:7547–7551.

119. Suematsu S, Matsusaka T, Matsuda T, et al. Generation of plasmacytomas with the chromosomal translocation t(12;15) in interleukin 6 transgenic mice. Proc Natl Acad Sci USA 1992;89:232–235.

120. Kawano M, Hirano T, Matsuda T, et al. Autocrine generation and essential requirement of BSF-2/IL-6 for human multiple myelomas. Nature 1988;332:83–85.

121. Klein B, Zhang X-G, Jourdan M, et al. Paracrine rather than autocrine regulation of myeloma-cell growth and differentiation by interleukin-6. Blood 1989;73:513–526.

122. Freeman GJ, Freedman AS, Rabinowe SN, et al. Interleukin 6 gene expression in normal and neoplastic B cells. J Clin Invest 1989;83:1512–1518.

123. Schwab G, Siegall CB, Aarden LA, Neckers LM, Nordan RP. Characterization of an interleukin-6-mediated autocrine growth loop in the human multiple myeloma cell line, U266. Blood 1991;77:587–593.

124. Scala G, Kuang YD, Hall RE, Muchmore AV, Gyenheim JJ. Accessory cell function of human B cells. I. Production of both interleukin-1 like activity and an interleukin-1 inhibitory factor by EBV-transformed human B cell line. J Exp Med 1985;159:1637–1652.

125. Scala G., Quinto I, Ruocco MR, et al. Expression of an exogenous interleukin 6 gene in human Epstein-Barr virus B cells confers growth advantage and in vivo tumorigenicity. J Exp Med 1990;172:61–68.

126. Yee C, Biondi A, Wang XH, et al. A possible autocrine role

for interleukin-6 in two lymphoma cell lines. Blood 1989; 74:798–804.

127. Biondi A, Rossi V, Bassan R, et al. Constitutive expression of the interleukin-6 gene in chronic lymphocytic leukemia. Blood 1989;73:1279–1284.

128. Oster W, Cicco NA, Klein H, et al. Participation of the cytokines interleukin 6, tumor necrosis factor-α, and interleukin-1β secreted by acute myelogenous leukemia blasts in autocrine and paracrine leukemia growth control. J Clin Invest 1989;84:451–457.

129. Bataille R., Jourdan M, Zhang X-G, Klein B. Serum levels of interleukin 6, a potent myeloma cell growth factor, as a reflect of disease severity in plasma cell dyscrasias. J Clin Invest 1989;84:2008–2011.

130. Zhang XG, Klein B, Bataille R. Interleukin-6 is a potent myeloma-cell growth factor in patients with aggressive multiple myeloma. Blood 1989;74:11–13.

131. Ludwig H, Nachbaur DM, Fritz E, Krainer M, Huber H. Interleukin-6 is a prognostic factor in multiple myeloma. Blood 1991;77:2794–2795.

132. Klein B, Wijdenes J, Zhang X-G, et al. Murine anti-interleukin-6 monoclonal antibody therapy for a patient with plasma cell leukemia. Blood 1991;78:1198–1204.

133. Suzuki H, Yasukawa K, Saito T, et al. Anti-human interleukin-6 receptor antibody inhibits human myeloma growth in vivo. Eur J Immunol 1992;22:1989–1993.

134. Sato K, Tsuchiya M, Saldanha J, et al. Reshaping a human antibody to inhibit the interleukin 6-dependent tumor cell growth. Cancer Res 1993;53:851–856.

135. Siegall CB, Chaudhary VK, FitzGerald DJ, Pastan I. Cytotoxic activity of an interleukin-6-Pseudomonas exotoxin fusion protein on human myeloma cells. Proc Natl Acad Sci USA 1988;85:9738–9742.

136. Kreitman RJ, Siegall CB, FitzGerald DJP, Epstein J, Barlogie B, Pastan I. Interleukin-6 fused to a mutant form of Pseudomonas exotoxin kills malignant cells from patients with multiple myeloma. Blood 1992;79:1775–1780.

CHAPTER 35

ROLE OF CYTOKINES IN THE PROCESS OF TUMOR ANGIOGENESIS

S. Joseph Leibovich

The development and growth of solid tumors beyond an initial nidus of slowly dividing transformed cells is believed to be critically dependent on the establishment within the tumor of new microvascular blood vessels, the process of tumor angiogenesis (1–8). These newly forming vessels are required to supply nutrients, gases, and the means for rapid removal of metabolic waste products involved in the extensive proliferation and growth of transformed cells that occur during rapid expansion and three-dimensional growth of solid tumors. A critical consequence of this hypothesis is that inhibition of the process of tumor angiogenesis might interfere with the growth of tumors, implying that pharmacological modulation of tumor angiogenesis might provide a therapeutic modality for the treatment of developing tumors (5, 9–14).

The process of angiogenesis is complex, and only in the last decade or so has a clearer, albeit fragmentary, understanding of the cellular and the molecular interactions involved in the control of new blood vessel formation begun to develop. Much of this understanding has, in fact, come about from studies of the rapid and aggressive angiogenesis that occurs in the growth of certain solid tumors. It is now apparent, however, that angiogenesis is a process that occurs in many critical normal situations, including embryogenesis, organogenesis, normal growth and development, various stages of the female menstrual cycle, and the process of wound repair. Angiogenesis in all these situations is essential to host survival, and it is precisely regulated by normal cellular homeostatic mechanisms; new blood vessels develop and regress in a strictly regulated manner.

In the process of embryogenesis, angiogenesis is rigorously controlled and developmentally regulated (15–18). In wound repair, specific host cells induced and activated at the site of injury produce the angiogenic stimuli that induce formation of new blood vessels and formation of granulation tissue (19–21). As injury resolves and inflammatory cells successfully remove the injurious stimuli, the signals that stimulate angiogenesis disappear, and normal homeostatic control of the microvasculature is reestablished. In many disease states, however, particularly in fibroproliferative diseases such as rheumatoid arthritis, lung fibrosis, and liver fibrosis, the development of new blood vessels occurs in an inappropriate manner (22–24). The inappropriate formation of granulation tissue results in local damage, loss of specialized structures, and ultimately, fibrosis. The synovial pannus in rheumatoid arthritis, for example, consists of a proliferating, invasive granulation tissue that, in the active phases of the disease, invades and degrades cartilage and bony structures of diarthrodial joints.

The ultimate example of this inappropriate angiogenesis is that which occurs in the development of solid tumors. Transformed cells that form incipient tumors elude and subvert the normal host defense inflammatory and wound healing mechanisms that have evolved to detect and to counteract invasion by foreign organisms, as well as altered or transformed self-cells. By inducing angiogenesis, which is essential to normal wound repair, the incipient tumors mimic proliferating granulation tissue, and they utilize this critical stage of the normal host response to injury to establish their own growth. Because the stimuli for induction of angiogenesis in tumors persist, angiogenesis persists. The new blood vessels then continuously supply the metabolic requirements of the proliferating tumor cells, thus enabling and facilitating their growth.

Solid tumors use a number of strategies to induce the vascular supply they need to establish and to promote their growth (22,23) including the following. (a) Direct production of angiogenic cytokines and growth factors by the transformed cells, which includes the production of oncogene products related to many of the growth factors and cytokines. (b) Decreases in the production of inhibitory factors that are normally involved in vascular homeostasis (26). This process includes inactivation or loss of function of suppressor genes that control the production of angiogenesis inhibitors (25,26). (c) Production of cytokines and chemical mediators that are chemoattractants for monocytes, macrophages, lymphocytes, and mast cells, and that infiltrate the developing tumor and behave in a manner analogous to their behavior in wound repair (27–32). (d) Production, either by the tumor cells or by stromal cells associated with the tumor, of enzymes that modulate basement membrane and induce the release of stored or cryptic growth factors from a normally inaccessible depot (32–38). Tumors have therefore developed a panoply of mechanisms to subvert and to utilize normal host responses to establish and to promote their own parasitic growth as a result of induction of angiogenesis.

I review the nature of the cellular and the molecular interactions that occur in the process of angiogenesis. I emphasize that, in addition to the production of angiogenic factors by tumor cells, normal host cells that infiltrate the tumors also have important roles in the control of tumor angiogenesis, in a manner analogous to their role in inflammation and granulation tissue formation in the wound healing process. The angiogenic stimulators and inhibitors that modulate and control the growth of the new blood vessels are discussed. Although these substances include polypeptide growth factors and cytokines, extracellular matrix constituents, and both high and low molecular weight nonpeptide substances, only growth factors and cytokines are discussed in detail (Table 35–1).

THE ANGIOGENIC CASCADE

In normal mature adults, angiogenesis is a rare event that occurs only in certain specialized situations, such as dur-

TABLE 35–1   CYTOKINES AND GROWTH FACTORS IMPLICATED IN THE ANGIOGENIC CASCADE

Growth factors
  Fibroblast growth factors (aFGF, bFGF, related oncogenes)
  Vascular endothelial growth factor (VEGF)
  Platelet-derived growth factor-BB (PDGF-BB)
  Angiogenin
  Transforming growth factor-α (TGF-α)
  Epidermal growth factor (EGF)
  Transforming growth factor-β
  Platelet-derived endothelial cell growth factor (PD-ECGF)
  Hepatocyte growth factor/scatter factor (HGF/SF)
  Colony-stimulating factors (M-CSF, GM-CSF)
Cytokines
  Tumor necrosis factor-α (TNF-α)
  Interleukin-1 (IL-1)
  IL-2
  IL-3
  IL-4
  IL-6
  IL-8
  Interferon-γ (IFN-γ)

ing the female reproductive and menstrual cycle. In the absence of injury, microvascular blood vessels are extremely long-lived: the endothelial cells that line the microvasculature have a half-life of months to years (37,38). The target vessels within the microvasculature for angiogenic factors are the postcapillary venules and the small venules (39,40). These vessels consist of endothelial cells surrounded by basal lamina, with associated pericytes and smooth muscle cells. These cells lie within the basal lamina of the vessels, and they form intimate attachments with the extraluminal surfaces of the endothelial cells (41,42). In response to angiogenic signals, a series of changes in the cells of the vessel wall occurs, thus initiating the angiogenic process. These changes can be arbitrarily divided into "early" and "late" events. They form a cascade that results in the formation of new vessels from old. A diagramatic formulation of this angiogenic cascade is shown in Fig. 35–1.

Early events in the angiogenic cascade

Early events in the initiation of angiogenesis include the following. (a) Modification of intercellular junctions between adjacent endothelial cells (43,44) and modulation of junctions between endothelial cells and adjacent peri-

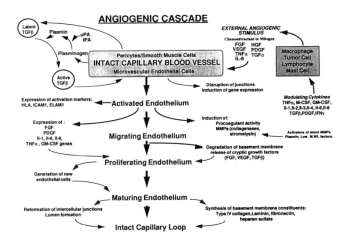

Figure 35–1 The angiogenic cascade. The principal features of the angiogenic process, beginning with an intact vessel in the microvasculature and resulting in a newly formed capillary loop, are described in the text.

cytes or smooth muscle cells occur (39,40,43). These changes prime the endothelial cells for the subsequent events of migration and proliferation. (b) Changes in the intercellular and cell-matrix adhesive properties of the endothelial cells occur; changes in the interactions between cytoskeletal constituents, cell surface adhesion molecules, such as integrin, immunoglobulin supergene, and selectin families, and components of the extracellular matrix occur (44–47). (c) Modulation of the proteolytic phenotype of the endothelial cells occurs, enabling these cells to begin to degrade extracellular matrix constituents, including basal lamina components, and to migrate away from the parent vessel (32,48,49). This process initiates the formation of a neovascular bud, and it may also induce localized release of cryptic growth factors from the basal lamina. (d) Induction of endothelial cell gene expression for certain cytokines and growth factors involved in subsequent stages of the angiogenic process occurs (50–53). These initial stages of the angiogenic cascade can proceed without endothelial cell proliferation, resulting in the formation of a capillary bud that will not continue to grow unless the subsequent steps in the cascade are allowed to continue (54).

Late events in the angiogenic cascade

Following the early migratory events that initiate formation of capillary buds, later events in the development of newly forming micro-vessels include the following. (a) Expression of specific cytokines and growth factors within endothelial cells in the newly forming capillary buds occurs (50–53,55–57). Expression of these cytokines and growth factors may be important in the autocrine or paracrine control of the growth and proliferation of the endothelial cells required for elongation of growing vessels following initial budding and migratory events. (b) Mobilization of cryptic growth factors from basement membrane depots occurs (58,59). (c) Vessel elongation by proliferation of endothelial cells occurs (60,61). (d) Vessel maturation occurs, with re-establishment of the basal lamina (62) and lumen formation. (e) Anastomosis of developing vascular buds occurs with other growing buds or pre-existing vessels to form intact capillary loops that allow for perfusion and transport of blood (47,62,63). Once mature capillaries form, they may stabilize and persist, mature into larger vessels, such as arterioles, venules, and ultimately arteries and veins, or regress and disappear. The phenomenon of neovascular regression accounts for the well-described change in color from red to white of maturing scar tissue. The factors that control the maturation of capillaries to larger vessels, and those that control their regression and disappearance are complex and poorly understood.

In this chapter, the involvement of cytokines and growth factors in induction and progression of this angiogenic cascade are addressed. Within this conceptual view of the angiogenic cascade, it is possible to incorporate the numerous diverse and often confusing data in the literature relative to the roles of certain cytokines and growth factors in the process of angiogenesis. In addition to factors that have direct inducing effects on the cells of the microvasculature, thus influencing the initial steps of the angiogenic process, there are also numerous factors that may have important roles in the sequential events that occur within the newly forming capillaries. These factors are induced within the cells of the microvasculature by initiation of the angiogenic cascade.

Some factors may have indirect roles in the angiogenic cascade. These indirect factors may function either by inducing immigration of cells, such as monocytes and macrophages, lymphocytes, or mast cells, to the site where angiogenesis is to be initiated, or by activating these cells to produce their own direct-acting angiogenic factors. In some cases, the indirect actions of these factors may be in contrast to their direct actions in the microvasculature, complicating our understanding of their roles in the angiogenic process. Indirect induction of angiogenesis may, however, be an extremely important function of certain cytokines and growth factors, and it is discussed in detail.

ANGIOGENIC GROWTH FACTORS AND CYTOKINES

The involvement of diffusible chemical mediators of the angiogenic process was first demonstrated by Greenblatt and Shubik (64). Subsequently, in a series of pioneering studies, Folkman and coworkers (7,11,20,65–67) demonstrated that tumors produce soluble factors that stimulate the growth of new blood vessels in a variety of in vivo and in vitro test systems. This activity was originally termed *tumor angiogeneic factor (TAF)* (68). TAF has since been studied in detail, and the angiogenic activity within it was found to consist in part of the heparin-binding polypeptide, basic fibroblast growth factor (bFGF) (69). The FGFs are not specific to tumors, and they are widely distributed and expressed in embryonic, developing, and mature animals and humans. The properties of the FGFs and their role in the angiogenic process are considered in detail. Although the FGFs were among the first of the angiogenic growth factors and cytokines to be clearly characterized, several other growth factors and cytokines have been shown to be important angiogenic inducers or to have important roles in control and progression of the angiogenic cascade (see Table 35–1). These factors include those that act directly on microvascular endothelial cells, as well as those that modulate the microvasculature via effects on other cell types, such as lymphocytes, monocytes/macrophages, mast cells, smooth muscle cells, keratinocytes, myofibroblasts, and pericytes. These factors are discussed in detail.

Assays of angiogenic factors

Development of assays to study the angiogenic process has been crucial to the major advances that have taken place in our understanding of angiogenesis in the past two decades. In vivo assays either modify vascular growth in amenable vascularized tissues or induce neovascularization into normally avascular tissues. Each assay has its advantages and shortcomings, and interpretation of results obtained using these assays must bear these shortcomings in mind. The process of angiogenesis consists of a cascade of cellular and humoral events that begin at the level of the intact microvasculature, and they result ultimately in the formation of new functional capillary loops. In vitro assays using cultured endothelial cells have been designed to analyze several critical stages of the angiogenic cascade. Because these assays illuminate the roles of these factors in the initiation or the progression of the angiogenic cascade, the principal aspects of the most commonly used in vivo and in vitro assays that have led to these advances are summarized.

CORNEAL BIOASSAY OF ANGIOGENESIS: The cornea of the eye, in common with certain other important anatomical structures, such as the vitreous of the eye and the cartilages, normally lacks blood vessels. The cells within the structures thus rely on diffusion of nutrients and gases from the aqueous humor, the surrounding scleral microvasculature, and the air for their metabolic needs. Avascular structures, in particular cartilage, have been studied extensively in recent years in an attempt to

isolate and to characterize antiangiogenic substances (i.e., substances that are responsible for inhibiting the ingrowth of blood vessels) (6,10,13,14). The study of cartilage-derived and other antiangiogenic factors has been discussed in recent reviews (7,11,12,14), and these factors are not discussed in detail herein. In 1974, Gimbrone and colleagues (70) developed a corneal implantation technique that involves surgical creation of a small pocket extending from near the center of the rabbit cornea to a distance of 1 to 2 mm from the limbal plexus. By implanting test tissues, cells, extracts, or purified factors within this pocket and by observing the ingrowth of new blood vessels from the limbal vasculature toward the implant over the course of several days, the angiogenic potency of these test agents can be determined. This model has been extended for use in the mouse and the rat (71,72).

There are certain important caveats that must be borne in mind when interpreting results obtained using this technique. First, although the cornea is normally avascular, implantation can induce inflammation. The infiltrating inflammatory cells, such as macrophages, can produce their own angiogenic factors (71,72–75). Care must be taken to ensure that such infiltration of inflammatory cells does not occur at any stage during the assay. Second, the corneal stroma is sandwiched on the external surface by the corneal epithelium, from which it is separated by a thick basement membrane structure, termed *Bowman's layer*, and on the internal aspect by the corneal endothelium, from which it is separated by another basement membrane structure, termed *Descemet's membrane*. These basement membranes may both serve as depots for the storage of growth factors such as the FGFs, which can be released by disruption of the basement membranes (57–59). Implanted substances in the cornea probably do not act in isolation, and care must be taken in the interpretation of results obtained using this model (76,77). Finally, with regard to the mode of delivery of test substances within the cornea, it is important to consider the nature of the carrier system used to deliver the substance within the cornea. Several sustained-release polymer systems have been developed for the continuous slow delivery of reagents from implanted pellets of these materials (78,79). These systems include Hydron (a poly-hydroxy-methylmethacrylate), Elvax (an ethylene-vinyl-acetate copolymer), and methyl cellulose. Characterization of the release kinetics of growth factors from these polymer systems within the cornea has rarely been rigorously undertaken. Nevertheless, despite these reservations, the rabbit or the rat cornea still remain the test systems of choice for demonstration of in vivo activity of putative angiogenic molecules.

EMBRYONIC CHICK CHORIOALLANTOIC MEMBRANE BIOASSAY: The second assay that has been used extensively in the study of angiogenesis, and which has been particularly useful in the assay of fractions during the purification of putative angiogenic factors, is the developing chick chorioallantoic membrane (CAM). The chorioallantois originates as a small diverticulum protruding from the tail gut into the chorionic cavity of the developing chick embryo, and it is comprised of an outer vascularized mesoderm and an inner endodermal monolayer. The mesoderm subsequently fuses with the chorionic ectoderm, which lies beneath the egg shell membrane, to form the CAM during days 4 to 5 of embryonic development. The CAM serves primarily as an embryonic lung (80). Progressive expansion of this surface, which includes microvessel angiogenesis, accommodates the gas exchange requirements of the developing embryo.

Accompanying the rapid growth of the CAM during development is the rapid growth of the CAM microvasculature. The intrinsic rate of angiogenesis within the CAM is maximal at days 10 to 11; by day 12, endothelial proliferation diminishes and cytodifferentiation begins (81). The CAM provides an amenable substrate for the application of putative angiogenic substances, which can modulate and influence the rate and pattern of vascular growth within the membrane. In the initial assay system, a window was cut in the shell of the developing eggs, exposing an area of the CAM. Subsequent assay development utilized an ex ovo shelless culture system; eggs are cracked at day 3 following fertilization into culture, and they are allowed to develop in vitro (82,83). In this system, the developing yolk sac (vitelline) membrane has also been used as a substrate for angiogenesis studies (84). This ex ovo system facilitates the assay by greatly reducing nonspecific reactions on the CAM induced by fragments of egg shell. The egg assay has the advantage over the corneal system of relative ease of set-up. Nevertheless, certain caveats apply to interpretation of results obtained in this system. First, the CAM is an avian rather than a mammalian system, and substances may have anomolous effects that are not relevant in mammals or humans. Second, the CAM and the yolk sac are prone to nonspecific inflammatory responses, and care must be taken to ensure that induced responses are not inflammatory in nature, inducing angiogenesis indirectly (85,86).

OTHER IN VIVO BIOASSAYS FOR ANGIOGENESIS:

A variety of additional in vivo systems have been used to assay for induction of angiogenesis, albeit not in a general manner. These systems include the hamster cheek pouch implant model (87), the subhepatic sponge implant (88), and the polyvinyl alcohol disk implant angiogenesis system (89). The hamster cheek pouch is extremely prone to nonspecific inflammation, because it has a large population of resident macrophages within it. The sponge implants all mimic wound healing and granulation tissue responses, and it is difficult to distinguish direct effects of factors from indirect effects medi-

ated by recruitment or activation of nonvascular cell types. Each of these assays has specific utility, but neither has been generally adopted as the assay of choice for the demonstration of angiogenesis.

ENDOTHELIAL CELL MIGRATION ASSAY:

Migration of endothelial cells is a critical early event in the process of angiogenesis. Microvascular endothelial cells respond to angiogenic stimuli by undergoing distinct morphological reorganization, as a result of activation of the cellular cytoskeletal motility apparatus. The activated cells migrate toward the source of the angiogenic stimulus, resulting in formation of a capillary bud. This chemoattraction of angiogenic substances for endothelial cells has been used extensively as an in vitro model of angiogenesis (90–93). Several variations of the technique have been developed. The most common technique involves determining the migration of endothelial cells across a porous filter in a multi-well Boyden chamber. Migration of endothelial cells in monolayer culture under agarose in a modified Ouchterlony assay has also been used, as has the endothelial monolayer "wounding" assay (94).

ENDOTHELIAL CELL PROLIFERATION ASSAY:

Proliferation of endothelial cells is also a vital process in the formation of new blood vessels; it generates the new cells that enable continued elongation of the capillary buds that develop following the initial challenge of a microvessel by an angiogenic stimulus. Both large vessel and microvascular endothelial cell cultures have been used extensively to assay for factors that modulate endothelial cell proliferation (7,27,57). This assay has been particularly useful in the measurement of activity during the purification of putative endothelial cell growth factors and angiogenic factors from a variety of tissues and cells (68,69,95,96). Microvascular endothelial cell cultures, from brain, adrenal gland, omentum, and other sources, have also been used extensively as target cells in the assay of endothelial cell growth factors. The development of techniques for the culture of microvascular endothelial cells provided an important tool for the study of putative angiogenic factors, and it enabled considerable progress to be made in our understanding of the angiogenic process.

ENDOTHELIAL CELL PROTEASE PRODUCTION:

To migrate away from the pre-existing microvasculature, endothelial cells must either reorganize or degrade components of the basement membrane and the extracellular matrix. Degradation of basement membrane components by endothelial cells has been shown to be mediated by production of various proteolytic enzymes, including urokinase, tissue-type plasminogen activator, and matrix metalloproteinases (MMPs). These enzymes are normally synthesized as precursor proenzymes in inactive form (98). Activation of these precursors is complex. Proteolytic activation has been demonstrated in some studies, whereas nonproteolytic activation mechanisms have also been demonstrated (99). In addition to control of production of active proteases at the level of activation of proenzymes, endothelial cells also produce high levels of inhibitors of proteolytic enzymes, including plasminogen-activator inhibitor types 1 and 2 (PAI-1, PAI-2) and tissue inhibitors of metalloproteinases (TIMP) (8–10). The nonstimulated endothelial cell phenotype has been reported to be characterized by low plasminogen activator and matrix metalloproteinase production and high PAI-1 and TIMP production, thus supporting a nonproteolytic phenotype (103). Stimulation of endothelial cells with growth factors such as FGF and VEGF, or with cytokines such as tumor necrosis factor-α (TNF-α) or interleukin-1 (IL-1), changes the phenotype of endothelial cells from nonproteolytic to proteolytic by up-regulating transcription and translation of proteases, while down-regulating the production of PAI-1 or TIMP.

Measurement of the production of collagenases by endothelial cells has been used as an in vitro assay for angiogenic substances. These assays are commonly based on the degradation in vitro of either reconstituted type 1 collagen fibrils or reconstituted basement membrane (type IV) collagen by conditioned media from endothelial cell cultures (38,48,49,105). Activation of latent proteases using trypsin or plasmin may be required for these assays. More sophisticated analysis involves zymography, the electrophoretic separation of media constituents on polyacrylamide gels containing the enzyme substrate. Quantitation and apparent molecular size of the active enzymes can then be determined by allowing in situ degradation of the substrate protein to occur in the gels (102,103). The presence of inhibitors such as PAI-1 and TIMP can also be demonstrated using this system.

IN VITRO CAPILLARY FORMATION BY ENDOTHELIAL CELLS CULTURED ON EXTRACELLULAR MATRICES:

As discussed earlier, the process of angiogenesis involves reorganization of migrating and proliferating endothelial cells into tubes that can ultimately act as conduits for the transport of blood. Endothelial cells cultured in vitro generally form monolayers at confluence that assume a characteristic cobblestone appearance. When maintained at confluence for extended periods, these monolayers often exhibit a phenomenon referred to as "sprouting," wherein cells begin spontaneously to grow above the monolayer in a manner that has been postulated to be analogous to the sprouting of capillary buds in vivo (106,107). The effects of certain angiogenic substances on this in vitro sprouting phenomenon have been studied. Growth of endothelial cells on extracellular matrix components has also been studied

extensively in recent years, and considerable insight regarding the role of the extracellular matrix in the formation of microvessels has been achieved (104,108–110). Endothelial cells cultured on type 1 collagen will initially form a monolayer, but over the course of several days, they gradually invade the gel and reorganize within it to form tube-like structures that resemble capillaries. The endothelial cells form intracellular and intercellular junctions and an internal lumen. The tube-like structures form basement membrane on their outside, and they are a close in vitro analog of forming capillaries in vivo. The process of tube formation on type 1 collagen can be greatly accelerated, either by plating the cells in a sandwich of collagen, so that the cells are covered top and bottom by the collagen fibrillar matrix, or by treating the endothelial monolayers on the collagen gel with certain growth factors and cytokines (111). These factors greatly accelerate invasion of the matrix by the cells, and they promote their reorganizational ability within the gels.

In contrast to endothelial cells cultured in type 1 collagen gels, endothelial cells cultured on matrices containing basement membrane collagen, such as Matrigel, rapidly organize on the gel into a stable, reticulated, branching network of capillary-like tubes (108,109). Formation of this network can be modulated by certain cytokines, possibly as a result of the induction of proteases in the endothelial cells, which interfere with the cell–matrix interactions required for the reorganizational events involved in the formation of the mature tubes. Studies of the formation of capillary-like tubes on extracellular matrices provide valuable insights into the interactive events that are required to occur between the endothelial cells, their cytoskeletal, transmembrane adhesion proteins, and the extracellular matrix in the formation of new blood vessels.

INTERACTIONS IN VITRO BETWEEN ENDOTHELIAL CELLS AND OTHER CELL TYPES:

Although the principal cell type forming the tubular structure of the microvasculature is the endothelial cell, smooth muscle cells and pericytes are also present, albeit in much fewer numbers. These cells have important roles in the control of microvascular tone, and they may also have a role in the control of angiogenesis. Pericytes are generally found associated intimately with endothelial cells, lying within the bounding basement membrane of the microvasculature. Pericytes, although often difficult to visualize morphologically, possess extended cellular processes that form junctional complexes with numerous endothelial cells (112). On the basis of coculture experiments of endothelial cells with pericytes, it has recently been suggested that the interactions between these cells maintain the endothelial cells in a quiescent state (113–115). At least part of this quiescence may be mediated by localized production of transforming growth factor-β

(TGF-β) by the pericytes. This interaction may be modulated by proteolytic enzymes, such as plasmin, and this modulation may be extremely important in the angiogenic cascade. Similar considerations may also apply to smooth muscle cell–endothelial interactions. Cytokines, growth factors, and chemical mediators that modulate the function of pericytes or smooth muscle cells may thus modulate endothelial cell function, and possibly angiogenesis, by modulating the nature of the interactions between these cell types. These interactions are amenable to study in vitro, and they should prove to be a fruitful area of research.

Angiogenic growth factors

FIBROBLAST GROWTH FACTORS: The family of FGFs consists of at least nine closely related gene products (116–118). Of these products, only two are found normally in mature mammals and humans: acidic-FGF (aFGF) and basic FGF (bFGF). The other forms are expressed in a developmentally regulated sequence during embryogenesis and fetal development (119,120), or they are expressed as oncogene products by certain transformed cells (121,122). Both aFGF and bFGF consist of single polypeptide chains that lack classic secretory peptide signal sequences (117). bFGF is synthesized in three different molecular weight forms as a result of initiation of translation at three alternative initiation codons in the gene sequence (123). Similar size heterogeneity is also observed with aFGF (117,118). The largest form is the 22.5-kd chain, and it contains a nuclear targeting signal within its N-terminal domain (124); the two smaller forms (20.5 and 17 kd) do not contain this signal. Nuclear targeting of FGF may be critical for its mitogenic effects.

FGFs have an extremely high affinity for heparin (7,69,95). In early studies of the role of mast cells in tumor angiogenesis, it was observed that heparin markedly promoted the migration of endothelial cells (125,126). Subsequently, heparin affinity was used to purify angiogenic growth factors from conditioned media of the Walker carcinoma (125,126), and these factors were shown to be identical to the endothelial cell mitogens characterized independently as FGF (117). This heparin affinity of the FGFs is used routinely in the purification of heparin-binding growth factors, of which the FGFs form one subclass.

Acidic FGF and bFGF are widely distributed in mature mammals and humans. Several studies have been performed to localize FGFs in various tissues and cells, using both light and electron microscopic immunohistochemical techniques. When localization of FGFs has been possible, the predominant sites FGF has been found are the cell cytoplasm and the nucleus (127,128). Localization of FGF in vascular basement membranes has also been reported, and FGF has been demonstrated to be present in association with the heparan sulfate proteoglycans of the extracellular matrix of endothelial cells cultured in vitro (57–59). This FGF can be released in active form by treatment with heparinase (59). These studies have given rise to the concept that extracellular matrices, basement membranes in particular, may serve as a depot for growth factors, maintaining them in an inactive or a cryptic form. Perturbation of the basement membrane could then result in localized release of bioactive growth factors.

Because aFGF and bFGF do not possess secretory signal sequences and they cannot be secreted by the classic secretory pathway, it is not understood how these forms of FGF are released by the cells into the basement membrane (130). It has been suggested that release of FGF by cells is associated with cellular injury (131). Similar observations have been made previously in connection with the release of IL-1 from macrophages; IL-1 release was shown to parallel release of the cytoplasmic enzyme, lactate dehydrogenase (132). Migrating endothelial cells in culture in the phogokinetic track assay described originally by Albrecht-Buehler (91) also deposit a trail of FGF as they migrate, which has been equated with FGF release from the cells (133). This release is likely related to the cytoplasmic budding and vesiculation associated with migration of endothelial cells in this assay (91). Despite our lack of understanding of the mechanisms of FGF release from cells, high affinity cell surface receptors for the various forms of FGF are widely distributed (134), suggesting a role for extracellular FGF. In addition, cell surface heparan sulfate proteoglycan may also have a role in presentation and stabilization of FGF to high-affinity receptors. Although aFGF and bFGF proteins are widely distributed, mRNA for these proteins is rarely found in nonperturbed systems in mature adults. Nonproliferating endothelial cells in culture do not express mRNA for FGF (135). Stimulation by treatment with exogenous FGF, however, rapidly induces expression of FGF mRNA by endothelial cells. It is not yet known whether this induction of FGF within the cells is required for the biological action of the exogenously added FGF.

Expression of FGF has been studied in several tumors (136–138). In tumors expressing FGF, the protein is generally found intracellularly, in cytoplasmic and nuclear locations. FGF binding sites are also generally found associated with the neovasculature in the areas of rapid blood vessel growth (139), again associated with the endothelial cells. These observations support the notion that FGF may have an important role as an autocrine or a paracrine mediator of angiogenesis, with its induction in endothelial cells being important for the control of endothelial cell proliferation.

Although the FGFs were the first angiogenic growth factors to be purified and characterized, the in vivo mechanism of their angiogenic effects is not entirely clear. In the cornea of rabbits and rats, FGF induces ingrowth of new blood vessels at a level of approximately 5 to 10 ng/slow release implant (96,140). It has been observed that the nature of the slow delivery polymer system is critical to the effects observed in the cornea with FGF (141). It has been suggested that at least low-grade infiltration of the cornea by monocytes/macrophages is required for the induction of angiogenesis, and that when this infiltration is absent, no angiogenic effect is observed. Similar induction of secondary cell types by bFGF has also been observed in the CAM assay (86).

Several oncogene products in the FGF family have been characterized (i.e., KGF, Int-2, hst/KS3, FGF5). Some of these products are secreted proteins that, in contrast to aFGF and bFGF, possess secretory signal sequences. The role of these oncogene products in tumor-related angiogenesis is not clear. It has been suggested that neovascularization in the development of a murine fibrosarcoma is associated with a switch from a non-exported intracellular FGF to an exported form, in a multi-step sequence (142). This switch has been postulated as a critical stage in the development of this solid tumor. Tumor cell secretion of FGF does not, however, appear to be a general phenomenon in vascularizing tumors.

PLATELET-DERIVED GROWTH FACTORS:

PDGFs consist of two primary gene products (PDGF-A and PDGF-B), and each has a molecular weight of approximately 16 to 18 kd (143). The active PDGF molecules consist of dimers of the A and B chains crosslinked by interchain disulfide crosslinks (144). A-A, B-B, and A-B dimers have been observed (145). PDGF was first discovered as a platelet-derived mitogenic activity that stimulated the growth of vascular smooth muscle cells, and it constituted the major mitogenic activity in serum for a variety of mesenchymal cell types (141). PDGF has since been shown to be produced by a variety of normal and transformed cell types (144,147). In addition to the primary A- and B-chain transcripts, post-translational modifications involving proteolytic cleavage of N- and C-terminal peptides, as well as alternative splicing from the initial nuclear mRNA transcripts, results in considerable microheterogeneity of the mature PDGF molecules (143,144). At least two classes of transmembrane high affinity cell surface receptors for PDGF isoforms have been defined and cloned (148–150). These receptors have been termed the α- and the β-receptors. α-receptors appear to bind the PDGF A chain exclusively, whereas the β-receptor binds both A and B chains, albeit with different affinities (143,151). The α- and β-receptors are differentially expressed in different cell types, and regulated expression may account for the distinct responsiveness of various cell types to PDGF preparations (143,147,152,153).

Although endothelial cells from human umbilical veins and large blood vessels do not express PDGF receptors (154–156), it has been reported that certain strains of microvascular endothelial cells do express PDGF receptors, and they respond mitogenically to PDGF (157–159). These cells include microvascular endothelial cells derived from human adipose tissue, human carcinoid tumors, rat brain, and rat liver. In addition, expression of PDGF α-receptors has been demonstrated in vivo on microvascular endothelial cells in certain distinct locations. For example, in malignant glioma that secrete PDGF, hyperproliferating microvascular endothelial cells growing near the secreting glioma cells express both PDGF B-chain protein and mRNA for the PDGF receptor (160). Human malignant glioblastoma multiforme capillary endothelial cells express PDGF receptors (160). A role for PDGF as an autocrine or a paracrine modulator of microvascular cells involved in neovascularization has been proposed on the basis of this evidence.

In the chick CAM assay of angiogenesis, it has been reported that PDGF-BB, but not PDGF-AA, induced an angiogenic response (161). This response was accompanied by little inflammation. In vitro PDGF-BB was found to be a potent chemoattractant for rat brain capillary endothelial cells, whereas PDGF-AA had less effect. In our hands, all three forms of PDGF (i.e., AA, AB, and BB), obtained as recombinant proteins, elicited clear, but weak angiogenic responses in the rat cornea (Leibovich SJ, et al., unpublished observations). These responses were accompanied in all experiments, however, by a low level of monocytic infiltration, suggesting the additional possibility of an indirect mode of action for the PDGF-induced angiogenic response. This indirect mode of action can be mediated in a variety of ways. PDGF has been shown to be chemotactic for monocytes (161), although these data have been questioned (163). The important role for monocytes and macrophages in the induction of angiogenesis is well established, and it has been discussed in detail in recent reviews (19,72,75,146). PDGF also affects smooth muscle cells; it stimulates their migration, growth, and synthesis of interstitial collagenase (MMP-1) and PAI-1 (164–169). Modulation of smooth muscle cells can lead to modification of the interactions between these cells and microvascular endothelial cells, as well as to their synthesis and production of endothelial cell mitogens (167). Recently, in an in vitro capillary tube–forming model of angiogenesis involving coculture of myofibroblasts and microvascular fragments from rat epididymal fat pads, PDGF-BB was shown to stimulate endothelial cell tube formation by stimulating myofibroblast proliferation, as well as their production of type 1 collagen and an endothelial cell growth factor distinct from PDGF (170). The endothelial cells in the microvascular fragments did not express PDGF receptors, clearly indicating the indirect nature of the PDGF response in this system.

Several tumors have been shown to express PDGF isoforms (143,147,160,173,174). The v-sis oncogene product p$^{28v\text{-}sis}$, the transforming product of the simian sarcoma virus, is closely related to the PDGF B-chain (171). Numerous transformed cell lines, such as fibrosarcomas, glioblastomas, and osteosarcomas, have been shown to express c-sis mRNA (143,147,175,176). Whether the protein product of the c-sis gene is involved in the angiogenic cascade in tumors is not yet clear.

VASCULAR ENDOTHELIAL GROWTH FACTOR: Vascular endothelial growth factor (VEGF), also referred to as vascular permeability factor (VPF) or vasculotropin, is a heparin-binding dimeric polypeptide consisting of two identical subunits with apparent molecular masses of 20 to 23 kd (176–179). Four different homodimeric species of VEGF have been demonstrated, formed by alternative splicing from the initial mRNA transcript. The monomeric forms have 121, 165, 189, or 206 amino acids, respectively (177). In contrast to FGF-1 and FGF-2, all four forms of VEGF contain a hydrophobic leader sequence characteristic of secreted proteins (176). The two smaller forms are found as soluble, secreted proteins; the two larger forms, however, are bound to heparin-containing proteoglycans at the cell surface or to components of basement membranes (180,181). VEGF was originally identified in the conditioned media of folliculostellate cells (179), as well as tumor cell lines, including the human HL-60 and U937 myelomonocytic cell lines (178,180). VEGF is a potent mitogen for endothelial cells, and it potently stimulates vascular permeability (182). VEGF has little mitogenic activity for either fibroblasts or smooth muscle cells, which do not appear to express the receptors for this factor (183). VEGF bears a significant sequence and structural homology to PDGF; preservation of the eight cysteine pairs is found in both the A- and the B-chains of PDGF (178,180).

The fact that VEGF is in part a secreted endothelial cell–specific mitogen strongly suggests a potential role for this factor in the process of angiogenesis. In vivo, VEGF has been shown to induce angiogenesis in rat and rabbit corneal bioassays, as well as in the CAM assay (176–179). It induces human endothelial cell chemotaxis, and it stimulates endothelial cell collagenase (MMP-1) production in vitro (184). Production of TIMP was, however, unchanged in these cells. Other matrix metalloproteinases that might be involved in the degradation of basement membrane constituents were not induced. Expression of endothelial cell tissue–type plasminogen activator and urokinase-type plasminogen activator was, however, induced by VEGF in microvascular endothelial cells, as was PAI-1 (185). Expression of VEGF has been demonstrated in the ovarian corpus luteum and in the developing brain, and it appears to correlate with the development of blood vessels in these tissues (176,183). High affinity binding sites for VEGF are found in endothelial cells, but not on other cell types in adult tissue sections (183). Abundant

VEGF mRNA is expressed in several normal tissues, and it is temporally related to the growth of microvessels in a variety of proliferating tissues (176).

Several transformed cell lines express VEGF mRNA and secrete VEGF protein (187,188). Several human tumors also express VEGF mRNA at high levels (189–191). These tumors include capillary hemangioblastomas and the highly vascularized glioblastoma multiforme (191, 192). Although oncogene products related closely to VEGF have not yet been identified, transfection of the secretable forms of VEGF into Chinese hamster ovary cells results in the acquisition by these cells of the ability to form tumors in nude mice (193). Recently, it has been demonstrated that inhibition of VEGF in vivo using a specific monoclonal antibody resulted in inhibition of growth in nude mice of three human tumor cell lines: rhabdomyosarcoma, glioblastoma multiforme, and leiomyosarcoma (194). This effect was suggested to be due to the inhibition of angiogenesis in these tumors and to indicate an important role for this secreted endothelial cell mitogen in the process of angiogenesis. In addition to its potential as a direct-acting angiogenic factor, VEGF may also have a role as an autocrine or a paracrine factor in the process of angiogenesis. Although there is often a correlation between expression of VEGF and growth of new microvessels, expression of VEGF has also been correlated in several tumors with the presence of necrobiosis within the tumor mass (195). This finding suggests a complex and multifunctional role for VEGF in vascular and tumor biology.

ANGIOGENIN: Angiogenin, a 14.1 kd single chain polypeptide, was isolated originally from conditioned media of the HT29 human adenocarcinoma cell line (196,197), and it was named on the basis of its ability to induce an angiogenic response on the CAM. Angiogenin has also been reported to induce angiogenesis in the cornea. Angiogenin is a secreted protein that shows a high degree of homology to pancreatic ribonuclease; it has a 68% amino acid sequence homology and conserved essential active site residues. Angiogenin is inactive in standard ribonuclease assays, but it expresses a unique ribonucleolytic activity toward ribosomal and transfer RNAs that appears to be required for its angiogenic activity (198). Angiogenin reportedly does not induce endothelial cell proliferation, migration, or protease production. However, high affinity binding sites have been demonstrated on several types of endothelial cells, including bovine brain capillary, calf pulmonary artery, bovine aorta, cornea, and adrenal cortex capillary endothelial cells (199,200). In cultured endothelial cells, angiogenin induces a transient intracellular increase in 1,2-diacyglycerol and activation of phospholipase A$_2$. In vascular smooth muscle cells, angiogenin induces activation of phospholipase C and rapid cholesterol esterification (201). Angiogenin has been shown to support endothelial cell as well as fibroblast cell adhesion in culture (201), and it has also been shown recently to be an actin-binding protein (203).

Studies of the distribution of mRNA for angiogenin in developing rats showed no correlation with sites of rapid microvascular growth; rapidly growing liver showed little expression, and adult liver showed the greatest expression (204). In regenerating liver and in human colon cancer, mRNA levels for angiogenin are related to the degree of cell replication and differentiation (205). It has been noted that the angiogenic response induced by angiogenin in the cornea and the CAM is accompanied by an influx of inflammatory cells. These observations, combined with the lack of effect of angiogenin on endothelial cell migration and proliferation, suggest that the angiogenic effects of angiogenin may be indirect rather than direct (85).

EPIDERMAL GROWTH FACTOR AND TRANSFORMING GROWTH FACTOR-α:

EGF is a small, single chain 6-kd polypeptide, isolated originally from mouse salivary glands on the basis of its ability to stimulate precocious tooth eruption and eyelid opening in newborn mice (206). EGF is found normally in the salivary glands, saliva, and milk (207,208), as well as in urine, where it was originally termed *urogastrone* (209). EGF is expressed by cells in various adult tissues. It is a broad-range mitogen for epithelial cells, as well as for a variety of mesenchymal and nonmesenchymal cells (209). The effects of EGF are mediated via a single cell surface receptor that is broadly expressed on most known cell types (210). Several proteins have been identified that closely resemble EGF in their amino acid sequence, and they appear to mediate their effects by binding to the same EGF receptor. These proteins include TGF-α, amphiregulin, and the vaccinia virus growth factor (VVGF) (209). In addition, several growth factor receptors and cell surface adhesion molecules, including the "selectin" family and the LDL-receptor, contain multiple regions with homology to EGF within their extracellular multidomain structures (211).

TGF-α was first described as a mitogen secreted by transformed fibroblasts that reversibly transformed normal cells from an anchorage-dependent phenotype to an anchorage-independent one, with the ability to form colonies in soft agar with a greatly lowered serum requirement (212). TGF-α has been shown to be produced by monocytes and macrophages following activation (213,214), and it is also a product of numerous transformed and tumor cells (212). Both EGF and TGF-α are produced as large, precursor integral membrane glycoproteins, from which the mature growth factors are cleaved (215,216). TGF-α is also found in a cell-associated form that is biologically active.

Both EGF and TGF-α have been reported to stimulate

angiogenesis in vivo in the hamster cheek pouch assay; TGF-α requires 0.3 to 1 μg to induce this response, whereas approximately 10 μg EGF is required (87). The drawbacks of the hamster cheek pouch model of angiogenesis were discussed, with particular reference to the presence of high levels of resident and inducible macrophages in this system. EGF and TGF-α both stimulate proliferation of bovine pulmonary endothelial cells in culture (87,216). Although EGF and TGF-α modulate the proteolytic phenotype of several cell types, effects in the in vitro capillary forming assays using endothelial cells have not been reported (97). Expression of TGF-α by various transformed cells and tumors, however, suggests that further investigation of the role of this factor in tumor-induced angiogenesis is warranted.

TRANSFORMING GROWTH FACTOR-β:

TGF-β was first characterized as a factor produced by transformed cells that acted in concert with EGF to induce clonal anchorage-independent growth of normal rat kidney epithelial cells in soft agar (217). TGF-β has since been shown to be produced by a large range of normal cell types, as well as by transformed cells, and it is believed to have important roles in the control of cellular proliferation, gene expression, and synthesis of extracellular matrix (218). The active forms of TGF-β consist of two polypeptide chains of approximately 11.5 to 12.5 kd, crosslinked by intermolecular disulfide bonds. At least five forms of TGF-β have been described (TGF-β_{1-5}) (219). TGF-β_1 and TGF-β_2 are the most abundant forms in normal adults, and they exist primarily as homodimers, although the TGF-$\beta_{1,2}$ heterodimer has been observed in porcine platelets (220). The other forms are expressed in a regulated manner during embryonic and fetal development and growth (221). A number of factors that are closely related to TGF-β are also expressed during development and growth, including the inhibins, the activins, and the bone morphogenetic proteins (BMPs) (218). These factors have been designated as the TGF-β supergene family.

In normal situations, TGF-β is found in high concentrations in bone, spleen, and in the α-granules of platelets, from which it is released as a result of platelet activation (222). This release from platelets may have a role in the process of inflammation and wound repair, during which vascular injury results in platelet activation, adhesion, and release of α-granule constituents. TGF-β is also produced by activated macrophages (224), lymphocytes (223), and smooth muscle cells (225). Smooth muscle cell and pericyte TGF-β is normally produced in inactive form as a precursor complexed with a latency-inducing binding protein (114,115,226,227). Proteolytic cleavage of latent TGF-β by enzymes, such as plasmin, may have a role in controlling the effects of latent TGF-β locally produced in the microvasculature. Numerous transformed cells have also been shown to produce TGF-β (218). The TGF-β produced by transformed cells in developing tumors may have several roles in the control of tumor angiogenesis.

TGF-β has been shown to have a number of important effects that implicate it as an important participant in the process of angiogenesis. These include direct effects on endothelial cells and smooth muscle cells, as well as indirect effects mediated by induction and modulation of cells, such as monocytes, macrophages, lymphocytes, and pericytes. In terms of its direct effects on endothelial cells, TGF-β₁ has been shown to be a potent inhibitor of endothelial cell proliferation and to antagonize the mitogenic effects of the FGFs on these cells (228,229). At low concentrations (200–500 pg/mL), TGF-β₁ induced endothelial cells cultured on type 1 collagen gels to reorganize and form capillary-like tubes (104,230). At higher concentrations (5–10 ng/mL), however, TGF-β₁ inhibited invasion, and it antagonized phorbol-ester–induced invasion of these gels (104,231). TGF-β stimulates the production of extracellular matrix and basement membrane constituents by endothelial cells (228,229), it depresses their production of matrix metalloproteinases, and it up-regulates their production of protease inhibitors, such as TIMP and PAI-1 (100). These direct biphasic effects of TGF-β on endothelial cells suggest an important role for this growth factor in the "late," maturational events of the angiogenic process, with induction of basement membrane deposition, capillary lumen formation, and acquisition of capillary morphology. Factors that modulate the number of pericytes and smooth muscle cells, or their production of active TGF-β, could therefore have an important role in controlling angiogenesis.

Although TGF-β has several direct effects on angiogenesis that suggest a role in the late, maturation processes of vessel formation, TGF-β also has important effects on extravascular cells that may be important for the regulation of angiogenesis in inflammation, wound repair, and tumor growth. TGF-β is a potent chemoattractant for monocytes and macrophages at femtomolar concentrations (232,233). Release of TGF-β by cells at the extravascular site where angiogenesis is to be induced could thus induce migration of monocytes from the circulation. These monocytes might then be activated to express their own angiogenic factors (232,233), and thus initiate and participate in the angiogenic cascade. At higher concentrations, TGF-β acts as an activating agent for monocytes and macrophages, and it induces their expression of IL-1, TNF-α, and other cytokines. Although TGF-β induces gene expression of cytokines, as well as their expression of integrins and collagenase (234), at high concentrations it also inhibits the production of oxygen radicals (235). Oxygen radical production by monocytes and macrophages is normally a process that occurs very rapidly as a result of activation of the cell membrane–associated oxidase system and the cellular respiratory burst, following challenge of the cells with an activating agent, such as endotoxin (236). The effects of TGF-β on the production of nitric oxide by monocytes/macrophages has not yet been reported. However, nitric oxide has a critical role in monocyte/macrophage–induced angiogenesis; it acts in concert with cytokines such as TNF-α and IL-8 (237).

Induction of monocyte/macrophage chemotaxis at low concentration, combined with the monocyte/macrophage activating effects at higher concentrations, may account at least in part for the potent angiogenic effect of TGF-β in the corneal bioassay (233,238–240). In this assay, TGF-β induces a potent angiogenic response, accompanied by monocyte/macrophage infiltration into the corneal stroma. The indirect angiogenic activity of TGF-β mediated by monocyte/macrophage recruitment and activation is distinct from the direct effects of TGF-β on endothelial and smooth muscle cells, in which an important role in inducing cessation of endothelial cell proliferation, maturation of the forming vessel, and capillary morphogenesis is likely. TGF-β has also been shown to have effects on angiogenesis in the CAM (241), where it appears to have an effect on several cell types.

PLATELET-DERIVED ENDOTHELIAL CELL GROWTH FACTOR: Platelet-derived endothelial cell growth factor (PD-ECGF) is a homodimeric, non-glycosylated 45-kd protein found in platelets (242). PD-ECGF, like bFGF, aFGF, and IL-1, has no signal peptide sequence, and it does not appear to be a secretory protein (243–245). PD-ECGF does not bind to heparin, and its action is not potentiated by it. PD-ECGF was originally described on the basis of stimulation of the incorporation of ³H-thymidine as a platelet-derived mitogen that stimulated a variety of endothelial cells, but not fibroblasts (242). PD-ECGF was also shown to stimulate endothelial cell, but not smooth muscle cell, chemotaxis in vitro (244). In vivo, PD-ECGF induced angiogenesis on the chick CAM (246). In addition to being found in platelets, PD-ECGF is found in the connective tissue cells of human placenta, and it is also produced by human foreskin fibroblasts, squamous carcinoma cells, and anaplastic thyroid carcinoma cells (244,247). PD-ECGF is not secreted by these cells, but it is retained intracellularly. Recently, it has been shown that human PD-ECGF is homologous to the *Escherichia coli* enzyme thymidine phosphorylase (248,249), and that the thymidine phosphorylase activity of PD-ECGF is responsible for its apparent endothelial cell mitogenicity, via modulation of intracellular thymidine concentrations and homeostasis. The mechanism by which PD-ECGF modulates angiogenesis in the CAM are unclear, but it has been suggested that this effect may be indirect (249). Angiogenic effects of PD-ECGF in the cornea have not been described. Modulation of wound repair responses by administration of PD-ECGF has, however, been reported (250).

HEPATOCYTE GROWTH FACTOR: Hepatocyte growth factor (HGF), a mitogen characterized in normal serum (251,252), is identical to a cytokine termed *scatter factor* (SF) that is secreted by fibroblasts, vascular smooth muscle cells, and leukocytes (253–255). HGF stimulates epithelial cell motility, and it disperses cohesive epithelial cell colonies (256). HGF (SF) is a basic, heparin-binding glycoprotein composed of two polypeptide chains, a heavy 58-kd chain, and a light 31-kd chain. It has significant homology with plasminogen (257).

Recently, HGF has been shown to induce inflammation-free angiogenesis in the in vivo corneal bioassay in rats, as well as in a murine bioassay involving induction of growth of new blood vessels from subcutaneous tissue into an implanted solid gel of basement membrane (Matrigel) (258). In vitro, HGF stimulates endothelial cell proliferation, chemotaxis, and chemokinesis (259). It promotes migration of endothelial cells from carrier beads to flat surfaces, and it induces capillary-like tube formation in vitro (260). It has also been reported that HGF induces endothelial cell expression of plasminogen activators (261). The receptor for HGF, which has been identified as the c-met oncogene product (262), is expressed by endothelial cells, and immunoreactive c-met protein is present in the endothelial cells and the pericytes of blood vessel walls (258). Because HGF is apparently produced by stromal cells located outside the vessel wall, it has been suggested that it may act as paracrine mediator in the angiogenic cascade (258).

COLONY-STIMULATING-FACTORS: The CSFs, M-CSF, GM-CSF, and G-CSF, were discovered as factors that stimulated proliferation and differentiation of hematopoietic progenitor cells in bone marrow cell suspensions to form colonies of mature granulocytes or macrophages in semisolid agar cultures (263,266). M-CSF has been shown to stimulate macrophage colony formation; GM-CSF stimulates formation of both macrophages and granulocytes. Direct angiogenic effects of M-CSF and GM-CSF have not been reported; however, GM-CSF stimulates macrophages to produce a variety of cytokines that might be important in the angiogenic cascade. These cytokines include IL-1, IFN-γ, TNF-α, and IL-6. GM-CSF is also a direct chemoattractant for monocytes (267–270). By virtue of their ability to increase macrophage numbers, induce macrophage recruitment and differentiation, and stimulate macrophage cytokine expression, the CSFs may have a role in the indirect induction of angiogenesis. GM-CSF is produced by fibroblasts, macrophages, activated T cells, and endothelial cells, predominantly following antigenic or endotoxin challenge. TNF-α and IL-1 both up-regulate GM-CSF expression by endothelial cells (268–

270). Endothelial cells also respond to challenge by the CSFs by expressing inducible cytokines, including IL-6 (269). This finding again suggests a potential role for the CSFs in the angiogenic cascade. Both GM-CSF and G-CSF stimulate migration and proliferation of human endothelial cells, although much less potently that bFGF and TNF-α (272). Direct induction of angiogenesis in in vivo models has not been reported.

Angiogenic cytokines

TUMOR NECROSIS FACTOR-α: TNF-α is a single-chain polypeptide synthesized primarily, although not exclusively, by activated monocytes and macrophages. TNF-α is a 17-kd polypeptide that is released from these cells (273); it is also a cell-associated 26-kd polypeptide that retains an N-terminal extension (274). TNF-α was characterized independently in at least two contexts. First, as cachectin, the macrophage-derived factor found in the serum of infected animals that induced the marked cachexia that characterizes severe bacterially infected animals (275); second, as the macrophage-derived factor produced in bacillus Calmette-Guerin–primed animals in response to endotoxin that induced the regression of certain susceptible experimental tumors, such as the meth-A chemically induced sarcoma in rats (276). TNF-α has also been shown to be an endogenous pyrogen involved in the febrile response (277). In contrast to its effects as a cachectic and a cytotoxic factor, TNF-α has been shown to be a potent angiogenic factor; it induces angiogenesis in the corneal bioassay and the chick CAM at nanogram levels (278,279). This angiogenic effect appears to be mediated by direct effects of TNF-α on microvascular endothelial cells, which are activated, induced to migrate, and assume a proteolytic phenotype in response to this cytokine (278). At higher concentrations, TNF-α induces an inflammatory response in the cornea, which may also contribute to the induction of angiogenesis (278,279).

TNF-α is a pleitropic mediator that has multiple roles in inflammation, wound repair, infection, and the host response to cell transformation and tumor development (280). Cellular receptors for TNF-α are broadly distributed on many cell types, and they mediate the responses of these cells to this factor. At least two receptor classes, the p60 (apparent molecular weight, 60 kd) and the p80 (apparent molecular weight, 80 kd), have been demonstrated and cloned (281,282). Shed forms of these receptors have been demonstrated in the circulation, and they may have a role as inhibitors of TNF-α (283). TNF-α, as its name implies, has been implicated as an important factor in the host response to tumors, and it is believed to be involved in macrophage-mediated killing of tumor cells (284). Certain tumor cells in culture are clearly susceptible to killing by TNF- α; however, the majority of tumor cell types are not. In vivo administration of TNF-α causes regression of certain tumor types (276,285). It seems likely, however, even in the case of the meth-A sarcoma, which was used as the target tumor for isolation and purification of TNF-α, that the mechanism of induction of tumor regression is not via a direct cytotoxic effect on the tumor cells, but rather via an effect on the tumor microvasculature (286,287).

TNF-α has been shown to have several effects on vascular endothelial cells in culture (288,289). These effects include induction of migration; induction of expression of activation markers, such as the histocompatability complex type I antigens and the cell surface adhesion molecules ICAM-1 and ELAM-1; induction of gene expression for PDGF isoforms, IL-1 and GM- CSF; induction of expression of procoagulant activity and of matrix metalloproteinases; and suppression of expression of thrombomodulin and TIMP. In the case of certain types of endothelial cells, such as those from human umbilical vein, TNF-α has been shown to inhibit cell proliferation and to antagonize the mitogenic effects of FGF on these cells (279). However, mitogenesis of dermal and other microvascular endothelial cells is not inhibited in the same way (290,291).

Although TNF-α is generally not cytotoxic to endothelial cells directly, cytotoxic effects on endothelium have been observed in the presence of activated neutrophils that produce oxygen radicals (292,293). In vivo, it has been suggested that TNF-α induces tumor regression in susceptible tumors by activating the tumor microvasculature and by inducing the expression of endothelial cell tissue factor and a coagulative phenotype (276,286,287, 294), resulting in intravascular coagulation within the tumor. This coagulation in turn induces the necrosis and the secondary inflammation responsible for inducing tumor regression. In contrast to its effects as an antitumor agent, TNF-α also acts as an angiogenic agent by inducing the growth of new blood vessels.

Because tumor angiogenesis is believed to have a critical role in establishing the growth of solid tumors, this effect of TNF-α seems to be paradoxical, because it might serve to establish the growth of tumors rather than to cause their regression. This paradox was first noted in the effects of macrophages on tumor growth; macrophages have a role both in establishing tumor growth and development and in inducing tumor regression (29). The angiogenic effects of TNF-α are apparently mediated by direct effects on endothelial cells, as are the antitumor effects. We have suggested that these effects may be closely related, hinging on the mode of delivery of TNF-α to the endothelial cells (19). Intravascular delivery, with presentation to the luminal surface of the endothelial cells, might induce a polarized expression of endothelial cell activation markers, resulting in the induction of in-

travascular coagulation. Such a delivery would occur when TNF-α was injected into the circulation, or when monocytes are activated within the vasculature prior to diapedesis. However, when monocytes are recruited to migrate from the circulation to extravascular sites by chemoattractants, produced either as a result of tissue injury or as products of transformed cells, delivery of TNF-α would be from the extravascular locus to the abluminal side of the endothelial cells. This process could then induce polarized expression of endothelial cell activation markers, including metalloproteinases, on the abluminal side of the microvessels, enabling the cells to migrate and to degrade basement membrane and extracellular matrix constituents.

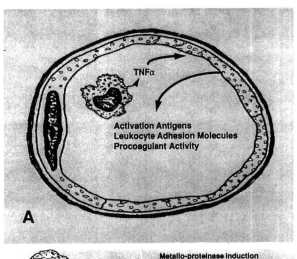

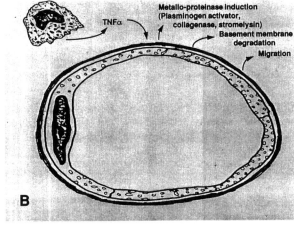

Figure 35–2 (A) Effect of intraluminal delivery of TNF-α (an angiogenic cytokine) by a monocyte in the vessel on microvascular endothelial cells. Polarized activation of the luminal aspect of the cell, with induction of expression of activation antigens, adhesion molecules, and procoagulant activity, may result in leukocyte adhesion and intravascular coagulation. (B) Effect of extravascular delivery of TNF-α produced by an extravasated monocyte/macrophage on microvascular endothelial cells. Polarized activation of the abluminal surface of the cells, with expression of plasminogen activator and matrix metalloproteinases, may initiate angiogenesis by enabling localized degradation of basement membrane constituents and extracellular matrix.

As discussed, these are critical early events in angiogenesis. This scenario is shown diagramatically in Fig. 35–2.

All tissues and organs have intrinsic populations of tissue macrophages that took residence within them during development (295). These macrophages are present prior to chemotactic recruitment of monocytes from the circulation. They are normally quiescent, but they can be activated by local environmental stimuli, including endotoxin, immune complexes, and cytokines, such as the IFNs, IL-2, the CSFs, TGF-β, as well as local oxygen and lactate concentrations. These local macrophages may be extremely important in the induction of angiogenesis in wound repair, as well as in tumor growth. Recently, we demonstrated that the inducible nitric oxide synthase pathway is required for generation of angiogenic activity by human monocytes (131). The nature of the interaction between the nitric oxide–synthase products and the angiogenic cytokines is not yet clear, but it is under active investigation.

INTERLEUKIN-1: At least three closely related forms of IL-1 have been characterized: IL-1α, IL-1β, and the IL-1 receptor antagonist (IL-1Ra) (296). IL-1 is produced primarily by activated monocytes and macrophages, but it is also expressed at much lower levels by keratinocytes, astrocytes, B lymphocytes, kidney mesangial cells, and activated endothelial cells (297). IL-1 is a pleitropic mediator that has several important roles in inflammation and the immune response. IL-1α and IL-1β are single-chain polypeptides of approximately 17.5 kd molecular weight, and they are synthesized as precursor molecules that are cleaved to yield the mature forms. The IL-α precursor has 271 amino acids, and it yields a 153 amino acid mature form. The IL-1β precursor has 269 amino acids, and it also yields a mature form of 153 amino acids. The IL-1β precursor is cleaved by a specific protease that appears to be confined to cells of the myelomonocytic lineage (298). The various forms of IL-1 do not have hydrophobic leader sequences that are generally associated with secretory proteins, although they do have potential membrane anchoring sequences (299,300). The precursor forms are not secreted from cells, but they accumulate in the cytoplasm. As discussed earlier for the FGFs, the mechanism by which these cytokines are released from cells have not yet been clarified. It has been suggested that their release is associated with cellular injury (132). It is interesting in this context that no accumulation of IL-1 is detectable in serum during inflammatory and immune responses, suggesting that IL-1 functions as an autocrine or a paracrine mediator in these processes.

In contrast to TNF-α, with which IL-1 shares many biological effects (288,289), IL-1 does not appear to exhibit marked angiogenic activity in corneal or CAM bioassays. Reports of angiogenic effects of IL-1 in the cornea have been presented (301,302), but relatively high concentrations of IL-1 were implanted, and the presence of edema and an inflammatory infiltrate was reported. Induction of angiogenesis in the rabbit cornea was found to depend on the use of Elvax as the slow delivery system (302), and it was likely associated with induction of inflammation. In our hands, IL-1 induced only a mild angiogenic response in rat corneas at doses greater than 200 ng/implant, and this response was clearly associated with an influx of monocytes/macrophages. It is not clear why TNF-α and IL-1 differ so markedly in their angiogenic potency because both have numerous effects on endothelial cells that would seem to implicate them in the early stages of the angiogenic cascade (288). Both up-regulate expression of endothelial cell activation markers, including human leukocyte antigens and ICAM-1; both alter endothelial cell proteolytic phenotype, inducing expression of procoagulant activity, plasminogen activator, and matrix metalloproteinases; and both induce expression of PDGF. IL-1 also stimulates mitogenesis of smooth muscle cells by inducing expression of PDGF-AA, which then acts as a self-stimulatory growth factor for these cells (303). As discussed earlier, these effects appear to be involved in the early stages of the angiogenic cascade, leaving as a puzzle why IL-1 does not appear to have a prominent role in the induction of the angiogenic cascade in vivo.

INTERLEUKIN-2: Direct induction of angiogenesis by IL-2 has not been observed. However, IL-2 may be involved indirectly in the induction of monocyte/macrophage activation and expression of angiogenic factors, such as TNF-α, IL-8, and others (304,305). Thus, IL-2 may, in certain situations, have an indirect role in the angiogenic response as part of the cytokine network involved in the control of monocyte/macrophage activity.

INTERLEUKIN-3: IL-3 is a 15 to 17 kd, 133 amino acid single-chain polypeptide produced primarily by activated T lymphocytes, but it may also be made by activated natural killer (NK) cells and mast cells (306,307). Normally, IL-3 is produced only following immunological stimulation, and it is involved in stimulating growth and differentiation of hematopoietic stem cells and mast cells. Although IL-3 has not been reported to have any direct angiogenic effects in cornea, CAM, or endothelial cell cultures, it may have indirect effects as part of the hematopoietic network of cytokines and growth factors. For example, IL-3 stimulates production of monocytes/macrophages from bone marrow precursors (307), and the role of these cells in the process of angiogenesis is well established. IL-3 may also stimulate megakaryocytes, resulting in increased levels of circulating platelets. Platelets have also been implicated in certain situations as contributors to the angiogenic process (308). In addition, IL-3 may also have a role by stimulating mast cells, which have been shown in numerous studies to have a facilitating role in angiogenesis (20,30–32,125). In endothelial cells, IL-3 induces expression of IL-6 (264), which has been shown to be expressed transiently in vivo in newly forming blood vessels (310). The significance of this observation in the process of angiogenesis is not yet clear.

INTERLEUKIN-4: IL-4 is a 15 to 19 kd, 129 amino acid polypeptide produced by various T cell, thymocyte populations, and by certain non-T, non-B cells (311). IL-4 induces proliferation of immunoglobulin M (IgM)–activated B cells, activated T cells, and NK cells. Direct effects of IL-4 in in vivo angiogenesis assays have not been described; however, IL-4 has been shown to be a potent mitogen for capillary endothelium (312). IL-4 regulates IL-8 gene expression by blood monocytes and endothelial cells (313). The role of IL-8 in angiogenesis has recently been studied (314–316). IL-4 inhibits endothelial cell expression of ICAM-1 induced by IL-1, TNF-α, and IFN-γ, and it inhibits ELAM-1 expression induced by IL-1 or TNF-α.

INTERLEUKIN-6: IL-6 is a 21 to 26 kd single-chain polypeptide produced by a wide variety of cells (317). It is produced as a precursor of 212 amino acids, and mature IL-6 in humans consists of 184 amino acids. IL-6 is produced by activated T and B lymphocytes and monocytes/macrophages (318), and its expression can be induced in fibroblasts, mesangial cells, keratinocytes, and endothelial cells (319). IL-6 is a pleiotropic mediator with *in vitro* effects ranging from stimulation of proliferation of T cells, mesangial cells, and keratinocytes, through inhibition of proliferation of various transformed cell lines (320). IL-6 also induces maturation of megakaryocytes, macrophage differentiation of myeloid leukemic cell lines, and production of acute-phase proteins by hepatocytes (329). Transient IL-6 expression has been demonstrated in newly forming blood vessels during embryonic development in mice (310), and this expression is downregulated when angiogenesis ceases. Although the function of this expression of IL-6 in newly growing vessels is unclear, it has been suggested that this transient expression indicates a role for IL-6 in angiogenesis, in addition to its role in the development of myeloid and lymphoid hematopoietic cells. The effects of IL-6 in in vivo corneal and CAM bioassays have not been reported. In vitro IL-6 has been reported to inhibit endothelial cell growth (322), although others have reported no effects on endothelial cell growth (323). However, IL-6 is produced by endothelial-like Kaposi's sarcoma cells, and these cells respond proliferatively to addition of exogenous IL-6 (324).

INTERLEUKIN-8: IL-8, previously known as monocyte-derived neutrophil chemotactic factor (MDNCF) (325) or neutrophil-activating factor (NAF) (326), is an 8 kd heparin-binding polypeptide that has been shown recently to induce an angiogenic response in the rat cornea and to induce endothelial cell migration and proliferation in vitro (314–316,327). IL-8 is major product secreted product by activated monocytes and macrophages (329–331). It is also produced by stimulated neutrophils, lymphocytes, fibroblasts, keratinocytes, hepatocytes, and melanocytes, as well as by vascular endothelial cells and several tumor cell lines (329–331). IL-8 has several effects on endothelial cells in culture that suggest that it may be an important angiogenic mediator (133,314,315). It stimulates endothelial cell proliferation, and it induces migration of endothelial cells in the modified Boyden chamber bioassay. The angiogenic activity produced by activated macrophages is contributed in part by macrophage-derived IL-8, which appears to be a much more abundantly expressed protein than, for example, IL-1 and TNF-α (314,315).

IL-8 is a mediator of leukocyte recruitment, accumulation, and activation in inflammatory reactions (328,332), but it also suppresses adhesion of neutrophils to cytokine-activated endothelial cell monolayers (333). This effect may be important in distinguishing between the inflammatory response, during which adhesion of neutrophils to endothelium is required, and the granulation tissue formation stage of the response to injury, during which microvascular budding and angiogenesis take place without adhesion of leukocytes. In wound repair, monocytes/macrophages extravasate and accumulate at a later stage than neutrophils. It may be that as these cells become activated and express IL-8 outside the vasculature, this inhibitory effect of IL-8 on leukocyte adhesion enables the angiogenic process to proceed without the interference of adhering leukocytes. Similar considerations may apply in relation to tumor angiogenesis. Expression of IL-8 is also induced in vascular endothelial cells by agents such as endotoxin, IL-1, and TNF-α (330). IL-8 may therefore act as an autocrine or a paracrine factor in the control of endothelial cell function in angiogenesis. Additional studies of this cytokine are required to clarify its role in the angiogenic cascade.

INTERFERON-γ: IFN-γ is a single-chain polypeptide composed of 127 to 134 amino acids; the variable size is due to cleavage of C-terminal residues from a 143 amino acid chain (334,335). Variable glycosylation gives rise to IFN-γ forms of 25 and 20 kd, with a minor 15.5 kd form (336). IFN-γ is produced primarily by a subset of T lymphocytes (Th1 subtype) and by NK cells (334). Its production by these cells is regulated by antigenic challenge, by certain lectins, and by cytokines such as IL-2. Receptors for IFN-γ are widely and ubiquitously distrubuted on almost all cell types (334,337). IFN-γ has an important role as a primer and an activator of monocytes and macrophages (336). When these cells are treated with IFN-γ, they become greatly sensitized to activation by subsequent challenge (e.g., by endotoxin), and they express the genes for several cytokines, including IL-1, TNF-α, and IL-8. Induction of the nitric oxide–generating enzyme, nitric oxide-synthase, is also primed by IFN-γ, at least in murine macrophages (339). Comparable data in human monocytes has not yet been found. Induction of the L-arginine–dependent nitric oxide-synthase pathway in monocytes has been shown to be critical for generation of monocyte/macrophage–derived angiogenic activity; inhibition of this pathway abrogates the production of angiogenic activity, despite the continued production of angiogenic cytokines, including TNF-α and IL-8 (133). IFN-γ also primes vascular endothelial cells, inducing effects that are similar to those observed in macrophages (340). IFN-γ inhibits proliferation of endothelial cells (341,342), and it blocks the formation of capillary tube-like structures in vitro (341). The effects of IFN-γ as a macrophage and an endothelial cell primer suggest a potentiating secondary role for this cytokine in the process of angiogenesis, in addition to a possible direct role in vessel homeostasis.

CONCLUSIONS

Angiogenesis seems to be critically involved in the rapid expansion and growth of solid tumors. Tumors modulate angiogenesis either directly by producing angiogenic factors that induce the local microvasculature, or indirectly by inducing host cells such as monocytes/macrophages, lymphocytes, and mast cells to infiltrate the tumor and to produce their own direct-acting angiogenic factors. The angiogenic factors produced by tumor cells do not differ from those produced in other situations in which angiogenesis is prominent, such as embryogenesis, wound repair, and chronic fibroproliferative responses. However, the normal controls that limit angiogenesis in these situations are subverted. Several growth factors, cytokines, and their related oncogene products have been shown to participate in the process of angiogenesis. Growth factors involved include the FGFs, PDGF, VEGF, EGF, TGF-α, TGF-β, PD-ECGF, angiogenin, HGF, and the CSFs. Cytokines involved include TNF-α, IL-1, IL-2, IL-3, IL-4, IL-6, IL-8, and IFN-γ.

Some of these factors may act as initiators of the angiogenic cascade, inducing certain critical "early" events in the target microvasculature; these events include disruption of intercellular junctions, induction of expression of endothelial cell activation antigens and a proteolytic phenotype, and initiation of endothelial cell migration in a directional manner. Following these "early" events, the angiogenic cascade proceeds with autocrine and paracrine expression of growth factor and cytokine genes within the cells of the developing capillary bud. Growth factors may also be released from basement membrane depots as a result of controlled endothelial cell–mediated degradation. Endothelial cells than proliferate, generating the new cells required for elongation of the developing capillary bud. Subsequent maturation, with synthesis of basement membrane and extracellular matrix, establishment of a lumen, and formation of capillary loops, completes the process of angiogenesis.

To initiate the angiogenic cascade, angiogenic growth factors and cytokines delivered from an extravascular source are required. Progression of the angiogenic cascade then requires controlled sequential induction and suppression of expression of a series of growth factor and cytokine genes by endothelial cells, pericytes, and smooth muscle cells of the microvasculature. These cells in turn modulate the interactions of these cells, with each other and with the extracellular matrix, leading to the formation of new functional capillary loops. Understanding the mechanism and features of the autocrine and the paracrine events involved in the formation of new blood vessels may lead to rational approaches to therapeutic modulation of this critical process.

REFERENCES

1. Folkman J. What is the evidence that tumors are angiogenesis-dependent? J Natl Cancer Inst 1989;81:570–576.

2. Ide AG, Baker NH, Warren SL. Vascularization of the Brown-Pierce rabbit epithelioma transplant as seen in the transplant ear chambers. Am J Roentgen Radiother 1939; 42:891–899.

3. Folkman J, Long D, Becker F. Growth and metastasis of tumor in organ cultures. N Engl J Med 1963;16:453–463.

4. Folkman J. Tumor angiogenesis. Adv Cancer Res 1985; 43:175–205.

5. Folkman J. What is the evidence that tumors are angiogenesis dependent? J Natl Cancer Inst 1990;82:4–6.

6. Folkman J. Anti-angiogenesis: new concept of therapy of solid tumors. Ann Surg 1972;175:409–416.

7. Klagsbrun M, Folkman J. Angiogenesis. In: Sporn MB, Roberts AB, eds. Peptide growth factors and their receptors, vol 2. Berlin: Springer Verlag, 1990:549–586.

8. Folkman J. Tumor angiogenesis: therapeutic implications. N Engl J Med 1971;285:1182–1186.

9. Gimbrone MA, Leapman SB, Cotran RS, Folkman J. Tumor dormancy in vivo by prevention of neovascularization. J Exp Med 1972;136:261–276.

10. Eisenstein R, Sorgente N, Soble L, Miller A, Keuttner KE. The resistance of certain tissues to invasion: penetrability of explanted tissues by vascularized mesenchyme. Am J Pathol 1973;73:765–774.

11. Folkman J. Angiogenesis and its inhibitors. In: DeVita DJ Jr, Hellman S, Rosenberg SA, eds. Important advances in oncology. Philadelphia: JB Lippincott, 1985:42–62.

12. Kerbel RS. Inhibition of tumor angiogenesis as a strategy to

circumvent acquired resistance to anti-cancer therapeutic agents. BioEssays 1991;13:31–36.

13. Brem S, Folkman J. Inhibition of tumor angiogenesis mediated by cartilage. J Exp Med 1975;141:427–438.

14. Moses MA, Langer R. Inhibitors of angiogenesis. Bio-Technology 1991;9:630–634.

15. Risau W, Breier G, Drexler H, Schnurch H. Vasculogenesis, angiogenesis and endothelial cell differentiation during embryonic development. In: Feinberg RM, Sherer GK, Auerbach R. eds. The development of the vascular system. Basel: Karger, 1991:58–68.

16. Folkman J. Toward an understanding of angiogenesis: search and discovery. Perspect Biol Med 1985;29:10–36.

17. Pardanaud L, Yassine F, Dieterlenlievre F. Relationship between vasculogenesis, angiogenesis and hematopoiesis during avian ontogeny. Development 1989;105:473–485.

18. Benharroch D, Birnbaum D. Biology of the fibroblast growth factor gene family. Isr J Med Sci 1990;26:212–219.

19. Leibovich SJ, Wiseman DM. Macrophages, angiogenesis and wound repair. In: Barbul A, Pines E, Caldwell M, Hunt TK, eds. Growth factors and other aspects of wound healing: biological and clinical implications. New York: Alan R. Liss 1988:131–148.

20. Whalen FW, Zetter BR. Angiogenesis. In: Cohen K, Deigelmann R, Lindblad W, eds. Wound healing: biochemical and clinical aspects. Philadelphia: WB Saunders, 1992: 77–95.

21. Hunt TK, Banda MJ, Silver IA. Cell interactions in post-traumatic fibrosis. In: Evered D, Whelan J, eds. Fibrosis. A CIBA Foundation Symposium, vol 114, London: Pitman, 1985:127–158.

22. Blood CH, Zetter BR. Tumor interactions with the vasculature: angiogenesis and tumor metastasis. Biochim Biophys Acta 1990;1032:89–118.

23. Schor AM, Schor SL. Tumor angiogenesis. J Pathol 1983; 141:385–413.

24. Bouck N. Angiogenesis: a mechanism by which oncogenes and tumor suppressor genes regulate tumorigenesis. In: Benz CC, Liu ET, eds. Oncogenes and tumor suppressor genes in human malignancies. Boston: Kluwer Academic, 1993:359–371.

25. Bouck N. Tumor angiogenesis: the role of oncogenes and tumor suppressor genes. Cancer Cells 1990;2:179–185.

26. Rastinejad F, Polverini PJ, Bouck N. Regulation of the activity of a new inhibitor of angiogenesis by a cancer suppressor gene. Cell 1989;56:345–355.

27. Polverini PJ, Leibovich SJ. Induction of neovascularization in vivo and endothelial cell proliferation in vitro by tumor-associated macrophages. Lab Invest 1984;51:635–642.

28. Polverini PJ, Leibovich SJ. Effect of macrophage depletion on growth and neovascularization of hamster buccal pouch carcinomas. J Oral Pathol 1987;16:436–441.

29. Evans R. Host cells in transplantable murine tumors and their possible revelance to tumor growth. J Reticuloendothel Soc 1979;26:427–437.

30. Kessler DA, Langer RS, Pless NA, et al. Mast cells and tumor angiogenesis. Int J Cancer 1976;18:703–709.

31. Roche WR. The nature and significance of tumor-associated mast cells. J Pathol 1986;148:175–182.

32. Young JD, Liu CC, Butler G, et al. Identification, purification and characterization of a mast cell-associated cytotoxic factor related to tumor necrosis factor. Proc Natl Acad Sci USA 1987;84:9175–9179.

33. Goslen JB, Eisen AZ, Bauer EA. Stimulation of skin fibroblast collagenase production by a cytokine derived from basal cell carcinomas. J Clin Invest 1985;85:161–164.

34. Stopeeli MP, Verde P, Grimaldi G, Locatelli E, Blasi F. Increase in urokinase plasminogen activator mRNA synthesis in human carcinoma cells is a primary effect of the potent tumor promoter, phorbol myristate acetate. J Cell Biol 1986;102:1235–1241.

35. Stetler-Stevenson WG. Type-IV collagenases in tumor invasion and metastasis. Cancer Metastasis Rev 1990;9:289–303.

36. Bonfil RD, Medina PA, Gomez DE, et al. Expression of gelatinase/type IV collagenase in tumor necrosis correlates with cell detachment and tumor invasion. Clin Exp Metastasis 1992;10:211–220.

37. Hobson B, Denekamp J. Endothelial proliferation in tumors and normal tissues: continuous labelling studies. Br J Cancer 1984;49:405–413.

38. Denekamp J. Angiogenesis, neovascular proliferation and vascular pathophysiology as targets for cancer therapy. Br J Radiol 1993;66:181–196.

39. Ausprunk DH, Folkman J. Migration and proliferation of endothelial cells in preformed and newly formed blood vessels during tumor angiogenesis. Microvasc Res 1977;14: 53–65.

40. Phillips GD, Whitehead RA, Knighton DR. Initiation and pattern of angiogenesis in wound healing in the rat. Am J Anat 1991;192:257–262.

41. Sims DE. The pericyte. A review. Tissue Cell 1986;18:153–174.

42. Bar TH, Wolff JR. The formation of capillary basement membranes during internal vascularization of the rat's cerebral cortex. Z Zellforsch 1972;133:231–248.

43. Schwartz SM, Heimark RL. Control of growth of vessel wall cells by inhibition. In: Edgington T, Ross R, Silverstein SS, eds. Perpectives in inflammation, neoplasia and vascular biology. New York: Alan R. Liss 1987:195–205.

44. Ingber DE. Mechanochemical switching between growth and differentiation during fibroblast growth factor-stimulated angiogenesis in vitro: role of extracellular matrix. J Cell Biol 1989;109:317–330.

45. Ingber DE. Fibronectin controls capillary endothelial cell growth by modulating cell shape. Proc Natl Acad Sci USA 1990;87:3579–3583.

46. Madri J, Pratt B, Tucker A. Phenotypic modulation of endothelial cells by transforming growth factor-β depends upon the composition and organization of the extracellular matrix. J Cell Biol 1988;106:1375–1384.

47. Gamble JR, Matthias LJ, Meyer G, et al. Regulation of in vitro capillary tube formation by anti-integrin antibodies. J Cell Biol 1993;121:921–943.

48. Rifkin DB, Gross JL, Moscatelli D, Jaffe E. Proteases and angiogenesis: production of plasminogen activator and collagenase by endothelial cells. In: Nossel H, Vogel HJ, eds. Pathobiology of the endothelial cell. New York: Academic Press, 1982:191–197.

49. Pepper MS, Vassalli JD, Orci L, Montesano R. Proteolytic

balance and capillary morphogenesis in vitro. In: Steiner R, Weisz PB, Langer R, eds. Angiogenesis: key principles. Basel: Birkhauser Verlag, 1992:137–145.

50. Sarma V, Wolf FW, Marks RM, Shows TB, Dixit VM. Cloning of a novel tumor necrosis factor-alpha-inducible primary response gene that is differentially expressed in development and capillary-tube-like formation in vitro. J Immunol 1992;148:3302–3312.

51. Gerritsen ME, Bloor CM. Endothelial cell gene expression in response to injury. FASEB J 1993;7:523–532.

52. Bauer J, Margolis M, Schreiner C, et al. In vitro model of angiogenesis using a human endothelium-derived permanent cell line—contributions of induced gene expression, G-proteins and integrins. J Cell Physiol 1992;153:437–449.

53. Liaw L, Schwartz SM. Comparison of gene expression in bovine aortic endothelium in vivo versus in vitro. Arteriosclerosis Thrombosis 1993;13:985–993.

54. Sholley MM, Fergusen GP, Seibel HR, Montour JL, Wilson JD. Mechanisms of neovascularization. Vascular sprouting can occur without proliferation of endothelial cells. Lab Invest 1984;51:624–634.

55. Libby P, Ordovas JM, Auger KR, Robbins AH, Birinyi LK, Dinarello CA. Endotoxin and tumor necrosis factor induce interleukin-1 gene expression in adult human vascular endothelial cells. Am J Pathol 1986;124:179–185.

56. Okanura K, Sato Y, Matsuda T, et al. Endogenous basic fibroblast growth factor-dependent induction of collagenase and interleukin-6 in tumor necrosis factor-treated human microvascular endothelial cells. J Biol Chem 1991;266:19162–19165.

57. Vlodavski I, Folkman J, Sullivan R, et al. Endothelial cell-derived basic fibroblast growth factor; synthesis and deposition into subendothelial extracellular matrix. Proc Natl Acad Sci USA 1987;84:2292–2296.

58. Baird A, Ling N. Fibroblast growth factors are present in the extracellular matrix produced by endothelial cells in vitro: implications for a role of heparinase-like enzymes in the neovascular response. Biochem Biophys Res Commun 1985;126:358–364.

59. Bashkin P, Doctrow S, Klagsbrun M, Suahn CM, Folkman J, Vlodavski I. Basic fibroblast growth factor binds to subendothelial extracellular matrix and is released by heparanase and heparin-like molecules. Biochemistry 1989;28:1737–1743.

60. Ausprunk DH, Folkman J. Migration and proliferation of endothelial cells in preformed and newly formed blood vessels during tumor angiogenesis. Microvasc Res 1977;14:53–65.

61. Folkman J, Haudenschild CH. Angiogenesis in vitro. Nature (London) 1980;288:551–556.

62. Konerding MA, VanAckern C, Steinberg F, Streffer C. Combined morphological approaches in the study of network formation in tumor angiogenesis. In: Steiner R, Weisz PB, Langer R, eds. Angiogenesis: key principles. Basel: Birkhauser Verlag, 1992:40–58.

63. Paweletz N, Knierim M. Tumor-related angiogenesis. Crit Rev Oncol Hematol 1989;9:197–242.

64. Greenblatt M, Shubik P. Tumor angiogenesis: transfilter diffusion studies in the hamster by the transparent chamber technique. J Natl Cancer Inst 1968;41:111–124.

65. D'Amore PA, Klagsbrun M. Angiogenesis: factors and mechanisms. In: Sirica AE, ed. The pathobiology of neoplasia. New York: Plenum Press, 1989:513–531.

66. Klagbrun M, D'Amore PA. Regulators of angiogenesis. Ann Rev Physiol 1991;53:217–239.

67. Gullino PM. Angiogenesis factor(s). In: Baserga R. ed. Handbook of experimental pharmacology, vol 57. New York: Springer-Verlag, 1981:427–449.

68. Folkman J, Merler E, Abermathy C, Williams G. Isolation of a tumor factor responsible for angiogenesis. J Exp Med 1971;133:275–288.

69. Shing Y, Folkman J, Sullivan R, Butterfield C, Murray J, Klagsbrun M. Heparin affinity: purification of a tumor-derived capillary endothelial cell growth factor. Science 1984;223:1296–1299.

70. Gimbrone MA Jr, Cotran RS, Folkman J. Tumor growth neovascularization: an experimental model using rabbit cornea. J Natl Cancer Inst 1974;52:413–427.

71. Polverini PJ, Cotran RS, Gimbrone MA Jr, Unanue E. Activated macrophages induce neovascular proliferation. Nature (London) 1977;269:804–806.

72. Polverini PJ. Macrophage-induced angiogenesis: a review. In: Sorg C, ed. Macrophage-derived cell regulatory factors. Basel: Karger, 1989:54–73.

73. Koch AE, Polverini PJ, Leibovich SJ. Induction of neovascularization by activated human monocytes. J Leukocyte Biol 1986;39:233–238.

74. Polverini PJ. Macrophage-induced angiogenesis: a review. In: Sorg C, ed. Macrophage-derived cell regulatory factors: cytokines, vol 1. Basel: karger, 1989:54–73.

75. Sunderkotter C, Goebeler M, Schulze-Osthoff K, Bhardwaj R, Sorg C. Macrophage-derived angiogenesis factors. Pharmacol Therapeut 1991;51:195–216.

76. Wilting J, Christ B. A morphological study of the rabbit corneal assay. Ann Anat 1992;174:549–556.

77. Sunderkotter C, Roth J, Sorg C. Immunohistochemical detection of bFGF and TNF-alpha in the course of inflammatory angiogenesis in the mouse cornea. Am J Pathol 1990;137:511–515.

78. Langer R. Delivery systems for angiogeneis stimulators and inhibitors. In: Steiner R, Weisz PB, Langer R, eds. Angiogenesis: key principles. Basel: Birkhauser Verlag, 1992:327–330.

79. Langer R, Moses S. Biocompatible controlled release polymers for delivery of polypeptides and growth factors. J Cell Biochem 1991;45:340–345.

80. Hamilton HL. In: Lilly's development of the chick, ed 3. New York: Rinehart and Winston, 1965.

81. Ausprunck DH, Knighton DR, Folkman J. Differentiation of vascular endothelium in the chick chorioallantois. Dev Biol 1974;38:237–248.

82. Auerbach R, Kubai L, Knighton D, Folkman J. A simple procedure for the long term cultivation of chicken enbryos. Dev Biol 1974;41:391–394.

83. Vu MT, Smith CF, Burger PC, Klintworth GK. Methods in laboratory investigation: an evaluation of methods to quantitate the chick chorioallantoic membrane assay in angiogenesis. Lab Invest 1985;53:499–508.

84. Taylor EM, Weiss JB. The chick vitelline membrane as a new test system for angiogenesis and antiangiogenesis. Int J Microcirc 1984;3:337–342.

85. Wilting J, Christ B, Bokeloh M. A modified chorioallantoic membrane (CAM) assay for qualitative and quantitative study of growth factors—studies on the effects of carriers, PBS, angiogenin, and bFGF. Anat Embryol 1991;183:259–271.

86. Takahashi K, Maksto N. Development, differentiation and proliferation of macrophages in the yolk sac. Tissue Cell 1993;25:351–362.

87. Screiber AB, Winkler ME, Derynck R. Transforming growth factor-alpha: a more potent angiogenic mediator than epidermal growth factor. Science 1986;232:1250–1253.

88. Thomson JA, Andersen JD, DiPietro JM, et al. Site-directed neovessel formation in vivo. Science 1988;241:1349–1352.

89. Fajardo LF, Kowalski J, Kwan HH, Prionas SD, Allison AC. Methods in laboratory investigation: the disc angiogenesis sytem. Lab Invest 1988;58:718–724.

90. Zetter BR. Migration of capillary endothelial cells is stimulated by tumor-derived factors. Nature (London) 1980;285:41–43.

91. Albrecht-Buehler G. Autonomous movement of cytoplasmic fragments. Proc Natl Acad Sci USA 1980;77:6639–6643.

92. Jozaki K, Marucha PT, Despens AW, Kreutzer DL. An in vitro model of cell migration—evaluation of vascular endothelial cell migration. Anal Biochem 1990;190:39–47.

93. Mignatti P, Morimoto T, Rifkin DB. Basic fibroblast growth factor released by single, isolated cells stimulates their migration in an autocrine manner. Proc Natl Acad Sci USA 1991;88:11007–11011.

94. Kleinsoyer C, Beretz A, Cazanave JP, Driot F, Maffrand JP. Behavior of confluent endothelial cells after irradiation—modulation of wound repair by heparin and acidic fibroblast growth factor. Biol Cell 1990;68:231–238.

95. Lobb RR, Fett JW. Purification of two distinct growth factors from bovine neural tissue by heparin affinity chromatography. Biochemistry 1984;23:6295–6299.

96. Thomas KA, Rios-Candelore M, Gimenez-Gallego G, et al. Pure brain-derived acidic fibroblast growth factor is a potent angiogenic vascular endothelial cell mitogen with sequence homology to interleukin-1. Proc Natl Acad Sci USA 1985;82:6409–6413.

97. Mullins DE, Rifkin DB. Induction of proteases and protease inhibitors by growth factors. In: Sporn MB, Roberts AB, eds. Peptide growth factors and their receptors, vol 2. Berlin: Springer-Verlag, 1990:481–507.

98. Okada Y, Morodomi T, Enghild JJ, et al. Matrix metalloproteinase-2 from human rheumatoid synovial fibroblasts—purification and activation of the precursor and enzymic properties. Eur J Biochem 1990;194:721–730.

99. Taylor CM, Weiss JB, Lye RH. Raised levels of latent collagenase activating angiogenesis factor (ESAF) are present in actively growing human intracranial tumors. Br J Cancer 1991;64:164–168.

100. Saksela O, Moscatelli D, Rifkin DB. The opposing effects of basic fibroblast growth factor and transforming growth factor-beta on the regulation of plasminogen activator activity in capillary endothelial cells. J Cell Biol 1987;105:957–963.

101. Loskutoff DJ. Regulation of PAI-1 gene expression. Fibrinolysis 1991;5:197–206.

102. Herron GS, Werb Z, Dwyer K, Banda MJ. Secretion of metalloproteinases by stimulated capillary endothelial cells. I. Production of procollagenase and prostromelysin exceeds expression of proteolytic activity. J Biol Chem 1986;261:2810–2813.

103. Herron GS, Banda MJ, Clark EJ, Gavrilovic J, Werb Z. Secretion of metalloproteinases by stimulated capillary endothelial cells. II. Expression of collagenase and stromelysin activities is regulated by endogenous inhibitors. J Biol Chem 1986;261:2814–2818.

104. Pepper MS, Vassalli JD, Orci L, Montesano R. Biphasic effect of transforming growth factor-β1 on in vitro angiogenesis. Exp Cell Res 1993;204:356–363.

105. Gross JL, Moscatelli D, Rifkin DB. Increased capillary endothelial cell protease activity in response to angiogenic stimuli in vitro. Proc Natl Acad Sci USA 1983;80:2623–2627.

106. Cotta-Pereira G, Sage H, Bornstein P, Ross R, Schwartz SM. Studies of morphological atypical (sprouting) cultures of bovine aortic endothelial cells. Growth characteristics and connective tissue protein synthesis. J Cell Physiol 1980;102:183–191.

107. Smith P. The effect of passage number on the stimulation by hypoxia of growth and sprouting activity in cultured aortic endothelium from the rat. Int J Exp Pathol 1990;71:479–484.

108. Madri JA, Pratt BM. Angiogenesis. In: Clark RAF, Henson PM, eds. The molecular and cellular biology of wound repair. Boston: Plenum Press, 1988:337–358.

109. Kubota Y, Kleinman HK, Martin GR, Lawley TJ. Role of laminin and basement membrane in the morphological differentiation of human endothelial cells into capillary-like structures. J Cell Biol 1988;107:1589–1598.

110. Montesano R, Mouron R, Orci L. Vascular outgrowth from tissue explants embedded in fibrin or collagen gels: a simple in vitro model of angiogenesis. Cell Biol Int Rep 1985;9:869–875.

111. Montesano R, Vassali JD, Baird A, Guilleman R, Orci L. Basic fibroblast growth factor induces angiogenesis in vitro. Proc Natl Acad Sci USA 1986;83:7297–7301.

112. Mazanet R, Franzini-Armstrong C. Scanning electron microscopy of pericytes in rat red muscle. Microvasc Res 1982;23:361–369.

113. Schor AM, Canfield AE, Sutton AB, Allen TD, Sloan P, Schor SL. The behavior of pericytes in vitro: relevance to angiogenesis and differentiation. In: Steiner R, Weisz PB, Langer R, eds. Angiogenesis: key principles. Basel: Birkhauser Verlag, 1992:167–178.

114. Antonelli-Orlidge A, Saunders KB, Smith ER, D'Amore PA. An activated form of transforming growth factor-beta is produced by co-cultures of endothelial cells and pericytes. Proc Natl Acad Sci USA 1989;86:4544–4548.

115. Sato Y, Rifkin DB. Inhibition of endothelial cell movement by pericytes and smooth muscle cells: activation of a latent transforming growth factor-β1-like molecule by plasmin during coculture. J Cell Biol 1989;109:309–315.

116. Miyamoto M, Naruo K, Seko C, Matsumoto S, Kondo T, Kurokawa T. Molecular cloning of a novel cytokine cDNA encoding the ninth member of the fibroblast growth factor family, which has a unique secretory property. Mol Cell Biol 1993;13:4251–4259.

117. Gospodarowicz D. Fibroblast growth factors. In: Aggarwal BB, Gutterman JU, eds. Human cytokines: handbook for basic and clinical research. Boston: Blackwell Scientific Publications, 1992:329–352.

118. Thomas KA. Fibroblast growth factors. FASEB J 1987;1: 434–440.

119. Hebert JM, Basilico C, Goldfarb M, Haub O, Martin GR. Isolation of cDNAs encoding four mouse FGF family members and characterization of their expression patterns during embryogenesis. Dev Biol 1990;138:454–463.

120. Haub O, Goldfarb M. Expression of fibroblast growth factor-5 gene in the mouse embryo. Development 1991; 112:397–406.

121. Aaronson SA. Growing families of fibroblast growth factors and receptors. Jpn J Cancer Res 1993;84:1326–1327.

122. Brem H, Klagsbrun M. The role of fibroblast growth factors and related oncogenes in tumor growth. Cancer Treat Res 1992;63:211–231.

123. Florkiewicz RZ, Sommer A. Human basic fibroblast growth factor gene encodes four polypeptides: three initiate translation from non-AUG codons. Proc Natl Acad Sci USA 86:3978–3981.

124. Imamura T, Engleka K, Zhan X, et al. Recovery of mitogenic activity of a growth factor mutant with a nuclear translocation sequence. Science 1990;249:1567–1570.

125. Azizkhan R, Azizkhan J, Zetter B, Folkman J. Mast cell heparin stimulates migration of capillary endothelial cells in vitro. J Exp Med 152:931–944.

126. Thornton S, Mueller S, Levine E. Human endothelial cells: use of heparin in cloning and long term serial cultivation. Science 1983;222:623–625.

127. Sano H, Engleka K, Mathern P, et al. Co-expression of phosphotyrosine-containing proteins, platelet-derived growth factor B and fibroblast growth factor-1 in situ in synovial tissues of patients with rheumatoid arthritis and adjuvant or streptococcal cell wall arthritis. J Clin Invest 1993;91:553–565.

128. Bouche G, Gas N, Prats H. Basic fibroblast growth factor enters the nucleolus and stimulates the transcription of ribosomal genes in ABAE cells undergoing G0-G1 transition. Proc Natl Acad Sci USA 1987;84:6770–6775.

129. Funakoshi Y, Matsudo S, Uryu K, Fujita H, Okumura N, Sakamoto M. An immunohistochemical study of basic fibroblast growth factor in the developing chick. Anat Embryol 1993;139:570–579.

130. D'Amore P. Modes of FGF release in vivo and in vitro. Cancer Metastasis Revs 1990;9:227–238.

131. Gajdusek CM, Carbon S. Injury-induced release of basic fibroblast growth factor from bovine aortic endothelium. J Cell Physiol 1989;139:570–579.

132. Hogquist KA, Unanue ER, Chaplin DD. Release of IL-1 from mononuclear phagocytes. J Immunol 1991;147: 2181–2186.

133. Leibovic SJ, Polverini PJ, Fong TW, Harlow LA, Koch AE. Production of angiogenic activity by human monocytes requires an L-arginine/nitric oxide-synthase-dependent effector mechanism. Proc Natl Acad Sci USA 1994 (in press).

134. Korhonen J, Partanen J, Eerola E, et al. Five FGF receptors with distinct expression patterns. In: Steiner R, Weisz PB,

135. Weich HA, Iberg N, Klagsbrun M, Folkman J. Transcriptional regulation of basic fibroblast growth factor expression in capillary endothelial cells. J Cell Biochem 1991;47: 158–164.

136. Takahashi JA, Mori H, Fukumoto M, et al. Gene expression of fibroblast growth factors in human gliomas and meningiomas: demonstration of cellular source of basic fibroblast growth factor mRNA and peptide in tumor tissues. Proc Natl Acad Sci USA 1990;87:5710–5714.

137. Moscatelli D, Presta M, Joseph-Silverstein J, Rifkin DB. Both normal and tumor cells produce basic fibroblast growth factor. J Cell Physiol 1986;129:273–276.

138. Yoshitake Y, Nishikawa K. Distribution of fibroblast growth factors in cultured tumor cells and their transplants. In Vitro Cell Dev Biol Animal 1992;28A:419–428.

139. Herblin WF, Gross JL. Binding sites for basic fibroblast growth factor on solid tumors are associated with the vasculature. In: Steiner R, Weisz PB, Langer R, eds. Angiogenesis: key principles. Basel: Bookhauser Verlag, 1992: 214–218.

140. Shing Y, Folkman J, Haudenschild C, Lund D, Grum R, Klagsbrun M. Angiogenesis is stimulated by a tumor-derived endothelial cell growth factor. J Cell Biochem 1985; 29:275–287.

141. Knighton DR, Phillips GD, Fiegel VD. Wound healing angiogenesis: indirect stimulation by basic fibroblast growth factor. J Trauma 1990;30:5134–5144.

142. Kandel J, Bossey-Wetzel E, Radvanyi F, Klagsbrun M, Folkman J, Hanahan D. Neovascularization is associated with a switch to the export of bFGF in the multistep development of fibrosarcoma. Cell 1991;66:1095–1104.

143. Raines EW, Bowen-Pope DF, Ross R. Platelet-derived growth factor. In: Sporn MB, Roberts AB, eds. Peptide growth factors and their receptors, vol 1. Berlin: Springer-Verlag, 1990:173–262.

144. Antoniades HN, Hunkapiller MW. Human platelet-derived growth factor (PDGF): amino terminal amino acid sequence. Science 1983;220:963–965.

145. Hart CE, Bailey M, Curtis DA, et al. Purification of PDGF AB and PDGF BB from human platelet extracts and the identification of all three PDGF dimers in human platelets. Biochemistry 1990;29:166–172.

146. Ross R, Glomset JA, Kariya B, Harker L. A platelet-dependent serum factor that stimulates the proliferation of arterial smooth muscle cells in vitro. Proc Natl Acad Sci USA 1974;71:1207–1210.

147. Deuel T, Kawaha RS. Platelet-derived growth factor. In: Aggarwal BB, Gutterman JU, eds. Human cytokines. Cambridge: Blackwell Scientific Publications, 1992:300–328.

148. Yarden Y, Escobedo JA, Kuang WJ, et al. Structure of the receptor for platelet-derived growth factor helps define a family of closely related growth factor receptors. Nature (London) 1986;323:226–232.

149. Claesson-Welsh L, Eriksson A, Westermark B, Heldin CH. Cloning and expression of human platelet-derived growth factor alpha and beta receptors. Peptide Growth Factors [C] 1991;198:72–77.

150. Gronwald RGK, Grant EJ, Haldeman BA, et al. Cloning and expression of a cDNA coding for the human platelet-de-

rived growth factor receptor: evidence for more than one receptor class. Proc Natl Acad Sci USA 1988;85:3435–3439.

151. Herren B, Rooney B, Weyer KA, Iberg N, Schmid G, Pech M. Dimerization of extracellular domains of platelet-derived growth factor receptors—a revised model of receptor-ligand interactions. J Biol Chem 1993;268:15088–15095.

152. Coats, SR, Olson JE, Pledger WJ. Rapid induction of competence formation is PDGF-isoform specific. J Cell Biochem 1992;48:242–247.

153. Mauro A, Bulfone A, Turco E, Schiffer D. Co-expression of platelet-derived growth factor-B (PDGF) chain and PDGF-B type receptor in human gliomas. Child Nerv Syst 1991; 7:432–436.

154. Haudenschild CC, Zahniser D, Folkman J, Klagsbrun M. Human vascular endothelial cells in culture: lack of response to serum growth factors. Exp Cell Res 1976;98:175–181.

155. Bowen-Pope DF, Ross R. Platelet-derived growth factor. II. Specific binding to cultured cells. J Biol Chem 1982;1257:5161–5171.

156. Kazlauskas A, DiCorleto PE. Cultured endothelial cells do not respond to a platelet-derived growth factor-like protein in an autocrine manner. Biochim Biophys Acta 1985;846:405–412.

157. Beitz JG, Kim I, Calabresi P, Frackelton AR Jr. Human microvascular endothelial cells express receptors for platelet-derived growth factor. Proc Natl Acad Sci USA 1991;88:2021–2025.

158. Smits A, Hermansson M, Nister M, et al. Rat brain capillary endothelial cells express functional PDGF B-type receptors. Growth Factors 1989;2:1–8.

159. Heldin P, Pertoft H, Nordlinder H, Heldin CH, Laurent TC. Differential expression of platelet-derived growth factor alpha and alpha receptors on fat storing cells and endothelial cells of rat liver. Exp Cell Res 1991;193:364–369.

160. Hermansson M, Nister M, Betsholtz C, Heldin CH, Westermark B, Funa K. Endothelial cell hyperplasia in human glioblastoma: co-expression of mRNA for platelet-derived growth factor (PDGF) B chain and PDGF receptor suggests autocrine growth stimulation. Proc Natl Acad Sci USA 1988;85:7748–7752.

161. Risau W, Drexler H, Mironov V, et al. Platelet-derived growth factor is angiogenic in vivo. Growth Factors 1992; 7:261–266.

162. Deuel TF, Senior RM, Huang JS, Griffin GL. Chemotaxis of monocytes and neutrophils to platelet-derived growth factor. J Clin Invest 1982;69:1046–1049.

163. Graves DT, Grotendorst GR, Antoniades HN, Schwartz CJ, Valente AJ. Platelet-derived growth factor is not chemotactic for human peripheral blood monocytes. Exp Cell Res 1989;180:497–503.

164. Grotendorst GR, Chang T, Seppa HEJ, Kleinman HK, Martin GR. Platelet-derived growth factor is a chemoattractant for vascular smooth muscle cells. J Cell Physiol 1982;113:261–266.

165. Hwang DL, Latus LJ, Levran A. Effects of platelet-contained growth factors (PDGF, EGF, IGF-1, and TGF-beta) on DNA synthesis in porcine aortic smooth muscle cells in culture. Exp Cell Res 1992;200:358–360.

166. Kondo T, Konighi F, Inui H, Inagami T. Differing signal transductions elicited by 3 isoforms of platelet-derived growth factor in vascular smooth muscle cells. J Biol Chem 1993;268:4458–4464.

167. Sato Y, Hamanaka R, Ono J, Kawana M, Rifkin DB, Takaki R. The stimulatory effect of PDGF on vascular smooth muscle cell migration is mediated by the induction of endogenous basic FGF. Biochim Biophys Acta 1991;174:1260–1266.

168. Sperti G, Vanleewven R, Maseri A, Kluft C. Platelet-derived growth factor increases plasminogen activator inhibitor-1 activity and messenger RNA in rat cultured vascular smooth muscle. In: Fibrinolysis, in tissue remodelling, and in development. Ann NY Acad Sci 1992;677:178–180.

169. Yanagi H, Sasaguri Y, Sugama K, Morimatsu M, Nagase H. Production of tissue collagenase (matrix metalloproteinase-1) by human aortic smooth muscle cells in response to platelet-derived growth factor. Atherosclerosis 1991;91:201–216.

170. Sato N, Beitz JG, Kato J, et al. Platelet-derived growth factor indirectly stimulates angiogenesis in vitro. Am J Pathol 1993;142:1119–1129.

171. Robbins KC, Antoniades HN, Devare SC, Hunkapiller MW, Aaronson SA. Structural and immunological similarities between simian sarcoma virus gene product(s) and human platelet-derived growth factor. Nature (London) 1983;305:605–608.

172. Chung CK, Antoniades HN. Expression of c-sis/platelet-derived growth factor-b, insulin-like growth factor 1 and transforming growth factor β messenger RNAs in primary human gastric carcinomas. In vivo studies with in situ hybridization and immunocytochemistry. Cancer Res 1992; 52:3453–3459.

173. Nister H, Heldin CH, Wasteson A, Westermark B. A platelet-derived growth factor analog produced by a human clonal glioma cell line. Proc Natl Acad Sci USA 1984;81:926–930.

174. Sariban E, Sitaras NM, Antoniades HN, Kufe DW, Pantazis P. Expression of platelet-derived growth factor (PDGF)-related transcripts and synthesis of biologically active PDGF-like proteins by human malignant epithelial cells. J Clin Invest 1988;82:1157–1164.

175. Fleming TP, Matsui T, Heidaran MA, Molloy CJ, Antri PJ, Aaronson SA. Demonstration of an activated platelet-derived growth factor autocrine pathway and its role in human tumor cell proliferation in vitro. Oncogene 1992;7:1355–1359.

176. Ferrara N, Houck K, Jakeman L, Leung DW. Molecular and biological properties of the vascular endothelial growth factor family of proteins. Endocr Rev 1992;13:18–32.

177. Houck KA, Ferrara N, Winer J, Cachianes G, Li B, Leung DW. The vascular endothelial growth factor family: identification of a fourth molecular species and characterization of alternative splicing of RNA. Mol Endocrinol 1991;5:1806–1814.

178. Keck PJ, Hauser SD, Krivi G, et al. Vascular permeability factor, an endothelial cell mitogen related to PDGF. Science 1989;246:1309–1312.

179. Plouet J, Schilling J, Gospodarowicz D. Isolation and characterization of a newly identified endothelial mitogen produced by AtT-20 cells. EMBO J 1989;8:3801–3806.

180. Leung DW, Cachianes G, Kuang WJ, Goeddel DV, Ferrara N. Vascular endothelial growth factor is a secreted endothelial mitogen. Science 1989;246:1306–1308.

181. Houck KA, Leung DW, Rowland AM, Winer J, Ferrara N. Dual regulation of vascular endothelial growth factor bioavailability by gentic and proteolytic mechanisms. J Biol Chem 1992;267:26031–26037.

182. Senger D, Galli JS, Dvorak AM, Perruzzi AC, Harvey VS, Dvorak HF. Tumor cells secrete a vascular permeability factor which promotes ascites fluid accumulation. Science 1983;219:983–985.

183. Jakeman LB, Winer J, Bennett BL, Altar CA, Ferrara N. Binding sites for vascular endothelial growth factor are localized on endothelial cells in adult rat tissues. J Clin Invest 1992;89:244–253.

184. Unemori EN, Ferrara N, Bauer EA, Amento, EP. Vascular endothelial growth factor induces interstitial collagenase expression in human endothelial cells. J Cell Physiol 1992;153:557–562.

185. Pepper MS, Ferrara N, Orci L, Montesano R. Vascular endothelial growth factor (VEGF) induces plasminogen activators and plasminogen activator inhibitor 1 in microvascular endothelial cells. Biochem Biophys Res Commun 1991;181:902–906.

186. Phillips HS, Hains J, Leung DW, Ferrara N. Vascular endothelial growth factor is expressed in rat corpus luteum. Endocrinology 1990;127:965–967.

187. Senger DR, Perruzzi CA, Feder J, Dvorak HF. A highly conserved vascular permeability factor secreted by a variety of human and rodent cell lines. Cancer Res 1986;46:5629–5632.

188. Rosenthal R, Megyesi JF, Henzel WJ, Ferrara N, Folkman J. Conditioned medium from mouse sarcoma 180 cells contains vascular endothelial growth factor. Growth Factors 1990;4:53–59.

189. Berse B, Brown LF, Van De Water L, Dvorak HF, Senger DR. Vascular permeability factor (vascular endothelial growth factor) gene is expressed differentially in normal tissues, macrophages and tumors. Mol Biol Cell 1992;3:211–220.

190. Yeo KT, Wang HH, Nagy JA, et al. Vascular permeability factor (vascular endothelial growth factor) in guinea pig and human tumor and inflammatory effusions. Cancer Res 1993;53:2912–2918.

191. Plate KH, Breier G, Weich HA, Risau W. Vascular endothelial growth factor is a potential tumor angiogenesis factor in human gliomas in vivo. Nature (London) 1992;359:845–848.

192. Berkman RA, Merrill MJ, Reinhold WC, et al. Expression of the vascular permeability factor/vascular endothelial growth factor gene in central nervous system neoplasms. J Clin Invest 1993;91:153–159.

193. Ferrara N, Winer J, Burton T, et al. Expression of vascular endothelial growth factor does not promote transformation but confers a growth advantage in vivo to Chinese hamster ovary cells. J Clin Invest 1993;91:163–170.

194. Jin Kim K, Li B, Winer J, et al. Inhibition of vascular endothelial growth factor induced angiogenesis suppresses tumor growth in vivo. Nature (London) 1993;362:841–844.

195. Phillips HS, Armani MP, Stavrou D, Ferrari N, Westphal

M. Intense focal expression of vascular endothelial growth factor mRNA in human intracranial neoplasms: associations with regions of necrosis. Int J Oncol 1993;2:913–919.

196. Fett JW, Strydom DJ, Lobb RF, et al. Isolation and characterization of angiogenin, an angiogenic protein from human carcinoma cells. Biochemistry 1985;24:5480–5486.

197. Fox EA, Riordan JF. The molecular biology of angiogenin. In: Chein S, ed. Molecular biology of the cardiovascular system. Philadelphia: Lea and Fabiger, 1990:139–154.

198. Shapiro R, Vallee BL. Human placental ribonuclease inhibitor abolishes both angiogenic and ribonucleolytic activities of angiogenin. Proc Natl Acad Sci USA 1987;84:8783–8787.

199. Badet J, Soncin F, Guitton JD, Lamare O, Cartwright T, Barritault D. Specific binding of angiogenin to pulmonary artery endothelial cells. Proc Natl Acad Sci USA 1989;86:8427–8431.

200. Chamoux M, Dehouck MP, Fruchart JC, Spik G, Montreuil J, Ceachelli R. Characterization of angiogenin receptors on bovine brain capillary endothelial cells. Biochem Biophys Res Commun 1991;176:833–839.

201. Bicknell R, Vallee BL. Angiogenin activates endothelial cell phospholipase C. Proc Natl Acad Sci USA 1988;85:5961–5965.

202. Somin F. Angiogenin supports endothelial and fibroblast cell adhesion. Proc Natl Acad Sci USA 1992;89:2232–2236.

203. Hu GF, Strydom DJ, Fett JW, Riordan JF, Vallee BL. Actin is binding protein for angiogenin. Proc Natl Acad Sci USA 1993;90:1217–1221.

204. Weiner HL, Weiner LH, Swain J. The tissue distribution and developmental expression of the messenger RNA encoding angiogenin. J Cell Physiol 1987;102:267–277.

205. Bresaker RS, Toribara NW, Weiner HL, Raper SE, Swain JL, Kim YS. Angiogenin messenger RNA levels are related to degree of cell replication and differentiation in the regenerating rat liver and in human colon cancer cells. Clin Res 1988;36:129A.

206. Cohen S. Isolation of a mouse submaxillary gland protein accelerating incisor eruption and eyelid opening in the newborn animal. J Biol Chem 1962;237:1555–1562.

207. Carpenter G, Cohen S. Epidermal growth factor. Ann Rev Biochem 1979;48:193–216.

208. Kasselberg AG, Orth DN, Gray ME, Stahlman MT. Immunocytochemical localization of human epidermal growth factor/urogastrone in several human tissues. J Histochem Cytochem 1985;33:315–322.

209. Das M, Pengaraju M, Samanta A. Epidermal growth factor. In: Aggarwal BB, Gutterman JU, eds. Human cytokines: handbook for basic and clinical research. Cambridge: Blackwell Scientific Publications, 1992:365–382.

210. Lee DC, Han KM. Expression of growth factors and their receptors in development. In: Sporn MB, Roberts AB, eds. Peptide growth factors and their receptors, vol 1. Berlin: Springer-Verlag, 1990:611–654.

211. Mills A. Modelling the carbohydrate recognition domain of human E-selectin. FEBS Lett 1993;319:5–11.

212. Todaro GJ, Fryling C, DeLarco JE. Transforming growth factors produced by certain human tumor cells: polypeptides that interact with epidermal growth factor receptors. Proc Natl Acad Sci USA 1980;77:5258–5262.

213. Madtes DK, Raines EW, Sakariassen KS, et al. Induction of transforming growth factor-α in activated alveolar macrophages. Cell 1988;53:285–293.

214. Rappolee DA, Mark D, Banda MG, Werb Z. Wound macrophages express TGFβ and other growth factors in vivo: analysis by mRNA phenotyping. Science 1988;241:708–712.

215. Scott J, Urdea M, Quiroga M, et al. Structure of a mouse submaxillary messenger RNA encoding epidermal growth factor and seven related proteins. Science 1983;221:236–240.

216. Derynck R, Roberts AB, Winkler ME, Chen EY, Goeddel DV. Human transforming growth factor-alpha: precursor studies and expression in E. Coli. Cell 1984;38:287–297.

217. Roberts AB, Anzaro MA, Lamb LC, Smith JM, Sporn MB. New class of transforming growth factors potentiated by epidermal growth factor. Proc Natl Acad Sci USA 1981;78:5339–5343.

218. Roberts AB, Sporn MB. The transforming growth factor-βs. In: Sporn MB, Roberts AB, eds. Peptide growth factors and their receptors, vol 1. Berlin: Springer-Verlag, 1990:419–472.

219. Roberts AB, Kim SJ, Noma T, et al. Multiple forms of TGF-beta: distinct promoters and differential expression. CIBA Foundation Symposium 1991;157:7–15.

220. Cheifetz S, Weatherbee JA, Tsang MLS, et al. The transforming growth factor-beta system: a complex pattern of cross reactive ligands and receptors. Cell 1987;48:409–415.

221. Pelton RW, Saxena B, Jones M, Moses HL, Gold LI. Immunohistochemical localization of TGF-beta1, TGF-beta2, and TGF-beta3 in the mouse embryo—expression patterns suggest multiple roles during embryonic development. J Cell Biol 1991;115:1091–1105.

222. Assoian RK, Sporn MB. Type-beta transforming growth factor in human platelets: release during platelet degranulation and action in vascular smooth muscle cells. J Cell Biol 1986;102:1217–1223.

223. Kehrl JH, Wakefield LM, Roberts AB, et al. Production of transforming growth factor beta by human T-lymphocytes and its potential role in the regulation of T cell growth. J Exp Med 1986;163:1037–1050.

224. Assoian RK, Fleurdelys BE, Stevenson HC, et al. Expression and secretion of type beta transforming growth factors by activated human macrophages. Proc Natl Acad Sci USA 1987;84:6020–6024.

225. Majesky MW, Reidy MA, Twardzik DR, Schwartz SM. Production of type-1 transforming growth factor-beta (TGFβ1) during repair of arterial injury. FASEB J 1989;3:A398.

226. Dennis PA, Rifkin DB. Cellular activation of latent transforming growth factor-beta requires binding to the cation-independent mannose-6-phosphate insulin-like growth factor type II receptor. Proc Natl Acad Sci USA 1991;88:580–584.

227. Flaumenhaft R, Abe M, Sato Y, et al. Role of the latent TGF-beta binding protein in reactivation of latent TGF-beta. J Cell Ciol 1993;120:995–1002.

228. Baird A, Durkin T. Inhibition of endothelial cell proliferation by type-beta transforming growth factor: interaction with acidic and basic fibroblast growth factors. Cancer Res 1983;43:3281–3286.

229. Frater-Schroder M, Muller G, Birchmeier W, Bohlen P. Transforming growth factor-beta inhibits endothelial cell proliferation. Biochem Biophys Res Commun 1986;137:295–302.

230. Madri JA, Pratt BM, Tucker A. Phenotypic modulation of endothelial cells by transforming growth factor-β depends upon the composition and organization of the extracellular matrix. J Cell Biol 1988;106:1375–1384.

231. Muller G, Behrens J, Nussbaumer U, Bohlen P, Birchmeier N. Inhibitory action of transforming growth factor-β in endothelial cells. Proc Natl Acad Sci USA 1987;84:5600–5604.

232. Wahl SM, Hunt DA, Wakefield LM, et al. Transforming growth factor-beta (TGF-beta) induces monocyte chemotaxis and growth factor production. Proc Natl Acad Sci USA 1987;84:5788–5792.

233. Wiseman DM, Polverini PJ, Kamp DW, Leibovich SJ. Transforming growth factor-beta (TGFβ) is chemotactic for human monocytes and induces their expression of angiogenic activity. Biochem Biophys Res Commun 1988;157:793–800.

234. Wahl SM, Allen JB, Weeks BS, Wong HL, Klotman PC. Transforming growth factor-β enhances integrin expression and type IV collagenase secretion in human monocytes. Proc Natl Acad Sci USA 1993;90:4577–4581.

235. Tsunawaki S, Sporn MB, Ding A, Nathan C. Deactivation of macrophages by transforming growth factor-β. Nature (London) 1988;334:260–262.

236. Tauber AI. Phagocyte NADPH-oxidase. In: Greenwald RA, ed. Handbook of methods for oxygen radical research. Florida: CRC Press, 1987:143–148.

237. Quaglino D, Nanney LB, Kennedy R, Davidson J. Transforming growth factor-beta stimulates wound healing and modulates extracellular matrix gene expression in pig skin. 1. Excisional wound model. Lab Invest 1990;63:307–319.

238. Cromack DT, Porrasreyes B, Purdy JA, Pierce GF, Mustoe TA. Acceleration of tissue repair by transforming growth factor-beta1—identification of in vivo mechanisms of action with radiotherapy induced specific healing deficits. Surgery 1993;113:36–42.

239. Lynch SE, Colvin RB, Antoniades HN. Growth factors in wound healing—single and synergistic effects on partial thickness porcine skin wounds. J Clin Invest 1989;84:640–646.

240. Phillips GD, Whitehead RA, Stone AM, Ruebel MW, Goodkin ML, Knighton DR. Transforming growth factor-β (TGFβ) stimulation of angiogenesis—an electron microscopic study. J Submicrosc Cytol 1993;25:149–155.

241. Yang EY, Moses HL. Transforming growth factor-beta-1-induced changes in cell migration, proliferation and angiogenesis in the chick chorioallantoic membrane. J Cell Biol 1990;111:731–741.

242. Miyazono K, Okabe T, Urabe A, Takaku F, Heldin CH. Purification and properties of an endothelial cell growth factor from human platelets. J Biol Chem 1987;262:4098–4103.

243. Miyazono K, Heldin CH. High yield purification of platelet-derived endothelial cell growth factor: structural char-

acterization and establishment of a specific antiserum. Biochemistry 1989;28:1704–1710.

244. Usuki K, Heldin NE, Miyazono K, et al. Production of platelet-derived endothelial cell growth factor by normal and transformed human cells in culture. Proc Natl Acad Sci USA 1989;81:7427–7431.

245. Miyazono K, Heldin CH. Platelet-derived endothelial cell growth factors. In: Sporn MB, Roberts AB. Peptide growth factors and their receptors, vol 2. Berlin: Springer-Verlag, 1990:125–133.

246. Ishikawa F, Miyazone K, Hellman U, et al. Identification of angiogenic activity and the cloning and expression of platelet-derived endothelial cell growth factor. Nature (London) 1989;338:557–562.

247. Usuki K, Norberg L, Larsson E, et al. Localizatoin of platelet-derived endothelial cell growth factor in human placenta and purification of an alternatively processed form. Cell Regul 1990;1:577–596.

248. Usuki K, Saras J, Waltenberger J, et al. Platelet-derived endothelial cell growth factor has thymidine phosphorylase activity. Biochem Biophys Res Commun 1992;184:1311–1316.

249. Finnis C, Dodsworth N, Pollitt CE, Carr G, Sleep D. Thymidine phosphorylase activity of platelet-derived endothelial cell growth factor is responsible for endothelial cell mitogenicity. Eur J Biochem 1993;212:201–210.

250. Mustoe T, Pierce G, Morishima C, Deuel T. Growth factor-induced acceleration of tissue repair through direct and inductive activities in a rabbit dermal ulcer model. J Clin Invest 1991;87:694–703.

251. Weidner KM, Arakaki N, Hartmann G, et al. Evidence for the identity of human scatter factor and human hepatocyte growth factor. Proc Natl Acad Sci USA 1991;88:7001–7005.

252. Miyazawa K, Tsubuchi H, Naka D, et al. Molecular cloning and sequence analysis of cDNA for human hepatocyte growth factor. Biochem Biophys Res Commun 1989;163:967–973.

253. Stoker M, Perryman M. An epithelial scatter factor released by embryo fibroblasts. J Cell Sci 1985;77:209–223.

254. Stoker M, Gherardi E, Perryman M, Gray J. Scatter factor is a fibroblast-derived modulator of epithelial cell mobility. Nature (London) 1987;327:239–242.

255. Rosen EM, Goldberg ID, Kacinski BM, Buckholz T, Vinter DW. Smooth muscle releases an epithelial cell scatter factor which binds to heparin. In Vitro Cell Dev Biol 1989;25:163–173.

256. Gherardi E, Gray J, Stoker M, Perryman M, Furlong R. Purification of scatter factor, a fibroblast-derived basic protein that modulates epithelial interactions and movement. Proc Natl Acad Sci USA 1989;86:5844–5848.

257. Nakamura T, Nishizawa T, Hagiya M, et al. Molecular cloning and expression of human hepatocyte growth factor. Nature (London) 1989;342:440–443.

258. Grant DS, Kleinman HK, Goldberg ID, et al. Scatter factor induces blood vessel formation in vivo. Proc Natl Acad Sci USA 1993;90:1937–1941.

259. Rosen EM, Meromsky L, Setter E, Vinter DW, Goldberg ID. Purified scatter factor stimulates epithelial and vascular endothelial cell migration. Proc Soc Exp Biol Med 1990;195:34–43.

260. Rosen EM, Jaken S, Carley W, et al. Regulation of motility in bovine brain endothelial cells. J Cell Physiol 1991;146:325–335.

261. Rosen EM, Grant D, Kleinman H, et al. Scatter factor stimulates migration of vascular endothelium and capillary-like tube formation. In: Goldberg ID, Rosen EM, eds. Cell motility factors. Basel: Birkhauser Verlag, 1991:76–88.

262. Bottaro DP, Rubin JS, Faletto DL, et al. Identification of the hepatocyte growth factor receptor as the c-met proto-oncogene product. Science 1991;251:802–804.

263. Metcalf D. The molecular control of cell division, differentiation, commitment and maturation in hemopoietic cells. Nature (London) 1989;339:27–30.

264. Sachs L. The molecular control of blood cell development. Science 1987;238:1374–1379.

265. Crosier PS, Garnick MB, Clark SC. Granulocyte-macrophage colony stimulating factor. In: Aggarwal BB, Gutterman JU, eds. Human cytokines: handbook for basic and clinical research. Boston: Blackwell Scientific Publications, 1992:238–252.

266. Stanley ER. Colony stimulating factor-1. In: Aggarwal BB, Gutterman JU, eds. Human cytokines: handbook for basic and clinical research. Boston: Blackwell Scientific Publications, 1992: 196–220.

267. Mantovani A, Bussolino F, Dejana E. Cytokine regulators of endothelial cell function. FASEB J 1992;6:2591–2599.

268. Broudy VC, Kaushansky K, Segal GM, Harlan JM, Adamson JW. Tumor necrosis factor-α stimulates human endothelial cells to produce granulocyte/macrophage colony-stimulating factor. Proc Natl Acad Sci USA 1986;83:7467–7471.

269. Holzman LB, Marks RM, Dixit VM. A novel immediate early response gene of endothelium is induced by cytokines and encodes a secreted protein. Mol Cell Biol 1990;10:5830–5838.

270. Bagby GC, Shaw G, Heinrich MC, et al. Interleukin-1 stimulation stabilizes GM-CSF messenger RNA in human vascular endothelial cells—preliminary studies of the role of the 3′ AU rich motif. Biol Hematopoiesis 1990;352:233–239.

271. Sachs L. Angiogenesis—cytokines as part of a network. In: Steiner R, Weisz PB, Langer R, eds. Angiogenesis: key principles. Basel: Birkhauser Verlag, 1992:20–22.

272. Bussolino F, Wang JM, Defilippi P et al. Granulocyte- and granulocyte-macrophage-colony stimulating factors induce human endothelial cells to migrate and proliferate. Nature (London) 1989;337:471–473.

273. Aggarwal BB, Kohr WJ, Hass PE, et al. Human tumor necrosis factor production, purification and characterization. J Biol Chem 1985;260:2345–2354.

274. Kriegler M, Perez C, deFay K, Albert I, Lu S. A novel form of TNF/cachectin is a cell-surface cytotoxic transmembrane protein: ramifications for the complex physiology of TNF. Cell 1988;53:45–53.

275. Beutler B, Cerami A. Cachectin and tumor necrosis factor as two sides of the same biological coin. Nature (London) 1986;320:584–588.

276. Carswell EA, Old LJ, Kassel RL, Green S, Fiore N, Williamson B. An endotoxin-induced serum factor that causes necrosis of tumors. Proc Natl Acad Sci USA 1975;72:3666–3670.

277. Dinarello CA. The endogenous pyrogens in host defense interactions. Hosp Pract 1989;24:111–115.

278. Leibovich SJ, Polverini PJ, Shepard HM, Wiseman DM, Shively V, Nuseir N. Macrophage-induced angiogeneis is mediated by tumour necrosis factor-α. Nature (London) 1987;329:630–632.

279. Frater-Schroder M, Risau W, Hallmann P, Gautschi R, Bohlen P. Tumor necrosis factor type-α, a potent inhibitor of endothelial cell growth in vitro, is angiogenic in vivo. Proc Natl Acad Sci USA 1987;84:5277–5281.

280. Aggarwal DB. Tumor necrosis factor. In: Aggarwal BB, Gutterman JU, eds. Human cytokines: handbook for basic and clinical research. Boston: Blackwell Scientific Publications, 1992:270–286.

281. Loetscher H, Pan Y-CE, Lahm HW, et al. Molecular cloning and expression of the human 55kD tumor necrosis factor receptor. Cell 1990;61:351–359.

282. Schall TJ, Lewis M, Koller KJ, et al. Molecular cloning and expression of a receptor for human tumor necrosis factor. Cell 1990;61:361–370.

283. Seckinger P, Isaaczs D, Dayer JM. Purification and biological characterization of a specific tumor necrosis factor inhibitor. J Biol Chem 1989;264:1966–1973.

284. Engelmann H, Novick D, Wallach D. Two tumor necrosis factor-binding proteins purified from human urine. Evidence for immunological cross reactivity with cell-surface tumor necrosis factor receptors. J Biol Chem 1990;265:1531–1536.

285. Teng MN, Park BH, Keoppen HKW, Tracey KJ, Fendly BM, Schreiber H. Long term inhibition of tumor growth by tumor necrosis factor in the absence of cachexia or T-cell immunity. Proc Natl Acad Sci USA 1991;88:3535–3539.

286. Robertson PA, Ross HJ, Figlin RA. Tumor necrosis factor induces hemorrhagic necrosis of a sarcoma. Ann Intern Med 1989;111:682–684.

287. Denekamp J. Vascular attack as a therapeutic strategy for cancer. Cancer Metastasis Rev 1990;9:267–282.

288. Le J, Vilcek J. Tumor necrosis factor and interleukin-1: cytokines with multiple overlapping biological activity. Lab Invest 1987;56:234–248.

289. Pober JS, Cotran SR. The role of endothelial cells in inflammation. Physiol Rev 1990;70:427–451.

290. Meyrick B, Christman B, Jesmok G. Effects of recombinant tumor necrosis factor-alpha on cultured pulmonary artery and lung microvascular endothelial cells. Am J Pathol 1991;138:93–101.

291. Detman M, Imcke E, Ruszczak Z, Orfanos CE. Effects of recombinant tumor necrosis factor-alpha on cultured microvascular endothelial cells derived from human dermis. J Invest Dermatol 1990;95:5219–5222.

292. Clark IA, Thumwood CM, Chaudhri G, Lowden WB, Hunt NH. Tumor necrosis factor and reactive oxygen species: implications for free-radical induced tissue injury. In: Halliwell B, ed. Oxygen radicals and tissue injury. Proceedings of an Upjohn Symposium. Fed Am Soc Exp Biol 1988:122–129.

293. Ward PA, Varani J. Mechanisms of neutrophil-mediated killing of endothelial cells. J Leukocyte Biol 1990;48:97–102.

294. Persidsky Y, Frolov A. Reactions of microvascular endo-
thelial cells to tumor necrosis factor in vivo. In: Steiner R, Weisz PB, Langer R, eds. Angiogenesis: key principles. Basel: Birkhauser Verlag, 1992:432–435.

295. Ginsel LA. Origin of macrophages. In: Horton MA, ed. Blood cell biochemistry, vol 5. New York: Plenum, 1993:87–113.

296. Dower SK. Interleukin-1. In: Aggarwal BB, Gutterman JU, eds. Human cytokines: handbook for basic and clinical research. Boston: Blackwell Scientific Publications, 1992:46–80.

297. Dinarello CA. Interleukin-1. Rev Infect Dis 1984;6:51–95.

298. Block RA, Kronheim SR, Sleath PR. Activation of IL-1β by co-induced protease. FEBS Lett 1989;81:7907–7911.

299. Auron PE, Webb AC, Rosenwasser L, et al. Nucleotide sequence of the human monocyte interleukin-1 precursor cDNA. Proc Natl Acad Sci USA 1984;81:7907–7911.

300. March CJ, Mosley B, Larsen A, et al. Cloning, sequence and expression of two distinct human interleukin-1 complementary cDNAs. Nature (London) 1985;315:641–647.

301. Prendergast RA, Lutty GA, Dinarello CA. Interleukin-1 induces corneal neovascularization. Invest Ophthalmol Vis Sci 1987;28(suppl):100.

302. Ben Ezra D, Hemo I, Maftzir G. In vivo angiogenic activity of interleukins. Arch Ophthalmol 1990;108:573–576.

303. Raines EW, Dower SK, Ross R. IL-1 mitogenic activity for fibroblasts and smooth muscle cells is due to PDGF-AA. Science 1989;243:393–396.

304. Kovacs EJ. Fibrogenic cytokines: the role of immune mediators in the development of scar tissue. Immunol Today 1991;12:17–23.

305. Kovacs EJ, Neuman JE. Selective induction of PDGF-A chain and B chain gene expression in rat peritoneal macrophages by interleukin-2. In: Meltzer MM, Mantovani A, eds. Cellular and cytokine networks in tissue immunity. New York: John Wiley and Sons, 1991:307–312.

306. Schrader JW, Clark-Lewis I, Leslie KB, Ziltener HJ. Interleukin-3. In: Aggarwal BB, Gutterman JU, eds. Human cytokines: handbook for basic and clinical research. Boston: Blackwell Scientific Publications, 1992:98–112.

307. Schrader JW, Clark-Lewis I, Crapper RM, et al. The physiology and pathology of pan-specific hemopoietin (IL-3). In: Schrader JW, ed. Interleukin-3: the pan-specific hemopoietin. Lymphokines, vol 15. New York: Academic Press, 1988:281–311.

308. Knighton DR, Hunt TK, Thakral KK, Goodson WH III. Role of platelets and fibrin in the healing sequence. Ann Surg 1982;196:379–388.

309. Hiraizumi Y, Transfeldt EE, Kawahara V, Sung JH, Knighton D, Fiegel VD. In vivo angiogenesis by platelet-derived wound healing formula in injured spinal cord. Brain Res Bull 1993;30:353–357.

310. Motro B, Itin A, Sachs L, Keshet E. Pattern of interleukin-6 gene expression in vivo suggests a role for this cytokine in angiogenesis. Proc Natl Acad Sci USA 1990;87:3092–3096.

311. De Vries JE. Interleukin-4. In: Agggarwal BB, Gutterman JU, eds. Human cytokines: handbook for basic and clinical research. Boston: Blackwell Scientific Publications, 1992:111–129.

312. Toi M, Harris AL, Bicknell R. Interleukin-4 is a potent mi-

togen for capillary endothelium. Biochem Biophys Res Commun 1991;174:1287–1293.

313. Standiford D, Strieter PM, Kasahara K, Kunkel SL. Disparate regulation of interleukin-8 gene expression from blood monocytes, endothelial cells and fibroblasts by interleukin-4. Biochem Biophys Res Commun 1990;171:531–536.

314. Koch AE, Polverini PJ, Kunkel SL, et al. Interleukin- 8 as a macrophage-derived mediator of angiogenesis. Science 1992;258:1798–1801.

315. Streiter RM, Kunkel SL, Elner VM, et al. Interleukin-8: a corneal factor that induces neovascularization. Am J Pathol 1992;141:1279–1284.

316. Hori Y, Fan TPD. Interleukin-8 stimulates angiogenesis in rats. Inflammation 1993;17:135–143.

317. Taga T, Kishimoto T. Interleukin-6. In: Aggarwal BB, Gutterman JU, eds. Human cytokines: handbook for basic and clinical research. Boston: Blackwell Scientific Publications, 1992: 141–167.

318. Hirano T, Kishimoto T. Interleukin-6. In: Sporn MB, Roberts AB, eds. Peptide growth factors and their receptors, vol 1. Berlin: Springer-Verlag, 1989:633–665.

319. Helle M, Boeije L, Pascualsalcedo D, Aarden L. Differential induction of interleukin-6 production by monocytes, endothelial cells and smooth muscle cells. Bacterial Endotoxins 1991;367:61–71.

320. Bendtzen K. Interleukin-1, interleukin-6 and tumor necrosis factor in infection, inflammation and immunity. Immunol Lett 1988;19:183–192.

321. Kishimoto T. The biology of interleukin-6. Blood 1990;74:1–10.

322. May LT, Torcia G, Cozzolino F, et al. Interleukin-6 gene expression in human endothelial cells: RNA start sites, multiple IL-6 proteins, and inhibition of proliferation. Biochem Biophys Res Commun 1989;159:991–998.

323. Podor TJ, Jirik FR, Loskutoff DJ, Carson DA, Lotz M. Human endothelial cells produce IL-6. Lack of responses to exogenous IL-6. Ann NY Acad Sci 1989;557:374–385.

324. Miles SA, Rezai AR, Salazar-Gonzalez JF, et al. AIDS Kaposi sarcoma-derived cells produce and respond to interleukin-6. Proc Natl Acad Sci USA 1990;87:4068–4072.

325. Schroder JM, Morowietz E, Christophers E. Purification and partial biochemical characterization of a human monocyte-derived neutrophil activating peptide that lacks interleukin-1 activity. J Immunol 1987;139:3474–3483.

326. Peveri P, Waltz A, Dewald B, Baggioloni M. A novel neutrophil activating factor produced by human mononuclear phagocytes. J Exp Med 1988;167:1547–1559.

327. Elner VM, Streiter RM, Pavilack MA, et al. Human corneal interleukin-8. IL-1 and TNF-induced gene expression and secretion. Am J Pathol 1991;139:977–988.

328. Matsushima K. Oppenheim JJ. Interleukin-8 and MCAF. Novel inflammatory cytokines inducible by IL-1 and TNF. Cytokine 1989;1:2–13.

329. Koch AE, Kunkel SL, Burrows JC, et al. Synovial tissue macrophage as a source of the chemotactic cytokine Il-8. J Immunol 1992;147:2187–2195.

330. Zacchariae CO, Matsushima K. Interleukin-8. In: Aggarwal BB, Gutterman JU, eds. Human cytokines: handbook for basic and clinical research. Boston: Blackwell Scientific Publications, 1992:181–195.

331. Kristensen MS, Paludan K, Larsen CG, et al. Quantitative determination of IL-1β induced IL-8 mRNA levels in cultured human keratinocytes, dermal fibroblasts, endothelial cells and monocytes. J Invest Dermatol 1991;97:506–510.

332. Thelen M, Peveri P, Kesnen P, von Tschamer V, Walz A, Baggiolini M. Mechanism of neutrophil activation by NAF, a novel monocyte-derived peptide agonist. FASEB J 1988;2:2702–2706.

333. Gimbrone MA, Obins MS, Brock AF, et al. Endothelial interleukin-8: a novel inhibitor of leukocyte-endothelial interactions. Science 1990;246:1601–1603.

334. Gray PW. Interferon-γ. In: Aggarwal BB, Gutterman JU, eds. Human cytokines: handbook for basic and clinical research. Boston: Blackwell Scientific Publications, 1992:30–45.

335. Nathan C, Yoshida R. Cytokines: interferon-gamma. In: Gallin JI, Goldstein IM, Snyderman R, eds. Inflammation: basic principles and clinical correlates. New York: Raven, 1988:229–251.

336. Rinderknecht E, O'Connor BH, Rodriguez H. Natural human interferon-γ. J Biol Chem 1984;259:6790–6797.

337. Aguet M, Dembic Z, Merlin G. Molecular cloning and expression of the human interferon-gamma receptor. Cell 1988;55:273–280.

338. Nathan C, Yoshida R. Cytokines: interferon-gamma. In: Gallin JI, Goldstein IM, Snyderman R, eds. Inflammation: basic principles and clinical correlates. New York: Raven, 1988:229–251.

339. Xie Q, Cho HJ, Calaycay J, et al. Cloning and characterization of inducible nitric oxide synthase from mouse macrophages. Science 1992;256:225–228.

340. Pober JS, Cotran RS. Cytokines and endothelial cell biology. Physiol Rev 1990;70:427–451.

341. Tsuruoka N, Sugiyama M, Tawaragi Y, et al. Inhibition of in vitro angiogenesis by lymphotoxin and interferon-gamma. Biochem Biophys Res Commun 1988;155:429–435.

342. Friesel R, Komoriya A, Maciag T. Inhibition of endothelial cell proliferation by gamma interferon. J Cell Biol 1987;104:689–696.

CHAPTER 36

CYTOKINE MODULATION OF RADIATION INJURY

Michael A. Doukas and Vincent S. Gallicchio

There are currently four cytokine factors approved for human use and available for the treatment of oncology therapy–associated neutropenia or modulation of tumor growth. These 4 cytokines, granulocyte-macrophage colony-stimulating factor (GM-CSF), granulocyte-colony stimulating factor (G-CSF), interleukin-2 (IL-2), and interferon-α (IFN-α), are merely the first of more than two dozen identified or cloned cytokines. A number of these are, by virtue of in vitro cell culture or animal data, potential modulators of radiation damage to either normal tissues or malignant tumors. In the first instance, a desirable decrease in normal tissue damage to radiation, or radioprotection, can allow for an improvement in the risk–benefit ratio of those toxic therapies which include radiotherapy. The normal tissue with the greatest sensitivity (in addition to germinal tissue, which does not affect morbidity/mortality) to radiation is hematopoietic tissue, followed by the gastrointestinal tract and the lung (1).

Due to the focal targeting of malignant tissue in the conventional use of radiotherapy, dangerous general hematopoietic depression is unusual because of the dispersed nature of the hematopoietic "organ" (2). However, the increasing use of combined chemotherapy plus conventional radiotherapy and the many protocols incorporating total body irradiation (TBI) in bone marrow transplantation (BMT) make attempts at radioprotection of normal tissues, especially marrow, desirable. Furthermore, the intrinsic or acquired radioresistance of malignant tumors has led to a search for pharmacological

means of sensitizing these tumors to radiation. The biology of normal and malignant tissues and the elucidation of the role of growth factors in their survival and growth make a variety of cytokines potential candidates for pharmacological protection or sensitization, respectively.

TUMOR AND NORMAL TISSUE CYTOKINE ELABORATION

Before embarking on a description of the effects of the pharmacological administration of cytokines, we briefly review the physiological responses of normal and tumor tissues to irradiation. Such responses include induction of specific genes as a part of the lethal and repair responses to irradiation; radiation-induced growth factors and cytokines are an important component of this response (3–5). The autocrine, paracrine, and endocrine effects of these cytokines on irradiated normal and tumor tissues may be a guide to the most desirable pharmacological interventions attempted clinically.

Many normal tissues and tumors elaborate cytokines constitutively (6,7). The role of these factors in tumorigenesis and angiogenesis is reviewed extensively in Chapters 34 and 35; their role in hematopoiesis (and therefore critical to any potential hematological radioprotection) is reviewed in Chapter 12. Irradiation of cell types that are known constituents of the bone marrow microenvironment, or "stroma," provokes an increased elaboration of CSF and ILs, specifically GM-CSF and M-CSF (marrow stroma), IL-6 (fibroblasts), and IL-1 (macrophages) (8–11). Irradiation of liver and large bowel also causes transforming growth factor-β (TGF-β) expression (12–14). The normal cell types involved in these immunohistochemical studies of TGF-β were hepatocytes, deformed bowel crypts and epithelium, vessel walls, and associated inflammatory cells (lymphocytes and macrophages).

Cytokine release of growth factors from irradiated endothelial cells in vitro is also reported, specifically platelet-derived growth factor (PDGF) and fibroblast growth factor (FGF) (15,16). Normal peripheral blood monocytes express increased levels of tumor necrosis factor (TNF) RNA transcripts in a time and irradiation dose-dependent manner (17). Protein kinase C is hypothesized to be required for the induction of this increased TNF gene expression (18). Finally, irradiated alveolar macrophages exhibit enhanced production and release of TGF-α and TGF-β as compared with control samples (19). Tumor cell lines also produce cytokines when irradiated, specifically TNF-α (HL-60, U937, human sarcoma), and IL-1 and FGF (HeLa cell line) (17,18,20,21).

It is clear from these studies that normal tissues and tumors may elaborate cytokines as part of the response to irradiation. These cytokines may influence local cellular growth and cause remote (endocrine) effects on other tissues (Table 36–1). The decreased survival of irradiated mice when pretreated with an antibody to the IL-1 receptor strongly suggests a protective role for endogenously generated IL-1 (22). Thus, certain cytokine responses are desirable with regard to normal tissue repair. However, other responses may be undesirable if protectant to the tumor or if they enhance the damage to normal tissues. This latter possibility may be true of those cytokines now believed to mediate late irradiation damage to lung, liver, and blood vessels (14,15,19), several specific examples for which preliminary data exists.

Certain cytokine effects of undetermined clinical significance are also described. It has only recently been appreciated that irradiation of marrow stroma confers a long-lasting effect on hematopoiesis by virtue of altered cytokine elaboration (23). Long-term bone marrow cultures (LTBMC) established one year after sublethal irradiation of mice generate granulocytes in which significant enhancement of superoxide-anion production is evident. This effect was also seen when stromal layers irradiated in vitro were reseeded with normal bone marrow progenitors; the effect, therefore, is mediated by the stroma. Increased production of granulocyte superoxide anions was correlated with increased CSF elaboration; neutralizing antibodies to GM-CSF blocked the bulk of the stromal-derived CSF activity. Whether this chronic priming of granulocyte metabolic function is clinically desirable is unknown. The complex and interlocking cascade of

TABLE 36–1 CYTOKINES ELABORATED IN RESPONSE TO IONIZING RADIATION

Cytokine	Tissue	Reference
GM-CSF	Marrow stroma	(9,10)
M-CSF	Marrow stroma	(9,10)
IL-6	Fibroblasts	(11)
IL-1	Macrophages, HeLa cells	(12) (23)
TGF	Liver, large bowel, alveolar macrophages	(13,15) (14) (20)
FGF	Endothelium, HeLa cells	(16,17) (23)
PDGF	Endothelium	(16)
TNF	Monocytes, U937; HL-60; human sarcoma	(18) (18,19) (22)

known endogenous secondary cytokine responses naturally evokes caution when considering the use of exogenous, pharmacological doses of single or combination cytokines for the purpose of either normal tissue protection or tumor sensitization.

IMMUNOMODULATORS—EARLY ATTEMPTS AT RADIATION INJURY MODULATION

The therapeutic efficacy of cytoreductive therapy for cancer is hypothesized to be related to dose intensity (24,25). Total body irradiation or combined modality chemoradiotherapy are aggressive modalities in which hematological or gastrointestinal toxicity limits dose. Therapeutically, however, regimens for allogeneic (and, to a lesser extent, autologous) bone marrow transplantation utilize TBI at dosages of 1,000 to 1,575 cGy (plus concomitant chemotherapy), which exceeds marrow tolerance (26). Hematological rescue is therefore required, and it is achieved by transplantation of totipotent hematopoietic stem cells.

Animal models of whole body irradiation established

the potential of rescuing mice subjected to a lethal dose of radiation with an infusion of syngeneic marrow cells, and this model system has been used in a variety of preclinical BMT studies (27). This preclinical model established the first threshold-limiting irradiation dose as hematological in nature. Additional work with the immunomodulatory agent, bacterial lipopolysaccharide (LPS) or endotoxin, revealed that in lieu of marrow transplantation, radioprotection could be achieved by LPS pretreatment (28–30).

Radioprotection has been subsequently reported with other immunomodulatory agents, including mycobacterium bovis strain BCG, glucan, streptococcus pyrogenes OK-432, muramyl dipeptide Ivastimul, AS101, and lithium salts (31–38). These agents were given prior to irradiation; a few agents were studied in both pre- and postirradiated states. These studies served as a starting point to define better optimal methods of radioprotection and to investigate basic hematopoiesis. These goals have come together, in that it is understood, in the case of LPS and possibly other agents, that their principal mode of activity is via a cascade of secondary cytokine release (39). This cascade is perhaps best described for LPS, which may be acting principally, although not exclusively, via IL-1 and TNF. When these two factors were cloned and became available in quantity, it was found that both agents alone afford radioprotection (40,41). Of greater interest perhaps were studies that show these two cytokines act cooperatively and that blockade of both by appropriate specific antibodies unmasks a radiosensitizing effect of LPS, presumably due to another induced cytokine (42). The authors hypothesize that this sensitizing cytokine is TGF-β, because this cytokine, when administered alone, mimics the radiosensitization of LPS plus antibody to both TNF and IL-1 receptor.

Other cytokines induced as a part of the acute-phase response may also be candidates for this LPS effect. Appropriate testing with neutralizing antibodies to these candidate cytokines will hopefully result in broader elucidation of the in vivo cytokine cascades relevant to LPS modulation and the resultant cytokine interactions. Combinations of cytokines already being examined in preclinical models may enhance the desired therapeutic effect or they could conversely provoke antagonistic effects.

CYTOKINE MODULATION OF RADIATION INJURY TO NORMAL TISSUES

The desired aim of pharmacological manipulation (drug or cytokine) of host normal tissue is reduction of radiation damage. Radiosensitization by certain factors is reported, however (42), and it must be considered a possi-

bility when evaluating the newer cytokines being described. To add to the complexity of potential cytokine use is the issue of interactions; certain factors used alone will radiosensitize, yet paradoxically in combination with a second cytokine, they will provide synergistic or additive radioprotective effects (43).

Several cautionary notes should be made regarding currently approved cytokines. The decision process of Food and Drug Administration (FDA) approval for GM-CSF and G-CSF utilized a number of "surrogate markers" of desirable clinical response; chief among these markers of biological response were increases in absolute neutrophil count (ANC) or time to ANC recovery (44). Also measured were days of hospitalization, incidence of infection/antibiotic usage, mucositis severity, and other factors. Although many of these markers at first inspection would appear to be of distinct patient benefit or to enhance quality of life, they may not directly address the issue of influence on survival or potential cure due to criticisms leveled at the study designs. The most quoted surrogate marker, the ANC, is subject to scientific concerns relating to neutrophil kinetics (circulating neutrophils are a tiny fraction of total body neutrophils) and qualitative neutrophil function (44,45). Finally, the trials involving GM-CSF and G-CSF utilized chemotherapy treatments alone, the agents were administered after the anticancer therapy, and tumor stimulation by these agents remains a theoretical concern in some cancers (46–49). These issues involving clinical use of cytokines have been reviewed and are presented in Table 36–2 (50).

A definition of the intent of protection is therefore in order. *Webster's* defines "protect" as to "shield from that which would injure." The term is derived from *protogere*, literally "to cover in front" (51), which implies that radioprotection specifically refers to some intervention prior to therapy. An appropriate term for an intervention after radiation (or chemotherapy) treatment would be *myelorestorative*, as coined by Neta and Oppenheim (39). Furthermore, the term *radioprotection* has drawn fire because no proof currently exists that hematopoietic or other stem cells are protected; rather, their subsequent proliferation via proposed, but unproved, mechanisms appears to be accelerated in the recovery phase after the radiation insult (52). We will, however, continue to use the term *radioprotection* in an operational sense for the salutary use of cytokines prior to irradiation insult.

Interleukin-1 and tumor necrosis factor

IL-1 was the first cytokine demonstrated to produce radioprotection (40). Intraperitoneal injection of 2,000 U recombinant IL-1 (333 ng protein, containing less than 4 pgm LPS) 20 hours before a lethal dose (LD) of irradiation to C57BL6 mice (950 cGy produced 100% death in control mice within 17 days [i.e., LD 100/17]) resulted in 75 to 90% survival. This treatment with IL-1 increased bone marrow cellularity and endogenous spleen colony-forming units (CFU-S) (53). This study also determined that the time of injection was important, because the protective effect decreased to survival percentages of 30 and 12.5% respectively, if IL-1 was administered 4 hours or 45 hours before irradiation. Also, the degree of IL-1–induced radioprotection was influenced by the strain of mice used (53). The timing of IL-1 administration was also addressed in another study in which human IL-1 was administered to C3H/HeN mice (54). The optimum time for radioprotection was observed to be from 25 to 4 hours before LD 100/14 (800 cGy) irradiation. The optimum time with a higher radiation dose (900 cGy) appeared to be from 4 to 7 hours before irradiation.

This group also evaluated the radioprotective effect of other cytokines, in particular, TNF-α, although much higher doses were required compared with IL-1 (TNF-α, 5–7.5 μg or 48,000–72,000 U IL-1, 0.075–0.5 μg). The combination of IL-1 and TNF-α had a synergistic effect on providing protection from lethal irradiation (41). Administration of 100 ng IL-1 plus 5 μg TNF-α 20 hours before lethal irradiation in B6D2F1 mice (1,150 cGy, LD$_{100/30}$) produced a survival percentage of 60% when compared with IL-1 alone (26%) and TNF-α (6%). When murine TNF-α was administered intravenously (2 μg, 52,000 U) 20 hours before a sublethal exposure to BALB/c mice (750 cGy), the absolute neutrophil counts (PMN) were 10-fold greater in the TNF-treated group compared with control mice 20 days after irradiation. The number of progenitors in both bone marrow and spleen were also significantly greater in the TNF-treated groups both 10 and 20 days after irradiation (55). Similar results for IL-1 were reported from this laboratory; B6C3F1 mice receiving IL-1 24 hours prior to 200- cGy irradiation had accelerated recovery of circulating leukocyte and platelet counts and increasing numbers of erythroid (CFU-E/E-BFU), myeloid (CFU-GM), and megakaryocyte (CFU-Meg) progenitors compared with control mice (56).

In normal, healthy, nonirradiated mice, a single dose of IL-1 (2,800 U) administered intravenously induced a 50% decrease in marrow-derived CFU-GM and splenic CFU-S 12 hours following injection (57). This coincided with a four-fold increase in splenic CFU-GM and a 5-fold increase in blood leukocyte counts. We reported that IL-1 administered in vivo induced profound changes in marrow and splenic erythroid, myeloid, and megakaryocyte hematopoietic progenitor cells (56). However, the effects on erythroid progenitors attributed to IL-1 may have been indirect because systemic levels of prostaglandin E series in these IL-1–treated mice were found to be elevated significantly compared with control mice. Furthermore, the erythropoietic response observed in IL-1–treated mice could be abrogated by prior treatment of mice with indo-

TABLE 36–2 ISSUES THAT BEAR ON THE EMPIRICAL USE OF COLONY-STIMULATING FACTORS AS MYELOPROTECTIVE AGENTS

Disease characteristics
  Dose-response relationship
  Therapeutic goals
Host characteristics
  Age
  Prior therapy
  General medical status
Treatment characteristics
  Incidence of neutropenia
  Duration of neutropenia
  Depth of neutropenia
  Goal of therapy
Cytokine characteristics
  Side effects
  Cost
  Schedule
  Effects on tumor cells
  Effects on other effector cells or other cytokine-secreting cells

Reproduced by permission from Schuchter LM, ed. The current status of toxicity protectants in cancer therapy. Philadelphia: WB Saunders, 1992.

methacin, an effective inhibitor of endogenous prostaglandin synthesis. The altered state of hematopoietic response following sepsis, chronic inflammation, or endotoxin, with subsequent protective response to irradiation, could be in part a response to altered prostaglandin levels, especially with regard to radiation effects on stromal cells (58). However, a study comparing IL-1, IL-1 plus indomethacin, and indomethacin alone produced no significant difference in survival in mice receiving 950 cGy (53).

Use of an antibody to the IL-1 receptor in vivo was capable of blocking the radioprotective effect of IL-1. In these studies, the IL-1 receptor antibody had only a moderate capability of reducing circulating CSF. This observation supports the hypothesis that systemic CSFs have a minor role in providing radioprotection (22). Use of the IL-1 receptor antibody has also been used in relation to determining the relationship between IL-1 and the c-kit ligand, stem-cell factor (SCF), in inducing radioprotection because administration of either alone provides radioprotection. IL-1 receptor antibody can reduce the radioprotective effect of SCF by 60% (59). These studies demonstrate that endogenous IL-1 is necessary for SCF radioprotection.

Several studies have attempted to identify the mechanism by which IL-1 induces radioprotection. One suggested mechanism is that IL-1 administered in vivo stimulates stem-cell proliferation such that resting hemato-poietic progenitor cells are placed in cell cycle, thus making them less irradiation-sensitive (60–63). More recently, evidence has been presented demonstrating that within 6 hours after IL-1 injection, there is an increase in murine bone marrow cell–derived manganese superoxide dismutase (MnSOD) (64). In this study, pretreatment with IL-1 also protected bone marrow long- term culture-initiating cells capable of reconstituting irradiated stromal cultures. This effect was correlated with elevated levels of MnSOD. Human cell lines associated with high basal MnSOD RNA levels were found to be highly radioresistant compared with cell lines that had low levels and which were radiosensitive. In a cell line (A375) with low baseline MnSOD levels, IL-1 treatment in vitro resulted in increased MnSOD protein levels and concomitant radioprotection. These studies suggest that the antioxidant enzyme MnSOD may be important in the mechanism by which IL-1 induces radioprotection.

Additional studies have investigated the relationship between IL-1–induced radioprotection in systems in which the stated objective was enhanced hematopoietic recovery. For example, IL-1 has been shown to improve the capacity of allogeneic bone marrow cells to rescue animals receiving lethal TBI (65,66). These studies suggested that IL-1 may improve stem-cell survival in these systems by enhancing marrow stem-cell engraftment, by reducing the development of graft-versus-host disease, or by promoting microenvironmental support.

IL-1–induced radioprotection has also been investigated in tumor-bearing animals because it is known that rodent tumors significantly influence the hematopoietic condition of their hosts. Studies have indicated that the radioprotective effect of IL-1 was significantly reduced when administered to murine hosts containing either Lewis lung or EMT-6 tumors (67). In another study using head and neck tumor models, use of IL-1 still provided radioprotection (68). An explanation for these discrepant results may relate to strain specificity of the tumor hosts because in the former study, Balb/c mice served as the host. The radiosensitivity in Balb/c mice may have been altered in these tumor-bearing animals, in contrast to the latter study that compared C57BL/Ka with C3H/Km mice (68). The implications of strain differences in IL-1–induced radioprotection requires additional study. In mice bearing certain tumors (e.g., Lewis lung, EMT-6) associated with expanded hematopoiesis and high serum prostaglandin E levels, IL-1 does not radioprotect (69). Furthermore, interference with prostaglandin production by indomethacin did not alter the stimulated marrow state or restore the radioprotective ability of IL-1.

Although IL-1 has been recognized to be a potent inducer of radioprotection, with the focus of many investigations being placed upon the hematopoietic system, IL-1 has also been demonstrated to provide radioprotection of the gastrointestinal system; studies demonstrated IL-1 protection of intestinal crypt cells of mice (70) and murine intestinal stem cells (71). These studies indicate that IL-1 promotes increased survival, as opposed to altering the repopulation kinetics of intestinal cells.

GM-CSF and G-CSF

GM-CSF and G-CSF are glycoprotein molecules of relatively low molecular weight that are part of the cytokine network that regulates production and metabolic function of granulocytes and macrophages (72). The early description of in vitro culture systems of hematopoietic colony growth, dependent on the addition of exogenous diffusible factors termed *colony-stimulating activities* (73), marked the onset of the search for specific hematopoietic regulatory molecules. Laborious purification work led to cloning and subsequent generation of large quantities of these factors (74,75) for research and ultimately clinical use. The precise physiological role of these cytokines remains controversial; certain data favor a role for G-CSF in normal steady-state hematopoiesis (76). It has been hypothesized that GM- CSF is a locally produced and acting factor that therefore enhances local host defenses (72). In vitro marrow cultures, however, do not rule out a local role via marrow stroma in physiological steady-state hematopoiesis by GM-CSF (77). Although distinct biochemical, physiological, and clinical toxicity differences exist between these cytokines, they both induce neutrophilia in vivo and they have been used, almost interchangeably, by clinicians for a wide range of clinical causes of neutropenia (72,78). For this reason, and because a proportion of studies compare and contrast the utility and role of both GM-CSF and G-CSF, they are discussed together.

Early interest in the potential role of CSFs in radioprotection was a result of the observations that LPS (79) and, later, IL-1 and TNF-α (80) administration in vivo induced the appearance of CSFs. Later work in vitro confirmed and expanded these data by showing that IL-1 exposure to endothelial cells, fibroblasts, and marrow stromal cells resulted in elaboration of GM-CSF, G-CSF, and M-CSF (81–83). Similar results with TNF-α were also reported for endothelial cells in which GM-CSF was induced (84). A role for CSFs was thus hypothesized as a part of the aforementioned cytokine cascades provoked by the known radioprotectants, IL-1 and TNF-α.

In vitro studies have established a radioprotective effect for GM- CSF and G-CSF (85). This study utilized the in vitro colony growth assays for erythroid (erythroid, burst-forming unit, BFU-E) and granulocyte/macrophage progenitors (CFU-GM) exposed to varying sublethal doses of irradiation after 24 hours' incubation with these cytokines. Although truly pure populations of progenitors were not attainable, these human hematopoietic progenitors were highly depleted of lymphocytes, monocyte/macrophages, and differentiating myeloid and erythroid cells by the isolation procedures used. This study design decreased the possibility that the CSF effects were indirectly mediated (i.e., any effect seen on radiation sensitivity of the hematopoietic progenitors was presumptively a direct cytokine-progenitor cell effect).

Both GM-CSF and G-CSF decreased the radiation sensitivity and enhanced survival of GM-CFU. The radiation survival curves established a salutary effect of GM-CSF and G-CSF at and above the doses of 500 and 15 ng/mL, respectively. The improvement on the radiation survival curves of E-BFU were less impressive, although still significant, for GM-CSF. The radiation survival curves for E-BFU preincubated with G-CSF showed a trend toward sensitization, but this trend was not significant. Additional experiments with fractionated radiation showed that cytokine preincubation allowed progenitors to repair sublethal radiation damage. In marked contrast to subsequent in vivo work, GM-CSF was more effective in radioprotection than IL-1.

In a study by Neta and colleagues (53) comparing the effects of several cytokines administered to mice 20 hours prior to lethal irradiation, GM-CSF and G-CSF given alone conferred no protective effect. However, either CSF, when given in conjunction with a suboptimal radioprotective dose of IL-1, synergized and re-established radioprotection comparable to that achieved by an optimal IL-1 dose alone (41). This synergism was lost, however, at supralethal (1,150 cGy) radiation levels. A subsequent report by this group established that both CSFs conferred no effect on survival when administered to mice 1 to 3 hours after irradiation (86). In contrast, Talmadge and associates (87) reported both protective (preirradiation) and restorative (postirradiation) effects of GM-CSF. This study utilized lethal gamma-irradiation as opposed to the sublethal x-irradiation of the prior negative studies. Use of GM-CSF either 20 hours before or daily for 15 days beginning after lethal irradiation prolonged survival as compared with saline control; however, all mice ultimately succumbed in the pretreatment group. The posttreatment group and a group receiving both pre- and postirradiation GM-CSF had a modest 20% survival.

A subsequent experiment established improved survival in mice receiving both GM-CSF and a suboptimal dose of marrow cells in a murine bone marrow transplant model, as opposed to either intervention alone. Following their prior in vitro work, Uckun and colleagues (88) reported a definite protective effect of G-CSF in vivo. This murine study established radioprotection with G-CSF administered 24 hours or 30 minutes prior to gamma-irradiation; optimum radioprotection was achieved when the same total dose was administered in two divided doses both 24 hours and 30 minutes before irradiation. Little or

no radioprotection was seen, however, with supralethal radiation levels, nor did postirradiation G-CSF administration have any survival effect. The G-CSF protection related only to marrow hematopoiesis; pathological changes seen in the gut and the spleen with TBI were not affected. The finding that a single dose 30 minutes prior to irradiation confers hematopoietic protection is important because expansion of marrow progenitors could not occur within this time frame. Presumably cellular metabolic events could be the mechanism of protection with this dosage timing. The authors suggest that both alteration of progenitor cell cycling and the capacity to repair radiation damage are at issue in explaining the maximal efficacy of the split dosing regimen (88).

The major difference in this work and that of Neta and associates (41) is the escalation of G-CSF dose to 4 μg/animal, where protection is first noted, to the optimal dose of 40 μg/animal (88). Both studies agree on a lack of effect at and below 2 μg/animal. Whether the relatively high G-CSF doses elicit secondary cytokine release as the mechanism of radioprotection is unknown. Waddick and coworkers (89) subsequently extended their in vivo work and established radioprotection with GM-CSF, in addition to G-CSF. In contrast to their prior in vitro data (85), G-CSF was significantly more effective in vivo than GM-CSF. G-CSF and GM-CSF had no additive or synergistic activity when given together; in fact, GM-CSF given simultaneously or before G-CSF greatly attenuated the radioprotective effects of G-CSF.

Other animal data support a role for CSF use after irradiation with a myelorestorative intent. A murine study of varying doses and times of administration of G-CSF after LD$_{95/30}$ irradiation arrived at optimal conditions of 1 mg/kg given 2 hours after irradiation, and survival was not significantly different than a syngeneic BMT recipient group (90). In the murine model, both GM-CSF and G-CSF were found to significantly enhance hematopoietic recovery when administered for 10 days after a modest dose of irradiation (43). A study of G-CSF alone, but with different dose schedules, emphasized the need to begin therapy with this cytokine shortly (2 hr) after completion of irradiation, as well as the superiority of twice a day versus once daily dosing (91). Schuening and colleagues (92) conducted a study of allogeneic transplantation in dogs; animals received G-CSF for 10 days after TBI. G-CSF treatment significantly accelerated time to recovery of neutrophils, monocytes, and lymphocytes. Graft failure was low in both the treated group and the historical control animals. A trend toward greater incidence of graft-versus-host disease was noted, however, in the G-CSF group.

Clinical use of GM-CSF and G-CSF has been primarily in chemotherapy-induced marrow suppression. However, radiation therapy was included in two of the five different treatment groups (76% of all patients received 1200–1440 cGy TBI) included in the autologous BMT study, which led to FDA approval for GM-CSF (46). This work had been preceded by studies of primates undergoing TBI/autologous BMT with GM-CSF support (93). The human GM-CSF group was shown in this randomized, double-blind BMT trial to have an improved clinical outcome, as evidenced by earlier neutrophil recovery, fewer infections, and decreases in antibiotic use and hospital stay. Another similar study in the autologous BMT setting largely confirmed these findings (94). This study, in contrast to the former, was more homogenous: all patients were diagnosed with lymphoma and were treated at one medical center with one of two protocols; however, only 43% of the patients received radiation therapy (1,200 cGy TBI) as a part of their therapy. Neither study showed a statistically significant effect on survival with GM-CSF use.

Reports are now appearing regarding the use of CSFs in the setting of conventional fractionated radiation only or combined conventional chemotherapy plus radiotherapy protocols. Marks and associates (95) reported a patient with medulloblastoma undergoing craniospinal irradiation who was successfully treated with G-CSF for neutropenia. Although the patient had received prior heavy chemotherapy, the patient at the outset of radiotherapy had normal hematological values, which diminished over the subsequent 2 to 3 weeks. Use of G-CSF resulted in a significant increase in neutrophil count, and it allowed for completion of radiation with continued red cell and platelet transfusion support. Fushiki and colleagues (96) reported preliminary data on 12 leukopenic patients receiving G-CSF with radiotherapy alone or combination radiation and chemotherapy, with recovery of white counts despite continuation of therapy. Two additional studies suggest possible chemotherapy intensification with G-CSF use in combined chemoradiotherapy protocols for sarcoma and head and neck carcinoma (97,98). Also, GM-CSF was given to patients in the uncontrolled ^{60}cobalt radiation accident in Brazel (99); four of eight evaluable patients survived.

One final study deserves mention as an example of potential cytokine and radiation interactions. The Southwest Oncology Group (SWOG) reported more than 200 patients treated with combined chemotherapy and chest radiation therapy for limited-stage small-cell carcinoma of the lung (100). The GM-CSF arm received six cycles of chemotherapy, and the salient feature of the trial was 45 Gy chest radiotherapy in 25 fractions, resulting in overlap of GM-CSF administration with radiation. The study was closed due to increased toxocity in the GM-CSF arm, including grade 3/4 dyspnea, pneumonia, and an increase in infections, days febrile, and incidence of thrombocytopenia. These outcomes were despite reduction in incidence of granulocytopenia in the GM-CSF arm. These outcomes lend caution to the consideration of protocols featuring concomitant cytokine use and radiotherapy, and they are in accordance with untoward toxicities reported with concurrent chemotherapy and CSFs (101,102).

Although certain trials have reported decreases in mucositis with CSFs, these have been largely chemotherapy trials (103). No effect on mucositis by CSFs has been noted to date in protocols including radiotherapy (46,94). Likewise, no increase in tumor growth was noted in Phase I trails of these agents (74). This was a theoretical concern, due to reports of CSF receptors on certain tumors (72,104,105).

Considerable data support the use of CSFs with radiation therapy containing treatment regimens; clinical information to date has focused exclusively on myelorestorative usage. The mechanisms of CSF effects remain unknown; possibilities include alteration of hematopoietic progenitor cell cycle status, induction of DNA repair mechanisms, and generation of free radical scavengers, as has been proposed for IL-1 and TNF (33).

Interleukin-6

As part of the investigation of the cytokine cascades initiated by IL-1 (and by implication, LPS, among others), release of IL-6 in response to IL-1 from a variety of cell types that are known constituents of the marrow microenvironment has been described (106–108). This cytokine has proliferative effects on hematological progenitors, and it may be active at an early, pluripotent progenitor level (109). Because IL-6 is less toxic than IL-1 or TNF, possible replacement of the latter is clinically attractive if radioprotection is maintained by IL-6. Early work confirmed that detectable levels of serum IL-6 were induced by IL-1 administration; peak titers occurred 2 to 4 hours after intraperitoneal administration of IL-1 (43). An antibody to IL-1 receptor reduced this in vivo induction of IL-6 by IL-1 by 96 to 98% (22). Doses of up to 1,000 ng/mouse IL-6 given 20 hours before sublethal irradiation were not protective, however, and in fact were radiosensitizing (43). As with prior work by this group on CSFs, suboptimal doses of IL-1 plus IL-6 conferred greater radioprotection than that seen by the suboptimal dose of IL-1 alone. The authors present the hypothesis that IL-6 suppresses endogenous production of IL-1 as the cause of IL-6 radiosensitization when given alone. A follow-up study utilizing an anti-IL-6 blocking antibody revealed that (a) IL-6 contributes to innate radiation resistance because the antibody increased mortality in irradiated mice, and (b) IL-1 and TNF radioprotection is mediated to a major extent via IL-6 because the blocking antibody almost abrogated the protective effect of these cytokines along with circulating IL-6 levels in the serum (110). This finding contrasts with the lack of protection by IL-6 alone (43), and it suggests that IL-6 protective effects require the presence of other cytokines. In contrast with preirradiation use of IL-6, use of this cytokine after sublethal irradiation does confer accelerated multilineage hematopoietic recovery (111). This myelorestorative capacity of IL-6 was also noted in a primate model, although platelet recovery only was enhanced; there was no discernible effect on granulocyte recovery (112).

Interferons

Interferons (α, β, γ) are biological response modifiers with antiviral and antitumor activity (113). Biological effects include modulation of the cell cycle (114,115) and cell growth inhibition (116). These agents also have antitumor effects; IFN-α is FDA-approved on the basis of clinical trials in patients with hairy-cell leukemia, although it was also investigated with other cancers (117). IFN-γ is used in the treatment of chronic granulomatous disease (it is FDA-approved for this indication), and it is also under investigation for malignancy (117).

The known induction of IFN release secondary to LPS (118) provided the basis for early examination of IFN as a mediator of LPS radioprotection. Early work revealed a lack of effect of IFN-γ when given prior to $LD_{100/30}$–irradiated mice (53). A study of the effect of anti-IFN-γ antibody on LPS-induced radioprotection likewise found no effect (119). Several groups, however, had shown improved survival of mice treated after irradiation with partially purified preparations of IFN (i.e., fibroblast-derived, IFN-α, IFN-β) (120,121) or inducers of endogenous IFN production (122). This myelorestorative effect was later confirmed with recombinant IFN-α given as a single dose 1 to 3 hours after a $LD_{95/30}$ dose of irradiation (86). This enhancement of survival contrasts with the reports of tumor sensitization.

Other cytokines

A variety of other cytokines have been examined, albeit with largely negative results, conflicting results, or simply less data currently available. In vitro experiments with IL-2 and IL-3 have shown no protective action; IL-2 showed a trend toward sensitization, although this effect was not statistically significant (85,123). Recently, however, Waddick and Uckan (124) showed enhanced radiation repair capacity of myeloid progenitors without evidence of altered radiation sensitivity. IL-2 in vivo was reported to have no protective effect (53), whereas IL-3 administered after irradiation in primates enhanced hematopoietic recovery (89).

More recent studies reported from this laboratory demonstrated in vitro that basic fibroblast growth factor

(bFGF), in addition to inducing early day-12 CFU-S and committed hematopoietic progenitors, also provided radioprotection of murine or human hematopoietic progenitor cells (125). Dose escalation of irradiation from 0.5 to 5 Gy was studied in the presence or absence of dose-escalated bFGF (0.1–100 ng/mL). For example, 5 Gy irradiation in the presence of 0.5 ng/mL bFGF produced 60% survival, compared with 0% survival in the absence of bFGF. These studies have been extended to in vivo experiments, and the results are described in Fig. 36–1. Preliminary data also support a role for FGF in the induction of radiation repair mechanisms in cultured endothelial cells (126). It is hypothesized that radiation induces endothelial FGF, which acts in an autocrine fashion; the capacity of different sections of the vascular system to respond in this manner may paradoxically correlate with late vascular changes leading to organ injury (3).

Stem-cell factor is the product of the steel (sl) locus of the mouse, and it is the ligand for the c-kit tyrosine kinase receptor encoded by the white spotting (W) locus of the mouse. The biological properties of SCF demonstrate that the action of SCF is on very primitive cell populations, which have been described as stem-cell populations. The action of SCF on these early progenitors suggest that it may act as a radioprotective agent, similar to IL-1 using murine (127) or dog (128) models, although studies described earlier demonstrated that endogenous IL-1 is necessary for the full SCF radioprotective effect (59). Recent data suggest that the synergism of IL-1 and SCF relate to IL-1 induction of mRNA and subsequent cell surface expression of the SCF receptor (c-kit). Secondary cytokine release by SCF alone was not seen (59). Administration of a neutralizing antibody to SCF results in complete loss of

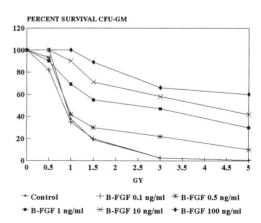

Figure 36–1 Effect of bFGF administered intraperitoneally in vivo 24 hours prior to whole body irradiation (950 cGy) in C57BL6 mice. Animals were killed and femoral marrow cells were plated for granulocyte-macrophage progenitors (CFU-GM). Each point represents an average of 5 animals; values are expressed as percent control.

LPS and IL-1 radioprotective effect; when given alone to sublethally irradiated mice (LD $_{50/30}$), there was a marked increase in mortality (129). This finding is very similar to previous work with antibodies directed against IL-1 receptor, TNF, or IL-6 (42,110), and it adds SCF to the constellation of cytokines contributing either to innate radiation resistance or to obligatory hematopoietic stem-cell support. Finally, IL-4 and leukemia inhibitory factor have also been reported to enhance the survival of irradiated mice when administered after irradiation (130). The mechanisms for their myelorestorative effects are unknown.

In addition to the aforementioned proposed role of TGF-β in late irradiation tissue injury, TGF-β has been reported to increase radiation lethality in mice when administered before or after irradiation (131). The authors reviewed and hypothesized which of the several known effects of TGF-β may explain this phenomenon (39). TGF-β may also have a role in the overall effects of LPS. The combined administration of anti-IL-1 receptor and anti-TNF antibodies in LPS-treated animals results in radiosensitization, as previously noted (42). LPS-induced TGF-β has been proposed as a candidate mediator of this effect (3).

Combination therapies

As the number of hematopoietic cytokines has grown, so has the number of combinations attempted to maximize in vitro progenitor support and proliferation. This approach has in the past few years extended into preclinical models of radioprotection/myelorestorative attempts. In a postirradiation treatment model with dogs, addition of IL-1 to erythropoietin (EPO) added little to the effects of EPO alone, and addition of GM-CSF to EPO likewise was considered not helpful (132). A previously discussed article showed actual antagonism between GM-CSF and G-CSF in a radioprotection model when GM-CSF was administered prior to G- CSF (89). The combination of IL-6 plus G-CSF after irradiation enhances murine marrow progenitor recovery, as compared with either treatment alone (133). Canine survival was not improved when combining SCF and G-CSF after irradiation (128). The combinations of multiple cytokines (and any secondary cytokine cascades triggered) may, as has been shown so far, elicit antagonistic or no salutary effects. In vitro combinations do not appear reliably predictive of in vivo effects.

Finally, of some interest is the data on the combination of SCF and the stable free radical, tempol, which were shown to act synergistically in radioprotection of mice (134). In a similar vein, the protein kinase C activator, bryostatin 1, enhances the radioprotective effect of GM-CSF (135), and the GM- CSF/IL-3 fusion protein PIXY 321 (136). The combination of the aminothiol WR-2721 [S-2(3-aminopropylamino)-ethyl phosphoronic acid; ethiofos; gammaphos], a potent radioprotectant, and G-CSF conferred enhanced survival in irradiated (LD$_{50/30}$) mice with greater than additive activity, as measured by the dose reduction factor (DRF) of the various treatments (Fig. 36–2) (137). This extensive study included the biological markers of peripheral blood counts and marrow and splenic hematopoietic progenitor pool sizes, which correlated with animal survival. These latter three combination trials are intriguing because the mechanisms of a cytokine plus another pharmacological agent may be quite different, and they may confer clinically useful synergistic radioprotection.

CYTOKINE MODULATION OF RADIATION INJURY TO MALIGNANT TUMORS

As previously noted, cytokines are important in tumorigenesis (see Chapter 34) and angiogenesis (see Chapter 35); the latter is critical to the ingrowth of new vessels to support the proliferating tumor mass. Radiation can alter gene expression and production of growth factors (138). Cytokines that alter cell cycle status or metabolic mechanisms of radiation repair in a manner that sensitizes malignant cells are potential candidates for clinical trials to test for improved irradiation effect.

As with the radioprotection literature, initial interventions in radiosensitization utilized several nonspecific immunomodulators. These attempts included use of BCG (139,140), anaerobic *Corynecbacterium* (141,142), and muramyl-tripeptide (143). Results with these agents were

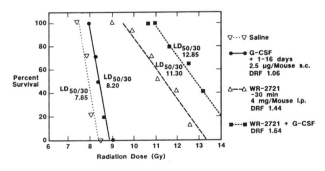

Figure 36–2 Effect of saline, G-CSF, WR-2721, and WR-2721 plus G-CSF treatments on survival of irradiated mice. C3H/HeN mice were administered WR-2721 (4 mg/mouse, IP) 30 minutes before ^{60}Co irradiation and G-CSF (2.5 μg/mouse/day, SC) on days 1 to 16 after irradiation. Each data point represents results obtained from 30 mice.

variable, and they did not appear clinically useful in combination with radiotherapy, in part due to serious side effects. Intratumoral injection resulted in one study in an improvement in radiation sensitivity (144). These variable results led to cytokine investigations when these factors became available.

Interferon

Interferon testing as a potential radiosensitizer of tumor began in the early 1980s, utilizing partially purified cell culture–derived IFNs. An early in vitro report utilizing murine fibroblast–derived IFN 2 hours prior to irradiation of murine 3T3 cells revealed enhancement of radiation response due to a reduction in the shoulder of the survival curve, with no effect on the slope (145). Human IFN had no effect. This report was followed by similar data utilizing human fibroblast–derived IFN (partially purified IFN-β) against HeLA cells (cervical cancer cell line) and WI-38- CT-I cells (a transformed fibroblast line) (146). A study performed using both partially purified human IFN-α and IFN-β on a human bronchogenic carcinoma cell line showed radiosensitization and intrinsic growth inhibition with IFN-β, but not IFN-α (147).

When the IFNs became available in recombinant form, Chang and Keng (148) tested IFN-α, IFN-β, and IFN-γ against human hypernephroma cells, with different periods of preincubation prior to irradiation. IFN-α and IFN-β were associated with modest cell growth inhibition; IFN-γ had the most potent effect. These activities were reflected in the relative efficacy of these agents as radiosensitizers. The test IFNs were present during irradiation, along with the preincubation exposure in these studies. The sensitizing effect, in addition to being IFN subtype–dependent, was radiation dose–and IFN exposure time–dependent. The longest preincubation (29 hr) had the most potent effect. These studies showed a greater accumulation of cells in the G_2-M phase of the cell cycle in the IFN/radiation–treated group 24 and 48 hours after irradiation, as compared with either treatment alone.

Although confirming the radiosensitizing effect of pretreatment with IFN-α against a small-cell carcinoma cell line, Kardamakis and associates (149) found no alteration in the distribution of cells in the phases of cell cycle measured 24 and 72 hours after irradiation. One mouse study with IFN-α/β given after irradiation showed enhanced survival in animals bearing P388 leukemia cells, as opposed to animals receiving either treatment alone (120). This enhancement was felt to be a result of radioprotection of normal tissue and concomitant radiosensitization of the tumor. More recently, a Phase I/II trial of radiation with or without natural IFN-α given before the radiotherapy sessions for patients with inoperable nonsmall-cell lung cancer was reported (150). Although a small study

(20 patients) and with essentially equal responses (5/10 partial responses [PRs] with radiotherapy alone, 6/10 PRs with combination therapy), it was noted that administration of the combination was laborious and toxic. The combined radiotherapy/IFN patients suffered early radiological changes of pulmonary injury in the majority, and 4 of 10 patients suffered severe esophagitis not seen in the radiotherapy-only arm. Severe mucositis and esophagitis was also noted by several other groups with combined therapy or prior (recent) treatment with IFN followed by TBI plus chemotherapy in a bone marrow transplant protocol (151,152). A Phase I/II trial of IFN-β is planned by the Radiation Therapy Oncology Group (RTOG) for advanced local nonsmall-cell lung cancer.

Despite encouraging preclinical results, clinical IFN administration has been associated with significant toxicities. Optimization of the combination of IFN and radiotherapy in animal models and subsequently humans will require additional carefully controlled studies.

Tumor necrosis factor

Tumor necrosis factor is a cytokine with intrinsic antitumor effects that can act as a growth factor with certain normal cell types (153). A part of TNFs antitumor capacity (in addition to direct effects on tumor cells) relates to its promotion of thrombosis (154), resulting in tumor microvascular obliteration and subsequent hemorrhagic necrosis (155). Early work with recombinant human TNF-α as a potential enhancer of radiotherapy revealed no activity in vitro, but there was a delay in in vivo tumor regrowth with the combination of radiotherapy followed by TNF greater than that seen with either treatment alone (156). Certain conclusions of this study are tempered by the use of human TNF in a murine tumor and model system, as well as administration of TNF after the irradiation dose. Another in vitro study utilized human recombinant TNF against a battery of human carcinomas (157). Synergistic (4 cell lines) or additive (3 cell lines) antitumor effect was seen with the combination of TNF and irradiation. The maximum effects were observed when tumor cell line exposure to TNF preceded irradiation by 4 to 12 hours. The authors hypothesize that the cooperative effects relate to the observation that TNF-induced hydroxyl radical production requires several hours, is not noted in TNF-resistant lines (158), and may interact favorably with the radiation-induced free radical production, which is also an intermediate of DNA damage (159).

Another study investigated postirradiation human TNF use in a murine model (160). This study confirmed that augmentation of antitumor effect with the combination occurred at a higher (800 cGy) radiation dose, with no overt toxicity. These encouraging results, coupled to data on hematopoietic radioprotection, should lead to investigations of dose scheduling and simultaneous examination of both radiosensitization of tumor and radioprotection of normal tissue. Human Phase I clinical trials are in progress with radiotherapy plus TNF (4).

Epidermal growth factor

Recent work by Sutherland and colleagues (138) with EGF has added this cytokine to the small family of potential radiosensitizers. The first in vitro observation of this effect was shown with a human squamous-cell carcinoma line; the best result was noted when EGF was present after as opposed to before and during irradiation (161). A reduction in the shoulder region of cell survival curves and decreased plating efficiency were associated with this enhanced radiosensitivity. A subsequent study of 4 human squamous carcinoma cell lines concluded that EGF-related radiosensitization was dependent on EGF receptor density (162). A model utilizing one of these cell lines grown as spheroids indicates a role for cell-to-cell interactions (163) and cell cycle in the radiosensitizing effect (164). The work of this group is reviewed in detail by Sutherland and colleagues (138). This group has elicited this radiosensitizing effect in 3 of 4 squamous-cell lines derived from a variety of tumor sites (i.e., vulva, cervix, tongue), whereas a preliminary study with human breast adenocarcinoma cells and EGF revealed a lack of radiosensitization (165). A broader survey of tumor cell types may elicit a distinct category of tumor types responsive to EGF.

SUMMARY

Considerable data suggest a potential role for cytokine modulation of radiation injury in either a protective/supportive role (of normal tissues) or a sensitizing (of tumor) role. Additional elucidation of the secondary cytokine cascades sometimes triggered and of the interactions in vivo between the various cytokines will hopefully lead to rational use, dosing, and scheduling of these factors. Questions of clinical efficacy must await the results of carefully crafted and executed controlled, randomized human trials.

REFERENCES

1. Adams GE. Current topics: lethality from acute and protracted radiation exposure in man. Int J Radiat Biol 1984; 46:209–217.

2. Plowman PN. The effects of conventionally fractionated, extended portal radiotherapy on the human peripheral blood count. Int J Radiat Oncol Biol Phys 1983;9:829–839.

3. Hallahan DE, Haimovits-Friedman A, Kufe DW, Fuks Z,

Weichselbaum RR. The role of cytokines in radiation oncology. In: DeVita VT, Hellman S, Rosenberg SA, eds. Important advances in oncology 1993. Philadelphia: JB Lippincott, 1993:71–80.

4. Weichselbaum RR, Beckett MA, Hallahan DE, Kufe DW, Vokes EE. Molecular targets to overcome radioresistance. Semin Oncol 1992;19(suppl 11):14–20.

5. Weichselbaum RR. Cellular and molecular aspects of human tumor radioresistance. In: DeVita VT Jr, Hellman S, Rosenberg SA, eds. Important advances in oncology 1991. Philadelphia: JB Lippincott, 1991:73–83.

6. Yamamura M, Modlin RL, Ohmen JD, Moy RL. Local expression of antiinflammatory cytokines in cancer. J Clin Invest 1993;91:1005–1010.

7. Pekarek LA, Weichselbaum RR, Beckett MA, Nachman J, Schreiber H. Footprinting of individual tumors and their variants by constitutive cytokine expression patterns. Cancer Res 1993;53:1978–1981.

8. Gualtieri RJ. Consequences of extremely high doses of irradiation on bone marrow stromal cells and the release of hematopoietic growth factors. Exp Hematol 1987;15:952–957.

9. Albaerico TA, Ihle JN, Liang CM, McGrath HE, Quesenberry PJ. Stromal growth factor production in irradiated lectin exposed long-term murine bone marrow cultures. Blood 1987;69:1120–1127.

10. Brach MA, Grub HJ, Kaisho T, Asano Y, Hirano T, Herrmann F. Ionizing radiation induces expression of interleukin 6 by human fibroblasts involving activation of nuclear factor-kB. J Biol Chem 1993;268:8466–8472.

11. Ansel J, Luger TA, Kock A, Hochstein D, Green I. The effect of in vitro UV irradiation on the production of IL-1 by murine macrophages and P388D$_1$ cells[1]. J Immunol 1984; 133:1350–1355.

12. Anscher MS, Crocker IR, Jirtle RL. Transforming growth factor-β1 expression in irradiated liver. Radiat Res 1990; 122:77–85.

13. Canney PA, Dean S. Transforming growth factor beta: a promoter of late connective tissue injury following radiotherapy? Br J Radiol 1990;63:620–623.

14. Jirtle RL, Anscher MS. The role of TGF-β1 in the pathogenesis of radiation-induced hepatic fibrosis. In: Dewey WC, Edington M, Fry FJM, Hall EJ, Whitmore GR, eds. Radiation research: a twentieth-century perspective, vol II. San Diego: Academic Press, 1992:821–823.

15. Witte L, Fuks Z, Haimovitz-Friedman A, Vlodavsky I, Goodman DS, Eldor A. Effects of irradiation on the release of growth factors from cultured bovine, porcine, and human endothelial cells. Cancer Res 1989;49:5066–5072.

16. Haimovitz-Friedman A, Vlodavsky I, Chaudhuri A, Witte L, Fuks Z. Autocrine effects of fibroblast growth factor in repair of radiation damage in endothelial cells. Cancer Res 1991;51:2552–2558.

17. Sherman ML, Datta R, Hallahan DE, Weichselbaum RR, Kufe DW. Regulation of tumor necrosis factor gene expression by ionizing radiation in human myeloid leukemia cells and peripheral blood monocytes. J Clin Invest 1991;87: 1794–1797.

18. Hallahan DE, Virudachalam S, Sherman ML, Huberman E, Kufe DW, Weichselbaum RR. Tumor necrosis factor gene expression is mediated by protein kinase C following acti-

vation by ionizing radiation. Cancer Res 1991;51:4565–4569.

19. Rubin P, Finkelstein J, Shapiro D. Molecular biology mechanisms in the radiation induction of pulmonary injury syndromes: interrelationship between the alveolar macrophage and the septal fibroblast. Int J Radiat Oncol Biol Phys 1992;24:93–101.

20. Hallahan DE, Spriggs DR, Beckett MA, Kufe DW, Weichselbaum RR. Increased tumor necrosis factor α mRNA after cellular exposure to ionizing radiation. Proc Natl Acad Sci USA 1989;86:10104–10107.

21. Kramer M, Sachsenmaier C, Herrlich P, Rahmsdorf HJ. UV irradiation-induced interleukin-1 and basic fibroblast growth factor synthesis and release mediate part of the UV response. J Biol Chem 1993;268:6734–6741.

22. Neta R, Vogel SN, Plocinski JM, Tare NS, Benjamin W, Chizzonite R, Pilcher M. In vivo modulation with anti-interleukin-1 (IL-1) receptor (p80) antibody 35F5 of the response to IL-1. The relationship of radioprotection, colony-stimulating factor, and IL- 6. Blood 1990;76:57–62.

23. Gaitan S, Tejero C, Humphreys ER, Lord BI. A relationship between residual stromal damage in hematopoietic tissue and the functional activity of granulocytes. Exp Hematol 1993;21:1227–1232.

24. DeVita VT. Principles of chemotherapy. In: DeVita VT, Hellman S, Rosenberg SA, eds. Cancer: principles and practice of oncology, ed 4. Philadelphia: JB Lippincott, 1993: 276–292.

25. Hewitt HB, Wilson CW. A survival curve for mammalian leukaemia cells irradiated in vivo: implications for the treatment of mouse leukaemia by whole body irradiation. Br J Cancer 1959;13:69–75.

26. Chopra R, Goldstone AH. Modern trends in bone marrow transplantation for acute myeloid and acute lymphoblastic leukemia. Curr Opin Oncol 1992;4:247–258.

27. Martin PJ. Animal experimentation relevant to human marrow transplantation. Curr Opin Oncol 1992;4:239–246.

28. Mefford RB, Henkel DT, Loeffer JB. Effect of pyromen on survival of irradiated mice. Proc Soc Exp Biol Med 1953; 83:54–63.

29. Smith WW, Alderman IM, Gillespe RF. Increased survival in irradiated animals treated with bacterial endotoxins. Am J Physiol 1957;191:124–130.

30. Ainsworth EJ, Chase HB. Effect of microbial antigens on irradiation mortality in mice. Proc Soc Exp Biol Med 1959; 102:483–485.

31. Behling UH. The radioprotective effect of bacterial endotoxin. In: Nowotny A, ed. Beneficial effects of endotoxin. New York: Plenum Press, 1983:127–148.

32. Patchen ML, D'Alesandro MM, Brook I, Blakely WF, MacVittie TJ. Glucan: mechanisms involved in its radioprotective effect. J Leukocyte Biol 1987;42:95–105.

33. Talmadge JE. Therapeutic potential of cytokines and peptides in irradiation-induced myelosuppression. In: Dewey WC, Edington M, Fry RJM, Hall EJ, Whitmore GF, eds. Radiation research: a twentieth-century perspective, vol II. San Diego: Academic Press, 1992:834–838.

34. Vacek A, Rotkovska D, Bartonickova A. Radioprotection of hemopoiesis conferred by aqueous extract from chlorococ-

cal algae (Invastimul) administered to mice before irradiation. Exp Hematol 1990;18:234–237.

35. Kalechman Y, Albeck M, Oron M, et al. Radioprotective effects of the immunomodulator AS101. J Immunol 1990; 145:1512–1517.

36. Vacek A, Sikulova J, Bartonickova A. Radiation resistance in mice increased following chronic application of lithium carbonate. Acta Radiol Oncol 1982;21:325–330.

37. Gallicchio VS, Chen MG, Watts TD, Gamba-Vitalo C. Lithium stimulates the recovery of granulopoiesis following acute radiation injury. Exp Hematol 1983;11:553–563.

38. Gallicchio VS, Chen MG, Watts TD. Ability of lithium to accelerate the recovery of granulopoiesis after subacute radiation injury. Acta Radiol Oncol 1984;23:361–366.

39. Neta R, Oppenheim JJ. Radioprotection with cytokines—Learning from nature to cope with radiation damage. Cancer Cell 1991;3:391–396.

40. Neta R, Douches S, Oppenheim JJ. Interleukin-1 is a radioprotector. J Immunol 1986;136:2483–2485.

41. Neta R, Oppenheim JJ, Douches SD. Interdependence of the radioprotective effects of human recombinant interleukin-1α, tumor necrosis factor α, granulocyte colony-stimulating factor, and murine recombinant granulocyte-macrophage colony stimulating factor. J Immunol 1988;140:108–111.

42. Neta R, Oppenheim JJ, Schreiber RD, Chizzonite R, Ledney GD, MacVittie TJ. Role of cytokines (Interleukin 1, tumor necrosis factor, and transforming growth factor β) in natural and lipopolysaccharide-enhanced radioresistance. J Exp Med 1991;173:1177–1182.

43. Tanikawa S, Nakai I, Tsuneoka K, Nara N. Effects of recombinant granulocyte colony-stimulating factor (rG-CSF) and recombinant granulocyte-macrophage colony-stimulating factor (rGM-CSF) on acute radiation hematopoietic injury in mice. Exp Hematol 1989;17:883–888.

44. Zoon KC, Cohen RB, Gerrard T. Regulatory issues involved in hematopoietic growth factor approval. Semin Oncol 1992;19:432–440.

45. Athens JW. Granulocytes monocytes. In: Lee GR, Bithell TC, Foerster J, Athens JW, Lukens JN, eds. Wintrobe's clinical hematology, ed 9. Philadelphia: Lean & Febiger, 1993:223–266.

46. Nemunaitis J, Rabinowe SN, Singer JW, et al. Recombinant granulocyte-macrophage colony-stimulating factor after autologous bone marrow transplantation for lymphoid cancer. N Engl J Med 1991;324:1773–1778.

47. Crawford J, Ozer H, Stokker R, et al. Reduction by granulocyte colony-stimulating factor of fever and neutropenia induced by chemotherapy in patients with small-cell lung cancer. N Engl J Med 1991;325:164–170.

48. Avalos BR, Gasson JC, Hedvat C, et al. Human granulocyte colony-stimulating factor: biologic activities and receptor characterization on hematopoietic cells and small cell lung cancer cell lines. Blood 1990;75:851–857.

49. Baldwin GC, Gasson JC, Kaufman SE, et al. Non-hematopoietic tumor cells express functional GM-CSF receptors. Blood 1989;73:1033–1037.

50. Schuchter LM, Luginbuhl WE, Meropol NJ. The current status of toxicity protectants in cancer therapy. Semin Oncol 1992;19:742–751.

114. Watanabe Y, Sokawa Y. Effect of interferon on the cell cycle of Balb/C 3T3 cells. J Gen Virol 1978;41:411–415.

115. d'Hooghe C, Brouty-Boye D, Malaise E, Gresser I. Interferon and cell division XII. Prolongation by interferon of the intermitotic phase of mouse mammary tumor cells in vitro. Microcinematographic analysis. Exp Cell Res 1977; 105:73–77.

116. Pauker K, Cantell K, Henke W. Quantitative studies on viral interference in suspended L-cells. III. Effect of interfering viruses and interferon on the growth rate of cells. Virology 1962;17:324–334.

117. Baron S, Tyring SK, Fleischmann WR Jr, et al. The interferons: mechanisms of action and clinical applications. JAMA 1991;266:1375.

118. Younger JS, Stinebring WR. Interferon appearance stimulated by endotoxin, bacteria or viruses in mice pre-treated with Escherichia coli or infected with Mycobacterium tuberculosis. Nature 1965;208:456–458.

119. Neta R, Oppenheim JJ, Ledney GD, MacVittie TJ. Role of cytokines in innate and LPS-enhanced radioresistance. In: Dewey WC, Edington M, Fry FJM, Hall EJ, Whitmore GF, eds. Radiation Research: a twentieth-century perspective, vol II. San Diego: Academic Press, 1992;830–833.

120. Borden EC, Sidky YA. Interferon (IFN)-α/β and irradiation (XRT): protection against lethality and augmentation of antitumor effects (abstract A1536). Proc Am Assoc Cancer Res 1989;30:387.

121. Ortaldo JR, McCoy JL. Protective effects of interferon in mice previously exposed to lethal irradiation. Radiat Res 1980;81:262–266.

122. Talas M, Fedorenko B, Batkai L, Stoger I. Interferon production by and radioprotective effect of poly I:C and tilorone in mice exposed to helium alpha irradiation. Acta Microbiol Hung 1985;32:225–231.

123. Gallicchio VS, Hulette BC, Messino MJ, Gass C, Bieschke MW, Doukas MA. Effect of various interleukins (IL-1, IL-2, and IL-3) on the in vitro radioprotection of bone marrow progenitors (CFU-GM and CFU-MEG). J Biol Resp Mod 1989;8:479–487.

124. Waddick KG, Uckun FM. Effects of recombinant interleukin-3 and recombinant interleukin-6 on radiation survival of normal human bone marrow progenitor cells. Radiat Oncol Invest 1993;1:34–40.

125. Gallicchio VS, Hughes NK, Hulette BC, DellaPuca R, Noblitt L. Basic fibroblast growth factor (B-FGF) induces early- (CFU-S) and late-stage hematopoietic progenitor cell colony formation (CFU-gm, CFU-meg, and BFU-e) by synergizing with GM-CSF, Meg-CSF, and erythropoietin, and is a radioprotective agent in vitro. Int J Cell Clon 1991; 9:220–232.

126. Haimovitz-Friedman A, Vlodavsky I, Chadhuri A, Witte L, Fuks Z. Autocrine effects of fibroblast growth factor in repair of radiation damage in endothelial cells. Cancer Res 1991;51:2552–2558.

127. Zsebo KM, Smith KA, Hartley CA, Greenblatt M, Cooke K, Rich W, McNiece IK. Radioprotection of mice by recombinant rat stem cell factor. Proc Natl Acad Sci USA 1992; 89:9464–9468.

128. Schuening FG, Appelbaum FR, Deeg HJ, Sullivan-Pepe M, Graham TC, Hackman R. Effects of recombinant canine stem cell factor, a c-kit ligand, and recombinant granulo-cyte colony-stimulating factor on hematopoietic recovery after otherwise lethal total body irradiation. Blood 1993; 81:20–26.

129. Neta R, Williams D, Selzer F, Abrams J. Inhibition of c-kit ligand/steel factor by antibodies reduces survival of lethally irradiated mice. Blood 1993;81:324–327.

130. Neta R, Wong GHW, Pilcher M. LIF and IL-4 used after lethal irradiation protect mice from death (abstract.) Lymphokine Res 1990;9:568.

131. Neta R, Oppenheim JJ, Schreiber RD, Chizzonite R, Ledney GD, MacVittie TJ. Role of cytokines (interleukin 1, tumor necrosis factor and transforming growth factor β) in natural and lipopolysaccharide-enhanced radioresistance. J Exp Med 1991;173:1177–1182.

132. Selig C, Nothdurft W, Kreja L, Fliedner M. Influence of combined treatment with Interleukin 1 and erythropoietin or GM-CSF and erythropoietin on the regeneration of hemopoiesis in the dog after total body irradiation—a preliminary report. Behring Inst Mitt 1991;90:86–92.

133. Patchen ML, Fischer R, MacVittie TJ. Effects of combined administration of interleukin-6 and granulocyte colony-stimulating factor on recovery from radiation-induced hemopoietic aplasia. Exp Hematol 1993;21:338–344.

134. Liebmann J, DeLuca AM, Epstein A, Steinberg S, Morstyn G, Mitchell JB. Protection from lethal irradiation by the combination of stem cell factor and tempol. Radiat Res 1994;137:400–404.

135. Grant S, Pettit GR, McCrady C. Effect of Bryostatin 1 on the in vitro radioprotective capacity of recombinant granulocyte-macrophage colony-stimulating factor (rGM-CSF) toward committed human myeloid progenitor cells (CFU-GM). Exp Hematol 1992;20:34–42.

136. Grant S, Traylor RS, Pettit GR, Lin PS. The macrolytic lactone protein kinase C activator, bryostatin 1, either alone, or in conjunction with recombinant murine granulocyte-macrophage colony-stimulating factor, protects Balb/c and C3H/HeN mice from the lethal in vivo effects of ionizing radiation. Blood 1994;83:663–667.

137. Patchen ML, MacVittie TJ, Souza LM. Postirradiation treatment with granulocyte colony-stimulating factor and pre-irradiation WR-2721 administration synergize to enhance hemopoietic reconstitution and increase survival. Int J Radiat Oncol Biol Physiol 1992;22:773–779.

138. Sutherland RM, Ausserer WA, Grant TD, et al. Regulatory polypeptide factors, signal transduction and radiation response. In: Dewey WC, Edington M, Fry FJM, Hall EJ, Whitmore GF, eds. Radiation research: a twentieth-century perspective, vol II. San Diego: Academic Press, 1992: 824–829.

139. Haddow A, Alexander P. An immunological method of increasing the sensitivity of primary sarcomas to local irradiation with x-rays. Lancet 1964;1:452–457.

140. Dubois JB, Serrou B. Treatment of the mouse Lewis tumor by the association of radiotherapy and immunotherapy with bacillus Calmette-Guerin. Cancer Res 1976;36:1731–1734.

141. Milas L, Hunter N, Withers HR. Combination of local irradiation with systemic application of anaerobic corynebacteria in therapy of a murine fibrosarcoma. Cancer Res 1975;35:1274–1277.

142. Milas L, Hunter N, Stone HB, Withers RH. Corynebacte-

produce granulocyte colony-stimulating factor and macrophage colony- stimulating factor. Blood 1988;71:430–435.

84. Sieff CA, Tsai S, Faller DV. Interleukin 1 induces cultured human endothelial cell production of granulocyte-macrophage colony-stimulating factor. J Clin Invest 1987;79:48–51.

85. Uckun FM, Gillis S, Souza L, Song CW. Effects of recombinant growth factors on radiation survival of human bone marrow progenitor cells. Int J Radiat Oncol Biol Physiol 1989;16:415–435.

86. Neta R, Oppenheim JJ. Cytokines in therapy of radiation injury. Blood 1988;72:1093–1095.

87. Talmadge JE, Tribble H, Pennington R, et al. Protective, restorative, and therapeutic properties of recombinant colony-stimulating factors. Blood 1989;73:2093–2103.

88. Uckun FM, Souza L, Waddick KG, Wick M, Song CW. In vivo radioprotective effects of recombinant human granulocyte colony-stimulating factor in lethally irradiated mice. Blood 1990;75:638–645.

89. Waddick KG, Song CW, Souza L, Uckum FM. Comparative analysis of the in vivo radioprotective effects of recombinant granulocyte colony stimulating factor (G-CSF), recombinant granulocyte-macrophage CSF, and their combination. Blood 1991;77:2364–2372.

90. Sureda A, Valls A, Kadar E, et al. A single dose of granulocyte colony stimulating factor modifies radiation induced death in $B_6D_2F_1$ mice (abstract #631). Exp Hematol 1993; 21:1605–1607.

91. Tanikawa S, Nose M, Aoki Y, Tsuneoka K, Shikita M, Nara N. Effects of recombinant human granulocyte colony-stimulating factor on the hematologic recovery and survival of irradiated mice. Blood 1990;76:445–449.

92. Schuening GF, Storb R, Goehle S, et al. Recombinant human granulocyte colony-stimulating factor accelerates hematopoietic recovery after DLA-identical littermate marrow transplants in dogs. Blood 1990;76:636–640.

93. Niehuis AW, Donahue RE, Karlsson S. Recombinant human granulocyte-macrophage stimulating factor (GM-CSF) shortens the period of neutropenia after autologous bone marrow transplantation in a primate model. J Clin Invest 1987;80:573–577.

94. Advani R, Chao NJ, Horning SJ, et al. Granulocyte- macrophage colony-stimulating factor (GM-CSF) as an adjunct to autologous hemopoietic stem cell transplantation for lymphoma. Ann Intern Med 1992;116:183–189.

95. Marks LB, Friedman HS, Kurtzbert J, Oakes WJ, Hockenberger BM. Reversal of radiation-induced neutropenia by granulocyte colony-stimulating factor. Med Pediatr Oncol 1992;20:240–242.

96. Fushiki M, Ono K, Takahashi M, Abe M. Clinical effects of recombinant human granulocyte colony-stimulating factor on neutropenia induced by irradiation (abstract A91). Radiat Oncol Biol Physiol 1989;17(suppl 1):162.

97. Brachman D, Haraf D, Weichselbaum R, McEvilly J, Luckett P, Vokes E. Granulocyte-colony stimulating factor (G-CSF) and concomitant accelerated chemoradiotherapy for advanced head and neck cancer (HNC): a dose-escalation study (abstract A905). Proc Am Soc Clin Oncol 1993; 12:280.

98. Womer RB, Daller RT, Miser A, Miser J. G-CSF allows dose intensification by interval reduction in pediatric sarcomas (abstract A351). Proc Am Soc Clin Oncol 1993;12:138.

99. Butturini A, Gale RP, Lopes DM, et al. Use of recombinant granulocyte-macrophage colony stimulating factor in the Brazil radiation accident. Lancet 1988;2:471–474.

100. Bunn PA Jr, Crowley J, Hazuka M, Tolley R, Livingston R. The role of GM-CSF in limited stage SCLC: a randomized phase III study of the Southwest Oncology Group (SWOG) (abstract A974). Proc Am Soc Clin Oncol 1992;11:292.

101. Meropol NJ, Miller LL, Korn EL, et al. Severe myelosuppression resulting from concurrent administration of granulocyte colony-stimulating factor and cytotoxic chemotherapy. J Natl Cancer Inst 1994;84:1201–1203.

102. Robert NJ, Taylor SG, Bowker B, et al. Phase I study of dose escalation of cyclophosphamide, adriamycin, and 5 FU with GM- CSF in metastatic breast cancer: an ECOG protocol. Proc Adj Ther Breast Cancer 1992:79.

103. Gabrilove JJ, Jakubowski A, Scher H, et al. Effect of granulocyte colony-stimulating factor on neutropenia and associated morbidity due to chemotherapy for transitional-cell carcinoma of the urothelium. N Engl J Med 1988;318: 1414–1422.

104. Baldwin GC, Gasson JC Kaufman SE, et al. Non-hematopoietic tumor cells express functional GM-CSF receptors. Blood 1989;73:1033–1037.

105. Berdel WE, Danhauser-Riedl S, Doll M, Herrmann F. Effect of hematopoietic growth factors on the growth of non-hematopoietic tumor cell lines. In: Mertelsmann R, Herrmann F, eds. Hematopoietic growth factors in clinical applications. New York: Marcel Dekker, 1990:339–362.

106. Van Damme J, Opdenakker G, Simpson RJ, et al. Identification of the human 26-kD protein, interferon β_2 (IFN-β_2), as a B-cell hybridoma/plasmacytoma growth factor induced by interleukin-1 and tumor necrosis factor. J Exp Med 1987;165:914.

107. Sironi M, Breviario F, Poserpio P, et al. IL-1 stimulates IL-6 production in endothelial cells. J Immunol 1989;142:549.

108. Bauer J, Ganter U, Geiger T, et al. Regulation of interleukin-6 expression in cultured human blood monocytes and monocyte-derived macrophages. Blood 1988;72:1134.

109. Kishimoto T. The biology of interleukin-6 (review article). Blood 1989;74:1–10.

110. Neta R, Perlstein R, Vogel SN, Ledney GD, Abrams J. Role of interleukin 6 (IL-6) in protection from lethal irradiation and in endocrine responses to IL-1 and tumor necrosis factor. J Exp Med 1992;175:689–694.

111. Patchen ML, MacVittie TJ, Williams JL, Schwartz GN, Souza LM. Administration of interleukin-6 stimulates multilineage hematopoiesis and accelerates recovery from radiation-induced hematopoietic depression. Blood 1991; 77:472–480.

112. MacVittie TJ, Farese AM, Patchen ML, Myers LA. Comparative therapeutic efficacy of combination recombinant human IL-6 and IL-3 cytokine protocols in a primate model of radiation-induced marrow aplasia (abstract A592). Exp Hematol 1993;21:1171.

113. Mossman KL, Hill LT, Dritschilo A. Utility of interferons in clinical radiotherapy. J Natl Med Assoc 1982;74:1083–1087.

114. Watanabe Y, Sokawa Y. Effect of interferon on the cell cycle of Balb/C 3T3 cells. J Gen Virol 1978;41:411–415.

115. d'Hooghe C, Brouty-Boye D, Malaise E, Gresser I. Interferon and cell division XII. Prolongation by interferon of the intermitotic phase of mouse mammary tumor cells in vitro. Microcinematographic analysis. Exp Cell Res 1977; 105:73–77.

116. Pauker K, Cantell K, Henke W. Quantitative studies on viral interference in suspended L-cells. III. Effect of interfering viruses and interferon on the growth rate of cells. Virology 1962;17:324–334.

117. Baron S, Tyring SK, Fleischmann WR Jr, et al. The interferons: mechanisms of action and clinical applications. JAMA 1991;266:1375.

118. Younger JS, Stinebring WR. Interferon appearance stimulated by endotoxin, bacteria or viruses in mice pre-treated with Escherichia coli or infected with Mycobacterium tuberculosis. Nature 1965;208:456–458.

119. Neta R, Oppenheim JJ, Ledney GD, MacVittie TJ. Role of cytokines in innate and LPS-enhanced radioresistance. In: Dewey WC, Edington M, Fry FJM, Hall EJ, Whitmore GF, eds. Radiation Research: a twentieth-century perspective, vol II. San Diego: Academic Press, 1992;830–833.

120. Borden EC, Sidky YA. Interferon (IFN)-α/β and irradiation (XRT): protection against lethality and augmentation of antitumor effects (abstract A1536). Proc Am Assoc Cancer Res 1989;30:387.

121. Ortaldo JR, McCoy JL. Protective effects of interferon in mice previously exposed to lethal irradiation. Radiat Res 1980;81:262–266.

122. Talas M, Fedorenko B, Batkai L, Stoger I. Interferon production by and radioprotective effect of poly I:C and tilorone in mice exposed to helium alpha irradiation. Acta Microbiol Hung 1985;32:225–231.

123. Gallicchio VS, Hulette BC, Messino MJ, Gass C, Bieschke MW, Doukas MA. Effect of various interleukins (IL-1, IL-2, and IL-3) on the in vitro radioprotection of bone marrow progenitors (CFU-GM and CFU-MEG). J Biol Resp Mod 1989;8:479–487.

124. Waddick KG, Uckun FM. Effects of recombinant interleukin-3 and recombinant interleukin-6 on radiation survival of normal human bone marrow progenitor cells. Radiat Oncol Invest 1993;1:34–40.

125. Gallicchio VS, Hughes NK, Hulette BC, DellaPuca R, Noblitt L. Basic fibroblast growth factor (B-FGF) induces early- (CFU-S) and late-stage hematopoietic progenitor cell colony formation (CFU-gm, CFU-meg, and BFU-e) by synergizing with GM-CSF, Meg-CSF, and erythropoietin, and is a radioprotective agent in vitro. Int J Cell Clon 1991; 9:220–232.

126. Haimovitz-Friedman A, Vlodavsky I, Chadhuri A, Witte L, Fuks Z. Autocrine effects of fibroblast growth factor in repair of radiation damage in endothelial cells. Cancer Res 1991;51:2552–2558.

127. Zsebo KM, Smith KA, Hartley CA, Greenblatt M, Cooke K, Rich W, McNiece IK. Radioprotection of mice by recombinant rat stem cell factor. Proc Natl Acad Sci USA 1992; 89:9464–9468.

128. Schuening FG, Appelbaum FR, Deeg HJ, Sullivan-Pepe M, Graham TC, Hackman R. Effects of recombinant canine stem cell factor, a c-kit ligand, and recombinant granulo-cyte colony-stimulating factor on hematopoietic recovery after otherwise lethal total body irradiation. Blood 1993; 81:20–26.

129. Neta R, Williams D, Selzer F, Abrams J. Inhibition of c-kit ligand/steel factor by antibodies reduces survival of lethally irradiated mice. Blood 1993;81:324–327.

130. Neta R, Wong GHW, Pilcher M. LIF and IL-4 used after lethal irradiation protect mice from death (abstract.) Lymphokine Res 1990;9:568.

131. Neta R, Oppenheim JJ, Schreiber RD, Chizzonite R, Ledney GD, MacVittie TJ. Role of cytokines (interleukin 1, tumor necrosis factor and transforming growth factor β) in natural and lipopolysaccharide-enhanced radioresistance. J Exp Med 1991;173:1177–1182.

132. Selig C, Nothdurft W, Kreja L, Fliedner M. Influence of combined treatment with Interleukin 1 and erythropoietin or GM-CSF and erythropoietin on the regeneration of hemopoiesis in the dog after total body irradiation—a preliminary report. Behring Inst Mitt 1991;90:86–92.

133. Patchen ML, Fischer R, MacVittie TJ. Effects of combined administration of interleukin-6 and granulocyte colony-stimulating factor on recovery from radiation-induced hemopoietic aplasia. Exp Hematol 1993;21:338–344.

134. Liebmann J, DeLuca AM, Epstein A, Steinberg S, Morstyng G, Mitchell JB. Protection from lethal irradiation by the combination of ste cell factor and tempol. Radiat Res 1994;137:400–404.

135. Grant S, Pettit GR, McCrady C. Effect of Bryostatin 1 on the in vitro radioprotective capacity of recombinant granulocyte-macrophage colony-stimulating factor (rGM-CSF) toward committed human myeloid progenitor cells (CFU-GM). Exp Hematol 1992;20:34–42.

136. Grant S, Traylor RS, Pettit GR. Lin PS. The macrolytic lactone protein kinase C activator, bryostatin 1, either alone, or in conjunction with recombinant murine granulocyte-macrophage colony-stimulating factor, protects Balb/c and C3H/Hen mice from the lethal in vivo effects of ionizing and radiations. Blood 1994;83:663–667.

137. Patchen ML, MacVittie TJ, Souza LM. Postirradiation treatment with granulocyte colony-stimulating factor and pre-irradiation WR-2721 administration synergize to enhance hemopoietic reconstitution and increase survival. Int J Radiat Oncol Biol Physiol 1992;22:773–779.

138. Sutherland RM, Ausserer WA, Grant TD, et al. Regulatory polypeptide factors, signal transduction and radiation response. In: Dewey WC, Edington M, Fry FJM, Hall EJ, Whitmore GF, eds. Radiation research: a twentieth-century perspective, vol II. San Diego: Academic Press, 1992: 824–829.

139. Haddow A, Alexander P. An immunological method of increasing the sensitivity of primary sarcomas to local irradiation with x-rays. Lancet 1964;1:452–457.

140. Dubois JB, Serrou B. Treatment of the mouse Lewis tumor by the association of radiotherapy and immunotherapy with bacillus Calmette-Guerin. Cancer Res 1976;36:1731–1734.

141. Milas L, Hunter N, Withers HR. Combination of local irradiation with systemic application of anaerobic corynebacteria in therapy of a murine fibrosarcoma. Cancer Res 1975;35:1274–1277.

142. Milas L, Hunter N, Stone HB, Withers RH. Corynebacte-

rium parvum: effect on radiocurability of murine tumors. Cancer Immunol Immunother 1978;5:109–117.

143. Saiki I, Milas L, Hunter N, Fidler IJ. Treatment of experimental lung metastasis with local thoracic irradiation followed by systemic macrophage activation with liposomes containing muramyl tripeptide. Cancer Res 1986;46:4966–4970.

144. Plesnicar S, Rudolf Z. Combined BCG and irradiation treatment of skin metastases originating from malignant melanoma. Cancer 1982;50:1100–1106.

145. Dritschilo A, Mossman K, Gray M, Sreevalsan T. Potentiation of radiation injury by interferon. Am J Clin Oncol 1982;5:79–82.

146. Namba M, Yamamoto S, Tanaka H, Kanamori T, Nobuhara M, Kimoto T. In vitro and in vivo studies on potentiation of cytotoxic effects of anticancer drugs or cobalt 60 gamma ray by interferon on human neoplastic cells. Cancer 1984; 54:2262–2267.

147. Gould MN, Kakria RC, Olson S, Borden EC. Radiosensitization of human bronchogenic carcinoma cells by interferon beta. J Interferon Res 1984;4:123–128.

148. Chang AYC, Keng PC. Potential of radiation cytotoxicity by recombinant interferons, a phenomenon associated with increased blockage at the G_2-M phase of the cell cycle. Cancer Res 1987;47:4338–4341.

149. Kardamakis D, Gillies NE, Souhami RL, Beverley PCL. Recombinant human interferon alpha-2b enhances the radiosensitivity of small cell lung cancer in vitro. Anticancer Res 1989;9:1041–1044.

150. Maasilta P, Holsti LR, Halme M, Kivisaari L, Cantell K, Mattson K. Natural alpha interferon in combination with hyperfractionated radiotherapy in the treatment of non-small cell lung cancer. Int J Radiat Oncol Biol Physiol 1992;23:863–868.

151. Cottler-Fox M, Torrisi J, Spitzer TR, Deeg HJ. Increased toxicity of total body irradiation in patients receiving interferon for leukaemia. Lancet 1990;1:174.

152. Torrisi J, Berg C, Bonnem E, Dritschilo A. The combined use of interferon and radiotherapy in cancer management. Semin Oncol 1986;13(suppl. 2):78–83.

153. Sugarman BJ, Aggarwal BB, Hass PE, Figari IS, Palladino MA, Shepard HM. Recombinant human tumor necrosis factor-α: effects on proliferation of normal and transformed cells in vitro. Science 1985;230:943–945.

154. Nawroth PP, Stern DM. Modulation of endothelial cell hemostasis properties by tumor necrosis factor. J Exp Med 1986;163:740–745.

155. Old LJ. Antitumor activity of microbial products and tumor necrosis factor. In: Bonavida B, Gifford GE, Kirchner H, Old LJ, eds. Tumor necrosis factor/cachectin and related cytokinesis. Basel, Switzerland: Karger, 1988:7–19.

156. Sersa G, Willingham V, Milas L. Anti-tumor effects of tumor necrosis factor alone or combined with radiotherapy. Int J Cancer 1988;42:129–134.

157. Hallahan DE, Beckett MA, Kufe D, Weichselbaum RR. The interaction between recombinant human tumor necrosis factor and radiation in 13 human tumor cell lines. In J Radiat Oncol Biol Physiol 1990;19:69–74.

158. Yamauchi T, Kuriyama H, Watanabe N, Neda Hiroshi, Maeda M, Niitsu Y. Intracellular hydroxyl radical production induced by recombinant human tumor necrosis factor and its implication in the killing of tumor cells in vitro. Cancer Res 1989;49:1671–1675.

159. Repine JB, Pfenninger OW, Talmage DW, Berger EM, Pettijohn DE. Dimethyl sulfoxide prevents DNA nicking mediated by ionizing radiation or iron/hydrogen peroxide-generated hydroxyl radical. Proc Natl Acad Sci USA 1981; 78:1001–1003.

160. Leonard MP, Jeffs RD, Gearhart JP, Coffey DS. Recombinant human tumor necrosis factor enhances radiosensitivity and improves animal survival in murine neuroblastoma. J Urol 1992;148:743–746.

161. Kwok TT, Sutherland RM. Enhancement of sensitivity human squamous carcinoma cells to radiation by epidermal growth factor. J Natl Cancer Inst 1989;81:1020–1024.

162. Kwok TT, Sutherland RM. Differences in EGF related radiosensitization of human squamous carcinoma cells with high and low numbers of EGF receptors. Br J Cancer 1991;64:251–254.

163. Kwok TT, Sutherland RM. Epidermal growth factor modification of radioresistance related to cell-cell interactions. Int J Radiat Oncol Biol Physiol 1991;20:315–318.

164. Kwok TT, Sutherland RM. Cell cycle dependence of epidermal growth factor induced radiosensitization. Int J Radiat Oncol Biol Physiol 1992;22:525–527.

165. Schlappack OK, Hill RP. Lack of radiosensitization of human breast cancer cells (MDA 468) by epidermal growth factor (abstract). Annual Mtg Radiat Res So New Orleans, LA, 1990.

PART **6**

ROLE OF CYTOKINES IN ORGAN SPECIFIC DISEASES

CHAPTER 37

ROLE OF CYTOKINES
IN LUNG-RELATED DISEASES

Roger Spragg, Cecelia Smith, Robert Smith, and Stephen Wasserman

The numerous disorders affecting the lung and the myriad of cytokines identified in pulmonary disease in samples of blood, bronchial lavage fluid, or lung tissue and cells make an encyclopedic review of this topic impossible within the confines of a single chapter. We chose to highlight three conditions to illustrate the potential cytokines possess for mediating widely varying, clinically relevant common disorders. These examples are meant to provide a framework for understanding the breadth and importance of cytokines in the expression of disordered lung function. Adult respiratory distress syndrome (ARDS), interstitial fibrotic lung disease, and asthma illustrate the spectrum of diseases and patterns of cytokines operative in lung pathobiology.

ADULT RESPIRATORY
DISTRESS SYNDROME

ARDS is a constellation of clinical findings as a consequence of injury to the alveolar-capillary membrane resulting in a marked increase in permeability to water, solutes, and plasma proteins. This syndrome has been reported to occur after both local pulmonary injuries and systemic insults (1). Risk factors for ARDS include shock, trauma, infection, disseminated intravascular coagulation, anaphylaxis, cardiopulmonary bypass, transfusion reactions, exposure to certain drugs or toxins, central ner-

vous system disease, aspiration, pancreatitis, and uremia. The probability for development of ARDS increases proportionately with the number of risk factors; rarely can no trigger be identified.

Operational definitions of ARDS vary slightly. Many investigators define the syndrome to be lung edema that occurs over less than seven days, is present in the absence of pulmonary vascular pressures sufficient to be the primary cause of pulmonary edema, and is diffuse in nature as reflected by panlobar infiltrates on chest radiographs. In the presence of such edema, shunting of pulmonary blood flow and diminished lung compliance are common. The resistance of the pulmonary vasculature to blood flow is often increased, and airway resistance is also significantly increased (2).

Acute and chronic stages of ARDS exist (3). Early alveoli fill with proteinaceous fluid containing red blood cells, neutrophils, macrophages, and cell fragments. Type I epithelial cells are focally destroyed, and endothelial cells are swollen. Interstitial edema occurs, and cuffs of edema are seen around bronchioles and vessels. Hyalin membranes composed of fibrin strands and plasma proteins are seen predominately in alveolar ducts. The number of polymorphonuclear leukocytes (PMNs) seen in capillaries is markedly increased; extravasated PMNs are seen in the interstitium and the alveoli (4). A more chronic stage of acute lung injury is apparent after 1 to 2 weeks. Cuboidal epithelial cells closely resembling Type II cells cover the surfaces of alveoli and alveolar ducts. Proliferation of pericytes and fibroblasts occurs, and plasma cells, histiocytes, and lymphocytes are seen in the interstitium. Intravascular microthrombi are common (5). The acinar architecture of the lung is replaced by thick layers of fibrotic tissue, in a pattern centered on alveolar ducts (6). Fibrosis commences within the first few days, when procollagen III peptide can be identified in bronchoalveolar lavage (BAL) fluid or serum (7,8); by 10 days, total lung collagen is increased two- to threefold (9).

Analysis of both pulmonary tissue and BAL fluid from patients with ARDS suggests that a variety of mediators of inflammation may contribute to the lung injury. Lavage fluid contains 1 to 10 mg protein/mL, representing all classes of serum proteins (10). PMNs, normally less than 2% of cells in BAL, may reach more than 90%, and total cell yield is increased. Analysis of BAL also reveals the presence of a variety of soluble mediators of inflammation. A central challenge to understanding the mechanisms that contribute to acute lung injury is to decipher the information presented in studies of BAL fluid, particularly the roles of the individual mediators that have been identified in that fluid. It is attractive to implicate proinflammatory cytokines identified in BAL fluid from patients with ARDS as contributing to the development or persistence of the syndrome. However, rigorous definition of the participation of specific cytokines will require use of strategies that selectively and specifically remove or antagonize the activity of individual mediators. Neutralizing antibodies may prove to be useful for analyzing and treating the clinical syndrome and for investigating animal models, whereas genetic manipulations may aid in understanding mediator participation in animal models. Unfortunately, no single such model is accepted as truly representative of the syndrome, and the capacity of specific mediators to cause tissue injury varies widely between species.

The role of tumor necrosis factor (TNF) in septic shock has received much attention, and interest has also focused on its role in acute lung injury. TNF-α, in particular, can induce production of interleukin-1 (IL-1) by vascular endothelium (11), increase endothelial permeability in vitro (12), stimulate mononuclear phagocytes and alveolar macrophages to induce PMN chemotaxis (13), and cause PMN degranulation and respiratory burst activity (14,15). In animals, both TNF-α and TNF-β appear in the circulation early after induction of septicemia (16), their levels correlate with the severity of lung injury, and infusion of TNF-α results in pulmonary lesions similar to those of ARDS (17,18). In humans, elevated TNF-α levels have often been found in the plasma of patients at risk for ARDS and with established disease, but levels were not correlated with the presence or severity of lung injury. The brief duration of monocyte or macrophage TNF-α release following exposure to bacterial endotoxin may explain why elevated blood levels are not consis-

tently noted. Alternatively, local production of TNF-α by lung mononuclear phagocytes in ARDS may be substantially greater than production by circulating cells (19), and its substantial elevation in BAL, but not blood, has been reported in patients with ARDS (20,21). For example, elevated BAL TNF-α was found in approximately half the at-risk patients and half with established disease; no correlation was found between TNF levels in BAL or blood and severity of ARDS (20). Confounding interpretation is the observation that elevated levels of TNF inhibitors (soluble TNF receptors I and II) are present in the lungs of patients with ARDS, and that TNF recovered from patients with ARDS may be biologically inactive (21).

IL-1 is the proinflammatory cytokine most often grouped pathophysiologically with TNF. Studies have demonstrated a broad spectrum of IL-1 effects relevant to ARDS, including activation of vascular endothelium with induction of procoagulant activity and up-regulation of leukocyte adhesion molecules, induction of fibroblast proliferation, and activation of phagocytes (22–24). Antigenic levels of IL-1 are increased in BAL fluid, but not in plasma, of patients with ARDS compared with normal subjects, and, in contrast to TNF, they remain elevated into the later stages of disease (21). An inhibitor of IL-1 biological activity is present in normal BAL fluid and is increased in BAL from patients with ARDS (25), thus obscuring the relevance of increased antigenic levels of IL-1 in ARDS.

Examination of lung tissue from patients at risk for, or who have died with, ARDS (3,4) and of BAL from patients with ARDS (26–28) confirms a marked influx of PMN into the lung and suggests that products of PMN may participate in initiation or propagation of the lung pathology. However, ARDS can occur in profoundly neutropenic patients (29), suggesting that products of PMN may not always be necessary. Nevertheless, release or production of substances chemotactic for PMN, such as IL-8, may contribute to neutrophil influx during the initial stages of acute lung injury (30). IL-8 is perhaps the best studied member of a proinflammatory supergene family of mediators that includes GRO-α, GRO-β, GRO-γ, ENA-8, and RANTES (31,32). IL-8 is a potent neutrophil chemoattractant produced by many cells of the lung, including Type II epithelial cells, fibroblasts, endothelial cells, and macrophages. Macrophage expression of IL-8 can be induced by bacterial lipopolysaccharide (LPS), TNF, or IL-1. Locally produced IL-1 or TNF may subsequently induce neighboring Type II pneumocytes, fibroblasts, and endothelial cells to synthesize and secrete IL-8. Thus, a cascade of mediator release resulting in a powerful chemotactic signal at the alveolar level may be initiated by the alveolar macrophage.

Thus, IL-8 produced at the alveolar level could participate in recruitment of PMN that contribute to the pulmonary inflammation that characterizes the early phase of ARDS. In 29 consecutive at-risk patients (i.e., severe pancreatitis, severe multiple trauma, or perforated bowel) sampled within 72 hours of the onset of symptoms, 7 progressed (within 6–72 hours after sampling) to development of ARDS (33). IL-8 concentrations in BAL (but not serum) were significantly higher in those in whom ARDS developed. No significant elevation in BAL PMN content was seen, suggesting that sampling had been performed prior to significant PMN recruitment, or that non-PMN–dependent mechanisms were dominant initially.

In 7 of 8 patients with established ARDS, BAL IL-8 levels were significantly increased, but levels were not increased in BAL from 4 of 5 patients at risk or 11 without risk for ARDS (34). In contrast, serum levels of IL-8 were not elevated in patients with ARDS, but they were increased in four of five patients at risk for ARDS. Similar elevations in plasma IL-8 levels have been reported in patients during the first 24 hours after severe trauma who were at risk for development of ARDS (35). IL-8 levels have also been shown to be significantly elevated in patients with ARDS (36), and they correlated with percent BAL PMN. Approximately 70% of the BAL chemotactic activity for PMN fluid could be removed by anti-IL-8 antibodies. Thus, BAL IL-8 levels are frequently elevated in patients who are identified prospectively as being at risk for ARDS, or in patients with established ARDS. Consistent with a proposed local role of IL-8 in the development of ARDS, serum levels do not appear to correlate with the development or presence of ARDS.

In patients with established ARDS, additional substances known to attract PMN are present in the inflamed lung. Leukotriene B_4 (LTB$_4$)-active (37) components of the complement system (38), monokines, fragments of coagulation proteins (39), fragments of elastin and collagen (40,41), oxidized α_1-proteinase inhibitor (α_1-PI) (42,43), and chemotactic bacterial products (e.g., formulated peptide f-met-leu-phe) can be present in the lung and can participate in attracting neutrophils. Recruitment of PMN may be assisted by activation of complement in the setting of acute lung injury (44). C5a, or its active metabolite, C5a$_{des\ arg}$, may result in intravascular aggregation of leukocytes, with sequestration in the pulmonary vasculature and resultant pulmonary injury. In addition, neutrophil proteases, particularly cathepsin G, have the ability to cleave platelet basic protein or its derivative, β-thromboglobulin, into neutrophil-activating peptide-2, NAP-2 (45–47). This 70 amino acid polypeptide shares substantial homology with IL-8, and it competes for the same receptor (48,49). Elevated levels of NAP-2 have been found in BAL fluid from patients with ARDS, as well as those with congestive heart failure, and they may contribute to PMN migration into those fluids (50).

An additional vascular event that may promote adherence of PMN to lung endothelial cells is expression by those cells of adhesion molecules, including ICAM-1 and ELAM-1. The former is constitutively expressed, and expression is increased following stimulation with IL-1, TNF, or interferon-γ (IFN-γ) (51), whereas the latter appear after such exposure (52). The CD11/CD18 complex on PMN has increased expression after exposure of cells to IL-1 or TNF, and it may be the recognition site for ICAM-1. Finally, although endothelial cell IL-8 released in response to inflammatory mediators is chemotactic for PMNs, it may cause inhibition of PMN-endothelial cell adhesion (53).

Neutrophils in the lungs of patients with ARDS are likely to release highly reactive reduced oxygen species, such as superoxide (O_2) or hydrogen peroxide (H_2O_2). Breath condensate gathered from intubated patients with newly developed ARDS has been shown to contain five-fold more H_2O_2 than that of critically ill patients without ARDS (54). Evidence for the direct participation of oxidants in acute lung injury comes from the discovery that α_1PI function in BAL from patients with ARDS is markedly diminished, due in part to oxidation of a critical methionine residue (27). After oxidative inactivation of α_1PI, the unopposed activity of neutrophil elastase present in the alveolus may contribute to tissue injury (42,55). Oxidative modification of proteins that have migrated into the alveolus may generate factors chemotactic for PMN (56). In addition, HuNE and a variety of other PMN and macrophage proteases may also contribute to acute lung injury (57–59).

In some patients with acute, severe ARDS, there is rapid reconstitution of alveolar structure and function, whereas others proceed through a process of alveolar filling and remodeling that prolongs the illness and can result in death. The evolution of lung injury from the acute inflammatory stage to a fibroproliferative phase marked by obliteration of normal architecture, fibrin deposition in the alveolus, and proliferation of new capillaries and mesenchymal cells is poorly understood. In contrast to BAL fluid from acutely ill patients without ARDS, fluid obtained from patients within three days of onset of ARDS showed markedly stimulated migration and proliferation of lung fibroblasts in vitro (60). The ARDS BAL fluid contained only small amounts of native 29 kd platelet-derived growth factor (PDGF), although a 14-kd polypeptide was identified, which reacted with anti-PDGF antibodies and competed with native PDGF for its receptor. The same investigators found culture conditions such that fibroblast proliferation required the coordinate presence of PDGF, epidermal growth factor (EGF), and insulin, and they showed that ARDS BAL fluid possessed all 3.

In addition to the presence of growth-promoting factors in the lungs of patients with ARDS, there is evidence to suggest that the mesenchymal cells exhibit an enhanced proliferative phenotype. Fibroblasts isolated from intra-alveolar granulation tissue present in the lungs of patients dying with late-stage ARDS, but not those from normal lungs, were found to proliferate in medium devoid of growth factors. The genes encoding the proto-oncogenes, c-fos and c-jun, were constituitively expressed in cells from ARDS lungs, but not in those from control lungs (61). Despite this enhanced proliferative phenotype, the fibroblasts from ARDS lungs did not appear transformed, and they responded normally to the addition of peptide growth factors. Lavage fluid from most patients with ARDS also appears to promote angiogenesis (62), and it contains basic fibroblast growth factor (bFGF), a recognized endothelial cell growth factor, as well as a novel 150-kd polypeptide that stimulates migration and attachment of endothelial cells.

Despite the intensity of the late-stage fibrotic response, survivors of ARDS demonstrate remarkable recovery when examined 12 to 24 months later (63). This observation suggests that as lungs afflicted by ARDS heal, a mechanism may be activated that terminates the fibroproliferative response. In support of this possibility, BAL fluid recovered from patients recovering from ARDS initiated apoptosis in endothelial cells and death, but not necrosis in fibroblasts (64). Thus, both initiation and termination of the fibrotic stage of ARDS appears to be closely regulated, and an understanding of the factors controlling this process may lead to a greatly improved understanding of the mechanisms of lung repair in ARDS and in other lung diseases. Our understanding of ARDS suggests that of the important cytokines in its expression, IL-1, IL-8, and TNF must be assigned central roles.

INTERSTITIAL LUNG DISEASE

The term *interstitial lung disease* (ILD) is generic for a heterogeneous group of disorders defined by the presence of fibrosis in the interstitium and shared histological features (i.e., thickening of the interstitium and destruction of alveoli, terminal airways, and vessels) (65,66). Known etiologies include occupational and environmental inhalants: inorganic dusts (i.e., silica, asbestos, beryllium, hard metal dusts), organic dusts (pigeon breeder's lung), gases, fumes, vapors, and aerosols. Drugs (bleomycin), poisons (paraquat), radiation, and infectious agents can each cause interstitial fibrosis. Collagen vascular diseases (lupus, rheumatoid arthritis), vasculitides (Wegener's granulomatosis), and inherited disorders (neurofibromatosis) have also been associated with pulmonary fibrosis. Idiopathic pulmonary fibrosis (IPF), sarcoidosis, and histiocytosis X (65) are several interstitial lung diseases of unknown etiology. Pathologically, IPF is characterized by an increase in lung matrix due to fibroblast deposition of matrix macromolecules (66). The numbers and spatial re-

lationships of lung parenchymal and inflammatory cells present within the interstitium are also altered, eventuating in airspace fibrosis, alveolar collapse, and development of honeycombed lung (66).

The interstitial lung diseases can be clinically divided into acute or chronic categories based on the duration of symptoms and rate of progression of respiratory impairment (66). Examples of acute disease include ARDS and Hamman-Rich disease, both of which manifest as diffuse alveolar damage. Chronic disease has various patterns, the most common being usual interstitial pneumonia (UIP). Less common patterns include bronchiolitis obliterans with organizing pneumonia (BOOP) and desquamative interstitial pneumonia (DIP) (66).

Using IPF as an example, the typical clinical features include progressive breathlessness on exertion, digital clubbing, a restrictive ventilatory defect with reduced gas exchange (i.e., low arterial partial pressure of oxygen), and a chest radiograph demonstrating widespread diffuse reticulonodular shadows, particularly in the lung bases and periphery (67). On high resolution computed tomograph (HRCT) (a more sensitive means of imaging the lung for interstitial lung disease), the finding of a ground-glass pattern correlates with a cellular process, whereas a reticular pattern indicates fibrosis.

The prognosis for patients with the various interstitial lung diseases depends on the underlying etiology. Fifty percent of patients with IPF die within five years of the date of diagnosis (67,68).

Theories of fibrogenesis/granuloma formation

Damage to endothelial or epithelial cells can be the initial step leading to fibrosis. There is an influx of inflammatory and immune cells into the interstitium and alveolar spaces, and the infiltrating cells release mediators that stimulate collagen production by fibroblasts (69). In IPF and asbestosis, there is ultrastructural evidence of both epithelial and endothelial cell injury from the earliest stages of disease (70). Epithelial cell damage without an ability to repair is associated with fibrogenesis (71). In other diseases of pulmonary fibrosis, endothelial cell injury precedes inflammation and fibrosis (72).

Granulomas are characteristic lesions associated with sarcoidosis and other interstitial lung diseases. Granulomas are comprised of a central collection of inflammatory cells and a peripheral rim of fibroblasts and scar tissue (73). One hypothesis to explain this lesion is a variation in cytokine secretion between the center and the periphery of the granuloma (74). Gradients of fibrogenic activity (greatest at the rim) and inflammatory activity (greatest at the core) may exist. Production of IL-1 and IL-6 by fibroblasts in the center of a developing granuloma augment local inflammatory events, whereas at the periphery, the fibroblasts would be exposed to other cytokines, which induce collagen production.

Cells and cytokines associated with inflammation and fibrogenesis

A variety of cells are involved in inflammation and fibrogenesis of interstitial lung disease (Table 37–1). Alveolitis seen early is associated with lymphocytes, plasma cells, and macrophages. Increased numbers of neutrophils, eosinophils, and mast cells are also seen in BAL of patients with interstitial lung diseases (65). In sarcoido-

sis, a lymphocyte alveolitis is thought to cause the characteristic disease alterations (75). The presence of neutrophils and eosinophils in the lavage of patients with IPF is associated with a lesser response to glucocorticoids than if lymphocytes are present (76).

Macrophages/monocytes

Alveolar macrophages are seen in alveolar spaces and in the interstitium in biopsy specimens of patients with interstitial pulmonary fibrosis (69). Alveolar macrophages harvested by lavage from the lungs of patients with interstitial lung disease proliferate 2- to 15-fold faster than in

TABLE 37–1 CYTOKINES ASSOCIATED WITH INTERSTITIAL LUNG DISEASES

Disease	Effector Cell	Cytokines
IPF	Macrophage	IL-1, IL-8, PDGF, TGF-β, IGF-1, TNF-α
	Lymphocyte	IFN-γ
	Mast cell	TGF-β
	Epithelial cell	TGF-β, MCP-1, TNF-α
Sarcoidosis	Lymphocyte	IL-2, IFN-γ
	Macrophage	IL-1, PDGF, IGF1, TNF-α
Asbestosis	Macrophage	IL-1, PDGF, IGF-1, TNF-α, MFF
	Mast cell	TGF-β
CTD	Macrophage	IL-8, PDGF, TNF-α
Scleroderma	Macrophage	IGF-1
	Epithelial cell	MCP-1, TNF-α
Bleomycin toxicity	Macrophage	IL-1, PDGF, TNFα, MCP-1
	Lymphocyte	IL-2
	Mast cell	TGF-β
	Fibroblast	TGF-β
	Endothelial cell	TGF-β
Silicosis	Macrophage	IL-1, IGF-1, MFF, TNF-α, Type 2 epithelial cell growth factor
	Lymphocyte	IFN-γ
Radiation toxicity	Mast cell	TGF-β
Hypersensitivity pneumonitis	Macrophage	PDGF
BOOP	Macrophage	PDGF

CTD = connective tissue disease; BOOP = bronchiolitis obliterans with organizing pneumonia.

normal control patients (77). When stimulated, they secrete IL-8 and neutrophil chemotactic factors (78,79), TNF-α (80), and IL-1 (81). Alveolar and tissue macrophages in IPF (82) release factors that stimulate lung fibroblast proliferation and collagen synthesis, including fibronectin, PDGF, and insulin-like growth factor-1 (IGF-1) (83). Alveolar macrophages isolated from patients with IPF also express fibrogenic and regulatory cytokines, including TGF-β, PDGF, IL-1, and TNF-α (80,81,83,84). In pneumoconiosis, the cytokines involved include macrophage fibrogenic factor (MFF), IL-1, fibronectin, and tissue necrosis factor (85).

Various substances thought to cause pulmonary fibrosis can also stimulate macrophages to release cytokines. Cultured macrophages from bleomycin-exposed rats release cytokines mitogenic for fibroblasts (86), whereas asbestos induces release of PDGF (87). Growth factor activity due to TNF-α was detected in alveolar macrophages from BAL of patients with various connective tissue diseases, and it was higher and accompanied by fibronectin and PDGF in those with pulmonary disease (88). Macrophages attached to a plastic substrate in vitro spontaneously produce PDGF, and addition of organic or inorganic particles significantly increases the fibroblast-stimulating activity (89).

There is some evidence of discoordinate regulation of cytokine genes in interstitial lung disease. Alveolar macrophages from patients with various interstitial lung diseases produce more PDGF-β but not more TGF-β or human leukocyte antigen-DR-α (HLA-DR-α) mRNA than those from control subjects (90). Addition of IFN-γ causes PDGF-β and HLA-DR-α but not TGF-β levels to increase.

Although cytokine release can be observed in controlled settings, a specific cytokine's role in fibrogenesis may be misinterpreted, because the response seen in vivo may relate to the specific cells or tissue compartment exposed to an activating stimulus. For example, pulmonary fibrosis after exposure to long asbestos fibers appears unrelated to alveolar macrophages, and it is probably caused by fiber penetration into the peribronchiolar tissue, where interstitial macrophage activation may occur (91).

In human studies, alveolar macrophages harvested from patients with IPF and sarcoidosis showed measurable fibroblast growth factor activity, whereas macrophages from control subjects did not (92). Macrophages from patients with pneumoconiosis (93), sarcoidosis (92), and scleroderma (94) have all been found to release IGF-α. Normal alveolar macrophages do not bind IGF-1, whereas macrophages activated in vitro by chrysotile asbestos or LPS, or those obtained from individuals with interstitial lung disease, do (95). Individuals with pneumoconioses (asbestos, coal, or silica) have macrophage-dominated alveolitis. Macrophages from these individuals

release IGF-1, but less than that released in patients with IPF (96).

Alveolar macrophages exposed acutely to asbestos release TNF-α but not IL-1β, IL-6, or granulocyte-macrophage colony-stimulating factor (GM-CSF), whereas alveolar macrophages from individuals exposed to asbestos for more than 10 years secrete enhanced amounts of IL-1β, TNF-α, and IL-6 (97). Alveolar macrophages can also generate TNF-α through Fc receptor (FcR) modulation (98), or after exposure to chrysotile asbestos (99). Bleomycin also mediates cytokine production. TNF-α can be detected as early as 4 hours, and IL-1β by 8 hours after bleomycin exposure. TGF-β is also increased (100). As in asbestosis, alveolar macrophages from patients with IPF have increased mRNA for TNF-α and IL-1β. In IPF, in vitro levels of TNF-α correlate with the number of neutrophils in BAL. Finally the inorganic particles, chrisotile, crocidolite, amosite asbestos, and silica, stimulate IL-1β and TNF-α release, and they up-regulate their respective mRNAs in macrophages of monocytes, whereas macrophages from most patients with sarcoidosis spontaneously release TNF and IL-1. The relative release of the individual cytokines were correlated (101).

The alveolar macrophages in IPF can also participate in neutrophilic inflammation. The macrophage can indirectly recruit neutrophils via secretion of stimulatory cytokines (i.e., IL-1 or TNF) to induce nonimmune cells to generate IL-8, or directly via IL-8 synthesis (see discussion of ARDS). IL-8 mRNA expression by human alveolar macrophages from patients with IPF, fibrosis secondary to connective tissue disease, or sarcoidosis, or in normal subjects, correlates with the percent of neutrophils in BAL (102). The role of neutrophils in lung injury has been discussed.

Lymphocytes

Macrophages and lung T lymphocytes from patients with sarcoidosis and fibrosing alveolitis spontaneously release IFN-γ (103,104), which can augment an inflammatory response and suppress collagen production. IFN-γ activates macrophages and T cells, stimulates endothelial cells to express ICAM-1, and induces HLA-DR expression on antigen-presenting cells and epithelial cells (69). HLA-DR expression is found on macrophages, endothelial cells, and epithelial Type 2 cells in fibrosing alveolitis (105). Because IFN-γ can inhibit fibroblast collagen production, impaired IFN-γ release might be a potentiating factor in the pathogenesis of fibrosing lung diseases. Lymphocyte IFN-γ production has been shown to be impaired in 56% of patients with various fibrosing lung disorders. Low IFN-γ levels correlated with deterioration of lung function, and those with higher levels of circulating IFN-γ more frequently responded to corticosteroids (106).

Mast cells

Increased numbers of pulmonary mast cells are found in rodent models of pulmonary fibrosis produced by a diverse group of etiological agents, including bleomycin (107), radiation (108), and asbestosis (109). Electron microscopic studies of tissue from patients with IPF show mast-cell degranulation in areas of fibrosis (110). The release of mast-cell histamine and tryptase occurs in IPF and correlates with fibrosis (111). However, bleomycin-induced lung fibrosis can occur in mast-cell–deficient mice (112).

Endothelial cells/epithelial cells

Endothelial cells produce mediators such as TGF-β, heparin-binding growth factors (113), and PDGF (114), which appear to interact with mesenchymal cells and connective tissue beneath the basement membrane. Expression of endothelial leukocyte adhesion molecules (ELAM), which bind neutrophils, is enhanced by the cytokines IFN-γ, TNF-α, and IL-1 (115). In vitro exposure of rat pulmonary artery endothelial cells to bleomycin caused a dose-dependent increased secretion of TGF-β, which specifically increased collagen synthesis of rat lung fibroblasts (116). Endothelial cells express mRNA for monocyte chemotactic protein-1 (MCP-1) (117), and they secrete IL-8 after stimulation by IL-1 and TNF (118).

Fibroblasts

In the development of pulmonary fibrosis, there is an increase in fibroblast numbers, their proliferation rate (119), and the production of collagen (120). Fibroblasts participate in the inflammatory response. They can stimulate lymphocyte proliferation (121), enhance the survival of eosinophils (122), and amplify the production of mediators by other cells. Lung fibroblasts secrete IL-1 in response to the synergistic actions of IL-1 and TNF-α (123), and they spontaneously release GM-CSF (122).

Both TGF-β_1 and TGF-β_2 similarly alter the morphology and the cytoskeleton of rat lung fibroblasts, but TGF-β_1 is more potent in inhibiting fibroblast growth and colony formation (124). TGF-β also stimulates synthesis of procollagen and fibronectin, and it inhibits collagenase secretion by lung fibroblasts (125,126). Bleomycin-treated rat lung fibroblasts have increased transcription of TGF-β mRNA, total cellular mRNA for TGF-β, and type I procollagen mRNA; those producing the greatest amount of Type I collagen have the greatest response (127). Normal human lung fibroblast cell line steady-state FGF-β expression is increased 602% by TGF-β and 108% by PDGF (128). The two growth factors independently modulate FGF-β gene expression, and they simultaneously modify lung fibroblast FGF-β protein production.

Murine lung fibroblasts have been divided into two major subpopulations defined by the expression of Thy$_1$. After treatment with IFN-γ, high levels of class I major histocompatibility complex (MHC) expression are seen in both, but only Thy$_1$ cells display class II MHC and present antigen to T-lymphocyte clones (129). This subset of fibroblasts may be involved primarily in promoting chronic lung inflammation. Thy$_1$, but not Thy$_1$-positive fibroblasts, produce IL-1α (121), and after treatment with TNF-α, they increase IL-1α mRNA. Both Thy$_1$-positive and fibroblasts have receptors for IL-1, and both increase collagen synthesis after exposure to IL-1 (130).

IL-6 and IL-8 are also synthesized by human lung fibroblasts. IL-6 synthesis is up-regulated by IL-1 and TNF-α (131), whereas IL-8 production by fibroblasts is dependent on alveolar macrophage generation of IL-1 and TNF.

Network of cytokines

In pulmonary fibrosis, there appears to be a network of interacting cytokines with bidirectional communication. IL-1, TNF, IFN-γ, and IL-6 all have important roles in this communication (74). IL-1, TNF, IFN-γ individually stimulate quiescent fibroblasts to proliferate, whereas IFN-γ inhibits proliferation of rapidly proliferating fibroblasts. When combined, these cytokines have quantitatively and qualitatively different effects. IL-1 and TNF in combination inhibit growth and synergistically stimulate prostaglandin E$_2$ (PGE$_2$) production, which inhibits fibroblast proliferation. When IFN-γ and TNF are combined, a synergistic inhibition of fibroblast proliferation, not mediated by PGE$_2$, occurs. As individual cytokines, IL-1 and TNF in serum-free conditions stimulated fibroblast production of Types 1 and 3 collagen, whereas IFN-γ did not. In the presence of serum, IL-1, TNF, and IFN-γ each inhibits the production of Types 1 and 3 collagen. Combining IL-1 and TNF caused fibroblasts to produce less collagen, and IFN-γ cancelled the stimulatory effects of IL-1 or TNF seen in serum-free media.

In summary, individual cytokines were stimulatory, whereas cytokines in combination tended to inhibit collagen production (74). Similarly, monocyte chemotactic protein-1 (MCP-1) production by fibroblasts appears to require macrophage synthesis of IL-1 or TNF (117). Studies of monocytes and macrophages suggest that the secretion of IL-1β, TNF-α, and PGE$_2$ are mechanistically linked after bleomycin. Thus, TNF-α stimulates IL-1β secretion (131,132), and IL-1β stimulates PGE$_2$ secretion (133). PGE$_2$ is a negative regulator of IL-1β (134) and TNF-α (135). Therefore, bleomycin stimulation of TNF-α secretion causes release of IL-1β, which augments production of PGE$_2$. PGE$_2$ secretion, in an autocrine manner, then down-regulates TNF-α secretion (135). Bleomycin stimulation results in greater release of IL-1β and TNF-α than of IL-6 and PGE (136). A shift toward cytokines that have the ability to cause growth and stimulation may therefore have a role in initiation of fibrosis. On the basis of animal models of lung injury (bleomycin-induced fibrosis and silicosis), TNF is involved in a scheme of cytokine activation in which a sequence of signals, each dependent on its antecedent, is required for the evolving injury. Inhibiting the action of one cytokine, TNF-α, halts the progression of injury (137,138).

Animal models of fibrosis

Animal models have been utilized to study the kinetics of cytokine production in conjunction with fibrogenesis and to locate the source of specific cytokine production. In a rat model of bleomycin-induced pulmonary fibrosis, total lung TGF-β is elevated prior to peak collagen synthesis (73). It was first localized in bronchiolar epithelial cells and alveolar macrophages, whereas later it was noted extracellularly at sites of collagen deposition (139). In bleomycin-responding mouse strains, TNF-α and TGF-β mRNA are increased in the lungs; they peaked on day 7 and then returned toward normal. This time course parallels that of β-actin, but it precedes that of collagens I and III. Only alveolar macrophages from responding mice secreted IL-1, whereas TNF-α was increased in both alveolar macrophages and interstitial cells, the latter after the increase in matrix protein mRNA expression was already instituted (140). The kinetics of secretion was different for these different cell types; a delay was seen in the secretion of TNF-α by interstitial cells.

A lupus-prone mouse model was used to study the role of TNF-α in autoimmune pulmonary inflammation. The development of fibrosis and alveolitis was associated with an increase in the level of lung TNF-α mRNA. Injection of anti-TNF antibodies markedly inhibited the development of pulmonary inflammation (141).

Human BAL, peripheral blood, and lung biopsy analysis

The presence and amount of cytokines in the BAL of patients with various interstitial lung diseases have been assessed. In 12 of 40 patients with IPF secondary to connective tissue disease, BAL cells had increased IFN-γ production (104). A comparable result was observed in patients with sarcoidosis. In contrast, BAL cells from 22 patients with sarcoidosis, 14 patients with IPF, and 10 control subjects did not differ in production of TNF-α, IL-1α, and IL-1β, (142). A few patients from both disease groups had inhibitory activity against IL-1 and TNF-α.

Immunohistochemistry, in-situ hybridization, and monoclonal antibodies have been used to study the location of particular cytokines in lung biopsy specimens. Among patients with IPF, intracellular TGF-β was found to be widespread in bronchiolar epithelial cells, alveolar macrophages, and hyperplastic Type II pneumocytes. The extracellular form of TGF-β was localized to the subendothelial matrix of bronchiolar epithelium and Type II pneumocytes. Lung sections without inflammation or fibrosis did not stain for TGF-β (143). In patients with IPF, TGF-β was demonstrated in areas of the biopsy that contained activated fibroblasts. Alveolar macrophages and epithelial cells in these biopsies expressed TGF-β mRNA (143,144). In advanced IPF, bronchiolar epithelial cells, epithelial cells of honeycomb cysts, and hyperplastic type II pneumocytes had intracellular staining for TGF-β. Extracellular TGF-β localized to the lamina propria of bronchioles and subepithelial regions of honeycomb cysts in areas of dense fibroconnective tissue deposition (143,144). The close approximation of extracellular to intracellular TGF-β suggests that epithelial cells are the primary source of TGF-β in IPF. In IPF and scleroderma, there is widespread staining of epithelial cells, particularly hyperplastic type II pneumocytes for TNF-α (145). Only patients with IPF express MCP-1 in pulmonary epithelial cells, whereas patients and normal subjects display it in monocytes/macrophages, vascular endothelial cells, and smooth muscle cells (146).

To assess their clinical utility, serum levels of three markers of cell-mediated immunity (soluble CD$_8$, soluble IL-2 receptors, and neopterin) and TNF were measured in 20 patients with IPF, 20 normal subjects, and 12 patients with sarcoidosis (147). Levels were lowest in normal subjects, but no difference was noted in levels between the 2 disease groups. Only 30% of all patients with lung disease had measurable circulating levels of TNF. There was no correlation between TNF levels, soluble IL-2 receptors, or soluble CD$_8$ and clinical, radiological, and physiological measures of disease activity or with clinical outcomes after a mean follow-up of 23 months (147). Plasma TGF-β levels in normal subjects and in 41 patients before and after ongoing high-dose chemotherapy and autologous bone marrow transplantation for advanced breast cancer were quantitated and shown to predict the development of lung fibrosis or hepatic veno-occlusive disease (148). Pretransplantation, TGF-β levels were significantly higher in those patients in whom fibrosis developed.

Inhibitors of fibrosis

There is a growing body of evidence that IFN-γ, substances that stimulate IFN-γ, cytokine receptor antagonists, or monoclonal antibodies to specific cytokines can block or modify the progression of fibrosis. Several animal models lend insight into this exciting potential therapy for these diseases.

Treatment with polyinosinic-polycytidylic acid (Poly IC), an inducer of IFNs, in a mouse model of bleomycin-induced lung fibrosis inhibited half the volume of lung collagen accumulation (149). Direct use of recombinant murine IFN-γ also significantly reduced the number of fibroblasts and collagen accumulation in the lungs of bleomycin-treated mice (150). Administration of IL-1 receptor antagonist (IL-1RA) to mice in both bleomycin-induced pulmonary fibrosis and silicosis completely prevented formation of collagen-rich nodules and collagen deposition, and it decreased the severity of damage even when given after challenge (150). Similarly, silica-induced collagen deposition was almost completely prevented by anti-TNF antibody, and it was significantly increased by continuous infusion of mouse recombinant TNF (137).

ASTHMA

Asthma presents a pathobiological picture and a cytokine profile that are markedly different from pulmonary fibrosis and ARDS. We attempt to elucidate the interactions between cytokines and cells important to the expression of clinical asthma, the implications for their interactions in the pathogenesis and treatment of this disorder, and contrast asthmatic inflammation with that identified in ARDS and IPF.

Asthma as an inflammatory disease

Although clinically characterized as a disease manifest as reversible bronchial obstruction with cough or wheeze accompanied by hyperresponsiveness of the airways to a variety of irritant triggers, the current concept of asthma is that of a unique inflammatory response responsible for the characteristic pathophysiological and clinical manifestations (151,152). This inflammatory picture is manifest as infiltration of the airways by CD4$^+$-activated T lymphocytes, eosinophils, and a modest increase in the number of submucosal and epithelial mast cells. In addition, a subbasement membrane deposition of collagen, presumably from activated myofibroblasts, is accompanied by desquamation of the airway epithelium, as well as hypertrophy and hyperplasia of mucous glands, mucous-secreting cells, and smooth muscle (153). These pathological changes have been recognized for more than 100 years (154). Such findings were initially reported in patients dying of asthma, and they are currently known to be present in patients with newly diagnosed asthma (155). Inflammatory changes are more intense in patients

with chronic asthma. Importantly, the degree and type of inflammation is similar in patients with atopic or nonatopic triggers of asthma (156).

The sequence and pathophysiology of this inflammatory cascade has been elucidated in studies of allergen bronchoprovocation in atopic individuals. Allergic individuals, when challenged with antigen, develop an acute bronchoconstrictive event and recover spontaneously, only to manifest a second, more prolonged and persistent bronchoconstriction (157). During the early phase, histamine, prostaglandin D_2, leukotrienes C_4, and platelet-activating factor release are accompanied by increased mucous secretion; 6 to 24 hours later, a brisk infiltration of eosinophils is added (158), and an influx of CD4 T lymphocytes can be appreciated at 24 to 48 hours (159). The lymphocytes in the airway in atopic asthma express mRNA for IL-3, IL-4, IL-5, and GM-CSF, a pattern that has been characterized as the Th2 phenotype (160). In lavage fluid of patients with chronic symptomatic asthma, TNF, GM-CSF, and IL-6 have been identified (161). Walker and colleagues (162) demonstrated elevated lavage levels of IL-2 and IL-5 in nonallergic asthmatics and IL-4 and IL-5 in allergic asthmatics. The late-phase antigen-induced asthmatic inflammation is also accompanied by exacerbation of nonspecific bronchial hyperresponsiveness (163), and similar findings may be induced in animal models by direct installation of IL-2 into the airway (164). Thus, the pathological characteristics of asthma and the resultant physiological aberrations appear to be directly linked to the inflammatory changes that occur in asthma.

Cells and cytokine networks in asthma

As noted previously, evidence exists for the release of cytokines into the airways of patients with both atopic and nonatopic asthma (Table 37–2). The mechanism, whereby cytokines participate in the genesis of inflammation's complex expression, are still being unravelled. Nonetheless, several important cytokine interactions and cascades have been described for cells known to be important in the genesis of asthma. In addition, specific cellular sources of cytokines in this disorder have been elucidated, and the interplay of the effect of cytokines on various cell types and of the recruitment and addition of cytokine synthesis and secretion by cells recruited into the airway and activated by allergic processes permit an increasingly sophisticated understanding of the induction and maintenance of asthma.

One of the central cells in the expression of asthma is the mast cell. This cell, by virtue of its possession of high-affinity receptors for immunoglobulin E (IgE) antibody; its unique intracellular granules containing peptides, proteins, amines, and proteoglycans; its ability to remodel its

TABLE 37–2 CYTOKINES ASSOCIATED WITH ASTHMA

Il-3	Mast cell and basophil growth; eosinophil longevity and activation
Il-4	IgE production; endothelial adhesion receptor expression; mast-cell growth; induction of Th2 lymphocytes
IL-5	Eosinophil growth, migration, activation, and longevity
IL-9	Mast-cell growth
IL-10	Mast-cell growth; suppression of Th1 lymphocytes
GM-CSF	Growth, longevity, and activation of eosinophils

IL= interleukin; IgE = immunoglobulin E; GM-CSF = granulo-cyte-macrophage colony-stimulating factor.

cell membrane and to generate lipid mediators; and its ability to be stimulated to synthesize and to secret cytokines make it a centrally important cell in the genesis of allergic asthma. Moreover, the ability of the mast cell to be stimulated by a variety of histamine-releasing factors generated from lymphocytes and mononuclear leukocytes extends the involvement of this cell to non-IgE–mediated processes as well (165). The vasoactive mediators include histamine, prostaglandin D$_2$, leukotriene C$_4$, and platelet-activating factor, as well as adenosine liberated during the metabolism of adenosine triphosphate. The latter is known to interact with A2 receptors on the mast-cell surface to augment ongoing mediator release (166).

In addition, mast cells release a variety of potent enzymes, including tryptase, proteoglycans (such as heparin), and chemoattractant molecules, particularly those directed toward eosinophil migration. More recently, the ability of mast cells to synthesize cytokines, particularly TNF-α and IL-4, has been documented (167). To date, it has been conclusively demonstrated that mast cells generate these cytokines in response to IgE-mediated signals, but it is also likely that such triggers as histamine releasing factors or other inflammatory molecules may mediate IL-4 production.

IL-4 has a uniquely important role in the allergic phenotype, and its genesis by mast cells is particularly cogent. Recently, the other cell bearing high affinity receptors for the IgE molecule, the human basophil, has also been demonstrated to release IL-4 (168). Mast-cell growth is regulated by IL-3, IL-4, IL-9, IL-10, and the kit ligand

(169,170). These molecules lead to growth from undifferentiated pleuripotential stem cells of mast cells that contain specific granules and possess high-affinity receptors for IgE. It is highly likely that the presence of these cytokines in the airway in asthma leads to the proliferation of mast cells noted in this disorder.

Eosinophils

Regulation of eosinophils by cytokines is intimate, direct, and critical. For eosinophils to participate in asthma, they must first be generated in the bone marrow, recruited from the peripheral circulation, and allowed to migrate into the lung epithelium and into the airway lumen. Eosinophil growth and development is under the regulation of 3 cytokines: most importantly, IL-5, as well as IL-3 and GM-CSF (171–174). All these cytokines prolong eosinophil survival by delaying apoptosis. Moreover, these molecules interact with the eosinophil to induce its activation phenotype, and to prime the eosinophil for increased superoxide production, oxygen metabolism, and leukotriene and PAF generation, as well as granule release.

In addition to supporting eosinophil growth and development, IL-3, IL-5, and GM-CSF, as well as other less well-characterized chemokines, such as lymphocyte chemoattractant factor and RANTES, have been shown to attract eosinophils to inflammatory sites (175), and antibody to IL-5 suppresses eosinophil accumulation in inflammatory processes (176). To accumulate in tissue, eosinophils must adhere to vascular endothelium to migrate through it and into the lung. Eosinophil adherence and ingress appear to be regulated by cytokines, in that their adherence appears to rely on L-selectin and VLA-4. The latter molecule is found on human eosinophils, but not neutrophils, and it enables the cell to adhere to vascular endothelial-expressed VCAM-1 (177). IL-5 selectively enhances the surface expression of adhesion molecules of eosinophils, and IL-4 is particularly effective in up-regulating endothelial VCAM-1 (178). Once eosinophils have migrated into the tissue, their ability to be activated is also modulated by a variety of cytokines, including TGF-β, which up-regulates 5-lipoxygenase activity, whereas IL-1, IL-3, IL-5, and GM-CSF modulate the ability of eosinophils to respond to a variety of other signals (171). Human eosinophils, once activated, can express a variety of inflammatory cytokines, including TNF-α, macrophage inflammatory protein-1α (179), TGF-β (180), as well as GM-CSF and IL-5 (181,182).

In addition to the vasoactive mediators LTC$_4$ and PAF (which the eosinophil shares with the mast cell), the eosinophil can release a variety of toxic granular constituents. For example, the eosinophil major basic protein, eosinophil cationic peptide, eosinophil-derived neurotoxin, and eosinophil peroxidase likely participate in damaging airway epithelium. It is probable that the major basic protein is directly toxic to epithelia and causes its desquamation in asthma (183). These findings suggest a critical effector cell function for the eosinophil in asthma (184).

Lymphocytes and other lung cells

Other cells within the airway can respond to or generate cytokines. For example, airway epithelial cells are capable of generating IL-3, IL-6, and IL-8, as well as GM-CSF, G-CSF, and TNF-α (185). Finally, the classic identification of activated T lymphocytes in asthma is also associated with the generation of a unique family of cytokines. This latter family is increasingly held to be of critical importance in asthma. The mechanism whereby lymphocytes are recruited to the airway remains somewhat controversial. However, it has recently been demonstrated that activated CD4 cells will migrate in response to MIP-1α (186), a product of eosinophils (179), and it is known that one mechanism of lymphocyte homing involves lymphocyte surface VLA-4 that recognizes specific molecules on endothelium. Many studies report a tight correlation between lymphocytes, eosinophils, specific cytokines, and bronchial hyperreactivity (154,187).

The cytokine profile in asthma is a unique one, and it is associated with a lymphocyte phenotype termed *Th2*. This phenotype is characterized by the production of IL-4, IL-5, and IL-10, as well as by the absence of IFN-γ and IL-2. Such a phenotype has been identified in atopic disease and in allergen-induced reactions (188,189). It is thought that a reciprocal relationship exists between the generation of Th1 lymphocytes (producing IFN-γ and IL-2) and Th2 lymphocytes. IL-10 produced by the Th2 cells suppresses Th1 responses, and IFN-γ produced by TH1 cells suppresses Th2 cells (190). A close association has been demonstrated between activation of T lymphocytes in asthma and increased serum and BAL concentrations of IL-5, as well as with accompanying airway hyperreactivity (176,191,192). The role of the Th2 cytokines to engender allergic inflammation is supported by the fact that IL-4 (the defining interleukin of a Th2 response) is the cytokine central to the genesis of an IgE response (193).

Integration of cytokine network in the expression of asthma

Recruitment and activation of Th2-type lymphocytes and production of their unique family of cytokines (i.e., IL-3, -4, -5, -10) work in concert to increase production of IgE (IL-4), to enhance the adhesion of IL-4 and recruitment and activation of IL-3,5, GM-CSF eosinophils, to growth and differentiation of mast cells (IL-3, -4, -9, -10), and thus to histological expression of asthmatic inflammation. The concerted effect of vasoactive and spasmogenic mediators, along with chemoattractant molecules, active enzymes, and the unique granular products of mast cells and eosinophils, leads to the characteristic physiological picture associated with asthma.

More recent studies have demonstrated correlations with the severity of asthma, the number of eosinophils, the number of lymphocytes, and the genesis of IL-5, thus tying together in a coherent story the asthmatic state. Therapeutic initiatives support this understanding. For example, glucocorticoid therapy of asthma is associated with declines in airway fluid levels of IL-4 and IL-5, whereas IFN-γ therapy suppresses levels of IgE (194,195), presumably by counteracting the effect of IL-4. Thus, our current understanding of asthma gives relevance to the concept of Th2 lymphocytes, and it underscores the ability of unique cytokine networks to participate in the genesis of specialized inflammatory cascades and the expression of disease. The inflammatory processes induced by Th2 cells and prominently expressed in asthma contrast greatly with the fibrosis and neutrophilic infiltrates seen in IPF and ARDS. It is apparent, therefore, that histological expression of lung injury and clinical pathophysiology of disease can be differentially regulated by activation of unique families of cytokines. A complete understanding of the interacting cytokine networks should permit appreciation of novel disease states and permit the tailoring of unique, aggressive, and effective therapies for disorders currently poorly understood and ineffectively treated.

REFERENCES

1. Spragg RG, Smith RM. Biology of acute lung injury. In: Crystal RG, West JB, eds. The lung: scientific foundations. New York: Raven, 1990:2003–2017.
2. Wright PE, Bernard GR. The role of airflow resistance in patients with the adult respiratory distress syndrome. Am Rev Respir Dis 1989;139:1169–1174.
3. Bachofen M, Weibel ER. Structural alterations of lung parenchyma in the adult respiratory distress syndrome. Clin Chest Med 1982;3:35–56.
4. Schlag G, Voigt WH, Schnells G, Glatzl A. Vergleichende Untersuchungen der Ultrastruktur von menschlicher Lunge und Skeletmuskulatur im Schock. II. Anaesthesist 1977;26:612–622.
5. Zapol WM, Jones R. Vascular components of ARDS. Clinical pulmonary hemodynamics and morphology. Am Rev Respir Dis 1987;136:471–474.
6. Pratt PC, Vollmer RT, Shelburne JD, Crapo JD. Pulmonary morphology in a multihospital collaborative extracorporeal membrane oxygenation project. Am J Pathol 1979; 95:191–214.
7. Farjanel J, Hartmann DJ, Guidet B, Luquel L, Offenstadt G. Four markers of collagen metabolism as possible indicators of disease in the adult respiratory distress syndrome. Am Rev Respir Dis 1993;147:1091–1099.
8. Hallgren R, Samuelsson T, Laurent TC, Modig J. Accumulation of hyaluronan (hyaluronic acid) in the lung in adult

respiratory distress syndrome. Am Rev Respir Dis 1989; 139:682–687.

9. Zapol WM, Trelstad RL, Coffey JW, Tsai I, Salvador RA. Pulmonary fibrosis in severe acute respiratory failure. Am Rev Respir Dis 1979;119:547–554.

10. Holter JF, Weiland JE, Pacht ER, Gadek JE, Davis WB. Protein permeability in the adult respiratory distress syndrome loss of size selectivity of the alveolar epithelium. J Clin Invest 1986;78:1513–1522.

11. Libby P, Ordovas JM, Auger KR, Robbins AH, Birinyi LK, Dinarello CA. Endotoxin and tumor necrosis factor induce interleukin-1 gene expression in adult human vascular endothelial cells. Am J Pathol 1986;124:179–185.

12. Goldblum SE, Sun WL. Tumor necrosis factor-alpha augments pulmonary arterial transendothelial albumin flux in-vitro. Am J Physiol 1990;258:L57–L67.

13. Harmsen AG, Havell EA. Roles of tumor necrosis factor and macrophages in lipopolysaccharide-induced accumulation of neutrophils in cutaneous air pouches. Infect Immun 1990;58:297–302.

14. Bajaj MS, Kew RR, Webster RO, Hyers TM. Priming of human neutrophil functions by tumor necrosis factor: enhancement of superoxide anion generation, degranulation, and hemotaxis to chemoattractants C5a and F-Met-Leu-Phe. Inflammation 1992;16:241–250.

15. Laudanna C, Miron S, Berton G, Rossi F. Tumor necrosis factor-alpha/cachectin activates the $O_2(-)$-generating system of human neutrophils independently of the hydrolysis of phosphoinositides and the release of arachidonic acid. Biochem Biophys Res Commun 1990;166:308–315.

16. Leeper-Woodford SK, Carey PD, Byrne K, et al. Tumor necrosis factor. Alpha and beta subtypes appear in circulation during onset of sepsis-induced lung injury. Am Rev Respir Dis 1991;143:1076–1082.

17. Tracey KJ, Beutler B, Lowry SF, et al. Shock and tissue injury induced by recombinant human cachectin. Science 1986;234:470–474.

18. Stephens KE, Ishizaka A, Larrick JW, Raffin TA. Tumor necrosis factor causes increased pulmonary permeability and edema. Comparison to septic acute lung injury. Am Rev Respir Dis 1988;137:1364–1370.

19. Rich EA, Panuska JR, Wallis RS, Wold CB, Leonard ML, Ellner JL. Dyscoordinate expression of tumor necrosis factor-alpha by human blood monocytes and alveolar macrophages. Am Rev Respir Dis 1989;130:1010–1016.

20. Hyers TM, Tricomi SM, Dettenmeier PA, Fowler AA. Tumor necrosis factor levels in serum and bronchoalveolar lavage fluid of patients with the adult respiratory distress syndrome. Am Rev Respir Dis 1991;144:268–271.

21. Suter PM, Suter S, Girardin E, Roux-Lombard P, Grau GE, Dayer JM. High bronchoalveolar levels of tumor necrosis factor and its inhibitors, interleukin-1, interferon, and elastase, in patients with adult respiratory distress syndrome after trauma, shock, or sepsis. Am Rev Respir Dis 1992;145:1016–1022.

22. Schleef RR, Bevilacqua MP, Sawdry M, Gimbrone MA Jr. Cytokine activation of the vascular endothelium. Effects on tissue-type plasminogen activator and type 1 plasminogen activator inhibitor. J Biol Chem 1988;263:5797–5803.

23. Bevilacqua MP, Pober JS, Wheeler ME, Cotran RS, Gimbrone MA. Interleukin-1 activation of the vascular endothelium: effects on procoagulant activity and leukocyte adhesion. Am J Pathol 1985;121:393–403.

24. Schmidt JA, Mizel SB, Cohen D, Green I. Interleukin-1, a potential regulator of fibroblast proliferation. J Immunol 1982;128:2177–2182.

25. Siler TM, Swierkosz JE, Hyers TM, Fowler AA, Webster RO. Immunoreactive interleukin-1 in bronchoalveolar lavage fluid of high-risk patients and patients with the adult respiratory distress syndrome. Exp Lung Res 1989;15:881–894.

26. Lee CT, Fein AM, Lippman M, Holtzmann H, Kimbel P, Wienbaum G. Elastolytic activity in pulmonary lavage fluid from patients with adult respiratory distress syndrome. N Engl J Med 1981;304:192–206.

27. McGuire WW, Spragg RG, Cohen AB, Cochrane CG. Studies on the pathogenesis of the adult respiratory distress syndrome. J Clin Invest 1982;69:543–553.

28. Weiland JE, Davis WB, Holter JF, Mohammed JR, Dorinsky PM, Gadek JE. Lung neutrophils in the adult respiratory distress syndrome: clinical and pathophysiologic significance. Am Rev Respir Dis 1986;133:218–225.

29. Ognibene FP, Martin SE, Parker MM, et al. Adult respiratory distress syndrome in patients with severe neutropenia. N Engl J Med 1986;315:547–551.

30. Kunkel SL, Standiford T, Kasahara K, Strieter RM. Interleukin-8 (IL-8): the major neutrophil chemotactic factor in the lung. Exp Lung Res 1991;17:17–23.

31. Geiser T, Dewald B, Ehrengruber MU, Clark-Lewis I, Baggiolini M. The interleukin-8-related chemotactic cytokines GRO alpha, GRO beta, and GRO gamma activate human neutrophil and basophil leukocytes. J Biol Chem 1991;268:15419–15424.

32. Neoson PJ, Kim HT, Manning WC, Goralski TJ, Krensky AM. Genomic organization and transcriptional regulation of the RANTES chemokine gene. J Immunol 1993;151:2601–2612.

33. Donnelly SC, Strieter RM, Kunkel SL, et al. Interleukin-8 and development of adult respiratory distress syndrome in at-risk patient groups. Lancet 1993;341:643–647.

34. Torre D, Zeroli C, Giola M, et al. Levels of interleukin-8 in patients with adult respiratory distress syndrome (letter). J Infect Dis 1993;167:505–506.

35. Hoch RC, Rodriguez R, Manning T, et al. Effects of accidental trauma on cytokine and endotoxin production. Crit Care Med 1993;21:839–845.

36. Miller EJ, Cohen AB, Nagao S, et al. Elevated levels of NAP-1/interleukin-8 are present in the airspaces of patients with the adult respiratory distress syndrome and are associated with increased mortality. Am Rev Respir Dis 1992;146:427–432.

37. Stephenson AH, Lonigro AJ, Hyers TM, Webster RO, Fowler AA. Increased concentrations of leukotrienes in bronchoalveolar lavage fluid of patients with ARDS or at risk for ARDS. Am Rev Respir Dis 1988;138:714–719.

38. Hetland G, Johnson E, Aasebo U. Human alveolar macrophages synthesize the functional alternative pathway of complement and active C5 and C9 in vitro. Scand J Immunol 1986;24:603–608.

39. Senior RM, Skogen WF, Griffin GL, Wilner GD. Effects of fibronogen derivatives upon the inflammatory response.

Studies with human fibronopeptide B. J Clin Invest 1986; 77:1014–1019.

40. Senior RM, Griffin GL, Mecham RP. Chemotactic activity of elastin-derived peptides. J Clin Invest 1980;66:859–862.

41. Riley DJ, Berg RA, Soltys RA, et al. Neutrophil response following intratracheal instillation of collagen peptides intorat lungs. Exp Lung Res 1988;14:549–563.

42. Cochrane CG, Spragg R, Revak SD. Pathogenesis of the adult respiratory distress syndrome. Evidence of oxidant activity in bronchoalveolar lavage fluid. J Clin Invest 1983; 71:754–761.

43. Stockley RA, Shaw J, Afford SC, Morrison HM, Burnett D. Effect of alpha-1-proteinase inhibitor on neutrophil chemotaxis. Am J Respir Cell Mol Biol 1990;2:163–170.

44. Hammerschmidt DE, Weaver LJ, Hudson LD, Craddock PR, Jacob HS. Association of complement activation and elevated plasma-C5a with adult respiratory distress syndrome. Pathophysiological relevance and possible prognostic value. Lancet 1980;1:947–949.

45. Car BD, Baggiolini M, Walz A. Formation of neutrophil-activating peptide 2 from platelet-derived connective-tissue-activating peptide III by different tissue proteinases. Biochem J 1991;275:581–584.

46. Cohen AB, Stevens MD, Miller EJ, Atkinson MA, Mullenbach G. Generation of the neutrophil-activating peptide-2 by cathepsin G and cathepsin G-treated human platelets. Am J Physiol 1992;293:L249–L256.

47. MacArthur CK, Miller EJ, Cohen AB. A peptide secreted by human alveolar macrophages releases neutrophil granule contents. J Immunol 1987;139:3456–3462. (Published erratum appears in J Immunol 1988;140:1713).

48. Leonard EJ, Yoshimura T, Rot A, et al. Chemotactic activity and receptor binding of neutrophil attractant/activation protein-1 (NAP-1) and structurally related host defense cytokines: interaction of NAP-2 with the NAP-1 receptor. J Leukocyte. Biol 1991;49:258–265.

49. Walz A, Dewald B, von Tscharner V, Baggiolini M. Effects of the neutrophil-activating peptide NAP-2, platelet basic protein, connective tissue-activating peptide III and platelet factor 4 on human neutrophils. J Exp Med 1989;170: 1745–1750.

50. Cohen AB, Stevens MD, Miller EJ, et al. Neutrophil-activating peptide-2 in patients with pulmonary edema from congestive heart failure or ARDS. Am J Physiol 1993; 264:L490–L495.

51. Pober JS, Gimbrone MA Jr, Lapierre LA, et al. Overlapping patterns of activation of human endothelial cells by interleukin 1, tumor necrosis factor, and immune interferon. J Immunol 1986;137:1893–1896.

52. Bevilacqua MP, Pober JS, Mendrick DL, Cotran RS, Gimbrone MA Jr. Identification of an inducible endothelial-leukocyte adhesion molecule. Proc Natl Acad Sci USA 1987;84:9238–9242.

53. Gimbrone MA Jr, Obin MS, Brock AF, et al. Endothelial interleukin-8: a novel inhibitor of leukocyte-endothelial interactions. Science 1989;246:1601–1603.

54. Baldwin SR, Simon RH, Grum CM, Ketai LH, Boxer LA, Devall LJ. Oxidant activity in expired breath of patients with adult respiratory distress syndrome. Lancet 1986; 1:11–14.

55. Johnson D, Travis J. The oxidative inactivation of human

alpha 1-proteinase inhibitor: further evidence for methionine at the reactive center. J Biol Chem 1979;254:4022–4026.

56. Petrone DA, English DK, Wong K, McCord JM. Free radicals and inflammation: superoxide-dependent activation of a neutrophil chemotactic factor in plasma. Proc Natl Acad Sci USA 1980;77:1159–1163.

57. Werb Z, Gordon S. Secretion of a specific collagenase by stimulated macrophages. J Exp Med 1975;142:346–360.

58. McDonald JA, Kelley DG. Degradation of fibronectin by human leukocyte elastase. Release of biologically active fragments. J Biol Chem 1980;255:8848–8858.

59. Gadek JE, Fells GA, Wright DG, Crystal RG. Human neutrophil elastase functions as a type III collagen collagenase. Biochem Biophys Res Commun 1980;95:1815–1822.

60. Snyder LS, Hertz MI, Peterson MS, et al. Acute lung injury. Pathogenesis of intraalveolar fibrosis. J Clin Invest 1991; 88:663–673.

61. Chen B, Polunovsky V, White J, et al. Mesenchymal cells isolated after acute lung injury manifest an enhanced proliferative phenotype. J Clin Invest 1992;90:1778–1785.

62. Henke C, Fiegel V, Peterson M, et al. Identification and partial characterization of angiogenesis bioactivity in the lower respiratory tract after acute lung injury. J Clin Invest 1991;88:1386–1395.

63. Alberts WM, Priest GP, Moser KM. The outlook for survivors of ARDS. Chest 1983;84:272–274.

64. Polunovsky VA, Chen B, Henki C, et al. Role of mesenchymal cell death in lung remodeling after injury. J Clin Invest 1993;92:388–397.

65. Crystal RG, Gadek JE, Ferrans VJ, Fulmer JD, Line BR, Hunninghake GW. Interstitial lung disease: current concepts of pathogenesis, staging, and therapy. Am J Med 1981;70:542–568.

66. Crouch E. Pathobiology of pulmonary fibrosis. Am J Physiol 1990;259:L159–L184.

67. Crystal RG, Fulmer JD, Roberts WC, Moss ML, Line BR, Reynolds HY. Idiopathic pulmonary fibrosis: clinical, histologic radiographic, physiologic, scintigraphic, cytologic, and biochemical aspects. Ann Intern Med 1976;85:769–788.

68. duBois RM. Idiopathic pulmonary fibrosis. Ann Rev Med 1993;44:441–450.

69. Sheppard MN, Harrison NK. Lung injury, inflammatory mediators, and fibroblast activation in fibrosing alveolitis. Thorax 1992;47:1063–1074.

70. Corrin B, Dewar A, Rodriguez-Rogin R, Turner-Warwick M. Fine structural changes in cryptogenic fibrosing alveolitis and asbestosis. J Pathol 1985;147:107–119.

71. Terzaghi M, Nettesheim P, Williams ML. Repopulation of denuded tracheal grafts with normal, preneoplastic, and neoplastic epithelial cell populations. Cancer Res 1978;38: 4546–4553.

72. Harrison NK, Myers AR, Corrin B, et al. Structural features of interstitial lung disease in systemic sclerosis. Am Rev Respir Dis 1991;5:221–229.

73. Thrasher DR, Briggs DD Jr. Pulmonary sarcoidosis. Clinics in chest medicine 1982:537–563.

74. Elias JA, Freundlich B, Kern JA, Rosenbloom J. Cytokine

networks in the regulation of inflammation and fibrosis in the lung. Chest 1990;97:1439–1445.

75. Line BR, Hunninghake GW, Keogh BA, Jones AE, Johnston GS, Crystal RG. Gallium-67 scanning to stage the alveolitis of sarcoidosis: correlation with clinical studies, pulmonary function studies, and bronchoalveolar lavage. Am Rev Respir Dis 1981;123:440–446.

76. Rudd RM, Haslam PL, Turner-Warwick M. Cryptogenic fibrosing alveolitis: relationship of pulmonary physiology and bronchoalveolar lavage to response to treatment and prognosis. Am Rev Respir Dis 1981;124:1–8.

77. Bitterman PB, Saltzman LI, Adelberg S, Ferrans VJ, Crystal RG. Alveolar macrophage replication. One mechanism for the expansion of the mononuclear phagocytic population in the chronically inflamed lung. J Clin Invest 1984;74: 460–469.

78. Merrill WW, Vaegel GP, Mathay RA, Reynolds HA. Alveolar macrophage derived chemotactic factor. Kinetics of in vitro production and partial characterization. J Clin Invest 1980;65:268–276.

79. Carre PC, Mortenson RL, King TE, Noble PW, Sable CL, Riches WH. Increased expression of the interleukin-8 gene by alveolar macrophages in idiopathic pulmonary fibrosis. J Clin Invest 1991;88:1802–1810.

80. Gosset P, Perez T, Cassalle P, et al. Increased TNF secretion by alveolar macrophages from patients with rheumatoid arthritis. Am Rev Respir Dis 1991;143:593–597.

81. Nagai S, Aung H, Takeuchi M, Kusume K, Izumi T. IL-1 and IL-1 inhibitory activity in the culture supernatants of alveolar macrophages from patients with interstitial lung diseases. Chest 1991;99:674–680.

82. Rennard SI, Hunninghake GW, Gadek JE, Fales H, Crystal RG. Production of fibronectin by human alveolar macrophages: mechanism for recruitment of fibroblasts to sites of tissue injury in interstitial lung disease. Proc Natl Acad Sci USA 1981;78:7147–7151.

83. Martinet Y, Rom WN, Gratendorst GR, Martin GR, Crystal RG. Exaggerated spontaneous release of platelet derived growth factor by alveolar macrophage from patients with idiopathic pulmonary fibrosis. N Engl J Med 1987;317: 202–209.

84. Raghou R. Role of transforming growth factor-β in repair and fibrosis. Chest 1991;99:61S–65S.

85. Heppleston AG. Minerals, fibrosis, and the lung. Environ Health Perspect 1991;94:149–168.

86. Phan SH, Kunkel SL. Inhibition of bleomycin-induced pulmonary fibrosis by nordihydroguiaretic acid. The role of alveolar macrophage activation and mediator release. Am J Pathol 1986;124:343–352.

87. Bonner JC, Osorniovargas AR, Badgett AM, Brody AR. Differential proliferation of rat lung fibroblasts induced by the platelet-derived growth factor—AA, factor-AB, and factor-BB isoforms secreted by rat alveolar macrophages. Am J Respir Cell Mol Biol 1991;5:539–547.

88. Thornton SC, Robbins JM, Penny R, Breit SN. Fibroblast growth factors in connective tissue disease associated interstitial lung disease. Clin Exp Immunol 1992;90:447–452.

89. Bauman MD, Jetten AM, Bonner JC, Jumar RK, Bennett RA, Brody AR. Secretion of a platelet-derived growth factor homologue by rat alveolar macrophages exposed to particulates in vitro. Eur J Cell Biol 1990;51:327–334.

90. Shaw RJ, Benedict SH, Clark RAF, King TE. Pathogenesis of pulmonary fibrosis in interstitial lung disease. Am Rev Resp Dis 1991;143: 167–173.

91. Adamson IYR, Bowden DH. Pulmonary reaction to long and short asbestos fibers is independent of fibroblast growth factor production by alveolar macrophages. Am J Pathol 1990;137:523–529.

92. Bitterman PB, Adelberg S, Crystal RG. Mechanisms of pulmonary fibrosis. Spontaneous release of the alveolar macrophage-derived growth factor in the interstitial lung disorders. J Clin Invest 1983;72:1801–1813.

93. Rom WN, Bitterman PB, Rennard SI, Canatin A, Crystal RG. Characterization of the lower respiratory tract inflammation of nonsmoking individuals with interstitial lung disease associated with chronic inhalation of inorganic dusts. Am Rev Respir Dis 1987;136:1429–1434.

94. Rossi GS, Bitterman PB, Rennard SI, et al. Evidence of chronic inflammation as a component of the interstitial lung disease associated with progressive systemic sclerosis. Am Rev Respir Dis 1985;131:612–617.

95. Rom WN, Paakko P. Activated alveolar macrophages express the insulin-like growth factor-I receptor. Am J Respir Cell Mol Biol 1991;4:432–439.

96. Rom WN. Relationship of inflammatory cell cytokines to disease severity in individuals with occupational inorganic dust exposure. Am J Ind Med 1991;19:15–27.

97. Perkins RC, Scheule RK, Hamilton R, Gomes G, Freidman G, Holian A. Human alveolar macrophage cytokine release in response to in vitro and in vivo asbestos exposure. Exp Lung Res 1993;19:55–65.

98. Kim JW, Wierda WG, Kim YB. Immobilized IgG immune complex induces secretion of tumor necrosis factor-a by porcine alveolar macrophages. Am J Respir Cell Mol Biol 1991;5:249–255.

99. Ouellet S, Yang H, Aubin RA, Hawley RG, Wenckebach GF, Lamaire I. Bidirectional modulation of TNA-α production by alveolar macrophages in asbestos-induced pulmonary fibrosis. J Leukocyte Biol 1993;53:279–286.

100. Scheule RK, Perkins RC, Hamilton R, Holian A. Bleomycin stimulation of cytokine secretion by the human alveolar macrophage. Am J Physiol 1992;262:L386–L391.

101. Pueringer RJ, Schwartz DA, Dayton CS, Gilbert SR, Hunninghake GW. The relationship between alveolar macrophage TNF, IL-1, and PGE$_2$ release, alveolitis, and disease severity in sarcoidosis. Chest 1993;103:832–838.

102. Lyynch JP III, Standiford TJ, Rolfe MW, Kunkel SL, Strieter RM. Neutrophilic alveolitis in idiopathic pulmonary fibrosis. Am Rev Respir Dis 1992;145:1433–1439.

103. Robinson BWS, McLemore TL, Crystal RG. Gamma interferon is spontaneously released by alveolar macrophages and lung T lymphocytes in patients with pulmonary sarcoidosis. J Clin Invest 1985;75:1488–1495.

104. Robinson BW, Rose AH. Pulmonary gamma interferon production in patients with fibrosing alveolitis. Thorax 1990;45:105–108.

105. Kradin RL, Divertis MB, Colvin RB. Usual interstitial pneumonitis is a T-cell alveolitis. Immunol Immunopathol 1986;40:224–235.

106. Prior C, Haslam PL. In vivo levels and in vitro production of interferon-γ in fibrosing interstitial lung diseases. Clin Exp Immunol 1992;88:280–287.

107. Gogo T, Befus D, Low R, Bienenstock J. Mast cell heterogeneity and hyperplasia in bleomycin-induced pulmonary fibrosis of rats. Am Rev Respir Dis 1984;130:797–802.

108. Watanabe S, Watanabe K, Ohishe T, Aiba M, Kageyama K. Mast cells in the rat alveolar septa undergoing fibrosis after ionizing radiation. Lab Invest 1974;5:555–567.

109. Wagner MN, Edwards RE, Moncrieff CB, Wagner JC. Mast cells and inhalation of asbestos in rats. Thorax 1984; 39:539–544.

110. Kawanami O, Ferrans VJ, Fulmer JD, Crystal RG. Ultrastructure of pulmonary mast cells in patients with fibrotic lung disorders. Lab Invest 1979;40:717–734.

111. Broide D, Smith CM, Wasserman S. Mast cells and pulmonary fibrosis. Identification of a histamine releasing factor on bronchoalveolar lavage fluid. J Immunol 1990;145:1838–1844.

112. Mori H, Kawada K, Zhang P, Uesugi Y, Sakamoto O, Koda A. Bleomycin-induced pulmonary fibrosis in genetically mast cell-deficient WBB6F1-W/Wv mice and mechanism of the suppressive effect of tranilast, an antiallergic drug inhibiting mediator release from mast cells, on fibrosis. Int Arch Allergy Appl Immunol 1991;95:195–201.

113. Roche WR, Beasley R, Williams J, Holgate ST. Subepithelial fibrosis in the bronchi of asthmatics. Lancet 1989;1:520–524.

114. Starksen NF, Harsh GR, Gibbs VC, Williams LT. Regulated expression of the platelet-derived growth factor-α chain gene in microvascular endothelial cells. J Biol Chem 1987; 262:14381–14384.

115. Pober JS. Cytokine-mediated activation of vascular endothelium. Am J Pathol 1988;133:426–433.

116. Phan SH, Gharaee-Kermani M, Wolber F, Ryan US. Stimulation of rat endothelial cell transforming growth factor-β production by bleomycin. J Clin Invest 1991;87:148–154.

117. Kunkel SL, Standiford T, Kasahara K, Strieter RM. Stimulus specific induction of monocyte chemotactic protein-1 (MCP-1) gene expression. In: Westwick J, et al. Chemotactic cytokines. New York: Plenum Press, 1991:65–71.

118. Kunkel SL, Standiford T, Kasahara K, Strieter RM. Interleukin-8 (IL-8): the major neutrophil chemotactic factor in the lung. Exp Lung Res 1991;17:17–23.

119. Jordana M, Schulman J, McSharry C, et al. Heterogeneous proliferative characteristics of human adult lung fibroblast lines and clonally-derived fibroblasts from control and fibrotic human lung. Am Rev Respir Dis 1988;138:579–584.

120. Piguet PF. Cytokines involved in pulmonary fibrosis. Int Rev Exp Pathol 1993;34B:173–181.

121. Phipps RP, Penney DP, Keng P, Silvera M, Harkins S, Derdak S. Immune functions of subpopulations of lung fibroblasts. Immunol Res 1990;9:275–286.

122. Vancheri C, Gauldie J, Bienenstock J, et al. Human lung fibroblast-derived granulocyte-macrophage colony stimulating factor (GM-CSF) mediates eosinophil survival in vitro. Am J Respir Cell Mol Biol 1989;1:280–295.

123. Elias JA, Reynolds MM, Kotloff RM, Kern JA. Fibroblast interleukin-1β synthesis: stimulation by recombinant interleukin-1 and tumour necrosis factor. Proc Natl Acad Sci USA 1989;86:6171–6175.

124. Kalter VG, Brody AR. Receptors for transforming growth factor-β (TGF-β) on rat lung fibroblasts have higher affinity for TGF-β₁ than for TGF-β₂. Am J Respir Cell Mol Biol 1991;4:397–407.

125. Ignotz R, Massague J. Transforming growth factor-β stimulates the expression of fibronectin and collagen and their incorporation into the extracellular matrix. J Biol Chem 1986;261:4337.

126. Overall CM, Wrana JL, Sodek J. Independent regulation of collagenase, 72 kDa progelatinase and metallo-proteinase inhibitor expression in human fibroblasts by transforming growth factor-β. J Biol Chem 1989;264:1860–1869.

127. Breen E, Shull S, Burne S, et al. Bleomycin regulation of transforming growth factor-β mRNA in rat lung fibroblasts. Am J Respir Cell Mol Biol 1992;6:146–152.

128. Goldsmith KT, Gammon RB, Garver RI. Modulation of bFGF in lung fibroblasts by TGF-β and PDGF. Am J Physiol 1991;261:L378–L385.

129. Phipps RP, Penney DP, Keng P, et al. Characterization of two major populations of lung fibroblasts: distinguishing morphology and discordant display of thy₁ and class II MHC. Am J Respir Cell Mol Biol 1989;1:65–74.

130. Derdak S, Penney DP, Keng P, Gelch ME, Brown D, Phipps RP. Differential collagen and fibronectin production by Thy₁⁺ and Thy₁⁻ lung fibroblast subpopulations. Am J Physiol 1992;263:L283–L290.

131. Dinarello CA, Cannon JG, Wolff SM, et al. Tumor necrosis factor (cachectin) is an endogenous pyrogen and induces production of interleukin 1. J Exp Med 1986;6:1433–1450.

132. Raghu G, Kavanagh T. The human lung fibroblast: a multifaceted target and effector cell. In: Selman Lama M, Barrios R, eds. Interstitial pulmonary diseases: selected topics. Boca Raton, FL: CRC Press, 1991:1–34.

133. Censini S, Bartalini M, Tagliabue A, Boraschin D. Interleukin 1 stimulates production of LTC4 and other eicosanoides by macrophages. Lymphokine Res 1989;8:107–114.

134. Knudsen PJ, Dinarello CA, Strom TB. Prostaglandins posttranscriptionally inhibit monocyte expression of interleukin 1 activity by increasing intracellular cyclic adenosine monophosphate. J Immunol 1986;137:3189–3194.

135. Scales WE, Chensue SW, Otterness I, Kunkel SL. Regulation of monokine gene expression; prostaglandin E₂ suppressea tumor necrosis factor but not interleukin-1α or β-mRNA and cell-associated bioactivity. J Leukocyte Biol 1989;45:416–421.

136. Zhang Y, Lee TC, Guillemin B, Yu MC, Rom WN. Enhanced IL-1 beta and tumor necrosis factor-α release and messenger RNA expression in macrophages from idiopathic pulmonary fibrosis or after asbestos exposure. J Immunol 1993;150:4188–4196.

137. Piguet PF, Collart MA, Grau GE, Sappino AP, Vassalli P. Requirement of tumour necrosis factor for development of silica-induced pulmonary fibrosis. Nature 1990;344:245–247.

138. Piguet PF, Collart MA, Grau GE, Kapanci Y, Vassalli P. Tumor necrosis factor/cachetin plays a key role in bleomycin-induced pneumopathy and fibrosis. J Exp Med 1989;170:655–663.

139. Khalil N, Bereznay O, Sporn M, Greenberg AH. Macro-

phage production of transforming growth factor β and fibroblast collagen synthesis in chronic pulmonary inflammation. J Exp Med 1989;170:727–737.

140. Phan SH, Kunkel SL. Lung cytokine production in bleomycin-induced pulmonary fibrosis. Exp Lung Res 1992;18:29–43.

141. Deguchi Y, Kishimoto S. Tumour necrosis factor/cachectin plays a key role in autoimmune pulmonary inflammation in lupus-prone mice. Clin Exp Immunol 1991;85:392–395.

142. De Rochemonteix-Galve B, Dayer JM, Junod AF. Fibroblast-alveolar cell interactions in sarcoidosis and idiopathis pulmonary fibrosis: evidence for stimulatory and inhibitory cytokine production by alveolar cells. Eur Respir J 1990;3:653–664.

143. Khalil N, O'Connor RN, Unruh HW, et al. Increased production and immunohistochemical localization of transforming growth factor-β in idiopathic pulmonary fibrosis. Am J Respir Cell Mol Biol 1991;5:155–162.

144. Broekelmann TJ, Limper AH, Colby TV, McDonald JA. Transforming growth factor β_1 is present at sites of extracellular matrix gene expression in human pulmonary fibrosis. Proc Natl Acad Sci USA 1991;88:6642–6646.

145. Nash JR, McLaughlin PJ, Butcher D, Corrin B. Expression of tumour necrosis factor-α in cryptogenic fibrosing alveolitis. Histopathology 1993;22:343–347.

146. Antoniades HN, Neville-Godlen J, Galanopoulos T, Kradin RL, Valente AJ, Graves DT. Expression of monocyte chemoattractant protein 1 in mRNA in human idiopathis pulmonary fibrosis. Proc Natl Acad Sci USA 1991;89:5371–5375.

147. Meliconi R, Lalli E, Borzi RM, et al. Idiopathic pulmonary fibrosis: can cell mediated immunity markers predict clinical outcome? Thorax 1990;45:536–540.

148. Anscher MS, Peters WP, Reisenbichler H, Petros WP, Jirtle RL. Transforming growth factor-β as a predictor of liver and lung fibrosis after autologous bone marrow transplantation for advanced breast cancer. N Engl J Med 1993;328:1592–1598.

149. Hyde DM, Giri SN. Polyinosinic-polycytidylic acid, an interferon inducer, ameliorates bleomycin-induced lung fibrosis in mice. Exp Lung Res 1990;16:533–546.

150. Piguet PF, Vesin C, Grau GE, Thompson RC. Interleukin 1 receptor antagonist (IL-1ra) prevents or cures pulmonary fibrosis elicited in mice by bleomycin or silica. Cytokine 1993;5:57–61.

151. Holgate SB. The role of inflammatory processes in airway hyperresponsiveness. Oxford: Blackwell Scientific, 1989.

152. Kay AB. Allergy and inflammation. London: Academic Press, 1987.

153. Hogg JC. Pathology of asthma. In: Middleton E, Reed CE, Adkinson NF, Yuninger JW, Bosse WW, eds. Allergy principles and practice, ed 4. St. Louis: CV Mosby, 1993:1215–1224.

154. Holgate S. Mediator and cytokine mechanisms in asthma. Thorax 1993;48:103–109.

155. Laitinen LA, Laitinen A, Haahtela T. Airway mucosal inflammation even in patients with newly diagnosed asthma. Am Rev Respir Dis 1993;147:697–704.

156. Bentley AM, Naestrelli P, Saetta M, et al. Activated T-lymphocytes and eosinophils in the bronchial mucosa in es-

ocyanate-induced asthma. J Allergy Clin Immunol 1992;89:821–829.

157. Booij-Noord H, de Vries K, Sluiter JH, et al. Late bronchial obstructive reaction to experimental inhalation of house dust extract. Clin Allergy 1972;2:43.

158. Beasley R, Roche WR, Roberts JA, Holgate ST. Cellular events in the bronchi in mild asthma and after bronchial provocation. Am Rev Respir Dis 1989;139:806–817.

159. Gonzalez MC, Diaz P, Galleguillos FR, Ancic P, Cromwell O, Kay OB. Allergen-induced recruitment of bronchoalveolar helper and suppressor T-cells in asthma. Am Rev Respir Dis 1987;136:600–604.

160. Ricci M, Rossi O, Bertoni M, Matucci A. The importance of Th-2 like cells in the pathogenesis of airway allergic inflammation. Clin Exp Allergy 1993;23:360–369.

161. Broide DH, Lotz M, Cuomo AJ, Coburn DA, Federman OC, Wasserman SI. Cytokines in symptomatic asthma airways. J Allergy Clin Immunol 1992;89:958–967.

162. Walker C, Bode E, Boer L, Hansel TT, Blaser K, Virchow JC. Allergic and non-allergic asthmatics have distance patterns of T-cell activation and cytokine production in peripheral blood and bronchoalveolar lavage. Am Rev Respir Dis 1992;148:109–115.

163. Cartier A, Thomson NC, Frith MB, Roberts R, Hargreave FE. Allergen-induced increase in bronchial responsiveness to histamine. J Allergy Clin Immunol 1982;70:170–177.

164. Renzi PM, Sapienza S, Du T, Wang NS, Martin JG. Lymphokine-induced airway hyperresponsiveness in the rat. Am Rev Respir Dis 1991;143:375–379.

165. Alam R. Novel concepts in allergy and asthma: interleukins and other cytokines as mediators. Insights Allergy 1991;6:1–8.

166. Marquardt DC, Walker LL, Wasserman SI. Adenosine receptors on mouse bone marrow derived mast cells: functional significance and regulation by aminophylline. J Immunol 1984;133:932–937.

167. Plaut M, Pierce JH, Watson CJ, Hanley-Hyde J, Nordan RP, Paul WE. Mast cell lines produce lymphokines in response to cross-linkage of FcERI or to calcium ionophores. Nature 1989;339:64–67.

168. Brunner T, Heusser CH, Dakinden CA. Human peripheral blood basophils primed by IL-3 produce IL-4 in response to immunoglobulin E receptor stimulation. J Exp Med 1993;177:605–611.

169. Stevens RL, Austen KF. Recent advances in the cellular and molecular biology of mast cells. Immunol Today 1989;10:381–386.

170. Quesniaus VFJ. Interleukins 9,10,11 and 12 and kit-ligand: a brief overview. Res Immunol 1992;43:385–400.

171. Fabian I, Kletter Y, Mor S, et al. Activation of human eosinophil and neutrophil functions by hoemopoietic growth factors IL-1, IL-3, IL-5 and GM-CSF. Br J Haematol 1992;80:137–143.

172. Rothenberg ME, Owen WF, Silberstien DS, et al. Human eosinophils have prolonged survival, enhanced functional properties and become hypodense when exposed to human interleukin 3. J Clin Invest 1988;81:1986–1992.

173. Silberstein DS, Owen WF, Gasson JC, et al. Enhancement of eosinophil cytotoxicity and leukotriene synthesis by bio-

synthetic granulocyte-macrophage colony-stimulating factor. J Immunol 1986;137:3290–3294.

174. Ohnishi T, Sur S, Collins DS, Fish JE, Gleich GJ, Peters SP. Eosinophil survival activity identified as interleukin-5 is associated with eosinophil recruitment and degranulation and lung injury twenty four hours after segmental antigen lung challenge. J Allergy Clin Immunol 1983;92:607–615.

175. Resnick MB, Weller PF. Mechanisms of eosinophil recruitment. Am J Respir Cell Mol Biol 1993;8:349–355.

176. Van Oosterhout AJM, Ladenios C, Savelkoul HF, et al. Effect of anti-IL-5 and IL-5 on airway hyperreactivity and eosinophils in guinea pigs. Am Rev Respir Dis 1993;147:548–552.

177. Neeley SP, Hamann KJ, White SR, Barenowski SL, Burch RA, Left AR. Selective regulation of expression of surface adhesion molecules MAC-1, L-selectin and VLA-4 on human eosinophils and neutrophils. Am J Respir Cell Mol Biol 1993;8:633–639.

178. Schleimer RP, Sterbinsky SA, Kaiser S, et al. IL-4 induces adherence of human eosinophils and basophils but not neutrophils to endothelium: association with expression of VCAM-1. J Immunol 1992;148:1086–1092.

179. Costa JJ, Matossian K, Resnick MC, et al. Human eosinophils can express the cytokines tumor necrosis factor-α and macrophage inflammatory protein-1α. J Clin Invest 1993;91:2673–2684.

180. Ohno I, Lea RG, Flanders KC, et al. Eosinophils in chronically inflamed human upper airway tissues express transforming growth factor β-1 gene. J Clin Invest 1992;89:1662–1668.

181. Broide DH, Paine MM, Firestein GS. Eosinophils express interleukin 5 and granulocyte macrophage colony stimulating factor mRNA at sites of allergic inflammation in asthmatics. J Clin Invest 1992;90:1414–1420.

182. Moqbel R, Hamid Q, Ying S, et al. Expression of mRNA and immunoreactivity for the granulocyte macrophage colony stimulating factor in activated human eosinophils. J Exp Med 1991;174:749–852.

183. Gleich GJ. The eosinophil and bronchial asthma's current understanding. J Allergy Clin Immunol 1990;85:422–436.

184. Gleich GJ, Flavakan NA, Fujisawa T, Vanhoutte PM. The eosinophil as a mediator of damage to respiratory epithelin. A model for bronchial hyperreactivity. J Allergy Clin Immunol 1988;81:776–781.

185. Devalia JL, Davies RJ. Airway epithelial cells and mediators of inflammation. Respir Med 1993;87:405–408.

186. Taub DD, Conlin K, Lloyd AR, Oppenheim JJ, Kelvin DJ. Preferential migration of activated CD4+ and CD5+ T cells in response to MIP-1α and MIP-1β. Science 1993;260:355–358.

187. Berman JS, Weller PF. Airway eosinophils and lymphocytes in asthma. Am Rev Respir Dis 1992;145:1246–1248.

188. Kay AB, Ying S, Varney V, et al. Messenger RNA expression of the cytokine gene cluster, interleukin 3, 4, 5 and granulocyte macrophage colony stimulating factor, in allergen-induced last phase cutaneous reactions in atopic subject. J Exp Med 1991;173:775–778.

189. Wierenga EA, Snoek M, de Groot C, et al. Evidence for compartmentalization of functional subsets of CD 4 + T lymphocytes in atopic patients. J Immunol 1990;144:4651–4656.

190. Zlotnik A, Moore KW. Interleukin 10. Cytokine 1991;3:366–371.

191. Corrigan CJ, Haczku A, Gemou-Engesaeth V, et al. CD4 T-lymphocyte activation in asthma is accompanied by increased serum concentrations of interleukin-5. Am Rev Respir Dis 1993;147:540–547.

192. Djukankovic R, Roche WR, Wilson JW, et al. State of the art: Mucosal inflammation in asthma. Ann Rev Respir Dis 1990;142:434–457.

193. Callard RE. Immunoregulation by interleuken 4 in man. Br J Haematol 1991;78:293–299.

194. Robinson D, Hamid Q, Ying S, et al. Prednisolone treatment in asthma is associated with modulation of bronchoalveolar lavage cell interleukin 4, interleukin 5 and interferon γ cytokine gene expression. Am Rev Respir Dis 1993;148:401–406.

195. Boquniewicz M, Jaffe HS, Izn A, et al. Recombinant gamma interferon in treatment of patients with atopic dermatitis and elevated IgE levels. Am J Med 1990;88:365–369.

CHAPTER **38**

ROLE OF CYTOKINES IN SYSTEMIC CAPILLARY LEAK SYNDROME

Larry C. Casey

The systemic capillary leak syndrome is divided into two types; idiopathic and iatrogenic. The iatrogenic form is a complication of interleukin-2 (IL-2) and lymphokine-activated killer cell (LAK) infusion, which are used for cancer therapy. The idiopathic systemic capillary leak syndrome, also known as Clarkson's disease, was first described in 1960 (1).

CLINICAL MANIFESTATIONS

Clinical features of the side effects of IL-2 infusion

Systemic capillary permeability develops in all patients treated with IL-2 and LAK cells (2). The increased vascular permeability begins to occur within the first 24 hours after starting IL-2 transfusion. The characteristic feature is accumulation of extracellular fluid, manifested by the development of ascites, peripheral edema, hydrothorax, and pulmonary edema. Erythematous skin eruptions are also common. The systemic toxicity of IL-2 and LAK cell infusion limits the therapy. These toxic side effects can be reversed by stopping the IL-2 infusion.

Clinical features of Clarkson's disease

The patient that Clarkson described was a young woman who presented with unexplained periodic profound hypovolemic episodes with peripheral edema. Since this original description, only approximately 24 patients have been reported. Although underlying mechanisms are unknown and therapy is empiric, recent evidence has implicated cytokines as mediators of the capillary permeability. The characteristic feature of the idiopathic systemic capillary leak syndrome is sudden, but reversible, capillary permeability. There may be a shift in intravascular volume by as much as 70%, and the patient presents in hypovolemic shock. During attacks, water, electrolytes, and plasma proteins of molecular weight less than 900 kd are lost from the intravascular space into the interstitial space (3). The loss of intravascular fluid causes hemoconcentration, with increases in red blood cell, white blood cell, and platelet counts. The hematocrit level generally parallels the severity of the attack. Because of the profound loss of intravascular volume, the patient often presents in shock, with oliguria and prerenal azotemia.

Fluid and proteins return to the intravascular space during the recovery phase. There may be volume overload during the recovery phase, when large volumes of fluid are used as treatment during the shock phase. Pulmonary edema may occur during the recovery phase. One interesting feature of this syndrome is that the lung vasculature is spared during the acute permeability phase (4), suggesting the presence of regional differences in endothelial cell permeability.

PATHOPHYSIOLOGY OF IL-2–INDUCED ENDOTHELIAL CELL PERMEABILITY

Interleukin-2 is a 133 amino acid polypeptide secreted by lymphocytes and natural killer cells, and it has a variety of immunological functions, the most notable being the ability to promote proliferation and maturation of activated T cells. Other biological activities attributed to IL-2 include (a) stimulation of proliferation of activated and natural killer cells and tumor-infiltrating lymphocytes, as well as enhancement of the ability of these cytotoxic lymphocytes to kill target cells; (b) stimulation of proliferation and maturation of activated helper T cells; (c) induction of IL-2 receptors on T cells; (d) stimulation of proliferation of antibody producing B-cells; (e) induction of secretion of interferon-γ (IFN-γ) and tumor necrosis factor-α (TNF-α) and TNF-β by peripheral blood monocytes; (f) stimulation of the rate of synthesis of c-myc RNA and transferrin receptors; and (g) activation of neutrophils.

IL-2 and LAK cell infusion causes systemic capillary leak

In vitro culture of lymphocytes with IL-2 leads to the generation of LAK cells (5). LAK cells are capable of lysing a variety of tumor cells. In mice, the adoptive transfer of LAK cells, in conjunction with multiple injections of IL-2, causes regression of established metastatic tumors (6). Recent clinical trials using LAK cells and IL-2 treatment have been completed. Although tumor regression in response to IL-2 and LAK cell infusion appear promising, this therapy causes significant side effects. Systemic capillary leak develops in all patients; which is reversible after stopping the IL-2 infusion. One major difference between IL-2–induced systemic capillary leak and Clarkson's disease is that IL-2 infusion causes pulmonary edema, whereas the lung is spared in Clarkson's disease.

Mediators of IL-2–induced capillary permeability

The mediators of the iatrogenic form of the systemic capillary permeability syndrome are related to the infusion of IL-2. Whether this effect of IL-2 is direct or indirect remains unclear. Although infusion of IL-2 causes capillary permeability, and cessation of the infusion reverses the permeability, this effect may not be directly mediated by IL-2. The strongest evidence supporting a secondary mediator is that IL-2–induced capillary permeability does not develop in nude (athymic) mice, mice that were previously irradiated, or mice pretreated with cyclophosphamide (7, 8). These studies suggest that activated lymphocytes are required for IL-2–induced capillary permeability, and that IL-2 alone is insufficient.

Damle and Doyle (9) studied the effect of cytokines alone, supernatants from LAK cells, or LAK cells alone on transendothelial albumin flux. they found that IL-1, IL-2, IL-3, IL-4, IL-6, TNF, IFNγ, granulocyte-macrophage colony-stimulating factor (GM-CSF), M-CSF or 10-fold concentrated culture supernatant from LAK cells did not increase endothelial cell permeability to albumin. In this study, IL-1 and TNF increased endothelial cell expression of leukocyte adhesion molecules, but not endothelial cell permeability. Other investigators have found direct effects of IL-2 and TNF on endothelial cell permeability. These data suggests that cytokines alone may not be solely responsible for the permeability, and that the expression of leukocyte adhesion molecules may not be directly linked to endothelial permeability. However, expression of leukocyte adhesion molecules may still have an important role.

Expression of leukocyte adhesion molecules may facilitate adherence of leukocytes to endothelium, leading to changes in permeability. Co-culture of endothelial cells with LAK cells causes endothelial cell permeability in direct proportion of the number of added LAK cells (9). Furthermore, adherence of LAK cells to endothelium was inhibited by monoclonal antibodies to one of the adhesion molecules, CD11a. Monoclonal antibodies to CD11a blocked LAK cell–induced endothelial monolayer permeability (9). IL-2 did not directly induce expression of leukocyte adhesion molecules on endothelial cells; instead, IL-2 induced the synthesis of other cytokines, notably TNF, and TNF may be responsible for the up-regulation of leukocyte adhesion molecules.

IL-2 Induces endothelial cell activation

It has been shown previously that cytokines, especially TNF and IL-1, induce endothelial expression of leukocyte adhesion molecules (10). Expression of leukocyte adhesion molecules allows tight binding of polymorphonuclear leukocytes to the endothelium, resulting in further damage caused by the release of oxygen free radicals or proteases. Monoclonal antibodies to leukocyte adhesion molecules were recently shown to prevent polymorphonuclear (PMN) adhesion to endothelium and endothelial cell damage.

To determine whether IL-2 causes expression of leukocyte adhesion molecules on endothelium during IL-2 infusion, skin biopsies were obtained after the infusion of IL-2 (11). These biopsies showed endothelial cell expression of leukocyte adhesion molecules; however, incubation of IL-2 with umbilical vein endothelial cells in vitro did not induce expression of leukocyte adhesion molecules (9). Both TNF and IL-1 induce expression of leukocyte adhesion molecules on umbilical vein endothelial cells, and because IL-2 induces TNF synthesis, the authors (9) postulated that the increased expression of leukocyte adhesion molecules during IL-2 infusion was the result of IL-2–induced TNF synthesis. However, other investigators have found direct effects of IL-2 on endothelial cells.

TNF mediates edema by ICAM-1 – and CD18-dependent mechanisms

TNF induces expression of cell surface adhesion molecules, such as the intercellular adhesion molecule (ICAM-1) and the endothelial cell adhesion molecule (ELAM-1; currently referred to as E-selectin). Expression of these endothelial cell adhesion molecules is a critical factor in the binding of leukocytes to the vessel wall at the site of inflammation. Because adherent cells are capable of producing greater amounts of oxidants than nonadherent PMNs, adhesion of PMN to endothelium may be essential for mediating injury.

TNF prestimulation of the pulmonary vascular bed causes neutrophil uptake in the lung, a process that is dependent in part on the expression of ICAM-1 antigen on endothelial cells, as well as on the binding of ICAM-1 to CD18 integrin on neutrophils (12). Activation of neutrophils sequestered in the TNF-primed lungs resulted in marked alterations of pulmonary hemodynamics and fluid balance, characterized by vasoconstriction, increased capillary hydrostatic pressure, increased vascular permeability, and fulminant pulmonary edema (12). Thus, cytokines activate endothelial cells and neutrophils, leading to adherence of the PMNs to the endothelium; a second neutrophil-activating stimulus after the PMNs are adherent causes severe microvascular injury.

Neutrophil adherence to activated endothelial cells potentiates LTB₄ production

LTB_4 is a potent mediator in the inflammatory process. LTB_4 mediates PMN chemotaxis and degranulation and it induces production of oxygen radicals. PMNs adherent to TNF-activated endothelial cells have a 3-fold greater production of LTB_4 than nonadherent PMNs (13). Anti-ICAM-1, anti-ELAM-1, and CD18 monoclonal antibodies (mAbs) each inhibit approximately 40 to 60% of the PMN adherence to TNF-activated endothelial cells, and the mAbs also decreased LTB_4 production (13). Thus, following adherence to activated endothelium, PMNs synthesize greater quantities of leukotrienes, which may enhance the inflammatory response.

IL-2 induces edema by causing vasoconstriction independent of lymphocytes

Ferro and colleagues (14) investigated the ability of IL-2 to induce edema in isolated buffer–perfused lungs. Edema occurred 30 to 60 minutes after IL-2 infusion. Edema formation was dependent on pulmonary vasoconstriction, not increased microvascular permeability. The evidence supporting this conclusion was based on the following observations: (a) the increase in lung weight correlated with the increase in capillary pressure; (b) papaverine (a vasodilator) prevented both the increase in capillary pressure and the increase in weight gain; and (c) the capillary filtration coefficient was unchanged after IL-2 infusion. Thus, pulmonary vasoconstriction was an essential component of IL-2–induced pulmonary edema.

Thromboxane A_2 (TxA_2) is a potent vasoconstrictor, and it has a central role in mediating the pulmonary hypertension seen in acute lung injury (15). IL-2 infusion into the isolated perfused lung caused the appearance of increased concentrations of thromboxane B_2, the stable product of TxA_2 (14). Furthermore, pretreatment with a selective thromboxane synthetase inhibitor inhibited both the IL-2–induced increase in pulmonary artery pressure and the increase in lung weight (14).

These data demonstrate that IL-2 causes TxA_2 synthesis, which leads to vasoconstriction and hydrostatic edema, not a direct change in endothelial cell permeability. Furthermore, because these changes occurred in an isolated perfused lung system, they were independent of the presence of circulating lymphocytes or neutrophils.

Cytokines increase endothelial cell permeability

TNF, IL-1, and IL-2 may all increase endothelial cell permeability. TNF can mediate endothelial cell injury by one of several different mechanisms. TNF or its induced secondary mediators may directly affect endothelial cell function; alternatively, there is a neutrophil-dependent pathway. In support of the direct pathway, TNF is known to induce increased permeability both in vivo and in vitro. Furthermore, TNF induces the release of other inflammatory mediators, such as platelet-activating factor, IL-1, GM-CSF, and reactive oxygen species, which may contribute to the increased permeability. The second pathway involving PMNs may be the result of TNF-induced augmentation of PMN activation, resulting in the release of oxygen radicals and arachidonic acid metabolites. The release of oxidants, in particular H_2O_2, can directly increase vascular endothelial permeability (16). TNF also mediates PMN adhesion to endothelial cells by increasing expression of leukocyte adhesion molecules, thereby promoting cell-to-cell contact and enhancing PMN activation.

A third mechanism by which TNF may contribute to endothelial cell injury is by increasing the susceptibility of endothelial cells to oxidants. TNF can interfere with the intracellular oxidant buffering capacity so that cells become more sensitive to oxidant-mediated injury. TNF causes a reduction in endothelial cell intracellular glutathione, which makes the cells more sensitive to the effects of H_2O_2 (16). In these studies, endothelial permeability failed to increase in response to TNF, even at 4 ng/mL (100 U/mL). However, this same concentration of TNF was able to prime endothelial cell monolayers, rendering them more susceptible to exposure to H_2O_2. These changes were associated with changes in the shape of the endothelial cells, with redistribution of cytoskeletal actin filaments, and not just from cytolysis (16).

Downey and associates (17) studied the effect of IL-2 on cultured endothelial cell permeability. They found that IL-2 (500–25,000 U/mL) increased the steady-state transfer rate of ^{125}I-albumin across bovine pulmonary artery endothelial cell monolayers. The increase in albumin transfer was dose-dependent, and it occurred within 4 hours of the addition of IL-2. They found similar results using human umbilical vein endothelial cells. They also found that incubation of endothelial cells with IL-2 resulted in upregulation of expression if IL-2 receptors on the endothelial cells. Thus, IL-2 may directly induce endothelial cell activation.

Royall and colleagues (18) quantitated the movement of radiolabeled macromolecules of various sizes across bovine endothelial monolayers. They found that both TNF and IL-1 increased endothelial monolayer permeability in a dose- and time-dependent manner; maximal increases occurred between 12 and 24 hours.

IL-2 directly affects endothelial cell morphology

Bucana and co-workers (19) used electron microscopy to determine whether IL-2 directly affects bovine endothelial cell morphology. They found that IL-2 caused endothelial cells to retract and elongate, leading to enlarged gaps between cells reverted to their "normal" morphology within 6 to 12 hours after the removal of IL-2 from the culture medium. Similar results were obtained after incubating fresh bovine aortas with IL-2. Thus, IL-2 directly causes endothelial cell contraction, with widening of the gap junctions.

Cytokine-mediated changes in endothelial cell cytoskeleton organization

A structure–function relationship exists between endothelial cell barrier function and cytoskeletal organization. Agents that disrupt actin filaments cause increased permeability (20). Similarly, agents that stabilize actin filaments prevent the increase in endothelial permeability (21). The treatment of endothelial cells with TNF causes a rearrangement of F-actin (22). Following treatment with TNF, the peripheral actin bands become either more or less distinct, whereas the central stress fibers become more prominent and numerous. Intercellular gaps also appear. Depolymerization of F-actin to monomeric G-actin is also accompanied by new G-actin synthesis. Inhibition of new G-actin synthesis (by cycloheximide) amplified the decrease in F-actin and enhanced endothelial permeability. Agents that stimulate actin polymerization and filamentogenesis, especially at interendothelial cell junctions, are expected to limit or to prevent permeability, whereas agents that cause microfilament dissembly and reorganization promote permeability.

The role of F-actin rearrangement in IL-2–induced endothelial cell permeability was evaluated by Welbourn and associates (23). Phalloidin, a derivative of *Amanita phalloides,* binds to F-actin, enhances its polymerization, and reduces macromolecular flux across endothelial cell monolayers. Pulmonary edema, developed in rats treated with IL-2 infusion, and bronchoalveolar lavage fluid contained increased protein levels and neutrophils. Phalloidin treatment significantly reduced lung edema and protein leakage, but it did not prevent sequestration of neutrophils in the lung. These findings suggest that the changes in F-actin organization, which are responsible for the permeability, are independent of the expression of leukocyte adhesion molecules. Furthermore, these data suggest that IL-2 causes interendothelial gaps to widen via F-actin depolymerization.

Cytokine alteration of endothelial cell extracellular matrix contributes to permeability

TNF decreases collagen and fibronectin synthesis, and it induces expression of metalloproteinases that degrade collagen, laminin, and other extracellular matrix proteins. These changes in synthesis and degradation of extracellular matrix proteins may contribute to TNF-induced increases in endothelial cell permeability. To examine this hypothesis, Partridge and associates (24) designed a series of elegant experiments. They grew endothelial cells on semipermeable membranes, stimulated them with TNF, and then removed the cells from the membrane.

Fresh endothelial cells were then seeded onto the extra-cellular matrix–coated membrane and tested for permeability using ^{125}I-albumin. When the original cells, used to initially synthesize the extracellular matrix, were treated with TNF, the second monolayer had increased permeability to ^{125}I-albumin, compared with cells grown on matrix synthesized by untreated cells. These results suggest that exposure of endothelial cells to TNF caused the endothelial cells to modify synthesis of their extracellular matrix so that fresh endothelial cells formed a more permeable membrane.

TNF did not cause a decrease in the synthesis of total extracellular matrix proteins (24); however, there was a marked decrease in matrix-bound fibronectin. Because fibronectin is an important determinant of endothelial adhesion to the subendothelial matrix via the integrin receptors, its loss may contribute to TNF-induced morphological changes and monolayer permeability.

PATHOPHYSIOLOGY OF CLARKSON'S DISEASE

Possible mediators of Clarkson's disease

The mediators responsible for the idiopathic systemic capillary permeability syndrome remain unknown, although IL-2 has been implicated. A number of different pathways have been investigated (25). Although some reports suggest complement activation, this has not been a consistent finding. Immune complexes are not present. Low levels of plasma prekallikrein levels, modest elevation of histamine levels, and increased arachidonic acid metabolism by the lipoxygenase pathway have each been reported in individual patients, but these have not been consistent findings. Atrial natriuretic factor is known to cause hemoconcentration and increased capillary permeability, but in the one patient in whom this factor was measured, it was not elevated.

Clarkson's disease-associated paraproteinemia

The only consistent abnormal laboratory data in patients with the idiopathic form of the systemic capillary leak syndrome is the presence of an abnormal paraprotein (i.e., immunoglobulin [IgG] gammopathy) (3). It is generally thought that this abnormal paraprotein in some way causes endothelial cell contraction, with widening of the gap junctions. Monoclonal IgG gammopathy either exists or develops in most of the patients with this syndrome; however, four patients have been described with the syndrome who did not have paraproteinemia. Fur-

thermore, the partially purified paraprotein failed to alter endothelial cell permeability. Thus, the paraprotein may represent a marker of the disease, and it may not be a mediator.

IL-2 receptor expression in patients with Clarkson's disease

The IL-2 receptor is a protein that mediates the action of IL-2. Normal testing T and B lymphocytes do not express these receptors; however, following immune stimulation and proliferation of T lymphocytes, the expression of IL-2 receptors on the T lymphocytes change. First, there is an increased number of IL-2 recptors expressed on the cell surface; second, IL-2 receptors are shed from the surface of the cell. Soluble IL-2 receptors are of lower molecular weight (10 kd) than the membrane-bound form (55 kd), suggesting that the receptors may be proteolytically cleaved from the membrane; however, the mechanisms regulating their cleavage from the membrane are still under investigation.

Recently, Cicardi and associates (26) evaluated the role of cytokines as mediators of the idiopathic form of the systemic capillary leak syndrome. Although they failed to detect circulating levels of IL-1 or IL-2, they did find an increase in Tac-positive mononuclear cells and an increase in circulating levels of the soluble IL-2 receptor. Antibodies to the Tac antigen recognize the β-chain of the IL-2 receptor. Thus, peripheral blood mononuclear cells from patients with the idiopathic form of the systemic capillary leak syndrome consistently express IL-2 receptors. In general, expression of IL-2 receptors is induced on T lymphocytes following mitogen or antigen activation. Thus, the authors postulated that IL-2 receptor expressing T lymphocytes are induced in response to an unknown signal in the idiopathic systemic capillary leak syndrome (26). Because peripheral blood mononuclear cells express IL-2 receptors in response to IL-2, they suggested that cytokines are produced during episodes of increased vascular permeability in the idiopathic systemic capillary permeability syndrome. However, because neither IL-1 nor IL-2 were detected, and because other cytokines were not measured, the role of cytokines as mediators of this syndrome remains speculative.

In addition to Clarkson's disease, plasma levels of IL-2 receptor are elevated in patients with leukemia (especially hairy-cell leukemia), lymphoma, transplant rejection, viral infections (including acquired immunodeficiency syndrome), and systemic lupus erythematosus. These diseases are not associated with a systemic capillary leak. Thus, levels of IL-2 receptor may be useful in characterizing the activity of these different diseases, but they may not be directly responsible for permeability.

CURRENT THERAPY

Current therapy of IL-2–induced capillary permeability

If the systemic capillary leak syndrome is the result of IL-2 infusion, then stopping the IL-2 infusion reverses the permeability. However, this limits the effectiveness of use of IL-2 and LAK cell infusion for treating metastatic cancer. Future efforts may be directed at preventing IL-2–induced capillary permeability. Currently, the most promising approaches appear to be inhibiting IL-2 production of TNF. Inhibition of TNF by mAbs to TNF or by infusion of TNF-soluble receptors both appear promising. Another approach is to use drugs known to inhibit TNF synthesis. One such drug is pentoxifylline, which is an inhibitor of phosphodiesterase, and it is known to inhibit endotoxin-induced TNF synthesis. Pretreatment of patients with pentoxifylline decreases the side effects of IL-2 infusion (27). The potential limitation of inhibition of TNF production is that TNF may be an important component of the antitumor effect of IL-2–LAK cell infusion. Thus, although blocking TNF production may decrease systemic side effects, it may also decrease therapeutic benefits. A future approach could be to develop drugs that stabilize F-actin and prevent is depolymerization. This approach might decrease the permeability, but not the antitumor effects, of IL-2.

Current therapy of Clarkson's disease

In patients with the idiopathic form of the systemic capillary leak syndrome, the current approach to therapy is initial volume resuscitation. Although this is a sound approach in theory, it may have little effect on the outcome. Because of the macromolecular permeability, colloids offer no benefit over crystalloids. Excessive volume resuscitation may result in pulmonary edema during the recovery phase. Diuretics may be necessary, but death from pulmonary edema has been described.

β_2-agonists and other drugs that increase cAMP are beneficial in a number of models of pulmonary edema. Drugs that increase cAMP are thought to cause endothelial cell relaxation, which produces a decrease in the size of the interendothelial cell junctions, or to effect leukocyte adhesion. On the basis of the data presented, the beneficial role of drugs that increase cAMP may be related to its effect of decreasing interendothelial cell junctions or by inhibiting expression of leukocyte adhesion molecules.

A number of drugs have been used to try to prevent the acute attacks associated with Clarkson's disease (25). The class of drugs most commonly used are β_2-agonists. Many but not all patients treated with β_2-agonists have had a decrease in the frequency of the attacks. Some drugs that appear to have no benefit include ketotifen, danazol, epsilon amino caproic acid, nonsteroidal anti-inflammatory drugs, atropine, anti-histamines (type I and II), tranexamic acid, and cromoglycate (25).

In the future, efforts to modulate endothelial gap formation should be considered. Other approaches to preventive therapy might include cytokine antagonists, cytokine receptor blockers, or inhibitors of F-actin depolymerization.

REFERENCES

1. Clarkson B, Thompson D, Horwith M, Luckey E. Cyclical edema and shock due to increased capillary permeability. Am J Med 1960;29:193–216.

2. Rosenberg S, Lotze M, Muul L, et al. Observations on the systemic administration of autologous lymphokine-activated killer cells and recombinant interleukin 2. N Engl J Med 1985;313:1485.

3. Atkinson J, Waldmann T, Stein S, et al. Systemic capillary leak syndrome and monoclonal IgG gammapathy. Medicine 1977;56:225–239.

4. George C, Regnier B, Le Gall J, Gostinne H, Carlet J, Rapin M. Hypovolemic shock with edema due to increased capillary permeability. Intensive Care Med 1978;4:159–163.

5. Grimm E, Robb R, Roth J, et al. Lymphokine-activated killer cell phenomenon. Evidence that IL-2 is sufficient for direct activation of peripheral blood lymphocytes into lymphokine-activated killer cells. J Exp Med 1983;158:1356.

6. Mule J, Shu S, Schwarz S, Rosenberg S. Adoptive immunotherapy of established pulmonary metastasis with LAK cells and recombinant interleukin 2. Science 1984;225:1487.

7. Rosenstein M, Ettinghausen S, Rosenberg S. Extravasation of intravascular fluid mediated by systemic administration of recombinant interleukin 2. J Immunol 1986;137:1735–1742.

8. Mole J, Shu J, Rosenberg S. The antitumor efficacy of lymphokine-activated killer cells and recombinant interleukin-2. Immunol 1985;135:646–52.

9. Damle N, Doyle L. IL-2 activated human killer lymphocytes but not their secreted products mediate increase in albumin flux across cultured endothelial monolayers: Implications for vascular leak syndrome. J Immunol 1989;142:2660–2669.

10. Pober J, Bevilacqua M, Mendrick D, Lapierre L, Fiers W, Gimbrone M. Two distinct monokines, interleukin 1 and tumor necrosis factor, each independently induce biosynthesis and transient expression of the same antigen on the surface of cultured human vascular endothelial cells. J Immunol 1986;136:1680.

11. Cotran R, Pober J, Gimbrone M, et al. Endothelial activation during interleukin 2 immunotherapy: A possible mechanism for the vascular leak syndrome. J Immunol 1987;139:1883–1888.

12. Lo S, Everitt J, Gu J, Malik A. Tumor necrosis factor mediates experimental pulmonary edema by ICAM-1 and CD18-dependent mechanisms. J Clin Invest 1992;89:981–1005.

13. Ishii Y, Lo S, Malik A. Neutrophil adhesion to TNF-activated endothelial cells potentiates leukotriene B4 production. J Cell Physiol 1992;153:187–195.

14. Ferro T, Johnson A, Everitt J, Malik A. IL-2 induces pulmonary edema and vasoconstriction independent of circulating lymphocytes. J Immunol 1989;142:1916–1921.

15. Casey LC, Fletcher JR, Zmudka M, Ramwell PW. Prevention of endotoxin induced pulmonary hypertension in primates by the use of a selective thromboxane synthetase inhibitor, OKY 1581. J Pharm Exp Ther 1982;222:441–446.

16. Ishii Y, Partridge C, Del Vecchio P, Malik A. Tumor necrosis factor mediated decrease in glutathione increases the sensitivity of pulmonary vascular endothelial cells to H_2O_2. J Clin Invest 1992;89:794–802.

17. Downey G, Ryan U, Hayes B, and Friedman M. Interleukin 2 directly increases albumin permeability of bovine and human vascular endothelium in vitro. Am J Respir Cell Mol Biol 1992;7:58–65.

18. Royall J, Berkow R, Beckman J, Cunningham M, Matalon S, Freeman B. Tumor necrosis factor and interleukin 1 alpha increase vascular endothelial permeability. Am J Physiol 1989;257:L399–410.

19. Bucana C, Trial J, Papp A, Wu K. Bovine aortic endothelial cell incubation with interleukin 2: morphological changes correlate with enhanced vascular permeability. Scan Microsc 1988;2:1559–1566.

20. Shasby D, Shasby S, Sullivan J, Peach M. Role of endothelial cell cytoskeleton in control of endothelial permeability. Circ Res 1982;51:657–661.

21. Phillips P, Lum H, Malik A, Tsan M. Phallacidin prevents thrombin-induced increases in endothelial permeability to albumin. Am J Physiol 1989;257:C562–C567.

22. Goldblum S, Ding X, Campbell-Washington J. TNF-alpha induces endothelial cell F-actin depolymerization, new actin synthesis, and barrier dysfunction. Am J Physiol 1993;264:C894–C905.

23. Welbourn R, Goldman G, Kobzik L, Valeri C, Hechtman H, Shepro D. Attenuation of IL-2-induced multisystem organ edema by phalloidin and antamanide. J Appl Physiol 1991;70:1364–1368.

24. Partridge C, Horvath C, Del Vecchio P, Phillips P, Malik A. Influence of extracellular matrix in tumor necrosis factor induced increase in endothelial permeability. Am J Physiol 1992;263:L627–L637.

25. Teelucksingh S, Padfield P, Edwards C. Systemic capillary leak syndrome. Q J Med 1990;277:515–524.

26. Cicardi M, Gardinali M, Bisiani G, Rosti A, Allavena P, Agostoni A. The systemic capillary leak syndrome. Appearance of interleukin-2-receptor-positive cells during attacks. Ann Intern Med 1990;113:475–477.

27. Edwards M, Heniford B, Klar E, Doak K, Miller F. Pentoxifylline inhibits interleukin-2-induced toxicity in C57BL/6 mice but preserves antitumor efficacy. J Clin Invest 1992;90:637–641.

CHAPTER 39

ROLE OF CYTOKINES
IN BLOOD-BRAIN BARRIER DAMAGE

Mohammad K. Sharief

The concept of a blood-brain barrier was initiated by Paul Ehrlich's discovery in 1885 that intravenous injection of an acidic dye (coerulein-s) into animals caused vital staining of all organs except the brain (1). The first systematic experiment to document the blood-brain barrier was performed in 1913 by Goldman (2), who showed that the brains of experimental animals were stained only after the dye had been injected into the cerebrospinal fluid (the liquid that bathes the brain and the spinal cord), but not into the blood stream. Approximately 50 years later, electron microscopy confirmed these observations at the ultrastructural level (3), where overlapping edges of brain capillary endothelial cells were observed to be sealed together by tight junctions. Intravenously injected tracer proteins were observed to remain in the capillary lumens without penetrating the cerebral endothelium, whereas markers injected into the cerebrospinal fluid eventually penetrated into the brain side of the interendothelial junctions, but they did not pass through to the capillary lumen (3).

The term *blood-brain barrier* refers to a series of structural and functional barriers located at the interfaces of brain and blood and of blood and cerebrospinal fluid. Due to the barrier, the chemical composition of brain and the cerebrospinal fluid remain relatively stable, compared with that of other body tissues. Within the central nervous system, however, free traffic between extracellular fluid and cerebrospinal fluid is assumed because of the absence of tight junctions between ventricular ependymal cells.

In the normal state, the blood-brain barrier maintains the brain within a protected environment, relatively free from circulating micro-organisms or biologically active molecules that may alter normal synaptic transmission. Invasion of the brain by viruses, for example, appears to require a sequence of events involving extraneural tissues, blood, and the various components of the blood-brain barrier. This may explain why viral meningitis and encephalitis in humans are relatively rare, even though infections with viruses that have the potential to cause neurological disease are common. Presumably, only by eluding each of these barriers in sequence can an invading agent gain access to the central nervous system.

STRUCTURE OF THE BLOOD-BRAIN BARRIER

The central nervous system is relatively isolated from systemic immune responses in the absence of disease, and there are indeed several differences between the central nervous system and the majority of peripheral sites. First, lymph drainage from the brain to the peripheral lymph nodes is not well defined, although experiments have shown that macromolecules deposited within the brain can reach deep cervical lymph nodes. Second, classic antigen-presenting cells, the dendritic leukocytes that reside in almost all tissues of the body, are absent from the brain.

Third, major histocompatibility complex (MHC) antigens, which have a key role in generation and propagation of the immune response, are not expressed at detectable levels in healthy unactivated central nervous system tissue, apart from endothelial cells. Finally, proteins and cells of blood are relatively excluded from the central nervous system under normal conditions by the blood-brain barrier.

The term *blood-brain barrier* is generally applied to describe the overall exclusionary interfaces between circulating blood at one side, and the extracellular as well as the cerebrospinal fluid space at the other side (4). These interfaces include the epithelium of the choroid plexus, the endothelial cells of cerebral capillaries, the plasma membrane and the adventitia (Rouget cells) of the blood vessels, the layer of cells lining the arachnoid membrane, and the foot processes of astrocytes (5) (Fig. 39–1).

Brain capillary endothelial cells differ from those located elsewhere in the body (except for the kidneys) in that they contain tight junctions that seal the cells together, have few pinocytic vesicles, and have no fenestrations or transendothelial channels. Cerebral endothelial cells have more mitochondria than other types of endothelium, indicating high energy requirement. Together with adjacent astrocytes, cerebral capillary endothelium transports organic molecules as well as inorganic electrolytes from the blood plasma to the central nervous system. Plasma constituents can travel via pinocytotic vesicles into the narrow space between the albuminal side of the endothelia and the basement membrane. The intricate network of the basement membrane is passed by restricted diffusion in either direction, and the extracellular space of the parenchyma can thus be cleared by reversed pinocytosis.

In experimental animals, barrier changes may be detected by examining cerebrospinal fluid or brain capillary endothelial cells for intravenously injected radiolabeled markers, dyes, or marker proteins that normally do not pass the barrier. Changes in the blood-brain barrier can be detected in the clinical laboratory by examining the cerebrospinal fluid for increased concentrations of plasma proteins. In routine work, the integrity of the blood-brain barrier is usually evaluated by calculating the cerebrospinal fluid-to-serum albumin quotient (Q_{alb}), which is one of the best chemical indicators of barrier damage (6). It is noteworthy, however, that measurement of Q_{alb} represents an approximation to blood-brain breakdown, because it commonly measures breakdown of the blood-cerebrospinal fluid barrier. The choroid plexus, in particular, has no significant blood-tissue barrier function.

PATHOLOGICAL ALTERATIONS IN THE BLOOD-BRAIN BARRIER

There is considerable evidence that alterations of the blood-brain barrier are important in the pathogenesis of several diseases of the central nervous system, such as bacterial or viral infections, as well as inflammatory diseases of the nervous system. Pathological features of altered brain capillary endothelium include changes in cell volume, increased vesicular transport, and widening of tight junctions.

In inflammatory diseases, immunological injury is strongly implicated in disruption of the blood-brain barrier, primarily through secretion of cytokines that stimulate proliferation or other metabolic activities of the basic barrier components. The brain contains few immune cells and it lacks organized lymphoid tissue. Lymphocytes do not usually appear within the central nervous system, except when the blood-brain barrier is disrupted. Lymphocytes may pass through the capillary endothelium via altered tight junctions or by direct damage to cerebral endothelium. The consequences of minor vascular injury are far more serious in the central nervous system than in other organs because of barrier dysfunction, and they may even lead to death.

In infections of the central nervous system, viruses may be carried across the endothelial cells in infected leukocytes. This mechanism of invasion may be facilitated by cytokine-induced endothelial damage. Some viruses infect cerebral vascular endothelial cells prior to infection

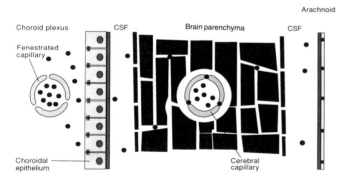

Figure 39–1 The blood-brain barrier. Protein particles are represented by •. As demonstrated, there are three barriers, each characterized by different permeability and flux conditions: (1) the blood-brain barrier (circulating blood/extracellular space); (2) the blood-cerebrospinal fluid (CSF) barrier (circulating blood/CSF space); and (3) the parenchymal cell membrane barrier (extracellular space/intracellular space). The essential anatomical structures of the blood-brain barrier are (*a*) the endothelia of arterioles, capillaries, and venules; (*b*) the epithelial cells and the basement membrane of the choroid plexus; and (*c*) the layer of cells lining the arachnoid membrane. (Modified by permission from Leibowitz S, Hughes RAC. Immunity and the blood brain barrier. Immunology of the nervous system. London: Edward Arnold Ltd, 1983:1–9.)

of the adjacent glia and neurones, and this mechanism, as will be discussed, also involves cytokine-induced damage.

CYTOKINE REGULATION OF ENDOTHELIAL CELLS

After considerable research into the location and the properties of the blood-brain barrier (7), it was established by electron microscopy that its principal site is the endothelial cell layer of blood capillaries supplying the brain (8). Endothelial cells have long been viewed as a passive lining of blood vessels endowed essentially with negative properties (e.g., being nonreactive to blood components). It is now well established that these cells, which gate the traffic of molecules and cells across the blood-brain barrier, have an active role in homeostasis, inflammatory reactions, and immunity. In addition to responding rapidly to agonists such as histamine and thrombin, endothelial cells, after exposure to cytokines, undergo profound alterations of function that involve gene expression and protein synthesis.

Cytokine regulation of endothelial cell function was thoroughly discussed in Chapter 7. I focus on the interaction between the cytokine network and the cerebral capillary endothelial cells. This interaction is now widely regarded as a major mechanism involved in disruption of the blood-brain barrier. Almost all recent research work has centered on three cytokines: tumor necrosis factor-α (TNF-α), interleukin-1 (IL-1), and IL-2. I therefore deal with the effect of these cytokines on the blood-brain barrier.

BLOOD-BRAIN BARRIER DAMAGE IN MULTIPLE SCLEROSIS

Multiple sclerosis is an inflammatory and demyelinating disease of the central nervous system that is a major cause of neurological disability in young adults. The disease follows a chronic recurrent course and it has several well-established immunological aberrations that involve B lymphocytes and various subsets of T lymphocytes (9).

There is considerable evidence that alterations of the blood-brain barrier might be important in the pathogenesis of multiple sclerosis (10–12). Initial observations that early plaques of multiple sclerosis usually develop around small cerebral blood vessels have long been considered to be an important clue to the pathogenesis of this disease (13,14). This notion has recently received new impetus from Gd-enhanced magnetic resonance imaging, (MRI) which shows foci of blood-brain barrier leakage as an early detectable change in the central nervous system of patients with multiple sclerosis (15). Furthermore, there is now direct evidence that these foci are inflammatory in origin (16), raising the important suggestion that they might represent the primary lesion in multiple sclerosis.

Immunocytological studies in multiple sclerosis brains have demonstrated that damage of blood vessels of acute plaques was closely associated with the presence of activated macrophages and other inflammatory cells (16). In addition, deposition of complement, as well as immunoglobulin G (IgG) and IgM, but not IgA, was detected in all acute plaques examined (16). Such a finding suggests that damage to the blood-brain barrier in early multiple sclerosis plaques is due to inflammatory changes, which are probably mediated by activated immune cells. The presence of IgM in these plaques further emphasizes the acute association.

Blood-brain barrier and cytokines in multiple sclerosis

It is now well known that oligodendrocytes and cerebral endothelial cells are selectively damaged in multiple sclerosis lesions, whereas astrocytes are spared and may be proliferative (17). Cytokines may exert selective effects on glial cells, and they usually have a stimulatory effect on astrocytes, whereas, in contrast, they appear to have a deleterious effect on oligodendrocytes and endothelial cells (18,19). The importance of the cytokine network in multiple sclerosis is thoroughly discussed in Chapter 12, and I focus on the role of cytokines in the disruption of blood-brain barrier in patients with multiple sclerosis. Special attention is paid to the role of IL-2 and TNF-α in this mechanism.

IL-2 AND BLOOD-BRAIN BARRIER DAMAGE

A role for IL-2 has been implicated in the pathogenesis of a number of central nervous system diseases, including multiple sclerosis. Evidence for this role has emanated from studies on tissues from multiple sclerosis plaques (20–22) and on serum and cerebrospinal fluid samples from patients with multiple sclerosis (23–25). IL-2 receptor (IL-2R)–bearing lymphocytes have been detected in the perivascular infiltrate in multiple sclerosis brain lesions, and an in vivo relationship of IL-2 and soluble IL-2 (sIL-2) receptor to blood-brain barrier impairment has recently been reported in patients with active multiple sclerosis. In the following sections, I discuss the pathological effects of IL-2 on the blood-brain barrier in active multiple sclerosis.

Effect of recombinant IL-2 on the blood-brain barrier

Pathological studies have consistently shown that administration of recombinant IL-2 leads to disruption of the blood-brain barrier (26,27), a finding that could be relevant in the context of pathophysiological changes seen in patients with multiple sclerosis. Clinical studies have also shown that administration of recombinant IL-2 to patients with cancer who had no evidence of central nervous system involvement may result in disruption of the blood-brain barrier (28). Recombinant IL-2 preparations are not glycosylated, and they differ very slightly in amino acid sequence from native IL-2, but they have identical biological activities (29).

It could be argued that pathological and clinical adverse reactions of recombinant IL-2 may merely represent some coincidental findings that do not necessarily implicate IL-2 in the damage observed in endothelial cells. However, firm evidence that human endothelial cells are directly affected by IL-2 has recently been provided (30). Such evidence is mainly based on the fact that human vascular endothelial cells express significant levels of functional IL-2 receptors, both of low and high affinity. Therefore, IL-2 may directly affect human endothelial cells both in vitro and in vivo.

Correlation of IL-2 and sIL-2R with blood-brain barrier impairment

In patients with multiple sclerosis, a significantly higher incidence of blood-brain barrier damage was reported in patients who had high cerebrospinal fluid levels of IL-2 or sIL-2R (Table 39–1). Some authors sought to exclude pas-

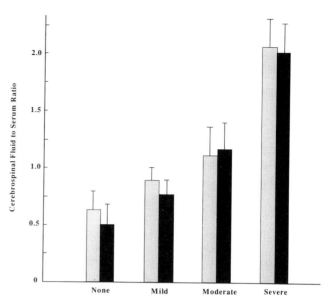

Figure 39–2   Correlation of intrathecal levels of IL-2 (□) and sIL-2R (■) (expressed as cerebrospinal fluid-to-serum ratio) with the degree of blood-brain barrier damage in patients with active multiple sclerosis. Values depict means ± standard error of the mean. (Reproduced with permission from Sharief MK, Hentges R, Ciardi M, Thompson EJ. In vivo relationship of interleukin-2 and soluble IL-2 receptor to blood-brain barrier impairment in patients with active multiple sclerosis. J Neurol 1993;240:46–50.)

sive transudation of IL-2 or sIL-2R from the systemic circulation through damaged barriers by calculating cerebrospinal fluid-to-serum ratios to correct for any passive leakage from the systemic to the intrathecal compartment. Such correction confirmed that intrathecal levels of IL-2 and sIL-2R significantly correlated with barrier impairment (Fig. 39–2).

TABLE 39–1   NUMBER (AND %) OF PATIENTS WITH MULTIPLE SCLEROSIS WHO SHOWED SIGNS OF BLOOD-BRAIN BARRIER DAMAGE RELATED TO THE PRESENCE OF IL-2 AND sIL-2R IN THE CEREBROSPINAL FLUID (CSF)

Condition of Blood-brain Barrier[a]	CSF IL-2		CSF sIL-2R	
	Absent	Present	Normal	High
Intact (n = 41)	22 (54%)	19 (46%)	12 (29%)	29 (71%)
Damaged (n = 69)	8 (12%)	61 (88%)[b]	9 (13%)	60 (87%)[c]

[a]As evaluated by CSF-to-serum albumin quotient; values > 5.8×10^{-3} indicate barrier damage.
[b]$p < 0.0001$.
[c]$p < 0.0005$.
Modified from Sharief MK. The importance of interleukin-2 and its soluble receptor in patients with MS and other inflammatory diseases of the central nervous system. PhD thesis, University of London, 1992.

Possible mechanisms of IL-2–related blood-brain barrier damage

Several mechanisms have been proposed to explain the effect of IL-2 on cerebral endothelial cells. First, cerebral endothelial damage may result from a direct effect of IL-2 on endothelial cells, which results in a local Shwartzman reaction (i.e., focal thrombosis, hemorrhage, or inflammation). Second, endothelial damage could result from a direct cell-to-cell interaction between endothelial cells and IL-2–activated lymphocytes or vasoactive factors elaborated from IL-2–activated cells (32). Several studies have clearly demonstrated that IL-2–induced capillary leak is due to cell-mediated injury to the endothelium (32), and a three-dimensional ultrastructural model of target cell killing by IL-2–activated killer cells has already been presented (33). In addition, Watts and others (27) attributed blood-brain barrier disruption to the presence of arachidonic acid and its oxidative products (e.g., prostaglandins, thromboxanes, and leukotrienes), which could be released by IL-2–activated lymphocytes.

A third mechanism to explain a putative IL-2 effect on the blood-brain barrier may be IL-2–enhanced production of other cytokines, particularly IL-1 and TNF-α (34). Both IL-1 and TNF-a have profound proinflammatory effects on endothelial cell functions (35), and they could cause endothelial cell damage. The role and possible mechanisms of TNF-α–mediated blood-brain barrier damage are presented.

TNF-α AND BLOOD-BRAIN BARRIER DAMAGE

It has been reported that newly formed multiple sclerosis plaques contain T lymphocytes and macrophages at their active edge (36). Both cell types secrete TNF-α, a pleiotropic cytokine with a wide variety of biological functions on a broad range of cells. TNF-α is well recognized as an important mediator of several inflammatory and immunological responses in a number of tissues, including the central nervous system, and its effects on neural cells are therefore widely studied. TNF-α–mediated responses within the central nervous system include (a) enhancement of class I MHC antigen expression on astrocytes and oligodendrocytes (37), (b) enhancement of class II MHC expression on astrocytes through its synergistic interaction with other cytokines (38), (c) induction of intracellular adhesion molecule-1 (ICAM-1) on human fetal astrocytes (39), (d) proliferation of adult astrocytes (40), (e) induction of other cytokine production by astrocytes (41), and (f) lysis of oligodendrocytes, which produce

myelin in the central nervous system, as well as direct damage to myelin sheaths (18).

TNF-α has already been identified in multiple sclerosis brain lesions (42). Moreover, independent research groups have provided evidence that TNF-α levels in cerebrospinal fluid reflect disease activity in multiple sclerosis (43,44). There is increasing evidence that TNF-α is capable of causing vascular endothelial damage, both in experimental animals and in humans. Effects of TNF-α on endothelial cells that are relevant to multiple sclerosis include modulation of endothelial cell functions, resulting in vascular endothelial damage, and an increase in vascular endothelial permeability, which leads to vascular leak syndrome.

Correlation of TNF-α with blood-brain barrier impairment

Recent work has established that high cerebrospinal fluid levels of TNF-α in active multiple sclerosis are significantly associated with a higher incidence of barrier damage (45), as measured by the cerebrospinal fluid/serum albumin ratio (Fig. 39–3). Moreover, a significant association was detected between the presence of TNF-α and the degree of barrier damage; low intrathecal TNF-α levels were detected in patients with mild barrier impairment, whereas high levels were associated with severe barrier damage (Fig. 39–4). This finding further extends recent reports (43) of endothelial cell immunoreactivity for TNF-α at the edge of acute multiple sclerosis lesions,

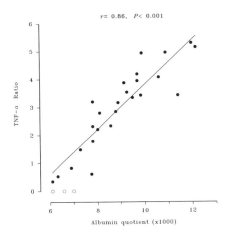

Figure 39–3 Correlation of cerebrospinal fluid (CSF)/ serum ratio of TNF-α with barrier damage (as expressed by CSF/serum albumin ratio) in patients with active multiple sclerosis. *Open circles* depict patients who had detectable TNF-α levels in serum but not CSF samples. Values of CSF/serum albumin ratio above 5.8×10^3 indicate barrier damage. (Reproduced with permission from Sharief MK, Thompson EJ. In vivo relationship of tumor necrosis factor-α to blood-brain barrier damage in patients with active multiple sclerosis. J Neuroimmunol 1993;38:27–34.

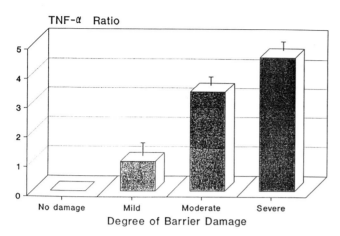

Figure 39–4   Correlation of intrathecal level of TNF-α (expressed as cerebrospinal fluid to serum ratio) with the degree of blood-brain barrier damage in patients with active multiple sclerosis. Values represent means ± standard error of the mean. (Reproduced with permission from Sharief MK, Hentges R. Association between tumor necrosis factor-α and disease progression in patients with multiple sclerosis. N Eng J Med 1991;325:467–472.

and it suggests that TNF-α may be related to the pathogenesis of barrier damage.

A putative TNF-α–induced disruption of the blood-brain barrier could result from several mechanisms. TNF-α causes increased vascular permeability by inducing morphological and structural changes of endothelial cells through a direct toxic effect. It also down-regulates endothelial cell expression of thrombomodulin, and it causes enhanced procoagulant activity that promotes intravascular coagulation and capillary thrombosis. In addition, TNF-α changes the propensity of endothelial cells to bind neutrophils, possibly contributing to the intense margination response that is observed in vivo following infusion of the cytokine (46).

Furthermore, leukocytes, particularly neutrophils, adherent to endothelial cells are stimulated by TNF-α to increase biosynthesis and release of reactive superoxide intermediates and arachidonic acid metabolites. Indeed, 100 U/mL TNF-α, a concentration readily attainable in cerebrospinal fluid of patients with active multiple sclerosis, stimulate eosinophils and other cells to damage human endothelial cells in vitro (47). However, the precise mechanisms of interaction between TNF-α and cellular elements in multiple sclerosis brain lesions are not clearly identified.

THE DYNAMICS OF TNF-α AND IL-2 IN BLOOD-BRAIN BARRIER DAMAGE

As seen in Fig. 39–5, intrathecal levels of TNF-α, as well as those of IL-2 and sIL-2R, correlate with the severity of barrier damage. However, intrathecal TNF-α levels in

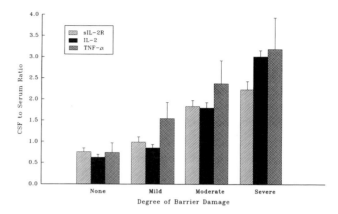

Figure 39–5   Relationship of intrathecal levels of IL-2, sIL-2R, and TNF-α with the degree of blood-brain barrier impairment in 110 patients with active multiple sclerosis. Values represent means ± standard error of the mean.

individual grades of barrier damage show a standard deviation much larger than that of IL-2 or sIL-2R. This finding may suggest that blood-brain barrier damage in active multiple sclerosis is more closely related to intrathecal levels of IL-2 and sIL-2R than to intrathecal levels of TNF-α, although further pathological studies are required to establish the relative importance of these cytokines in barrier damage.

Because the precise relationship between barrier impairment and both IL-2 and TNF-α levels is crucial in understanding the pathophysiology of blood-brain barrier changes in multiple sclerosis, multivariate statistical procedures, including discriminant analysis, were employed to analyze cytokine levels together, not one at a time (48). Because IL-2, sIL-2R, and TNF-α could be interrelated, considering them simultaneously in statistical analysis will incorporate important information about their relationships with each other and with blood-brain barrier impairment. Thus, the relative relations of intrathecal levels of IL-2, sIL-2R, and TNF-α to barrier impairment in multiple sclerosis were tested by multivariate analysis of variance combined with discriminant analysis. As shown in Table 39–2, the relationship between barrier impairment and cerebrospinal fluid concentration of Il-2 was stronger than the relationship between barrier impairment and cerebrospinal fluid TNF-α concentrations.

The positive correlation between blood-brain barrier disruption and cerebrospinal fluid levels of IL-2 and TNF-α may be relevant to the pathological endothelial abnormalities induced by TNF-α. Although detection of elevated levels of IL-2 and TNF-α in the cerebrospinal fluid may merely reflect the presence of activated T cells or macrophages, earlier pathological evidence suggests that some IL-2–associated conditions of blood-brain barrier damage may be causally related to high cerebrospinal fluid levels of TNF-α. As discussed, activated astrocytes, oligodendrocytes, and other microglial cells synthesize

TABLE 39–2 MULTIVARIATE ANALYSIS OF VARIANCE AND DISCRIMINANT ANALYSIS OF THE RELATIONSHIP BETWEEN CEREBROSPINAL FLUID (CSF) CYTOKINES AND BLOOD-BRAIN BARRIER IMPAIRMENT IN 110 PATIENTS WITH ACTIVE MULTIPLE SCLEROSIS.

CSF Variable (n)	F Value	P Value
Interleukin-2 (80)	14.1	< 0.0001
Tumour necrosis factor-α (68)	11.9	< 0.001
Soluble IL-2 receptor (89)	6.8	< 0.003

and secrete IL-2. Therefore, intrathecal production of this cytokine can generate and potentiate inflammatory immune responses through subsequent induction of other inflammatory mediators, including TNF-α.

High concentrations of TNF-α are not always critical in mediating blood-brain barrier disruption in patients with active multiple sclerosis. Recent studies (48) reported that IL-2–induced barrier disruption could develop in the absence of TNF-α reactivity, suggesting that other mediators may be involved in this process. IL-1β has been suggested to cause disruption of blood-brain barrier in experimental animals (49). In addition, IL-1β was reported to initiate meningeal inflammation without a concomitant increase in TNF-α levels (50). However, no consistent IL-1β reactivity is detected in the cerebrospinal fluid of patients with multiple sclerosis despite severe barrier disruption. It is tempting, therefore, to suggest that IL-1β is not associated with blood-brain barrier impairment in multiple sclerosis patients, although the influence of subclinical levels of IL-1β cannot be excluded.

CORRELATION OF TFN-α WITH INTRACELLULAR ADHESION MOLECULE-1

Adhesion of inflammatory cells to vascular endothelium is essential for their migration into inflamed tissues. In multiple sclerosis, cellular infiltration leading to demyelination denotes specific recognition between the immune system and its target membrane, myelin, and it is probably preceded by lymphocyte-endothelial recognition. Data has recently accumulated showing that the prelude to lymphocyte infiltration in autoimmune demyelination is adhesion to central nervous system endothelium (51). Endothelial cells lining the postcapillary venules and the microcirculation express several adhesion molecules, both constitutively and in response to inflammatory mediators, including TNF-α (52). Thus, detection of adhesion molecule expression in vivo at sites of acute inflammation has been used to infer functional activation of

the endothelium at these settings (53). Indeed, treatment with monoclonal antibody against certain adhesion molecules abrogates the development of experimental allergic encephalomyelitis (EAE) by blocking the entry of lymphocytes and monocytes to the brain (54).

Intercellular adhesion molecule-1 (ICAM-1, CD54), a molecule bound to the cell surface membrane, is an important early marker of immune activation and response (55), including production of inflammatory vascular injury in vivo (56). The expression of ICAM-1, which may confer adhesivity for lymphocytes, is detected in several organs, including human neuronal cells and cerebral endothelium (57). Moreover, up-regulation of ICAM-1 on central nervous system endothelia has been documented in the active lesions of EAE (58), although the up-regulating signal has not been fully characterized.

The normal constraints of human biopsy or autopsy procedures invariably restrict evaluation of ICAM-1 expression in patients with multiple sclerosis. Therefore, the recent detection of free circulating ICAM-1 (cICAM-1) in human sera (59) improved the prospects for investigating the dynamics of ICAM-1 in vivo in patients with active multiple sclerosis. Recently, serum and cerebrospinal fluid levels of free cICAM-1 have been shown to correlate with both TNF-α levels and blood-brain barrier disruption in patients with active multiple sclerosis (60).

The blood-brain barrier, which is formed by specialized endothelial cells, regulates the interaction between the immune and the central nervous systems. In the normal brain, there is very limited lymphocyte traffic, but lymphocyte infiltration is critical for the pathogenesis of autoimmune demyelination (51). A crucial early step in mounting an effective inflammatory or immune response is promotion of leukocyte adhesion to the vascular endothelium before they can migrate chemotactically to the appropriate microenvironment (61).

It has been recently reported that adhesion molecules are expressed on human blood-brain barrier and cerebrovascular cells (62). Because active multiple sclerosis lesions are commonly associated with cerebral endothelial damage, it is reasonable to suggest that ICAM-1 may act as a homing signal in central nervous system inflammation seen in this disease. In addition, the adhesive interactions between inflammatory cells and the functional adhesion molecules expressed on endothelial cells may result in activation of inflammatory cells prior to their migration into the intrathecal compartment, further underlying the potential importance of ICAM-1 in the regulation of central nervous system inflammation. Whether the release of cICAM-1 preceded or occurred during disruption of the blood-barrier is not yet clear, but it is currently the subject of further longitudinal studies. Preliminary evidence (54), however, suggests that several adhesion molecules are generally up-regulated in multiple sclerosis; no specific role of ICAM-1 was found in pathogenesis.

BLOOD-BRAIN BARRIER AND CYTOKINES IN BACTERIAL MENINGITIS

The discovery of the cytokine network has increased our understanding of the inflammatory processes within the intrathecal compartment, and it has provided a new theoretical basis to explain pathogenesis, progression, and complications of bacterial meningitis. Although inflammation in bacterial meningitis is largely limited to neuronal and vascular structures within the subarachnoid space, profound alterations in intracranial physiology are known to occur, particularly those regulating cerebral endothelial and blood-brain barrier functions. Damage to

cerebrovascular cells may lead to increased local vascular resistance, thrombus formation, or even brain infarction. Moreover, damage of blood-brain barrier in meningitis results in an increase in cerebrovascular permeability, and it may consequently induce potentially fatal brain edema (63).

As discussed, several cytokines, particularly TNF-α have an important role in modulating endothelial cells functions. Of relevance to meningitis, TNF-α results in vascular endothelial damage, alteration of endothelial homeostasis, and an increase in vascular permeability, leading to vascular leak syndrome. Some of the proinflammatory effects of TNF-α were reported to be influenced by IL-1 (64), although recent evidence suggests that TNF-α mediated blood-brain barrier damage is dissociated from the effect of IL-1 (65).

High levels of TNF-α and IL-1β are often detected in cerebrospinal fluid of patients with bacterial, particularly gram-negative, meningitis, but they are usually undetectable in aseptic meningitis at the time of diagnosis (66,67). High cerebrospinal fluid TNF-α and IL-1β concentrations could also be seen in gram-positive meningitis, in which some components of pneumococcal cell wall are comparable to lipopolysaccharide/endotoxin of *Haemophilus influenzae* in inducing release of TNF-α and IL-1β (68). There are usually higher cerebrospinal fluid levels of TNF-α and IL-1β in bacterial meningitis compared with serum levels, suggesting local release of these cytokine within the intrathecal compartment. In the central nervous system, TNF-α and Il-1β could be released at multiple sites; TNF-α is produced by macrophages and mono-

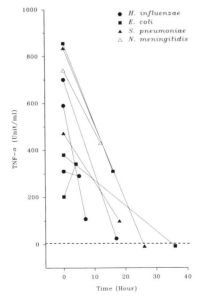
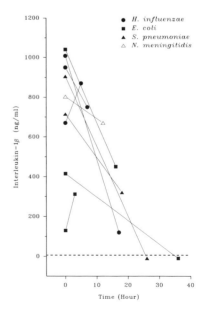

Figure 39–6 Repeat levels of cerebrospinal fluid TNF-α (**A**) and IL-1β (**B**) following antibiotics therapy in three patients with *Haemophilus influenzae,* two patients with *Streptococcus pneumoniae,* three patients with *Escherichia coli,* and a patient with *Neisseria meningitidis meningitis.* (Reproduced with permission from Sharief MK, Ciardi M, Thompson EJ. Blood-brain barrier damage in patients with bacterial meningitis: association with tumor necrosis factor-α but not interleukin-1β. J Infect Dis 1992;166:350–358.)

cytes in response to a variety of infectious stimuli that include bacterial endotoxic and components of bacterial cell wall. It is also synthesized by lymphocytes, natural killer cells, astrocytes, and microglial cells of the brain. Similarly, IL-1β could be produced by astrocytes, microglial cells, and cerebral vascular cells. Intrathecal cytokine concentrations in bacterial meningitis decrease promptly following antibiotic treatment (Fig. 39–6).

Impairment of blood-brain barrier in bacterial meningitis

The importance of TNF-α and IL-1 in disruption of the blood-brain barrier was further characterized by Sharief and co-workers (65) who studied serum and cerebrospinal fluid of patients afflicted with bacterial meningitis. All patients with bacterial meningitis had abnormally high Q_{alb}, which suggests barrier impairment. Cerebrospinal fluid concentration of TNf-α in patients with bacterial meningitis significantly correlated with blood-brain barrier damage (as measured by Q_{alb}) (Fig. 39–7), whereas IL-1β concentrations in the same group of patients failed to correlate with Q_{alb}. Nevertheless, evidence for synergistic activity between Il-1β and TNF-α was detected in patients with bacterial meningitis: patients who had detectable concentrations of both TNF-α and Il-1β in cerebrospinal fluid demonstrated higher Q_{alb} values than matching patients who had isolated increases of TNF-α (Fig. 39–7).

Intrathecal levels of TNF-α in bacterial meningitis also seem to be proportional to the degree of blood-brain barrier disruption (Fig. 39–8), suggesting that TNF-α may be related to the pathogenesis of barrier damage in this condition. TNF-α–induced disruption of the blood-brain bar-

rier could result from several mechanisms. TNF-α causes an increase in vascular permeability by inducing morphological and structural changes of endothelial cells through a direct toxic effect. It also down-regulates endothelial cell expression of thrombomodulin, and it causes enhanced procoagulant activity that promotes intravascular coagulation and capillary thrombosis. As mentioned earlier, leukocytes adherent to endothelial cells are stimulated by TNF-α to increase biosynthesis and release of reactive superoxide intermediates and arachidonic acid metabolites.

IL-1β was also suggested to cause disruption of the blood-brain barrier in experimental meningitis (69). In addition, IL-1β was reported to initiate meningeal inflammation without a concomitant increase in TNF-α (50). However, a correlation between IL-1β and cerebrospinal fluid indexes of meningeal inflammation or blood-brain barrier damage was not observed in patients with bacterial meningitis (65), although evidence of synergy between TNF-α and IL-1β was noticed.

Additional support for the central role of TNF-α in mediating blood-brain barrier injury was provided by Quagliarello and others (49). These workers demonstrated that compared with intracesternal challenge of IL-1β alone, combined IL-1β and anti-TNF antibody challenge caused a significant reduction in both meningeal inflammation and blood-brain barrier permeability in ex-

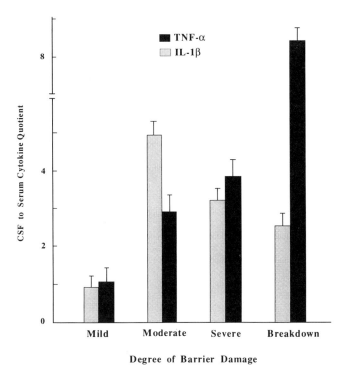

Figure 39–8   Correlation of intrathecal levels of TNF-α and IL-1β (expressed as cerebrospinal fluid to serum quotient) to the degree of blood-brain barrier damage in patients with bacterial meningitis. Values represent means ± standard error of the mean.

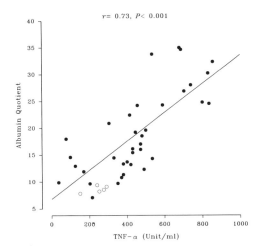

Figure 39–7   Relationship between blood-brain barrier (expressed as albumin quotient) and TNF-α in cerebrospinal fluid from patients with bacterial meningitis. Patients with no detectable TNF-α are not included. Patients who have no detectable levels of IL-1β are depicted as (○).

perimental meningitis. This finding suggests that the biological effect of IL-1β may be related to intrathecal production of TNF-α, which may synergistically participate in the observed in vivo effects. In agreement with experimental models, clinical studies have provided evidence that cerebrospinal fluid concentrations of IL-1β did not correlate with indexes of meningeal inflammation (70) in patients with bacterial meningitis.

It must be emphasized, however, that endothelial damage should not be considered a result solely of overproduction of TNF-α, thereby ignoring the complex interactions between cytokines and other mediators, such as prostaglandins and leukotrienes. Ongoing research of these and other mediators will provide further insight into the pathogenesis of meningeal inflammation in bacterial meningitis. Nonetheless, TNF-α appears to be an important mediator of blood-brain barrier damage, and this fact could have important therapeutic implications because TNF-α–dependent endothelial toxicity is strongly inhibited by heparin or corticosteroids, and biosynthesis of TNF-α is inhibited by dexamethasone. Reassessment of treatment strategies in bacterial meningitis to down-regulate production of TNF-α may provide more effective therapeutic modalities.

BLOOD-BRAIN BARRIER AND CYTOKINES IN HUMAN IMMUNODEFICIENCY VIRUS INFECTION

Neurological complications are a very significant feature of human immunodeficiency virus (HIV) infection at all stages, ranging from HIV seropositivity to acquired immune deficiency syndrome (AIDS)–related complex and full-blown AIDS. Approximately 10% of patients with HIV infection present neurologically (71), whereas approximately 70% of patient with AIDS have some evidence of neurological involvement; this figure may extend to 80% if pathological data are also taken into consideration.

One of the most important neurological complications is HIV encephalitis, also known as AIDS-dementia complex, which is caused by direct HIV infection within the brain. However, the precise pathogenesis of brain inflammation and injury has not been clearly defined, and although HIV has been demonstrated within macrophages and multinucleate giant cells, its localization within glial cells and neurons has not been demonstrated convincingly. The amount of virus detected in some brain lesions is not proportionate to the degree of pathological damage, and some brain regions with significant damage (e.g., spinal cord) contain little or no HIV Similarly, humorally mediated immune mechanisms are not significantly involved in the pathogenesis of central nervous system inflammation or injury (72).

It is therefore likely that indirect mechanisms, such as release of cytokines, may have an important role in mediating brain inflammation in HIV infection. Indeed, there is now increasing evidence that TNF-α, which is a central mediator of inflammation, has a crucial role in the development of AIDS, as discussed in Chapter 28. In brief, TNF-α enhances replication of HIV, and it induces expression of a wide array of inflammatory cytokines. Moreover, TNF-α selectively kills HIV-infected cells, probably through a direct cytotoxic effect, and it is currently implicated in the pathogenesis of most clinical and pathological features of AIDS.

Impairment of the blood-brain barrier is another important pathogenetic feature that contributes to brain damage in infection with HIV. The detection of viral antigen in cerebral endothelial cells (73) fueled speculations that viral entry into the central nervous system may be through the blood-brain barrier. It follows that HIV infection of endothelial cells may alter the integrity of the blood-brain barrier, thereby augmenting neurological dysfunction. Indeed, several investigators have reported significant impairment of the blood-brain barrier in HIV brain inflammation, which ranged form 27% in early infections (74) to 79% in more advanced stages (75). In addition, changes in cerebral perfusion occur early in the course of HIV infection (76), and HIV-seropositive patients appear to be at increased risk of cerebral ischemia and infarction.

The notion that TNF-α is released within the intrathecal compartment in HIV-1 infection of the central nervous system is supported by in vitro studies, which demonstrated that viral challenge of astrocytes induces TNF-α release (77). Indeed, cerebrospinal fluid TNF-α levels were reported to be more elevated in patients with HIV-1 encephalopathy than in healthy HIV-1–seropositive patients (78) and they are also high in patients with HIV-1 encephalopathy or opportunistic central nervous system infections (79). Intrathecal production of TNF-α may also result from release by macrophages, which are abundant in brain lesions, as well as by microglial cells. Due to the inflammatory changes mediated by TNF-α on human cerebral endothelial cells, it is likely that a TNF-α–induced cerebrovascular disturbance may lead to brain damage in HIV-infected patients. Intrathecal release of TNF-α in these patients has been reported to correlate with signs of disruption of the blood-brain barrier (Fig. 39–9). Moreover, TNF-α levels correlated with the degree of barrier impairment, suggesting that this cytokine may be related to the pathogenesis of barrier damage in HIV-1 infection (Fig. 39–10).

Recent studies (79) reported no relationship between IL-1β level and blood-brain barrier damage. Although IL-1β may precipitate blood-brain barrier damage in experimental animals (49), it seems that the effects of TNF-α on

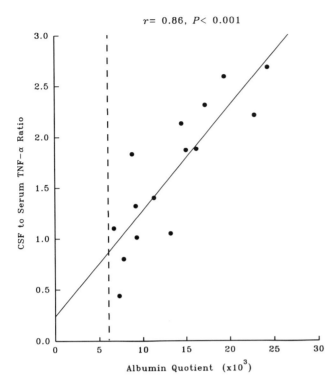

r= 0.86, P< 0.001

Figure 39–9 Correlation of intrathecal levels of TNF-α (expressed as cerebrospinal fluid [CSF] to serum ratio) with albumin quotient in 15 HIV-1–seropositive patients who had detectable TNF-α in CSF and serum. *Vertical interrupted line* represents the cut-off value of albumin quotient in normal subjects. (Reproduced with permission from Sharief MK, Ciardi M, Thompson EJ, et al. Tumor necrosis factor-α mediates blood-brain barrier damage in HIV-1 infection of the central nervous system. Mediat Inflam 1992;1:162–168.)

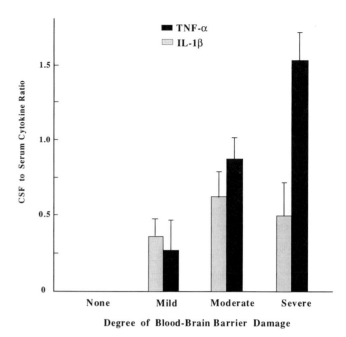

Figure 39–10 Correlation of intrathecal levels of TNF-α and Il-1β (expressed as cerebrospinal fluid to serum ratios) with the degree of blood-brain barrier damage in 31 HIV-1–seropositive patients. Values represent means ± standard error of the mean. (Reproduced with permission from Sharief MK, Ciardi M, Thompson EJ, et al. Tumor necrosis factor-α mediates blood-brain barrier damage in HIV-1 infection of the central nervous system. Mediat Inflam 1992;1:162–168.)

human cerebral endothelium can be dissociated from the presence of IL-1β. In support of this notion, Saukkonen and others (80) reported a role for TNF-α in the generation of inflammation and tissue damage, whereas IL-1b failed to provide a significant meningeal response in experimental animals. It must be emphasized, however, that endothelial damage should not be considered a result solely of overproduction of TNF-α, thereby ignoring the complex interactions between cytokines and other mediators, such as prostaglandins and leukotrienes. Studies of these and other mediators should provide a further insight into the pathogenesis of brain inflammation in HIV infection.

OVERVIEW ON CYTOKINE-MEDIATED BLOOD-BRAIN BARRIER DAMAGE

Findings presented in this chapter argue for a putative role for IL-2 and TNF-α in disruption of the blood-brain barrier in inflammatory and infective diseases of the central nervous system. However, it must be emphasized that cerebral endothelial damage should not be considered a result solely of overproduction of IL-2 and TNF-α, thereby ignoring the complex interaction between cytokines and other mediators, such as prostaglandins and leukotrienes. Ongoing studies of these and other mediators will undoubtedly provide additional insight into the pathogenesis of barrier damage in diseases of the central nervous system. Moreover, regulation of TNF-α expression is exceedingly complex, and it can be controlled at both the transcriptional and the post-transcriptional level. As a result, induction of TNF-α release should not be linked only to an IL-2 effect, thereby excluding the influence of other members of the cytokines network.

In vivo damage to the blood-brain barrier could be more precisely detected by MRI with gadolinium-DTPA enhancement. Unfortunately, no study to date has evaluated the relationship between cytokine levels and MRI-detected blood-brain barrier damage. Nonetheless, available evidence indicates that IL-2 and TNF-α are related to cerebral endothelial impairment in several diseases of the central nervous system.

REFERENCES

1. Ehrlich P. Das Sauerstaff: bedurfris des organismus. Berlin: Eine Farbenanalytische Studie. 1885:69–72.

2. Goldmann GE. Vitalfarbung am zentral nerven system abhn preuss akad wiss. Berlin: Eimer, 1913.

3. Reese TS, Karnovsky MJ. Fine structural localization of a blood-brain barrier to exogenous peroxide. J Cell Biol 1967;34:207–217.

4. Felgenhauer K. The blood-brain barrier redefined. J Neurol 1986;233:193–194.

5. Leibowitz S, Hughes RAC. Immunity and the blood brain barrier. Immunology of the nervous system. London; Edward Arnold Ltd, 1983;1–9.

6. Tibbling G, Link H Ohman S. Principles of albumin and IgG analyses in neurological diseases. Establishment of reference values. Scan J Clin Lab Invest 1977;37:285–390.

7. Bradbury MWB. The developing experimental approach to the idea of blood-brain barrier. Ann NY Acad Sci USA 1986;481:137–141.

8. Reese TS, Feder N, Brightman MW. Electron microscopic study of the blood-brain and blood-cerebrospinal fluid barriers with microperoxidase. J Neuropathol Exp Neurobiol 1971;30:137–138.

9. Tourtelotte WW. The cerebrospinal fluid in multiple sclerosis. In: Koetsier JC, ed. Handbook of clinical neurology, vol 3 (47): demyelinating diseases. Amsterdam; Elsevier Science Publishers, 1985:79–130.

10. James PB. Multiple sclerosis or blood-brain barrier disease. Lancet 1989;1:46.

11. Kermode AG, Thompson AJ, Tofts P, et al. Breakdown of the blood-brain barrier precedes symptoms and other MRI signs of new lesions in multiple sclerosis. Pathogenic and clinical implications. Brain 1990;113:1477–1489.

12. Koopmans RA, Li DK, Oger JF, Mayo J, Paty DW. The lesion of multiple sclerosis: imaging of acute and chronic stages. Neurology 1989;39:959–963.

13. Dawson JW. This histology of disseminated sclerosis. Trans R Soc Edinb 1916;50:517–740.

14. Lumsden CE. The neuropathology of multiple sclerosis. In: Vinken PJ, Bruyn GW, eds. Handbook of clinical neurology. Amsterdam: North-Holland Publishing;1970:217–309.

15. Hawkings CP, Mackenzie F, Tofts P, du Boulay EP, McDonald WI. Patterns of blood-brain barrier breakdown in inflammatory demyelination. Brain 1991;114:801–810.

16. Gay D, Esiri M. Blood-brain barrier damage in acute multiple sclerosis plaques. An immnocytological study. Brain 1991;114:557–572.

17. Raine CS. Demyelinating diseases. In: Davies RL, Robertson DM, eds. Textbook of neuropathology. Baltimore: Williams & Wilkins, 1990:568–492.

18. Selmaj KW, Raine CS. Tumour necrosis factor mediates myelin and oliodendrocyte damage in vitro. Ann Neurol 1988;23:339–346.

19. Scolding NJ, Jones H. Compston DAS, Morgan BP. Oligodendrocyte susceptibility to injury by T-cell perforin. Immunology 1990;70:6–14.

20. Bellamy AS, Calder VL, Feldmann M, Davidson AN. The distribution of interleukin-2 receptor bearing lymphocytes in multiple sclerosis: evidence for a key role of activated lymphocytes. Clin Exp Immunol 1985;61:248–256.

21. Cuzner ML, Hayes GM, Newcombe J, Woodroofe MN. The nature of inflammatory components during demyelination in multiple sclerosis. J Neuroimmunol 1988;20:203–209.

22. Hofman FM, von Hanwehr RI, Dinarello CA, et al. Immunoregulatory molecules and IL-2 receptors identified in multiple sclerosis brain. J Immunol 1986;136:3239–3245.

23. Adachi K, Kumamoto T, Araki S. Elevated soluble interleukin-2 receptor levels in patients with active multiple sclerosis. Ann Neurol 1990;28:687–691.

24. Gallo P, Piccinno M, Pagni S, et al. Immune activation in multiple sclerosis: study of IL-2, sIL-2R, γ-IFN levels in serum and CSF. J Neurol Sci 1989;92:9–15.

25. Kittur SD, Kittur DS, Soncrant TT, et al. Soluble interleukin-2 receptors in cerebrospinal fluid from individuals with various neurological disorders. Ann Neurol 1990;28:168–173.

26. Elison MD, Povlishock JT, Merchant RE. Blood-brain barrier dysfunction in cats following recombinant interleukin-2 infusion. Cancer Res 1987;47:5765–5770.

27. Watts RG, Wright JL, Atkinson LL, Merchant RE. Histopathological and blood-brain barrier changes in rats induced by an intracerebral injection of human recombinant interleukin-2. Neurosurgery 1989;25:202–208.

28. Saris SC, Rosenberg SA, Friedman RB, Rubin JT, Barba D, Oldfield EH. Penetration of recombinant interleukin-2 across the blood-cerebrospinal fluid barrier. J. Neurosurg 1988;69:29–34.

29. Roche Pharmaceutical. Recombinant IL-2 investigational drug brochure. Nutley, NJ: Roche Pharmaceuticals, 1989.

30. Hicks C, Cooley MA, Panny R. Investigation of interleukin-2 receptors on human endothelial cells. Growth Factors 1991;5:201–208.

31. Sharief MK, Hentges R, Ciardi M, Thompson EJ. In vivo relationship of interleukin-2 and soluble IL-2 receptor to blood-brain barrier impairment in patients with active multiple sclerosis. J Neurol 1993;240:46–50.

32. Damel NK, Doyle LV. Il-2 activated human killer lymphocytes but not their secreted products mediate increase in albumin flux across cultured endothelial monolayers: implications for vascular leak syndrome. J Immunol 1989;142:2660–2669.

33. Iwasaka K. Infiltrative and cytolytic activities of lymphokine-activated killer (LAK) cells against a human glioma mass: ultrastructural analysis using a three-dimensional multicellular spheroid model. Arch Jpn Chir 1990;59:39–54.

34. Mier JW, Vachino G, van der Meer JW, et al. Induction of circulating tumour-necrosis factor (TNF-alpha) as the mechanism for the febrile response to interleukin-2 (IL-2) in cancer patients. J Clin Immunol 1988;8:426–436.

35. Convay EM, Bach R, Rosenberg RD, Konigsberg WH. TNF enhances expression of tissue factor mRNA in endothelial cells. Thromb Res 1989;53:231–241.

36. Hauser SL, Bhan AK, Gilles F, et al. Immunohistological analysis of the cellular infiltrate in multiple sclerosis lesions. Ann Neurol 1986;19:578–587.

37. Lavi E, Suzumura A, Murasko DM, Murray EM, Silberberg DH, Weiss SR. Tumor necrosis factor induces expression

of MHC class I antigens on mouse astrocytes. J Neuroimmunol 1988;18:245–253.

38. Massa PT, Schmipl A, Wecker E, ter Meulen V. Tumor necrosis factor amplifies virus-mediated Ia induction on astrocytes. Proc Natl Acad Sci USA 1987;84:7242–7245.

39. Forhman EM, Forhman TC, Dustin ML, et al. The induction of intracellular adhesion molecule I expression on human fetal astrocytes by interferon-γ, TNF-α, lymphotoxin, and IL-1: relevance to intracerebral antigen presentation. J Neuroimmunol 1989;23:117–124.

40. Selmaj KW, Farooq M, Norton WT, Raine CS, Brosnan CF. Proliferation of astrocytes in vitro in response to cytokines. A primary role for tumor necrosis factor. J Immunol 1990; 144:129–135.

41. Frei K, Malipiero UV, Leist TP, Zinkernagel RM, Schwab ME, Fontana A. On the cellular source and function of interleukin-6 produced in the central nervous system in viral diseases. Eur J Immunol 1989;19:689–694.

42. Selmaj K, Raine CS, Cannella B, Brosnan C. Identification of lymphotoxin and tumor necrosis factor in multiple sclerosis. J Clin Invest 1991;87:949–954.

43. Sharief MK, Hentges R. Association between tumor necrosis factor-α and disease progression in patients with multiple sclerosis. N Engl J Med 1991;325:467–472.

44. Tsukada N, Miyagi K, Matsuda M, Yanagisawa N, Yone K. Tumor necrosis factor and interleukin-1 in the CSF and sera of patients with multiple sclerosis. J Neurol Sci 1991; 102:230–234.

45. Sharief MK, Thompson EJ. In vivo relationship of tumor necrosis factor-α to blood-brain barrier damage in patients with active multiple sclerosis. J Neuroimmunol 1993;38: 27–34.

46. Beutler B, Cerami A. The biology of cachectin/TNF. A primary mediator of the host response. Ann Rev Immunol 1989;7:625–655.

47. Slungaard A, Vercellotti GM, Walker G, Nelson RD, Jacob HS. Tumor necrosis factor α/cachectin stimulates eosinophil oxidant production and toxicity towards human endothelium. J Exp Med 1990;171:2025–2041.

48. Sharief MK. The importance of interleukin-2 and its soluble receptor in patients with MS and other inflammatory diseases of the central nervous system. PhD thesis, University of London, 1992.

49. Quagliarello VJ, Wispelwey B, Long WJ, Scheld WM. Recombinant human interleukin-1 induces meningitis and blood-brain barrier injury in the rat. Characterization and comparison with timor necrosis factor. J Clin Invest 1991; 87:1360–1366.

50. Ramilo O, Saez-Llorens X, Mertsola J, et al. Tumor necrosis factor-α/cachectin and interleukin 1β initiate meningeal inflammation. J Exp Med 1990;172:497–507.

51. Cross AH, Cannella B, Brosnan CF, Raine CS. Homing to central nervous system vasculature by antigen-specific lymphocytes. I. Localization of 14C-labeled cells during acute, chronic, and relapsing experimental allergic encephalomyelitis. Lab Invest 1990;63:162–170.

52. Singer SJ. Intercellular communication and cell-cell adhesion. Science 1992;255:1671–1677.

53. Cotran RS, Gimbrone MA, Bevilacqua MP, Mendrick DL, Pober JS. Induction and detection of a humanendothelial activation antigen in vivo. J Exp Med 1986;164:661–667.

54. Yednock TA, Cannon C, Fritz LC, Sanchez-Madrid F, Steiman L, Karin N. Prevention of experimental autoimmune encephalomyelitis by antibodies against α4β1 integrin. Nature 1992;356:63–66.

55. Makgoba MW, Sanders, ME, Ginther GE, et al. ICAM-1 a ligand for LFA-1-dependent adhesion of B, T, and myeloid cells. Nature 1988;331:86–88.

56. Argenbright LW, Barton RW. Interactions of leukocyte integrins with intercellular adhesion molecule 1 in the production of inflammatory vascular injury in vivo. The Shwartzman reaction revisited. J Clin Invest 1992;89:259–272.

57. Birdsall HH. Induction of ICAM-1 on human neural cells and mechanisms of neutrophil-mediated injury. Am J Pathol 1991;139:1341–1350.

58. Cannella B, Cross AH, Raine CS. Upregulating and coexpression of adhesion molecules correlate with relapsing autoimmune demyelination in the central nervous system. J Exp Med 1990;172:1521–1524.

59. Rothlein R, Mainolfi EA, Czajkowski M, Marlin AD. A form of circulating ICAM-1 in human serum. J Immunol 1991;147:3788–3793.

60. Sharief MK, Noori MA, Ciardi M, Cirelli A, Thompson EJ. Increased levels of circulating ICAM-1 in serum and cerebrospinal fluid of patients with active multiple sclerosis. Correlation with TNF-α and blood-brain damage. J Neuroimmunol 1993;43:15–22.

61. Osborn L. Leukocytes adhesion to endothelium in inflammation. Cell 1990;62:3–6.

62. Rossler K, Neuchrist C, Kitz, K, Schiner O, Kraft D, Lassmann H. Expression of leucocyte adhesion molecules at the human blood-brain barrier. J Neurosci Res 1992; 31:365–374.

63. Tunkle AR, Scheld WM. Alterations of blood-brain barrier in bacterial meningitis: in vivo and in vitro models. Pediatr Infect Dis J 1989;8:911–918.

64. Pober JS, Gimbrone MA, Lapierre LA, et al. Overlapping patterns of activation of human endothelial cells by interleukin 1, tumour necrosis factor, and immune interferon. J Immunol 1986;137:1893–1896.

65. Sharief MK, Ciardi M, Thompson EJ. Blood-brain barrier in patients with bacterial meningitis: association with tumor necrosis factor-α but not interleukin-1β. J Infect Dis 1992; 166:350–358.

66. Arditi M, Manogue KR, Caplan M, Yogev R. Cerebrospinal fluid cachectin/tumor necrosis factor-α and platelet-activating factor concentrations and severity of bacterial meningitis in children. J Infect Dis 1990;162:139–147.

67. McCracken GH Jr, Mustafa MM, Ramilo O, Olsen KD, Risser RC. cerebrospinal fluid interleukin-1β and tumor necrosis factor concentrations and outcome from neonatal gram-negative enteric bacillary meningitis. Pediatr Infect Dis J 1989;8:155–159.

68. Smith AL. Neurologic sequelae of meningitis. N Engl J Med 1988;319:1012–1013.

69. Vecht CJ, Keohane C, Menon RS, Henzen-Logmand SC, Punt CJ, Stoter G. Acute fatal leukoencephalopathy after interleukin-2 therapy. N Engl J Med 1990;323:1146–1147.

70. Poser CM, Paty DW, Scheinberg L, et al. New diagnostic criteria for multiple sclerosis: guidelines for research protocols. Ann Neurol 1983;13:227–231.

71. Lavy RM, Bredesen DE, Rosenblum ML. Neurological manifestations of the acquired immunodeficiency syndrome (AIDS): experience at UCSF and review of the literature. J Neurosurg 1985;62:475–495.

72. Lenhardt TM, Wiley CA. Absence of humorally mediated damage within the central nervous system of AIDS patients. Neurology 1989;39:278–280.

73. Wiley CA, Schrier RD, Nelson JA, Lampert PW, Oldstone MBA. Cellular localization of human immunodeficiency virus infection within the brains of acquired immune deficiency syndrome patients. Proc Natl Acad Sci USA 1986; 83:7089–7093.

74. Price RW, Brew B, Sidtis J, Rosenblum M, Scheck AC, Cleary P. The brain in AIDS: central nervous HIV-1 infection and AIDS dementia complex. Science 1988;239:586–592.

75. Brew BJ, Bhalla RB, Fleisher M, et al. Cerebrospinal fluid beta2 microglobulin in patients infected with human immunodeficiency virus. Neurology 1989;39:830–834.

76. Felgenhauer K, Luer W, Poser S. Chronic HIV encephalitis. J Neuroimmunol 1988;20:141–144.

77. Lieberman AP, Pitha PM, Shin HS, Shin ML. Production of tumor necrosis factor and other cytokines by astrocytes stimulated with lipopolysaccharide or a neurotropic virus. Proc Natl Acad Sci USA 1989;86:6348–6352.

78. Perez VL, Janssen R, Spira T, et al. Presence of tumor necrosis factor in the cerebrospinal fluid of AIDS patients with HIV encephalopathy. Montreal: 5th International Conference on AIDS 1989;WCP87 (abstract).

79. Sharief MK, Ciardi M, Thompson EJ, et al. Tumor necrosis factor-α mediates blood-brain barrier damage in HIV-1 infection of the central nervous system. Mediat Inflam 1992; 1:162–168.

80. Saukkonen K, Sande S, Cioffe C, et al. The role of cytokines in the generation of inflammation and tissue damage in experimental Gram-positive meningitis. J Exp Med 1990; 171:439–445.

CHAPTER 40

ROLE OF CYTOKINES IN HEPATIC AND HEPATOBILIARY DISEASES

Tilo Andus and Axel Holstege

The liver is the largest organ in the body (1,500 gm), and it provides a large number of essential functions for the organism. It is made up of different liver cell populations (i.e., hepatocytes, Kupffer cells, fat-storing cells, endothelial cells, pit cells, and biliary epithelial cells), which form multiple microenvironments, such as the sinusoids, the space of Disse, the extracellular matrix, and the biliary canalicular spaces (Fig. 40–1; Table 40–1) (1). It is the center for metabolism of nutrients and drugs, and it has a key role in the unspecific immune system by harboring Kupffer cells and the majority of all macrophages. The liver is the site of synthesis for many different metabolites, and it produces most of the plasma proteins.

All these functions of the liver must be coordinated and regulated in response to metabolic changes and minor or major injuries. This regulation is accomplished by metabolites, the autonomous nerve system, the endocrine system, and by cytokines, which form a complex network of mediator molecules. In the liver, hepatocytes, endothelial cells, Kupffer cells, and fat-storing cells produce cytokines (2).

Cytokines and the liver interact in several ways: (a) extrahepatically produced cytokines enter the liver via portal or arterial blood, cause changes of the hepatic intermediary metabolism, or induce a hepatic defense reaction;

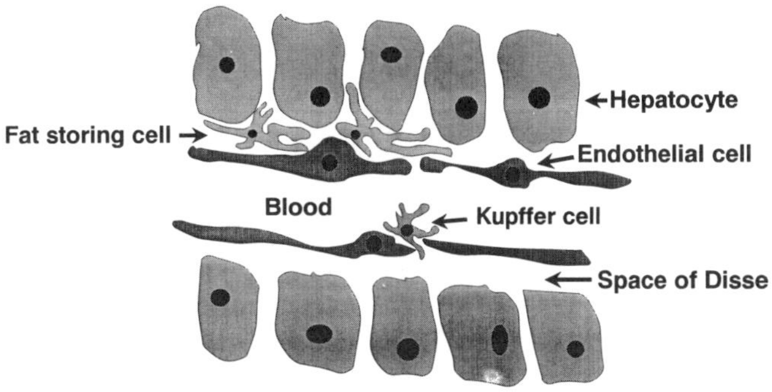

Figure 40–1 The liver sinusoid and the different cell types involved.

TABLE 40–1 CELLULAR COMPOSITION OF THE LIVER

	Part of cell number (%)	Part of liver volume (%)
Cells	100	84.1
Hepatocytes	60	77.8
Endothelial cells	30	2.8
Kupffer cells	10	1.4
Fat-storing cells	<5	1.4
Extracellular space		15.9
Sinusoids		10.6
Space of Disse		4.6
Bile canaliculi		0.4

(b) intrahepatically produced cytokines leave the liver and transmit information to extrahepatic organs; and (c) intrahepatically produced cytokines interact in a paracrine or autocrine manner with other hepatic cells. During the last 5 years, an increasing number of publications about these interactions have appeared (2–5). These studies have led to a better understanding of the interactions between parenchymal and nonparenchymal liver cells and of the pathogenesis of several liver diseases. We focus on the role of cytokines in pathogenesis and therapy of chronic and acute viral hepatitis, acute liver failure, autoimmune hepatitis, alcoholic hepatitis, fibrosis, cirrhosis, liver regeneration, and liver cancer.

CHRONIC VIRAL HEPATITIS

Viral hepatitis is a viral infection that predominantly affects the liver. Currently, five different hepatotropic viral agents are known (Table 40–2). All hepatitis viruses can induce an acute necroinflammatory infection of the liver, which is clinically characterized by nonspecific flu-like symptoms, jaundice, itching, fatigue, fever, and abdominal discomfort in the right upper quadrant. Histologically, acute viral hepatitis reveals hepatocellular necrosis, degeneration and regeneration of hepatocytes, sinusoidal cell activation, and inflammation. Hepatitis B (HBV), C, and D infection, in addition, can lead in a certain percentage of infected patients to chronic hepatitis, which in turn can result in fibrosis and cirrhosis of the liver.

Cytokines and pathogenesis of viral hepatitis

Depending on the interaction between the hepatitis virus and the host response, there is a wide spectrum of different clinical courses of viral hepatitis. Hepatitis B infection, for example, can lead to a moderate acute infection;

TABLE 40–2 FORMS OF VIRAL HEPATITIS

Virus	Transmission	Characteristics
Hepatitis A	Fecal-enteral	Acute, self-limited
Hepatitis B	Parenteral	Chronic in approximately 10%
Hepatitis C	Parenteral	Often chronic
Hepatitis D	Parenteral	Chronic, requires hepatitis B virus for replication
Hepatitis E	Fecal-enteral	Endemic in Asia, Africa, and Central America; self-limited

to severe, fulminant liver failure; to an asymptomatic chronic form of hepatitis; to hepatocellular cirrhosis; or to carcinoma. HBV mutants have been found to be associated with fulminant hepatitis (6). However, differences in the immunological host response are thought to be major factors that determine the course of the hepatitis infection (6). In chronic viral hepatitis, the cell-mediated immune response remains strong enough to cause hepatocellular necrosis, but it is insufficient to clear the hepatitis virus (7). Lysis of infected hepatocytes by cytotoxic T lymphocytes reactive against the hepatitis B core antigen seems to be important for elimination of the virus.

Cytokines are key mediators for regulation of the host response to all kinds of infections. They are involved in both specific and nonspecific immune responses. In patients with chronic viral hepatitis, several alterations have been found with respect to the production and action of cytokines. These alterations seem to be involved in the impaired clearance of HBV, which occurs in 10% of infected patients, resulting in chronic infection.

The actions of interferons (IFNs) have been studied most extensively because IFNs are potent antiviral agents produced by cells in response to viral infection (8) and because IFN-α is used as a therapeutic agent in chronic viral hepatitis. IFNs have several antiviral actions. One action is induction of human leukocyte antigens (HLA) (9–11) and the RING genes, which process viral proteins and allows them to associate with HLA antigens and to induce cytotoxic T lymphocytes (12,13). In addition to IFNs, interleukin-1 (IL-1) (14) and tumor necrosis factor (TNF) (15) also induce HLA antigens in hepatocytes. The presentation of antigenic structures of the hepatitis B core protein linked to HLA class I antigens is very important for targeting of cytotoxic T lymphocytes to virally infected hepatocytes (10). Optimal binding of cytotoxic T cells to antigens on their target cells also requires interaction of adhesion molecules on T cells (e.g., LFA-1) with their counter-receptors on the antigen-presenting or target cells (e.g., ICAM-1). During hepatitis B infection, ICAM-1 expression is up-regulated on hepatocytes (16), probably by IFN-γ, which is produced by liver-infiltrating memory T lymphocytes (17). This effect is supported by in vitro studies, which showed that IFN-γ induces expression of the adhesion molecule ICAM-1 on HepG2 cells, whereas IFN-α, IL-1, IL-6, and TNF had no effect (18,19). These findings suggest that induction of ICAM-1 on hepatocytes by IFN-γ is another important step of the host response against hepatitis virus infection.

In acute HBV infection, IFN-α is produced in large amounts (20,21). Patients with chronic HBV infection, however, have deficient IFN-α and IFN-β production in peripheral blood cells (22–26) and in the liver (21,27), in which mononuclear cells produce most of the IFN-α and IFN-γ (28). The number of hepatocytes containing hepatitis B core antigen correlates inversely with the proportion of neighboring sinusoidal cells that express IFN-α (21). This finding and in vitro experiments (29) indicate that the HBV core protein inhibits production of IFN-β. In contrast, the hepatitis B-X protein stimulates production of IFN-β (27).

IFN-γ production is induced by hepatitis B core antigen and hepatitis E antigen, but not by hepatitis surface antigen (30). Increased production of hepatitis B core antigen–specific IFN-γ at the time of acute exacerbations indicates that IFN-γ induced by hepatitis B core antigen has a role in hepatocellular injury of patients with chronic hepatitis B (31). IFN-γ production in peripheral blood mononuclear cells from patients with chronic active hepatitis is impaired by a prostaglandin-mediated mechanism (32). Little is known about the effect of hepatitis C virus on IFN production. It seems that hepatitis C virus induces IFNs, because hepatitis C infection of chimpanzees leads to induction of HLA class I antigens and IFN-inducible genes (33).

HBV modulates not only production of but also the cellular response to IFN. Cells transfected in vitro with HBV obtain a defective response to IFN (34). This modulation occurs at the postreceptor level, because IFN-α receptors (35,36) and IFN-γ receptors (37,38) are neither up-regulated nor down-regulated in viral hepatitis. The blunted response to IFN is due to the terminal protein of HBV, which inhibits the cellular response to IFN-α and IFN-γ by inhibiting activation of a critical transactivating protein, known as E, which is normally activated after binding of IFN to its cell surface receptor (6,39). Strong expression of this protein in liver biopsies is associated with unresponsiveness to IFN treatment (40).

In addition to the IFNs, several other cytokines have been studied in patients with viral hepatitis. IL-2 and its receptor are key factors for T-cell activation (41). Because IL-2 induces IL-2 receptor and IL-2 receptor is shed into the circulation, measurement of increased concentrations of soluble IL-2 receptors and IL-2 are markers for T-cell activation. Soluble IL-2 receptor concentrations in serum are elevated in patients with acute viral hepatitis A and B (42,43), but not in those with hepatitis non-A and non-B (43). Studies of IL-2 and IL-2 receptor synthesis in patients with chronic HBV infection are conflicting. Some studies report decreased (44–46), increased (43,47), or unchanged (48) production and serum concentrations of IL-2 and IL-2 receptors in patients with chronic HBV. Thus, additional studies are required to assess if and how production of IL-2 and its receptor are modified by hepatitis viruses.

Data are also conflicting with regard to IL-1. IL-1 is a pleiotropic cytokine that exerts several immune functions, including helper activity for lymphocyte activation. Production of IL-1 was found to be reduced (49–53) or elevated in peripheral blood mononuclear cells from patients with chronic HBV infection (45). Additional studies are needed to examine the role of IL-1 in chronic hepatitis. Reduced production of IL-1 could contribute to some of the defective immune functions seen in patients with viral hepatitis, such as reduced lymphocyte transformation (54,55).

TNF and IL-1 are both proinflammatory cytokines with a similar spectrum of actions. They act synergistically in several ways (56,57). TNF is cytotoxic to many tumor cells. In perfused livers, it induces superoxide anion production by Kupffer cells (58), and it inhibits mitochondrial respiration of hepatocytes in primary cultures (59). TNF-α synthesis by stimulated peripheral blood mononuclear cells of patients with chronic hepatitis is increased (60). There was a significant correlation between TNF-α production and histologically assessed disease activity in patients with chronic persistent hepatitis or chronic active hepatitis (60). An immunohistological study showed that TNF-α is produced and secreted by infiltrating mononuclear cells in focal inflammatory areas of the livers of patients with chronic hepatitis B and C (61). In addition, both types of TNF receptors are up-regulated during chronic inflammation of hepatocytes, sinusoidal endothelial cells, bile duct epithelial cells, and mononuclear inflammatory cells (62). These findings show that TNF-α production is increased in chronic liver disease locally and systemically, and that the increased TNF-α production is related to the activity of liver inflammation.

IL-6 is another pleiotropic cytokine that induces multiple systems, such as acute-phase protein synthesis by hepatocytes, maturation of B lymphocytes for immunoglobulin synthesis, and coactivation of T cells (63). One study described impaired IL-6 production by lipopolysaccharide (LPS)-stimulated peripheral blood mononuclear cells in patients with chronic HBV (64). This finding is in contrast to other studies that indicated increased IL-6 production with or without stimulation by IL-2 (65,66) or LPS as well as elevated IL-6 serum levels in patients with hepatitis B and C (65). Using immunohistochemical techniques, elevated IL-6 production was found in mononuclear cells infiltrating portal areas in chronic hepatitis (67). Increased IL-6 production could explain the hypergammaglobulinemia often observed in chronic hepatitis (68). Expression of IL-6 on the cell surface is sufficient to endow them with receptors for HBV (69,70). This process may allow HBV particles to enter IL-1–expressing extrahepatic cells, such as bone marrow cells (71) and peripheral blood cells (72,73).

From these and other studies it can be concluded that cytokines (especially IFNs) have an important role in the pathophysiology of chronic viral hepatitis. However, the wide spectrum of different courses of disease, the different methodologies, and the multiple interactions of the cytokine network led to sometimes conflicting results, which does not allow us to determine exactly the role of the different cytokines studied. The high prevalence and morbidity of chronic hepatitis, however, has urged investigators to undertake multiple trials using cytokines for the treatment of hepatitis B and C despite the still somehow unclear effect of IFNs.

Treatment of chronic viral hepatitis with cytokines

Multiple immunomodulatory and antiviral drugs have been studied in patients with chronic hepatitis, but only IFNs (i.e., IFN-α2a, IFN-α2b, IFN-α1n, and IFN-β) have clearly proved to ameliorate the course of chronic hepatitis B and hepatitis C (74–78). Optimal dose and duration of therapy is still under investigation. Usually, 5 to 10 million U IFN are given subcutaneously three times a week for 12 to 16 weeks in patients with HBV (79,80), and 3 to 5 million U are given 3 times a week for 6 to 12 months in patients with hepatitis C (81–83). A positive response is characterized by disappearance of hepatitis e antigen, DNA, and RNA; a transient increase in serum transaminase levels at approximately 8 weeks occurs (only in hepatitis B) as infected cells are lysed (84). This exacerbation is thought to represent immune clearance of HBV-infected hepatocytes. This spike is followed by normalization of serum transaminase levels and clinical and histological improvement and elimination of the virus (85). A similar percentage of patients with chronic hepatitis D also responded to IFN therapy in some small studies (86,87).

Unfortunately, only approximately 30 to 40% of patients with hepatitis B (81) and 45 to 50% of patients with hepatitis C (78,82,83,88) respond to this treatment, and approximately half of the responders relapse within 6 months, resulting in an overall long-term response rate of approximately 20 to 25% (78,79,82,83,89). Recently a lower relapse rate was found in hepatitis C after 10 million U IFN-α2b was administered six times a week for two weeks, followed by 3 times a week for 12 weeks (90). Several factors have been identified to be associated with higher or lower probability of response to IFN treatment. Female sex, high serum transaminase levels, good compliance, recent infection, and low HBV DNA (79) or HCV RNA (91) are factors associated with good response, whereas homosexuality, human immunodeficiency virus infection, oriental race, and infection early in life are factors associated with low response rates (79). Moreover, human leukocyte antigen (HLA) type may be associated with the response to IFN (92). The degree of variability in the amino terminal region of the E2/NS1 protein of hepatitis C virus presumably correlates with responsiveness to IFN therapy in viremic patients (93). In patients with hepatitis C who respond to IFN therapy, higher levels of IFN-inducible proteins could be detected than in nonresponders, indicating that the effect of IFN is impaired in nonresponders (94).

The relatively low rate of response to IFN therapy led to trials using short-term pretreatment with glucocorticoids in an attempt to increase the response rate. In two studies, there was no better response, but there was an increase in side effects (75,95). Another more recent, large study, however, found a better and quicker response after steroid withdrawal and subsequent IFN therapy (96). In patients with hepatitis C, prednisolone pretreatment seems to reduce relapse rates after response to IFN therapy (97). Trials with combinations of IFN-α with acyclovir (98,99), vidarabin (100,101), zidovudine (102,103), levamisole (102), and IFN-γ (104) were not successful in enhancing the response rate.

IFN has multiple actions in vivo, such as blocking of viral assembly and replication (105,106), improvement of T-lymphocyte proliferation (107) and activation (44), and induction of HLA antigen expression (10,108). Treatment with IFN-α leads to normalization of elevated transforming growth factor-β (TGF-β$_1$), which is involved in the production of extracellular matrix proteins, and to reduction of serum procollagen type III peptide, a marker for hepatic fibrosis (109), suggesting an antifibrotic effect in patients with chronic hepatitis. Furthermore, it interacts with many other cytokines (e.g., IFN-α). It induces IFN-γ production in peripheral blood mononuclear cells of HBV carriers, suggesting that IFN- α enhances the cellular immune response against HBV by augmenting the endogenous production of IFN-γ (110). Because of these multiple actions, it is hard to assess which of its actions are essential for its therapeutic effect.

Treatment with IFN is commonly associated with side effects (84,111,112). After the first injection of IFN, an influenza-like syndrome develops; high fever, chills, malaise, weakness, and muscle aches typically begin 4 to 6 hours after injection, and they last 6 to 12 hours. These side effects are dose-related and they decrease during the following injections. During IFN treatment, fatigue, muscle aches, headaches, poor appetite, weight loss, hair loss, anxiety, psychotic or depressive disturbances, bone-marrow suppression, and autoimmune diseases may develop. These side effects are highly individual. Most of these side effects are reversible when IFN treatment is stopped.

Another therapeutic approach for chronic viral hepatitis is the use of IL-2. Pilot studies with recombinant human IL-2 for treating chronic type B hepatitis showed some clinical improvement (113–116); however, larger trials are lacking. Treatment with IL-2 results in enhanced release of antibodies against hepatitis B surface antigen (117), which can be helpful for immunization of immunodeficient nonresponders to hepatitis B vaccination (118).

In conclusion, IFN-α is the only effective therapy for chronic viral hepatitis B or C. The low response rate, combined with a high relapse rate and common side effects, strongly demand improvements. Combination of IFN therapy with other cytokines, such as IL-2 or TNF, which impairs HBV gene expression in transgenic mice (119), may improve clearance. Furthermore, it remains to be shown that treatment with IFN improves survival and morbidity in the long term (120), because little is known about the long-term course after IFN treatment (121).

ACUTE VIRAL HEPATITIS AND FULMINANT LIVER FAILURE

Recently, first studies indicated that IFN-α therapy of acute hepatitis C may prevent the development of chronic hepatitis in some patients (77,122–124), whereas there is no evidence that IFN-α therapy is helpful in acute HBV (84,125).

In fulminant liver failure, serum concentrations of cytokines, such as hepatocyte growth factor (HGF) (126) and IL-6 (127), are extremely elevated. It was suggested that the outcome in fulminant hepatic failure can be predicted by measuring serum human HGF concentrations (128). Both cytokines can be produced by many different cells, and both are predominantly cleared by the liver (129–131). The strong elevation of their plasma levels probably is the result of increased synthesis by activated hepatocytes (i.e., HGF) (132), renal cells (i.e., HGF), or blood cells (i.e., HGF, IL-6) and endothelial cells (i.e., IL-6), in combination with a reduced clearance. Elevated serum concentrations of HGF stimulate DNA synthesis in hepatocytes (133–135), indicating that HGF contributes to regeneration of hepatocytes in vivo (129,136). Other cytokines that are elevated in fulminant hepatic failure, however, may be detrimental. In vitro experiments with rat hepatocyte cultures indicated that IL-1 has an inhibitory effect on hepatocyte DNA synthesis. Furthermore, TNF indirectly induces hepatocellular damage by serine proteases, which are possibly activated by this cytokine in vivo (137).

CYTOKINES IN AUTOIMMUNE HEPATITIS, PRIMARY BILIARY CIRRHOSIS, AND SCLEROSING CHOLANGITIS

Classic autoimmune type 1 "lupoid" chronic active hepatitis is characterized by antinuclear antibodies, liver membrane antibodies, and smooth muscle antibodies. A second subgroup of autoimmune-type chronic active hepatitis is characterized by anti-liver kidney–microsomal antibodies, which are directed against a specific cytochrome P450 isoenzyme. Autoimmune hepatitis develops in a subgroup of these patients after infection with hepatitis C (138). A third subgroup of autoimmune-type chronic active hepatitis is identified by autoantibodies to a soluble cytoplasmic liver antigen (139). Disturbances in the immune network are believed to be the key step in the pathogenesis of autoimmune liver diseases (140,141). There are several lines of evidence indicating that cytokines have an important role in the pathogenesis of these diseases. (a) Treatment of chronic viral hepatitis B or C with IFNs induces autoantibodies in a high percentage of the patients, and, in some susceptible patients, it leads to autoimmune-type hepatitis (111,142–144) or to other autoimmune diseases, such as thyroid diseases with autoantibodies (112,145). This effect may be mediated by the induction of HLA class II antigens, because blocking the action of IFN can prevent induction of HLA class II antigens in IL-2–stimulated BALB/c mice (146). (b) Autoimmune-type chronic active hepatitis benefits from immunosuppressive therapy, such as corticosteroids or colchicine, which suppress the production of cytokines (147). (c) The production of cytokines such as TNF and IFN and their receptors has been shown to be altered in patients with autoimmune hepatitis (148–150), primary biliary cirrhosis (151–155), primary sclerosing cholangitis (151), and in animal models (156,157). (d) Cytokines are involved in other autoimmune diseases (158).

CYTOKINES IN ALCOHOLIC HEPATITIS

Alcoholic liver disease has been an important health problem for many centuries (159). A number of questions with respect to the pathogenesis of alcoholic liver disease remains unanswered. The roles of cytokines have been studied in the last few years quite extensively, and they have been summarized in recent excellent reviews (160–162).

In alcoholic hepatitis, serum levels (28,163–168) and production of IL-1 (153,163,165,169), TNF (28,153,164, 165,170), IL-6 (153,165–167), IL-8 (160,168), and TGF-β (171,172) by peripheral blood cells (169,170) has been found to be elevated. Further studies demonstrated increased intrahepatic concentrations of IL-1, IL-6, TGF-β, TNF, and TNF receptors (62,160,171,172). Increased TNF serum levels correlated with increased mortality (28,164), suggesting an important role of TNF in the pathogenesis of alcoholic hepatitis and a prognostic value of TNF determination.

There are several factors that are thought to be responsible for the increase in cytokine production during alcoholic hepatitis. Alcohol intake increases gut permeability, allowing substances such as LPS, which is a strong inducer of cytokines such as IL-1, TNF, and IL-6, to enter the circulation (173,174). In addition, ethanol impairs the function of the hepatic reticuloendothelial system (174). Alcohol does not stimulate cytokine production in vitro, but rather it depresses the production of IL-1 and TNF (170,175). This effect is in accordance with the finding that chronic but not acute administration of alcohol stimulated cytokine synthesis in animal models (175, 176). Additional factors that may influence cytokine production in alcoholic hepatitis are IgA deposits present in liver sinusoids (177), which have been shown to stimulate IL-6 and TNF (166,178,179); reduced glutathione levels in alcoholic hepatitis (180); and reduced prostaglandin E production in alcoholics (181).

Our knowledge about the role of increased cytokine production in the pathogenesis of alcoholic hepatitis is limited. Several experimental models of liver injury, such as the galactosamine model, clearly showed that TNF can cause liver cell injury or death (160). This effect may be mediated by mechanisms involving priming of the hepatocytes by inhibitors of protein synthesis, such as nitric oxide (182), in combination with the cytotoxic effect of high concentrations of TNF (160). Another mechanism may be inhibition of hepatocyte mitochondrial respiration (59). A better understanding of the role of cytokines in alcoholic hepatitis may be helpful for the treatment of patients with alcoholic liver disease.

CYTOKINES IN LIVER FIBROSIS AND LIVER CIRRHOSIS

Cytokines and pathogenesis of liver fibrosis and cirrhosis

Fibrosis and cirrhosis of the liver are common complications if chronic liver diseases such as chronic active viral hepatitis or chronic alcoholic hepatitis persist for many years. Because both viral hepatitis and chronic alcohol abuse are quite frequent findings in the populations of many countries, liver cirrhosis is a problem for many patients. Usually fibrosis is the result of a chronic inflammation, leading to inappropriate activation and proliferation of mesenchymal cells and accumulation of extracellular matrix. In cirrhosis, this process results in irreversible remodeling and destruction of the normal liver architecture and, finally, in chronic liver failure.

Fibrogenesis is regulated by a complex interaction between hepatic parenchymal and nonparenchymal cells, such as fat-storing cells (i.e., Ito cells, lipocytes, perisinusoidal cells, retinoid-storing cells), Kupffer cells, and hepatic endothelial cells, and the extracellular matrix, consisting of collagens, proteoglycans, fibronectin, laminin, tenascin, nidogen, and other matrix substances. Fat-storing cells are the most important cells that produce the extracellular matrix in the liver. Activation and transformation of these fat-storing cells into myofibroblast-like

cells are mediated by paracrine and autocrine loops involving TGF-β secreted by activated liver macrophages, endothelial cells, and disintegrated thrombocytes (Fig. 40-2) (183). Cytokines are the most powerful stimulators of fibrogenesis among the soluble factors studied. They are synthesized by hepatocytes, Kupffer cells, fat-storing cells, endothelial cells, and inflammatory cells invading from the circulation (184–187).

TGF-β is the most powerful fibrogenic cytokine studied thus far (187). Among the different subtypes, TGF-β$_1$ is the most extensively studied in fibrogenesis. TGF-β is secreted in a latent form, and it is activated extracellularly by plasmin or other proteases (188). TGF-β is produced by fat-storing cells (189) and other nonparenchymal cells (172,190,191) during fibrogenesis and regeneration in the liver. TGF-β mRNA concentrations and procollagen mRNA concentrations correlate in liver biopsies of patients with liver disease (171). TGF-β activates fat-storing cells, and it stimulates production of collagen, other extracellular matrix proteins (109,189,190,192–196), and its own mRNA in fat-storing cells (197). In addition, TGF-β inhibits the synthesis of matrix-degrading proteolytic enzymes (198,199). Secretion of TGF-β$_1$ by fat-storing cells is increased after activation and differentiation of fat-storing cells into myofibroblast-like cells (200). The secreted TGF-β from these activated cells is able to induce transformation of resting fat-storing cells into activated myofibroblast-like cells (200,201). This positive feedback mechanism may be relevant in self-perpetuation of liver fibrogenesis.

Platelet-derived growth factor (PDGF) is a potent growth factor. It is a 30-kd molecule consisting of two disulfide-linked peptide chains A and B, forming homodimers or heterodimers (202). PDGF is a strong inducer of fat-storing cell activation and proliferation (203,204). Furthermore, it can induce TGF-β production, and it is a chemotactic factor for smooth muscle cells (187,202). Finally, fat-storing cells release macrophage colony-stimulating factor after stimulation by PDGF and basic fibroblast growth factor (FGF), and they may therefore contribute to activation of resident Kupffer cells or infiltrating macrophages in inflammatory liver diseases (205).

In addition to TGF-β and PDGF, several other

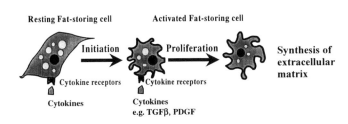

Figure 40–2   Role of cytokines in activation of fat-storing cells. (Modified with permission from Friedman SL. The cellular basis of hepatic fibrosis. Mechanisms and treatment strategies. N Engl J Med 1993;328:1828–1835.)

cytokines have been shown to express fibrogenic activities. Epidermal growth factor (EGF), basic FGF, TGF-α, IL-1, insulin-like growth factors I and II, and other cytokines also stimulate proliferation of fat-storing cells (187,204,206,207). TNF-α transforms Ito cells into myofibroblasts (201). In *Schistosoma japonicum*–infected mice, the development of hepatic fibrosis is critically dependent on IL-2 levels (208).

Not all cytokines act fibrogenically. IFN-γ inhibits proliferation and extracellular matrix protein expression in fat-storing cells in vitro (194,209). IFN-α and IFN-γ reduce collagen synthesis in human fibroblasts (210) and in *Schistosoma japonicum*–infected mice (211). Moreover, in patients with chronic hepatitis C, serum procollagen III peptide levels and TGF-β mRNA and procollagen-α_1(I) mRNA levels returned to normal after treatment with IFN-α (109,206), indicating an antifibrogenetic effect of IFN-α and IFN-γ. In contrast, C1-esterase inhibitor synthesis was increased in fat-storing cells by IFN-γ, suggesting that IFN-γ–stimulated fat-storing cells may enhance deposition of extracellular matrix proteins by inhibiting their degradation (212).

Cytokines and treatment of liver fibrosis and liver cirrhosis

The strong fibrogenetic effects of cytokines such as TGF-β and PDGF, and the antifibrogenetic effect of IFNs suggest that cytokine modulation may be helpful to prevent fibrogenesis. This hypothesis is supported by the observations of positive effects of IFN treatment on fibrogenesis (109,206). In an experimental model of liver fibrosis (induced by chronic treatment of rats with carbon tetrachloride), long-term dietary vitamin E supplementation resulted in a net inhibition of both hepatic TGF-β_1 and procollagen-α_2(I) mRNA levels (213). Furthermore, vitamin E supplementation down-modulated baseline levels of TGF-β_1 mRNA in the liver of untreated animals, suggesting that a dietary regimen rich in vitamin E may potentially interfere with both initiation and progression of the fibrosclerotic processes (213). Recently, in another animal model (i.e., the low-dose yellow phosphorus model in pigs), long-term administration of pentoxifylline (an inhibitor of the synthesis of PDGF, IL-6, and TNF) prevented the development of fibrosis in these animals (214).

Cytokines and complications of liver cirrhosis

There is preliminary evidence that cytokines may be involved in regulation of hepatic microvasculature and portal pressure in liver cirrhosis (215). The increased concentration of gut-derived LPS in the portal blood stimulates Kupffer cells and leads to synthesis of cyto-

kines, such as TNF and IL-1. These cytokines, in combination with prostaglandins, stimulate synthesis of inducible nitric oxide synthetase in hepatocytes (182,216,217) and Kupffer cells (218). Nitric oxide is a strong vasodilator; its role in portal hypertension and hyperdynamic circulation, however, remains to be further characterized (219).

Cytokines may be of diagnostic value, because elevated concentrations of IL-1 and IL-6 have been found to discriminate between spontaneous bacterial peritonitis and cirrhotic or malignant ascites without infection (220) and elevated soluble TNF receptors could discriminate between infected or malignant ascites and uncomplicated cirrhotic ascites (221).

CYTOKINES AND LIVER REGENERATION

The liver has an enormous capacity for regeneration. Because it consists of different cell types forming a highly organized, complex structure, liver regeneration must be a closely regulated process. Several cytokines are involved in this regulation (5,222–224).

HGF is the most potent cytokine (222,223); it stimulates proliferation of hepatocytes in vivo (225,226) and in vitro at picomolar concentrations (227). HGF is a heterodimeric protein consisting of 69- and 34-kd subunits, which are derived from a single molecule precursor cleaved by urokinase (228) and show structure homologies with plasminogen (223). HGF is produced in many organs (e.g., lung, kidney, brain, liver, thymus, and placenta). In the liver, fat-storing cells are the major site of synthesis (229,230), whereas no synthesis of HGF was found in hepatocytes. During the first two hours after partial hepatectomy, HGF plasma levels increase to concentrations that are well above the mitogenic range for hepatocytes in culture (231). This increase is followed by an increase in DNA synthesis in hepatocytes after 24 hours. Because HGF mRNA increased 3 to 6 hours after partial hepatectomy (232,233), the initial increase is more likely due to an impaired clearance of HGF by the damaged liver than to an increase in its synthesis (234). Induction of HGF synthesis is mediated by injurin, a 10- to 20-kd protein (235), and it is enhanced by growth hormone and insulin-like growth factor I (236). The HGF receptor, which is identical to the c-met proto-oncogene, is a 190-kd transmembrane protein that possesses tyrosine-kinase activity (237,238). In rat hepatocytes, 2 different receptors have been found (239). The c-met receptor is autophosphorylated on tyrosine after binding of HGF (237,238), followed by activation of phospholipase-C and an increase in inositol-1,4,5-triphosphate, 1,2-diacylglycerol and intracellular calcium concentrations in hepatocytes (224). The mitogenic effect of HGF is amplified by norepinephrine, which also is elevated in the plasma after hepatic injury (231), suggesting a combined action of these mediators. It was recently shown that HGF is able to stimulate the growth of nonparenchymal epithelial cells in vitro (240,241).

EGF and transforming growth factor-α (TGF-α), which both bind to the EGF receptor on hepatocytes, are also complete hepatocyte mitogens (242–247). However, plasma levels of EGF do not increase after partial hepatectomy, and TGF-α mRNA levels in hepatocytes and nonparenchymal liver cells increase later after injury when DNA synthesis of hepatocytes has already started (243,244,248). The action of EGF is inhibited by ethanol, prostaglandine synthesis inhibitors, and estrogen (2). Furthermore, inhibition of EGF by neutralizing antibodies did not prevent liver regeneration in vivo (249), indicating that EGF is not absolutely required for hepatocyte regeneration in vivo.

In contrast to TGF-α, TGF-β inhibits proliferation of hepatocytes (250–252). Furthermore, it impairs synthesis (253) and the proliferative effect of TGF-α in vitro (244,254) and in vivo (255,256). Its mRNA expression in regenerating liver reaches a peak after the major wave of hepatocyte cell division and mitosis has taken place and after peak expression of the *ras* proto-oncogenes (191). This finding suggests that TGF-β may function as the effector of an inhibitory paracrine loop activated during liver regeneration to prevent uncontrolled hepatocyte proliferation.

FGF is another cytokine that stimulates hepatocyte regeneration (257–259). Expression of FGF is increased in fat-storing cells and in oval cells 24 hours after partial hepatectomy (260,261). It reduces the inhibitory effect of TGF-β, and it may allow hepatocytes to proliferate despite low levels of TGF-β (258,260).

Inflammatory cytokines such as IL-1, IL-6, and TNF may also contribute to the complex regulation of hepatic regeneration. IL-1, and to a smaller extent, TNF-α and IFN-γ, stimulate the synthesis of HGF in human fibroblasts (262). This stimulation can be inhibited by TGF-β (262). Both IL-1 and IL-6 inhibit EGF-stimulated DNA synthesis in rat hepatocyte primary cultures (263), whereas IL-1 has no effect (264). In contrast, IL-6 stimulates proliferation of mouse hepatocytes in primary cultures in the presence and absence of EGF (265). TNF stimulates DNA synthesis in rat (266) and mouse (264) hepatocytes in primary culture. This effect is inhibited by TGF-β, IL-6, and IFN-γ. Because neutralizing TNF antibodies inhibit liver regeneration and IL-6 induction in rats after partial hepatectomy in vivo, TNF seems to be necessary for liver regeneration (267). The synthesis of both IL-1 (268) and IL-6 (269) is increased in Kupffer cells during liver regeneration.

Recently, a novel nonparenchymal liver cell–derived factor inhibiting hepatocyte proliferation was detected,

indicating that there are even more factors involved in liver regeneration (270). In addition, classic hormones, such as insulin, glucagon, and norepinephrine modulate liver regeneration positively or negatively in a dose- and time-dependent manner (224).

In conclusion, a regeneration of hepatocytes begins with priming of hepatocytes, which moves them from the G0 to the G1 phase of the cell cycle. HGF and norepinephrine are possible candidates to mediate this process, which leads to production of additional mitogens, such as EGF and TGF-α, and to induction of DNA synthesis in hepatocytes. Due to multiple interactions of endocrine, paracrine, and autocrine acting cytokines; other soluble mediators; and cellular matrix components, the exact mechanisms, however, still remain unknown.

CYTOKINES AND MALIGNANT TRANSFORMATION

Cytokines and pathogenesis of hepatocellular carcinoma

Hepatocellular carcinoma is one of the most frequent cancers worldwide. It is clearly associated with chronic hepatitis. Altered autocrine and paracrine regulation of cell growth by cytokines, proto-oncogenes, growth factors, and tumor suppressor genes is clearly implicated in carcinogenesis (271).

Due to its high mitogenic activity and because HGF serum concentrations are elevated in chronic hepatitis and liver cirrhosis (272), HGF was examined as a possible autocrine growth factor in hepatocellular carcinoma. However, transformation and expression of the HGF gene in hepatoma cell lines showed that HGF strongly inhibits the growth of hepatoma cell lines (273). HGF, however, stimulates angiogenesis (274), which may also be important for tumor growth. Insulin-like growth factor II (IGF-II) is another hepatic mitogen. Expression of IGF-II was found in precancerous and hepatocellular carcinoma tissues in woodchucks, rats, and humans (275–279). Transgenic mice experiments showed that expression of IGF-II mRNAs takes place at specific steps of liver cancer progression, both in early pretumorous lesions and in well-differentiated hepatocellular carcinomas (280,281). IGF-II is focally expressed in precancerous lesions, and it leads to intracellular retention in perinuclear compartments of a 15-kd IGF-II polypeptide (281).

TGF-α is a powerful autocrine mitogen for hepatocytes. It is also involved in hepatocarcinogenesis, because several hepatoma cell lines express TGF-α (282–284), expression of TGF-α in transgenic mice induces *c-myc* and multifocal hepatocellular carcinoma (285–288), patients with chronic HBV have immunoreactive TGF-α in virus-infected cells (289), and patients with hepatocellular carcinoma have high concentrations of TGF-α in their urine (290). The majority of liver tumors arising in TGF-α–transgenic mice have highly elevated concentrations of IGF-II RNA (286). TGF-β, which is a growth-inhibiting factor, seems also to be involved in carcinogenesis, because the carcinogen diethylnitrosamine induces resistance to TGF-$β_1$–dependent growth control (291) during carcinogenesis.

Cytokines and treatment of hepatocellular carcinoma

Treatment of patients with inoperable hepatocellular carcinoma with IFN-α (50 million U/m^2 3 times a week) led to objective tumor regression in 11 of 35 patients and to an increase in the median survival time from 7.5 to 14.5 weeks (292). IFN-α was superior to doxorubicin for the treatment of inoperable hepatocellular carcinoma (293). However, other studies showed no effect of IFN-α (294). IFN may be of even greater value in the prevention of hepatocellular carcinoma than in treatment, because in a large study, IFN-α reduced considerably the incidence of hepatocellular carcinoma in high-risk patients (295).

CONCLUSION

Cytokines are involved in the pathogenesis of many liver diseases. They are already in use and are helpful for the treatment of chronic hepatitis B and C. Additional therapeutic strategies involving cytokines or cytokine modulators (Table 40-3), will be available in the near future for the treatment of hepatic diseases. However, due to the complex interactions between different cytokines and

other soluble factors, our knowledge is still incomplete about their role in liver injury, regeneration, or even physiological processes, especially the important interactions between cytokines and extracellular matrix components in the different microenvironments of the liver. Exploration of these mechanisms will probably lead to great progress in understanding of the cellular biology and the management of liver diseases.

TABLE 40–3 CYTOKINE-MODULATING DRUGS

Available drugs	Possible future drugs
Corticosteroids	Antibodies against lipopolysaccharide
Colchicine	Antibodies against cytokines
Prostaglandins	Soluble cytokine receptors
Bile acids	Cytokine production blockers
Interferons	
Pentoxifyllin	
N-acetylcysteine	

REFERENCES

1. Alberts B, Bray D, Lewis J, Raff M, Roberts K, Watson JD. Molecular biology of the cell. New York: Garland, 1983.

2. Andus T, Bauer J, Gerok W. Effects of cytokines on the liver. Hepatology 1991;13:364–375.

3. Andus T, Palitzsch KD, Gross V, Schölmerich J. Metabolische und endokrine Funktionen der Zytokine. Dtsch Med Wochenschr 1993;118:306–313.

4. Rehermann B, Trautwein C, Böker KH, Manns MP. Interleukin-6 in liver diseases. J Hepatol 1992;15:277–280.

5. Ramadori G, Meyer zum Büschenfelde KH. Liver cells and cytokines. Curr Opin Gastroenterol 1993;9:359–366.

6. Foster GR, Thomas HC. Recent advances in the molecular biology of hepatitis B virus: mutant virus and the host response. Gut 1993;34:1–3.

7. Dudley FJ, Tox RA, Sherlock S. Cellular immunity and hepatitis associated (Australia) antigen liver diseases. Lancet 1972;1:723–726.

8. Samuel CE. Antiviral action of interferons. Virology 1991; 183:1–11.

9. Thomas HC, Pignatelli M, Scully LJ. Viruses and immune reactions in the liver. Scand J Gastroenterol 1985;114 (suppl):105–117.

10. Pignatelli M, Waters J, Brown D, et al. HLA class I antigens on the hepatocyte membrane during recovery from acute hepatitis B virus infection and during interferon therapy in chronic hepatitis B virus infection. Hepatology 1986;6:349–353.

11. Ramadori G, Mitsch A, Rieder H, Meyer zum Büschenfelde KH. Alpha- and gamma-interferon (IFN alpha, IFN gamma) but not interleukin-1 (IL-1) modulate synthesis and secretion of beta 2-microglobulin by hepatocytes. Eur J Clin Invest 1988;18:343–351.

12. Trowsdale J, Hanson I, Mockridge I, Beck S, Townsend A, Kelly A. Sequences encoded in the class III region of the MHC related to the ABC superfamily of transporters. Nature 1990;349:7412–7414.

13. Kelly AK, Powis SH, Glynne R, Radley E, Beck S, Trowsdale J. Second proteosome related gene in the human class II region. Nature 1991;353:667–688.

14. Yoshioka K, Fuji A, Tahara H, Arao M, Kakumu S. Recombinant human interleukin 1 alpha is cytotoxic for and increases surface expression of HLA-A,B,C antigens of a human hepatoma cell line, PLC/PRF/5. Immunobiology 1989;178:380–389.

15. Yoshioka K, Kakumu S, Tahara H, Arao M, Fuji A. Effect of interferon alpha, gamma, and tumor necrosis factor alpha on the HLA-A,B,C expression of cell lines derived from human liver. Liver 1989;9:14–19.

16. Volpes R, van den Oord JJ, Desmet VJ. Hepatic expression

of intercellular adhesion molecule-I (ICAM-1) in viral hepatitis B. Hepatology 1990;12:148–154.

17. Volpes R, van den Oord JJ, Desmet VJ. Memory T cells represent the predominant lymphocyte subset in acute and chronic liver inflammation. Hepatology 1991;13:826–829.

18. Volpes R, van den Oord JJ, Desmet VJ, Yap SH. Induction of intercellular adhesion molecule-1 (CD54) on human hepatoma cell line HepG2: influence of cytokines and hepatitis B virus-DNA transfection. Clin Exp Immunol 1992; 87:71–75.

19. Hu KQ, Yu CH, Vierling JM. Up-regulation of intercellular adhesion molecule 1 transcription by hepatitis B virus X protein. Proc Natl Acad Sci USA 1992;89:11441–11445.

20. Kato Y, Nakagawa H, Kobayashi K. Interferon production by peripheral lymphocytes in HBsAg positive liver disease. Hepatology 1987;6:645–647.

21. Nouri Aria KT, Arnold J, Davison F, et al. Hepatic interferon-alpha gene transcripts and products in liver specimens from acute and chronic hepatitis B virus infection. Hepatology 1991;13:1029–1034.

22. Pointrine A, Chousterman S, Chousterman M, Naveau S, Thang MN, Chaput JC. Lack of in vivo activation of the interferon system of HBsAg-positive chronic active hepatitis. Hepatology 1985;5:171–174.

23. Abb J, Zachoval R, Eisenburg J, Pape GR, Zachoval V, Deinhardt F. Production of interferon alpha and interferon gamma by peripheral blood leukocyte from patients with chronic hepatitis. J Med Virol 1985;16:171–176.

24. Ikeda T, Lever AM, Thomas HC. Evidence for a deficiency of interferon production in patients with chronic hepatitis B virus infection acquired in adult life. Hepatology 1986;6: 962–965.

25. Zachoval R, Abb J, Zachoval V, et al. Interferon alpha in hepatitis type B and non-A, non-B. Defective production by peripheral blood mononuclear cells in chronic infection and development of serum interferon in acute disease. J Hepatol 1988;6:364–368.

26. Twu JS, Lee CH, Lin PM, Schloemer RH. Hepatitis B virus suppresses expression of human beta interferon. Proc Natl Acad Sci USA 1988;85:252–256.

27. Twu JS, Schloemer RH. Transcriptional transactivation function of hepatitis B virus. J Virol 1989;63:3065–3071.

28. Bird GL, Sheron N, Goka AK, Alexander GJ, Williams RS. Increased plasma tumor necrosis factor in severe alcoholic hepatitis. Ann Intern Med 1990;112:917–920.

29. Whitten TM, Quets AT, Schloemer RH. Identification of the hepatitis B virus factor that inhibits expression of the beta interferon gene. J Virol 1991;65:4699–4704.

30. Wakita T, Kakumu S, Tsutsumi Y, Yoshioka K, Machida A, Mayumi M. Gamma-interferon production in response to hepatitis B core protein and its synthetic peptides in patients with chronic hepatitis B virus infection. Digestion 1990;47:149–155.

31. Takehara T, Hayashi N, Katayama K, Kasahara A, Fusamoto H, Kamada T. Hepatitis B core antigen-specific interferon gamma production of peripheral blood mononuclear cells during acute exacerbation of chronic hepatitis B. Scand J Gastroenterol 1992;27:727–731.

32. Fuji A, Kakumu S, Ohtani Y, Murase K, Hirofuji H, Tahara H. Interferon-gamma production by peripheral blood mononuclear cells of patients with chronic liver disease. Hepatology 1987;7:577–581.

33. Kato T, Esumi M, Yamashita S, Abe K, Shikata T. Interferon-inducible gene expression in chimpanzee liver infected with hepatits C virus. Virology 1992;190:856–860.

34. Onji M, Lever AM, Saito I, Thomas HC. Defective response to interferons in cells transfected with the hepatitis B virus genome. Hepatology 1989;9:92–96.

35. Dooley JS, Vergalla J, Hoofnagle JH, Zoon KC, Munson PJ, Jones EA. Specific binding of human alpha interferon to high-affinity cell-surface binding sites on peripheral blood mononuclear cells. J Lab Clin Med 1989;113:623–631.

36. Lau JY, Sheron N, Morris AG, Bomford AB, Alexander GJ, Williams R. Interferon-alpha receptor expression and regulation in chronic hepatitis B virus infection. Hepatology 1991;13:332–338.

37. Kakumu S, Yoshioka K, Fuji A, Tahara H. Interferon-gamma receptors on T cells in patients with chronic liver disease. Hepatogastroenterology 1988;35:158–161.

38. Lau JY, Morris AG, Alexander GJ, Williams R. Interferon-gamma receptor expression in chronic hepatitis B virus infection. J Hepatol 1992;14:294–299.

39. Foster GR, Ackrill AM, Goldin RD, Kerr IM, Thomas HC, Stark GR. Expression of the terminal protein region of hepatitis B virus inhibits cellular responses to interferons a and g and double-stranded RNA. Proc Natl Acad Sci USA 1991; 88:2888–2892.

40. Foster GR, Goldin RD, Hay A, McGarvey J, Stark GR, Thomas HC. Expression of the terminal protein of hepatitis B virus is associated with failure to respond to interferon therapy. Hepatology 1993;17:757–762.

41. Smith KA. Interleukin-2. Curr Opin Immunol 1992;4:271–276.

42. Müller C, Knoflach P, Zielinski CC. Soluble interleukin 2 receptor in acute viral hepatitis and chronic liver disease. Hepatology 1989;10:928–932.

43. Alberti A, Chemello L, Fattovich G, et al. Serum levels of soluble interleukin-2 receptors in acute and chronic viral hepatitis. Dig Dis Sci 1989;34:1559–1563.

44. Alexander GJ, Nouri Aria KT, Neuberger J, et al. In vitro effects of lymphoblastoid interferon on lymphocyte activation and cell-mediated cytolysis in patients with chronic hepatitis B virus infection. J Hepatol 1986;3(suppl 2): S269–S277.

45. Anastassakos C, Alexander GJ, Wolstencroft RA, et al. Interleukin-1 and interleukin-2 activity in chronic hepatitis B virus infection. Gastroenterology 1988;94:999–1005.

46. Masumoto T, Onji M, Ohta Y. Decreased interleukin-2 receptor beta chain expression by peripheral blood lymphocytes in chronic liver disease. J Gastroenterol Hepatol 1992;7:399–404.

47. Raptopoulou Gigi M, Orphanou Koumerkeridou H, Lagra F. Possible mechanisms underlying peripheral lymphocyte activation in chronic liver disease and asymptomatic HBsAg carriers. Allerg Immunopathol Madr 1989;17:145–148.

48. Kakumu S, Yoshioka K, Fuji A, Tahara H. Interleukin 2 receptor bearing T lymphocytes in patients with chronic liver disease. Gastroenterol Jpn 1988;23:408–413.

49. Kakumu S, Tahara H, Fuji A, Yoshioka K. Interleukin 1

alpha production by peripheral blood monocytes from patients with chronic liver disease and effect of sera on interleukin 1 alpha production. J Clin Lab Immunol 1988;26: 113–119.

50. Müller C, Godl I, Ahmad R, Wolf HM, Mannhalter JW, Eibl MM. Interleukin-1 production in acute viral hepatitis. Arch Dis Child 1989;64:205–210.

51. Müller C, Knoflach P, Zielinski CC. Reduced production of immunoreactive interleukin-1 by peripheral blood monocytes of patients with acute and chronic viral hepatitis. Dig Dis Sci 1993;38:477–481.

52. Yokota M, Sakamoto S, Koga S, Ibayashi H. Decreased interleukin 1 activity in culture supernatants of lipopolysaccharide stimulated monocytes from patients with liver cirrhosis and hepatocellular carcinoma. Clin Exp Immunol 1987;67:335–342.

53. Knudsen PJ, Strom RB, Zeldis JB. Hepatitis B virus blocks monocyte release of interleukin-1 in vitro (abstract). Gastroenterology 1986;90:1738.

54. Giustino V, Dudley FJ, Sherlock S. Thymus-dependent lymphocyte function in patients with hepatitis associated antigen. Lancet 1972;2:850–852.

55. Hanson G, Hoofnagle JH, Minuck GY, Purcell RH, Gerin JL. Cell-mediated immunity to hepatitis B surface antigen in man. Clin Exp Immunol 1984;57:257–262.

56. Dinarello CA, Wolff SM. The role of interleukin-1 in disease. N Engl J Med 1993;328:106–113.

57. Ruddle NH. Tumor necrosis factor (TNF-alpha) and lymphotoxin (TNF-beta). Curr Opin Immunol 1992;4: 327–332.

58. Bautista AP, Schuler A, Spolarics Z, Spitzer JJ. Tumor necrosis factor-alpha stimulates superoxide anion generation by perfused rat liver and Kupffer cells. Am J Physiol 1991; 261:G891–G895.

59. Stadler J, Bentz BG, Harbrecht BG, et al. Tumor necrosis factor alpha inhibits hepatocyte mitochondrial respiration. Ann Surg 1992;216:539–546.

60. Yoshioka K, Kakumu S, Arao M, Tsutsumi Y, Inoue M. Tumor necrosis factor alpha production by peripheral blood mononuclear cells of patients with chronic liver disease. Hepatology 1989;10:769–773.

61. Yoshioka K, Kakumu S, Arao M, et al. Immunohistochemical studies of intrahepatic tumour necrosis factor alpha in chronic liver disease. J Clin Pathol 1990;43:298–302.

62. Volpes R, van den Oord JJ, De Vos R, Desmet VJ. Hepatic expression of type A and type B receptors for tumor necrosis factor. J Hepatol 1992;14:361–369.

63. Heinrich PC, Castell JV, Andus T. Interleukin-6 and the acute phase response. Biochem J 1990;265:621–636.

64. Müller C, Zielinski CC. Interleukin-6 production by peripheral blood monocytes in patients with chronic liver disease and acute viral hepatitis. J Hepatol 1992;15:372–377.

65. Ren H, Zheng DF, Jia XP. Tumor necrosis factor and interleukin 6 in hepatitis C virus infection. Chung Hua Nei Ko Tsa Chih 1992;31:344–346, 381.

66. Kakumu S, Shinagawa T, Ishikawa T, Yoshioka K, Wakita T, Ida N. Interleukin 6 production by peripheral blood mononuclear cells in patients with chronic hepatitis B

67. Kakumu S, Fukatsu A, Shinagawa T, Kurokawa S, Kusakabe A. Localisation of intrahepatic interleukin 6 in patients with acute and chronic liver disease. J Clin Pathol 1992;45:408–411.

68. Triger DR, Wright R. Hypergammaglobulinemia in liver disease. Lancet 1973;1:1494–1496.

69. Neurath AR, Strick N, Sproul P. Search for hepatitis B virus cell receptors binding sites for interleukin-6 on the virus envelope protein. J Exp Med 1992;175:461–469.

70. Neurath AR, Strick N, Li YY. Cells transfected with human interleukin 6 cDNA acquire binding sites for the hepatitis B virus envelope protein. J Exp Med 1992;176:1561–1569.

71. Zeldis JB, Mugishima H, Steinberg HN, Nir E, Gale RP. In vitro hepatitis B virus infection of human bone marrow cells. J Clin Invest 1986;78:411–417.

72. Romet-Lemonne JL, McLane MF, Elfassi E, Haseltine WA, Azocar J, Essex M. Hepatitis B virus infection in clutured human lymphoblastoid cells. Science 1983;221:667–669.

73. Pontisso P, Poon MC, Tiollais P, Bréchot C. Detection of hepatitis B virus DNA in mononuclear blood cells. Br Med J 1984;288:1563–1566.

74. Greenberg HB, Pollard RB, Lutwick LI, Gregory PB, Robinson WS, Merigan TC. Effect of human leucocyte interferon on hepatitis B virus infection in patients with chronic active hepatitis. N Engl J Med 1976;295:517–522.

75. Perillo RP, Schiff ER, Davis GL, et al. A randomized controlled trial of interferon alfa-2b alone and after prednisone withdrawal for the treatment of chronic hepatitis B. N Engl J Med 1990;323:295–301.

76. Hoofnagle JH, Peters M, Mullen KD, et al. Randomized, controlled trial of recombinant human alpha-interferon in patients with chronic hepatitis B. Gastroenterology 1988; 95:1318–1325.

77. Ohnishi K, Nomura F, Nakano M. Interferon therapy for acute posttransfusion non-A, non-B hepatitis: response with respect to anti-hepatitis C virus antibody status. Am J Gastroenterol 1991;86:1041–1049.

78. Perillo RP. Interferon in the management of chronic hepatitis B. Dig Dis Sci 1993;38:577–593.

79. Sherlock S, Dooley J. Chronic hepatitis. In: Sherlock S, Dooley J, eds. Diseases of the liver and biliary system, ed 9. London: Blackwell Scientific Publications, 1993:293–321.

80. Davis GL. Chronic hepatitis. In: Kaplowitz N, ed. Liver and biliary diseases. Baltimore: Williams & Wilkins, 1993:289–299.

81. Hoofnagle JH, Mullen KD, Jones DB, et al. Treatment of chronic non-A, non-B hepatitis with recombinant human alpha interferon. A preliminary report. N Engl J Med 1986; 315:1575–1578.

82. Davis GL, Balart LA, Schiff ER, et al. Treatment of chronic hepatitis C with recombinant interferon alfa. A multicenter randomized, controlled trial. Hepatitis Interventional Therapy Group. N Engl J Med 1989;321:1501–1506.

83. Di Bisceglie AM, Martin P, Kassianides C, et al. Recombinant interferon alfa therapy for chronic hepatitis C. A randomized, double-blind, placebo-controlled trial. N Eng J Med 1989;321:1506–1510.

84. Dusheiko G, Hoofnagle JH. Hepatitis B. In: McIntyre N,

Benhamou JP, Bircher J, Rizzetto M, Rodes J, eds. Oxford textbook of clinical hepatology. Oxford: Oxford Medical Publications, 1991:571–592.

85. Omata M, Ito Y, Yokosuka O, et al. Histological changes of the liver by treatment of chronic non-A, non-B hepatitis with recombinant leukocyte interferon alpha. Comparison with histological changes in chronic hepatitis B. Dig Dis Sci 1989;34:330–337.

86. Rosina F, Pintus C, Rizzetto M. Long-term interferon treatment of chronic hepatitis D: a multicentre Italian study. J Hepatol 1990;11(suppl 1):S149–S150.

87. Hopf U, Neuhaus P, Lobeck H, et al. Follow-up of recurrent hepatitis B and delta infection in liver allograft recipients after treatment with recombinant interferon-alpha. J Hepatol 1991;13:339–346.

88. Marcellin P, Boyer N, Giostra E, et al. Recombinant human alpha-interferon in patients with chronic non-A, non-B hepatitis: a multicenter randomized controlled trial from France. Hepatology 1991;13:393–397.

89. Tine F, Magrin S, Craxi A, Pagliaro L. Interferon for non-A, non-B hepatitis: a meta-analysis of randomized clinical trials. J Hepatol 1991;13:192–199.

90. Iino S, Hino K, Kuroki T, Suzuki H, Yamamoto S. Treatment of chronic hepatitis C with high-dose interferon alpha-2b. Dig Dis Sci 1993;38:612–618.

91. Hagiwara H, Hayashi N, Mita E, et al. Quantitative analysis of hepatitis C virus RNA in serum during interferon alfa therapy. Gastroenterology 1993;104:877–883.

92. Giacchino R, Nocera A, Timitilli A, et al. Association between HLA class I antigens and response to interferon therapy in children with chronic HBV hepatitis. Arch Virol 1992;4(suppl):281–283.

93. Okada S, Akahane Y, Suzuki H, Okamoto H, Mishiro S. The degree of variability in the amino terminal region of the E2/NS1 protein of hepatitis C virus correlates with responsiveness to interferon therapy in viremic patients. Hepatology 1992;16:619–624.

94. Giannelli G, Antonelli G, Fera G, Dianzani F, Schiraldi O. 2',5'-Oligoadenylate synthetase activity as a responsive marker during interferon therapy for chronic hepatitis C. J Interferon Res 1993;13:57–60.

95. Fevery J, Elewaut A, Michielsen P, et al. Efficacy of interferon alfa-2b with or without prednisone withdrawal in the treatment of chronic viral hepatitis B. A prospective double-blind Belgian-Dutch study. J Hepatol 1990;11:S108–S112.

96. Takano S, Omata M, Yokosuka O, Imazeki F, Ohto M. Effects of antiviral agents on chronic hepatitis B. Analysis using Cox proportional hazard model. Dig Dis Sci 1992;37:1633–1643.

97. Liaw YF, Sheen IS, Lin SM, Chen TJ, Chu CM. Effects of prednisolone pretreatment in interferon alfa therapy for patients with chronic non-A, non-B (C) hepatitis. Liver 1993;13:46–50.

98. Berk L, de Man RA, Housset C, Berthelot P, Schalm SW. Alpha lymphoblastoid interferon and acyclovir for chronic hepatitis delta. Prog Clin Biol Res 1991;364:411–420.

99. Berk L, Schalm SW, de Man RA, et al. Failure of acyclovir to enhance the antiviral effect of alpha lymphoblastoid interferon on HBe-seroconversion in chronic hepatitis B. A multi-centre randomized controlled trial. J Hepatol 1992;14:305–309.

100. Schalm SW. Treatment of chronic viral hepatitis anno 1990. Scand J Gastroenterol 1990;178(suppl):111–118.

101. Gracia G, Smith CI, Weissber JI, et al. Adenid arabinoside monophosphate (vidarabine phosphate) in combination with human leukocyte interferon in the treatment of chronic hepatitis B (abstract). Ann Intern Med 1987;107:278–285.

102. Fattovich G, Giustina G, Brollo L, et al. Therapy for chronic hepatitis B with lymphoblastoid interferon-alpha and levamisole. Hepatology 1992;16:1115–1119.

103. Janssen HL, Berk L, Heijtink RA, ten Kate FJ, Schalm SW. Interferon-alpha and zidovudine combination therapy for chronic hepatitis B: results of a randomized, placebo-controlled trial. Hepatology 1993;17:383–388.

104. Di Bisceglie AM, Rustgi VK, Kassianides C, et al. Therapy of chronic hepatitis B with recombinant human alpha and gamma interferon. Hepatology 1990;11:266–270.

105. Hayashi Y, Koike K. Interferon inhibits hepatitis B virus replication in transfected viral DNA. J Virol 1989;63:2936–2940.

106. Qian C, Camps J, Maluenda MD, Civeira MP, Prieto J. Replication of hepatitis C virus in peripheral blood mononuclear cells. Effect of alpha-interferon therapy. J Hepatol 1992;16:380–383.

107. Ishikawa T, Kakumu S, Yoshioka K, et al. Effects of interferon-alpha treatment of hepatitis B virus antigen-specific immunologic responses in patients with chronic hepatitis B. Liver 1993;13:95–101.

108. Franco A, Barnaba V, Natali P, Balsano C, Musca A, Balsano F. Expression of class I and class II major histocompatibility complex antigens on human hepatocytes. Hepatology 1988;8:449–454.

109. Castilla A, Prieto J, Fausto N. Transforming growth factors beta 1 and alpha in chronic liver disease. Effects of interferon alfa therapy. N Engl J Med 1991;324:933–940.

110. Katayama K, Hayashi N, Takehara T, et al. Effects of alpha-interferon on gamma-interferon production of peripheral blood mononuclear cells in hepatitis B virus carriers. J Clin Immunol 1992;12:347–352.

111. Mayet WJ, Hess G, Gerken G, et al. Treatment of chronic type B hepatitis with recombinant alpha-interferon induces autoantibodies not specific for autoimmune chronic hepatitis. Hepatology 1989;10:24–28.

112. Lisker Melman M, Di Bisceglie AM, Usala SJ, Weintraub B, Murray LM, Hoofnagle JH. Development of thyroid disease during therapy of chronic viral hepatitis with interferon alfa. Gastroenterology 1992;102:2155–2160.

113. Nishioka M, Kagawa H, Shirai M, Terada S, Watanabe S. Effects of human recombinant interleukin-2 in patients with chronic hepatitis B: a preliminary report. Am J Gastroenterol 1987;82:438–442.

114. Onji M, Kondoh H, Horiike M, et al. Effect of recombinant interleukin 2 on hepatitis B e antigen positive chronic hepatitis. Gut 1987;28:1648–1652.

115. Minuk GY, Lafreniere R. Interleukin-1 and interleukin-2 in chronic type B hepatitis. Gastroenterology 1988;94:1094–1096.

116. Kuroki T. Therapy with interleukin 2 for chronic viral hepatitis. Nippon Rinsho 1992;50:1984–1989.

117. Kakumu S, Fuji A, Tahara H, Yoshioka K, Sakamoto N. Enhancement of antibody production to hepatitis B surface antigen by interleukin 2. J Clin Lab Immunol 1988;26:25–27.

118. Meuer S, Dumann H, Meyer zum Büschenfelde KH, Köhler H. Low-dose interleukin-2 induces systemic immune responses against HBsAg in immunodeficient non-responders to hepatitis B vaccination. Lancet 1989;1:15–18.

119. Gilles PN, Fey G, Chisari FV. Tumor necrosis factor alpha negatively regulates hepatitis B virus gene expression in transgenic mice. J Virol 1992;66:3955–3960.

120. Tinè F, Liberati A, Craxi A, Almasio P, Pagliaro L. Interferon treatment in patients with chronic hepatitis B: a meta-analysis of the published literature. J Hepatol 1993;18:154–162.

121. Carreno V, Castillo I, Molina J, Porres JC, Bartolomé J. Long-term follow-up of hepatitis B chronic carriers who responded to interferon therapy. J Hepatol 1992;15:102–106.

122. Hagiwara H, Hayashi N, Kasahara A, et al. Three cases of posttransfusion hepatitis C treated with interferon-alpha. Confirmation of a carrier state by detection of hepatitis C virus RNA after interferon therapy. Dig Dis Sci 1992;37:631–634.

123. Yamamoto H, Hayashi E, Nakamura H, Kimura Y, Ito H, Kambe H. Interferon therapy for non-A, non-B hepatitis: a pilot study and review of the literature. Hepatogastroenterology 1992;39:377–380.

124. Genesca J. Interferon alfa in acute posttransfusion hepatitis C: a randomized, controlled trial. Gastroenterology 1992;103:1702–1703.

125. Sanchez Tapias JM, Mas A, Costa J, et al. Recombinant alpha 2c-interferon therapy in fulminant viral hepatitis. J Hepatol 1987;5:205–210.

126. Gohda E, Tsubouchi H, Nakayama H, et al. Purification and partial characterization of hepatocyte growth factor from plasma of a patient with fulminant hepatic failure. J Clin Invest 1988;81:414–419.

127. Sun Y, Tokushige K, Isono E, Yamauchi K, Obata H. Elevated serum interleukin-6 levels in patients with acute hepatitis. J Clin Immunol 1992;12:197–200.

128. Tsubouchi H, Kawakami S, Hirono S, et al. Prediction of outcome in fulminant hepatic failure by serum human hepatocyte growth factor. Lancet 1992;340:307.

129. Appasamy R, Tanabe M, Murase N, et al. Hepatocyte growth factor, blood clearance, organ uptake, and biliary excretion in normal and partially hepatectomized rats. Lab Invest 1993;68:270–276.

130. Liu KX, Kato Y, Narukawa M, et al. Importance of the liver in plasma clearance of hepatocyte growth factors in rats. Am J Physiol 1992;263:G642–G649.

131. Castell JV, Geiger T, Gross V, et al. Plasma clearance, organ distribution and target cells of interleukin-6/hepatocyte-stimulating factor in the rat. Eur J Biochem 1988;177:357–361.

132. Tomiya T, Nagoshi S, Fujiwara K. Significance of serum human hepatocyte growth factor levels in patients with hepatic failure. Hepatology 1992;15:1–4.

133. Tsubouchi H, Hirono S, Gohda E, et al. Clinical significance of human hepatocyte growth factor in blood from patients with fulminant hepatic failure. Hepatology 1989;9:875–881.

134. Gohda E, Yamasaki T, Tsubouchi H, et al. Biological and immunological properties of human hepatocyte growth factor from plasma of patients with fulminant hepatic failure. Biochim Biophys Acta 1990;1053:21–26.

135. Strain AJ, Ismail T, Tsubouchi H, et al. Native and recombinant human hepatocyte growth factors are highly potent promoters of DNA synthesis in both human and rat hepatocytes. J Clin Invest 1991;87:1853–1857.

136. Tsubouchi H, Hirono S, Gohda E, et al. Human hepatocyte growth factor in blood of patients with fulminant hepatic failure. I. Clinical aspects. Dig Dis Sci 1991;36:780–784.

137. Nagaki M, Muto Y, Ohnishi H, Moriwaki H. Significance of tumor necrosis factor (TNF) and interleukin-1 (IL-1) in the pathogenesis of fulminant hepatitis: possible involvement of serine protease in TNF-mediated liver injury. Gastroenterol Jpn 1991;26:448–455.

138. Bianchi FB. Autoimmune hepatitis: the lesson of the discovery of hepatitis C virus. J Hepatol 1993;18:273–275.

139. Manns M, Meyer zum Büschenfelde KH, Arnold W. The diagnostic value of immunologic findings in the differentiation of chronic liver diseases. Leber Magen Darm 1988;18:290–295.

140. Meyer zum Büschenfelde KH, Lohse AW, Manns M, Poralla T. Autoimmunity and liver disease. Hepatology 1990;12:354–363.

141. Meyer zum Büschenfelde KH, Poralla T. Immunology and autoimmune liver diseases. Curr Opin Gastroenterol 1992;8:380–387.

142. Silva MO, Reddy KR, Jeffers LJ, Hill M, Schiff ER. Interferon-induced chronic active hepatitis? Gastroenterology 1991;101:840–842.

143. Fattovich G, Betterle C, Brollo L, et al. Autoantibodies during alpha-interferon therapy for chronic hepatitis B. J Med Virol 1991;34:132–135.

144. Shindo M, Di Bisceglie AM, Hoofnagle JH. Acute exacerbation of liver disease during interferon alfa therapy for chronic hepatitis C. Gastroenterology 1992;102:1406–1408.

145. Chung YH, Shong YK. Development of thyroid autoimmunity after administration of recombinant human interferon-alpha 2b for chronic viral hepatitis. Am J Gastroenterol 1993;88:244–247.

146. Himeno H, Saibara T, Onishi S, Yamamoto Y, Enzan H. Administration of interleukin-2 induces major histocompatibility complex class II expression on the biliary epithelial cells, possibly through endogenous interferon-gamma production. Hepatology 1992;16:409–417.

147. Miller LC, Kaplan MM. Serum interleukin-2 and tumor necrosis factor-alpha in primary biliary cirrhosis: Decrease by colchicine and relationship to HLA-DR4. Am J Gastroenterol 1992;87:465–470.

148. Lobo Yeo A, Mieli Vergani G, Mowat AP, Vergani D. Soluble interleukin 2 receptors in autoimmune chronic active hepatitis. Gut 1990;31:690–693.

149. Franco A, Barnaba V, Ruberti G, Benvenuto R, Balsano C, Musca A. Liver-derived T cell clones in autoimmune chronic active hepatitis: accessory cell function of hepatocytes expressing class II major histocompatibility complex

molecules. Clin Immunol Immunopathol 1990;54:382–394.

150. Schlaak J, Löhr H, Gallati H, Meyer zum Büschenfelde KH, Fleischer B. Elevated IL-4 production by liverinfiltrating T cells in autoimmune hepatitis. Hepatology 1992;16:64A.

151. Spengler U, Möller A, Jung MC, et al. T lymphocytes from patients with primary biliary cirrhosis produce reduced amounts of lymphotoxin, tumor necrosis factor and interferon-gamma upon mitogen stimulation. J Hepatol 1992; 15:129–135.

152. Menendez JL, Girón JA, Manzano L, et al. Deficient interleukin-2 responsiveness of T lymphocytes from patients with primary biliary cirrhosis. Hepatology 1992;16:931–936.

153. Tilg H, Wilmer A, Vogel W, et al. Serum levels of cytokines in chronic liver diseases. Gastroenterology 1992;103:264–274.

154. Broome U, Eriksson LS, Sundin U, Sundqvist KG. Decreased in vitro production of tumor necrosis factor in primary biliary cirrhosis patients. Scand J Gastroenterol 1992;27:124–128.

155. Krams SM, Martinez OM, Villanueva JC, et al. Molecular and cellular mediators involved in the pathogenesis of primary biliary cirrhosis. Hepatology 1992;16:60A.

156. Magilavy DB, Rothstein JL. Spontaneous production of tumor necrosis factor alpha by Kupffer cells of MRL/lpr mice. J Exp Med 1988;168:789–794.

157. Magilavy DB, Foys KM, Gajewski TF. Liver of MRL/lpr mice contain interleukin-4-producing lymphocytes and accessory cells that support the proliferation of Th2 helper T lymphocyte clones. Eur J Immunol 1992;22:2359–2365.

158. Brennan FM, Feldmann M. Cytokines in autoimmunity. Curr Opin Immunol 1992;4:754–759.

159. Salaspuro M. Epidemiological aspects of alcohol and alcoholic liver disease, ethanol metabolism, and pathogenesis of alcoholic liver injury. In: McIntyre N, Benhamou JP, Bircher J, Rizzetto M, Rodes J, eds. Oxford textbook of clinical hepatology. Oxford: Oxford Medical Publications 1993:791–809.

160. McClain C, Hill D, Schmidt J, Diehl AM. Cytokines and alcoholic liver disease. Semin Liver Dis 1993;13:170–182.

161. Paronetto F. Immunologic reactions in alcoholic liver disease. Semin Liver Dis 1993;13:183–195.

162. Mendenhall CL. Alcoholic liver disease. Curr Opin Gastroenterol 1993;9:397–404.

163. McClain CJ, Cohen DA, Dinarello CA, et al. Serum interleukin-1 (IL-1) activity in alcoholic hepatitis. Life Sci 1986; 39:1479–1485.

164. Felver ME, Mezey E, McGuire M, et al. Plasma tumor necrosis factor alpha predicts decreased long-term survival in severe alcoholic hepatitis. Alcohol Clin Exp Res 1990;14:255–259.

165. Khoruts A, Stahnke L, McClain CJ, Logan G, Allen JI. Circulating tumor necrosis factor, interleukin-1 and interleukin-6 concentrations in chronic alcoholic patients. Hepatology 1991;13:267–276.

166. Deviere J, Content J, Denys C, et al. High interleukin-6 serum levels and increased production by leucocytes in alcoholic liver cirrhosis. Correlation with IgA serum levels and lymphokines production. Clin Exp Immunol 1989;77: 221–225.

167. Hill DB, Marsano L, Cohen D, Allen J, Shedlofsky S, McClain CJ. Increased plasma interleukin-6 concentrations in alcoholic hepatitis. J Lab Clin Med 1992;119:547–552.

168. Richardet JP, Dehoux M, Mal F, et al. Influence of corticosteroids (CS) on plasma cytokines concentrations in patients with severe alcoholic hepatitis (HA): results of a randomized study (abstract). J Hepatol 1993;18:1232.

169. Deviere J, Content J, Denys C, et al. Excessive in vitro bacterial lipopolysaccharide-induced production of monokines in cirrhosis. Hepatology 1990;11:628–634.

170. McClain CJ, Cohen DA. Increased tumor necrosis factor production by monocytes in alcoholic hepatitis. Hepatology 1989;9:349–351.

171. Annoni G, Weiner FR, Zern MA. Increased transforming growth factor-beta 1 gene expression in human liver disease. J Hepatol 1992;14:259–264.

172. Milani S, Herbst H, Schuppan D, Stein H, Surrenti C. Transforming growth factors beta 1 and beta 2 are differentially expressed in fibrotic liver disease. Am J Pathol 1991;139:1221–1229.

173. Bode C, Kugler V, Bode JC. Endotoxemia in patients with alcoholic and non-alcoholic cirrhosis and in subjects with no evidence of chronic liver disease following acute alcohol excess. J Hepatol 1987;4:8–14.

174. Bjarnason I, Ward K, Peters TJ. The leaky gut of alcoholism: possible route of entry for toxic compounds. Lancet 1984;1:179–182.

175. Honchel R, Ray MB, Marsano L, et al. Tumor necrosis factor in alcohol enhanced endotoxin liver injury. Alcohol Clin Exp Res 1992;16:665–669.

176. D'Souza NB, Bagby CJ, Nelson S, et al. Acute alcohol infusion suppresses endotoxin induced serum tumor necrosis factor. Alcohol Clin Exp Res 1989;13:295–298.

177. Van de Wiel A, Delecroix DL, Van Hattum J, et al. Characteristics of serum IgA and liver IgA deposits in alcoholic liver disease. Hepatology 1987;7:95–99.

178. Devière J, Vaerman JP, Content J, et al. IgA triggers TNF alpha secretion by monocytes. A study in normal subjects and patients with alcoholic liver cirrhosis. Hepatology 1991;13:670–675.

179. Devière J, Content J, Denys C, et al. Immunoglobulin A and interleukin 6 form a positive secretory feedback loop. A study of normal subjects and alcoholic cirrhotics. Gastroenterology 1992;103:1296–1301.

180. Peristeris P, Clark B, Gatii S, et al. N-acetylcysteine and glutathione as inhibitors of tumor necrosis factor production. Cell Immunol 1992;140:390–399.

181. Maxwell WJ, Keting JJ, Hogan FP, et al. Prostaglandin E2 and leukotriene B4 synthesis by peripheral leucocytes in alcoholics. Gut 1989;30:1270–1274.

182. Curran RD, Billiar TR, Stuehr DJ, et al. Multiple cytokines are required to induce hepatocyte nitric oxide production and inhibit total protein synthesis. Ann Surg 1990;212:462–469.

183. Friedman SL. The cellular basis of hepatic fibrosis. Mechanisms and treatment strategies. N Engl J Med 1993;328:1828–1835.

184. Feder LS, Todaro JA, Laskin DL. Characterization of inter-

leukin-1 and interleukin-6 production by hepatic endothelial cells and macrophages. J Leukocyte Biol 1993;53:126–132.

185. Itoh Y, Okanoue T, Morimoto M, et al. Functional heterogeneity of rat liver macrophages: interleukin-1 secretion and Ia antigen expression in contrast with phagocytic activity. Liver 1992;12:26–33.

186. Emilie D, Navratil E, Devergne O, et al. Monokine gene expression in normal human liver: selective involvement of the portal compartment. Liver 1992;12:34–41.

187. Lissoos TW, Davis BH. Pathogenesis of hepatic fibrosis and the role of cytokines. J Clin Gastroenterol 1992;15:63–67.

188. Sporn MB, Roberts AB. Transforming growth factor-beta: recent progress and new challenges. J Cell Biol 1992;119:1017–1021.

189. Nakatsukasa H, Nagy P, Evarts RP, Hsia CC, Marsden E, Thorgiersson SS. Cellular distribution of transforming growth factor-beta 1 and procollagen types I, III, and IV transcripts in carbon tetrachloride-induced rat liver fibrosis. J Clin Invest 1990;85:1833–1843.

190. Meyer DH, Bachem MG, Gressner AM. Modulation of hepatic lipocyte proteoglycan synthesis and proliferation by Kupffer cell-derived transforming growth factors type beta 1 and type alpha. Biochem Biophys Res Commun 1990;171:1122–1129.

191. Braun L, Mead JE, Panzica M, Mikumo R, Bell GI, Fausto N. Transforming growth factor beta mRNA increases during liver regeneration: a possible paracrine mechanism of growth regulation. Proc Natl Acad Sci USA 1988;85:1539–1543.

192. Roberts AB, Sporn MB, Assoian RK, et al. Transforming growth factor type-beta: rapid induction of fibrosis and angiogenesis in vivo and stimulation of collagen formation in vitro. Proc Natl Acad Sci USA 1986;83:4167–4171.

193. Czaja MJ, Weiner FR, Flanders KC, et al. In vitro and in vivo association of transforming growth factor-beta1 with hepatic fibrosis. J Cell Biol 1989;108:2477–2488.

194. Ramadori G, Knittel T, Odenthal M, Schwögler S, Neubauer K, Meyer zum Büschenfelde KH. Synthesis of cellular fibronectin by rat liver rat-storing (Ito) cells: regulation by cytokines. Gastroenterology 1992;103:1313–1321.

195. Meyer DH, Krull N, Dreher KL, Gressner AM. Biglycan and decorin gene expression in normal and fibrotic rat liver: cellular localization and regulatory factors. Hepatology 1992;16:204–216.

196. Schwögler S, Odenthal M, Meyer zum Büschenfelde KH, Ramadori G. Alternative splicing products of tenascin gene distinguish rat liver fat storing cells from arterial smooth muscle cells and skin fibroblasts. Biochem Biophys Res Commun 1992;185:768–775.

197. Casini A, Pinzani M, Milani S, et al. Regulation of extracellular matrix synthesis by transforming growth factor beta 1 in human fat-storing cells. Gastroenterology 1993;105:245–253.

198. Sporn MB, Roberts AB, Wakefield LM, de Crombrugghe B. Some recent advances in the chemistry and biology of transforming growth factor-beta. J Cell Biol 1987;105:1039–1045.

199. Clément B, Loréal O, Levavasseur F, Guillouzo A. New challenges in hepatic fibrosis. J Hepatol 1993;18:1–4.

200. Bachem MG, Meyer D, Melchior R, Sell KM, Gressner AM. Activation of rat liver perisinusoidal lipocytes by transforming growth factors derived from myofibroblastlike cells. A potential mechanism of self perpetuation in liver fibrogenesis. J Clin Invest 1992;89:19–27.

201. Bachem MG, Sell KM, Melchior R, Kropf J, Eller T, Gressner AM. Tumor necrosis factor alpha (TNF alpha) and transforming growth factor beta 1 (TGF beta 1) stimulate fibronectin synthesis and the transdifferentiation of fat-storing cells in the rat liver into myofibroblasts. Virchows Arch [B] 1993;63:123–130.

202. Heldin CH, Westermark B. Possible in vivo effect and clinical utility of platelet-derived growth factor and PDGF antagonists. Transplant Proc 1993;25:2074–2076.

203. Pinzani M, Knauss TC, Pierce GF, et al. Mitogenic signals for platelet-derived growth factor isoforms in liver fat-storing cells. Am J Physiol 1991;260:C485–C491.

204. Pinzani M, Gesualdo L, Sabbah GM, Abboud HE. Effects of platelet-derived growth factor and other polypeptide mitogens on DNA synthesis and growth of cultured rat liver fat-storing cells. J Clin Invest 1989;84:1786–1793.

205. Pinzani M, Abboud HE, Gesualdo L, Abboud SL. Regulation of macrophage colony-stimulating factor in liver fat-storing cells by peptide growth factors. Am J Physiol 1992;262:C876–C881.

206. Capra F, Casril M, Gabrielli GB, et al. Alfa interferon in the treatment of chronic viral hepatitis: effect on fibrogenesis serum markers. J Hepatol 1993;18:112–118.

207. Gressner AM, Brenzel A, Vossmeyer T. Hepatocyte-conditioned medium potentiates insulin-like growth factor (IGF) 1 and 2 stimulated DNA synthesis of cultured fat storing cells. Liver 1993;13:86–94.

208. Cheever AW, Xu Y, Sher A, Finkelman FD, Cox TM, Macedonia JG. Schistosoma japonicum-infected mice show reduced hepatic fibrosis and eosinophilia and selective inhibition of interleukin-5 secretion by CD4+ cells after treatment with anti-interleukin-2 antibodies. Infect Immun 1993;61:1288–1292.

209. Rockey DC, Maher JJ, Jarnagin WR, Gabbiani G, Friedman SL. Inhibition of rat hepatic lipocyte activation in culture by interferon-gamma. Hepatology 1992;16:776–784.

210. Jimenez SA, Freundlich B, Rosenbloom J. Selective inhibition of human diploid fibroblast collagen synthesis by interferons. J Clin Invest 1984;74:1112–1116.

211. Czaja MJ, Weiner FR, Takahashi S, et al. Gamma-interferon treatment inhibits collagen deposition in murine schistosomiasis. Hepatology 1989;10:795–800.

212. Schwögler S, Odenthal M, Knittel T, Meyer zum Büschenfelde KH, Ramadori G. Fat-storing cells of the rat liver synthesize and secrete C1-esterase inhibitor; modulation by cytokines. Hepatology 1992;16:794–802.

213. Parola M, Muraca R, Dianzani I, et al. Vitamin E dietary supplementation inhibits transforming growth factor beta 1 gene expression in the rat liver. FEBS Lett 1992;308:267–270.

214. Peterson TC. Pentoxifylline prevents fibrosis in an animal model and inhibits platelet-derived growth factor-driven proliferation of fibroblasts. Hepatology 1993;17:486–493.

215. McCuskey RS, Reilly FD. Hepatic microvasculature: dynamic structure and its regulation. Semin Liver Dis 1993;13:1–12.

216. Geller DA, Nussler AK, Di Silvio M, et al. Cytokines, endo-

toxin, and glucocorticoids regulate the expression of inducible nitric oxide synthase in hepatocytes. Proc Natl Acad Sci USA 1993;90:522–526.

217. Nussler AK, Di Silvio M, Billiar TR, et al. Stimulation of the nitric oxide synthase pathway in human hepatocytes by cytokines and endotoxin. J Exp Med 1992;176:261–264.

218. Gaillard T, Mulsch A, Klein H, Decker K. Regulation by prostaglandin E2 of cytokine-elicited nitric oxide synthesis in rat liver macrophages. Biol Chem Hoppe Seyler 1992; 373:897–902.

219. Vallance P, Moncada S. Hyperdynamic circulation in cirrhosis: a role for nitric oxide? Lancet 1991;337:776–778.

220. Andus T, Schölmerich J. Spontaneous bacterial peritonitis in patients with liver cirrhosis and ascites—new insights using cytokine and cytokine receptor analysis in ascites. Can J Gastroenterol 1992;6:141–146.

221. Andus T, Gross V, Holstege A, et al. High concentrations of soluble tumor necrosis factor receptors in ascites. Hepatology 1992;16:749–755.

222. Michalopoulos GK, Zarnegav R. Hepatocyte growth factor. Hepatology 1992;15:149–155.

223. LaBrecque DR. Hepatocyte growth factor—how do I know thee? Let me count the ways. Gastroenterology 1992; 103:1686–1691.

224. Moshage H, Yap SH. Molecular and cellular biology of the liver. Curr Opin Gastroenterol 1993;9:367–373.

225. Francavilla A, Starzl TE, Porter K, et al. Screening for candidate hepatic growth factors by selective portal infusion after canine Eck's fistula. Hepatology 1991;14:665–670.

226. Ishiki Y, Ohnishi H, Muto Y, Matsumoto K, Nakamura T. Direct evidence that hepatocyte growth factor is a hepatotrophic factor for liver regeneration and has a potent antihepatitis effect in vivo. Hepatology 1992;16:1227–1235.

227. Higuchi O, Nakamura T. Identification and change in the receptor for hepatocyte growth factor in rat liver after partial hepatectomy or induced hepatitis. Biochem Biophys Res Commun 1991;176:599–607.

228. Naldini L, Tamagnone L, Vigna E, et al. Extracellular proteolytic cleavage by urokinase is required for activation of hepatocyte growth factor/scatter factor. EMBO J 1992;11: 4825–4833.

229. Schirmacher P, Geerts A, Pietrangelo A, Dienes HP, Rogler CE. Hepatocyte growth factor/hepatopoietin A is expressed in fat-storing cells from rat liver but not myofibroblast-like cells derived from fat-storing cells. Hepatology 1992;15:5–11.

230. Ramadori G, Neubauer K, Odenthal M, et al. The gene of hepatocyte growth factor is expressed in fat-storing cells of rat liver and is downregulated during cell growth and by transforming growth factor-beta. Biochem Biophys Res Commun 1992;183:739–742.

231. Lindroos PM, Zarnegar R, Michalopoulos GK. Hepatocyte growth factor (hepatopoietin A) rapidly increases in plasma before DNA synthesis and liver regeneration stimulated by partial hepatectomy and carbon tetrachloride administration. Hepatology 1991;13:743–750.

232. Kinoshita T, Hirao S, Matsumoto K, Nakamura T. Possible endocrine control by hepatocyte growth factor of liver regeneration after partial hepatectomy. Biochem Biophys Res Commun 1991;177:330–335.

233. Zarnegar R, Defrances MC, Kost KP, Lindroos P, Michalopoulos GK. Expression of hepatocyte growth factor mRNA in regenerating rat liver after partial hepatectomy. Biochem Biophys Res Commun 1991;177:559–565.

234. Tomiya T, Tani M, Yamada S, Hayashi S, Umeda N, Fujiwara K. Serum hepatocyte growth factor levels in hepatectomized and nonhepatectomized surgical patients. Gastroenterology 1992;103:1621–1624.

235. Matsumoto K, Tajima H, Hamanoue M, Kohno S, Kinoshita T, Nakamura T. Identification and characterization of "injurin," an inducer of expression of the gene for hepatocyte growth factor. Proc Natl Acad Sci USA 1992; 89:3800–3804.

236. Ekberg S, Luther M, Nakamura T, Jansson JO. Growth hormone promotes early initiation of hepatocyte growth factor gene expression in the liver of hypophysectomized rats after partial hepatectomy. J Endocrinol 1992;135:59–67.

237. Bottaro DP, Rubin JS, Faletto DL, et al. Identification of the hepatocyte growth factor receptor as the c-met proto-oncogene product. Science 1991;251:802–804.

238. Naldini L, Weidner KM, Vigna E, et al. Scatter factor and hepatocyte growth factor are indistinguishable ligands for the MET receptor. EMBO J 1991;10:2867–2878.

239. Arakaki N, Hirono S, Ishii T, et al. Identification and partial characterization of two classes of receptors for human hepatocyte growth factor on adult rat hepatocytes in primary culture. J Biol Chem 1992;267:7101–7107.

240. Joplin R, Hishida T, Tsubouchi H, et al. Human intrahepatic biliary epithelial cells proliferate in vitro in response to human hepatocyte growth factor. J Clin Invest 1992;90:1284–1289.

241. Johnson M, Koukoulis G, Matsumoto K, Nakamura T, Iyer A. Hepatocyte growth factor induces proliferation and morphogenesis in nonparenchymal epithelial liver cells. Hepatology 1993;17:1052–1061.

242. Skov Olsen P, Boesby S, Kirkegaard P, et al. Influence of epidermal growth factor on liver regeneration after partial hepatectomy in rats. Hepatology 1988;8:992–996.

243. Brenner DA, Koch KS, Leffert HL. Transforming growth factor-alpha stimulates proto-oncogene c-jun expression and a mitogenic program in primary cultures of adult rat hepatocytes. DNA 1989;8:279–285.

244. Mead JE, Fausto N. Transforming growth factor alpha may be a physiological regulator of liver regeneration by means of an autocrine mechanism. Proc Natl Acad Sci USA 1989; 86:1558–1562.

245. Rasmussen TN, Jorgensen PE, Almdal T, Kirkegaard P, Olsen PS. Stimulatory effect of epidermal growth factor on liver regeneration after partical hepatectomy in rats. Scand J Gastroenterol 1992;27:372–374.

246. Blanc P, Etienne H, Daujat M, et al. Mitotic responsiveness of cultured adult human hepatocytes to epidermal growth factor, transforming growth factor alpha, and human serum. Gastroenterology 1992;102:1340–1350.

247. Kokudo N, Kothary PC, Eckhauser FE, Raper SE. Transforming growth factor-alpha (TGF-alpha) improves hepatic DNA synthesis after hepatectomy in cirrhotic rats. J Surg Res 1992;52:648–655.

248. Evarts RP, Nakatsukasa H, Marsden ER, Hu Z, Thorgeirsson SS. Expression of transforming growth factor- alpha in

regenerating liver and during hepatic differentiation. Mol Carcinog 1992;5:25–31.

249. Vesey DA, Selden AC, Woodman AC, Hodgson HJ. Effect of in vivo administration of an antibody to epidermal growth factor on the rapid increase in DNA synthesis induced by partial hepatectomy in the rat. Gut 1992;33:831–835.

250. Wollenberg GK, Semple E, Quinn BA, Hayes MA. Inhibition of proliferation of normal, preneoplastic, and neoplastic rat hepatocytes by transforming growth factor-beta. Cancer Res 1987;47:6595–6599.

251. Carr BI, Hayashi I, Branum EL, Moses HL. Inhibition of DNA synthesis in rat hepatocytes by platelet-derived type beta transforming growth factor. Cancer Res 1986;46: 2330–2334.

252. Strain AJ, Frazer A, Hill DJ, Milner RD. Transforming growth factor beta inhibits DNA synthesis in hepatocytes isolated from normal and regeneration rat liver. Biochem Biophys Res Commun 1987;145:436–442.

253. Gohda E, Matsunaga T, Kataoka H, Yamamoto I. TGF-beta is a potent inhibitor of hepatocyte growth factor secretion by human fibroblasts. Cell Biol Int Rep 1992;16:917–926.

254. Jakowlew SB, Mead JE, Danielpour D, Wu J, Roberts AB, Fausto N. Transforming growth factor-beta (TGF-beta) isoforms in rat liver regeneration: messenger RNA expression and activation of latent TGF-beta. Cell Regul 1991;2: 535–548.

255. Russell WE, Coffey RJJ, Ouellette AJ, Moses HL. Type beta transforming growth factor reversibly inhibits the early proliferative response to partial hepatectomy in the rat. Proc Natl Acad Sci USA 1988;85:5126–5130.

256. Francavilla A, Azzarone A, Carrieri G, et al. Effect on the canine Eck fistula liver of intraportal TGF-beta alone or with hepatic growth factors. Hepatology 1992;16:1267–1270.

257. Houck KA, Zarnegar R, Muga SJ, Michalopoulos GK. Acidic fibroblast growth factor (HBGF-1) stimulates DNA synthesis in primary rat hepatocyte cultures. J Cell Physiol 1990;143:129–132.

258. Kan M, Huang JS, Mansson PE, Yasumitsu H, Carr B, McKeehan WL. Heparin-binding growth factor type 1 (acidic fibroblast growth factor): a potential biphasic autocrine and paracrine regulator of hepatocyte regeneration. Proc Natl Acad Sci USA 1989;86:7432–7436.

259. Kan M, Yan GC, Xu J, Nakahara M, Hou J. Receptor phenotype underlies differential response of hepatocytes and nonparenchymal cells to heparin-binding fibroblast growth factor type 1 (aFGF) and type 2 (bFGF). In Vitro Cell Dev Biol 1992;28A:515–520.

260. Presta M, Statuto M, Rusnati M, Dell'Era P, Ragnotti G. Characterization of a Mr 25,000 basic fibroblast growth factor form in adult, regenerating, and fetal rat liver. Biochem Biophys Res Commun 1989;164:1182–1189.

261. Marsden ER, Hu Z, Fujio K, Nakatsukasa H, Thorgeirsson SS, Evarts RP. Expression of acidic fibroblast growth factor in regenerating liver and during hepatic differentiation. Lab Invest 1992;67:427–433.

262. Matsumoto K, Okazaki H, Nakamura T. Up-regulation of hepatocyte growth factor gene expression by interleukin-1 in human skin fibroblasts. Biochem Biophys Res Commun 1992;188:235–243.

263. Nakamura T, Arakaki R, Ichihara A. Interleukin-1 beta is a potent growth inhibitor of adult rat hepatocytes in primary culture. Exp Cell Res 1988;179:488–497.

264. Satoh M, Yamazaki M. Tumor necrosis factor stimulates DNA synthesis of mouse hepatocytes in primary culture and is suppressed by transforming growth factor beta and interleukin 6. J Cell Physiol 1992;150:134–139.

265. Kuma S, Inaba M, Ogata H, et al. Effect of human recombinant interleukin-6 on the proliferation of mouse hepatocytes in the primary culture. Immunobiology 1990;180: 235–242.

266. Feingold KR, Soued M, Grunfeld C. Tumor necrosis factor stimulates DNA synthesis in the liver of intact rats. Biochem Biophys Res Commun 1988;153:576–582.

267. Akerman P, Cote P, Yang SQ, et al. Antibodies to tumor necrosis factor-alpha inhibit liver regeneration after partial hepatectomy. Am J Physiol 1992;263:G579–G585.

268. Goss JA, Mangino MJ, Flye MW. Kupffer cell autoregulation of IL-1 production by PGE2 during hepatic regeneration. J Surg Res 1992;52:422–428.

269. Goss JA, Mangino MJ, Flye MW. Prostaglandin E2 production during hepatic regeneration downregulates Kupffer cell IL-6 production. Ann Surg 1992;215:553–559.

270. Woodman AC, Selden CA, Hodgson HJ. Partial purification and characterisation of an inhibitor of hepatocyte proliferation derived from nonparenchymal cells after partial hepatectomy. J Cell Physiol 1992;151:405–414.

271. Rogler CE, Chisari FV. Cellular and molecular mechanisms of hepatocarcinogenesis. Semin Liver Dis 1992;12: 265–278.

272. Tsubouchi H, Niitani Y, Hirono S, et al. Levels of the human hepatocyte growth factor in serum of patients with various liver diseases determined by an enzyme-linked immunosorbent assay. Hepatology 1991;13:1–5.

273. Shiota G, Rhoads DB, Wang TC, Nakamura T, Schmidt EV. Hepatocyte growth factor inhibits growth of hepatocellular carcinoma cells. Proc Natl Acad Sci USA 1992;89:373–377.

274. Bussolino F, Di Renzo MF, Ziche M, et al. Hepatocyte growth factor is a potent angiogenic factor which stimulates endothelial cell motility and growth. J Cell Biol 1992; 119:629–641.

275. Su TS, Liu WY, Han SH, et al. Transcripts of the insulin-like growth factors I and II in human hepatoma. Cancer Res 1989;49:1773–1777.

276. Cariani E, Lasserre C, Seurin D, et al. Differential expression of insulin-like growth factor II mRNA in human primary liver cancers, benign liver tumors, and liver cirrhosis. Cancer Res 1988;48:6844–6849.

277. Cariani E, Seurin D, Lasserre C, Franco D, Binoux M, Brechot C. Expression of insulin-like growth factor II (IGF-II) in human primary liver cancer: mRNA and protein analysis. J Hepatol 1990;11:226–231.

278. Cariani E, Lasserre C, Kemeny F, Franco D, Brechot C. Expression of insulin-like growth factor II, alpha-fetoprotein and hepatitis B virus transcripts in human primary liver cancer. Hepatology 1991;13:644–649.

279. Norstedt G, Levinovitch A, Moller G, Eriksson LC, Andersson G. Expression of IGF I and IGF II mRNA during hepatic devleopment. Proliferation and carcinogenesis in the rat. Carcinogenesis 1988;9:209–213.

280. Cariani E, Dubois N, Lasserre C, Briand P, Brechot C. Insulin-like growth factor II (IGF-II) mRNA expression during hepatocarcinogenesis in transgenic mice. J Hepatol 1991; 13:220–226.

281. Schirmacher P, Held WA, Yang D, Chisari FV, Rustum Y, Rogler CE. Reactivation of insulin-like growth factor II during hepatocarcinogenesis in transgenic mice suggest a role in malignant growth. Cancer Res 1992;52:2549–2556.

282. Derynck R, Goeddel DV, Ullrich A, et al. Synthesis of messenger RNAs for transforming growth factors alpha and beta and the epidermal growth factor receptor by human tumors. Cancer Res 1987;47:707–712.

283. Liu C, Tsao MS, Grisham JW. Transforming growth factors produced by normal and neoplastically transformed rat liver epithelial cells in culture. Cancer Res 1988;48:850–855.

284. Luetteke NC, Michalopoulos GK, Teixido J, Gilmore R, Massague J, Lee DC. Characterization of high molecular weight transforming growth factor alpha produced by rat hepatocellular carcinoma cells. Biochemistry 1988;27: 6487–6494.

285. Jhappan C, Stahle C, Harkins RN, Fausto N, Smith GH, Merlini G. TGF alpha overexpression in transgenic mice induces liver neoplasia and abnormal development of the mammary gland and pancreas. Cell 1990;61:1137–1146.

286. Takagi H, Sharp R, Hammermeister C, et al. Molecular and genetic analysis of liver oncogenesis in transforming growth factor alpha transgenic mice. Cancer Res 1992;52: 5171–5177.

287. Lee GH, Merlino G, Fausto N. Development of liver tumors in transforming growth factor alpha transgenic mice. Cancer Res 1992;52:5162–5170.

288. Sandgren EP, Luetteke NC, Qiu TH, Palmiter RD, Brinster RL, Lee DC. Transforming growth factor alpha dramatically enhances oncogene-induced carcinogenesis in transgenic mouse pancreas and liver. Mol Cell Biol 1993;13: 320–330.

289. Hsia CC, Axiotis CA, Di Bisceglie AM, Tabor E. Transforming growth factor-alpha in human hepatocellular carcinoma and coexpression with hepatitis B surface antigen in adjacent liver. Cancer 1992;70:1049–1056.

290. Yeh YC, Tsai JF, Chuang L, et al. Elevation of transforming growth factor and its relationship to the epidermal growth factor and alpha-fetoprotein levels in patients with hepatocellular carcinoma. Cancer Res 1987;47:896–901.

291. Stenius U. Different inhibition of DNA synthesis by transforming growth factor beta and phenobarbital on GST-P-positive and GST-P-negative hepatocytes. Carcinogenesis 1993;14:159–161.

292. Lai CL, Lau JY, Wu PC, et al. Recombinant interferon-alpha in inoperable hepatocellular carcinoma: a randomized controlled trial. Hepatology 1993;17:389–394.

293. Lai CL, Wu PC, Lik ASF, et al. Recombinant alpha2 interferon is superior to doxorubicin for inoperable hepatocellular carcinoma: a prospective randomised trial. Br J Cancer 1989;60:928–933.

294. Kardinal CG, Moertel CG, Wieand HS, et al. Combined doxorubicin and alpha-interferon therapy of advanced hepatocellular carcinoma. Cancer 1993;71:2187–2190.

295. Oon CJ. Long-term survival following treatment of hepatocellular carcinoma in Singapore: evaluation of Wellferon in the prophylaxis of high-risk pre-cancerous conditions. Cancer Chemother Pharmacol 1992;31 (suppl):S137–S142.

CHAPTER 41

ROLE OF CYTOKINES IN PSORIASIS AND OTHER T-CELL–MEDIATED DISEASES

Brian J. Nickoloff

The field of cytokine research has been rapidly assimilated into the daily investigative activity of numerous clinician-scientists interested in the immunopathology of several skin diseases. It is highly likely that cytokines have an important role in maintaining cutaneous immunohomeostasis in normal skin and perpetuating disease activity in T-cell–mediated dermatoses. This "doubled-edged" sword–like nature of cytokines (i.e., they can protect the organism from environmental perturbations, and yet they contribute to or exacerbate a physiological response and aid in the creation of a pathological condition) challenges investigative skin biologists in unraveling key molecular mediators that participate in cytokine networks in the skin. In this chapter, I review advances made in dissecting cytokine networks in three different skin diseases. These three common T-cell–mediated disorders are psoriasis, atopic dermatitis, and allergic contact dermatitis.

PSORIASIS

Psoriasis is a very common skin disease that affects approximately 3% of individuals worldwide (1). Clinically, it is characterized by symmetrical scaling erythematous plaques that typically involve points of trauma, such as elbows, fingernails, and scalp. Histologically, psoriasis is characterized by hyperkeratosis, parakeratosis, acanthosis, tortuous and dilated blood vessels, and a mononu-

clear cell infiltrate, including T cells, monocyte/ macrophages, and dendritic cells. There are increased mast cells, but no eosinophils or plasma cells, and variable collections of neutrophils, particularly localized in or near the stratum corneum (2). Genetically, there appears to be two distinct subsets of patients. Christophers and Henseler reported that individuals with an "early onset" possess a linkage disequilibrium for human leukocyte antigens (HLA) B13, BW57, and CW6; whereas "late onset" patients are associated with HLA B27 and CW2 (3). In addition to tendency for psoriasis to run in families (4), there are numerous environmental triggering factors that can provoke or exacerbate skin lesions, including stress, streptococcal pharyngitis, lithium, and beta-blockers. Immunologically, a large number of abnormalities have been documented involving T cells and antigen-presenting cells (5). Perhaps the most compelling data supporting an important role for immunocytes in psoriasis is the clinically beneficial effects of compounds with immunomodulatory activity, such as cyclosporine, corticosteroids, vitamin D, methotrexate, ultraviolet irradiation, and anti-CD4 monoclonal antibody (6–12).

Despite this enormously complicated compendium of clinical characteristics of psoriasis, it is possible to provide a unifying explanation that highlights the role of cytokines in the etiopathophysiology of this disease (13). Although other mediators of inflammation/autoimmunity have been previously suggested as key participants, such as prostaglandins, cyclic AMP, and leukotrienes, none of these agents can induce a psoriatic lesion when given to a genetically predisposed individual. However, when interferon-γ (IFN-γ) is administered intradermally within clinically symptomless skin, a psoriatic lesion is produced that is clinically and pathologically indistinguishable from idiopathic lesions (14). Thus, there is good clinical evidence to encourage investigators to search for and sort out which cytokines are present and which cytokines are absent from psoriatic skin, and to compare and contrast this profile with normal skin.

Table 41–1 lists which cytokines have been detected in psoriatic lesions (15–24). As can be appreciated from a review of the articles cited in this table, numerous cytokines are present in either epidermal or dermal compartments of the lesional skin at the mRNA or protein level of detection using a wide variety of experimental approaches. The detection systems employed by psoriasis researchers include immunohistochemical staining to detect protein or various mRNA-based strategies, including Northern blot hybridization, in situ hybridization, or reverse-transcriptase polymerase chain reactions. Despite the different approaches, it is clear from these studies that there is crosstalk between various cell types across the epidermal/dermal basement membrane zone that involves cytokines (25). These cytokines are likely candidates for mediating the complex intercellular dialogue that involves growth regulation, adhesion molecule expression, and angiogenesis. All of these processes need to be highly coordinated in both a spatial and a temporal fashion for the skin to transform itself from being clinically symptomless (and apparently normal to the naked eye), into a thick, scaling, erythematous plaque. With respect to

TABLE 41–1   CYTOKINES DETECTED IN PSORIATIC LESIONS[a]

Cytokine	mRNA	Protein	Reference
IL-1α	No	Yes	(15)
IL-1β	Yes	Yes	(16,17)
IL-1 receptor antagonist protein	Yes	Yes	(18)
IL-6	Yes	Yes	(17,19)
IL-8	Yes	Yes	(20,21)
TNF-α	Yes	Yes	(21,22)
IFN-γ	Yes	Yes	(22,23)
MCP-1	Yes	Yes	(24)

[a]Other cytokine mRNAs that have been searched for and were undetectable by polymerase chain reaction are IL-4 and IL-5 (22).
IL = interleukin; TNF = tumor necrosis factor; MCP-1 = monocyte chemotactic protein.

cytokines and clinically symptomless skin, it has been recently discovered that such skin is not entirely normal despite its apparent resemblance to the skin of normal healthy individuals without psoriasis.

To investigate subtle molecular alterations that might predispose the skin to the development of a psoriatic lesion in symptomless skin of individuals genetically susceptible to psoriasis, we recently completed a study in collaboration with the laboratory of Dr. Robert Modlin at the University of California, Los Angeleos. Although it has been known for some time (26) that symptomless skin of psoriatic individuals can be induced to express the psoriatic phenotype after trauma (Koebner phenomenon), the molecular basis for this reaction was largely unexplored. When we obtained biopsies at least 10 cm away from an active psoriatic lesion, these symptomless skin samples revealed aberrant expression of endothelial cell leukocyte adhesion molecule-1 (ELAM-1), vascular cell adhesion molecule-1 (VCAM-1), and keratinocyte intercellular adhesion molecule-1 (ICAM-1) expression (22). None of these adhesion molecules are typically seen in normal skin obtained from healthy control individuals. Moreover, in four of five symptomless skin biopsies of psoriatic patients, there was prominent cytokine mRNA expression, including interleukin-1α (IL-1α), IL-1β, and tumor necrosis factor-α (TNF-α), with lesser increases in IFN-γ and granulocyte-macrophage colony-stimulating factor (GM-CSF) compared with normal donor skin samples. Thus, we suggested that these findings of aberrant adhesion molecule expression and cytokine production profiles may underlay the predisposition of symptomless skin to produce psoriatic lesion after trauma in these genetically predisposed individuals.

Another conclusion was reached during this study of active psoriatic patients that involved classification of the T-cell immune response. Because psoriasis has been shown to be cleared after allogeneic bone marrow transplantation (27), in addition to the previously mentioned response of this disease to immunomodulatory agents (6–12), CD4+ T cells have been clearly implicated in the pathogenesis of psoriasis. The division of CD4+ T cells into distinct functional subsets, such as Th1 and Th2, based on cytokine production profiles (28), provided us with the opportunity to explore whether the T-cell–mediated skin reaction was a Th1- or Th2-type response. To determine whether active untreated psoriatic plaques contained T cells, belonging to either a Th1 or Th2 subset, we subjected the biopsy samples to reverse transcriptase polymerase chain reactions for detection of various cytokine mRNAs (22). Type 1 cytokines that were probed for included IL-2 and IFN-γ; type 2 cytokine included IL-4, IL-5, and IL-10 mRNAs. Our results indicated that there was readily detectable Th1 cytokine mRNAs, but no Th2-type cytokine mRNAs. With a different set of patient samples, we also observed the same result in collaboration with Dr. David Fivenson at Henry Ford Hospital, Detroit, Michigan (20). The lack of crossover among Th1- and Th2-type cytokines in psoriasis is consistent with other skin diseases that could also be categorized into discrete T-cell subsets bearing lesions such as cutaneous T-cell lymphoma (29), leprosy (30), and atopic dermatitis (31,32).

The next question we asked is how does this Th1-type cytokine profile come about in our psoriatic patients. One possibility involved the choice of antigen-presenting cells that were directly responsible for interacting with the CD4+ T lymphocytes. To address this issue, we investigated what type of cytokine profiles were produced in vitro when T cells were activated by bacterial-derived superantigens and two different accessory cells (i.e., epidermal keratinocytes and dermal dendritic cells). Bacterial-derived superantigens were selected because it is well known that streptococcal pharyngitis is a frequent triggering factor for psoriatic skin lesions (33). The skin lesions are sterile, which suggested that there may be a diffusible product that could localize to skin and initiate an immune reaction (34). Indeed, when the bacterial-derived superantigen staphylococcal enterotoxin B (SEB) was used, T cells proliferated vigorously, both when IFN-γ–treated keratinocytes were used (35), and when dermal dendritic cells (36) were used as the antigen-presenting cell. After removal of the conditioned medium from various T-cell proliferations and examination of their cytokine production profiles at both the mRNA and the protein level (via commercially available enzyme-linked immunosorbent assay [ELISA]), it was observed that different cytokine profiles emerged, depending on whether keratinocytes or dermal dendritic cells were present. Using keratinocytes, the T cells responded to SEB by proliferating and producing IL-2, IL-4, and IL-5, but not significant levels of IFN-γ (37). However, when dermal dendritic cells were present, T-cell proliferation to SEB was also observed, and higher levels of IL-2 and IFN-γ were produced (Nestle FP, et al. unpublished observations). A likely cell surface molecule responsible for the Th1 versus Th2 immunoresponsiveness of the T cells is the CD28 ligand B7. IFN-γ–treated keratinocytes lack B7, whereas dermal dendrocytes strongly express B7 (36,38). B7 is a critically important costimulatory molecule expressed by antigen-presenting cells that can influence activation of specific T-cell subsets (39).

Thus, if we apply these in vitro results to our in vivo psoriasis results, it is suggested that if bacterial-derived superantigens have a role, then the immunodominant accessory cell in the skin of such lesions is the dermal dendritic cell. All of our in vitro experiments involved autologous combinations of T cells and accessory cells. We have previously suggested an important immunobiological role for dermal dendrocytes in psoriasis (40), and the current experimental results may explain the functional significance for the massive accumulation of factor XIIIa–positive dermal dendrocytes that are present in lesional skin. From our immunophenotyping of psoriatic lesions, we also determined that these factor XIIIa–positive dermal dendrocytes contained the cytokine, TNF-α (21). Because dermal dendrocytes are strategically poised between endothelial cells and epithelial cells (much like interstitial mesangial cells in the renal glomerulus), these cells can monitor changes in the local microenvironment, originating either endogenously via the blood stream or exogenously from the skin surface. Endogenous stimuli that may initiate a psoriatic lesion include human immunodeficiency virus-type 1 (HIV-1), lithium, or beta blockers (41,42). Exogenously derived stimuli that may damage intraepidermal free nerve endings releasing substance P and other immunomodulatory peptides can also be envisioned to provoke lesion formation (43,44). In any event, once the dermal dendrocyte releases TNF-α, there is a cytokine cascade that can amplify this signal, leading to induction of ELAM-1 and VCAM-1 on endothelial cells, as well as keratinocyte ICAM-1, transforming growth factor-α, and IL-8. Such a scenario is entirely consistent with all available in vitro and in vivo data, and it demonstrates an interactive cytokine network operative among several different cell types on both sides of the epidermal-dermal basement membrane zone.

In summary of this psoriasis-related research, it is clear that many advances at both the cellular and the molecular level are being made by investigative skin biologists. It is clear that cytokines provide important signals for the interaction among several different cell types, including endothelial cells, dermal dendritic cells, T lymphocytes, and keratinocytes. Further delving into the pathophysiological mechanisms that initiate and maintain psoriatic lesions may point to the cause or to the genetic mutations that are ultimately responsible for this common and intractable T-cell–mediated papulosquamous skin disease.

ATOPIC DERMATITIS

Similar to psoriasis, atopic dermatitis is a common, chronic skin disease that affects approximately 2% of the population, which includes a positive family history in many affected individuals (45). Unlike psoriasis, the skin of patients with atopic dermatitis is intensely pruritic, and it is often associated with allergies and extracutaneous involvement of other anatomical sites, including allergic rhinitis and asthma (46). Many immunological abnormalities have been documented within the lesional skin of patients with atopic dermatitis, and most investigators regard this disease as the result of immunological dysregulation. As in psoriasis, an important role for T lymphocytes was supported by the clinical improvement seen after cyclosporine therapy (47).

Within a lesion of atopic dermatitis, histological alterations include mild epidermal thickening (acanthosis), intercellular edema (spongiosis), and a mononuclear cell infiltrate composed of T lymphocytes, factor XIIIa–positive dermal dendrocytes, occasional eosinophils, and mast cells (48,49). Even though there is an influx of several types of immunocompetent cells into the skin, from a functional T-cell perspective, lesional skin sites possess a decreased cell-mediated immune response. There is reduced responsiveness to the poison ivy antigen, urushiol, anergy to varous intracutaneous skin tests with *Candida, Streptococcus,* and *Trichophyton* antigens; as well as a decreased ability to sensitize the individual with the low molecular weight haptendenitrochlorobenzene (50–54).

Another potential key observation in this disease is the significant perturbation of the barrier function of lesional skin, which may be directly responsible for promoting colonization by staphylococcal organisms and the establishment of a viscous cycle of chronic overactivation of inflammatory and immunological pathways (54). I believe an important advance in our understanding of these immunological alterations was the discovery that CD4+ T cells in patients with atopic dermatitis belonged to the Th2 type (55–58). Cytokines such as IL-4, IL-5, and IL-10 tend to inhibit cell-mediated immune reactions and promote humoral responses. Thus, the localized decrease in cell-mediated reactions noted, as well as the presence of eosinophils and plasma cells could result directly from the abundance of Th2-type cytokines produced by lesional T cells. Also, this cytokine profile could explain the increase in circulating and skin-associated immunoglobulin E (IgE) detected in these patients (59–61). The connection between atopic dermatitis and Th2-type T lymphocytes resulted from studies of various T-cell clones tested for their reactivity to various etiologically relevant allergens or antigens, such as the house dust mite (*Dermatophagoides pteronyssinus*). When these T-cell clones were stimulated in vitro and the supernatants were analyzed, it was observed that high levels of IL-4 and IL-5 were present, but not IFN-γ. When T-cell clones from patients with nonatopic dermatitis were studied, they predominantly produced IFN-γ and not IL-4. Thus, there appears to be an intrinsic (and perhaps a genetically determined) accumulation of Th2-type CD4+ T lymphocytes.

Another consequence of the local cellular constituents of atopic lesions containing Th2-type T cells is the increased expression of low affinity receptors for IgE (CD23) on the Langerhans cells (62,63), because it is known that IL-4 molecules may increase the antigen-binding capacity of these dendritic cells, and thereby stimulate T cells to proliferate and produce cytokines (64).

A therapeutically relevant upshot of the recognition that patients with atopic dermatitis possess predominantly Th2-type disease-producing T cells has been the clinical trials using the Th1-type cytokine IFN-γ (65, 66). Although it may seem that the last agent one would like to give to individuals with a T-cell–mediated disease is a potent cytokine such as IFN-γ, several reports have confirmed its efficacy. Cyclosporine (which suppresses IFN-γ production by T cells) (67) improves atopic dermatitis, and IFN-γ also improves this disease. Such somewhat confounding observations reveal our incomplete understanding of cytokine networks, and they emphasize the need to continue to explore antagonistic/synergistic interactions among different types of cytokines and their net immunologic effects on various disease processes arising from dysregulation of the immune system.

In summary of this atopic dermatitis–related research activity, lesional skin contains T cells belonging to the Th2-type profile of cytokine production. Although these CD4+ T cells are activated, the local microenvironment of the lesion is more geared toward humoral rather than cell-mediated immune reactions. The complex interplay between IgE-bearing Langerhans cells, T cells, and keratinocytes can apparently be successfully corrected by systemic administration of the Th1-type cytokine IFN-γ.

ALLERGIC CONTACT DERMATITIS

When a foreign low molecular weight molecule such as dinitrochlorobenzene or pentadecylcatechol (the active molecule on the leaf surface responsible for poison ivy reactions) comes in contact with the skin, there is initially an inductive phase called sensitization. Upon re-exposure to the same hapten, the skin reacts with an immune response during the so called elicitation or challenge phase. This cutaneous reaction is mediated by T lymphocytes, and it is generally referred to as allergic contact dermatitis. Such reactions are not just a nuisance to outdoor recreational activity, but they are also common causes of occupational-related disease activity. Skin lesions become clinically evident within 24 to 48 hours of repeated exposure to the hapten, and they manifest themselves as intensely pruritic, erythematous eruptions that are often accompanied by edema and vesiculation. Resolution of this reaction is generally spontaneous after removal of the inciting allergen, and it occurs within 3 to 4 weeks. Histologically, there is prominent nonrandom movement of memory CD4+ T cells from the blood vessels into the epidermis. This highly reproducible migration pathway is accompanied, and most likely guided by, the rapid appearance (within minutes or hours) of cytokines, adhesion molecules, and chemotactic polypeptides. Within the past several years, there have been many advances made in our understanding of the pathophysiology of allergic contact dermatitis reactions, which involve cytokines.

By taking sequential biopsies from the skin of previously sensitized individuals, before and after hapten exposure, a dynamic series of rapid molecular events could be synthesized into a coherent schema (68 69). Similar studies and conclusions have been made in our laboratory, as well as in other laboratories, and 2 years ago we put forward the novel hypothesis that epidermal keratinocytes have a key initiating immunological role in the reaction of the skin following contact with allergic haptens (70). The essence of our hypothesis is that keratinocytes, via their active participation in genesis and propagation of cytokine networks, are key immunocytes in a wide variety of responses of skin to allergens (71). In the past, keratinocytes were believed only to be passive inert targets of T-cell–mediated destruction. However, it is currently recognized that keratinocytes can respond to diverse epicutaneous stimuli and produce cytokines, adhesion molecules, and polypeptide chemotactic factors, which guide the nonrandom movement of immunocompetent memory T cells into the epidermis.

In terms of the cytokine network operative in the challenge phase of allergic contact dermatitis lesions, working in collaboration with Drs. Robert Modlin and John Hanifin, we obtained preliminary evidence to suggest that a Th2-type profile is dominant. By polymerase chain reaction analysis of lesional skin samples in the poison ivy dermatitis reaction, mRNAs coding for IL-4 and IL-10 were identified, but not IFN-γ. The presence of IL-10 is particularly intriguing because this may be the endogenous cyclosporine-like molecule that down-regulates the initial brisk immune response leading to spontaneous resolution of the allergic contact reaction. IL-10 is produced by keratinocytes in vitro (72), and its mRNA has also been detected very early in a murine model of allergic contact dermatitis (73,74). IL-10 has also been recognized to be capable of inhibiting the antigen-presenting capability of various cell types (75), including Langerhans cells (76).

Thus, it can be postulated that keratinocytes, as a result of their initial production of proinflammatory and positive immunomodulatory cytokines TNF-α and IL-1β, can not only stimulate the early phase of allergic contact dermatitis, but also, as a result of their production of the cytokine inhibiting factor IL-10, terminate such reactions. It is also possible that in certain disease states, such as psoriasis, the ongoing immune response characteristically seen in the upper portion of skin reflects a local deficiency of the keratinocyte-derived cytokine IL-10 (77). As monoclonal antibodies and cDNA probes become available for detection and measurement of IL-10 levels in normal and diseases skin, such a hypothesis can be tested directly.

It should be clear that many new concepts are rapidly emerging in the field of immunodermatology. The allergic contact dermatitis reaction is an excellent model system because one can begin with normal skin in healthy individuals and generate a predictable series of immunological events simply and rapidly. Given the availability of animal models for this reaction, rapid progress in our understanding of the cytokine network operative in this area can be expected (78). Ultimately, it is likely that the new insights generated by such clinical-pathological correlations will be applicable to therapeutic modalites for a large number of T-cell–mediated dermatoses beyond allergic contact dermatitis.

REFERENCES

1. Farber EM, Bright RD, Nall ML. Psoriasis. A questionnaire survey of 2,144 patients. Arch Dermatol 1968;98:248–253.
2. Cox AJ. Mast cells in psoriasis. In: Farber EM, Cox AJ, eds. Psoriasis. New York: Yorke Medical Books 1977:36–43.
3. Christopher E, Henseler T. Patient subgroups and the inflammatory pattern in psoriasis. Acta Derm Venereol 1989; 151:88–92.
4. Farber EM, Nall ML, Watson W. Natural history of psoriasis in 61 twin pairs. Arch Dermatol 1974;109:207–211.
5. Valdimarsson H, Baker BS, Jonsdottir I, Fry L. Psoriasis: a disease of abnormal keratinocyte proliferation induced by T lymphocytes. Immunol Today 1986;7:256–259.
6. Bos VD. The pathomechanisms of psoriasis. The skin immune system and cyclosporin. Br J Dermatol 1988;118: 141–155.
7. Muller K, Svenson M, Bendtzen K. 1 alpha 25-dihydroxy vitamin D3 and a novel vitamin D analogue MC903 are potent inhibitors of human interleukin-1 in vitro. Immunol Lett 1988;17:361–366.
8. Fry L. Immunointervention in skin disorders. J Autoimmun 1988;1:593–601.
9. Cormane RH, Hammerlinck F, Siddiqui AL. Immunologic implication of PUVA therapy in psoriasis vulgaris. Arch Dermatol Res 1979;265:245–267.
10. Morison WL. Phototherapy and photochemotherapy of skin disease. New York: Praeger Publishers, 1983:33–107.
11. Gibbons JJ, Lucas J. Immunomodulation by low-dose methotrexate. J Immunol 1989;142:1867–1873.
12. Nicholas JF, Chamaick N, Thivolet J, Wijdnes J, Morel P, Revillard JP. CD4 antibody treatment of severe psoriasis. Lancet 1991;338:321.
13. Nickoloff BJ. The cytokine network in psoriasis. Arch Dermatol 1991;127:871–884.
14. Fierlbeck G, Rasner G, Maler G. Psoriasis induced at injection site by recombinant gamma interferon. Arch Dermatol 1990;126:345–355.
15. Takematsu H, Suzuki R, Tagami H, Kumagai K. Interleukin-1 like activity in horny layer extracts: decreased activ-

ity in scale extracts of psoriasis and sterile pustular dermatoses. Dermatologica 1986;172:236–240.

16. Cooper KD, Hammerberg C, Baadsgaard O. IL-1 activity is reduced in psoriatic skin. Decreased IL-1α and increased nonfunctional IL-1β. J Immunol 1990;144:4593–4603.

17. Ohta Y, Katayama I, Funato T. In-situ expression of messenger RNA of interleukin-1 and interleukin-6 in psoriasis. Arch Dermatol Res 1991;283:351–356.

18. Hammerberg C, Arend WP, Fischer GJ, Cooper KD. Interleukin-1 receptor antagonist in normal and psoriatic epidermis. J Clin Invest 1992;90:571–583.

19. Grossman RM, Krueger J, Yourish D. Interleukin-6 is expressed in high levels in psoriatic skin and stimulates proliferation of cultured human keratinocytes. Proc Natl Acad Sci 1989;86:6367–6371.

20. Schroder JM, Christophers E. Identification of C5a and an anionic neutrophil-activity peptide (ANAP) in psoriatic scales. J Invest Dermatol 1986;87:53–58.

21. Nickoloff BJ, Karabin GD, Barker JN, Kunkel S, Sarma V, Dixit V. Cellular localization of interleukin-8 and its inducer, tumor necrosis factor-alpha in psoriasis. Am J Pathol 1991;138:129–140.

22. Uyemura K, Yamamura M, Fivenson DF, Modlin RL, Nickoloff BJ. The cytokine network in psoriasis is characterized by a T-helper type I cell mediated response. J Invest Dermatol 1994;101:701–705.

23. Barker J, Karabin G, Stoof T, et al. Detection of interferon gamma but not tumor necrosis factor-alpha mRNA in psoriatic epidermal sheets by polymerase chain reaction. J Dermatol Sci 1991;2:106–111.

24. Gillitzer R, Wolff K, Tong D, et al. MCP-1 mRNA expression in basal keratinocytes of psoriatic lesions. J Invest Dermatol 1993;101:127–131.

25. Gearing AJH, Fincham NJ, Bird CR, Camp RDR. Cytokines in skin lesions of psoriasis. Cytokine 1990;2:68–75.

26. Farber EM, Roth RJ, Asheim E, Eddy ED, Epinette WW. Role of trauma in isomorphic response in psoriasis. Arch Dermatol 1965;91:246–257.

27. Eedy DJ, Burrows D, Bridges JM, Jones FG. Clearance of severe psoriasis after allogeneic bone marrow transplantation. Br Med J 1990;300:908.

28. Mosmann TR, Cherwinski H, Bond MW, Giedlin MA, Coffman RL. Two types of murine helper T cell clones I. Definition according to profiles of lymphokine activities and secreted proteins. J Immunol 1986;136:2348–2357.

29. Saed G, Fivenson DP, Naidu Y, Nickoloff BJ. Mycosis fungoides and psoriasis exhibit a TH-1 type cell mediated response while Sezary syndrome expresses a TH-2 type response. J Invest Dermatol 1994;103:29–33.

30. Yamamura M, Ugemura K, Deans HJ, et al. Defining protective response to pathogens: cytokine profiles in leprosy lesions. Science 1991;254:277–279.

31. Wiererger EA, Sinuek M, Grout C, Kapsenberg ML. Evidence for compartmentalization of functional subsets of CD4+ lymphocytes in atopic dermatitis. J Immunol 1990;144:4651–4660.

32. Kay AB, Ying S, Verney V, et al. Messenger RNA expression of the cytokine gene cluster interleukin-3, IL-4, IL-5, and granulocyte/macrophage colony stimulatory factor in aller-

gen-induced late-phase reactions in atopic subjects. J Exp Med 1992;58:173–183.

33. Rosenberg EQ, Noah PW. The Koebner phenomenon and the microbial basis of psoriasis. J Am Acad Dermatol 1988; 18:151–158.

34. Nickoloff BJ, Mitra RS, Green J, Shimizu Y, Thompson C, Turka LA. Activated keratinocytes present bacterial-derived superantigens to T lymphocytes: relevance to psoriasis. J Dermatol Sci 1994;6:127–133.

35. Nickoloff BJ, Mitra RS, Green J, Thomspon CB, Turka LA. Accessory cell function of keratinocytes for superantigens: dependence on lymphocyte function associated antigen-1/intercellular adhesion molecule-1 interaction. J Immunol 1993;150:2148–2159.

36. Nestle FO, Zheng XG, Thompson CB, Turka LA, Nickoloff BJ. Characterization of dermal dendritic cells obtained from normal human skin reveals phenotypic and functionally distinctive subsets. J Immunol 1994;151:6535–6545.

37. Naidu YM, Nestle F, Turka LA, Thompson C, Nickoloff BJ. T lymphocytes activated by bacterial superantigens presented by keratinocytes secrete a TH-2 type cytokine profile (abstract). Clin Res 1993;41:256.

38. Nickoloff BJ, Mitra RS, Green J, Thompson C, Turka L, Shimizu Y. Discordant expression of CD28 ligands BB-1 and B7 on cultured keratinocytes and psoriatic cells invivo. Am J Pathol 1993;142:1029–1040.

39. Gajewski TF, Pinnas M, Wong T, Fitch FW. Murine TH-1 and TH-2 clones proliferate optimally in response to distinct antigen-presenting cell populations. J Immunol 1991; 140:1750–1758.

40. Nickoloff BJ, Griffiths CEM. Lymphocyte trafficking in psoriasis. A new perspective emphasizing the dermal dendrocyte with active dermal recruitment mediated via endothelial cells followed by intraepidermal T-cell activation. J Invest Dermatol 1990;95:35s–37s.

41. Mahoney SE, Duvic M, Nickoloff B, et al. HIV transcripts identified in HIV-related psoriasis and Kaposi's sarcoma lesions. J Clin Invest 1991;88:174–185.

42. Krueger GG, Bergstresser PR, Lowe NJ, Voorhees JJ, Weinstein GD. Psoriasis. J Am Acad Dermatol 1984;11: 937–947.

43. Farber EM, Nickoloff BJ, Fraki J. Stress, symmetry and psoriasis: the probable role of neuropeptides. J Am Acad Dermatol 1986;14:305–311.

44. Hosoi J, Murphy GF, Egan CL, et al. Regulation of Langerhans cell function by nerves containing calcitonin-gene related peptide. Nature. 1993;363:159–163.

45. Hanifin JM, Rajka G. Diagnostic features of atopic dermatitis. Acta Derm Veneral (Stockh) 1980;92:44–47.

46. Hanifin JM. Atopic dermatitis. J Am Acad Dermatol 1982; 6:1–13.

47. VanJoost TH, Stolz E, Henle F. Efficacy of low-dose cyclosporin in severe atopic skin disease. Arch Dermatol 1987;123:166–167.

48. Bos JD, Garderen KD, Krieg SR, Poulter LW. Different insitu distribution patterns of dendritic cells having Langerhans and interdigitating cell immunophenotype in psoriasis, atopic dermatitis and other inflammatory dermatoses. J Invest Dermatol 1986;87:358–361.

49. Cerio R, Griffths CEM, Cooper KD, Nickoloff BJ, Head-

ington JT. Characterization of factor XIIIa positive dermal dendritic cells in normal and diseased skin. Br J Dermatol 1989;121:421–431.

50. Cronin E, Bandman JH, Calnan CD. Contact dermatitis in the atopic. Acta Dermatol Veneral (Stockh) 1970;50: 183–187.

51. Eliot ST, Hanifin JM. Delayed cutaneous hypersensitivity and lymphocyte transformation: dissociation in atopic dermatitis. Arch Dermatol 1979;115:36–39.

52. Rogge JL, Hanifin JM. Immunodeficiencies in severe atopic dermatitis: depressed chemotaxies and lymphocyte transformation. Arch Dermatol 1976;112:1391.

53. Rees J, Friedman PS, Mathews JNS. Contact sensitivity to dinitrochlorobenzene is impaired in atopic subjects. Arch Dermatol 1990;126:1173–1175.

54. Ogawa H, Yoshiike T. A speculative view of atopic dermatitis: barrier dysfunction in pathogenesis. J Dermatol Sci 1993;5:197–204.

55. Wrerenga EA, Snick M, De Groot C. Evidence for compartmentalization of functional subsets of CD4+ T lymphocytes in atopic patients. J Immunol 1990;144:4651–4656.

56. Wierenga EA, Snoek M, Bos JD, Jansen HM, Kapsenberg ML. Comparison of diversity and function of house dust mite-specific T lymphocyte clones from atopic and non-atopic donors. Eur J Immunol 1990;20:1519–1526.

57. Vander Heijden FL, Wierenga EA, Bos JD, Kapsenberg ML. High frequency of IL-4 producing CD4+ allergen-specific T lymphocytes in atopic dermatitis lesional skin. J Invest Dermatol 1991;97:389–394.

58. Kay AB, Ying S, Varney V, et al. Messenger RNA expression of the cytokine gene cluster interleukin 3, IL-4, IL-5, and granulocyte/macrophage colony-stimulatory factor in allergen-induced late-phase cutaneous reactions in atopic subjects. J Exp Med 1991;173:775–783.

59. Champion RH, Parish WE. Atopic dermatitis. In: Champion RH, Burton JL, Ebling FJG, eds. Textbook of Dermatology Oxford: Blackwell Scientific Publications, 1991: 589–610.

60. Bruynzeel-Koomen C, Van Der Donk EMM, Bruynzeel PLB, Capron M, DeGast GC, Mudde GC. Associated expression of CD1 antigen and FC receptor for IgE on epidermal Langerhans cells from patients with atopic dermatitis. Clin Exp Immunol 1988;74:137–142.

61. Barker JNWN, Alegre VA, MacDonald DM. Surface-bound immunoglobulin E on antigen presenting cells in cutaneous tissue of atopic dermatitis. J Invest Dermatol 1988; 90:117–121.

62. Bruynzeel-Koomen C, Van Wicker DF, Toonstra J, Berrens L, Burynzeel PLB. The presence of IgE molecules on epidermal Langerhans cells in patients with atopic dermatitis. Arch Dermatol Res 1986;278:199–205.

63. Bieber TM, Rieger A, Neuchrist C. Induction of Fc R2/CD23 on human epidermal Langerhans cells by human recominant interleukin 4 and interferon. J Exp Med 1989; 170:309–314.

64. Bruynzeel-Koomen C. IgE on Langerhans cells: new insights into the pathogenesis of atopic dermatitis. Dermatologica 1986;172:181–183.

65. Boguniewicz M, Jaffe MS, Izu A. Recombinant gamma interferon in treatment of patients with atopic dermatitis and elevated IgE levels. Am J Med 1990;88:365–370.

66. Reinhold U. Wehrmann W, Kukel S, Kreysel HW. Recombinant interferon-gamma in severe atopic dermatitis. Lancet 1990;1:1282.

67. Abb J, Abb H. Effect of cyclosporin on human leukocyte interferon production. Selective inhibition of gamma interferon synthesis. Transplant Proc 1983;15:2380–2382.

68. Griffiths CEM, Nickoloff BJ. Keratinocyte intercellular adhesion molecule-1 expression precedes dermal T lymphocytic infiltration in allergic contact dermatitis (Rhus dermatitis). Am J Pathol 1989;104–105.

69. Griffiths CEM, Barker JNWN, Kunkel S, Nickoloff BJ. Modulation of leukocyte adhesion molecules, a cell chemotaxin (IL-8), and a regulatory cytokine (TNF-α) in allergic contact dermatitis (Rhus dermatitis). Br J Dermatol 1991;124:519–526.

70. Barker JNWN, Mitra RS, Griffiths CEM, Dixit VM, Nickoloff BJ. Keratinocyte as initiators of inflammation. Lancet 1991;337:211–214.

71. Nickoloff BJ, Turka LA. Keratinocytes: key immunocytes of the integument. Am J Pathol 1993;143:325–331.

72. Enk AH, Katz SI. Identification and induction of keratinocyte-derived UK-10, J Immunol 1992;149:92–95.

73. Enk AH, Katz SI. Early molecular events in the induction phase of contact sensitivity. Proc Natl Acad Sci USA 1992; 89:1398–1402.

74. Enk AH, Katz SI. Early events in the induction phase of contact sensitivity. J Invest Dermatol 1992;99 (suppl): 39s–41s.

75. Florentino DF, Zlotnik A, Vieira P, et al. IL-10 acts on the antigen presenting cell to inhibit cytokine production by TH-1 cells. J Immunol 1991;146:3444–3451.

76. Enk AH, Angeloni VL, Udey MC, Katz SI. Inhibition of Langerhans cell antigen presenting function by IL-10. J Immunol 1993;151:2390–2398.

77. Nickoloff BJ, Fivenson DP, Kunkel SL, et al. Keratinocyte interleukin-10 expression is up-regulated in tape-stripped skin, poison ivy dermatitis, and sezary syndrome, but not in psoriatic plaques. Clin Immunol Immunopathol 1994; 73:63–68.

78. Nickoloff BJ. Pathophysiology of cutaneous inflammation. Arch Dermatol Res 1992;284(suppl):10–1

PART 7

GENETIC MANIPULATIONS OF CYTOKINES

CHAPTER 42

GENE DELETION MODELS
TO UNDERSTAND CYTOKINE FUNCTIONS

Martin M. Matzuk

As has been discussed in previous chapters of this book, many cytokines affect a wide range of processes. In addition, an individual cytokine is often polyfunctional, having a remarkable range of biological activities. Determination of the many activities of a particular cytokine have come from studies both in vitro and in vivo. In this chapter, I discuss studies to date on the generation of mice deficient in a number of cytokines or cytokine receptors. Generation of mice deficient in a particular cytokine allows evaluation of the role of the cytokine in vivo, and in many cases, discovery of new functions of the cytokine. Although many of these cytokines I review have unrelated functions, this chapter is meant to be as inclusive as possible. Hopefully this chapter will complement the more extensive discussions of the individual cytokines presented in previous chapters.

GENERATION OF MAMMALIAN MODELS VIA GENETIC MANIPULATION

A number of approaches have been used to address the role of specific protein products in mammalian development using transgenic mice (1–6). Until recently, the three main approaches to examining the role of a specific gene product included overexpression of the transgene, alteration of gene function by expressing a mutant copy of the gene, and retroviral insertion into the gene of interest. The classic example of overexpression of a transgene involves increased production of rat growth hormone (rGH) under control of the mouse metallothionein I promoter (7). In this study, increased production of rGH outside the pituitary was used to confirm its important physiological and developmental role. Similarly, production of a mutant form of the murine pro-$\alpha 1$(I) collagen gene in transgenic mice altered development by disrupting normal collagen fibril synthesis and resulted in early death of the mice (8). Finally, retroviral insertion has been used in a number of cases to disrupt the gene of interest (9) and therefore mimic specific human diseases.

Since 1990, a number of mutant mice have been produced with the advent of gene targeting and embryonic stem (ES) cell technology (10,11). This powerful technology involves disruption of specific genes in embryonic stem cells via homologous recombination between an introduced vector that contains sequences homologous to the gene of interest and the endogenous ES cell gene. This technology allows one to answer questions via "loss of function" experiments as opposed to "gain of function" experiments with the standard transgenic technology described.

The steps involved in generation of these mice are illustrated in Fig. 42–1. These steps are briefly described herein, and readers who wish more information are re-

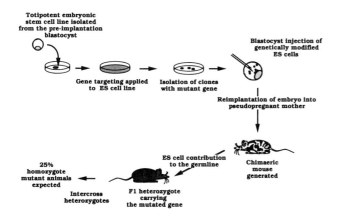

Figure 42–1 Generation of mutant mice via gene targeting in ES cells. (Modified with permission from Bradley A, Hasty P, Davis A, Ramirez-Solis R. Modifying the mouse: design and desire. Bio/Technology 1992;10:534–539.)

ferred to an excellent recent review (12). An important step in generating these mutant mice has been isolation of totipotent ES cell lines from the inner cell mass of blastocysts, which can contribute to all tissues, including the germline. The first isolation of ES cell lines and contribution of these totipotent cells to the germline came in the early 1980s from studies in Martin Evans laboratory (13, 14). Only recently, Bradley isolated ES ce**l** lines (AB1 and AB2.1) from 129Sv-derived blastocysts, which consistently contribute to the germline when grown under "appropriate" conditions (15–17). One major goal in these experiments is to maintain the totipotential nature of these ES cells by growing the cells in an environment that limits differentiation and genetically undesirable alterations. This growth can be achieved by growth in the presence of fetal calf serum supplemented with leukemia inhibitory factor (LIF) (6,18), or more easily on a monolayer of mitotically inactive fibroblast cells synthesizing LIF (SNL76/7 STO cell line) (15).

For the homologous recombination events, most gene targeting strategies utilize "replacement" vectors containing positive and negative selectable markers (19) with sequences homologous to the target gene flanking the positive marker. There are three commonly used positive selectable markers; the neomycin resistance gene, the hygromycin resistance gene, and the HPRT gene; and there are two commonly used negative selectable markers; the herpes simplex virus thymidine kinase gene and the diphtheria toxin gene. The positive selectable markers enrich for integration of the targeting vector into the ES cell genome, and the negative markers enrich for the homologous recombination event. ES cell clones containing the targeted event are identified by either Southern blot analysis (20) using external probes or by the polymerase

chain reaction (21). Cells from targeted clones are then injected into the blastocoel of 3.5-day-old blastocysts (usually from C57BL/6 matings) and reimplanted into pseudopregnant females to generate chimeric mice, which are a mixture of the injected ES cells and the inner cell mass (ICM) of the blastocyst (11). If the ES cells contribute to the germline, heterozygotes for the mutant allele can be obtained and intercrossed to obtain homozygotes with two copies of the targeted allele. These deficient mice are then worked-up biochemically, morphologically, and histologically to understand the role of the protein in mammals.

Why should we make a transgenic mouse with a targeted mutation/deletion in a gene of interest? Three main reasons are (a) to address the roles of specific protein products in mammalian development and oncogenesis; (b) to further understand mammalian development, including cell lineage development; and (c) to generate mammalian models for oncogenesis and other diseases, including developmental disorders. With respect to the latter, animal models are important both to understand the disease entity and to test new therapeutic regimens, including gene therapy approaches.

What are the advantages of making a mouse deficient in a protein of interest compared with more classic methods? Other methodologies to "block" production or activities of a protein have included use of an antisense approach and use of antibodies to the protein. In general, overexpression of antisense mRNA has not been very successful in ablating all of the mRNA coding for the protein of interest. In contrast, neutralizing antibodies, which could be injected into animals to block the activities of a secreted protein, may "soak up" the antigen of interest. However, in general, this approach is a very time- and cost-consuming approach that never truly answers the question of whether all of the activity is gone, especially if the secreted protein has autocrine or paracrine functions. In this scenario, the neutralizing antibody may not "see" the antigen before it exerts its actions. Furthermore, this approach cannot be easily adapted to address the role of a cytokine during embryonic development. Clearly, generation of a mouse with a null mutation is the only absolute means to answer the question of what happens in complete absence of the gene product. In addition, a null mouse allows determination of the essential role of a protein in development. Many cytokines can demonstrate effects on cells in vitro and in vivo, and in situ and immunohistochemical analysis can be used to demonstrate the expression of mRNA or protein in specific cell types and tissues. However, only a null mouse can determine the relevant/essential role of the protein and confirm postulated theories on these roles. Discussions of the generation of a number of cytokines and growth factor mutants follow (Table 42–1).

TABLE 42–1 MUTATIONAL ANALYSIS OF CYTOKINES AND GROWTH FACTORS

Cytokine/Cytokine Receptor Alterations*	Major Findings	Refs
IFN-γ/IFN-γ receptor	Reduced resistance to bacterial and viral infections	(25,26)
IL-2	Altered immune system function; ulcerative colitis-like condition	(29,30)
IL-4	Reduced serum immunoglobulin isotype level	(31)
TGF-β	Inflammatory disorder; death within 1 mo	(55,56)
BMP-5 (short ear)	Viable; skeletal and cartilage abnormalities	(66)
MIS	Males develop uteri; Leydig cell hyperplasia/tumors	(58)
Inhibin	Tumor suppressor role for inhibin; gonadal and adrenal tumors	(17,115)
Activin βB	Eye and reproductive abnormalities	(116)
TGF-α (waved-1)	Hair, hair follicle, eyelid, and eye abnormalities	(95,96)
LIF	Failure of uterus to allow blastocyst implantation	(99
TNF-α receptor, TNFRp55	Reduced resistance to bacterial infection; resistance to endotoxin/superantigen shock	(112)
IGF-II‡	Growth-deficiency; tissue-specific parental imprinting	(113,114)

*Names in parenthesis in this column refer to natural or induced mouse mutants with defects in that cytokine.
‡Not discussed in this chapter.

CYTOKINES OF THE IMMUNE SYSTEM

Interferon-γ/interferon-γ receptor

Interferon-γ (IFN-γ), a 146 amino acid glycoprotein that may form a dimer, is produced by activated T cells (both T-helper 1 [Th1] and cytotoxic suppressor cells) and natural killer (NK) cells. IFN-γ is released in response to a number of stimuli, and it has been shown to have an important immunomodulatory effect on multiple cells, including macrophages, NK cells, B cells, and CD4+T-helper 2 (Th2) cells (22,23). These responses are mediated via a unique IFN-γ receptor (24). IFN-γ has been implicated as the key cytokine involved in mounting a normal immune response to bacterial and viral pathogens. Among its functions is activation of macrophages to produce antimicrobial agents (e.g., nitric oxide), stimulation of cytotoxic activation of NK cells, induction of proliferation and lymphokine production by Th2 lymphocytes, and stimulation of antibody production by B lymphocytes. In addition, IFN-γ has been suggested to induce antitumor activity in macrophages, which may have important implications for therapeutic uses of IFN-γ in humans. Thus, absence of either IFN-γ or the IFN-γ receptor would be expected to have broad immunological effects on antipathogen and antitumor activity in mice.

Generation of IFN-γ-deficient mice by Dalton and colleagues (25) and INF-γ receptor-deficient mice by Huang and associates (26) proved the importance of IFN-γ-mediated signal transduction in these mentioned processes. Mice that lack IFN-γ activity via either mutation appear to be indistinguishable, and homozygotes develop normally, with no gross abnormalities. The immune systems of these mice also appear to be "set-up" normally. Thus, IFN-γ is apparently not necessary for development of any portion of the immune system. The growth of NK cells and other cytotoxic T cells appears to be normal. However, both groups found that IFN-γ is necessary for activation and stimulation of several immune system cell types. Antibodies are produced in the absence of IFN-γ activity, but antibody response in the IFN-γ receptor-deficient mice was reduced. Furthermore, although the NK cells can develop in the absence of IFN-γ, there is reduced NK cell differentiation and decreased activity of NK cells isolated from the spleen of the IFN-γ–deficient mice. More dramatic differences, however, were noted in the responses of macrophages and possibly neutrophils to pathogens. The majority of IFN-γ and IFN-receptor–deficient mice were killed by sublethal doses (sublethal for wild-type mice) of the intracellular bacteria *Listeria monocytogenes*, the mycobacterium *Mycobacterium bovis,* and the vaccinia virus, which replicated to 100- to 1,000-fold higher titers than control mice before killing them. Part of the pathogenicity of these infectious agents was likely secondary to impaired production of nitric oxide and other antimicrobial factors in macrophages, decreased presentation of major histocompatibility complex class II antigens on macrophages, and slightly reduced cytotoxic T lymphocytes, thus allowing increased viral replication.

Thus, IFN-γ appears to have important inducing roles in the host defenses against a variety of pathogens. Future studies with these mice will likely allow for greater understanding of IFN-γ in autoimmune diseases and as an anti-tumor agent.

Mice deficient in interleukins

The interleukins (ILs) are a group of immunomodulatory cytokines that are synthesized in a variety of cell types (27,28). More than 10 of these cytokines have been discovered, and many of these cytokines appear to have similar redundant effects on cells of the immune system in a number of in vitro assays. Therefore, analysis of their essential effects in vivo will require generation of mice deficient in individual ILs and eventually interbreeding of the IL-deficient mice to discover how much redundancy is present. Several IL-deficient mice have been generated, including mice deficient in IL-2, IL-3, IL-4, IL-6, IL-10, and the IL-8 receptor (29–32). Because only studies of IL-2– and IL-4–deficient mice have been published, the discussion is confined to studies of these two cytokines.

IL-2 has been suggested to be a critical autocrine and parocrine cytokine involved in T-cell and B-cell growth and differentiation, thymic maturation, and regulation of T-lymphocyte immune responses following antigen activation (27). Horak and colleagues (29) produced IL-2–deficient mice, and they showed that absence of IL-2 apparently does not alter the development of the thymus or affect thymocyte and peripheral T-lymphocyte subset composition. However, analysis of T-lymphocyte responses in vitro revealed a dramatic inability of the mutant T lymphocytes to induce immunoglobulin M (IgM) secretion in appropriately stimulated B cells. In addition, although IgM serum levels were normal in the IL-2–deficient mice, IgG1, IgG2a, and IgG2b levels were significantly higher in these mice. Later histological studies from these investigators (30) have shown that these alterations in Ig isotype levels may be secondary to a global dysregulation of B cells. Immature B cells are found in peripheral lymphoid organs, and mice that live past 10 weeks of age develop an inflammatory condition of their large intestine that greatly resembles ulcerative colitis in humans. Thus, generation of IL-2–deficient mice has suggested a possible pathway in the etiology of ulcerative colitis, and these mice may prove clinically important in the therapeutic treatment of ulcerative colitis and similar inflammatory bowel diseases.

In a similar manner, Kuhn and colleagues (31) generated mice deficient in the lymphoproliferative cytokine, IL-4. Similar to the IL-2 studies, IL-4–deficient mice survive embryonic life and apparently have normal T- and B-lymphocyte and lymphoid tissue development. However, analysis of serum antibody isotype levels revealed depressed IgG1 levels (one-sixth of control levels) and undetectable IgE levels. In addition, IgE induction in response to a parasite infection did not occur in the IL-4–deficient mice, and there was a suppressed IgG1 immune response after immunization in these mice. These results are fairly consistent with earlier studies in which mice were given anti-IL-4 antibodies (33) and shown to have suppressed IgE production, although the IgG1 responses in these studies were not as dramatic as those seen in the IL-4–deficient mice. Thus, these IL-4–deficient mice further reinforce the importance of IL-4 in parasitic infections, and they suggest that IL-4 may be useful in the treatment of patients with severe parasite infections, and antibodies or antagonists of IL-4 to IL-4 may be useful in the regulation of severe IgE-associated inflammatory/hypersensitivity reactions.

THE TRANSFORMING GROWTH FACTOR-β SUPERFAMILY

More than 20 members of the transforming growth factor B (TGF-β) superfamily have been discovered (34–53). These growth factors synthesized as prepropeptides and processed to dimeric proteins, are structurally related in their mature, active C-terminal region. These proteins are called by various nomenclature, depending on the assay system in which the proteins were discovered (and occasionally via the whim of the investigator). Among the mammalian members of this family are 2 inhibins (34), 3 activins (34), 3 TGF-βs (35–39), Müllerian inhibiting substance (MIS) (40–42), 7 bone morphogenetic proteins (BMPs) (these proteins also have other names) (43–48), 3 growth differentiation factors (GDFs) (their function may not have anything to do with their names) (49, 50), nodal (51), Vg-1–related protein (Vgr-2) (52), and dorsalin (53). Members of this family have been shown to have diverse functions in a variety of assay systems, ranging from regression of the Müllerian duct (MIS) (40–42) to mesoderm induction (activins) (34) to bone formation (BMPs) (43–47). These actions appear to be mediated through similar serine-threonine kinase transmembrane receptors (54). Many studies are currently addressing the roles of the cytokines via murine ES cells/gene targeting strategies. Several of these studies are described.

Transforming growth factor-β1

The TGF-β proteins are ubiquitous growth factors that have been implicated to have important functions in a wide range of processes, including adipogenesis, myogenesis, chondrogenesis, epithelial cell differentiation, and immune cell function. In addition, they have been shown to suppress tumor cell growth (39). There are three mammalian TGF-βs: TGF-β₁ (35), TGF-β₂ (36), and TGF-β₃ (37,38), which share more than 70% homology in their mature 112 amino C-terminal region. These three growth factors are often coexpressed in similar cell types, and they have similar actions on cell lines in vitro (35–39). To truly distinguish the individual functions of each of these three cytokines in vivo, genetic manipulation of the mouse must therefore be used, and eventually mice deficient in all three growth factors will need to be intercrossed to determine the level of redundancy of these three cytokines.

The first of these TGF-βs to be targeted was TGF-β₁. Doetschman and colleagues (55) at the University of Cincinnati and Karleson and colleagues (56) at the National Institutes of Health independently generated mice deficient in TGF-β₁. The constructs used to generate the mutation of the TGF-β₁ gene in ES cells were very different. The former group chose to target the 3′ region of the gene coding for the mature C-terminus, whereas the latter group targeted the 5′ region encoding the propeptide. In both cases, TGF-β₁ expression appeared to be eliminated, and similar findings were seen in mice deficient for TGF-β₁.

Genotyping of pups born from intercrosses of heterozygotes for the TGF-β₁ mutation revealed that less than one half of the expected TGF-β₁ homozygotes are born. It is unclear why the majority of TGF-β₁ homozygotes die during embryonic life, although the genetic background may influence this outcome. The remainder of the TGF-β₁–deficient mice that are born are found to die at approximately 3 to 4 weeks of age. Histological examination of these mice reveals multiorgan inflammatory infiltrates. The inflammation is seen primarily in the gastrointestinal, cardiovascular, and pulmonary systems, and it includes monocyte, lymphocyte, and neutrophil infiltration. These studies therefore suggest that TGF-β₁ is an important regulator of inflammatory cell responses and that these mice may be important mammalian models for future study of a number of inflammatory disorders. It will also be of interest to understand what function TGF-β₁ has during embryonic development and to determine the genetic modifiers that influence the embryonic lethality of TGF-β₋₁–deficient mice.

Müllerian inhibiting substance

Unlike many of the other members of this family that are expressed in many tissues and cell types, MIS expression is limited to both fetal and adult Sertoli cells of the male testis and the postnatal granulosa cells in the female ovaries (40–42). The major function of MIS (for which it is named) is to cause regression of the Müllerian duct during embryonic development in males. It is unknown what function MIS has in postnatal male and female gonads. Several studies have suggested, however, that MIS may act as an "antiproliferative" growth factor in the postnatal female reproductive tract. This hypothesis is derived from the finding that MIS can inhibit the growth of some reproductive tract carcinoma cell lines (including ovarian carcinoma cell lines) in vitro and in vivo (42,57). In addition, MIS has been postulated to have a role in the descent of the testes in the male (42).

To test these hypotheses, Behringer and associates (58) produced mice deficient in MIS. As might be expected from the limited expression of MIS, MIS-deficient mice are viable. In addition, MIS-deficient adult females are fertile, and adult males have descended testis (disproving one hypothesis); in vitro, motile sperm from these males are functionally normal. Consistent with its name, MIS-deficient males do not have regression of the Müllerian duct, which develops into a uterus in the males similar to the human syndrome known as persistent Müllerian duct syndrome. Thus, these males essentially have two reproductive tracts. In addition, the presence of the uterus in these males appears to result in blockage of sperm flow because the males can copulate with females but they cannot transfer sperm (which was found to be functionally normal in vitro, as described). An additional finding in these mice, which addresses the role of MIS in tumorigenesis, is the apparent development of Leydig-cell hyperplasia and tumors in the male mice. Thus, MIS appears to be a critical protein in male reproduction and testicular development.

Bone morphogenetic protein-5

A number of factors are involved in mammalian skeleton development. In 1988, Wozney and colleagues (43) at Genetics Institute described the first purification and cloning of several proteins and cDNAs that can induce bone formation in an in vivo assay system. Because of the assay system used, these proteins received the name bone morphogenetic proteins (BMPs). Since that time, other BMPs have been discovered (total, 7), and they have been shown to be members of the TGF-β superfamily (43–48). In addition, expression of these BMPs is not limited to bone (47,59–62), and several of these BMPs have high homology to *Drosophila* and *Xenopus* members of this family (63–65). Thus, absence of one of the BMPs could be expected to have a number of developmental defects, although the similarity (and possible redundancy) of function in the bone assay system suggests that one BMP could take the place of another BMP if temporal and spatial expression are appropriate.

Although no BMP mutation has been generated to date

via gene targeting strategies, it is noteworthy for this review to mention the first mutation of this group of proteins, which was identified via analysis of mice with radiation and chemical-induced mutations. Kingsley and colleagues (66) recently showed that the BMP-5 gene maps in the region of the mouse mutation, short ear, which was first identified more than 70 years ago (67). Via an extensive and elaborate study, several short ear mice were shown to have deletions of regions of the BMP-5 gene. In addition, mice that have large deletions limited to the BMP-5 locus are viable and fertile. Thus, BMP-5 is not essential for embryonic existence. However, because these short ear mice were identified on the basis of their ear phenotype, BMP-5 must have a role in skeleton/cartilage formation. Skeletal analysis of one mouse mutant, $se^{20\ Zb}$, in which there is a limited chromosomal deletion, including an exon encoding the active BMP-5 C-terminus, reveals short external ears and a frequent (50%) absence of the 13th pair of ribs. It is likely that this incomplete penetrance of rib formation is secondary to different genetic backgrounds, and the authors are likely to inbreed these mice to test this hypothesis. In addition, as more BMP-deficient mice arise, generation of mice deficient in multiple BMPs by interbreeding will undoubtedly occur. These studies will test whether the subtle phenotype of BMP-5 is due to the presence of other BMPs that supplant its function.

Inhibin

The inhibins are heterodimeric growth factors (α:βA or α:βB) that share a common β-subunit (βA or βB) with the activins (Fig. 42–2). Similar to the other members of this superfamily, these α-, βA-, and βB-subunits are synthesized as prepropeptides, and they are processed intracellularly to active dimers (34). The inhibins were discovered as gonadal, endocrine peptides (Sertoli cell and granulosa cell products) that fed back on the gonadotrophs of the pituitary to inhibit follicle-stimulating hormone (FSH) synthesis and secretion (34). Later studies suggested important paracrine and autocrine roles

of the inhibins in embryonic, extraembryonic (i.e., placenta), and adult tissues, including gonads, adrenal gland, and bone marrow (34,68–70).

To address the role of the inhibins in mammalian reproduction and development, we generated mice heterozygous and homozygous for a deletion on the inhibin α-subunit gene (17), which would abolish all inhibin activity (Fig. 42–3). Inhibin-deficient mice were viable, indicating that inhibin was not essential for embryonic development. However, gonadal sex-cord stromal tumors (99% penetrance) developed in the inhibin-deficient mice in both males and females. The predisposition of inhibin-deficient mice to tumors identified inhibin as a novel tumor suppressor, the first secreted protein that has this role.

Development of the sex cord-stromal tumors in the inhibin-deficient mice is rapidly followed by a severe wasting syndrome that mimics the cancer cachexia syndrome accompanying many human cancers (115). Proof that the cachexia is secondary to gonadal tumor formation comes from analysis of gonadectomized inhibin-deficient mice, which do not develop this cachexia. Thus, these studies suggest that inhibin-deficient mice are an important mammalian model for understanding cancer cachexia syndrome.

In addition to the synthesis of inhibin in the gonads and the placenta, inhibin subunit mRNAs or proteins are also detected at lower levels in the pituitary, adrenal gland, spleen, brain, and spinal cord (34,68). To address whether inhibin could function as a tumor suppressor in any of these tissues, we monitored the gonadectomized inhibin-deficient mice for the development of tumors. Ninety-nine percent (66 of 67) of the gonadectomized inhibin-deficient male and female mice developed adrenal cortical tumors, compared with 1 of 77 control mice (115). Thus, these studies identified inhibin as the first tumor suppressor with high specificity and high penetrance for the adrenal cortex. Future studies will evaluate

| | ACTIVIN | | | INHIBIN | |
	A	B	AB	A	B
Wild-Type	+	+	+	+	+
Δα /Δα	+	+	+	−	−
ΔβA /ΔβA	−	+	−	−	+
ΔβB /ΔβB	+	−	−	+	−
ΔβA /ΔβA ΔβB /ΔβB	−	−	−	−	−

Figure 42–3 Forms of the activins and the inhibins present in wild-type, α-subunit–deficient (Δα/Δα), βA-subunit–deficient (ΔβA/ΔβA), βB-subunit–deficient (ΔβB/ΔβB), and βA-subunit/ βB-subunit–deficient (ΔβA/ΔβA; ΔβB/ΔβB) mice.

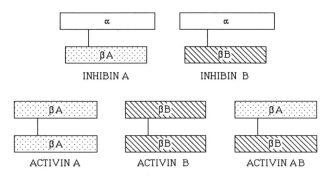

Figure 42–2 Structures of the inhibins and activins.

the various cytokines responsible for the severe wasting syndrome seen in these inhibin-deficient mice. In addition, these studies may have direct relevance for the studies of cancer cachexia syndrome and the development of gonadal and adrenal tumors in humans.

Activin βB

The activins are β-β dimers (βA:βA, βB:βB, or βA:βB) that share a common subunit with the α:β heterodimeric inhibins. Although the β-subunits are highly conserved between species, and active dimers of either βA or βB have similar in vitro activities, the βA and βB subunits share only 64% within a species (34). Although the activins were initially isolated from gonadal extracts and named for their ability to stimulate FSH production by the pituitary, the activin mRNAs and proteins have been shown to be present in a number of tissues during both embryonic (69,70) and adult (68) development, and activins have been shown to be active in many in vitro assays (34). In addition, activin B has been suggested to be a critical factor involved in mesoderm induction for the following reasons: (a) activin βB mRNA and protein has been shown to be present at the blastocyst stage in both mouse (70) and chick (71); (b) activins and activin receptors have been shown to be potent mesoderm-inducing factors in *Xenopus* explant experiments (72–75); and (c) injection of truncated activin receptor mRNA into *Xenopus* embryos can block mesoderm induction in a dominant-negative fashion (76).

To evaluate the role of activin βB during embryonic and reproductive development, Vassalli and Jaenisch (116) generated mice deficient in activin βB subunit, and therefore deficient in activin B, activin AB, and inhibin B (see Fig. 42–3). These mice are viable, suggesting that (a) activin B is not a mesoderm inducer in vivo; (b) activin A, which continues to be synthesized in these mice, may supplant the function of activin B; or (c) there is redundancy in the system, and other related or unrelated factors can overcome the loss of activin B. Although these βB-deficient mice are viable, they are not normal. The majority of the newborn mice (depending on the strain and the background) are born with their eyes open, which eventually progresses to trauma to the cornea. This phenotype, similar to the TGF-α phenotype, suggests a developmental defect in eye closure, which normally occurs at approximately day 16 of embryonic development. In addition, the reproductive capacity of female βB-deficient mice is greatly reduced, liveborn litters fail to survive postnatally (reason unclear). Thus, as hypothesized, activin βB is a critical protein involved in development and reproduction, but it is not essential for mesoderm induction. Analysis of mice deficient in all activin activity via crosses of activin βA– and activin βB–deficient mice

(see Fig 42–3) will evaluate further the roles of the activins during early mouse development.

OTHER PLEIOTROPIC CYTOKINES

Transforming growth factor-α

TGF-α shares structural homology to EGF (77). This structural homology is likely the reason for the functional similarity between TGF-α and EGF, and these two growth factors appear to interact with the same receptor to elicit similar, although apparently not identical, responses (77,78). Similar to the TGF-β family members, TGF-α is synthesized as a prepropeptide, which is processed extracellularly to a 50 amino acid secreted form with three disulfide bonds (79). However, unlike the TGF-βs, the precursor pro-TGF-α, which is membrane-bound, is also biologically active, and it can elicit responses on neighboring cells (80,81).

The expression pattern of TGF-α is widespread and diverse (82–90). Expression is noted in the preimplantation mouse embryo (82), the maternal decidua (83), the placenta (84), and later in embryonic development in a number of other tissues (84), including the kidney. These data suggest that TGF-α may function in the early stages of mouse development, in implantation or placental development, or at other places in mammalian development. Expression of TGF-α in the adult is widespread and ranges from expression in activated macrophages (85,86), the nervous system (87), the skin (88) to varying periods of mammary gland development (89,90). In addition, studies from overexpression of TGF-α in transgenic mice (91–93) demonstrate that TGF-α has an important role in epithelial cell growth in multiple systems; epithelial hyperplasia can be seen in mammary gland (91,92), colon (91), and skin (93) of these transgenic mice. In addition, TGF-α overexpression can be demonstrated in a number of transformed cell lines and human tumors (94). These studies suggest that it may be an important factor (possible initiator) in neoplastic transformation. Thus, TGF-α– deficient mice may be expected to result in any one of a number of phenotypes.

Two studies (95,96) have recently been reported in which waved-1, an apparent naturally occurring mouse TGF-α mutant, and TGF-α–deficient mice were analyzed. These TGF-α–deficient mice are healthy and fertile, which suggests that TGF-α does not have an essential role in reproduction (including implantation and placental development) and embryonic development. The major findings, and the clue that waved-1 represented a mutation in the TGF-α locus, was that TGF-α–deficient mice developed curly and wavy hair. This hair is demonstrated even at birth, in which the whiskers had a distinct curvature. Histological analysis of the skin suggests that the phenotype is caused by abnormal curvatures and arrangements of hair follicle bulbs and hair shafts. The bulbs were not perpendicular (and in some cases were parallel) to the muscle layer, and they were much closer to the underlying panniculus carnosus layer than in control mice. In addition, the majority of older TGF-α–deficient mice appear to develop corneal lesions. A number of the TGF-α–deficient mice are born with one or two of their eyelids open (which normally occurs at approximately day 16 of development), similar to the activin βB-deficient mice described above. This "eyelid-open" phenotype likely results in the inflammation and the eventual corneal ulceration that occurs in the adult mice. Thus, TGF-α–deficient mice have a limited number of phenotypic findings involving the skin. Absence of findings in other tissues could be secondary to a more important or redundant role of EGF or EGF-like factors in these tissues. Future studies will likely address the roles of TGF-α in tumor formation.

Leukemia inhibitory factor

LIF, a 190 amino acid secreted glycopeptide, received its name from its ability to induce differentiation of the M1 leukemia cell line into monocytes. However, like many of the cytokines described in this chapter, LIF has been shown to have a multitude of functions (97). As mentioned in the introduction, LIF has been used in in vitro culture systems to prevent ES cell differentiation (18). This approach suggests that LIF may be an important regulator of differentiation in the early embryo at about the time of implantation because ES cells are derived from cells of the inner cell mass of blastocysts. With regard to this point, LIF expression is induced in the uterine endometrial glands of mice on day 4 of pregnancy, which coincides with blastocyst implantation, suggesting that it may function as an antidifferentiation factor or directly in implantation in vivo (98). In addition to its effects on the M1 leukemia and ES cell lines, LIF has also been shown to regulate or to induce differentiation of other hematopoietic cell lines, including cells of erythroid, myeloid, and megakaryocyte lineages. LIF can prolong neuronal survival, increase acute-phase protein synthesis in hepatocytes, inhibits lipoprotein lipase activity and therefore fatty acid uptake in adipocytes, and alter bone remodeling via effects on osteoblasts (97). Thus, absence of LIF in mice would be expected to profoundly alter a number of in vivo processes.

Generation of LIF-deficient mice via a gene targeting strategy by Stewart and colleagues (99) resulted in mice that were viable, and both males and females were fertile.

Adults deficient in LIF, however, were approximately 75% of the body weight of sibling control mice. In addition, LIF-deficient females failed to get pregnant. This failure to get pregnant was demonstrated to be secondary to failure of blastocysts to implant into the uterus of homozygotes not expressing LIF. Recombinant LIF, however, given to 3-day pregnant homozygotes for 3 days, could allow implantation to occur in a limited number of females. Thus, these studies prove that LIF is a critical factor in at least allowing implantation to occur, and it is somehow involved in growth.

Why such a limited number of essential functions of LIF? One reason is that other factors, such as oncostatin-M and ciliary neurotrophic factor, which have primary and secondary structure similarities to LIF, may substitute for LIF at the LIF receptor. Alternatively, other cytokines that bind to similar cytokine receptors (e.g., IL-2–7, and granulocyte-macrophage colony-stimulating factor) and share the common transmembrane glycoprotein gp130 may supplement its role by eliciting a compensatory downstream signal. Thus, there may be cytokine redundancy at the LIF receptor or redundancy of function via similar signal transduction/cytokine receptor pathways (100). With regard to these points, it will be critical to interbreed mice deficient in LIF and other cytokinedeficient mice to determine if there is redundancy of function.

Tumor necrosis factor-α receptor, TNFRp55

Similar to a number of the cytokines described, tumor necrosis factor-α (TNF-α) has been demonstrated to have effects on multiple systems. TNF-α was initially discovered in 1975, and it was named for its ability to cause necrosis of tumors (101). Other studies demonstrated that TNF-α was identical to a macrophage-derived polypeptide called "cachectin," which was shown to cause cachexia (i.e., severe weight loss) (102). Macrophages are the major cell type of the immune system that produce TNF-α, although other immune system cell types, such as activated T-cells, NK cells, and mast cells, produce TNF-α at lower levels (102). In addition, TNF-α protein expression has been detected in brain, neural tube, and peripheral nerves of the developing nervous system (103). TNF-α is also expressed in the mammalian ovary (mainly granulosa cells) and from ovarian tumors (104,105). It has been postulated that ovarian TNF-α participates in follicular atresia because of its paracrine and autocrine effects on progesterone, androgen, and aromtase activities (106).

Multiple studies have addressed the roles of TNF-α. Use of anti–TNF-α antibodies has demonstrated (a) involvement of TNF-α in septic shock syndrome secondary to lipopolysaccharide or bacterial superantigens (10);

(b) the importance of TNF-α in the defense against bacteria, such as *Listeria* monocytogenes (107); and (c) alteration of the development of cachexia in mouse tumor models (108). Confirmation of a role for TNF-α in cachexia has come from experiments in which cells engineered to overexpress TNF-α have been injected into mice and shown to quickly produce a severe wasting syndrome (109). Studies have also suggested a role for TNF-α in obesity. Elevated TNF-α mRNA expression has been demonstrated in adipose tissue isolated from mouse and rat models of obesity and diabetes (110). Furthermore, arthritis develops in transgenic mice overexpressing TNF-α in macrophages, which suggests an important role of TNF-α in the pathogenesis of rheumatoid arthritis and other inflammatory disorders in humans (111).

To understand the physiological roles of TNF-α in mammals, Pfeffer and colleagues (112) generated mice deficient in one of the two TNF-α receptors, TNFRp55. TNF-α mediates its signals through a 55-kd receptor (TNFRp55) and a 75-kd receptor (TNFRp75). Signaling appears to be predominantly through TNFRp55; very little is known about the role of TNFRp75. Thus, the TNFRp55-disruption model was designed to address the role of TNF-α and to discriminate between functions of the two receptors. With respect to the immune system, the TNFRp55-deficient mice are found to act very similarly to what might be expected if this was the major receptor. TNFRp55-deficient mice are resistant to normally lethal doses of lipopolysaccharide and *Staphylococcus aureus* enterotoxin B. In addition, these mice are unable to defend against subinfectious levels of *Listeria* monocytogenes; they show titers more than 1,000-fold higher than control mice 6 days after inoculation. In contrast to these findings, thymocyte development and lymphocyte populations in spleen and thymus are normal. Furthermore, these TNFRp55-deficient mice show no phenotypic abnormalities or fertility problems up to 10 months of age when housed under pathogen-free conditions. The lack of any neurological or fertility deficients would suggest that either TNF-α has a minor role in these processes or these processes are mediated through the 75-kd receptor. It will be critical to examine mice deficient in TNFRp75, mice deficient in both receptors, or mice deficient in TNF-α to address these hypotheses. In addition, it will be interesting to intercross these mice with mouse diabetes/obesity models and mouse tumor models.

In conclusion, a number of cytokine and growth factor genes have been targeted in the mouse. Although these studies have led to a clearer understanding of the essential function of these cytokines in mammalian development, there are many puzzling results that await resolution. Future interbreeding experiments and analysis of other mutant mice will address questions such as redundancy and synergistic functioning.

REFERENCES

1. Palmiter RD, Brinster RL. Germ-line transformation of mice. Ann Rev Genet 1986;20:465–499.

2. Jaenisch R. Transgenic animals. Science 1988;240:1468–1474.

3. Hanahan D. Transgenic mice as probes into complex systems. Science 1989;246:1265–1275.

4. Westphal H, Grass P. Molecular genetics of development studied in the transgenic mouse. Annu Rev Cell Biol 1989;5:181–196.

5. Adams JM, Cory S. Transgenic models of tumor development. Science 1991;254:1161–1167.

6. Stewart TA. Models of human endocrine disorders in transgenic rodents. Trends Endocrinol Metab 1993;4:136–141.

7. Palmiter RD, Brinster RL, Hammer RE, et al. Dramatic growth of mice that develop from eggs microinjected with metallothionein-growth hormone fusion genes. Nature 1982;300:611–615.

8. Stacey A, Bateman J, Choi T, Mascara T, Cole W, Jaenisch R. Perinatal lethal osteogenesis imperfecta in transgenic mice bearing an engineered mutant pro-α1(I) collagen gene. Nature 1988;332:131–136.

9. Schnieke A, Harbers K, Jaenisch R. Embryonic lethal mutation in mice induced by retrovirus insertion into the α-1(1) collagen gene. Nature 1983;304:315–320.

10. Thomas KR, Capecchi MR. Site-directed mutagenesis by gene targeting in mouse embryo-derived stem cells. Cell 1987;51:503–512.

11. Bradley A. Production and analysis of chimeric mice. In: Robinson EJ, ed. Teratocarcinomas and embryonic stem cells: a practical approach. Oxford: IRL, 1987:113–151.

12. Bradley A, Hasty P, Davis A, Ramirez-Solis R. Modifying the mouse: design and desire. Bio/Technology 1992;10:534–539.

13. Evans MJ, Kaufman MH. Establishment in culture of puripotential cells from mouse embryos. Nature 1981;292:154–156.

14. Bradley A, Evans MJ, Kaufman MH, Robertson EJ. Formation of germ line chimeras from embryo-derived teratocarcinoma cell lines. Nature 1984;309:255–256.

15. McMahon AP, Bradley A. The Wnt-1 (Int-1) proto-oncogene is required for the development of a large region of the mouse brain. Cell 1990;62:1073–1085.

16. Soriano P, Montgomery C, Geske R, Bradley A. Targeted disruption of the c-src proto-oncogene leads to osteoporosis in mice. Cell 1991;64:693–702.

17. Matzuk MM, Finegold MJ, Su J-GJ, Hsueh AJW. α-Inhibin is a tumour-suppressor gene with gonadal specificity in mice. Nature 1992;360:313–319.

18. Williams RL, Hilton DJ, Pease S, et al. Myeloid leukemia inhibitory factor maintains the development potential of embryonic stem cells. Nature 1988;336:684–686.

19. Mansour SL, Thoma KR, Capecchi MR. Disruption of the proto-oncogene int-2 in mouse embryo-derived stem cells: a general strategy for targeting mutations to nonselectable genes. Nature 1988;336:348–353.

20. Ramirez-Solis R, Rivera-Perez J, Wallace JD, Wims M, Zherg H, Bradley A. Genomic DNA microextraction: a

method to screen numerous samples. Anal Biochem 1992; 201:331–335.

21. Kim H-S, Smithies O. Recombinant fragment assay for gene targeting based on the polymerase chain reaction. Nucleic Acid Res 1988;16:8887–8903.

22. Vilcek J. Interferons. In: Sporn MB, Roberts AB, eds. Peptide growth factors and their receptors II. Berlin: Springer-Verlag, 1990:3–38.

23. Williams JG, Jurkovich GJ, Maier RV. Interferon-γ: a key immunoregulatory lymphokine. J Surg Res 1993;54:79–93.

24. Aguet M, Dembic Z, Merlin G. Molecular cloning and expression of the human interferon-γ receptor. Cell 1988;55: 273–280.

25. Dalton DK, Pitts-Meek S, Keshav S, Figari IS, Bradley A, Stewart TA. Multiple defects of immune cell function in mice with disrupted interferon-γ genes. Science 1993;259: 1739–1742.

26. Huang S, Hendriks W, Althage A, et al. Immune response in mice that lack the interferon-γ receptor. Science 1993; 259:1742–1745.

27. Hatakeyama N, Taniguchi T. Interleukin-2. In: Sporn MB, Roberts AB, eds. Peptide growth factors and their receptors I. Berlin: Springer-Verlag, 1990:523–540.

28. Vitetta ES, Paul WE. Role of lymphokines in the immune system. In: Sporn MB, Roberts AB, eds. Peptide growth factors and their receptors II. Berlin: Springer-Verlag, 1990: 401–426.

29. Schorle H, Holtschke T, Hunig T, Schimpl A, Horak I. Development and function of T cells in mice rendered interleukin-2 deficient by gene targeting. Nature 1991;252: 621–624.

30. Sadlack B, Merz H, Schorle H, Schimpl A, Feller AC, Horak I. Ulcerative colitis-like disease in mice with a disrupted interleukin-2 gene. Cell 1993;75:253–261.

31. Kuhn R, Rajewsky K, Muller W. Generation and analysis of interleukin-4 deficient mice. Science 1991;254:707–710.

32. Rajewsky K. A phenotype or not: targeting genes in the immune system. Science 1992;256:483.

33. Finkelman FD, Katona IM, Urban JF, Snapper CM, Ohara J, Paul WE. Suppression of in vivo polyclonal IgE responses by monoclonal antibody to the lymphokine B-cell stimulating factor 1. Proc Natl Acad Sci USA 1986;83: 9675–9778.

34. Vale W, Hsueh A, Rivier C, Yu J. The inhibin/activin family of hormones and growth factors. In: Sporn MB, Roberts AB, eds. Peptide growth factors and their receptors II. Berlin: Springer-Verlag, 1990:211–248.

35. Derynck R, Jarrett JA, Chen EY, et al. Human transforming growth factor-β complementary DNA sequence and expression in normal and transformed cells. Nature 1985; 316:701–705.

36. de Martin R, Haendler B, Hofer-Warbinek R, et al. Complementary DNA for human glioblastoma-derived T cell suppressor factor, a novel member of the transforming growth factor-β gene family. EMBO J 1987;6:3673–3677.

37. Ten Dijke P, Hansen P, Iwata KK, Pieler C, Foulkes JG. Identification of another member of the transforming growth factor type β gene family. Proc Natl Acad Sci USA 1988;85:4715–4719.

38. Derynck R, Lindquist PB, Lee A, et al. A new type of trans-

39. Roberts AB, Sporn MD. The transforming growth factor-β's. In: Sporn MB, Roberts AB, eds. Peptide growth factors and their receptors I. Berlin: Springer-Verlag, 1990:419–472.

40. Cate RL, Mattaliano RJ, Hession C, et al. Isolation of the bovine and human genes for Mullerian inhibiting substance and expression of the human gene in animal cells. Cell 1986;45:685–698.

41. Picard J-Y, Benarous R, Guerrier D, Josso N, Kahn A. Cloning and expression of cDNA for anti-Mullerian hormone. Proc Natl Acad Sci USA 1986;83:5464–5468.

42. Cate RL, Donahue PK, MacLaughlin DT. Mullerian inhibiting substance. In: Sporn MB, Roberts AB, eds. Peptide growth factors and their receptors II. Berlin: Springer-Verlag, 1990:179–210.

43. Wozney JM, Rosen V, Celeste AJ, et al. Novel regulators of bone formation: molecular clones and activities. Science 1988;242:1528–1534.

44. Celeste AJ, Iannazzi JA, Taylor RC, et al. Identification of transforming growth factor-β members present in bone-inductive protein purified from bovine bone. Proc Natl Acad Sci USA 1990;87:9843–9847.

45. Ozkaynak E, Rueger DC, Drier EA, et al. OP-1 cDNA encodes an osteogenic protein in the TGF-β family. EMBO J 1990;9:2085–2093.

46. Celeste AJ, Taylor R, Yamaji N, Wang J, Ross J, Wozney J. Molecular cloning of BMP-8: a protein present in bovine bone which is highly related to the BMP-5/6/7 subfamily of osteoinductive molecules. J Cell Biochem 1992;(suppl) 16F:100.

47. Lyons K, Graycar JL, Lee A, et al. Vgr-1, a mammalian gene related to Xenopus Vg-1, is a member of the transforming growth factor β gene superfamily. Proc Natl Acad Sci USA 1989;86:4551–4558.

48. Lyons KM, Jones CM, Hogan BLM. The DVR gene family in embryonic development. Trends Genet 1991;7:408–412.

49. Lee SJ. Identification of a novel member (GDF-1) of the transforming growth factor-β superfamily. Mol Endocrinol 1990;4:1034–1040.

50. McPherron AC, Lee S-J. GDF-3 and GDF-9: two new members of the transforming growth factor-β superfamily containing a novel pattern of cysteines. J Biol Chem 1993; 268:3444–3449.

51. Zhou X, Sasaki H, Lowe L, Hogan BLM, Kuehn MR. Nodal is a novel TGF-β-like expressed in the mouse node during gastrulation. Nature 1993;361:543–547.

52. Jones CM, Simon-Chazottes D, Guenet J-L, Hogan BLM. Isolation of Vgr-2, a novel member of the transforming growth factor-β-related gene family. Mol Endocrinol 1992; 6:1961–1968.

53. Basler K, Edlund T, Jessel TM, Yamada T. Control of cell pattern in the neural tube: regulation of differentiation by dorsal-1, a novel TGF-β family member. Cell 1993;73:687–702.

54. Massague J. Receptors for the TGF-β family. Cell 1992; 69:1067–1070.

55. Schull MM, Ormsby I, Kier AB, et al. Targeted disruption

of the mouse transforming growth factor-β1 gene results in multifocal inflammatory disease. Nature 1992;359:693–699.

56. Kulkarni AB, Huh C-G, Becker D, et al. Transforming growth factor β1 null mutation in mice causes excessive inflammatory response and early death. Proc Natl Acad Sci USA 1993;90:770–774.

57. Chin T, Parry RL, Donahoe PK. Human Müllerian inhibiting substance inhibits tumor growth in vitro and in vivo. Cancer Res 1991;51:2101–2106.

58. Behringer RR, Feingold MJ, Cate RL. Müllerian inhibiting substance during mammalian sexual development. Cell 1994 (in press).

59. Lyons KM, Pelton RW, Hogan BLM. Patterns of expression of murine Vgr-1 and BMP-2a RNA suggest that transforming growth factor-β-like genes coordinately regulate aspects of embryonic development. Gene Dev 1989;3:1657–1668.

60. Lyons KM, Pelton RW, Hogan BLM. Organogenesis and pattern formation in the mouse: RNA distribution patterns suggest a role for bone morphogenetic protein-2A (BMP-2A). Development 1990;109:833–844.

61. Jones CM, Lyons KM, Hogan BLM. Involvement of bone morphogenetic protein-4 (BMP-4) and Vgr-1 in morphogenesis and neurogenesis in the mouse. Development 1991;111:531–542.

62. Ozkaynak E, Schnegelsberg PN, Opperman H. Murine osteogenic protein (OP-1): high levels of mRNA in kidney. Biochem Biophys Res Commun 1991;179:116–123.

63. Weeks DL, Melton DA. A maternal mRNA localized to the vegetal hemisphere in Xenopus eggs codes for growth factor related to TGF-β. Cell 1987;51:861–867.

64. Padgett RM, St. Johnston RD, Gelbert WM. A transcript from a Drosophilia pattern gene predicts a protein homologous to the transforming growth factor-β family. Nature 1987;325:81–84.

65. Wharton KA, Thomsen GH, Gelbart WM. Drosophilia 60A gene, another transforming growth factor β family member, is closely related to human bone morphogenetic proteins. Proc Natl Acad Sci USA 1991;83:9214–9218.

66. Kingsley DM, Bland AE, Grubber JM, et al. The mouse short ear skeletal morphogenesis locus is associated with defects in a bone morphogenetic member of the TGF-β superfamily. Cell 1992;71:399–410.

67. Lynch CJ. Short ears, an autosomal mutation in the house mouse. Am Nat 1921;55:421–426.

68. Meunier H, Rivier C, Evans RM, Vale R. Gonadal and extragonadal expression of inhibin α, βA, and βB subunits in various tissues predicts diverse functions. Proc Natl Acad Sci USA 1988;247–251.

69. Roberts VJ, Sawchenko PE, Vale W. Expression of inhibin/activin subunit messenger ribonucleic acids during rat embryogenesis. Endocrinology 1991;128:3122–3129.

70. Albano RM, Groome N, Smith JC. Activins are expressed in preimplantation mouse embryos and in ES and EC cells and are regulated on their differentiation. Development 1993;117:711–723.

71. Mitrani E, Ziv T, Thomsen G, Shimoni Y, Melton DA, Bril A. Activin can induce the formation of axial structures and is expressed in the hypoblast of the chick. Cell 1990;63:495–501.

72. Smith JC, Price BMJ, Van Nimmen K, Huylebroeck D. Identification of a potent Xenopus mesoderm-inducing factor as a homologue of activin A. Nature 1990;345:729–731.

73. Thomsen G, Woolf T, Whitman M, et al. Activins are expressed early in Xenopus embryogenesis and can induce axial mesoderm and anterior structures. Cell 1990;63:485–493.

74. Kondo M, Tashiro K, Fujii G, et al. Activin receptor mRNA is expressed early in Xenopus embryogenesis and the level of the expression effects the body axis formation. Biochem Biophys Res Commun 1991;181:684–690.

75. Mathews LS, Vale WE, Kintner CR. Cloning of a second type of activin receptor and functional characterization in Xenopus embryos. Science 1992;255:1702–1705.

76. Hemmati-Brivanlou A, Melton DA. A truncated activin receptor inhibits mesoderm induction and formation of axial structures in Xenopus embryos. Nature 1992;359:609–614.

77. Marquardt H, Hunkapiller MW, Hood LE, Todaro GJ. Rat transforming growth factor type 1: structure and relation to epidermal growth factor. Science 1984;223:1079–1082.

78. Ebner R, Derynck R. Epidermal growth factor and transforming growth factor-α: differential intercellular routing and processing of ligand-receptor complexes. Cell Regul 1991;2:599–612.

79. Derynck R, Goeddel DV, Ullrich A, et al. Synthesis of mRNAs for transforming growth factors α and β and the epidermal growth factor receptor by human tumors. Cancer Res 1987;47:707–712.

80. Bringman TS, Lindquist PB, Derynck R. Different transforming growth factor-α species are derived from a glycosylated and palmitoylated transmembrane precursor. Cell 1987;48:429–440.

81. Teixidó J, Wong ST, Lee DC, Massagué J. Generation of transforming growth factor-α from the cell surface by an O-glycosylation-independent multistep process. J Biol Chem 1990;265:6410–6415.

82. Rappolee DA, Brenner CA, Schultz R, Mark D, Werb Z. Developmental expression of PDGF, TGF-α and TGF-β genes in preimplantation mouse embryos. Science 1988;241:1823–1825.

83. Lee DC. Expression of rat transforming growth factor alpha mRNA during development occurs predominantly in the maternal decidua. Mol Cell Biol 1987;7:2335–2343.

84. Wilcox JN, Derynck R. Developmental expression of transforming growth factors alpha and beta in mouse fetus. Mol Cell Biol 1988;8:3415–3422.

85. Madtes DK, Raines EW, Sakariassen KS, et al. Induction of transforming growth factor-α in activated human alveolar macrophages. Cell 1988;53:285–293.

86. Rappolee DA, Mark DA, Banda MJ, Werb Z. Wound macrophages express TGF-α and other growth factor in vivo: analysis by mRNA phenotyping. Science 1988;241:708–712.

87. Wilcox JN, Derynck R., Localization of cells synthesizing transforming growth factor-alpha mRNA in the mouse brain. J Neurosci 1988;8:1901–1904.

88. Coffey RJ, Derynck R, Wilcox JN, et al. Production and autoinduction of transforming growth factor-α in human keratinocytes. Nature 1987;328:817–820.

89. Liscia DS, Merlo G, Ciardiallo F, et al. Transforming growth factor-α messenger RNA localization in the developing adult rat and human mammary gland by in situ hybridization. Dev Biol 1990;140:123–131.

90. Snedeker SM, Browth CF, Augustine RP. Expression and functional properties of transforming growth factor α and epidermal growth factor during mouse mammary ligand ductal morphogenesis. Proc Natl Acad Sci USA 1991;88: 8167–8171.

91. Matsui Y, Halter SA, Holt JT, Hogan BLM, Coffey RJ. Development of mammary hyperplasia and neoplasia in MMTV-TGFα transgenic mice. Cell 1990;61:1147–1155

92. Lee DC. Overexpression of TGFα in transgenic mice: induction of epithelial hyperplasia, pancreatic metaplasia, and carcinoma of the breast. Cell 1990;61:1121–1135.

93. Vassar R, Fuchs E. Transgenic mice provide new insights into the role of TGFα during epidermal development and differentiation. Gene Dev 1991;5:714–727.

94. Derynck R, Goeddel V, Ullrich A, et al. Synthesis of mRNAs for transforming growth factors α and β and the epidermal growth factor receptor by human tumors. Cancer Res 1987;47:707–712.

95. Mann GB, Fowler KJ, Gabriel A, Nice EC, Williams RL, Dunn AR. Mice with a null mutation of TGF-α gene have abnormal skin architecture, wavy hair, and curly whiskers and often develop corneal inflammation. Cell 1991;73: 249–261.

96. Luetteke NC, Qiu TH, Peiffer RL, Oliver P, Smithies O, Lee DC. TGF-α deficiency results in hair follicle and eye abnormalities in targeted and waved-1 mice. Cell 1993;73:263–278.

97. Hilton DJ. LIF: lots of interesting functions. Trend Biochem Sci 1992;17:72–76.

98. Bhatt H, Brunet LJ, Stewart CL. Uterine expression of leukemia inhibitory factor coincides with the onset of blastocyst implantation. Proc Natl Acad Sci USA 1991;88:11408–11412.

99. Stewart CL, Kaspar P, Brunet LJ, et al. Blastocyst implantation depends on maternal expression of leukaemia inhibitory-factor. Nature 1992;359:76–79.

100. Heath JL. Can there be life without LIF? Nature 1992; 359:17.

101. Carswell EA, Old LJ, Kassel RL, Green S, Fiore N, Williamson B. An endotoxin-induced serum factor that causes necrosis of tumors. Proc Natl Acad Sci USA 1975;72:3666–3670.

102. Beutler B, Cerami A. The biology of cachectin/TNF—a primary mediator of the host response. Annu Rev Immunol 1989;7:625–655.

103. Gendron RL, Nestel FP, Lapp WS, Baines MG. Expression of tumor necrosis factor alpha in the developing nervous system. Int J Neurosci 1991;60:129–136.

104. Zolti M, Meirom R, Shemesh M, et al. Granulosa cells as a source and target organ for tumor necrosis factor-α. FEBS Lett 1990;261:253–255.

105. Rubin SC, Hoskins WJ, Markman M, et al. Synergistic activity of tumor necrosis factor and interferon in a nude mouse model of human ovarian cancer. Gyn Oncol 1989; 34:353–356.

106. Sancho-Tello M, Perez-Roger I, Imakawa K, Tilzer L, Terranova PF. Expression of tumor necrosis factor-α in the rat ovary. Endocrinology 1992;130;1359–1364.

107. Nakane A. TNF in listeriosis. In: Beutler B, ed. Tumor necrosis factors: the molecules and their emerging role in medicine. New York: Raven, 1992:285–292.

108. Sherry BA, Gelin J, Forg Y, et al. Anticachectin/tumor necrosis factor-α antibodies alternate development of cachexia in tumor models. FASEB J 1989;3:1956–1962.

109. Oliff A, Defeo-Jones D, Boyer M, et al. Tumors secreting human TNF/cachectin induce cachexia in mice. Cell 1987; 50:555–563.

110. Hotamisligil GS, Shargill NS, Spiegelman BM. Adipose expression of tumor necrosis factor-α: direct role in obesity-linked insulin resistance. Science 1993;259:87–91.

111. Keffer J, Robert L, Cazlaris H, et al. Transgenic mice expressing human tumor necrosis factor: a predictive genetic model of arthritis. EMBO J 1991;10:4025–4031.

112. Pfeffer K, Matsuyama T, Kundig TM et al. Mice deficient for the 55 kd tumor necrosis factor receptor are resistant to endotoxic shock, yet succumb to L. monocytogenes infection. Cell 1993;73:457–467.

113. DeChiara TM, Robertson EJ, Efstratiadis A. Parental imprinting of the mouse insulin-like growth factor II gene. Cell 1991;64:849–859.

114. DiChiara TM, Efstratiadis A, Robertson EJ. A growth-deficiency phenotype in heteozygous mice carrying an insulin-like growth factor II gene disrupted by targeting. Nature 1990;345:78–80.

115. Matzuk MM, Feingold MJ, Mather JP, Krummen L, Lu H, Bradley H. Development of cancer cachexia-like syndrome and adrenal tumors in inhibin-deficient mice. Proc Natl Acac Sci USA 1994;91:8817–8821.

116. Vassalli A, Matzuk MM, Gardner HAR, Lee KF, Jaenisch R. Activin/inhibin βB subunit gene disruption leads to defects in eyelid development and female reproduction. Genes Dev 1994;8:414–427.

CHAPTER 43

SEVERE COMBINED IMMUNODEFICIENCY MOUSE MODEL FOR CYTOKINE THERAPY

Reiko Namikawa

During the past decade, we have learned about a wide variety of cytokines and their receptors. These molecules regulate the hematopoietic and immune systems by controlling proliferation, differentiation, and function. One of the goals of cytokine research is to develop new therapeutic modalities based on the biological activities of these molecules. Because these regulatory molecules have important roles not only in physiological but also in various pathological conditions, such as inflammatory and malignant diseases, they may prove to be applicable to a wide range of human diseases. Indeed, some of the cytokines are already proving their usefulness in the clinic. For example, hematopoietic growth factors, such as granulocyte colony-stimulating factor (G-CSF) and granulocyte-macrophage CSF (GM-CSF), are currently used to treat patients with bone marrow failure (1,2). As another example, the interferons (IFNs) have been approved for clinical use for various diseases, including viral hepatitis and cancer (3).

Preclinical in vivo testing of cytokines is usually performed in primates, which apart from its expense, may not necessarily show the full range of effects of human cytokines. The pathology of certain diseases may not be reproduced in animal models closely enough to draw conclusions that are directly applicable to humans. Clinical trials often require a long period to obtain statistically significant data because of the heterogeneity of patient populations. Given the potential clinical importance of these regulatory factors, a relevant animal model for cytokine therapy, which would be intermediate between the laboratory and the clinic, would provide a great tool for the rapid development of new therapeutic modalities.

Such a model was developed following the work of Bosma and colleagues (4), who found a strain of mouse with a spontaneous mutation resulting in deficiencies in both cellular and humoral immunity. This severe combined immunodeficient (SCID) mouse (C.B-17 *scid/scid*) could not reject xenogenic tissues, and it therefore appeared to be an ideal recipient for human tissue implantation. Indeed, the SCID mouse has given rise to a new strategy in creating an in vivo animal model with functional human cells and organs.

In this chapter, SCID models with human hematolymphoid function are reviewed as a result of focusing on the SCID-hu mouse model. The results of our recent study of the in vivo effects of human cytokines on human hematopoiesis are also presented.

SCID MOUSE MODEL RECONSTITUTED WITH HUMAN HEMATOLYMPHOID CELLS

Three different types of the SCID mouse model reconstituted with human hematolymphoid cells have been reported. One, called the hu-PBL-SCID model, was created by Mosier and colleagues (5) by transferring mature peripheral blood leukocytes (PBL) from normal human donors into SCID mice. It was reported that a transient engraftment of both T and B cells of human origin was observed after injection into the peritoneal cavities of SCID mice. Recent studies have demonstrated that injected human T cells migrate first into mouse abdominal lymph nodes (6–8). Human T cells with mature phenotypes (CD3+, TCR α/β+, CD4, or CD8 single–positive) are then primarily detected in peripheral blood, spleen, and peritoneal cavity. Human T cells isolated from the peripheral blood of hu-PBL-SCID mice were found to be unresponsive to stimuli by anti-CD3 antibody, phytohemagglutinin, or allogeneic cells, but they proliferated in response to exogenous interleukin-2 (IL-2) (9,10). The mechanisms underlying this anergy of human T cells remains unclear. It is possible, however, that peripheral tolerance can be induced in xenoreactive T cells in vivo, probably due to the lack of human antigen-presenting cells, which may also explain the lack of severe acute graft-versus-host disease in this model.

Attempts to reconstitute immunodeficient mice with human bone marrow cells have been performed by intravenous injection of human bone marrow cells. Triple mutant mice (*bg/nu/xid*) were used as a recipient in the initial report (11,12); the SCID mouse was then demonstrated to sustain human hematopoiesis when animals were treated with human mast-cell growth factor, a fusion protein of IL-3 and GM-CSF, or both (13). In *bg/nu/xid* mice, which carry deficiencies in T, B, natural killer (NK), and lymphokine activated killer (LAK) cell function, human macrophage progenitors have been demonstrated to migrate to the murine marrow and to be maintained in this environment for several months. However, no mature cells were detected in this system. In contrast, multiple lineage of human cells could be maintained in SCID mice with exogenous human cytokine treatment. Differentiated human cells of myeloid and lymphoid lineages could be found in the murine marrow. Inclusion of erythropoietin resulted in human red blood cells in the peripheral blood (13). The advantage of this system, in comparison with the SCID-hu mouse model described below, is that human adult bone marrow cells can be implanted; therefore, human fetal tissues are not required. The presence of highly potent human growth factors, which are required for engraftment and maintenance of human hematopoiesis, might be a problem when this system is applied to evaluate the effects of cytokines on human hematopoiesis.

The other model, the SCID-hu mouse, was created by surgical implantation of pieces of human fetal hematolymphoid organs. In our initial report, fetal thymus and lymph nodes were demonstrated to grow and to maintain their functional organ structures (14). Since then, significant improvements have been achieved in this system, which are described in detail.

All the models described herein use the SCID mouse as a recipient of human cells. However, there is a significant biological difference between a mouse injected with human cells, such as hu-PBL SCID, and one implanted with human organs, such as the SCID-hu mouse. In the former systems, human cells reside in a mouse organ environment, whereas human cells reside and function in a human stromal microenvironment in the latter.

SCID-hu MOUSE

The SCID-hu mouse is a heterochimeric small animal model designed to support proliferation and differentiation of human hematolymphoid cells in mouse. It can be created by surgical implantation of human fetal hematolymphoid organs into a SCID mouse. The advantage of transplanting human hematolymphoid organs is that all the elements necessary to maintain active human hematolymphopoiesis, including progenitor cells and stromal cells, are likely to be transplanted as a functional unit. The cellular interactions may be maintained thereafter. In these animals, human lymphoid and hematopoietic cells proliferate and differentiate in human microenvironments, such as the thymus and bone marrow. Given the complexity of the regulatory mechanisms surrounding hematolymphopoiesis, it would seem preferable to sustain human progenitor cells in a microenvironment of human origin. Human hematolymphopoiesis might then be regulated in a manner much more analogous to that found in humans. The effects of exogenously provided growth factors might be evaluated more precisely because they may act not only directly on progenitor cells but also on stromal elements, which consequently modulate hematolymphopoiesis.

Currently, we commonly use two types of SCID-hu mice to study human hematopoiesis and lymphopoiesis in vivo. SCID-hu-Thy/Liv mice created by cotransplantation of pieces of fetal thymus and fetal liver can sustain long-term human T-cell poiesis in the thymus, whereas SCID-hu-BM mice transplanted with pieces of fetal bone containing bone marrow elements can maintain active long-term human hematopoiesis in the grafts.

SCID-hu-Thy/Liv model

When a small fragment of human fetal thymus is engrafted beneath the SCID mouse kidney capsule, it is reproducibly vascularized and will thereafter grow. However, cortical thymocytes are usually depleted 3 months after implantation, indicating that long-lasting progenitor cells for T cells do not exist inside the graft.

Because the liver is one of the major hematopoietic organs in fetal life, fragments of fetal liver that contain both the hematopoietic precursors and the stromal microenvironment were implanted adjacent to human thymus fragments (Thy/Liv) (15). The histology of conjoint Thy/Liv grafts showed a thymic structure that was indistinguishable from normal human thymus for periods as long as 6 to 11 months after transplantation. The cortex was filled with cortical thymocytes, indicating active T-cell lymphopoiesis. The profile of CD4 and CD8 expression on these thymocytes was very similar to that found in normal fetal thymocytes. Human T cells with an appropriate CD4/CD8 subset distribution could also be found in the peripheral blood of these mice (16).

Thus, long-term human T-cell lymphopoiesis could indeed be introduced in the mouse by this approach. Even more surprisingly, long-term multilineage differentiation of human hematopoietic cells could be maintained in the Thy/Liv grafts. By implanting liver fragments that were allogeneic in the major histocompatibility complex (MHC) to the thymus fragments, it was confirmed that progenitor cells derived from the coimplanted fetal liver gave rise not only to T cells, but also to myelomonocytic cells in the thymus.

Several investigators demonstrated that this Thy/Liv model can serve as a unique tool for studying events involved in intrathymic differentiation and selection of T cells. Human T cells in the SCID-hu-Thy/Liv mice were shown to be phenotypically normal and functionally competent. T cells developed in Thy/Liv grafts in syngeneic combination of thymus and liver can respond to mitogens or allogeneic human cells in vitro (16). Clonal analysis of these T cells demonstrated that their repertoire was polyclonal, alloreactive, and as devoid of self-reactive cells as normal thymocytes (17). By creating animals with Thy/Liv constructs in allogeneic combination (i.e., thymus and liver from different donors), it is possible to study the mechanisms involved in tolerance induction and in the selection of T-cell repertoire. Vandekerckhove and colleagues (18,19) analyzed the influence of thymic selection on human T cell responsiveness and on the usage of TCR Vβ gene. Furthermore, it was demonstrated that bacterial superantigens could modulate the T-cell repertoire by inducing clonal deletion (20,21).

These studies indicated that the Thy/Liv grafts function for T-cell development in a biologically relevant manner. Therefore, it seems conceivable that this animal model can be used to examine the effects of various cytokines on intrathymic T-cell development.

SCID-hu-BM model

The SCID-hu-BM model was developed to introduce human hematopoietic function into the SCID mouse. Simple subcutaneous surgical implantation of pieces (ap-proximately $5 \times 5 \times 10$ mm) of fetal long bone (18–24 weeks old) containing active hematopoiesis resulted in a reproducible engraftment of functional human bone marrow (22).

The implantation process was associated with an immediate decrease in hematopoietic activity, followed by a rapid recovery by 6 weeks. The cellular composition of the hematopoietic cells in the grafts after recovery was analyzed by flow cytometry. First, the human origin of these cells was confirmed by staining with a monoclonal antibody MEM-43 (CD59), which reacts with all nucleated human cells (23). Most of the grafts contained more than 70% CD59+ human cells when analyzed before 20 weeks post-transplantation. In a series of experiments that required 168 bone grafts, 148 (88%) contained greater than 70% human cells. In these 148 bone grafts, the percentage of CD59+ cells was 88 ± 7% (mean ± a standard deviation) analyzed 8 to 12 weeks after transplantation. After longer periods of engraftment (> 20 wk), the human marrow space was progressively replaced by murine hematopoietic cells.

Cytological examination demonstrated that these bone marrow cells consisted of multilineage cells, including lymphoid, myeloid, blastoid, erythroid, and megakaryocytic cells in varying stages of differentiation, as observed in normal bone marrow. It was confirmed that the distribution of surface phenotypes in these cells was concordant with that found in normal fetal marrow cells. Most of the lymphoid cells were positive for the human pan-B cell marker, CD19, and they were positive for the pre-B cell marker CD10 as well. Approximately 20% of lymphoid cells were surface immunoglobulin (Ig)M+, and approximately 4% expressed IgM and IgD. Myeloid cell populations in varying degrees of differentiation (i.e., most immature [CD33+CD15−], intermediate [CD33+CD15+], and most mature [CD33^{lo}CD15+] myeloid compartments) (24) could be observed.

Thus, the implanted bones were able to sustain normal human B-cell differentiation, as well as myeloid cell differentiation. However, a slight difference was observed in the ratio between the cells of B lymphoid lineage and of myeloid lineage. The percentage of myeloid cell population in the grafts was lower than that of normal fetal bone marrow, and that of B lymphoid cells was higher. This finding indicates that either myelopoiesis is suppressed or lymphopoiesis is promoted in the human marrow after engraftment into mouse. It is possible that the cross-reactivity of endogenous murine cytokines may influence human lymphopoiesis or myelopoiesis in this regard.

Hematopoietic progenitor cell activity in the grafts was measured by in vitro colony-forming unit (CFU-C) assay as a function of time after implantation. Committed progenitor cells for both granulocyte-macrophage lineage (CFU-GM) and erythroid cells (BFU-E) recovered rapidly 4 weeks after implantation, and they reached a steady-state by 6 to 8 weeks, with comparable numbers of progenitor cells to normal fetal bone marrow cells (approximately 100 CFU-GM and 200 BFU-E/10^5 human hematopoietic cells). The standard level of CFU-C activity could be maintained at least until 20 weeks after transplantation, suggesting that more primitive progenitor cells with multipotent and self-renewing capacity were also implanted.

Although a reasonable amount of BFU-E activity was maintained in the grafts, the level of erythropoiesis in the grafted marrow was found to be significantly lower than in the normal marrow. When erythropoietic activity was indicated as the percentage of nucleated erythroid precursor cells in total nucleated hematopoietic cells, it was 3.4 ± 2.1% in the grafts in comparison with 27.6 ± 3.2% in normal marrow. We reasoned that this low erythropoietic activity might be due to the lack of human erythropoietin (EPO), because EPO is mainly produced in the kidney. Indeed, exogenously provided human EPO can restore erythropoietic activity in the grafts to the normal level.

In summary, human fetal bone grafts in the SCID mouse can maintain multilineage, long-term human hematopoiesis in a human marrow environment for approximately 20 weeks after implantation. No exogenous cytokine treatment is required for engraftment. The application of this model for evaluating various hematopoietic growth factors is described in the next section.

IN VIVO EFFECTS OF HUMAN CYTOKINES ON HUMAN HEMATOPOIESIS IN SCID-hu MICE

The in vivo effects of various hematopoietic growth factors were evaluated with the SCID-hu-BM mouse. The standard protocol employed for these experiments was as follows. SCID-hu-BM mice 8 to 10 weeks postimplantation were treated with recombinant human (rh) growth factors for either 7 or 14 days. Growth factors were given through an osmotic minipump (Alza 2001 or 2002) so that the factors could be delivered constantly and continuously during the period of treatment. At the end of treatment, cells in the human bone grafts were harvested and analyzed for cellular composition and progenitor cell activity.

Effects of single administration of hematopoietic growth factors

EFFECT OF rhEPO OF HUMAN ERYTHROPOIESIS: SCID-hu mice were treated with varying doses of rhEPO (5–40 U/day) for 7 days (22). The level of EPO activity was measured as the percentage of nucle-

ated erythroid precursor cells in total nucleated hematopoietic cells. The human origin of these erythroid lineage cells was also confirmed by staining with an antibody specifically reactive to human glycophorin A (GPA), a marker for erythroid lineage cells. As described, human erythropoietic activity in the grafts was significantly lower compared with that of normal fetal marrow, although a normal level of erythroid progenitor cell activity (BFU-E) was maintained. It was reported that mouse EPO crossreacts to human erythroid cells in vitro (25), but it may not be sufficient to induce differentiation of human erythroid lineage cells in vivo. In fact, by providing human EPO exogenously, human erythropoiesis was restored to the level observed in the normal marrow (Fig. 43–1). The percentages of nucleated human erythroid cells in the bone grafts increased in a dose-dependent fashion. Flow cytometric analysis of the cells revealed that both nucleated and enucleated GPA-positive human erythroid cell populations increased after treatment with EPO, indicating that proliferation and differentiation of erythroid precursor cells were induced.

EFFECT OF rhG-CSF ON HUMAN MYELOPOIESIS: SCID-hu mice were treated with varying doses (0.25–2.0 μg/day) of rhG-CSF for 7 days (26). As expected, G-CSF treatment induced a dramatic change in cellular composition in the human marrow. Histological examination demonstrated that bone marrow cellularity increased with the expansion of myeloid cell populations. A marked increase in myeloid cell population was observed by flow cytometry (Fig. 43–2), even at the lowest dose tested. Flow cytometric analysis and differential counting of marrow cells revealed that the neutrophilic

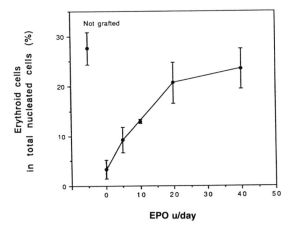

Figure 43–1   Effect of rhEPO on human erythropoiesis. SCID-hu mice were treated with varying doses of rhEPO for 7 days through osmotic minipumps. Erythropoietic activity in the human bone grafts was measured as the percentage of nucleated erythroid cells in total nucleated hematopoietic cells. Erythroid cells increase in a dose-dependent manner.

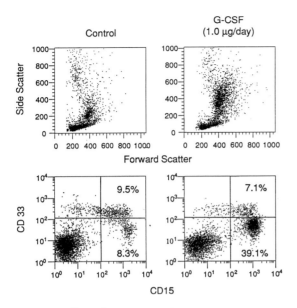

G-CSF
(1.0 µg/day)

Control

Figure 43–2 Effect of rhG-CSF on human myelopoiesis. SCID-hu mice were treated with rhG-CSF (1.0 µg/day) for 7 days through osmotic minipumps. Human bone marrow cells were analyzed by multiparameter flow cytometry. Scatter analysis (top panels) shows an increase of high-side scatter cells in treated samples. These cells correspond to the cells found in the lower right quadrant (CD33^{lo}CD15+) when stained with FITC-CD15 and PE-CD33 antibodies (lower panels).

granulocytes of later stages of differentiation were the major populations responding to rhG-CSF treatment. These cells were phenotypically CD33^{lo}CD15+ (24), as demonstrated in Fig. 43–2, and they were morphologically defined as metamyelocyte to band form of neutrophilic granulocytes.

Because G-CSF is known to induce emigration of mature granulocytes from bone marrow to circulation (27, 28), mouse peripheral blood was examined for human myeloid cells. The possible increase of human cell population in mouse blood was masked, however, by a huge increase of mouse granulocytes due to the crossreactivity of rhG-CSF on mouse hematopoiesis.

EFFECT OF rhIL-3 ON HUMAN HEMATOPOIESIS: Varying doses of rhIL-3 (1.2–12.0 µg/day) were administered for 14 days (26). It was shown that rhIL-3 treatment consistently induced an increase in E-BFU activity. The percentage of nucleated erythroid cells in the marrow was not increased, probably due to the lack of sufficient human EPO activity, as discussed. In contrast to rhG-CSF, rhIL-3 treatment increased eosinophilic lineage cells. Differential counting of marrow cells showed significant increases of eosinophilic granulocytes at all the doses tested, although a greater increase was shown at the highest dose. The effect of IL-3 on eosinophils was consistent with data from clinical trials, in which pronounced eosinophilia may develop in patients (29,30). IL-3–induced basophilia observed in monkeys (31,32) was not seen in SCID-hu mice nor in clinical trials.

EFFECT OF rhIL-6 ON HUMAN HEMATOPOIESIS: rhIL-6 (1.25–5.0 µg/day) was administered for 7 days (26). Unlike other factors described, rhIL-6 did not induce any significant changes in cellular composition in human bone marrow cells examined by flow cytometry and differential counting. Although IL-6 is known to induce platelet production in rodents (33,34) and primates (35), no evidence of increased human megakaryocytopoiesis was observed by histological examination. rhIL-6 was found to cause an increase in both CFU-GM and BFU-E activities.

Effects of combination treatment with human cytokines on human hematopoiesis in SCID-hu mice

On the basis of the results obtained by single administrations, we examined the effects of the growth factors when administered in combination (26). The combinations were chosen to have one factor acting on early progenitor cells (IL-3 or IL-6) and one of the lineage-restricted factors (G-CSF or EPO). Protocols used in these experiments are summarized in Table 43–1.

EFFECT OF SIMULTANEOUS TREATMENT WITH rhIL-6 AND rhEPO: When rhIL-6 (2.5 µg/day) was administered simultaneously in combination with rhEPO (20 U/day) for 7 days, the increase of erythroid cells induced by rhEPO was almost completely inhibited. No significant increase of erythroid cells was observed in bone grafts treated with rhEPO in combination with rhIL-6, whereas a single administration of rhEPO at this dose induced human erythropoiesis, as described. This unexpected inhibitory effect of rhIL-6 on EPO-induced erythropoiesis ws confirmed by an experiment with a fixed amount of rhEPO (20 U/day) in combination with varying doses of rhIL-6 (0.1–2.5 µg/day). Dose-dependent suppression of EPO-induced erythropoiesis was clearly demonstrated (Fig. 43–3). A possible explanation is that IL-6 may stimulate production of hematopoietic inhibitory factors from bone marrow stromal compartments, and thereby suppress erythropoiesis indirectly.

EFFECT OF SIMULTANEOUS TREATMENT WITH rhIL-6 AND rhG-CSF: SCID-hu mice were treated with rhG-CSF (0.25 µg/day) in combination with varying doses of rhIL-6 (1.25–5.0 µg/day) for 7 days. In this combination regimen, rhIL-6 showed a dose-dependent inhibitory effect on G-CSF–induced granulopoiesis. The percent of myeloid cells in the marrow treated with rhG-CSF along with rhIL-6 was significantly lower than

TABLE 43–1 EFFECTS OF COMBINATION CYTOKINE TREATMENTS
ON HUMAN HEMATOPOIESIS IN SCID-HU MICE

Combination	Protocol	Results
IL-6 + EPO	Simultaneous administration, 7 days	Suppression in EPO-induced erythropoiesis
IL-6 + G-CSF	Simultaneous administration, 7 days	Suppression in G-CSF–induced myelopoiesis
IL-3 + EPO	Sequential administration: IL-3, day 1–8; EPO, day 8–14	Enhancement of EPO-induced erythropoiesis
IL-3 + G-CSF	Sequential administration: IL-3, day 1–14; G-CSF, day 8–14	Increase in neutrophils and eosinophils

IL = interleukin; EPO = erythropoietin; G-CSF = granulocyte colony-stimulating factor.

that treated with rhG-CSF alone. The level of progenitors for myeloid cells (CFU-GM) was maintained, suggesting that the inhibitory effects of IL-6 may involve relatively differentiated stages of myeloid cells. Similarly to the inhibitory effect on EPO-induced erythropoiesis, this suppressive effect of IL-6 may be caused indirectly because IL-6 has been known to support myelopoiesis in vitro.

EFFECT OF SEQUENTIAL TREATMENT WITH rhIL-3 FOLLOWED BY rhEPO:

As described, a single administration of rhIL-3 increased BFU-E activity, and rhEPO induced proliferation and differentiation of ery-

throid cells in human marrow in SCID-hu mice. Therefore, we can predict that IL-3 may synergize with EPO on erythropoiesis. We treated SCID-hu mice with rhIL-3 (3 µg/day) for 7 days to allow an increase in committed progenitors; we then treated them with rhEPO (10 U/day) for the second week to induce maturation of erythroid cells. As expected, pretreatment with rhIL-3 significantly enhanced EPO-induced erythropoiesis (Fig. 43–4). The level of erythroid cell populations in the grafts treated with the combination of rhIL-3 and rhEPO was significantly higher than that in those treated with rhEPO alone.

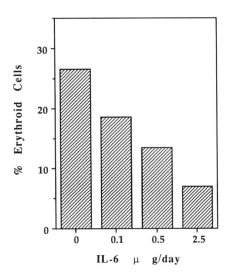

Figure 43–3 Effect of IL-6 on EPO-induced erythropoiesis. SCID-hu mice were treated with a fixed dose of rhEpo (20 U/day) in combination with varying doses of rhIL-6 for 7 days. Erythropoietic activity was measured as the percentage of nucleated erythroid cells in total nucleated hematopoietic cells. EPO-induced erythropoietic activity was suppressed by IL-6 in a dose-dependent fashion.

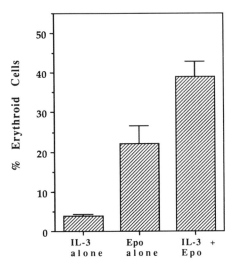

Figure 43–4 Effects of pretreatment with rhIL-3 on EPO-induced erythropoiesis. SCID-hu mice were treated with rhIL-3 (3 µg/day) for 7 days and then treated with rhEPO (10 U/day) for an additional 7 days. Erythropoietic activity was measured as the percentage of nucleated erythroid cells in total nucleated hematopoietic cells. The human bone grafts treated with IL-3 and EPO contained significantly higher levels of erythroid cell population in comparison with those treated with EPO alone for 7 days ($p = 0.0014$ by Student's t-test).

EFFECT OF SEQUENTIAL TREATMENT WITH rhIL-3 FOLLOWED BY rhG-CSF: To examine synergistic effects of IL-3 and G-CSF on myelopoiesis, SCID-hu mice were treated with rhIL-3 (3 μg/day) for 2 weeks in combination with rhG-CSF (1 μg/day) in the second week. By differential counting of marrow cells, a significant increase in both the neutrophilic and the eosinophilic granulocyte populations was noticed in the grafts treated with both factors. However, no additional increase of neutrophilic cells induced by G-CSF was observed following the addition of IL-3, and there was no augmentation by G-CSF of the increase in eosinophil population induced by IL-3. Thus, the combination of IL-3 and G-CSF in this treatment regimen resulted in an independent action of two cytokines. It is possible, however, that the synergistic effect may be observed with a lower dose of G-CSF because in vivo synergy of IL-3 and G-CSF has been reported in primates (36).

Effects of rhG-CSF on hematopoietic recovery after irradiation

In the experiments described, SCID-hu-BM mice were used at 8 to 10 weeks after implantation, when human hematopoiesis reaches a steady state (22). Thus, the effects of growth factors were analyzed in a "normal" hematopoietic state. Experiments to examine the effects of growth factors on damaged bone marrow were also performed, because growth factor treatments are often required in patients who have impaired hematopoietic activity after chemotherapy or radiotherapy. To mimic the clinical situation, SCID-hu mice were mildly irradiated (1 Gy). Immediately after irradiation, rhG-CSF treatment was initiated for 14 days. At the end of treatment, higher cellularity due to the increase of myeloid cell population was found in G-CSF–treated bone grafts compared with those receiving irradiation but no G-CSF treatment. It was also observed that rhG-CSF selectively increased the activity of committed progenitor cells for granulocytes (CFU-G) in treated marrow. Thus, rhG-CSF accelerated the recovery of myelopoiesis by stimulating proliferation and differentiation of myeloid progenitor cells that survived radiation exposure (37).

Discussion

We demonstrated that the SCID-hu mouse model could provide information on the effects of human cytokines on human hematopoiesis in vivo. As described, the effects of single or combination treatment of known growth factors have been analyzed either with the human marrow in a normal steady-state of hematopoiesis or with myelosuppressed marrow. Most of the results obtained from SCID-hu mice treated by single administrations of EPO, G-CSF, IL-3, or IL-6 were in accordance with those reported from clinical trials and animal experiments. Doses that showed significant effects on human hematopoiesis in SCID-hu mice approximated the ranges used in both clinical trials and in primate experiments (Table 43–2). Diverse modes of action of combination treatment, such as inhibitory, enhanced, or independent effects, have been demonstrated. These results suggest that the SCID-hu system is a

TABLE 43–2   COMPARISON OF THE DOSES USED IN SCID-hu MICE AND IN HUMANS OR PRIMATES

Factor	Dose in SCID-hu mice	Dose in humans/primates
G-CSF	0.25–2.0 μg/mouse/day (10–80 μg/kg/day)[a] (12.5–100 μg/m²/day)[b]	1–60 μg/kg/day (human, after chemotherapy [38,39]) 200 μg/m²/day (human, after chemotherapy [40])
IL-3	1.2–12.0 μg/mouse/day (48–480 μg/kg/day) (60–600 μg/m²/day)	30–500 μg/m²/day (human, normal [29,30]) 250–500 μg/m²/day (human, MDS[c] [41], AA [e] [42]) 3–100 μg/kg/day (Rhesus monkey [31,32,43,44])
IL-6	1.25–5.0 μg/mouse/day (50–200 μg/kg/day) (62.5–250 μg/m²/day)	30 μg/kg/day (Rhesus monkey [44]) 5–80 μg/kg/day (Cynomolgus monkey [35])

[a]Dose is calculated based on the mean mouse body weight as 25 gm.
[b]Dose is calculated based on the mean mouse body surface area as 200 cm².

relevant model for studying in vivo effects of human cytokines.

rhIL-6 inhibited EPO-induced erythropoiesis and G-CSF–induced myelopoiesis in SCID-hu mice. It is likely that these unexpected results are due to the indirect effect of IL-6. Taking the pleiotropic actions of IL-6 on various target cells into consideration (45–48), IL-6 may suppress hematopoiesis through stimulation of the production of hematopoietic inhibitory factors, such as TGF-β and TNF, from bone marrow stromal cells. These unexpected results, however, strongly suggest the importance of the relevant models in investigating the full range of in vivo effects of human cytokines for the following reasons. First, in vitro studies may not be able to reflect these indirect effects. Only in vivo systems can demonstrate the integrated outcome of elaborately regulated direct and indirect effects of pleiotropic factors, not only for IL-6, but also for other growth factors known to act in a pleiotropic fashion and to modulate the expression of other cytokines or their receptors. Second, the effects of cytokines may not necessarily be identical in different species. No suppressive effect of IL-6 on erythropoiesis in rodents has been previously reported (49), but the effects of IL-6 may differ among rodents, primates, and humans, because rhIL-6 did suppress erythropoiesis in cynomolgus monkeys (35). Concurrent anemia in certain disease states associated with elevated levels of IL-6 production, such as multiple myeloma (50) and rheumatoid arthritis (51), may also support our findings.

Thus, the SCID-hu model allows for creation of various experimental designs, depending on the questions to be answered. It will even be possible to study the effects of novel human cytokines on human hematolymphopoiesis. A caveat concerning this and other chimeric models is that in interpreting the results, one must consider the influence of endogenous mouse factors that may crossreact with human cells, such as IL-1 and IL-5.

POTENTIAL APPLICATIONS OF SCID-hu MOUSE MODEL TO DEVELOP CYTOKINE THERAPIES FOR HUMAN DISEASES

A SCID-hu mouse maintaining functional human lymphopoiesis and hematopoiesis could be used to create animal models for the study of human hematolymphoid disorders. It will be optimal, as a disease model, if human diseases can be reproducibly introduced into small animals in the context of functional human organs. Then, new therapeutic modalities can be evaluated in situations more closely analogous to the clinic. In this section, SCID-hu mouse models for the study of human infectious

diseases and human malignant diseases are introduced. The potential application of these models for studying the pathogenic or therapeutic roles of cytokines is also discussed.

Infection of human immune organs with human immunodeficiency virus

A basic premise underlying the experiments described herein is that the most useful animal model for human infectious diseases will be one in which infection by pathogenic agents for humans can occur in their natural hosts (i.e., human target organs). Pathology of viral infection found in patients may best be reproduced in this situation because viruses often have strict species and cell lineage specificities.

Human immunodeficiency virus (HIV) infection of human hematolymphoid organs in the SCID-hu mice has been well established and characterized (52–56). Infection of human CD4+ T cells and macrophages can be established either by direct injection of HIV into Thy/Liv grafts (52) or by intravenous injection of HIV into SCID-hu mice with fetal lymph node implants (55). The antiviral effects of AZT and ddI were demonstrated using these models (53–55), indicating that this model could be used for screening of potential antiviral compounds.

Researchers recently found that T cells in the infected thymus were accelerated toward apoptosis, or programmed cell death, which resulted in a rapid depletion of developing thymocytes (57). Although the mechanisms underlying this rapid depletion of thymocytes are not elucidated, it is possible that modulation of production of cytokines in the infected thymus may have an important role. The major target cell populations of HIV infection are CD4+ T cells and macrophages, the cell types which also have key roles in regulating the immune system. It is therefore conceivable that cytokines and monokines are involved in the pathology of HIV-infected individuals, but little is known about the role of cytokines in the processes of disease progression and the destruction of the immune system. SCID-hu mice infected with HIV may provide a unique opportunity to dissect the roles of cytokines, thereby developing new therapies.

Cytomegalovirus infection in SCID-hu mice

Human cytomegalovirus (CMV), a ubiquitous human virus, is an important pathogen of immunocompromised individuals. To establish an animal model for human CMV infection, SCID-hu mice implanted with various human fetal organs were examined. Among the organs tested, Thy/Liv conjoint implants were demonstrated to show reproducible and prolonged viral replication when infected with patient isolate of CMV. Histological examination revealed that the cell types that productively replicated CMV were mostly the epithelial cells located in the thymic medullary area. This epithelial cell compartment shares developmental origin of the pharyngeal pouch endoderm with the epithelial cells in submandibular salivary glands, known to be important sites of persistent replication of CMV in humans. With this model, it was demonstrated that a known anti-CMV compound, ganciclovir, suppressed replication of CMV (58).

CMV infection is one of the major problems of bone marrow transplantation patients. It has been reported that CMV infection occurs in approximately 60 to 70% of patients with allogeneic bone marrow transplantation who are CMV-seropositive prior to implantation or who receive CMV-seropositive marrow (59). In these patients, hematological abnormalities and impaired engraftment of marrow are frequently observed. Possible mechanisms of hematopoietic suppression could include induction of hematopoietic inhibitory factors or modulation of hematopoietic regulation caused by the infection of bone marrow elements with CMV (60). Because SCID-hu mice with human hematopoiesis are available, these questions can be directly addressed.

To study viral infection in conjunction with cytokine research is of particular interest, because many viral immune modulators have recently been discovered. Viruses pick up human cellular genes and incorporate them into their genome, perhaps because of the advantages for the infectivity and survival. These cellular genes include cytokines and their receptors. For instance, pox viruses carry the gene that encodes a protein mimicking the TNF receptor (61). Epstein-Barr virus contains a sequence homologous to IL-10 (62), and another herpes virus, CMV, has a product that binds to chemokines (63). The in vivo model for viral infection may provide a tool for understanding the role of these viral immune modulators, as well as the role of their cellular counterparts.

Human leukemia models

Human leukemias are highly lethal hematological malignancies characterized by abnormal proliferation and differentiation of hematopoietic progenitor cells. Despite recent advances in the identification of molecular events involved in leukemogenic processes, little is known about the regulatory mechanisms of proliferation and differentiation of human leukemias, due to the lack of suitable experimental systems. Many attempts have been made to create animal models of human leukemias using immune-deprived mice. However, the growth of human leukemia cells from patients in these animals was limited, probably because of the lack of a supportive environment or growth factors. Using the SCID-hu mouse as a leukemia model is therefore extremely advantageous because it can

provide a human bone marrow environment, the natural site where leukemia arises and proliferates.

Bone marrow cells from leukemia patients obtained at the time of diagnosis were directly injected into the pre-transplanted human fetal bone marrow in the SCID-hu mice. Cells from acute lymphoblastic leukemia (ALL) patients grew rapidly in the injected human marrow and spread into mouse marrow. In contrast, growth of myeloid leukemia cells was restricted in the human marrow, suggesting that they might require species-specific growth signals. The high frequency of successful propagation followed by establishment of serial in vivo passages with cells from myeloid leukemia patients clearly demonstrated the advantages of the SCID-hu mouse model (64).

Surface phenotypes and biological features of these leukemia cells growing in the SCID-hu mice were well maintained. Cells from acute myeloid leukemias (AML) or from chronic myeloid leukemia (CML) in blast crisis contained populations of varying degrees of differentiation toward myeloid cells, suggesting that the differentiative potential of myeloid leukemia cells from each patient was conserved in the SCID-hu mouse. Indeed, differentiation of promyelocytic leukemia cells growing in SCID-hu mice was demonstrated after treatment with all-trans-retinoic acid, a compound known to induce terminal differentiation of promyelocytic leukemia cells in patients (65,66).

Recently, the SCID mouse was shown to propagate human lymphoid leukemias (67,68,69) and myeloid leukemias (70,71). In contrast to the SCID-hu leukemia model, human leukemia cells grow in the murine hematopoietic organs in these systems. Different growth behaviors found in a SCID model and in the SCID-hu model suggest involvement of hematopoietic growth factors in engraftment of human leukemia cells. AML cells were reported to grow in SCID mouse marrow when human hematopoietic growth factors (a fusion protein of IL-3 and GM-CSF) were provided exogenously (72). In contrast, human myeloid leukemia cell lines dependent on either IL-3 or GM-CSF were demonstrated not to grow in the SCID mouse (71). These results suggest that the species-specific human cytokines, such as IL-3 and GM-CSF, are required for the proliferation of human leukemia cells in mouse. In the SCID-hu mouse model, however, growth and differentiation of human leukemia cells may be regulated by these factors, as well as by other regulatory molecules of human origin provided by bone marrow stromal elements.

More knowledge about regulation of normal and malignant hematopoiesis will lead to the development of new therapeutic modalities for leukemias. Modulation of differentiation or proliferation of leukemia cells by cytokines may provide new strategies for treating leukemias, such as IFN treatment of hairy-cell leukemia (73) and CML (74), in addition to the adjunctive roles of cytokines in current cytotoxic chemotherapies.

SUMMARY

I reviewed the SCID-hu mouse system with regard to human hematolymphoid organs and applications for cytokine research. This in vivo model may provide a useful preclinical tool for evaluating new therapeutic modalities with various hematopoietic growth factors and cytokines. Because the conclusions from such studies would be drawn from observations of human organs in vivo, it is likely that they will contribute relevant and meaningful insights into pathogenic and therapeutic roles for human cytokines in human disease states.

ACKNOWLEDGMENTS: The studies with SCID-hu mice presented herein were initiated at Stanford University with Drs. J. M. McCune, H. Kaneshima, M. Lieberman, and I. L. Weissman; they were then continued at SyStemix, Inc. The contributions of Drs. S. Kyoizumi and L. J. Murray are especially acknowledged for cytokine studies in SCID-hu mice. I would also like to acknowledge Drs. J. M. McCune and H. Kaneshima for scientific advice and continuous encouragement, the animal production group at SyStemix Inc. for excellent technical support, and Dr. D. Wylie for editorial assistance.

REFERENCES

1. Glaspy JA, Golde DW. Clinical trials of myeloid growth factors. Exp Hematol 1990;18:1137.

2. Metcalf D. Control of granulocytes and macrophages: molecular, cellular, and clinical aspects. Science 1991; 254:529.

3. Baron S, Tyring SK, Fleischmann WR, et al. The interferons. Mechanisms of action and clinical applications. JAMA 1991;266:1375.

4. Bosma GC, Custer RP, Bosma MJ. A severe combined immunodeficiency mutation in the mouse. Nature 1983; 301:527.

5. Mosier DE, Gulizia RJ, Baird SM, Wilson DB. Transfer of a functional human immune system to mice with severe combined immunodeficiency. Nature 1988;335:256.

6. Carlsson R, Martensson C, Kalliomaki S, Ohlin M, Borrebaeck CA. Human peripheral blood lymphocytes transplanted into SCID mice constitute an in vivo culture system exhibiting several parameters found in a normal humoral immune response and are a source of immunocytes for the production of human monoclonal antibodies. J Immunol 1992;148:1065.

7. Smith CIE, Abedi MR, Islam KB, Johansson MEB, Christensson B, Hammarstrom K. Humoral immunity in SCID mice reconstituted with cells from immunoglobulin-deficient or normal humans. Immunol Rev 1991;124:113.

8. Abedi MR, Christensson B, Islam KB, Hammarstrom L, Smith CIE. Immunoglobulin production in severe combined immunodeficient (SCID) mice reconstituted with human peripheral blood mononuclear cells. Eur J Immunol 1992;22:823.

9. Tary-Lehmann M, Saxon A. Human mature T cells that are anergic in vivo prevail in SCID mice reconstituted with human peripheral blood. J Exp Med 1992;175:503.

10. Simpson E, Farrant J, Chandler P. Phenotypic and functional studies of human peripheral blood lymphocytes engrafted in SCID mice. Immunol Rev 1991;124:98.

11. Kamel-Reid S, Dick JE. Engraftment of immune-deficient mice with human hematopoietic stem cells. Science 1988; 242:1706.

12. Dick JE. Immune-deficient mice as models of normal and leukemic human hematopoiesis. Cancer Cells 1991;3:39.

13. Lapidot T, Pflumio F, Doedens M, Murdoch B, Williams DE, Dick JE. Cytokine stimulation of multilineage hematopoiesis from immature human cells engrafted in SCID mice. Science 1992;255:1137.

14. McCune JM, Namikawa R, Kaneshima H, Shultz LD, Lieberman M, Weissman IL. The SCID-hu mouse: murine model for the analysis of human hematolymphoid differentiation and function. Science 1988;241:1632.

15. Namikawa R, Weilbaecher KN, Kaneshima H, Yee EJ, McCune JM. Long-term human hematopoiesis in the SCID-hu mouse. J Exp Med 1990;172:1055.

16. Krowka JF, Sarin S, Namikawa R, McCune JM, Kaneshima H. Human T cells in the SCID-hu mouse are phenotypically normal and functionally competent. J Immunol 1991; 146:3751.

17. Vandekerckhove BAE, Krowka JF, McCune JM, de Vries JE, Spits H, Roncarolo MG. Clonal analysis of the peripheral T cell compartment of the SCID-hu mouse. J Immunol 1991;146:4173.

18. Vandekerckhove BAE, Namikawa R, Bacchetta R, Roncarolo MG. Human hematopoietic cells and thymic epithelial cells induce tolerance via different mechanisms in the SCID-hu mouse thymus. J Exp Med 1992;175:1033.

19. Vandekerckhove BAE, Baccala R, Jones D, Kono DH, Theofilopoulos AN, Roncarolo MG. Thymic selection of the human T cell receptor Vβ repertoire in SCID-hu mice. J Exp Med 1992;176:1619.

20. Waller EK, Sen-Majumdar A, Kamel OW, Hansteen GA, Schick MR, Weissman IL. Human T-cell development in SCID-hu mice: Staphylococcal enterotoxins induce specific clonal deletions, proliferation, and anergy. Blood 1992;80: 3144.

21. Baccala R, Vandekerckhove BAE, Jones D, Kono DH, Roncarolo MG, Theofilopoulos AN. Bacterial superantigens mediate T cell deletions in the mouse severe combined immunodeficiency-human liver/thymus model. J Exp Med 1993;177:1481.

22. Kyoizumi S, Baum CM, Kaneshima H, McCune JM, Yee EJ, Namikawa R. Implantation and maintenance of functional human bone marrow in SCID-hu mice. Blood 1992;79: 1704.

23. Stefanova I, Hilgert I, Kristofova H, Brown R, Low MG, Horejsi V. Characterization of a broadly expressed human leucocyte surface antigen MEM-43 anchored in membrane through phosphatidylinositol. Mol Immunol 1989;26:153.

24. Terstappen LWMM, Loken MR. Myeloid cell differentiation in normal bone marrow and acute myeloid leukemia assessed by multidimensional flow cytometry. Analyt Cell Pathol 1990;2:229.

25. Shoemaker CB, Mitsock LD. Murine erythropoietin gene: cloning, expression, and human gene homology. Mol Cell Biol 1986;6:849.

26. Kyoizumi S, Murray LJ, Namikawa R. Preclinical analysis of cytokine therapy in the SCID-hu mouse. Blood 1993; 81:1479.

27. Tamura M, Hattori K, Nomura H, et al. Induction of neutrophilic granulocytosis in mice by administration of purified human granulocyte colony-stimulating factor (G-CSF). Biochem Biophys Res Commun 1987;142:454.

28. Ulich TR, Castillo JD, Souza L. Kinetics and mechanisms of recombinant human granulocyte-colony stimulating factor-induced neutrophilia. Am J Pathol 1988;133:630.

29. Ottman OG, Gancer A, Seipelt G, Eder M, Schultz G, Hoelzer D. Effects of recombinant human interleukin-3 on human hematopoietic progenitor and precursor cells in vivo. Blood 1990;76:1494.

30. Ganser A, Lindemann A, Seipelt G, et al. Effects of recombinant human interleukin-3 in patients with normal hematopoiesis and in patients with bone marrow failure. Blood 1990;76:666.

31. Wagemaker G, van Gils FCJM, Burger H, et al. Highly increased production of bone marrow-derived blood cells by administration of homologous interleukin-3 to rhesus monkeys. Blood 1990;76:2235.

32. Mayer P, Valent P, Schmidt G, Liehl E, Bettelheim P. The in vivo effects of recombinant human interleukin-3: demonstration of basophil differentiation factor, histamine-producing activity, and priming of GM-CSF-responsive progenitors in nonhuman primates. Blood 1989;74:613.

33. Ishibashi T, Kimura H, Shikama Y, et al. Interleukin-6 is a potent thrombopoietic factor in vivo in mice. Blood 1989; 74:1241.

34. Hill RJ, Warren MK, Levin J. Stimulation of thrombopoiesis in mice by human recombinant interleukin 6. J Clin Invest 1990;85:1242.

35. Asano S, Shibuya A, Hirano T, Kishimoto T, Takaku F, Akiyama Y. In vivo effects of recombinant human interleukin-6 in primates: stimulated production of platelets. Blood 1990;75:1602.

36. Krumwieh D, Weinmann E, Siebold B, Seiler FR. Preclinical studies on synergistic effects of IL-1, IL-3, G-CSF and GM-CSF in cynomolgus monkeys. Int J Cell Cloning 1990; 8(suppl 1):229.

37. Kyoizumi S, McCune JM, Namikawa R. Direct evaluation of radiation damage to human hematopoietic progenitor cells in vivo. Radiation Res 1994;137:76.

38. Gabrilove JL, Jakubowski A, Scher H, et al. Effect of granulocyte colony-stimulating factor on neutropenia and associated morbidity due to chemotherapy for transitional-cell carcinoma of the urothelium. N Engl J Med 1988;318:1414.

39. Morstyn G, Campbell L, Souza LM, et al. Effect of granulocyte colony stimulating factor on neutropenia induced by cytotoxic chemotherapy. Lancet 1988;1:667.

40. Ohno R, Tomonaga M, Kobayashi T, et al. Effect of granulocyte colony-stimulating factor after intensive induction therapy in relapsed or refractory acute leukemia. N Engl J Med 1990;323:871.

41. Ganser A, Seipelt G, Lindemann A, et al. Effects of recombinant human interleukin-3 in patients with myelodysplastic syndrome. Blood 1990;76:455.

42. Ganser A, Lindemann A, Seipelt G, et al. Effects of recombinant human interleukin-3 in aplastic anemia. Blood 1990;76:1287.

43. Geissler K, Valent P, Mayer P, et al. Recombinant human interleukin-3 expands the pool of circulating hematopoietic progenitor cells in primates—synergism with recombinant human granulocyte/macrophage colony-stimulating factor. Blood 1990;75:2305.

44. Geissler K, Valent P, Bettelheim P, et al. In vivo synergism of recombinant human interleukin-3 and recombinant human interleukin-6 on thrombopoiesis in primates. Blood 1992;79:1155.

45. Schindler R, Mancilla J, Endres S, Ghorbani R, Clark SC, Dinarello CA. Correlations and interactions in the production of interleukin-6 (IL-6), IL-1, and tumor necrosis factor (TNF) in human blood mononuclear cells: IL-6 suppresses IL-1 and TNF. Blood 1990;75:40.

46. Zhou D, Munster A, Winchurch RA. Pathologic concentrations of interleukin 6 inhibit T cell responses via induction of activation of TGF-β. FASEB J 1991;5:2582.

47. Van Bladel S, Libert C, Fiers W. Interleukin-6 enhances the expression of tumor necrosis factor on hepatoma cells and hepatocytes. Cytokine 1991;3:149.

48. Feldman GM, Ruhl S, Bickel M, Finbloom DS, Pluznik DH. Regulation of interleukin-4 receptors on murine myeloid progenitor cells by interleukin-6. Blood 1991;78:1678.

49. Pojda Z, Tsuboi A. In vivo effect of human recombinant interleukin 6 on hematopoietic stem cells and progenitor cells and circulating blood cells in normal mice. Exp Hematol 1990;18:1034.

50. Nachbaur DM, Herold M, Maneschg A, Huber H. Serum levels of interleukin-6 in multiple myeloma and other hematological disorders: correlation with disease activity and other prognostic parameters. Ann Hematol 1991;62:54.

51. Houssiau FA, Devogelaer J-P, Damme JV, Nagant de Deuxchaisnes C, Snick JV. Interleukin-6 in synovial fluid and serum of patients with rheumatoid arthritis. Arthritis Rheum 1988;31:784.

52. Namikawa R, Kaneshima H, Lieberman M, Weissman IL, McCune JM. Infection of the SCID-hu mouse by HIV-1. Science 1988;242:1684.

53. McCune JM, Namikawa R, Shih C-C, Rabin L, Kaneshima H. Suppression of HIV infection in AZT-treated SCID-hu mice. Science 1990;247:564.

54. Shih C-C, Kaneshima H, Rabin L, et al. Postexposure prophylaxis with zidovudine suppresses human immunodeficiency virus type 1 infection in SCID-hu mice in a time-dependent manner. J Infect Dis 1991;163:625.

55. Kaneshima H, Shih C-C, Namikawa R, et al. Human immunodeficiency virus infection of human lymph nodes in the SCID-hu mouse. Proc Natl Acad Sci USA 1991;88:4523.

56. McCune JM, Kaneshima H, Krowka J, et al. The SCID-hu mouse: a small animal model for HIV infection and pathogenesis. Annu Rev Immunol 1991;9:399.

57. Bonyhadi ML, Rabin L, Salimi S, et al. HIV induces thymus depletion in vivo. Nature 1993;363:728.

58. Mocarski ES, Bonyhadi M, Salimi S, McCune JM, Kaneshima H. Human cytomegalovirus in a SCID-hu mouse: thymic epithelial cells are prominent targets of viral replication. Proc Natl Acad Sci USA 1993;90:104.

59. Meyers JD, Fluornoy N, Thomas ED. Risk factors for cytomegalovirus infection after human marrow transplantation. J Infect Dis 1986;153:478.

60. Childs B, Emanuel D. Cytomegalovirus infection and compromise. Exp Hematol 1993;21:198.

61. Smith CA, Davis T, Wignall JM, et al. T2 open reading frame from the Shope Fibroma Virus encodes a soluble form of the TNF receptor. Biochem Biophys Res Commun 1991;176:335.

62. Vieira P, de Waal Malefyt R, Dang M, et al. Isolation and expression of human cytokine synthesis inhibitory factor (CSIF/IL-10) cDNA clones: homology to Epstein-Barr virus open reading frame BCRF1. Proc Natl Acad Sci USA 1991;88:1172.

63. Neote K, DiGregorio D, Mak JY, Horuk R, Schall TJ. Molecular cloning, functional expression, and signaling characteristics of a C-C chemokine receptor. Cell 1993,72:415.

64. Namikawa R, Ueda R, Kyoizumi S. Growth of human myeloid leukemias in the human marrow environment of SCID-hu mice. Blood 1993;82:2526.

65. Huang ME, Ye YI, Chen SR, et al. Use of all-trans-retinoic acid in the treatment of acute promyelocytic leukemia. Blood 1988;72:567.

66. Castaigne S, Chomienne C, Daniel MT, et al. All-trans retinoic acid as a differentiation therapy for acute promyelocytic leukemia. I. Clinical results. Blood 1990;76:1704.

67. Kamel-Reid S, Letarte M, Sirard C, et al. A model of human acute lymphoblastic leukemia in immune-deficient SCID mice. Science 1989;246:1597.

68. Cesano A, O'Connor R, Lange B, Finan J, Rovera G, Santoli D. Homing and progression patterns of childhood acute lymphoblastic leukemias in severe combined immunodeficiency mice. Blood 1991;77:2463.

69. Kamel-Reid S, Letarte M, Doedens M, et al. Bone marrow from children in relapse with pre-B acute lymphoblastic leukemia proliferates and disseminates rapidly in scid mice. Blood 1991;78:2973.

70. Sawyers CL, Gishizky ML, Quan S, Golde DW, Witte ON. Propagation of human blastic myeloid leukemias in the SCID mouse. Blood 1992;79:2089.

71. Cesano A, Hoxie JA, Lange B, Nowell PC, Bishop J, Santoli D. The severe combined immunodeficient (SCID) mouse as a model for human myeloid leukemias. Oncogene 1992;7:827.

72. Lapidot T, Sirard C, Vormoor J, Minden M, Hoang T, Dick JE. AML blast cells obtained from newly diagnosed patients engraft and proliferate in SCID mice in response to cytokines (abstract). Blood 1992;80(suppl 1):32a.

73. Saven A, Piro LD. Treatment of hairy cell leukemia. Blood 1992;79:1111.

74. Talpaz M, Kantarjian HM, McCredie K, Trujillo JM, Keating MJ, Gutterman J. Hematologic remission and cytogenetic improvement induced by recombinant human interferon alpha, in chronic myelogenous leukemia. N Engl J Med 1986;314:1065.

CHAPTER 44

CYTOKINE GENE THERAPY FOR CANCER

Barbara Pippen and Michael Lotze

The first approved clinical studies of gene transfer were conducted in the Surgery Branch of the National Cancer Institute (NCI), and they examined the safety and efficacy of retroviral-mediated transfer of the marker gene, bacterial neomycin phosphotransferase, in tumor infiltrating cells (TILs). We were able to show that TILs bearing the genetic marker could be detected by polymerase chain reaction (PCR) many months after adoptive transfer. Similarly, Brenner and colleagues (1) showed that bone marrow cells marked with the same retroviral vector could be detected in the periphery 3 months after transfer, as well as tumor cells presumably present in the transplanted bone marrow. Studies of retroviral transfer of the adenosine deaminase gene into children with that enzyme deficiency have also resulted in clinical improvement. These studies as well as murine models suggest the potential of gene therapy of cancer with the genetic delivery of immunological agents, including cytokines such as interleukin-2 (IL-2), IL-4, tumor necrosis factor (TNF), and other alternative immunological strategies, including introduction of requisite costimulatory signals, such as B7. Potential applications in transplantation include delivery of immunosuppressive cytokines, such as viral IL-10 or transforming growth factor-β (TGF-β) directly at the site of the transplanted organ or cell.

There are many ways tumor cells escape immune recognition. One potential mechanism is by inducing T-cell anergy. Activation of naive T cells requires at least two discrete signals: the direct interaction of the T-cell receptor with a major histocompatibility complex (MHC) peptide antigen complex, and often a second costimulatory signal, which can be a release of a soluble factor (e.g., IL-1 or IL-6) or a surface molecule (e.g., expression of the CD28 ligand, B7). Absence of the appropriate second signal in the presence of the MHC antigen complex can lead to T-cell anergy or unresponsiveness (2). One presumed mechanism for the tolerizing effects of tumor cells is lack of the second costimulatory signal, which leads to T-cell anergy (3). This tolerizing effect on T cells in the periphery is primarily against immunodominant epitopes, but not necessarily subdominant epitopes; therefore, T cells still exist in the circulation that could be stimulated to respond to these less immunogenic species.

Cytokines are largely paracrine, occasionally autocrine or endocrine, hormones that act primarily within the immune system. They are produced mainly by lymphocytes (lymphokines) and monocytes (monokines). These pleiotropic mediators can modulate and shape the quality and intensity of the immune responses, either activating and augmenting or alternatively suppressing some immunological events. Systemic anticancer therapy using these agents as biological modifiers presumably takes advantage of these immunostimulatory effects. Cytokine antitumor activity seems to be an antitumor effect in several ways: (a) direct inhibition of tumor growth (interferon-α [IFN-α]) (b) delivery of immune effectors to tumor sites (IL-2), (c) by effectively overcoming the anergy-inducing effects of tumor cells and allowing induction of new T-cell effectors, (d) by augmenting the effector function of T cells recognizing MHC-presented peptide epitopes on tumor cells, and (e) by direct antiproliferative effects. Cytokines can be delivered systemically (subcutaneous, intravenous), regionally (intraperitoneal, intralymphatic), or locally (intraarterial delivery, cytokine gene therapy). Some of the rationale for cytokine gene therapy is dictated by the notion that local delivery of cytokines most closely mimics the natural immune response and that many cytokines cannot be tolerated when administered at high systemic levels required for an effective response.

IL-2 transfection was used first as a means to deliver this cytokine locally (4). TNF transfection of tumors was initially tested to demonstrate its effects, but it was also "inadvertently" shown to delay tumor growth (5). The mature phase of cytokine gene therapy began in earnest only a few years ago, with the reports of Tepper and associates (6) of IL-4 transfection and those of Fearon and colleagues (7) with IL-2 transfection. Since then, virtually every available cytokine has been tested in murine tumor models, often before much of the biology of such cytokines was understood.

We sequentially review each of the cytokines tested, analyze their efficacy, and consider new approaches for the future. For all studies, we consider three separate and increasingly difficult objectives of cytokine gene delivery: type I studies—to abrogate establishment of tumor; type II—to immunize naive animals against wild-type tumor using local cytokine delivery along with irradiated transfected tumor vaccines; and type III—to treat animals with established tumors. Many of the studies performed to date have generated only minimal information about effects over a broad dose range, which makes it impossible to truly compare the efficacy of individual cytokines. Cytokines potentially useful in gene therapy are listed in Table 44–1, and the murine models are listed in Table 44–2.

INTERLEUKIN 2

The first biological agent reported in cytokine gene therapy was IL-2 (4). IL-2 is a growth factor that stimulates the proliferation of cytotoxic T cells (8), helper T cells (9), and natural killer (NK) cells (10), and it stimulates the cytolytic activity of both T and NK cells (known as lymphokine activated killer [LAK] activity) (11). These important effector cells of the immune system also have a significant role in cancer therapy. Bubenik and colleagues (4), in a pioneering study using retroviral transduction of fibroblasts with the IL-2 gene, showed that local production of IL-2 substantially inhibited the establishment and growth of human HeLa tumor cells in athymic BALB/c

mice. In addition, IL-2–activated splenocytes from these animals were cytotoxic for HeLa and other tumor targets, suggesting that LAK cells were important for the observed antitumor effects.

Subsequently, Fearon and co-workers (7) demonstrated that locally administered IL-2 could delay establishment and growth of two poorly immunogenic murine tumors, CT26 colon cancer and B16 melanoma. Decreased tumor progression was correlated with increased cytolytic T-cell function in treated animals, suggesting a possible T-helper deficiency in the antitumor response of untreated mice. Furthermore, long-term protective immunity to parental B16 cells could be generated by immunizing with the IL-2–transfected B16 tumor. Using the murine fibrosarcoma CMS-5, Gansbacher and associates (12) confirmed that local IL-2 administration via gene transfection of tumor cells could abrogate tumorigenicity as well as induce long-lasting protective immunity against subsequent challenge with the parental tumor cells.

Recently, Connor and co-workers (13) showed that IL-2 produced by transfected MBT-2 (a FANFT-induced murine bladder tumor) cells can be effectively used to treat C3H mice with pre-existing palpable bladder tumors. Seven days following intravesical instillation of parental 2×10^4 MBT-2 cells and then at weekly intervals (3×), mice were treated with 5×10^6 irradiated IL-2–secreting MBT-2 cells. Treatment delayed tumor progression by 20 days in two of five mice and resulted in complete tumor regression in three of five. These three mice remained tumor-free for more than 8 weeks, and they were resistant to subsequent challenge with parental MBT-2. Treatment of mice with IFN-γ–secreting cells, cisplatin, or a combination of either with IL-2–secreting tumors had individually a less pronounced effect in decreasing tumor growth or enhancing survival. When mice exhibiting long-term tumor regression were rechallenged with intravesicular instillation of parental MBT-2 cells, no tumor growth was observed in nine of nine mice tested, demonstrating that effective immunological memory had been established.

Tsai and associates (14) observed that induction of antitumor immunity by local IL-2 production seems to be most effective when this cytokine is secreted by the tumor cells, rather than by accesory carriers, such as fibroblasts. The BALB/c mouse mammary tumor line, 4T07, and an immortalized fibroblast line established from syngeneic mammary fatpads were both transfected with retroviral vectors encoding the cDNA for IL-2. A CTLL assay for IL-2 was used to demonstrate that 4TO7-IL-2 cells and IL-2–transfected fibroblasts secreted comparable amounts of IL-2 (1–3 ng/10^6 cells/24 hr and 3–6 ng/10^6 cells/24 hr, respectively). BALB/c mice were treated with 4T07 cells (3×10^5) coinjected with either 4T07-IL-2 cells (3×10^5) of IL-2–secreting fibroblasts (3×10^6). 4T07-IL-2 cells were found to induce active long-term immunity, and

TABLE 44–1   CYTOKINES TESTED IN GENE THERAPY OF CANCER

Cytokine	MW	Normal Cell Source	Target Cells	Effects
IL-1	17 kd; monomer	Macrophages	Most mammalian cells	Immunoaugmentation (inflammatory and hematopoietic)
IL-2	15 kd; monomer	T cells, LGL	T cells, B cells	Activates T cells, NK cells, and macrophages
IL-3	14–28 kd; monomer or homodimer	T cells	Myeloid cells	Hematopoietic growth factor; promotes growth of early myeloid progenitor cells
IL-4	20 kd; monomer	T cells, mast cells	T cells, B cells, eosinophils, endothelial cells, macrophages	Promotes IgE reactions; activates target cells; immunostimulation
IL-6	22–30 kd; monomer	Fibroblasts, T cells, endothelial cells	B cells	Augments inflammation; B-cell growth factor; augments polyclonal immunoglobulin production
IL-7	25 kd; monomer	Stromal cells (thymus and bone marrow)	T cells, B cells	Generates pre-B and pre-T cells; lymphocyte growth factor; lymphopoetin
IL-10	20 kd; homodimer	T cells, macrophages, monocytes, some tumors cells	B cells	Stimulates B cells; antiinflammatory; DTM inhibition; immunosuppression
IL-12	75 kd; heterodimer	Macrophages, B cells, (?) PMNs	NK cells, T cells	Stimulates IFN-γ production and proliferation and cytotoxicity of target cells; promotes Th1 cellular immune response
TGF-β	14 kd; monomer or heterodimer	Platelets, bone, some human cells	Most mammalian cells	Immunosuppression, wound healing, bone remodeling
TNF-α	17 kd; homodimer	T cells, macrophages	Most mammalian cells	Inflammation; immunoenhancing; tumoricidal; augments vascular thrombosis and tumor necrosis
IFN-γ	20–25 kd; homodimer	Th1 cells, NK cells	NK cells, macrophages, all cells	Stimulates target cells; induces MHC antigens and other proteins; antiviral antiproliferative, and immunomodulation
G-CSF	18–22 kd; monomer	Monocytes	Neutrophils	Differentiation of mature neutrophils; myeloid growth factor

IL = interleukin; TGF = transforming growth factor; TNF = tumor necrosis factor; G-CSF = granulocyte colony-stimulating factor; IFN = interferon.

TABLE 44–2　RESULTS OF CYTOKINE GENE THERAPY IN MURINE MODELS

Cytokine	Ref	Tumor	Strain	I*	II*	III*
IL-2	Bubenick, 1988 (4)	HeLa	nu/nu	X		
	Gansbacher, 1990 (12)	CMS-5	BALB/c	X	X	
	Fearon, 1990 (7)	CT26	BALB/c	X		
		B16	C57BL/6	X	X	
	Connor, 1993 (13)	MBT-2	C3H/HeJ	X	X	X
	Tsai, 1993 (14)	4TO7	BALB/c	X	X	
IL-3	Lord, 1993 (16)	Murine Line 1	BALB/c	X		
IL-4	Tepper, 1989 (6)	CT26	BALB/c	X	X	
	Golumbek, 1991 (24)	Renca	BALB/c	X	X	X
	Modesti, 1993 (25)	TS/A	BALB/c	X	X	
	Tepper, 1993 (22)	U87	nu/nu	X		
IL-6	Blankenstein, 1991 (29)	J558L	BALB/c			
	Sun, 1992 (30)	B16	C57BL/6	X		
	Porgador, 1992 (31)	D122	C57BL/6	X	X	
IL-7	Hock, 1991 (39)	J558L	Balb/c	X		
		TS/A		X		
G-CSF	Colombo, 1991 (58)	CMS-5	Balb/c	X		
IFN-γ	Watanabe, 1990 (42)	C1300	C57BL/6	X		
	Gansbacher, 1990 (43)	CMS-5	Balb/c	X	X	
	Restifo, 1992 (44)	MCA 101 MCA 102	C57BL/6	X		
	Porgador, 1992 (45)					
GM-CSF	Dranoff, 1993 (59)	B16 Lewis lung carcinoma WP-4	C57BL/6	X	X	
		RENCA CMS-5 CT-26	BALB/c			
TNF-α	Asher, 1991 (54)	MCA205	C57BL/6	X	X	
	Teng, 1991 (55)	1591-RE	nu/nu	X		
	Blankenstein, 1991 (29)	J558L	Balb/c	X		

*I = delay/inhibition of tumor establishment; II = vaccine/immunization effect; and III = therapy for pre-existing tumor.
IL = interleukin; G-CSF = granulocyte colony-stimulating factor; IFN = interferon; TNF = tumor necrosis factor.

they were able to both cause rejection of the immunizing tumor (by day 25, tumor incidence had been reduced from 100 to 0%), whereas the IL-2–secreting fibroblasts could not reduce tumorgenicity (by day 25, 100% of mice had nonregressing tumor). In a type II (vaccine) experiment, mice injected with 4T07-IL-2 cells coadministered with irradiated 4T07 were able to resist challenge with parental 4T07 on the contralateral side compared with control mice. Fourteen days after challenge, tumors developed in 12 of 13 untreated control mice (mean size, 234 ± 48 mm^3), and tumors developed in 10 of 12 control mice pretreated with irradiated tumor alone (mean size, 139 ± 37 mm^3); tumor developed in 2 of 10 4T07-IL-2–treated mice (mean size, 16 ± 11 mm^3).

Establishment of the technique of local cytokine delivery through genetic manipulation opened the way for the study of antitumor effects of other cytokines, such as IL-4, IFN-γ, TNF, GM-CSF, and IL-7. All these cytokines, as is true with virtually all immunostimulatory cytokines, can delay tumor establishment in vivo when delivered locally. Forni (personal communication) showed that multiple injections were superior to single immunization and that lower concentrations of IL-2 produced locally were superior in inducing an immune response, whereas higher doses were more effective in causing rejection of transfected tumor. Finally, for therapy, only approximately 20% of animals immunized after tumor implantation could generate an immune response capable of causing regression of established tumor.

INTERLEUKIN 3

IL-3 is a pluripotent hematopoietic growth factor. It increases maturation and development of cells of the myeloid lineage, and it has been used clinically to treat myelosuppression in patients who have received chemotherapy (15). Recently, Pulaski and colleagues (16) showed that expression of IL-3 by the BALB/c murine line 1 lung carcinoma could elicit tumor rejection by enhancing the development of CD4+-dependent cytotoxic T lymphocytes (CTL). TIL obtained from these tumors was shown to include CTL that developed similiarly to those observed for IL-2–producing tumors. mRNA for IL-2 was observed within the IL-3–producing tumors, but not within parental tumors, suggesting that IL-3 might elicit CTL indirectly by stimulating release of CTL growth factors from T-helper cells. Despite the presence of IL-2 and the role of T-helper cells in the development of cytolytic cells within the IL-3–secreting tumors, TIL isolated from tumors producing IL-2 and those producing IL-3 differed in their ability to induce nonspecific effector activity. TIL isolated from the IL-2–transfected tumors lysed YAC-1 very effectively, whereas TIL from the IL-3–transfected tumors did not. In a more recent article (17), this same group observed that IL-3 inhibits the development of nonspecific killer cells both in vitro and in vivo. Furthermore, this inhibition is dependent on the presence of IL-3 early in the development of nonspecific killer cells. Addition of IL-3 at the initiation of IL-2 stimulated culture; 1 day later, it had a

strong inhibitory effect on the generation of nonspecific killer cells, whereas addition of IL-3 on days 2 or 3 had little effect.

INTERLEUKIN 4

IL-4, a Th2 cytokine, was first characterized as a B-cell growth factor that induced isotype switching in B cells (18). IL-4 also serves as a T-cell growth factor, and, especially in mice, it enhances the cytolytic activity of T cells and NK cells (19). It also up-regulates expression of adhesion molecules, such as VCAM, which leads to binding and retention of macrophages, eosinophils, and neutrophils at sites of inflammation (20). In contrast to IL-2, IL-4 can activate and augment both antibody and T-cell responses, as well as nonspecific inflammation, making it a unique molecule for treating cancer.

Tepper and colleagues (6) transfected the IL-4 gene into two different murine tumor cell lines, the BALB/c plasmacytoma J558L and the mammary adenocarcinoma K4851. Multiple transfected cell lines that produced 0 to 5 U/mL/10^6 cells/48 hr were created. High IL-4–producing cells could elicit an antitumor effect in BALB/c mice. Early infiltrates at tumor inoculation sites lacked T cells and consisted mainly of eosinophils and macrophages. Furthermore, tumor formation was blocked when these IL-4 gene–transfected tumors were injected into athymic nude mice, suggesting that the observed initial antitumor effect was T-cell–independent.

Another report from this group (21) suggests that the mechanism of the immediate antitumor effect of IL-4 is eosinophil-dependent. C57BL/6 mice were depleted of eosinophils using MAb RB6-8C5, a monoclonal antibody that binds to surface antigens present on mature granulocytes (thus depleting neutrophils as well as eosinophils). Inoculation of such mice with both low (10,000 U/10^6 cells/48 hr) and high (20,000 U/10^6 cells/48 hr) IL-4–producing B16 tumor cells resulted in failed tumor growth in animals bearing high IL-4–producing tumor plus Mab RB6-8C5, whereas tumor formation was restored in animals bearing low IL-4 producers and MAb RB6-8C5. In both cases, addition of anti-IL-4 antibody restored tumorigenicity. The growth of implanted tumor was inversely correlated with eosinophilic inflammation at the tumor inoculation site.

A more recent report by the same group supports this observation (22). Yu and associates (22) report that there was significant inhibition of the growth of two glioma lines in nude mice when LT-1 (IL-4–secreting J558L) tumor cells were coadministered. Subcutaneous growth of the rat glioma cell line C6-BAG, when mixed with LT-1, was markedly inhibited compared with control mice during a 27-day observation period. Subcutaneous injections of U87 human glioma when mixed with LT-1 cells were completely rejected during a 34-day observation period, whereas very large tumors developed in contalateral control mice (U87 + J558L). Histological study of C6-BAG or U87 glioma + LT-1 tumor infiltrates three days after injection revealed tumor necrosis and an eosinophilic infiltrate containing occasional macrophages, whereas study of glioma + J558L control mice showed aggressive tumor growth without necrosis or infiltrate. In situ intracerebral administration of U87 glioma + LT1 cells also inhibited tumor growth compared with U87 + J558L control mice. By 9.5 weeks after implantation, all control animals were dead, whereas 6 of 12 (50%) animals receiving LT-1 cells survived. By week 13, 4 of 12 (33%) from the LT-1 group were healthy and neurologically normal. Hematoxylin and eosin staining of control brains 4 days after inoculation revealed glial tumor infiltrating into normal tissue, with a small necrotic area and no evidence of inflammatory response, whereas LT-1–treated brain showed that the majority of the tumor was necrotic, with granulocytic infiltrate throughout. Giemsa staining revealed tht this infiltrate consisted almost entirely of eosinophils. At 19 days and 7.5 weeks postimplant, U87/LT-1–treated brain was without evidence of tumor or inflammation, whereas control brain at 19 days showed a large ventral glial tumor made of pleomorphic cells with prominant nuclei, several of which were undergoing mitosis, and no evidence of necrosis or inflammatory infiltrate.

Blankenstein and coworkers (23) also introduced IL-4 locally into IL-4–dependent CT.4S cells to assess the function of IL-4 as an autocrine growth factor. IL-4–transfected CT.4S cells proliferated in the absence of exogenous IL-4 in vitro. In contrast to studies with other "autocrine" growth factors, such as IL-6, these cells were unable to grow in mice, which suggested that IL-4 induced local immune processes that inhibit the growth of CT.4S cells.

Golumbek and associates (24) reported similar findings using Renca (renal carcinoma) and CT26 (colon carcinoma) cell lines. Using IL-4–transfected tumor cells, they were able to show complete inhibition of tumor establishment, even at high tumor doses (2×10^7). Even though the early tumor infiltrate consisted primarily of macrophages and granulocytes, the sustained antitumor response was due to CD8+ T cells that were associated with long-lasting, tumor-specific immunity. Subsequent challenges with parental tumors were completely rejected. Furthermore, Renca tumor cells engineered to secrete large amounts of IL-4 caused regression of 6- to 9-day established tumors, demonstrating the efficacy of IL-4 in treating pre-established cancer. Administration of 15,000 U/10^6/24 hr was effective, whereas lower doses (3,300 U/10^6/24 hr) were not. Subsequently, it was found - that simple irradiation of this tumor also induced sim-

ilar antitumor effects (Pardoll D, personal communication).

Modesti and coworkers (25) showed that systemic IL-4–activated TS/A tumor rejection is a multicell-mediated reaction involving granulocytes, macrophages, and lymphocytes, which causes direct membrane and cytoplasmic damage to the tumor cell. In contrast to the study by Tepper and colleagues, IL-4–activated tumor rejection in their studies did not occur in T-cell–depleted mice. One possible reason for this discrepancy is the differing amount of IL-4 available locally. Modesti and coworkers suggest that the high amount of IL-4 used in the Tepper experiments resulted in a strong immediate nonspecific response that did not require T-cell effects.

INTERLEUKIN 6

IL-6 is produced by a wide variety of cells, such as T-helper 2 cells, macrophages, and monocytes and, similar to IL-1, it is a critical component in the acute-phase inflammatory response (26). IL-6 is also an inducer of B-cell maturation and proliferation, as well as T-cell maturation (27,28). The first report of local IL-6 genetic delivery to treat tumors was conducted by Blankenstein and associates (29). They showed that 500 U/mL IL-6 production by J558L tumors had no effect on tumor growth when injected into mice. In a separate report, IL-6–transfected B16 tumors were capable of causing slowed tumor growth when compared with control cells, and this delayed growth seems to be related to nonspecific inflammatory mechanisms (30). Local IL-6 production led to significant inhibition of tumor growth that was associated with a heavy inflammatory infiltrate. Tumor cell adhesion to matrix protein–coated plastic surfaces was enhanced with IL-6 genetic transfer, and it was associated with a reduction in tumor angiogenesis.

In a comprehensive study of the effect of local IL-6 on the Lewis lung carcinoma cell line D122, inhibition of tumor growth was inversely related to the amount of IL-6 produced by tumor cells (31). Tumor suppression was also observed in nude mice, although it was not as vigorous as in normal mice, suggesting that both T-cell–independent and –dependent antitumor mechanisms exist. Moreover, IL-6 production markedly activated the anti-D122 cytolytic activity of CTLs, and it also enhanced macrophage localization at tumor sites. IL-6 also inhibited the metastatic potential of the tumor, as determined by counting foci of lung metastases (control animals showed bulky metastases, whereas those receiving IL-6–transfected B16 showed fewer and more discrete metastases). Long-term immunity against local tumor growth and tumor metastasis was achieved against D122 parental tumors if recipient animals were immunized previously with irradiated IL-6–producing D122 cells. Long-term immunity was not observed in nude mice recipients, indicating that antitumor memory requires T cells.

INTERLEUKIN 7

IL-7 was originally described as a B-cell growth factor for early B cells (32). IL-7 also supports proliferation of mature CD4+ and CD8+ T cells (33–35), and it induces cytotoxic T-cell differentiation (36–38). Hock and associates (39) were able to show that IL-7 could induce substantial T-cell–dependent antitumor effects in a plastocytoma (J558L). The suppression of tumor growth was not apparent when nude mice were used as recipients. Depletion of CD8+ T cells in normal mice had no effect on tumor rejection, even though CD8+ cells were detected in tumor infiltrates. These results suggest that IL-7–induced anti-J558L immunity is dependent on the induction of CD4+ T cells. CR3+ cells, presumably macrophages, were also required for tumor suppression in addition to CD4+ T cells.

To confirm these results, the authors conducted similar experiments with local IL-7 production in a mammary adenocarcinoma cell line, TS/A. The mice injected with IL-7–producing TS/A cells remained tumor-free after four weeks. Tumors developed in control animals within two weeks. TS/A tumor cells grew in CD4+ cell–depleted mice, indicating a similar mechanism of tumor rejection as observed with J558L cells.

INTERFERON-γ

IFN-γ is a pleiotropic cytokine, produced primarily by Th1 cells and NK cells that induces the expression of MHC class I and class II antigens to enhance antigen presentation (40). IFN-γ also activates macrophages enhancing MHC molecule and Fc receptor expression; it also increases antibody-dependent cellular cytotoxicity, hydrogen peroxide and nitric oxide production, and monocyte tumoricidal activity, presumably secondary to TNF production (41). IFN-γ markedly enhances expression of TNF receptors on a variety of cell types; it has an important role in the inflammatory process, and it is required for the full development of cytotoxic T cells. Miyatake and coworkers (42) showed that local IFN-γ production using transfection techniques reduced establishment of the mouse neuroblastoma C1300 by augmentating antitumor immunity.

Gansbacher and associates (43) showed that local IFN-γ abrogates CMS-5 fibrosarcoma tumorigenicity and can induce strong long-lasting antitumor immunity. This in-

hibition of CMS-5 correlated with marked increase in the expression of MHC class I antigen (10- to 30-fold over control) in these otherwise low expressors of MHC antigen. Cytotoxicity assays using splenocytes from immune mice show that antitumor immunity was associated with enhanced specific CTL activity against the CMS-5 tumor. In addition, IFN-γ–secreting CMS-5 cells, but not unmodified tumor cells, were efficiently and specifically lysed by splenocytes from mice inoculated with the wild-type CMS-5 tumor.

Restifo and coworkers (44) suggested that the mechanism of local IFN-γ–induced antitumor immunity is due to enhanced antigen presentation associated with an increase in MHC class I antigen. Transduction of IFN-γ into either of the methylcholantrene-induced sarcomas, MCA 101 and MCA 102, converted these poor presenters of endogenously generated antigens into tumors capable of efficiently presenting antigens. IFN-γ–transfected MCA 101 expressing high levels of MHC class I, but not those with low level MHC class I expression, could induce antitumor CD8+ TILs in vivo. These results suggest that IFN-γ augments antitumor immunity by enhancing antigen presentation. In contrast, Porgador and associates (45) reported recently that IFN-γ–induced immunity in 3LL lung carcinoma results primarily from the induction of cytotoxic T cells. IFN-γ–producing 3LL tumor cells expressed high levels of MHC class I antigen; however, stronger antitumor immunity was found in those tumors that were high expressors of IFN-γ, which resulted in greater antitumor lytic activity.

TUMOR NECROSIS FACTOR α

TNF-α is produced primarily by macrophages, and it possesses potent direct and indirect antitumor effects. It enhances the function of monocytes and macrophages (46,47), increases neutrophil cytotoxic activation (48), and augments T-cell proliferation (49,50) and activation (14–16,51–53). MCA-205, murine sarcoma transfected to secrete TNF by Ascher and colleagues (54), showed significant reduction of tumor size after an initial (7–8 days) period of growth without apparent cachexia. TNF-producing MCA-205 admixed with parental cells also inhibited tumor growth in a similar manner, suggesting that paracrine production of TNF is sufficient for tumor regression. Anti-TNF monoclonal antibody abrogated the tumor growth inhibition mediated by local TNF. Tumor suppression required both CD4+ and CD8+ T cells because in vivo depletion of either subset inhibits tumor regression.

Blankenstein and associates (29), using a murine J558L plasmacytoma genetically engineered to secrete TNF, showed that 60% of animals with TNF-producing tumors completely suppressed tumor growth, whereas the remaining 40% exhibited significant growth delay compared with parental controls. Histological examination of the tumor infiltrate revealed an abundance of macrophages. Administration of anti-type 3 complement receptor (CR3), which inhibits inflammatory cell migration, abolished tumor suppression.

Finally, genetic transfer of plasmids carrying TNF genes into 1591-RE, a ultraviolet-induced murine skin tumor, by Teng and coworkers (55), leads to significant inhibition of tumor growth in mice. Injection of these TNF-producing tumor cells into nude mice also results in tumor growth suppression, suggesting that the TNF antitumor effect is T-cell–independent, a finding that confirms Blankenstein and colleagues observation. Teng and coworkers suggest that the ability of TNF to inhibit tumor growth in T-cell–deficient mice indicates that TNF may be useful for treating both "antigenic" and "nonantigenic" tumors.

GRANULOCYTE COLONY-STIMULATING FACTOR

Granulocyte colony-stimulating factor (G-CSF) was first identified by its ability to induce differentiation of the murine myelomonocytic leukemia cell line, WEHI-3B (56). G-CSF shows a restricted action; it primarily activates polymorphonuclear cells by stimulating neutrophilic granules and enhancing neutrophil migration to the site of cytokine production (57).

Colombo and associates (58) genetically engineered the murine colon adenocarcinoma C-26 to produce G-CSF to examine the role of neutrophils in antitumor immunity. Local G-CSF inhibited tumor growth by a mechanism that is T-cell–independent. Nude and NK-depleted mice, when injected with G-CSF–producing C-26 tumor cells, could still completely inhibit tumor growth. Histological studies confirm that the tumor infiltrate is comprised mainly of neutrophils. In contrast to other cytokines tested in this manner, the antitumor effect of G-CSF has not been shown to be paracrine, because admixture of parental with G-CSF–producing tumor resulted in rejection of G-CSF–transfected tumor cells, but not the parental tumor cells.

GRANULOCYTE-MACROPHAGE COLONY-STIMULATING FACTOR

Dranoff and coworkers (59) transfected a variety of murine tumors with cDNA for several cytokines (viral titers appear in parentheses). They observed that a combination of GM-CSF (300 ng/mL) and IL-2 (5,000 U/mL)–trans-

fected live B16 melanoma could generate potent systemic protection against wild-type tumor challenge; 8 of 10 survived 40 days and 6 of 10 survived without tumor until 100 days. A variety of other cytokines, including IL-2 alone and IL-4 (15 ng/mL), IL-6 (400 ng/mL), and IFN-γ (20 ng/mL), in combination with IL-2, resulted in rejection of initial tumor, but they could not induce significant long-term immunity. In addition, vaccination of irradiated GM-CSF alone transduced B16, CT-26, CMS-5, and RENCA tumor cells and resulted in complete suppression of wild-type tumor challenge compared with controls.

ROLE OF VARIOUS CELLULAR EFFECTORS IN INDUCING IMMUNITY

Although all the cytokines noted delayed growth of many tumor cell lines, not all resulted in long-term immunity. T-cell–mediated response against tumors seems to be crucial in the development of long-term immunity to rechallenge with tumor cells. Generation of memory T cells is required to maintain antitumor immunity initiated against the tumor in cytokine gene therapy, and it allows long-term resistance to tumor outgrowth. Local cytokine production at the site of tumor vaccine by cytokine gene transfer allows development of a variety of immunization protocols. Gansbacher and colleagues' (12) studies with IL-2 demonstrated that memory CTLs were generated, and these animals could reject a second dose of tumor cells. This ability of IL-2 to generate memory CTL was also observed by Fearon and associates (7) using a murine colon cancer, Connor and associates (13) using murine bladder tumor, and Tsai and colleagues (14) using a mouse mammary tumor.

Although the initial antitumor response associated with local IL-4 production was reported to be mediated primarily through eosinophils and macrophages, long-term immunity in studies by Golumbek and coworkers (24) was T-cell–dependent. We have observed that vaccination with syngeneic fibroblasts admixed with live or irradiated MC 38 (murine colon carcinoma) results in long-term immunity to parental tumor challenge (i.e., immune animals remain tumor-free 100 days after 10^5 tumor challenge). With TNF, only Asher and colleagues (54) have been able to show long-term immunity, which was related to the presence of CD4 and CD8 antitumor effector cells. Blankenstein and colleagues' (29) use of TNF in the J558L tumor demonstrated primarily a macrophage response against tumor, and Teng and coworkers (55) showed that inhibition of tumor growth was T-cell–independent and preserved in nude mice. No long-term immunity studies were reported.

IFN-γ was shown to be highly effective in generating long-term immunity to tumors, presumably due to its enhancement of effective antigen presentation and increased CTL activity. Restifo and associates (44) reported that increased MHC class I by IFN-γ could elicit CD8+ TIL that can then be used therapeutically to treat animals with established metastases. Porgador and associates (45) observed that IL-6 mediated long-term immunity against Lewis Lung carcinoma was achieved when animals were vaccinated with irradiated IL-6–transfected tumor. This effect was not observed in nude mice, again suggesting that such immunity is T-cell–dependent. GM-CSF–transfected tumor cells can induce long-term T-cell–dependent immunity in a variety of both live and irradiated tumor transfectant models, as described by Dranoff and coworkers (59). Studies of long-term immunity against tumor induced by IL-3, IL-7, and G-CSF have not been reported. Formal discussion about the relative efficacy of cytokines awaits more detailed study using a variety of cytokine doses and schedules.

CYTOKINE GENE THERAPY

The ultimate goal of cytokine cancer therapy research and human application is to stimulate host immunity to reject established tumors and induce a state of long-lived memory. Golumbek and associates (24) demonstrated the feasibility of implementing cytokine gene therapy to treat cancer by using IL-4 gene–transfected Renca cells as treatment for preadministered parental tumor. Studies in our laboratory support these findings. We showed that growth of preadministered MCA-105 tumor could be delayed up to 13 days with IL-4–transfected fibroblast immunization therapy (vaccines of 10^6 irradiated MCA-105 admixed with 10^6 fibroblasts producing > 4,000 U/mL/24 hr were administered on days 7, 10, and 14 after tumor inoculation). Tumor growth could be further decreased to a delay of up to 20 days by coadministration of 100,000 U IL-2 (b.i.d.) on days 10 to 14 after tumor inoculation.

Clinical application of cytokine cancer therapy is still in its infancy. Human clinical trials have concentrated on the use of exogenous cytokines to treat various tumors. Local IL-2 production from transfected tumor cells is being evaluated by Rosenberg and associates in patients with metastatic melanoma. They have observed that tumor regression can be achieved using this therapy. IFN-γ is also being evaluated at Memorial Sloan-Kettering Institute in patients with melanoma and renal-cell carcinoma.

IL-4 treatment of cancer patients has not been very effective because systemic IL-4 administration alone has not usually resulted in tumor regression (60). Furthermore, systemic delivery of IL-4 in combination with IL-2,

which is effective in cancer treatment, is associated with moderate to severe toxicities (61). The experience with IL-4 highlights the potential disadvantage of systemic cytokine administration, in which an ineffective amount of local cytokine exists to generate or to potentiate an immune response. Local administration of cytokine via gene transfection is therefore an attractive alternative in anticancer therapy because local paracrine production of cytokine may be sufficient for the host immune system to mount an antitumor response, and this type of administration circumvents systemic toxicities.

CURRENT CLINICAL PROTOCOLS

Currently, IL-2, TNF-α, IFN-γ, GM-CSF, and IL-4 gene therapies for a variety of cancers have been approved by the Recombinant DNA Advisory Committee, and they are in various stages of development for clinical trials (Table 44–3). IL-2 and TNF-α studies for the treatment of melanoma are being conducted by Steve Rosenberg at the NCI. Gansbacher is heading the IL-2 and IFN-γ clinical trials at the Memorial Sloan-Kettering Cancer Institute for patients with melanoma or renal-cell carcinoma. At St. Jude's, Brenner is overseeing an IL-2 clinical protocol in patients with neuroblastoma. Lotze and colleagues at the Pittsburgh Cancer Institute have begun IL-4 gene therapy for patients with metastatic melanoma, renal cell cancer, colorectal cancer, or breast cancer. This protocol ultimately will include both local IL-4 production (by cytokine gene transfection) and systemic administration of IL-2 protein.

IL-4–transfected cultured fibroblasts serve as the carrier of the IL-4 cDNA because the paracrine effects of IL-4 are sufficient to stimulate antitumor immunity. The fibroblast carrier has distinct advantages over direct transfection of tumor cells. Human fibroblast cells are easier to obtain and culture than many human tumor cells. In our hands, transfection of cytokine cDNA has also been less difficult with fibroblasts compared with tumor cells. We have successfully transfected both murine and human fibroblasts with the respective species-specific genes for IL-4, and we have shown that there is substantial production of IL-4. In vivo studies of MC 38 tumors in B6 mice have shown that tumor establishment can be suppressed and that nontumor-bearing mice exhibit long-lasting immunity to subsequent tumor challenge. In addition, vaccination experiments using irradiated tumor and IL-4–transfected fibroblasts have also resulted in long-lasting immunity. These results in mice suggest that IL-4 gene therapy is a potentially effective means of cancer treatment.

IL-4 is a potent effector molecule that demonstrates relatively mild toxicities when given systemically (i.e.,

TABLE 44–3   RAC SUBMITTED CYTOKINE GENE THERAPY PROTOCOLS

Cytokine	Protocol No.	Investigator	Institution	Date of RAC Approval (Submission)	Date of NIH Approval	Description
IL-2	9110-011	Rosenberg	NCI	10/7/91	10/15/91	Tumor vaccine to generate TILs
	9206-022 021	Gansbacher	MSKCC	6/2/92	8/14/92	Allogeneic HLA-A2 and melanoma vaccine
	9206-018	Brenner	St. Jude	6/1/92	8/14/92	Autologous neuroblastoma vaccine
		Tapas	U. of Illinois	7/13/93	Pending	Allogeneic melanoma immunization for patients with unresectable melanoma
		Cassileth	U. of Miami	12/22/92	Pending	Autologous tumor vaccine in limited stage small-cell lung cancer
IL-4	9209-033	Lotze	U. of Pittsburgh	9/15/92	2/5/93	Autologous skin fibroblasts admixed with tumor
IFN-γ	9306-043	Seigler	Duke	6/7/93	Pending	Autologous tumor cells for disseminated malignant melanoma
TNF	9007-003	Rosenberg	NCI	7/31/90	9/6/90	Autologous TILs
	9110-010	Rosenberg	NCI	10/7/91	10/15/91	Autologous cancer cells
GM-CSF	9303-040	Simons	Johns Hopkins	3/1/93	Pending	Autologous tumor cells for metastatic melanoma
IGF	9306-052	Hart	Case Western	6/8/93	Pending	Brain tumors, using episome-based antisense cDNA
	9306-044	Deisseroth	U. of Texas	6/7/93	Pending	Chemoprotection during therapy for ovarian cancer
	9306-045	Nabel	U. of Michigan	6/7/93	Pending	Immunotherapy by direct gene transfer

IL = interleukin; IFN = interferon; TNF = tumor necrosis factor; GM-CSF = granulocyte-macrophage colony-stimulating factor; IGF = insulin-like growth factor I.

vascular leak syndrome, oliguria, postural hypotension) (62). IL-4 is of particular interest in that it is able to stimulate host immunity at multiple sites and levels. First, IL-4 in vitro may enhance antigen presentation through up-regulation of MHC molecules, notably class I, as well as provide a costimulatory signal in the activation of T cells (63,64). Second, IL-4 is able to stimulate specific immunity by inducing B-cell maturation and production of antibodies (65). Furthermore, IL-4 can stimulate helper and cytotoxic T cells, which are important in the prolonged antitumor immune response, and it has been suggested as a key factor stimulating a Th2 response. Therapeutic effects have been demonstrated in vivo by Golumbek and colleagues (24), and Tepper and colleagues (6,22). Specific immunity is important for long-term memory response. Third, IL-4 can also recruit and activate non-specific effector cells, such as macrophages and eosinophils, which will contribute to the induction of an antitumor response. Tepper and colleagues (6) showed this early response in vivo in murine tumors. We have used IL-4–transfected fibroblasts to deliver this cytokine at sites of coadministered irradiated tumor or as a tumor vaccine.

FUTURE

Future gene therapy of cancer is likely to involve a combination of cytokines, either by mixed transfectants, such as the IL-2 and IL-4 combination implemented in murine models of Dranoff and associates (59), or by systemic administration of one cytokine and gene transfection of another, such as the combination of systemic IL-2 and IL-4 transfectants implemented by our group in murine models as well as planned clinical trials. Given the problems using tumor cells as cytokine carriers in human therapy, other possible syngeneic carriers, such as fibroblasts, keratinocytes, and myocytes, will likely be increasingly used. Alternatively, cytokine gene therapy could be used in conjunction with T cell costimulatory molecules, such as B7/BB1 (66). One can envision using B7/BB1-transduced tumor cells to overcome antitumor anergy in concert with cytokine-producing syngeneic fibroblasts as a means to activate and augment antitumor immunity. As precise interactions of various cytokines of the immune system become more understood, appropriate timing of cytokine administration during therapy will become more important.

REFERENCES

1. Brenner MK, Rill DR, Moin RC, et al. Gene-making to trace the origin of relapse after autologous bone-marrow transplantation. Lancet 1993;341:85–86.

2. Schwartz RH. A cell culture model to identify T-lymphocyte clonal origin. Science 1990;248:1349–1356.

3. Jenkins MK, Miller RA. Memory and anergy: challenges to traditional models of T-lymphocyte differentiation. FASEB J 1992;7:2428–2433.

4. Bubenik J, Voitenok NN, Kieler J, et al. Local administration of cells containing an inserted IL-2 gene and producing IL-2 inhibits growth of human tumors in nu/nu mice. Immunol Lett 1988;19:279–282.

5. Oliff A, Defeo-Jones D, Boyer M. Tumors secreting human TNF/cachectin induce cachexia in mice. Cell 1987;50:555–563.

6. Tepper RI, Pattengale PK, Leder P. Murine interleukin-4 displays potent anti-tumor activity in vivo. Cell 1989;57:503–512.

7. Fearon ER, Pardoll, DM, Itaya T, et al. Interleukin-2 production by tumor cells bypasses T-helper function in the generation of an antitumor response. Cell 1990;60:397–403.

8. Zubler RH, Erard F, Lee RK, et al. Mutant EL-4 thymoma cells polyclonally activate murine and human B cells via direct cell interaction. J Immunol 1985;134:3662–3668.

9. Fernadez-Botvan R, Sandis VM, Mosmann JR, Vitetta ES. Lymphokine-mediated regulation of the proliferative response of clones of T helper 1 and T helper 2 cells. J Exp Med 1988;168:543–558.

10. Cuturi MC, Anegon I, Sherman F, et al. Production of hematopoietic colony-stimulating factors by human natural killer cells. J Exp Med 1989;169:569–583.

11. Rosenberg SA, Lotze MT. Cancer immunotherapy using interleukin-2 activated lymphocytes. Annu Rev Immunol 1986;4:681–709.

12. Gansbacher B, Zier K, Daniels B, Cronin K, Bannerji R, Gilboa E. Interleukin-2 gene transfer into tumor cells abrogates tumorigenicity and induces protective immunity. J Exp Med 1990;172:1217–1224.

13. Connor J, Bannerji R, Soito S, Heston W, Fair W, Gilboa E. Regression of bladder tumors in mice treated with interleukin-2 gene modified tumor cells. 1993;177:1127–1134.

14. Tsai J, Gansbacher B, Tait L, Miller FR, Heppner GH. Induction of anti tumor immunity by interleukin-2 gene-transfected mouse mammary tumor cells versus transduced mammary stromal fibroblasts. J Natl Can Inst 1993;85:546–553.

15. Ganser A, Lindemann A, Seipelt G. Clinical effects of recombinant human interleukin-3. Am J Clin Oncol 1991;1:551–563.

16. Pulaski BA, McAdam AJ, Hutter EK, Bigger S, Lord EM, Frelinger JG. IL-3 enhances development of tumor reactive cytotoxic cells by a CD4 dependent mechanism. Cancer Res 1993;53:2112–2117.

17. McAdam AJ, Yeh KY, Pulaski BA, Freilinger JG, Lord EM. IL-3 inhibits the generation of non-specific killers by IL-2. J Immunother 1993;14:293–297.

18. Mosmann TR, Bond MW, Coffman RL, Ohara J, Paul WE. T-cell and most cell lines respond to B-cell stimulatory factor 1. PNAS 1986;83:5654–5658.

19. Paul WE, Ohara J. B-cell stimulating factor-1/interleukin-4. Annu Rev Immunol 1987;5:429–459.

20. Schleimer RP, Strbinsky SA, Kaiser J, et al. IL-4 induces adherence of human eosinophils and basophils but not neutrophils to endothelium. Association with expression of VCAM-1. J Immunol 1992;148:1086–1092.

21. Tepper RI, Coffman RL, Leder P. An eosinophil dependent mechanism for the anti-tumor effect of interleukin-4. Science 1992;257:548–551.

22. Yu JS, Mei MX, Chiocca A, Marhiza RL, Tepper RI. Treatment of glioma by engineered interleukin-4-secreting cells. Cancer Res 1993;53:3125–3128.

23. Blankenstein T, Li WA, Muller W, Diamenstein T. Retroviral interleukin-4 gene transfer into an interleukin-4-dependent cell live results in autocrine growth but not in tumorigenicity. Eur J Immunol 1990;20:935–938.

24. Golumbek PT, Lazenby AJ, Levitsky HI, et al. Treatment of established renal cancer by tumor cells engineered to secrete interleukin-4. Science 1991;254:713–716.

25. Modesti A, Masuelli L, Modice A, et al. Ultrastructural evidence of the mechanisms responsible for interleukin-4-activated rejection of a spontaneous murine adenocarcinoma. Int J Cancer 1993;53:988–993.

26. Hirano T. The biology of interleukin-6, In: Kishimoto T, ed. Interleukins: molecular biology and immunology, Chem Imunnol. 1992;51:153–180.

27. Kishimoto T. Factors affecting B cell growth and differentiation. Annu Rev Immunol 1985;3:133–157.

28. Lotze, MT, Jirik F, Kaboundis R, et al. BSF-2/IL-67 is a co-stimulant for human thymocytes and T lyphocytes. J Exp Med 1988;167:1253–1258.

29. Blankenstein T, San Z, Uberla K. Tumor suppression after tumor cell-targeted tumor necrosis factor gene transfer. J Exp Med 1991;173:1047–1052.

30. Sun WH, Kreisle RA, Phillips AW, Erschler WB. In vivo and in vitro characteristics of interleukin-6-transfected B16 melanoma cells. Cancer Res 1992;52:5412–5415.

31. Porgador A, Tzehoval E, Katz A. Interleukin-6 gene transfection into Lewis Lung carcinoma tumor cells suppresses the malignant phenotype and confers immunotherapeutic competence against parental metastic cells. Cancer Res 1992;52:3679–3686.

32. Namen AE, Schmierer AE, Mach CJ. B-cell precursor growth-promoting activity. Purification and characterization of a growth factor active on lymphocyte precursors. J Exp Med 1988;167:988–1002.

33. Morrissey PJ, Goodwin RG, Nordan RP, et al. Recombinant interleukin-7, pre-B cell growth factor has costimulatory activity on purified mature T-cells. J Exp Med 1989;169–707–716.

34. Chazen GD, Periera GM, LeGros G, Gillis S, Shevach EM. Interleukin-7 is a T cell growth factor. Proc Natl Acad Sci USA 1989;86:5923–5927.

35. Grabstein KH, Namen AE, Sharebeck K, Voica RF, Reed SG, Widmer MB. Regulation of T cell proliferation by IL-7. J Immunol 1990;144:3015–3020.

36. Lynch DH, Miller RE. Induction of murine lymphokine-activated killer cells by recombinant IL-7. J Immunol 1990; 145:1983–1990.

37. Alderson MR, Sassenfeld HM, Widmer MB. Interleukin 7 enhances cytolytic T lymphocyte generation and induces

38. Hickman CJ, Crim JA, Mostowski HS, Siegel JP. Regulation of human cytotoxic T lymphocytes development by IL-7. J Immunol 1990;145:2415–2420.

39. Hock M, Dorsch M, Diamanstein T, Blankenstein T. Interleukin 7 induces CD4+ T cell-dependent tumor rejection. J Exp Med 1991;174:1291–1298.

40. Carrel, S., Schmidt-Kessen A, Giuffre L. Recombinant interferon-gamma can induce the expression of HLA-DR and -DC or DR-negative melanoma cells and enhance the expression of HLA-ABC and tumor-associated antigens. Eur J Immunol 1985;15:118.

41. Tsujisaki M, Igarashi M, Sakaguchi K, et al. Immunochemical and functional analysis of HLA Class II antigens induced by recombinant immune interferon on normal epidermal melanocytes. J Immunol 1987;138:1310.

42. Miyatake S, Nishihara K, Kiruchi H, et al. Efficient tumor suppression by glioma-specific murine cytotoxic T lymphocytes transfected with interferon γ gene. J Natl Can Inst 1990;82:217–221.

43. Gansbacher B, Bannerji R, Daniels BK, Cronin K, Gilboa E. Retroviral vector-mediated gamma IFN gene transfer into human cells generates potent and long lasting antitumor immunity. Cancer Res 1990;50:7820–7825.

44. Restifo NP, Spiess PJ, Karp SE, Mule JJ, Rosenberg SA. A nonimmunogenic sarcoma-transduced with the cDNA for murine Interferon gamma elicits CD8+ T cells against the wild type tumor: correlation with antigen presentation capability. J Exp Med 1992;175:1423–1431.

45. Porgador A, Bannerji R, Watanabe Y, Feldman M, Gilboa E, Eisenbach L. Antimetastatic vaccination of tumor-bearing mice with two types of IFN-γ gene-inserted tumor cells. J Immunol 1993;150:1458–1470.

46. Philip R, Epstein L. Tumor necrosis factor as immunomodulator and mediator of monocyte toxicity induced by itself, gamma-interferon and interleukin-1. Nature 1986;323:86–89.

47. Talmadge, JE, Phillips EH, Schneider M, et al. Immunomodulatory properties of recombinant murine and human tumor necrosis factor. Cancer Res 1988;48:544–550.

48. Shalabay, MR, Aggarwal BB, Rinderknecht E, Svedersky P, Finkle BS, Palladino MA, Jr. Activation of human polymorphonuclear neutrophil functions by interferon-gamma and tumor necrosis factors. J Immunol 1985;135:2069–2073.

49. Scheurich P, Thoma B, Ucer U, Pfizenmaier K. Immunoregulatory activity of recombinant human tumor necrosis factor (TNF)-alpha: induction of TNF receptors on human T cells and TNF alpha mediated enhancement of T cell responses. J Immunol 1987;138:1186–1190.

50. Hackett, RJ, Davis LS, Lipsky PE. Comparative effects of tumor necrosis factor alpha and IL-1 beta on mitogen induced T cell activation. J Immunol 1988;140:2639–2644.

51. Ranges GE, Figari IS, Espevik T, Palladino MA. Jr. Inhibition of cytotoxic T cell development by transforming growth factor-beta and reversal by recombinant tumor necrosis factor-alpha. J Exp Med 1987;166:991–998.

52. Robinet E, Branelec D, Terminstelan AM, Blay JY, Gay F, Chouaib S. Evidence for tumor necrosis factor involvement

in the optimal induction of class I allospecific cytotoxic T cells. J Immunol 1990;144:4555–4561.

53. Owen-Schaub LB, Gutterman JU, Grimm AE. Synergy of tumor necrosis factor and interleukin-2 in the activation of human cytotoxic lymphocytes; effect of tumor necrosis factor alpha and interleukin-2 in the generation of human lymphokine-activated killer cell cytotoxicity. Cancer Res 1988;48:788–792.

54. Asher AL, Mule JJ, Kasid A, et al. Murine tumor cells transduced with the gene for tumor necrosis factor-alpha: evidence for immune effects of tumor necrosis factor against tumors. J Immunol 1991;146:3227–3234.

55. Teng MN, Park BH, Koeppen HK, Tracey KJ, Fendly BM, Schreiber H. Long-term inhibition of tumor growth by tumor necrosis factor in the absence of cachexia or T-cell immunity. Proc Natl Acad Sci USA 1991;88:3535–3539.

56. Nicola NA, Metcalf D, Matsumoto M, Johnson GR. Purification of a factor inducing differentiation in murine myelomonocytic leukemia cells: identification as granulocyte colony-stimulating factor (G-CSF). J Biol Chem 1983;258:9017–9025.

57. Nicola NA, Begley CJ, Metcalf D. Identification of the human analogue of a regulator that induces differentiation in murine leukaemic cells. Nature 1985;314:625–628.

58. Colombo MP, Ferrari G, Stoppacciaro A, et al. Granulocyte colony-stimulating factor gene transfer suppresses tumorigenicity of a murine adenocarcinoma in vivo. J Exp Med 1991;173:889–897.

59. Dranoff G, Jaffee E, Lazenby A, et al. Vaccination with irradiated tumor cells engineered to secrete murine granulocyte macrophage colony-stimulating factor stimulates potent, specific and long lasting anti tumor immunity. Proc Natl Acad Sci USA 1993;90:3539–3543.

60. Kawakami Y, Rosenberg SA, Lotze MT. Interleukin-4 promotes the growth of tumor infiltrating lymphocytes specific for human autologous melanoma. J Exp Med 1988; 168:2183–2191.

61. Lotze MT. Role of IL-4 in the antitumor response. In: Spitz H, ed. IL-4: structure and function. Boca Raton:CRC Press, 1992:237–262.

62. Rubin JT, Lotze MT. Acute gastric mucosal injury associated with the systemic administration of interleukin-4. Surgery 1992;111:274–280.

63. Lacey, DL, Erdmann JM, IL-1 and IL-4 modulate IL-1 receptor expression in a murine T cell line. J Immunol 1990;145: 4145–4153.

64. Aiello FB, Longo DL, Overton R, Takacs L, Durum SK. A role for cytokines in antigen presentation: IL-1 and IL-4 induce accessory functions of antigen-presenting cells. J Immunol 1990;144:2572–2581.

65. Paul WE. Interleukin-4/B-cell stimulatory factor I: 1 Lymphokine, many functions. FASEB J 1987;1:456.

66. Baskar S, Nabavi N, Glimcher LH, Ostrand-Rosenberg S. Tumor cells expressing MHC class II and B7 activation molecules stimulate potent tumor-specific immunity. J Immunother 1993;14:209–215.

CHAPTER 45

PHARMACOLOGICAL REGULATION OF THE PRODUCTION OF THE PROINFLAMMATORY CYTOKINES TNF-α AND IL-1β

Anthony C. Allison, John C. Lee and Elsie M. Eugui

Tumor necrosis factor-α (TNF-α) and interleukin-1β (IL-1β) are major cytokine products of monocyte-macrophage lineage cells. Although these two cytokines bind to different receptors, many (but not all) of the effects they elicit in various target cell types are the same. In general, these effects are proinflammatory and catabolic. From a teleological point of view, TNF-α and IL-1β appear to have been designed to recruit leukocytes into sites of microbial infection and tissue damage and prime them for activity, which are important physiopathological functions. However, excessive production of TNF-α and IL-1β, particularly over a long period, can have undesirable effects. In sites of inflammation, such as the synovial tissue of patients with rheumatoid arthritis, the intestinal mucosa in patients with Crohn's disease and ulcerative colitis, and the gingiva of patients with periodontal disease, continued release of TNF-α and IL-1β can produce swelling, pain, and discomfort, as well as erosion of cartilage and bone. TNF-α and IL-1β are major mediators of the hypotension, the disseminated intravascular coagulation, and the other manifestations of septic shock.

The clinical benefits that might result from inhibiting production or action of TNF-α and IL-1β are obvious. Attempts have been made to achieve this inhibition by use of monoclonal antibodies against the cytokines, recombinant soluble receptors, or recombinant IL-1 receptor antagonist (IL-1Ra). These experiments have provided valuable information about the roles of TNF-α and IL-1β in several experimental animal models of inflammation and septic shock. In some clinical trials, promising results have been obtained, although in other trials, the results have been disappointing. In any case, treatment requires large amounts of antibodies or recombinant proteins, which are expensive and difficult to use. The proteins must be administered by injection, and there is always the possibility that monoclonal antibodies will elicit anti-immunoglobulin responses.

For these reasons, several laboratories have initiated research programs directed toward identification of small molecules that inhibit production or effects of TNF-α and IL-1β. By "small molecule," we mean a synthetic organic compound with a relative molecular mass of 400 or less, which is not a natural product, such as a peptide, lipid, or sugar. A drug suppressing production of these cytokines might be useful as an anti-inflammatory agent lacking the gastrointestinal side effects of cyclo-oxygenase (Cox) inhibitors and the many side effects of glucocorticoids. Several isolated reports of compounds inhibiting production of TNF-α or IL-1β have been published. During the past few years, more systematic studies have identified drugs that inhibit production of both TNF-α and IL-1β at the levels of transcription or translation. We review currently available evidence on pharmacological regulation of TNF-α and IL-1β production. Complementary observations on IL-6, IL-10, and IL-1Ra are included. A brief account is given of mechanisms by which TNF-α and IL-1β exert inflammatory, catabolic, and procoagulant effects. Some of these effects are prevented by drugs such as glucocorticoids and cyclo-oxygenase inhibitors, which also have effects on production and activities of TNF-α and IL-1β.

PROINFLAMMATORY, CATABOLIC AND PROCOAGULANT EFFECTS OF TNF-α AND IL-1β

In this discussion, emphasis is placed on IL-1β as the major form of IL-1 released by activated cells of the monocyte-macrophage lineage. However, in some situations, IL-1α, derived mainly from other cell types, may predominate (e.g., in periodontal disease, where gingival epithelial cells produce IL-1α) (1). In bioassays using human cells, human IL-1α and IL-1β have equipotent activities, although some differences are observed when murine cells are used (2). TNF-α and IL-1β exert proinflammatory effects by inducing expression of adhesion molecules that recruit leukocytes, by priming leukocytes for oxidant production, and by inducing production of prostaglandins and other mediators of inflammation. They exert catabolic effects by inducing production of neutral metalloproteinases and plasminogen activators. They exert procoagulant effects by inducing endothelial cells to produce thromboplastin while down-regulating formation of plasminogen activators and thrombomodulin.

Induction of adhesion molecules

TNF-α and IL-1 induce production or expression of adhesion molecules by endothelial cells, thereby increasing recruitment of leukocytes into sites of microbial infection or inflammation (3). Both TNF-α and IL-1 induce expression on endothelial cells of E-selectin and ICAM-1, which, by binding LFA-1, recruits neutrophils, as well as of VCAM-1, which, by binding VLA-4, recruits monocytes and lymphocytes (4). Antibody against TNF-α was found to decrease recruitment of neutrophils following injection of immune complexes into the peritoneal cavity (5).

Induction of prostaglandin synthesis

Prostaglandins (PGs) are important mediators of inflammation and the pathogenesis of septic shock. PGE$_2$ from monocytes and fibroblasts and PGI$_2$ from endothelial cells are vasodilators, and they contribute to the heat, redness, and increased vascular permeability of inflammation. They are also co-mediators of pain. Vasodilatory prostaglandins are among the mediators of hypotension in septic shock. TNF-α and IL-1β induce synthesis of PGs in fibroblasts from rheumatoid synovial and periodontal tis-

sues and of PGI$_2$ in endothelial cells (6). IL-1α and IL-1β increase endogenous release of arachidonic acid in target cells, as well as stimulate synthesis of PGs from exogenously added arachidonic acid (7). IL-1–mediated stimulation of phospholipase A$_2$ activity is correlated with induction of cytosolic phospholipase A$_2$ (8). However, Cox undergoes irreversible selfinactivation, so that modulation of activity depends on continued synthesis of the enzyme (6).

Two genes encoding Cox, termed Cox-1 and Cox-2, have been cloned and expressed in functional form (9). The Cox-1 gene is expressed ubiquitously in vivo and in vitro, whereas the Cox-2 gene is expressed at very low levels in normal tissues in vivo and by quiescent cells in culture. However, IL-1 rapidly induces expression of the Cox-2 gene in cultured endothelial cells, with expression of the Cox-2 isoenzyme and production of prostacyclin. In unstimulated monocytes, the constituitive enzyme is Cox-1. Stimulation by lipopolysaccharide (LPS) has no effect on expression of the Cox-1 gene, but it rapidly induces a high level of expression of the Cox-2 gene (9). Cox-1 and Cox-2 transcripts have been found in synovia from patients with rheumatoid arthritis (10). Immunoprecipitation of in vitro labeled proteins from freshly explanted rheumatoid synovial tissues showed that synthesis of Cox-2 protein was markedly increased by IL-1β. In the presence of dexamethasone, Cox-2 mRNA was not increased by IL-1β. Other reports of stimulation by IL-1 of the expression of Cox-2 mRNA have been published (9,11). Thus, one of the proinflammatory effects of IL-1β is induction of expression of the Cox-2 gene, and one of the anti-inflammatory effects of glucocorticoids is suppression of the formation of Cox-2.

In some species, thromboxane produced by cells of the monocyte-macrophage lineage mediates pulmonary vasoconstriction and hypertension in septic shock (12). Thromboxane is one of the procoagulants responsible for disseminated intravascular coagulation in septic shock. The role of prostaglandins in bone erosion is discussed in the following section.

Degradation of cartilage and bone

Inflammatory responses are associated with degradation of cartilage and bone. In rheumatoid arthritis, proliferating pannus grows into and erodes articular cartilage and bone in the vicinity, with progressive joint destruction; there is also variable osteoporosis in the adjacent bones. In periodontal disease, erosion of alveolar bone, with consequent loss of teeth, is a major clinical problem. It is generally accepted that TNF-α and IL-1β induce in connective tissue cells production of neutral metalloproteinases, stromelysins, and collagenases that degrade both proteoglycan matrix and interstitial collagen in cartilage and bone (13). Addition of TNF-α, IL-1β, or IL-6 to organ cultures of rat fetal long bones augments catabolism, as shown by release of calcium, as well as fragments of proteoglycan and collagen, into the medium (14,15). When two or three of these cytokines are included in the culture medium, they have at least additive effects on bone resorption. Thus, all three cytokines are likely to contribute to bone erosion in rheumatoid arthritis and periodontal disease, and a drug inhibiting the production of all them might have clinical utility.

PGEs are co-mediators of bone catabolism induced by TNF-α, IL-1β, and IL-6. Cox inhibitors suppress IL-1–induced bone erosion in culture, although they vary markedly in potency in this assay; the most potent inhibitor of bone degradation identified thus far is ketorolac, which raises the possibility of use as a mouthwash to prevent alveolar bone erosion in periodontal disease (16). Classic Cox inhibitors such as indomethacin do not block bone resorption induced by parathyroid hormone, although the inhibitor of cytokine as well as prostaglandin production, SK&F 86002, does (17).

The mechanisms by which Cox inhibitors prevent IL-1–induced bone erosion are not fully understood. One factor that may be involved is the requirement for PGE$_2$ as a cofactor for IL-1–induced expression of plasminogen activators in cells of connective tissue type and their role in activation of neutral metalloproteinases. Prostromelysins and procollagenase are secreted as inactive proenzymes that are converted into active enzymes by proteolytic cleavage, or in other ways. The relatively broad-spectrum serine proteinase, plasmin, can initiate a cascade of proteolytic events, resulting in metalloproteinase activation (13). The narrower-spectrum serine esterases, urokinase-type and tissue-type plasminogen activators, convert plasminogen into plasmin. IL-1–induced expression of the genes for plasminogen activators requires PGE$_2$, which is inhibited by indomethacin and restored by adding PGE$_2$ (18); PGE$_2$ alone does not induce production of plasminogen activators (18).

Procoagulant effects of TNF-α

As discussed, TNF-α and IL-1 induce production of PGs. A PG released by activated cells of monocyte-macrophage lineage is thromboxane, which is procoagulant. LPS induces in these cells expression and activation of tissue factor, a potent procoagulant (19). TNF-α acts on endothelial cells to exert a net procoagulant effect (20). TNF-α increases expression on endothelial cells of tissue factor, which, in the presence of acidic phospholipids, initiates the extrinsic pathway of blood coagulation. TNF-α suppresses the release of tissue-type plasminogen activator and induces secretion of plasminogen activator inhibitor type I. TNF-α down-regulates thrombomodulin and

thereby impairs activation of protein C. Infusion of high doses of TNF-α in dogs resulted in microvascular thrombosis (21). Recombinant human TNF-α, administered as an intravenous bolus injection to healthy men, induced an early and short-lived increase in circulating levels of the activation peptide of factor X, followed by a prolonged increase in the plasma concentration of the prothrombin fragment F$_{1+2}$ (20). These findings show activation of factor X and prothrombin. There were no signs that the intrinsic pathway of blood coagulation was activated. Thus, a single injection of TNF-α elicited rapid and sustained activation of the common pathway of coagulation, probably through the extrinsic route. This effect of TNF-α could have an important part in the pathogenesis of disseminated intravascular coagulation in septicemia.

Increased production of oxidants

TNF-α primes neutrophils to produce more superoxide in response to other stimuli, including formylmethionine peptides, LPS, and immune complexes (22,23). This effect is normally a defence mechanism against micro-organisms, but oxidants can damage endothelial cells in respiratory distress syndromes (12). LPS and other bacteria also induce production of oxidants in cells of the monocyte-macrophage lineage (23); their role in activation of transcription factors is discussed.

Cytokines augment nitric oxide production

In the presence of interferon-γ (IFN-γ,), TNF-α and IL-1β augment production by endothelial cells of nitric oxide, a vasodilator. In experimental animals, an inhibitor of nitric oxide formation, NG-methyl-L-arginine, attenuates hypotension induced by TNF-α (24). Thus, nitric oxide may be one of the mediators of cytokine-induced hypotension in septic shock, but it is unlikely to be the only mediator (12). Species differences complicate interpretation (e.g., LPS-stimulated mouse macrophages produce nitric oxide, whereas human monocytes do not).

Role of IL-6 pathogenesis of inflammation and bone erosion

IL-6 stimulates production of hepatocytes of C-reactive protein and other acute-phase reactants (25), levels of which are positively correlated with the severity of rheumatoid arthritis (RA) (26). The role of IL-6 in the pathogenesis of RA is less well defined; however, the cytokine is a cofactor for T-lymphocyte differentiation (27) and in production of immunoglobulins by B lymphocytes in RA synovial tissue (28). Activated T lymphocytes (29) and immune complexes (30) are thought to contribute to the pathogenesis of RA. Moreover, IL-6 can act synergistically with IL-1 in augmenting bone erosion (15), which could contribute to joint destruction in RA, as well as alveolar bone erosion in periodontal disease. Hence, a useful property of a drug could be inhibition of the production of IL-6 as well as IL-1β and TNF-α.

ROLE OF CYTOKINES IN THE PATHOGENESIS OF INFLAMMATION AND SEPTIC SHOCK

A cytokine cascade or parallel mediation?

Evidence has been obtained for the existence of a cytokine cascade, involving sequentially TNF-α, IL-1β, IL-6, and IL-8 in the synovium of patients with RA. In cultures of RA synovial tissue and cells derived from it, neutralization of TNF-α with antibody decreases production of IL-1β (31), and neutralization of IL-1 with antibody or the IL-1Ra decreases production of IL-6 and IL-8 (32). Nevertheless, several effects of TNF-α occur independently of IL-1 (33), and several effects of IL-1 occur independently of IL-6 and IL-8. Administration of antibodies neutralizing TNF-α (34) or of IL-Ra (35) are reported to improve the clinical condition of patients with RA, confirming the importance of TNF-α and IL-1 in pathogenesis. However, the antibody and receptor antagonist are expensive and difficult to administer on a continuous basis. For these reasons, research has been directed toward identification of a small molecule that can inhibit, in a coordinate fashion, production by monocyte-macrophage lineage cells of TNF-α, IL-1β, and IL-6. Identification of compounds with the desired activities are reviewed in this chapter. In the section on the role of cytokines in septic shock, the question of parallel mediation is discussed further.

Effects of administration of TNF-α and IL-1 in humans

It has been ethically justified to inject TNF-α and IL-1 into humans to define their effects and maximal tolerated doses (e.g., using TNF-α for cancer therapy and using IL-1 to accelerate recovery of hematopoiesis following depletion of bone marrow precursors by chemotherapy or radiotherapy of patients with cancer). The information obtained provides insight into the role of these cytokines in the pathogenesis of septic shock. Because manifestations of this disorder vary in different experimental animal models, it is useful to have information on the major species for whom treatment of septic shock is intended.

Feinberg and colleagues (36) reported findings after

30-minute intravenous infusions of escalating doses of TNF-α to humans with disseminated cancers. The principal toxicities were constitutional symptoms, including fever, chills, headache, and fatigue, which increased in severity with dose. The maximum tolerated dose was 200 μg/m²; the dose-limiting toxicities were constitutional symptoms and hypotension. Following this dose, the level of TNF-α in the circulation was approximately 10 ng/mL. Counts of circulating granulocytes decreased, presumably because of induction of adhesion molecules and margination. TNF-α infusion increased circulating triglycerides and very low density lipoprotein. In this study, levels of circulating platelets decreased following TNF-α administration. Single injections of TNF-α (50 μg/m²) into normal humans activated the extrinsic pathway of blood coagulation, but it did not decrease platelet counts (20).

Low doses (1–10 ng/kg) of IL-1 injected into humans increased the numbers of circulating neutrophils and platelets; the number of hematopoietic stem cells was also increased (37). These effects were attributed to co-stimulation of the proliferation of stem cells and augmented release of leukocytes from the bone marrow into the circulation. High doses of IL-1 decreased the numbers of circulating neutrophils, presumably because the cytokine increases expression of adhesion molecules on endothelial cells, thereby augmenting binding and margination of neutrophils. Moderate doses of IL-1 also induced fever, joint and muscle aches, increased sensitivity to pain, and a state of lethargy. Higher doses of IL-1 (≥100 ng/kg) reduced appetite, induced gastrointestinal disturbances, and produced hypotension that could reach dangerous levels when more than 300 ng/kg was injected (38).

Cytokines in septic shock

A substantial body of literature on cytokines in septic shock has accumulated. It is reviewed in the context of gram-negative sepsis in Chapter 25 of this volume and of gram-positive sepsis in Chapter 24. In this chapter, available information is outlined in the context of formulating a strategy for preventing and treating septic shock by drugs inhibiting cytokine synthesis.

The pathogenesis of septic shock is complex, and it varies in different species of animals. For example, some animals are highly sensitive to LPS (e.g., humans, pigs, sheep, cows, goats, cats), whereas others are relatively resistant (e.g., baboons, dogs, rats, mice, rabbits) (39). Some animals have many macrophages within the pulmonary vasculature, which ingest a relatively high proportion of bacteria or other particles injected intravenously (e.g., pigs, sheep, cows, goats, cats). In these animals, pulmonary vasoconstriction, hypertension, and edema are characteristic features of sepsis. Humans, baboons, dogs, rats, mice, and rabbits have few pulmonary intravascular macrophages (39). In humans, the majority of injected particles are cleared in the liver and the spleen; only a small fraction are cleared in the lungs (40). Nevertheless, pulmonary hypertension develops in humans with the adult respiratory distress syndrome (39). In all animals, peripheral vasodilation and hypotension, which can be lethal, are features of septic shock.

Disseminated intravascular coagulation, with widespread deposition of fibrin in the microvasculature, is often observed in septic shock, and it is associated with the development of multiple organ failure (41). The mechanisms by which the clotting cascade is activated in septicemia are incompletely understood, but some are known. Bacterial products such as LPS act directly on monocytes to induce expression of tissue factor, which activates the extrinsic pathway of coagulation (19). Bacterial products also induce release from monocytes and macrophages of TNF-α, which acts on endothelial cells to exert a net procoagulant effect. In patients with sepsis, plasma levels of TNF-α are directly proportional to the extent of intravascular coagulation and fatal outcome (42,43). Hence, one of the roles of TNF-α in septic shock is activation of disseminated intravascular coagulation.

Several questions arise regarding the role of cytokines in septic shock. First, what concentrations of cytokines are released into the circulation at different times? Because cytokines released early (i.e., TNF-α and IL-1β) can induce production of those appearing later (i.e., IL-6 and IL-8), the next question is whether there is a cascade of cytokines (i.e., TNF-α inducing IL-1β, which in turn induces IL-6 and IL-8). If so, inhibiting production or effects of TNF-α alone should provide effective prevention or early treatment of septic shock. However, if TNF-α is only amplifying LPS-induced IL-1β production, but there is parallel induction of cytokines and mediation of their effects, it will be necessary to inhibit production of all cytokines contributing significantly to the pathogenesis of septic shock. There is evidence that TNF-α and IL-1β have a pathogenetic role in septic shock. As an academic exercise, it would be interesting to know the relative importance of late mediators of hemodynamic changes, disseminated intravascular coagulation, and metabolic disturbances (e.g., prostaglandins, leukotrienes, platelet-activating factor, activated complement components, kinins, histamine, nitric oxide). There are already indications that many late mediators are involved in septic shock; their relative importance varies from species to species (10). In general, it seems likely that combinations of many inhibitors of the production and effects of late mediators will be required to treat septic shock, and that efficacy in experimental animals may not be predictive of efficacy in humans. Relying on inhibition of a single mediator, such as nitric oxide, may not be justified.

The sequence of cytokines observed in the circulation of nonhuman primates following injections of high doses of LPS, or sublethal doses of *Escherichia coli*, is instructive (44,45) (Fig. 45–1). A large amount of TNF-α is released first; levels peak at 2 hours, and return to baseline by 4 hours. This effect is followed by a lower peak of IL-1β, which is maximal at 3 to 4 hours and it decreases more slowly than that of TNF-α. Still later, IL-6 and IL-8 are found in the circulation, where they remain much longer. In humans injected with small doses of LPS, similar but lower peaks of TNF-α and IL-6 have been observed, but IL-1β was usually undetectable (46,47); in one study, IL-1β was observed at a single time point after LPS infusion (48).

Administration of TNF-α to otherwise healthy nonhuman primates was found to induce cardiovascular collapse, multiorgan system failure, and death, similar to that seen in lethal septicemia and clinical septic shock. An early peak of circulating IL-1β and a later peak of IL-6 were observed; both were attenuated by giving the animals antibody against TNF-α (44). Neutralization of TNF-α also reduced hypoglycemia and hypertriglyceridemia, but it did not prevent a fatal outcome in animals given a high dose of LPS. These findings implicate TNF-α as a mediator of septic shock, acting in part by amplifying formation of IL-1β in response to LPS. However, they make it unlikely that TNF-α is the only important mediator of septic shock. Administration of an antibody against TNF-α also failed to prevent lethality after cecal ligation and puncture in mice (49). However, neutralization of TNF-α increased the survival of pigs injected with *E. coli* (50).

Injection of IL-1β into baboons was found to produce hypotension and other disorders similar to those pro-

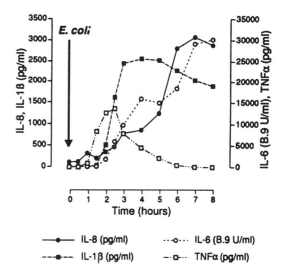

Figure 45–1 The sequence of cytokines in the circulation of the baboon *Papio anubis* following injection of *Escherichia coli* (Kenney J, unpublished observations).

duced by TNF-α, but less severe (51). These effects suggest that IL-1β could be another major mediator of septic shock. Consistent with that interpretation is the finding that administration of recombinant IL-1Ra to baboons during lethal *E. coli* septic shock attenuated the decrease in mean arterial blood pressure and cardiac output and improved survival (45). However, following an encouraging Phase II trial of IL-1Ra administration in patients with septic shock (52), the results of a Phase III trial were disappointing. This funding suggests that TNF-α (levels of which are unaffected by IL-1Ra administration) and other mediators exert effects through mechanisms independent of IL-1 (e.g., procoagulant effects). TNF-α is more toxic than IL-1 administered to baboons (44,51), presumably because it is not only inducing IL-1 production.

In humans with septic shock, high levels of TNF-α, IL-1, and IL-6 in the circulation are positively correlated with severe morbidity and a lethal outcome (42,43, 53,54). IL-6 is a major mediator of acute-phase responses; it induces production by hepatocytes of the proteins involved (25). Measurement of IL-6 levels in body fluids could provide a useful indication of the severity of the microbial challenge in sepsis, but it is not clear that IL-6 has a role in mediating hemodynamic and metabolic disturbances in shock. Starnes and associates (55) reported that treatment of rats with a monoclonal antibody against murine IL-6 improved survival in *E. coli* shock. However, administration of large doses of IL-6 to mice (45) or to dogs (56) had no hemodynamic or hematological effects. The general conclusion is that it is desirable to inhibit the production or the effects of both TNF-α and IL-1β to prevent or treat septic shock. Additional activities, such as inhibiting production of thromboplastin, would also be useful.

INHIBITORS OF CYTOKINE PRODUCTION

Agents that increase cyclic AMP levels suppress production of TNF-α but not IL-1β

Activated monocytes and macrophages produce PGs, notably PGE$_2$, which might provide feedback inhibition of cytokine production in vivo. E-type PGs bind to EP$_1$ receptors, which activate adenylate cyclase, and cAMP mediates many of their effects. Adrenalin binds to and activates β-adrenergic receptors, which also activate adenylate cyclase. Adrenalin circulating in septic shock might likewise act as a feedback inhibitor of cytokine production. Cyclic AMP phosphodiesterase inhibitors, in particular those active against the PDE-IV isozyme, which is present in human monocytes (57), would be expected to have similar effects on cytokine production. Reference PDE-IV inhibitors are rolipram and nitroquazone (57,58).

Evidence is accumulating for a differential effect of these agents on production of TNF-α and IL-1β.

Several groups of investigators have found that elevation of cAMP levels in human monocytes by activation of adenylate cyclase or inhibition of PDE suppresses LPS-induced TNF-α production, with little effect on IL-1β production (58–61). A typical experiment is shown in Fig. 45–2; Rolipram and nitroquazone inhibit TNF-α synthesis by LPS-activated monocytes, whereas inhibitors of other cAMP PDE isozymes have no significant effect (58). The nonselective PDE inhibitors, pentoxiphylline and isobutylmethyl xanthine (IBMX), were found to reduce steady-state levels of TNF-α mRNA and to suppress TNF-α production by LPS-stimulated monocytes and macrophages (59). Adding dibutyryl cAMP to LPS-stimulated murine macrophages lowered the rate of transcription of the TNF-α gene, decreased steady-state mRNA levels, and inhibited production of the cytokine (62). In the murine macrophage cell line, RAW264.7, Han and associates (63) found that pentoxiphylline blocked LPS-induced TNF-α mRNA accumulation, but it had no effect on reporter mRNA translation. In contrast, dexamathasone had little effect on mRNA accumulation, but it strongly impeded translational derepression. Pentoxiphylline also inhibited TNF-α, but not IL-1β, release from microglia, whereas dexamethasone inhibited production of both cytokines (64).

Beta-adrenergic agonists were also found to increase cAMP levels in THP-1 cells and to suppress production of TNF-α (65). Inhibition of TNF-α production was abolished by a β-adrenergic antagonist, but not by an α-adrenergic antagonist; the β-adrenergic agonist isoproterenol also inhibited TNF-α production.

Effects of elevating cAMP on the production of IL-1β have been less pronounced and consistent, depending on the cells used and the experimental conditions. It was initially reported that PGE$_2$ inhibits production of IL-1 by LPS-activated human monocytes (66). More recently, ev-

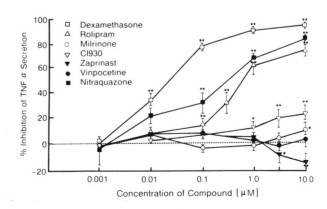

Figure 45–2 Suppression by dexamethasone and cyclic AMP phosphodiesterase (PDE-IV) inhibitors (rolipram, nitroquasone) of secretion of TNF-α by LPS-activated human monocytes. Inhibitors of other cAMP PDE isozymes had no effect on TNF-α secretion, whereas the inhibitor of cyclic GMP PDE zaprinast augmented secretion to some extent (58).

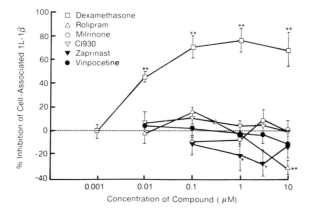

Figure 45–3 Dexamethasone suppresses synthesis of IL-1β by LPS-activated human monocytes, whereas inhibitors of cyclic AMP phosphodiesterases (including the type IV isozyme expressed in monocytes) had no effect. The inhibitor of cyclic GMP phosphodiesterase zaprinast augmented production of IL-1β to some extent. These observations are on cell-associated IL-1β; the effects of drugs on secreted IL-1β were comparable (58).

idence has been obtained that increased cAMP levels augment to some extent IL-1α and IL-1β gene expression and cytokine production in monocytes and macrophages (67,68). Others have found no significant effect of elevating cAMP levels, using PDE-IV inhibitors, on IL-1β production (58) (Fig. 45–3). However, increasing cAMP in monocytes can have some suppressive effect on secretion of IL-1β (58,67).

Elevating cyclic guanosine monophosphate (cGMP) levels by activating guanylate cyclase with sodium nitroprusside, adding exogenous cyclic nucleotides, or using zaprinast to inhibit cGMP-selective PDE-V somewhat augmented production of TNF-α in murine macrophages (58); this finding contrasts with the stronger suppressive effect of raising cAMP levels on TNF-α production (see Fig. 45–2). Exogenous dibutyryl cGMP had no effect on IL-1β production by human monocytes (67). One group

of investigators reported that increasing cGMP with SIN-1 inhibits IL-1β production by human mononuclear cells (60), whereas other investigators found that the PDE-V–selective inhibitor, zaprinast, somewhat augmented IL-1β secretion (58) (see Fig. 45–3).

In summary, agents elevating cAMP levels in cells of monocyte-macrophage lineage, including E-type PGs, β-adrenergic agonists, and cAMP phosphodiesterase type IV inhibitors, suppress production of TNF-α. They do not suppress production of IL-1β, but they may have some inhibitory effect on its secretion.

Effects of glucocorticoids on IL-1β production

Although glucocorticoids are among the most potent and widely used anti-inflammatory drugs, their mode of action is incompletely understood. The most popular theory has been that glucocorticoids induce formation of a group of proteins, collectively termed *lipocortins*, that inhibit phospholipase A₂ activity, thereby decreasing production of proinflammatory PGs and leukotrienes. However, when members of the lipocortin family were cloned, it became clear that they are present in rather high concentrations in many cell types, are not steroid-inducible, and are phospholipid-binding proteins rather than phospholipase inhibitors. Thus, the role of lipocortins as mediators of the anti-inflammatory effects of steroids is in doubt. An alternative explanation is that glucocorticoids inhibit formation of TNF-α, IL-1β, and other proinflammatory mediators (70).

It is generally accepted that glucocorticoids inhibit production of IL-1 by LPS-induced murine macrophages (17,71) and human monocytes (58,72,73), as well as by U937 human promonocytic cells (74,75). A representative experiment, showing suppression by dexamethasone of the production of IL-1α and IL-1β in LPS-stimulated human monocytes (73) is illustrated in Fig. 45–4A. There

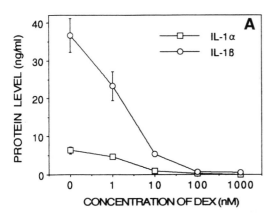

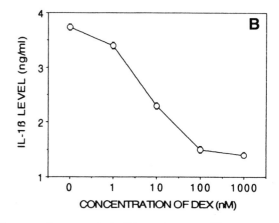

Figure 45–4 (A) Dose-dependent effect of dexamethasone (DEX) on the production of IL-1α and IL-1β by LPS-activated human monocytes. Cells were incubated with LPS for 24 hours, and cell-associated cytokines were measured by ELISA (73). (B) Dose-dependent inhibition by DEX of IL-1β secretion, under the same conditions.

is a consensus that dexamethasone decreases the steady-state level of IL-1β mRNA in LPS-activated human monocytes (72–74) (Fig. 45–5). Because many effects of glucocorticoids are exerted at the level of transcription, it was surprising to find that dexamethasone had no detectable effect on LPS-augmented transcription of the IL-1β gene in monocytes (72,73). However, dexamethasone markedly decreased the stability of IL-1β mRNA, as shown both by steady-state measurements and pulse labeling (73) (Table 45–1). Dexamethasone-induced instability of IL-1β mRNA required protein synthesis; a glucocorticoid antagonist blocked its effects.

In U937 cells primed with PMA and stimulated with LPS, dexamethasone was found to have some inhibitory effect on transcription of the IL-1β gene (75). However, in these cells, the transcription factors required for LPS-induced expression of the IL-1β gene are not already present, and protein synthesis is required for their induction: Dexamethasone may have been inhibiting formation of the transcription factors rather than the transcription process itself. In U937 cells, dexamethasone also decreased IL-1β mRNA stability (75).

To examine whether glucocorticoid treatment would accelerate degradation of all mRNAs containing an A+U–rich consensus sequence in the 3′-untranslated region, Fos mRNA was also investigated. In U937 cells, glucocorticoids had no effect on Fos mRNA stability under conditions during which IL-1β mRNA showed a marked decrease in stability (75). Thus, an A+U–rich sequence does not appear to be the common recognition target required for dexamethasone-induced mRNA degradation.

Because the glucocorticoid-induced lowering of IL-1β mRNA in LPS-treated monocytes paralleled the decrease in intracellular and secreted cytokine measured by immunoassay (see Figs. 45–4A, B), we concluded that glucocorticoids do not have a major effect on translational effi-

TABLE 45–1   EFFECT OF DEXAMETHASONE ON IL-1β mRNA STABILITY IN HUMAN MONOCYTES STIMULATED WITH LPS (73)

	Steady-State Accumulation		Pulse-Chase Labeling	
	K (hr⁻¹)*	Half-life (hr)†	K (hr⁻¹)	Half-life (hr)
Control	0.050	13.8	0.047	14.7
Dexamethasone	0.330	2.1	0.286	2.4
Actinomycin D	0.113	6.1	ND[b]	ND
Actinomycin D + dexamethasone	0.125	5.66	ND	ND

*The fractional degradative rate (K) was the slope of the linear regression line for logarithmically transformed observations.
†The half-life, $t_{1/2}$ = (ln 2/K), was calculated from the K value.
(Reproduced by permission from Amano Y, Lee SW, Allison AC. Inhibition by glucocorticoids of the formation of interleukin-1α, interleukin-1β and interleukin 6; mediation by decreased mRNA stability. Mol Pharmacol 1993;43:176–182.)

ciency or on secretion (73). Knudsen and associates (74) suggested that glucocorticoids decrease to some extent the efficiency of translation of the IL-1β message, and Kern and colleagues (72) postulated the existence of some inhibition of IL-1β secretion in human monocytes. The dose-response curves for dexamethasone-induced inhibition of intracellular and secreted IL-1β in LPS-induced monocytes reported by Molnar-Kimber and co-workers (58) (see Fig. 45–3) are also very similar, suggesting that there is no major effect on secretion. In an assay that discriminates between effects on IL-1β synthesis and secretion, dexamethasone inhibited production of IL-1β, with an IC$_{50}$ of 0.2 μmol/L, but it had little effect on secretion (76).

In summary, the principal mechanism by which glucocorticoids inhibit formation of IL-1β in monocytes is by decreasing the stability of its mRNA.

Effects of glucocorticoids on TNF-α production

Dexamethasone, in a dose-dependent manner, decreased LPS-induced production of TNF-α in mouse peritoneal macrophages, the RAW264.7 murine macrophage cell line (63), and in human monocytes (58) (see Fig. 45–2). Macrophage activation was found to induce an increase in the rate of transcription of the TNF-α gene and a concurrent increase in the efficiency with which TNF-α mRNA is translated (63); glucocorticoids partially inhibited TNF-α mRNA accumulation in LPS-activated RAW264.7

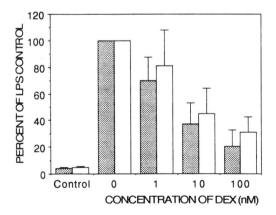

Figure 45–5   Dose-dependent inhibitory effect of DEX on steady-state levels of IL-1α (□) and IL-1β (■) mRNA in LPS-activated human monocytes (73). Observations made 18 hours after stimulation with LPS were normalized to mRNA levels in the LPS control in the absence of the drug (100%).

cells, but their major effect was to depress translation of the TNF-α mRNA produced. RAW264.7 cells were transfected with two constructs designed to assess post-transcriptional activation of TNF synthesis. In each construct, CAT transcription was driven by the SV40 late gene promoter. In construct A, the CAT-encoding sequence was followed by most of the human TNF-α 3′-untranslated region. In the control construct B, no TNF-α sequence was present. The presence of the TNF-α 3′-untranslated region permitted translational derepression to occur in cells containing construct A; dexamethasone inhibited this CAT expression, whereas pentoxiphylline did not. Cells transfected with construct A were not induced by LPS or suppressed by dexamethasone.

In summary, dexamethasone only weakly inhibits accumulation of TNF-α mRNA, but it strongly inhibits translational derepression. In LPS-activated human monocytes, the great majority of TNF-α protein is extracellular (only approximately 5% is intracellular); nevertheless, dose-response curves of dexamethasone inhibition of TNF-α in both compartments are comparable (58), so there is no obvious effect on secretion of the cytokine.

Fluroquinolone antibiotics

Fluorinated piperazinyl-substituted quinolone derivatives have a broad-spectrum antibacterial activity. Two of these agents, pefloxacin and ciprofloxacin, were found to decrease the amount of IL-1 (demonstrated by thymocyte comitogenic activity) in the supernatants of human monocytes stimulated by LPS (77). There was no effect of the antibiotics on intracellular IL-1 or on the expression of human leukocyte antigen-DR (HLA-DR). Thus, rather high concentrations of fluoroquinolone antibiotics (100 μg/mL) appear to inhibit release of IL-1 from LPS-activated cells. Whether this effect has any physiopathological significance remains to be demonstrated.

Clarithromycin

Clarithromycin is a macrolide antibiotic prepared by introducing a methoxy group at the 6-position of the erythromycin ring. Takeshita and coworkers (78) reported that clarithromycin inhibits production of IL-1 by LPS-stimulated murine peritoneal macrophages (significant inhibition at 3–10 μg/mL). Erythromycin was less active in this system. Clarithromycin did not inhibit Cox.

Tetrandrine

Tetrandrine, a bisbenzylisoquinoline analog, is a major alkaloid of the Chinese creeping plant *Stephania tetrandra*. It is reported to retard formation of fibrotic lesions of pulmonary silicosis in rats and humans. TNF-α stimulates fibroblast proliferation, and it is thought to be a mediator of fibrogenesis (79). Ferrante and colleagues (80) found that tetrandrine inhibits production of TNF-α by human monocytes stimulated with killed *Staphylococcus aureus*; the active concentration of tetrandrine was 0.1 to 5 μg/mL. Tetrandrine also inhibited IL-1 production by activated monocytes (81). Possibly, tetrandrine functions as an antioxidant, with effects analogous to those of isoquinolines (Table 45–4).

Morphine

It has been reported that morphine inhibits release of TNF-α from human peripheral blood mononuclear cell cultures (82). Pretreatment with naloxone did not affect the capacity of morphine to inhibit LPS-induced TNF-α release, although naloxone partially reversed the capacity of morphine to inhibit PHA-induced TNF-α release. The underlying molecular biology was not examined. Whether morphine is exerting effects analogous to those of apomorphine and norapamorphine (Table 45-4) remains to be established. This investigation concerned the possible role of opiate peptides as immunomodulators: side effects of opiates preclude clinical use in shock and inflammatory diseases.

Antirheumatic drugs

There have been several reports that long-acting antirheumatic drugs, including gold sodium thiomalate and auranofin, inhibit production of TNF-α and IL-1β by human peripheral blood monocytes (83–85). However, variation has been observed in responses of cells from healthy subjects and from patients with arthritis (84). Auranofin, chloroquine, and mycophenolic acid have been found to induce differentiation of human monocytes, as shown by surface markers (C3b and Fcγ receptors), as well as by production of lysozyme and lysosomal enzymes (86,87). As monocytes differentiate into macrophages, they produce less IL-1β and IL-6, and more IL-1Ra. Thus, induction of differentiation would be expected to exert an anti-inflammatory effect over a long period of treatment. Allison and Waters (86) postulate this as a mechanism by which long-acting antirheumatic drugs exert their effects. Antioxidants with similar actions are discussed.

IX 207,887

A group from the Sandoz Research Institute, Basel (88,89), reported development of a novel anti-inflammatory drug, IX 207,887. The chemical structure is (Z-10-methoxy-4H-benzo [4,5] cyclohepta [1,2b] thiophene-4-

yliden) acetic acid. IX 207,887 at a concentration of 60 μmol/L significantly decreased the concentration of IL-1 in the culture medium of LPS-stimulated human monocytes. The cytokine in cellular homogenates was not significantly decreased by the drug. It seems unlikely that this rather weak effect on secretion of IL-1 explains the in vivo anti-inflammatory activity of the drug (e.g., in suppressing adjuvant arthritis in rats [89], as well as efficacy in patients with rheumatoid arthritis [90]). IX 207,887 caused agranulocytosis in a number of patients, and Sandoz terminated the development of the compound because of its toxicity profile (91).

Tenidap

Tenidap (1-H-Indole-1-carboxamide, 5-chloro-2,3-dihydro-2-ono-3-[2-thienylcarbonyl]-[CAS]) is a potent Cox inhibitor with some capacity to inhibit 5-lipoxygenase in vitro (92). In patients with RA, Tenidap has activity expected of a Cox inhibitor, but it also decreases levels of C-reactive protein; this effect is attributed to inhibition of the production of IL-6, which induces production of C-reactive protein by hepatocytes (25). It was claimed that Tenidap inhibits production of IL-1 (93), but independent studies in several laboratories (including our own) have not shown inhibition of IL-1β or TNF-α production in LPS-activated human monocytes by Tenidap in clinically relevant concentrations (up to 30 μmol/L).

Naphthalenylpropenoic acid derivatives

Scientists of the Eisai Company, Tsukuba, Japan, synthesized a series of naphthalenylpropenoic acid derivatives that inhibit production of IL-1 in vitro and that show in vivo anti-inflammatory activity following oral administration. A prodrug designated E5090 was shown to be deacetylated to DA-E5090, which inhibits IL-1 formation by human monocytes in vitro (94,95). The structures of E5090 and DA-E5090 are shown in Fig. 45–6. Later, a series of 3-(4-hydroxy-1-naphthalenyl)-2-propenoic acids with improved oral bioavailability was described (96).

Human monocytes and rat peritoneal macrophages were stimulated with LPS, opsonized zymosan, or immune complexes. The active compounds were found to inhibit IL-1 production, measured by the LAF assay (IC$_{50}$,1.4–4.0 μmol/L). Northern blots showed that the drugs decrease steady-state concentrations of IL-1α and IL-1β mRNAs by mechanisms not yet defined. Oral dosage (50 mg/kg/rat) decreased production of IL-1 and PGE$_2$ in air pouches stimulated with carboxymethyl-cellulose-LPS. The size of the granuloma in the air pouch was also decreased. The drugs inhibited adjuvant arthritis in a dose-dependent manner. A very high concentration of the drugs (300 μmol/L) did not inhibit sheep seminal

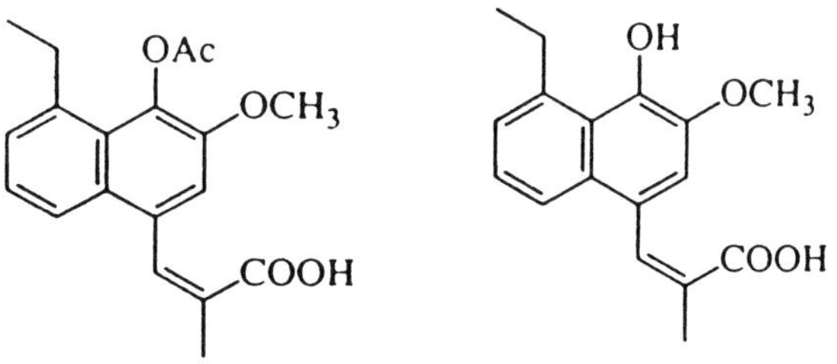

Figure 45–6 Chemical structures of E-5090 and the deacetylated metabolite DA-5090 (95).

vesicle Cox. These compounds were the first orally active inhibitors of IL-1 synthesis identified. Unfortunately, systemic toxicity has limited their clinical utility.

Bicyclic imidazoles as inhibitors of IL-1β and TNF-α formation

A group at the SmithKline Beecham Pharmaceutical Laboratories synthesized a novel group of antiinflammatory drugs by combining the structurally related pharmacophores of the Cox inhibitors, flumizole or tiflamizole, with the immunomodulatory agent, levamisole. This combination led to the class of fused bicyclic 2,3-dihydroimidazole [2,1-b] thiazolines (Fig. 45–7). SK&F 81114 was found to inhibit adjuvant arthritis in the rat. Replacement of a substituted phenyl ring in this compound with a 4-pyridyl ring gave SK&F 86002, with improved absorption and in vivo pharmacology. SK&F 86002 was found to inhibit synthesis of IL-1 in human monocytes (97); this compound was a more potent inhibitor of IL-1 production than products of its oxidative metabolism, the sulfoxide (SK&F 86096) or the sulfone (SK&F 104343).

A second series of bicyclic imidazoles was synthesized, replacing the cyclic sulfur-atom of the imidazothiazole with a methylene (CH$_2$) group to produce 6,7-dihydro-[5H]-pyrollo-[1,2-a]imidazoles (see Fig. 45–7). Of these, SK&F 105561 and its sulfoxide, SK&F 105809, have been most thoroughly investigated. The inactive prodrug SK&F 105809 is reductively metabolized to the sulfoxide SK&F 105561, which is a potent inhibitor of cytokine production in vitro, and it is also active in vivo. The active sulfide is, in turn, converted in vivo by oxidative metabolism to the inactive sulfone SK&F 105942. The lead imidazothiazoline SK&F 86002 and the lead imidazopyrrole SK&F 105561 are potent inhibitors of the production of TNF-α and IL-1β in LPS-stimulated human monocytes (Table 45–2).

Among the analogs of the two compounds tested, comparable IC$_{50}$s have been found for inhibition of both cytokines (Figs. 45–8A,B; Fig. 45–9), suggesting a similar

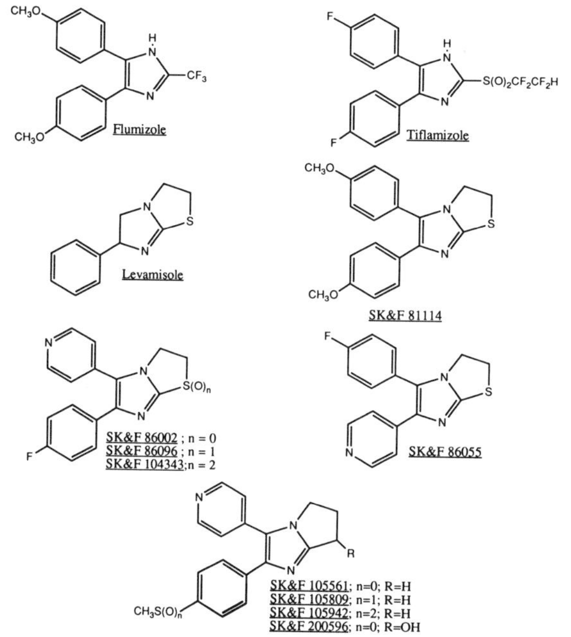

Figure 45–7 Chemical structures of bicyclic imidazoles (99).

TABLE 45–2 EFFECTS OF BICYCLIC IMIDAZOLES ON HUMAN PERIPHERAL BLOOD MONOCYTES

SK & F Compound No.	IC_{50} on Production			
	IL-1β*	TNF-α*	PGE_2[†]	LTB_4[†]
86002 (parent)	0.5	0.4	1	12
86096 (sulfoxide)	3.6	3.5	8	22
10343 (sulfone)	>5	5	14	14
105809 (prodrug)	Inactive	Inactive	Inactive	Inactive
105561 (sulfide)	2.7	3	0.1	2
105942 (sulfone)	Inactive	Inactive	Inactive	Inactive

*Freshly isolated human monocytes were treated with drugs for 1 hr before stimulation with 50 ng/mL LPS. After 16-hr culture, supernatants were recovered and assayed for cytokines by ELISA. IC_{50} values were determined from dose-response curves by regression analysis. Inactive = greater than 10 μmol/L.
[†]Human monocytes were stimulated by the calcium ionophore, A231987.
(Reproduced by permission from Lee JC, Badger AM, Griswold DE, et al. Bicyclic imidazoles as a novel class of cytokine biosynthesis inhibitors. Ann NY Acad Sci 1993;696:149–170.)

mechanism of action. This finding contrasts with independent regulation of transcription of the TNF-α and IL-1β genes (e.g., suppression of the former but not the latter by raising cAMP). SK&F 86002 and 105661 are weak inhibitors of cAMP phosphodiesterase, and they do not increase cAMP levels in unstimulated or LPS-stimulated human monocytes (17). It is unlikely that changes in cAMP levels contribute to their mode of action.

Concentrations of SK&F 86002 and 105661 required to suppress cytokine production in human monocytes inhibit the release of PGE_2 (98) (Table 45–2). Somewhat higher concentrations of the drugs also inhibit production of LTB_4 in monocytes activated by the calcium ionophore, A23187. However, among analogs of SK&F 86002, no correlation was found between potency as inhibitors of IL-1 synthesis and as inhibitors of PGE_2 or LTB_4 production (17).

SK&F 86002 and 105561 also inhibit production of IL-6 and IL-8 by human monocytes (17). When low concentrations of LPS were used to stimulate the cells, the IC_{50}s were comparable to those required for inhibition of TNF-α and IL-1β synthesis; when higher concentrations of LPS were used, more drug was required to inhibit IL-6 and IL-8 formation. However, the same drugs had no effect on formation of the IL-1Ra, granulocyte-macrophage colony-stimulating factor (GM-CSF), or IFN-α (17). Thus, the effect of the bicyclic imidazoles on induced cytokine formation in monocytes is selective.

SK&F 86002 also inhibited TNF-α production by LPS-stimulated, oil-elicited murine peritoneal macrophages

(17). However, the IC_{50} for mouse macrophages (5–8 μmol/L) was higher than that for human monocytes (0.5 μmol/L); complete inhibition of cytokine production was observed in human cells, but only 50% inhibition in mouse cells, in which the drug was used in nontoxic concentrations (see Figs. 45–8A,B). The effects of the drug in the mouse macrophage cell line, RAW264.7, were similar to those in murine peritoneal macrophages. In summary, the bicyclic imidazoles inhibit TNF-α production by both murine and human monocyte cultures. However, their potency as inhibitors is 5 to 10 times greater in human monocytes than in mouse primary macrophages or macrophage cell lines.

Inhibition by bicyclic imidazoles of IL-1β and TNF-α message translation

Lee and coworkers (17) analyzed the mechanism by which bicyclic imidazoles inhibit synthesis of TNF-α and IL-1β in human monocytes and THP-1 cells stimulated with LPS (0.5–1 μg/mL). Northern blots showed no effect of SK&F 86002 (5 μmol/L) on IL-1β mRNA, but there

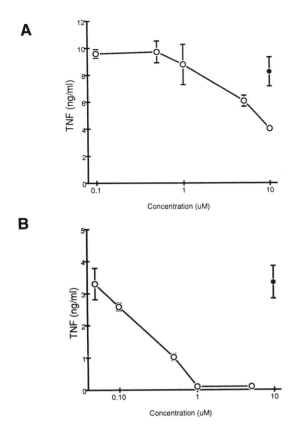

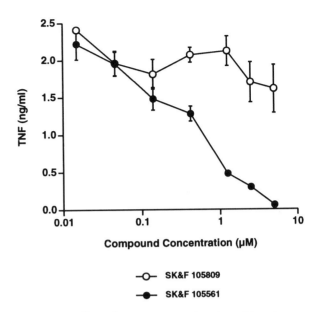

Figure 45–9   Effect of SK&F 105809 (prodrug ○) and SK&F 105561 (active metabolite, ●) on TNF production by human monocytes. TNF measured by ELISA in supernatants 18 hours after LPS stimulation (99).

Figure 45–8   (A) Effect of SK&F 86002 on TNF production in LPS-stimulated, oil-elicited murine peritoneal macrophages (99). (B) Effect of SK&F 86002 on TNF production in LPS-stimulated human monocytes measured by ELISA in culture supernatants 18 hours after stimulation (99). LPS control, *filled circles;* drug-treated, *open circles.*

was a 2-fold reduction in the level of TNF-α mRNA. In the same cells, Western blotting showed a 10-fold decrease in TNF-α protein and a 2-fold decrease in IL-1β protein. The transcript size and the ratio of intracellular to secreted proteins were unaffected by the drug. SK&F 86002 inhibited the rate of translation of IL-1β message, but it did not alter the half-life of the IL-1β, as measured by ³⁵S-methionine pulse chase.

In THP-1 cells, SK&F 86002 (1–5 μmol/L) had no effect on TNF-α mRNA levels, but it decreased TNF-α protein by almost 2-fold (17). These findings suggested that SK&F 86002 inhibits IL-1β and TNF-α synthesis at the translational level. To confirm this hypothesis, Lee and coworkers (17) compared the kinetics of action of SK&F 86002 with those of fast-acting inhibitors of transcription, actinomycin D, and those of translation, anisomycin. Parallel cultures of THP-1 cells were simultaneously activated with LPS, and individual cultures were treated with several inhibitors at various times after stimulation. All cultures were harvested 2.5 hours after LPS, and secreted TNF-α levels were measured by an enzyme-linked im-

munosorbent assay (ELISA). The results showed that the kinetics of action of SK&F 86002 coincided with those of anisomycin rather than those of actinomycin D, suggesting that SK&F 86002 inhibits a step close to the onset of TNF-α mRNA translation. Glucocorticoids also inhibit TNF-α production, mainly at the level of translation (63).

To examine directly the effect of the compounds on the efficiency of TNF-α mRNA translation, cytosolic extracts of human monocytes were fractionated on sucrose gradients. Fractions were analyzed by RNA polymerase chain reaction for TNF-α and cyclophilin. Quiescent monocytes contained a substantial amount of TNF-α mRNA, which was primarily associated with 43S preribosomal complexes. After activation, up-regulation of TNF-α mRNA was correlated with a proportional increase in TNF-α–specific message associated with polyribosomes. Treatment with active but not inactive analogs of the bicyclic imidazoles resulted in marked accumulation of TNF-α mRNA in the 43S complex-containing fractions, as well as a concomitant reduction in the polyribosome pool. Neither activation nor drug alone affected distribution of cyclophilin mRNA in the same fractions. These results suggest that initiation of TNF-α mRNA translation induced by activation is inhibited by the bicyclic imidazoles (Young et al, unpublished observations).

Chin and Kostura (76) found that human blood monocytes stimulated with low doses of LPS synthesize IL-1β, but they do not secrete it. Secretion can be induced by higher doses of LPS or heat-killed staphylococci. This assay can be used to discriminate between inhibitors of IL-1β synthesis and secretion. SK&F 86002 was found to be a potent inhibitor IL-1β secretion, suggesting that the drug affects events other than translation.

Bicyclic imidazoles in concentrations up to 10 μmol/L had no effect on production of IL-2 by murine T-cell hybridomas. The same concentrations of bicyclic imidazoles (SK&F 86002 and 104351) did not inhibit production of IL-2 or proliferation in human mixed leukocyte reactions or responses to specific antigen (17). Thus, the bicyclic imidazoles are not immunosuppressive for T cells, unlike cyclosporines and FK506. Their in vivo anti-inflammatory effects are unlikely to be due to immunosuppression.

The same mechanism may explain the inhibitory effect of SK&F 86002 and 105361 on parathyroid hormone (PTH)–induced bone resorption. In cultures of fetal rat long bones exposed to PTH, IL-1, or TNF-α resorption is increased, as shown by release of Ca, proteoglycan, and collagen degradation products into the culture media. In this system, SK&F 86002 (1 μmol/L) inhibited resorption, whereas Cox inhibitors (i.e., indomethacin, naproxen), 5-lipoxygenase inhibitors (i.e., phenidone), and dual CO/LO inhibitors were inactive (17). However, Cox inhibitors, notably ketorolac, efficiently block IL-1–induced resorption in this model (16).

Anti-inflammatory effects of bicyclic imidazoles

The effects of bicyclic imidazoles on production of cytokines in mice were analyzed. Following intraperitoneal injection of LPS, a peritoneal washout was recovered, and levels of TNF-α were measured by ELISA. SK&F 104343 (sulfone) showed greater potency in this assay (ED$_{50}$ for inhibition of TNF, 17 mg/kg/day orally) than SK&F 86002 (parental drug) and SK&F 105809 (17). With chronic dosing, the sulfone is the predominant form in vivo. Inhibition of cytokine production may contribute to the efficacy of the bicyclic imidazoles in collagen-induced arthritis and other chronic inflammatory models.

Because bicyclic imidazoles inhibit formation of PGs and leukotrienes in vivo as well as in vitro, it is not easy to interpret which effects are attributable to inhibition of TNF-α and IL-1β production or to inhibition of eicosanoid production. The question is interesting because it would be useful to know the in vivo effects of a drug that selectively inhibits TNF-α and IL-1β synthesis. The cytokines induce the formation of eicosanoids; therefore, there is a cascade.

Orally administered to mice, both SK&F 86002 and 105809 were found to inhibit arachidonic acid–induced inflammation, the edematous response, and neutrophil influx, as assayed by myeloperoxidase determination (99). Inhibition of leukotriene production is probably mainly responsible for preventing neutrophil recruit-

ment, although inhibition of TNF-α synthesis could contribute (5). Suppression of leukocyte infiltration was also shown in murine models of peritonitis induced by carrageenan or monosodium urate crystals (99).

SK&F 86002 (50 mg/kg/day, orally administered) significantly inhibited disease severity and acute-phase reactant response in collagen-induced arthritis in DBA/1 Sac J mice (100). Similar results were obtained with SK&F 105809 (101). This model is relatively insensitive to Cox inhibitors. A murine model of endotoxic shock was studied in which the animals are injected with LPS in combination with D-galactosamine. Oral administration of SK&F 86002 or SK&F 105809, 30 or 60 minutes before LPS injection, produced dose-dependent suppression of serum TNF-α levels (17,102) (Fig. 45–10A). This treat-

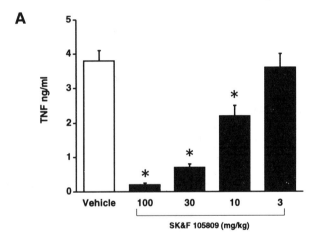

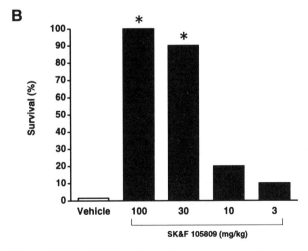

Figure 45–10 (A) Dose-dependent suppression of serum TNF levels in LPS-treated mice by oral administration SK&F 105809. Vehicle or drug was administered 0.5 hours before LPS challenge; TNF was measured by ELISA 1 hour after challenge. * = $p < 0.05$ by HSD test. (B) Protective effect of SK&F 105809 in LPS-D-galactosamine–induced shock. Vehicle or drug were administered orally 0.5 hour before LPS challenge, and survival was assessed 48 hours after challenge (99). * = $p < 0.05$ by Fisher's exact test.

ment increased the survival of mice in a dose-related manner, correlated with suppression of circulating TNF-α levels (Fig. 45–10B).

In summary, the bicyclic imidazoles represent a novel class of anti-inflammatory compounds with potent inhibitory effects on production of the proinflammatory cytokines TNF-α and IL-1β in vitro and in vivo. These effects are exerted mainly at the level of translation of the specific mRNAs. In addition, the bicyclic imidazoles are potent inhibitors of Cox and less potent inhibitors of 5-lipoxygenase. No immunosuppressive effects have been demonstrated. The bicyclic imidazoles are active in an acute model of septic shock and in models of acute and chronic inflammation in vivo. The clinical utility of the lead bicyclic imidazoles has been limited by toxicity, but analogs with better safety profiles may be found.

Inhibition by antioxidants of the transcription of genes for proinflammatory cytokines

Another strategy to identify small molecules able to inhibit production of TNF-α, IL-1β, and IL-6 is using antioxidants, which prevent activation of transcription factors required for induced expression of cytokine genes. Several reports were published on the inhibitory effects of antioxidants on production of individual cytokines by LPS-activated mouse peritoneal macrophages, human monocytes, THP-1 cells, and human whole blood (see Table 45–3). Eugui and colleagues (108) investigated the phenomenon systematically, comparing effects of different types of antioxidants on the production of TNF-α, IL-1β, and IL-6 in cultured human peripheral blood mononuclear (PBM) cells activated by LPS and in other ways. Some antioxidants, but not others, were found to be potent inhibitors of the production of all three cytokines.

The molecular basis of antioxidant-mediated inhibition was analyzed, showing that antioxidants can inhibit activation of transcription factors, NF-κB and AP-1, and transcription of cytokine genes. The in vitro observations were then confirmed by in vivo experiments in mice.

Initially, a series of compounds was tested for capacity to inhibit production of IL-1β in LPS-stimulated human PBM cultures. Tetrahydropapaveroline (THP), a tetrahydroisoquinoline derivative, was found to be a potent inhibitor of IL-1β production (IC$_{50}$, approximately 1.5 μmol/L) (Fig. 45–11). Because they are structurally related to THP, 10,11-dihydroxyaporphine (apomorphine) and norapomorphine were tested, and they were found to inhibit IL-1 production efficiently (see Table 45–4). The R(+) and R(−) stereoisomers of dihydroxyaporphine were equipotent in this assay, showing separation from dopamine agonist activity.

Antioxidants with widely different structures were then tested for capacity to inhibit production of IL-1β in LPS-activated human PBM. IL-1β released into culture supernatants, as well as cell-associated protein (cell lysates), were evaluated using a two-site ELISA assay. Several moderately lipophilic antioxidants, including butylated hydroxyanisole (BHA) and nordihydroguaiauretic acid (NDGA), were found to be potent inhibitors of IL-1β production (IC$_{50}$, ≤ 4 μmol/L) (see Table 45–4). NDGA is an inhibitor of 5-lipoxygenase and lipid peroxidation. However, another redox 5-lipoxygenase inhibitor, Zileuton, did not affect IL-1β formation, suggesting that 5-lipoxygenase products are not involved in the signal transduction system leading to cytokine production in LPS-activated monocytes.

The more hydrophilic antioxidants tested, ascorbic acid and trolox, had no effect on IL-1β production in concentrations up to 200 μmol/L. Mannitol, a hydroxyl radical scavenger, was inactive at a concentration of 100 μmol/L. The same was true of the physiological lipophilic antioxidant, α-tocopherol, as well as some classic antiox-

TABLE 45–3   INHIBITION BY ANTIOXIDANTS OF THE PRODUCTION OF TNF-α AND IL-1 IN MONOCYTES AND MACROPHAGES

Cells Used	Compound	Cytokine Tested	Ref
Murine macrophages	Butylated hydroxyanisole	TNF	(103)
Murine macrophages	Probucol	IL-1	(104)
THP-1	Probucol; α-tocopherol	IL-1β	(105)
Monocytes	N-acetylcysteine	TNF	(106)
Human whole blood	Dimethylsulfoxide; mannitol	IL-8	(107)

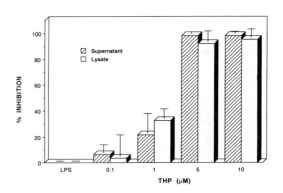

Figure 45–11 Dose-dependent inhibition by tetrahydropapaveroline (THP) of the production of IL-1β in human peripheral blood mononuclear cells activated by LPS. Means and standard errors of intracellular (lysate) and extracellular cytokines are shown (108).

TABLE 45–4   ANTIOXIDANTS VARY WIDELY IN POTENCY AS INHIBITORS OF CYTOKINE FORMATION

High Activity	IC$_{50}$ μmol/L
Butylated hydroxyanisole (BHA)	2.9
Tetrahydropapaveroline (THP)	1.0
Apomorphine	2.6
Norapomorphine	1.6
Nordihydroguaiauretic acid (NDGA)	1.3
Mepacrine	3.0

Low activity (insignificant inhibition in the range 50–200 μmol/L)

Ascorbic acid
α-tocopherol
Mannitol
Trolox
Butylated hydroxytoluene (BHT)
Quercetin
N,N'-diphenyl-p-phenylene diamine
Zileuton (5-lipoxygenase inhibitor)

(Reproduced by permission from Eugui EM, DeLustro B, Rouhafza S, et. al. Some antioxidants inhibit, in a coordinate fashion, the production of tumor necrosis factor-α, IL-1β and Il-6 by human peripheral blood mononuclear cells. International Immunol. 1994;6:409–422.)

idants (i.e., butylated hydroxytoluene [BHT], quercetin, and N,N'-diphenyl-p-phenylene diamine). N-acetylcysteine had some inhibitory effect (IC$_{50}$, 42 μmol/L), but this effect was much lower than that of several lipophilic antioxidants (see Table 45–4).

The question arose whether the inhibitory effect of THP is selective for the signaling pathway initiated by LPS, or whether it applies also to other effective inducers, such as silica and *Staphylococcus aureus,* Cowan I (Pansorbin). THP proved to be equally potent in the inhibition of IL-1β production with all inducers tested. The drug also inhibited IL-1β production using a weaker inducer, Zymosan. These observations show that THP can inhibit production of IL-1β by human PBM stimulated with several inducers. Similar observations were made with other antioxidants.

THP was also used to analyze the reversibility of the inhibitory effect. Adherent PBM were cultured with LPS and THP for 2 hours and repeatedly washed. Fresh medium containing the same amount of LPS was added, and the cultures were incubated overnight. Duplicate cultures were maintained with LPS and THP for the same period without washing. Removal of the drug did not reverse its inhibitory effect, so inhibition of IL-1β production by THP appears to be irreversible, at least until protein synthesis replaces inactivated molecules.

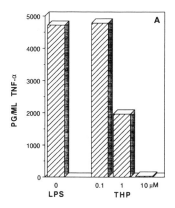

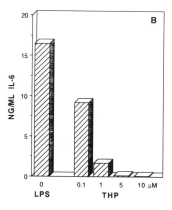

Figure 45–12   Dose-dependent inhibition by tetrahydropapaveroline (THP) of production of TNF-α and IL-6 by human peripheral blood mononuclear cells activated by LPS. Cytokines in the supernatant were assayed (108).

Tested in parallel with inhibition of cytokine synthesis, THP, 10,11-dihydroxyaporphine, and BHA did not inhibit protein synthesis, as shown by incorporation of labeled leucine. Emetine, which is structurally related to THP, strongly inhibited protein synthesis in parallel experiments using monocytes. BHA, THP, 10,11-dihydroxyaporphine, and NDGA were further tested for effects on production of TNF-α and IL-6 by LPS-stimulated human PBM. All three compounds were found to be approximately equipotent as inhibitors of the production of the three cytokines (Table 45–4; Fig. 45–12).

To ascertain whether this effect is exerted in all cell types, dermal fibroblasts and fibroblast-type cells from synovial tissue of patients with RA were studied. In these cells, IL-1 induces the production of IL-6. THP, BHA, 10,11-dihydroxyaporphine, and norapomorphine, in concentrations higher than required to inhibit totally the production of IL-6 in PBM, had no demonstrable effect on IL-6 production in fibroblasts (Fig. 45–13). Thus, antioxidant-mediated inhibition of cytokine production does not occur in all cell types.

Some of the compounds in Table 45–4 were selected for analysis of in vivo effects on cytokine production. Two

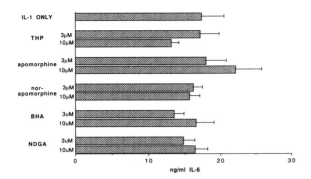

Figure 45–13 Lack of effect of antioxidants on production of IL-6 in human dermal fibroblasts induced by IL-1β (108).

different assays were used. In the first assay, IL-1β production was measured using elicited peritoneal cells from mice 4 hours after LPS challenge. The cytokine was measured in lysates of cells directly recovered from the peritoneal cavity (i.e., cell-associated IL-1β), as well as in the supernatants of cells after overnight culture (i.e., released IL-1β). Mice were pretreated with two doses of either THP or 10,11-dihydroxyaporphine (apomorphine, 50 mg/kg/dose) before LPS challenge (15 μg/mouse). The drugs were found to suppress production of IL-1β by 53 to 86%.

In the second assay, TNF-α and IL-1β were measured in serum following a lethal challenge with LPS (200 μg/mouse). Levels of TNF-α in circulating blood peak approximately 1.5 hours, and those of IL-1β 4 hours, after LPS injection Subcutaneous administration of a single dose of 10,11-dihydroxyaporphine (100 mg/kg) given 30 minutes before challenge inhibited TNF-α production by 95% (Fig. 45–14). Before IL-1β peak level, mice were given a second dose of dihydroxyaporphine (50 mg/kg), 2 hours after LPS and 2 hours before bleeding. This treatment reduced the circulating levels of IL-1β by 88% (Fig. 45–14). Thus, in vivo cytokine production is strongly inhibited by THP and dihydroxyaporphine.

Molecular biological effects of antioxidants

To analyze the mechanism by which antioxidants suppress cytokine formation, levels of cytokine mRNAs were determined in LPS-stimulated PBM (108). Previous studies had demonstrated that LPS markedly increases IL-1β mRNA. LPS also increases levels of TNF-α, IL-6, and IL-8 mRNAs in PBM. The antioxidants tested decreased TNF-α, IL-1β and IL-6 mRNA levels to baseline expression, but they had much less effect on IL-8 mRNA. Some of these effects are shown in Figs. 45–15 and 45–18.

To ascertain whether these effects are due to changes in transcription or changes in mRNA stability, nuclear transcription assays were performed. LPS markedly stimulated transcription of the IL-1β gene, and THP antago-

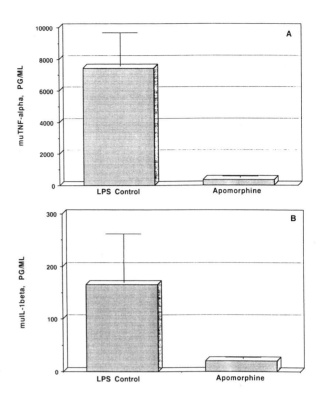

Figure 45–14 Apomorphine (10,11-dihydroxyaporphine) treatment of mice markedly decreases levels of TNF-α and IL-1β in the circulation of mice challenged with LPS (108).

nized the stimulatory effect of LPS on transcription (see Fig. 45–15). In view of observations that antioxidants decrease AP-1 activity, one of the reference messages studied was c-fos; however, no effect of THP on transcription of the c-fos gene could be detected (see Fig. 45–14).

The experiments described suggested that antioxidants inhibit LPS-stimulated transcription of some cytokine genes. To ascertain whether this inhibition is correlated with inhibited activation of transcription factors, electrophoretic mobility shift assays were performed. NF-κB and AP-1 were analyzed first because of reports that they are subject to redox regulation (109–113). As shown in Fig. 45–15, nuclear extracts of unstimulated PBM show NF-κB activity, which increases following LPS stimulation. Specificity of binding was shown by competition with unlabeled oligonucleotides. When PBM were treated with THP, in the presence or absence of LPS, nuclear NF-κB activity was markedly decreased or eliminated altogether. Similar observations were made with AP-1 (108). Thus, THP inhibited activation of NF-κB and AP-1 in intact cells, but it had no effect on the binding of these transcription complexes to cognate DNA recognition sequences. In cells treated with THP, no effect on several other transcription factors (i.e., SP-1, CRE, CTF/NF-1, OCT) could be demonstrated. Inhibition by antioxidants of the activation of transcription factors, including NF-κB and AP-1, could explain their suppression of cytokine gene transcription.

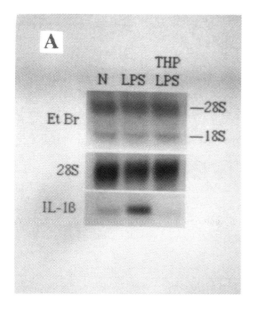

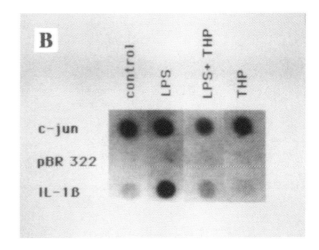

Figure 45–15 (A) Northern blot analysis of monocyte mRNA following treatment with LPS and THP (5 μmol/L) for 3 hours. Top panel ethidium bromide staining of RNA gel (Et Br); middle and bottom panels-blots probed with labeled 28S oligonucleotides and IL-1β cDNA; N-noninduced control (109). (B) Nuclear run-on assay of THP-treated and LPS-activated monocytes. Monocytes were cultured for 2 hours, and nuclei were isolated. mRNA transcripts were labeled with radioactive UTP and hybridized to cDNA immobilized on nitrocellulose membranes. LPS stimulated IL-1β gene transcription and THP decreased LPS-induced IL-1β transcription, but it did not affect c-jun transcription. pBR 322-negative control (108).

It is generally accepted that a c-fos serum responsive element and NF-κB have major roles in promoting expression of the IL-6 gene (25). At least one member of the NF-IL-6 transcription factor complex also associates with the p50 subunit of NF-κB (114). Evidence implicating κB

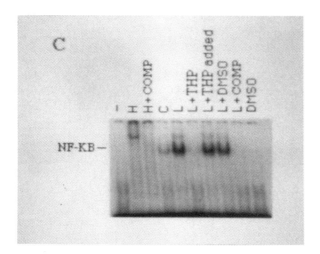

Figure 45–16 Gel mobility shift assays of monocyte nuclear extracts. Inhibition of NF-κB and binding to DNA sequences following LPS treatment in the presence of THP. LPS enhanced DNA binding activity, which was significantly decreased by THP treatment. I-labeled oligo alone; H-positive control with HeLa nuclear extract; C-no treatment; COMP-oligo competitor-competition showed sequence specificity of the DNA binding, L-LPS. Nuclear extracts were prepared 1 hour after treatment. THP decreased activation of the transcription factor, but it had no direct effect on DNA binding (108).

sequences in LPS-induced expression of the TNF-α gene in macrophages has also been presented (115,116). Less is known about regulation of the expression of the IL-1β gene, which is complicated by the fact that DNA sequences both proximal and distal to the transcription start site are involved (117). A phorbol myristate–responsive IL-1β enhancer element contains a DNA motif similar to that of the AP-1 binding site of the collagenase gene (117). The importance of NF-IL-6 transcription factors in activation of IL-1 has also been reported (117). The presence of a functional NF-κB site in the human IL-1β promoter has recently been described (118). Mutation of the NF-κB site in the context of the IL-1β promoter decreased the responsiveness of the promoter to LPS in human monocytic lineage cells. The authors conclude that the IL-1β gene may be considered as an important additional member of the family of cytokine genes regulated in part by the NF-κB/rel family of transcription factors (118). Thus, inhibition of NF-κB and AP-1 activation may contribute to the observed effect of antioxidants on transcription of the IL-1β gene, although specific internal deletions of sequences binding transcription factors will be required to establish their role.

Oxidants augment cytokine production

If antioxidants decrease cytokine production, it would be expected that oxidants can augment production of TNF-α and IL-1β. An experimentally convenient oxidant is H_2O_2, which, in concentrations not affecting cell viability, has effects on transcription factors and cytokine production. Sodium periodate, used in vitro, and alloxan and divicine, used in vivo, have oxidant effects. Chaudhri and Clark (103) found that secretion of TNF from mouse peritoneal macrophages exposed to LPS in vitro was increased in the presence of H_2O_2 or sodium periodate. Neither of these agents induced release of TNF in the absence of LPS. Both iron chelators and free radical scavengers inhibited this augmented secretion of TNF. Oxidant stress, produced by alloxan or divicine, increased levels of TNF in the circulation of mice.

Lee and Ilnicka (119) showed that oxidants promote LPS-induced cytokine gene expression in human cells of monocytic lineage. Nuclear extracts of U937 cells showed very little binding of AP-1 DNA sequences, and LPS induced only a low level of IL-1β mRNA. Exposure of U937 cells to H_2O_2 markedly increased AP-1 activity in nuclear extracts, as well as the amount of IL-1β mRNA induced by LPS (see Fig. 45–17). This does not necessarily mean that AP-1 elements are required for LPS responsiveness; other transcription factors subject to similar redox regulation may be involved. Examples of such transcription factors are TCF1(α) (111), the antioxidant response element (120), and the early growth 1 transcription factor (121). The experimental findings strongly suggest that transcription of the IL-1β gene is subject to redox regulation, but the transcription factors involved are not yet defined.

Suppression of cytokine synthesis by antioxidants

Several antioxidants were found to be potent inhibitors of the production of TNF-α and IL-1β in LPS-stimulated human PBM. The same concentrations of antioxidants were equally effective in the inhibition of cytokine production in PBM, regardless of the stimulus (i.e., LPS, staphylococci, silica, and Zymosan). Effects of antioxidants are not due to overall inhibition of protein synthesis, and they are gene-selective. The antioxidants do not affect transcription of the β-actin and the c-jun genes, and they actually increase production of the IL-1Ra, as well as of lysozyme and lysosomal enzymes in PBM. (87)

Remarkably, effects of the antioxidants are also cell-type selective. Antioxidants that are potent inhibitors of IL-6 production in PBM do not inhibit production of the same cytokine in dermal or synovial fibroblasts. The mechanisms stimulating IL-6 production are diverse (25), and presumably the transcription factors used in fibroblasts are less susceptible to redox regulation than those used in PBM. Other cell types should be studied, but the findings raise the possibility that selected antioxidants may be able to suppress the formation of proinflammatory cytokines in cells of the monocyte-macrophage lineage without major side effects.

Antioxidants show wide variation in potency as inhibitors of cytokine production. One of the most ac-

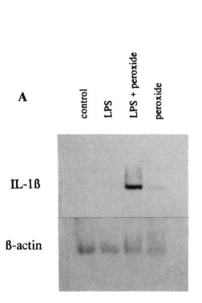

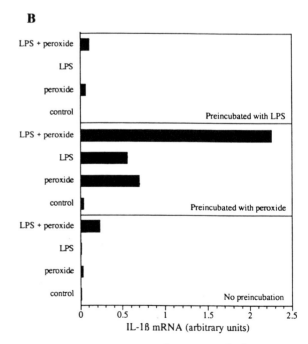

Figure 45–17 (A,B) Northern blot analysis of mRNA from the human promonocytic cell line U937. Neither LPS nor hydrogen peroxide alone induced IL-1β mRNA, but hydrogen peroxide primed the cells so that they responded to LPS by producing a high level of IL-1β mRNA and protein (119).

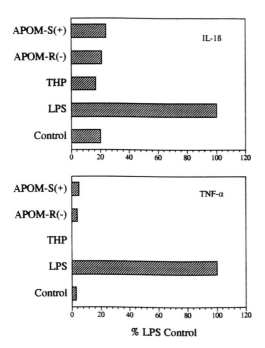

Figure 45–18 Northern blot analyses of cytokine mRNAs in human PBM (unstimulated, control), as well as LPS-stimulated cytokines in the absence of drugs and in the presence of tetrahydropapaveroline (5 μmol/L) or stereoisomers of apomorphine (APOM, 10 μmol/L). Densitometric scans are normalized to 28S rRNA, levels which were unchanged by LPS treatment (108).

tive compounds is THP, a tetrahydroisoquinoline. Two compounds with some structural relationship to THP, 10,11-dihydroxyaporphine (apomorphine) and norapomorphine, were also potent inhibitors. Because both stereoisomers of dihydroxyaporphine were equipotent as inhibitors of cytokine production, there was separation of this activity from dopamine agonist activity.

The classic antioxidants, BHA and NDGA, were strong inhibitors of cytokine production. NDGA is an inhibitor of 5-lipoxygenase and lipid peroxidation; however, zileuton, used in concentrations that inhibit 5-lipoxygenase activity, had no effect on cytokine production. This finding suggests that the antioxidant activity of NDGA, rather than its 5-lipoxygenase inhibitory activity, explains its effect on cytokine production. The common feature of the structurally diverse compounds with high activity listed in Table 45–4 is their capacity to function as antioxidants and moderate lipophilicity.

The water-soluble antioxidants, ascorbic acid and Trolox, were inactive, suggesting that the antioxidants have to function in a lipid environment. However, this must be a specialized microenvironment within target cells. The physiological membrane antioxidant, α-tocopherol, was ineffective as an inhibitor of cytokine production, as were several classic antioxidants listed in Table 45–4 (i.e., butylated hydroxytoluene, quercetin, N,N′diphenyl-p-phenylene diamine). Additional work is

necessary to define structure-activity relationships of inhibitors of cytokine production, the intracellular compartment in which they are active, and the mechanism by which they block activation of transcription factors.

Antioxidants augment expression of IL-1Ra

Coordinate inhibition by a drug of the production of TNF-α, IL-1β, and IL-6 in cells of the monocyte-macrophage lineage could obviously exert useful anti-inflammatory effects. An additional advantage could be if the drug also augments production of IL-1Ra. Waters and associates (87) found that some antioxidants known to be inhibitors of TNF-α, IL-1β, and IL-6 production increase production of IL-1Ra in cultures of human monocytes. The increase may not seem spectacular, but the amounts of IL-1Ra produced are more than 100 times those of IL-1β, and the ratio of production of IL-1β and IL-1Ra is substantially changed by the drugs.

It has been postulated that a balance between production of proinflammatory cytokines, such as TNF-α and IL-1β, and IL-1Ra has an important role in determining the course of RA (122). The same may be true of the arthritis associated with Lyme disease, caused by the bacterium *Borrelia burgdorferi*. Patients with high concentrations of IL-1Ra and low concentrations of IL-1β in synovial fluid had rapid resolution of attacks of arthritis, whereas patients with the reverse pattern of cytokine concentrations had long intervals to recover (123). Using drugs to manipulate the balance of production of cytokines and IL-1Ra in such a way as to have anti-inflammatory effects is a novel therapeutic strategy.

Effects of antioxidants in experimental animal models of septic shock

Chaudhri and Clark (103) made mice sensitive to LPS by low-level infection with malaria. Pretreatment with the antioxidant, BHA, or with the iron chelator, desferal, decreased TNF levels in the circulation following LPS challenge. BHA is a potent inhibitor of the production of both TNF-α and IL-1β by human monocytes (see Table 45–4). Nonaka and colleagues (124) found that following intraperitoneal injection of LPS, mice have increased lipid peroxide levels in the circulation (measured by peroxidase activity of hemoglobin). An antioxidant, 2-octadecylascorbic acid, decreased levels of circulating lipid peroxides, and it significantly increased the survival of mice injected with LPS. Calves are sensitive to induction by LPS infusion. The lazaroid tirilazad, mesylate, a 21 aminosteroid, was shown by Rose and Semrad (125) to mitigate clinical signs of endotoxemia in calves by attenuating hypoglycemia and preventing lactic acidosis. Tirilazad mesylate is an antioxidant that prevents iron-dependent lipid peroxidation (126). The protective effects of antioxidants in models of septic shock are likely to be due, at least in part, to inhibition of cytokine production.

IL-4 and IL-10

Some cytokines have been shown to inhibit production of TNF-α and IL-1β, and they are likely to be natural regulators of the production of proinflammatory cytokines. IL-4 was shown to inhibit the production of TNF-α, IL-1β, IL-6, IL-8, GM-CSF, and M-CSF human monocytes (127,128). IL-4 decreased steady-state levels of cytokine mRNAs, but it did not decrease class II MHC expression in these cells.

Human monocytes stimulated by LPS produce abundant IL-10, which is a relatively late product compared with the time of production of TNF-α, IL-1β, IL-6, IL-8, GM-CSF, and G-CSF (128). IL-10 added to cultures of LPS-stimulated human monocytes strongly suppressed production of TNF-α, IL-1α, IL-1β, IL-6, IL-8, GM-CSF, and G-CSF. Addition of IL-10 decreased steady-state levels of those cytokine mRNAs. IL-10 also decreased LPS-augmented class II MHC expression in the same cells. Thus, IL-10 could be an important natural regulator of the production of proinflammatory cytokines (129). Augmentation of the production of IL-10 by antioxidants could contribute to increased formation of IL-1Ra. Accelerating IL-10 formation could be a desirable mechanism of action of an anti-inflammatory drug for this reason, as well as the suppressive effect of IL-10 on the production of TNF-α and IL-1β and class II expression. Augmentation of the production of IL-4 or IL-13 (which likewise suppresses the synthesis of monocyte cytokines) is a less desirable effect because of induction of immunoglobulin E formation, which could favor allergic reactions.

A chronic inflammatory disease of the intestine develops in mice that have been genetically manipulated so that they cannot produce IL-10 (130). One extrapolation of these observations is that when IL-10–mediated inhibition of the production of TNF-α and IL-1β is removed, overproduction of the proinflammatory cytokines can lead to Crohn's disease and ulcerative colitis. If so, a drug inhibiting synthesis of those cytokines could be useful to treat chronic inflammatory bowel disease.

Augmentation of cytokine production by phosphatase inhibitors

In view of the importance of protein phosphorylation as a regulatory mechanism, it is likely to be involved in regulation of the formation of proinflammatory cytokines. The inhibitors of protein phosphatases 1 and 2A, okadaic acid and calyculin A, have been shown to augment pro-

duction of TNF-α, IL-1α, and IL-1β in human monocytes (131,132). In THP-1 cells stimulated by LPS or phorbol myristate acetate (PMA), levels of IL-1β mRNA are somewhat increased by okadaic acid, and they are further increased by staurosporin, an inhibitor of protein kinase C (119). Thus it seems unlikely that PMA augments expression of the IL-1β gene by activating PKC. Additional research is required to define the mechanism by which protein phosphorylation regulates cytokine expression. In principle, a selective inhibitor of phosphorylation might be used to suppress cytokine production, but obtaining selectivity may prove difficult.

PERSPECTIVES

During the past few years, anecdotal reports of inhibition of TNF-α and IL-1 synthesis by drugs have been replaced by systematic studies of natural and synthetic regulators of cytokine production. These studies have illuminated the mechanisms by which feedback regulation of cytokine production occurs, both locally and systemically. Circulating monocytes and tissue macrophages in healthy animals can be described as being in a neutral state. They can be activated into an inflammatory state by LPS, muramyl dipeptide, other microbial products, immune complexes, or activated complement components to become proinflammatory and procoagulant. LPS and other stimulants rapidly induce formation of TNF-α by activating transcription and increasing the efficiency of translation of TNF-α mRNA. Soon after TNF-α induction, synthesis of IL-1β is induced, and then IL-6 and IL-8 synthesis is induced. Synthesis of TNF-α is first turned off, whereas synthesis of IL-1β continues for a while; that of IL-6 and IL-8 continues longer. A local feedback regulator of TNF-α formation is PGE$_2$, which increases cAMP levels and thereby inhibits synthesis of TNF-α, but not that of IL-1β. A second local feedback regulator is IL-10, which is released by LPS-activated monocytes later than the aforementioned cytokines. IL-10 suppresses synthesis of TNF-α and IL-1β while stimulating formation of IL-1Ra.

Excess TNF-α and IL-1β released into the circulation, as in septic shock, trigger the release of systemic feedback inhibitors of their production. They induce release from the pituitary gland of corticotrophin-releasing factor, which in turn induces release into the circulation of ACTH and glucocorticoids (133). Glucocorticoids inhibit production of TNF-α and IL-1β, with little (if any) effect on transcription. Glucocorticoids decrease the stability of IL-1β mRNA and the efficiency of TNF-α mRNA translation. In septic shock, levels of circulating adrenalin also increase. Acting through β-adrenergic receptors, adrenalin increases cAMP levels in monocytes and macrophages, and it inhibits formation of TNF-α.

For prevention and treatment of septic shock, and for treatment of diseases with inflammatory pathogenesis, it is desirable to inhibit formation of both TNF-α and IL-1β. In periodontal disease and RA, inhibiting the synthesis of IL-6, a comediator of bone erosion, would also be desirable. Additional useful properties of a drug would be augmentation of formation of IL-1Ra and IL-10. This list of requirements excludes most known drugs. For example, pentoxyfylline and type IV cAMP phosphodiesterase inhibitors suppress formation of TNF-α, but not IL-1β. An inhibitor of the enzyme activating pro-IL-1β (134) would have no effect on TNF-α, IL-1α, or IL-6.

Two groups of compounds show that it is possible to inhibit selectively the formation of proinflammatory cytokines; one group exerts effects at the level of transcription, and the other at the level of translation. Stimulating cells of the monocyte-macrophage lineage into an inflammatory state involves activation of transcription factors and coordinate induction of the expression of genes for proinflammatory cytokines. Some antioxidants prevent activation of transcription factors required for coordinate expression of TNF-α, IL-1β, and IL-6 genes in response to stimulation of monocytes and macrophages by LPS and in other ways. These inhibitory effects are gene-selective: The same compounds can augment formation of IL-1Ra and lysosomal enzymes, whereas expression of most genes is unaffected. The effects of the antioxidants are also cell-type–selective; they inhibit IL-6 production in monocytes, but not in fibroblasts. A role of oxidant damage in inflammation and septic shock, in particular respiratory distress syndromes, has been postulated (12,40). Antioxidants could inhibit this type of tissue damage as well as induction of TNF-α and IL-1β gene expression.

Bicyclic imidazoles inhibit selectively the translation of TNF-α and IL-1β mRNAs. Doubtless other classes of drugs that coordinately inhibit cytokine production will be identified. In principle, they could provide the first successful treatment of septic shock, as well as novel therapies for inflammatory diseases free from the limiting side effects of glucocorticoids and Cox inhibitors. Clinical studies to be carried out during the next few years should establish whether the promise of drugs that suppress production of proinflammatory cytokines is fulfilled.

ACKNOWLEDGMENTS: We are indebted to Simon Lee, Barbara DeLustro, Sussan Rouhafza, Mariola Ilnicka, and other colleagues who contributed to our studies on inhibitors of cytokine production (listed in the primary publications), to K. Molnar-Kimber and J.S. Kenney for permission to use illustrations, and to Linda Miencier for preparation of the manuscript.

REFERENCES

1. Madada MP, Persson R, Kenney JS, Lee SW, Page RC, Allison AC. Measurement of interleukin-1α and -β in gingival crevicular fluid: implications for the pathogenesis of periodontal disease. J Periodont Res 1990;25:156–163.

2. Rodeke HH, Martin M, Topley N, Kaemer V, Resch K. Differential biological activities of human interleukin-1α and interleukin-1β. Eur Cytokine Net 1991;2:51–59.

3. Pober JS, Bevilacqua MP, Neudrido DL, Lapiere LA, Fiers W, Gimbrone MA. Two distinct monokines, interleukin-1 and tumor necrosis factor, each independently induce biosynthesis and transient expression of the same antigen on the surface of cultured human vascular endothelial cells. J Immunol 1986;136:1680–1687.

4. Elices M, Osborn L, Takada Y, et al. VCAM-1 on activated endothelium interacts with the leukocyte integrin VLA-4 at a site distinct from the fibronectin-binding site. Cell 1990;60:577–584.

5. Zhang Y, Rames BF, Jakschik BA. Neutrophil recruitment by tumor necrosis factor from mast cells in immune complex peritonitis. Science 1992;258:1957–1959.

6. Smith WL. Prostanoid biosynthesis and mechanism of action. Am J Physiol 1992;263:F181–F191.

7. Breviario F, Proserpio P, Bertocchi F, Lampugnani MG, Mantovani A, Dejana E. Interleukin-1 stimulates prostacyclin production by cultured human endothelial cells by increasing arachidonic acid mobilization and conversion. Arteriosclerosis 1990;10:129–134.

8. Lin LL, Lin AY, DeWitt DL. Interleukin-1α induces the accumulation of cytosolic phospholipase A_2 and the release of prostaglandin E_2 in human fibroblasts. J Biol Chem 1992;267:23451–23454.

9. Hla T, Ristimäki A, Appleby S, Barriocanal JG. Cyclooxygenase gene expression in inflammation and angiogenesis. Ann NY Acad Sci 1993;696:197–204.

10. Crofford LJ, Wilder RL, Ristimäki AP, Remmers EF, Epps HR, Hla T. Cyclooxygenase-1 and -2 expression in rheumatoid synovial tissues: effects of interleukin-1β, phorbol ester and corticosteroids. J Clin Invest 1994 (in press).

11. O'Banion MK, Winn VD, Young DA. cDNA cloning and functional activity of glycocorticoid-regulated inflammatory cyclooxygenase. Proc Natl Acad Sci USA 1992;89:4888–4892.

12. Olson NC, Dodam JR, Kruse-Elliott KT. Endotoxemia and gram-negative bacteremia in swine: chemical mediators and therapeutic considerations. J Am Vet Med Assoc 1992;200:1884–1893.

13. Matrisian LM. Metalloproteinases and their inhibitors in matrix remodeling. Trends Genet 1990;6:121–125.

14. MacDonald BR, Gowen M. Cytokines and bone. Br J Rheumatol 1992;31:149–155.

15. Ishimi Y, Miyaura C, Jin CH, et al. IL-6 is produced by osteoblasts and induces bone resorption. J Immunol 145:3297–3303.

16. Allison AC, Chin RC, Cheng Y. Cyclooxygenase inhibitors vary widely in potency for preventing cytokine-induced bone resorption. Ann NY Acad Sci 1993;696:303–306.

17. Lee JC, Badger AM, Griswold DE et al. Bicyclic imidazoles

as a novel class of cytokine biosynthesis inhibitors. Ann NY Acad Sci 1993;696:149–170.

18. Leizer T, Clarris BJ, Ash PE, Van Damme J, Saklatvala J, Hamilton J. Interleukin-1-beta and interleukin-1alpha stimulate the plasminogen activator activity and prostaglandin E_2 levels of human synovial cells. Arthritis Rheum 1987;30:562–566.

19. Prydz H, Allison AC. Tissue thromboplastin activity of isolated human monocytes. Thromb Hematosis 1978;39:582–591.

20. Van der Poll T, Büller HR, Tencate H, et al. Activation of coagulation after administration of tumor necrosis factor to normal subjects. N Engl J Med 1990;322:1622–1629.

21. Tracey KJ, Lowry SF, Fahey TJ III, et al. Cachectin/tumor necrosis factor induces lethal shock and stress hormone responses in the dog. Surg Gen Obstet 1987;164:415–422.

22. Shalaby MR, Aggarwal BB, Rinderknecht E, Svedersky LP, Palladino MA. Activation of human PMN functions by interferon and tumor necrosis factor. J Immunol 1985;135:2069–2073.

23. Johnston RB Jr. Enhancement of phagocytosis-associated oxidative metabolism as a manifestation of macrophage activation. In: Pick E, ed. Lymphokines, vol 3. New York: Academic Press, 1981;33–52.

24. Killbourn RG, Gross SS, Jubran A, et al. NG-methyl-L-arginine attenuates TNF-induced hypotension: implications for the involvement of nitric oxide. Proc Natl Acad Sci USA 1990;87:3629–3632.

25. Hirano T, Akira S, Taga T, Kishimoto T. Biological and clinical aspects of interleukin 6. Immunol Today 1990;11:443–449.

26. Dixon JS, Bird HA, Sitton NG, Pickup ME, Wright V. C-reactive protein in the serial assessment of disease activity in rheumatoid arthritis. Scand J Immunol 1984;13:39–44.

27. Takai Y, Wong GG, Clark SC, Burkoff SJ, Herrmann SH. B cell stimulatory factor-2 is involved in the differentiation of cytotoxic T lymphocytes. J Immunol 1988;140:508.

28. Nawata Y, Eugui EM, Lee SW, Allison AC. IL-6 is the principal factor produced by synovia of patients with rheumatoid arthritis that induces B-lymphocytes to secrete immunoglobulin. Ann NY Acad Sci 1989;557:230.

29. Gaston JSH, Strober S, Solvera JJ, et al. Dissection of the mechanisms of immune injury in rheumatoid arthritis using total lymphoid irradiation. Arthritis Rheum 1988;31:21–30.

30. Mannik M, Nardella FA, Self-associating IgG rheumatoid factors. In: Shiokawa Y, Abe T, Yamauchi Y, eds. New horizons in rheumatoid arthritis. Amsterdam: Excerpta Medica, 1983:124–130.

31. Brennan FM, Chantry D, Jackson A, Maini R, Feldmann M. Inhibitory effect of TNF-α antibodies on synovial cell interleukin-1 production in rheumatoid arthritis. Lancet 1989; 2:244.

32. Bertin PB, Kenney JS, Welch MR, Lindsley HB, Treves R, Allison AC. IL-1 inhibitors block IL-6 and IL-8 secretion by fragments of human rheumatoid arthritis synovium. Arthritis Rheum 1992;35(suppl):C189.33.

33. Beutler B. Tumor necrosis factors: the molecules and their emerging role in medicine. New York: Rowen Press, 1992:574.

34. Elliott MJ, Maini RN, Feldmann M, Williams RO, Brennan FM, Chu CQ. Treatment of rheumatoid arthritis with chimeric monoclonal antibodies to TNF-α: safety, clinical efficacy and control of the acute-phase response. J Cell Biochem 1993;17 suppl B:145.

35. Lebsack ME, Paul CC, Bloedow DC, et al. Subcutaneous IL-1 receptor antagonist in patients with rheumatoid arthritis. Arthritis Rheum 1991;34(suppl):545.

36. Feinberg B, Kurzrock R, Talpaz M, Blick M, Saks S, Gutterman JU. A phase 1 clinical trial of intravenously administered recombinant tumor necrosis factor alpha in cancer patients. J Clin Oncol 1988;6:1328–1334.

37. Tewari A, Buhles WC Jr, Starnes HF Jr. Preliminary report: effects of interleukin-1 on platelet counts. Lancet 1990; 336:712–714.

38. Smith JW II, Urba WJ, Steis RG, et al. Am Soc Clin Oncol 1990;9:717.

39. Dehring DJ. Sheep and pigs as animal models of bacteremia. In: Schlag G, Redl H, eds. The pathophysiology of shock, sepsis and organ failure. Berlin: Springer-Verlag 1993:1060–1075.

40. Buchanan JW, Wagner HN. Regional phagocytosis in man. In: Reichard SM, Filkins JP, eds. The reticuloendothelial system—a comprehensive treatise. New York: Plenum Press, 1985:147–170.

41. Marder VJ, Martin SE, Francis CW, Colman RW. Consumptive thrombo-hemorrhagic disorders. In: Colman RW, Hirsh J, Marder VS, Salzman EW, eds. Hemostasis and thrombosis: basic principles and clinical practice, ed 2. Philadelphia: J.B. Lippincott, 1987:975–1015.

42. Waage AP, Brandzaeg P, Haltenoten A, Kierulf P, Espevik T. The complex pattern of cytokines in serum from patients with meningococcal septic shock; association between interleukin-6, interleukin-1 and fatal outcome. J Exp Med 1989;169:333–338.

43. Girardin E, Gian GE, Dayer JM, et al. Tumor necrosis factor and interleukin-1 in the serum of children with severe infectious purpura. N Engl J Med 1988;319:397–400.

44. Fong Y, Tracey KJ, Moldawer LL, et al. Antibodies to cachectin/tumor necrosis factor reduce interleukin-1β and interleukin-6 appearance during lethal bacteremia. J Exp Med 1989;170:1627–1633.

45. Fischer E, Marano MA, van Zee et al. Interleukin-1 receptor blockade improves survival and hemodynamic performance in Escherichia coli septic shock, but fails to alter host responses to sublethal endotoxemia. J Clin Invest 1992;89:1551–1557.

46. Michie HR, Monogue KR, Spriggs DR, et al. Detection of circulating tumor necrosis factor after endotoxin administration. N Engl J Med 1988;318:1481–1486.

47. Fong Y, Marano MA, Moldawer LL, et al. The acute splanchnic and peripheral tissue metabolic response to endotoxin in man. J Clin Invest 1990;85:1896–1904.

48. Cannon JG, Tompkins RG, Gelfand JA, et al. Circulating interleukin-1 and tumor necrosis factor in septic shock and experimental endotoxin fever. J Infect Dis 1990;161:79–84.

49. Eskandari MK, Bolgos G, Miller C, Nguyen DT, De Forge LE, Remick DG. Antitumor necrosis factor antibody therapy fails to prevent lethality after cecal ligation and puncture or endotoxemia. J Immunol 1992;148:2724–2730.

50. Jesmok G, Lindsey C, Duerr M, Fournel M, Emerson T Jr. Efficacy of monoclonal antibody against human tumor necrosis factor in E. coli-challenged swine. Am J Pathol 1992; 141:1197–1207.

51. Fischer E, Morano MA, Barber A, et al. A comparison between the effects of interleukin 1α administration and sublethal endotoxemia in primates. Am J Physiol 1991;261: R442–452.

52. Fischer CJ, Jr, Slotman GJ, Opal S, Pribble J, Stiles D, Catalano M. Interleukin-1 receptor antagonist (IL-1ra) reduces mortality in patients with sepsis syndrome. Presented at the American College of Chest Physicians, San Francisco, CA, Nov 1991.

53. Debets JMH, Kampmeijer R, Van der Linden MPMH, Buurman WA, Van der Linden CJ. Plasma tumor necrosis factor and mortality in critically ill septic patients. Crit Care Med 1989;17:489–494.

54. Aarden LA Hybridoma growth factor. Ann NY Acad Sci 1989;557:192–199.

55. Starnes HF Jr, Pearce MK, Tewari JH, Yim JH, You JC, Abrams JS. Anti-IL-6 monoclonal antibodies protect against lethal Escherichia coli infection and lethal necrosis factor-α challenge in mice. J Immunol 1990;145:4185–4191.

56. Preiser JC, Schwarz D, van der Linden J, et al. Interleukin 6 administration has no acute hemodynamic or hematologic effect in the dog. Cytokine 1991;3:1–4.

57. Livi GP, Kmetz P, McHale MM, et al. Cloning and expression of cDNA for a human low-Km rolipram sensitive cyclic AMP phosphodiesterase. Mol Cell Biol 1990;10:2678–2686.

58. Molnar-Kimber KL, Yonno L, Heaslip RJ, Weichman BM. Differential regulation of TNF-α and IL-1β production from endotoxin stimulated human monocytes by phosphodiesterase inhibitors. Mediat Inflam 1992;1:411–417.

59. Renz H, Gong JH, Schmidt A, Nain M, Gemsa D. Release of tumor necrosis factor α from macrophages; enhancement and suppression are dose-dependently regulated by prostaglandin E₂ and cyclic nucleotides. J Immunol 1988;141: 2388–2393.

60. Endres S, Fuelle HJ, Sinha B, et al. Cyclic nucleotides differentially regulate the synthesis of tumor necrosis factor α and interleukin 1 beta by human mononuclear cells. Immunology 1991;72:56–60.

61. Semmler J, Wachtel H, Endres S. The specific type IV phosphodiesterase inhibitor rolipram suppresses tumor necrosis factor production by human mononuclear cells. Int J Immunopharmacol 1993;15:409–413.

62. Tannenbaum CS, Hamilton TA. Lipopolysaccharide induced gene expression in murine peritoneal macrophages is selectively suppressed by agents that elevate cAMP. J Immunol 1989;142:1274–1280.

63. Han J, Thompson P, Beutler B. Dexamethasone and pentoxyfylline inhibit endotoxin-induced cachectin-tumor necrosis factor synthesis at separate points in the signaling pathway. J Exp Med 1990;172:391–394.

64. Chao CC, Hu K, Close K, et al. Cytokine release from microglia: differential inhibition by pentoxyfylline and dexamethasone. J Infect Dis 1992;166:847–853.

65. Severn A, Rapson NT, Hunter CA, Liew FY. Regulation of tumor necrosis factor production by adrenaline and beta-adrenergic agonists. J Immunol 1992;148:3441–3445.

66. Knudsen PJ, Dinarello CA, Strom TB. Prostaglandins post-transcriptionally inhibit monocyte expression of interleukin 1 activity by increasing intracellular cyclic adenosine monophosphate. J Immunol 1986;137:3189–3194.

67. Hurme M. Modulation of interleukin-1β production by cyclic AMP in human monocytes. FEBS Lett 1990;263:35–37.

68. Kassis S, Lee JC, Hanna N. Effects of prostaglandins and cAMP levels on monocyte IL-1 production. Agents Actions 1989;27:274–276.

69. Brandwein SR. Regulation of interleukin 1 production by mouse peritoneal macrophages. J Biol Chem 1986;261: 8624–8632.

70. Allison AC, Lee SW. The mode of action anti-rheumatic drugs. I. Anti-inflammatory and immunosuppressive effects of glucocorticoids. Prog Drug Res 1989;33:63–81.

71. Snyder DS, Unanue ER. Corticosteroids inhibit murine macrophage Ia expression and interleukin-1 production. J Immunol 1982;129:1803–1805.

72. Kern JA, Lamb RJ, Reed JC, Daniele RP, Nowell PC. Dexamethasone inhibition of interleukin-1β production by human monocytes. J Clin Invest 1988;81:237–244.

73. Amano Y, Lee SW, Allison AC. Inhibition by glucocorticoids of the formation of interleukin-1α, interleukin-1β and interleukin-6; mediation by decreased mRNA stability. Mol Pharmacol 1993;43:176–182.

74. Knudsen PJ, Dinarello CA, Strom TB. Glucocorticoids inhibit transcriptional and posttranscriptional expression of interleukin 1 in U937 cells. J Immunol 1987;139:4129–4134.

75. Lee SW, Tsou AP, Chan H, et al. Glucocorticoids selectively inhibit the transcription of the IL-1β gene and decrease the stability of IL-1β mRNA. Proc Natl Acad Sci USA 1988;85:1204–1208.

76. Chin J, Kostura MJ. Dissociation of IL-1β synthesis and secretion in human blood monocytes stimulated with bacterial cell wall products. J. Immunol. 1993;151:5574–5585.

77. Roche Y, Fay M, Gougerot-Pocidalo MA. Effects of quinolones on interleukin-1 production in vitro by human monocytes. Immunopharmacology 13:99–109.

78. Takeshita K, Yamagichi I, Harada M, Otomo S, Nakagawa T, Mizushima Y. Immunological and anti-inflammatory effects of clarithromycin: inhibition of interleukin-1 production of mouse peritoneal macrophages. Drug Exp Clin Res 1989;15:527–533.

79. Piguet PF, Collart MA, Grau GE, Sappino AP, Vassalli P. Requirement of tumour necrosis factor for development of silica-induced pulmonary fibrosis. Nature (Lond) 1990; 344:245–247.

80. Ferrante A, Seow WK, Rowan-Kelly B, Thong YH. Tetrandine, a plant alkaloid, inhibits the production of tumor necrosis factor α (cachectin) by human monocytes. Clin Exp Immunol 1990;80:232–235.

81. Seow WK, Ferrante A, Li S-Y, Thong YH. Suppression of human monocyte interleukin-1 production by the plant alkaloid tetrandrine. Clin Exp Immunol 1989;75:47–51.

82. Chao CC, Molitor TW, Close K, Hu S, Peterson PK. Morphine inhibits the release of tumor necrosis factor in

human peripheral blood mononuclear cell cultures. Int J Immunopharmacol 1993;15:447–453.

83. Rordorf-Adam C, Lazdins J, Woods-Cook E et al. An assay for the detection of interleukin-1 synthesis inhibitors: effects of anti-rheumatic drugs. Drug Exp Clin Res 1989;15: 355–362.

84. Danis VA, Kulesz AJ, Nelson DS, Brooks PM. The effect of gold thiomalate and auranofin on lipopolysaccharide-induced interleukin-1 production by blood monocytes in vitro: variation in healthy subjects and patients with arthritis. Clin Exp Immunol 1990;79:335–340.

85. Chang D-M, Baptiste P, Schur PH. The effect of antirheumatic drugs on interleukin 1 (IL-1) activity and IL-1 inhibitor production by human monocytes. J Rheumatol 1990; 17:1148–1157.

86. Allison AC, Waters RV. Long-acting anti-rheumatic drugs induce differentiation of cells of the monocyte-macrophage lineage and alter expression of cytokines and IL-1 receptor antagonist. Agents Actions 1994 (in press).

87. Waters RV, Allison AC. Mycophenolic acid and some antioxidants induce differentiation of monocytic lineage cells and augment production of the IL-1 receptor antagonist (IL-1ra). Ann NY Acad Sci 1993;696:185–196.

88. Schnyder J, Cooper P, Mackenzie A. Modulation of secretory processes of phagocytes by IX207–887. Semin Immunopathol 1993;14:345–352.

89. Mackenzie AR. Pharmacological properties of IX 207–887. In: Lewis AJ, Furst DE, eds. Nonsteroidal anti-inflammatory drugs: mechanisms and chemical uses, ed 2. New York: Marcel Dekker, 1993; 391–410.

90. Dougados M, Combe B, Beveridge T, Bordeix I, Lallemand A, Amor B, Sany J. IX 207–887 in rheumatoid arthritis. Arthritis Rheum 1992;35:999–1006.

91. Carlson RP. Newer immunosuppressive drugs and other agents for the treatment of rheumatoid arthritis. Curr Opin Invest Drugs 1993;2:751–762.

92. Otterness IG, Carty TJ, Loose LD. Tenidap: a new drug for arthritis. In: Lewis AJ, Ackerman NR, Doherty NS, eds. Therapeutic approaches to inflammatory diseases. New York: Elsevier Press.

93. Otterness IG, Bliven ML, Downs JT, Natali EJ, Hanson DC. Inhibition of interleukin-1 synthesis by tenidap: a new drug for arthritis. Cytokine 1991;3:277–283.

94. Shirota H, Goto M, Hashida R, Yamatsu I, Katayama K. Inhibitory effects of E5110 on interleukin-1 generation from human monocytes. Agents Actions 1989;27:322–324.

95. Shirota H, Chiba K, Goto M, Yamatsu I, Katayama K. Pharmacological properties of E5090, an orally active inhibitor of interleukin-1 generation. In: Lewis AJ, Furst DE, eds. Nonsteroidal anti-inflammatory drugs: mechanisms and clinical uses, ed 2. New York: Marcel Dekker, 1993;411–425.

96. Tanaka M, Chiba K, Okita M, et al. A novel orally active inhibitor of IL-1 generation: synthesis and structure-activity relationships of 3-(4-hydroxy-1-naphthaonyl)-2-propenoic acid derivatives. J Med Chem 1992;35:4665–4675.

97. Lee JC, Griswold DE, Vott B, Hanna N. Inhibition of monocyte IL-1 production by the anti-inflammatory compound, SK&F 86002. Int J Immunopharmacol 1988;10:835–843.

98. Marshall PJ, Griswold DE, Breton J, et al. Pharmacology of the pyrroloimidazole, SK&F 105809. I. Inhibition of inflammatory cytokine production and of 5-lipoxygenase- and cyclooxygenase-mediated metabolism of arachidonic acid. Biochem Pharmacol 1991;42:813–824.

99. Griswold DE, Hoffstein S, Marshall PJ, Webb EF, Bender PE, Hanna N. Inhibition of inflammatory cell infiltration by bicyclic imidazoles SK&F 86002 and SK&F 104493. Inflammation 1989;13:727–739.

100. Griswold DE, Hillegas PC, Meunier PC, Di Martino MJ, Hanna N. Effect of inhibitors of eicosanoid metabolism in murine collagen-induced arthritis. Arthritis Rheum 1988; 31:1406–1412.

101. Hanna N, Marshal PJ, Newton J Jr, et al. Pharmacological profile of SK&F 105809, a dual inhibitor of arachidonic acid metabolism. Drug Ex Clin Res 1990;16:137–147.

102. Badger AM, Olivera DL, Talmadge JE, Hanna N. Protective effect of SK&F 86002, a novel dual inhibitor of arachidonic acid metabolism, in murine models of endotoxic shock: inhibition of tumor necrosis factor as a possible mechanism of action. Circ Shock 1989;27:51–61.

103. Chaudhri G, Clark IA. Reactive oxygen species facilitate the in vitro and in vivo lipopolysaccharide-induced release of tumor necrosis factor. J Immunol 1989;143:1290–1294.

104. Ku G, Doherty NS, Wolos JA, Jackson RL. Inhibition by probucol of interleukin 1 secretion and its implication in atherosclerosis. Am J Cardiol 1988;62:77B–81B.

105. Akeson AL, Woods CW, Mosher LB, Thomas CE, Jackson RL. Inhibition of IL-1β expression in THP-1 cells by probucol and tocopherol. Atherosclerosis 1991;86:261–270.

106. Peristeris P, Clark BD, Gatti S, et al. N-acetylcysteine and glutathione as inhibitors of tumor necrosis factor production. Cell Immunol 1992;140:390–399.

107. De Forge LE, Fantone JC, Kenney JS, Remick DG. Oxygen radical scavengers selectively inhibit interleukin 8 production in human whole blood. J Clin Invest 1992;90:2123–2129.

108. Eugui EM, DeLustro B, Rouhafza S, et al. Some antioxidants inhibit, in a co-ordinate fashion, the production of TNF-α, IL-1β and IL-6 by human peripheral blood mononuclear cells. Internat Immunol 1994;6:409–422.

109. Schreck R, Rieber P, Bauerle PA. Reactive oxygen intermediates as apparently widely used messengers in the activation of NFκB transcription factor and HIV-1. EMBO J 1991;10:2247–2258.

110. Israel N, Gougerat-Pocidalo M-A, Aillet F, Virelizier J-L. Redox status influences constitutive or induced NF-κB translocation and HIV long terminal repeat activity in human T and monocytic cell lines. J Immunol 1992;149: 3386–3393.

111. Ivanov B, Merkenschlager M, Ceredig R. Antioxidant treatment of thymic organ cultures decreases NF-κB and TCF1 (α) transcription factor activities and inhibits αβ T cell development. J Immunol 1993;151:4694–4704.

112. Devary Y. Gottlieb RA, Lau LF, Karin M. Rapid and preferential activation of the c-jun gene during the mammalian UV response. Mol Cell Biol 1991;11:2804–2811.

113. Datta R, Hallahan DE, Kharbanda SM, et al. Involvement of reactive oxygen intermediates in the induction of c-jun gene transcription by ionizing radiation. Biochemistry 1992;31:8300–8306.

114. Le Clair KP, Blanar MA, Sharp PA. The p50 subunit of NF-

κB associates with the NF-IL-6 transcription factor. Proc Natl Acad Sci USA 1992;89:8145–8149.

115. Shakhov AN, Collart MA, Vassali P, Nedospasov SA, Jongeneel CV. Kappa B-type enhancers are involved in lipopolysaccharide-mediated transcriptional activation of the tumor necrosis factor alpha gene in primary macrophages. J Exp Med 1990;171:35–47.

116. Sung SJ, Walters JA, Hudson J, Bimble JM. Tumor necrosis factor-α mRNA accumulation in human myelomonocytic cell lines. J Immunol 1991;147:2047–2054.

117. Shirakawa F, Saito K, Bonagura CA, et al. The human pro-interleukin β gene requires DNA sequences both proximal and distal to the transcription start site for tissue-specific induction. Mol Cell Biol 1993;13:1332–1344.

118. Hiscott J, Merois J, Garoufalis J, et al. Characterization of a functional NF-κB site in the human interleukin-1β promoter: evidence for a positive autoregulatory loop. Mol Cell Biol 1993;13:6231–6240.

119. Lee SW, Ilnicka M. Hydrogen peroxide primes pro-monocytic U937 cells to produce IL-1β. Ann NY Acad Sci 1994 (in press).

120. Nguyen T, Pickett CB. Regulation of rat glutathione 5-transferase Ya subunit gene expression. DNA-protein interaction at the antioxidant responsive element. J Biol Chem 1992;267:13535–13539.

121. Datta R, Taneja N, Sukhante VP, Querishi SA, Weichselbaum R, Kufe DW. Reactive oxygen intermediates target CC (A/T) 6 GG sequences to mediate activation of the early growth response 1 transcription factor gene by ionizing radiation. Proc Natl Acad Sci USA 1993;90:2419–2422.

122. Arend WP, Dayer JM. Cytokines and cytokine inhibitors or antagonists in rheumatoid arthritis. Arthritis Rheum 1990; 33:305–315.

123. Miller LC, Lynch EA, Isa S, Logan JW, Dinarello CA, Steere A. Balance of synovial fluid IL-1β and IL-1 receptor antagonist and recovery from Lyme arthritis. Lancet 1993;341: 146–148.

124. Nonaka A, Manabe T, Tobe T. Effect of a new synthetic free radical scavenger, 2-octadecyl ascorbic acid, on the mortality in mouse endotoxemia. Life Sci 1990;47:1933–1939.

125. Rose ML, Semrad SD. Clinical efficacy of tirilazad mesylate for treatment of endotoxemia in neonatal calves. Am J Vet Res 1992;53:2305–2310.

126. Braughler JM, Pregenzer JF, Chase JL, et al. Novel 21-aminosteroids as potent inhibitors of iron-dependent lipid peroxidation. J Biol Chem 1987;262:10438–10440.

127. Hart PH, Vitti GF, Burgess DR, Whitty GA, Piccoli DS, Hamilton JA. Potential anti-inflammatory effects of interleukin 4: suppression of human monocyte tumor necrosis factor-α, interleukin-1 and prostaglandin E₂. Proc Natl Acad Sci USA 1989;86:3803–3807.

128. te Velde AA, Huijbens RJF, Heije K, de Vries JE, Figdor CG. Interleukin 4 (IL-4) inhibits secretion of IL-1β, tumor necrosis factor-α and IL-6 by human monocytes. Blood 1990;76:1392–1397.

129. Malefyt R de W, Abrams J, Bennett B, Figdor CG, de Vries JE. Interleukin 10 (IL-10) inhibits cytokine synthesis by human monocytes: an autoregulatory role of IL-10 produced by monocytes. J Exp Med 1991;174:1209–1220.

130. Kuhn R, Löhler J, Rennick D, Rajewsky K, Müller W. Interleukin-10-deficient mice develop chronic entercolotis. Cell 1993;75:263–274.

131. Sung S, Walters JA, Fu SM. Stimulation of tumor necrosis factor α production in human monocytes by inhibitors of protein phosphatase 1 and 2A. J Exp Med 1992;176:897–901.

132. Sung S, Walters JA. Stimulation of interleukin-1α and interleukin-1β production in human monocytes by protein phosphatase 1 and 2A inhibitors. J Biol Chem 1993;268: 5802–5809.

133. Besedovsky H, del Rey A, Sorkin E, Dinarello CA. Immunoregulatory feedback between interleukin-1 and glucocorticoid hormones. Science 1986;233:652–654.

134. Thornberry NA, Bull HG, Calaycay JR, et al. A novel heterodimeric cysteine protease is required for interleukin-1β processing in monocytes. Nature (Lond) 1992;356: 768–774.

INDEX